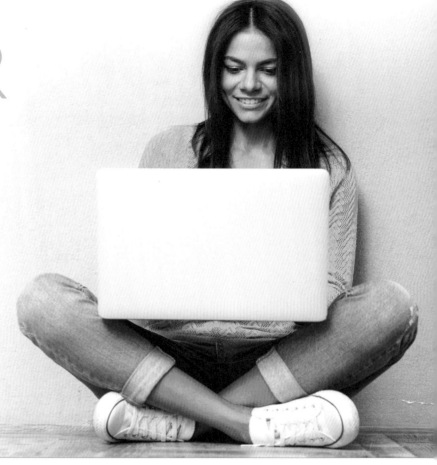

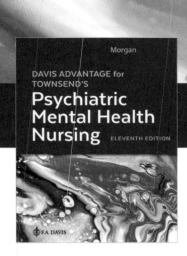

DAVIS ADVANTAGE for
TOWNSEND'S

Morgan

Psychiatric Mental Health Nursing ELEVENTH EDITION

F.A. DAVIS

TEXT

STEP #1
Build a solid foundation.

Communication Exercises let you practice your communication skills with vignettes and questions that prepare you for clinical and practice.

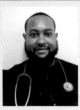

Communication Exercises

1. Hal, a patient on the psychiatric unit, has a diagnosis of schizophrenia. He lives in a halfway house, where last evening he began yelling that "aliens were on the way to take over our bodies! The message is coming through loud and clear!" The residence supervisor became frightened and called 911. As Hal was being admitted to the psychiatric unit, he told the nurse, "I'm special! I get messages from a higher being! We are in for big trouble!" How would the nurse respond appropriately to this statement by Hal?

Use of a passive rather than a directive communication approach, which offers the patient with paranoia the opportunity to make their own decisions about activities, treatment goals, and other aspects of care, helps establish trust while incorporating a patient-centered approach. For example, saying, "Would you like to attend group now?" is a less directive approach than saying "You need to go to group now."

Real Nurses, Real Advice shares helpful tips from practicing nurses to help you navigate clinical situations and provide the best possible care to your patients.

Quality and Safety Education for Nurses (QSEN) activities and content, highlighted with a special icon, help you attain the knowledge, skills, and attitudes required to fulfill the initiative's quality and safety competencies.

Real Nurses, Real Advice

"The anhedonia, psychomotor retardation, and anergia in acute depression can make assessment a challenge. It's important to offer hope to a client who may be uncertain about how to navigate their present state of deep depression and to remain diligent while not making the patient feel pressured to speak. Paraphrasing what the patient has said to you conveys understanding and provides validation. Open-ended questions encourage the patient to elaborate rather than just answer 'yes' or 'no.'"

—Larry Johnson, RN

 MOVIE CONNECTIONS

I Never Promised You a Rose Garden (schizophrenia)
• *A Beautiful Mind* (schizophrenia) • *The Fisher King* (schizophrenia) • *Bennie & Joon* (schizophrenia)
• *Out of Darkness* (schizophrenia) • *Conspiracy Theory* (paranoia) • *The Fan* (delusional disorder)
• *The Soloist* (schizophrenia) • *Of Two Minds* (schizophrenia)

Movie Connections list films that demonstrate conditions and behaviors you may not encounter in clinical.

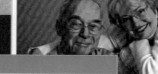

Table 24–2 | CARE PLAN FOR THE PATIENT WITH SCHIZOPHRENIA

NURSING DIAGNOSIS: DISTURBED SENSORY PERCEPTION: AUDITORY/VISUAL

RELATED TO: Panic anxiety, extreme loneliness, and withdrawal into the self

EVIDENCED BY: Inappropriate responses, disordered thought sequencing, rapid mood swings, poor concentration, disorientation

OUTCOME CRITERIA	NURSING INTERVENTIONS	RATIONALE
Short-Term Goal • Patient discusses content of hallucinations with nurse or therapist within 1 week. Long-Term Goals • Patient is able to define and test reality, reducing or eliminating the occurrence of hallucinations. *Note:* This goal may not be realistic for the individual with severe and persistent illness who has experienced auditory hallucinations for many	1. Observe for signs of hallucinations (listening pose, laughing or talking to self, stopping in midsentence). Ask, "Are you hearing something else?" Or "Are you hearing other voices?" 2. Avoid touching the patient without warning them that you are about to do so.	1. Early intervention may prevent aggressive response to command hallucinations. Because the patient may not recognize these voices as hallucinations, it is better to ask the patient about what they are hearing rather than use the word "hallucinations." 2. The patient may perceive touch as threatening and may respond in an aggressive manner.

Therapeutic Communication Icon identifies helpful interventions and guidance on how to speak with your patients. Look for this icon in Care Plan sections.

TEST YOUR CLINICAL REASONING AND CLINICAL JUDGMENT SKILLS

Sara, a 23-year-old single woman, has just been admitted to the psychiatric unit by her parents. They explain that over the past few months she has become increasingly withdrawn. She stays in her room alone but lately has been heard talking and laughing to herself.

Sara left home for the first time at age 18 to attend college. She performed well during her first semester, but when she returned after Christmas, she began to accuse her roommate of stealing her possessions. She started writing to her parents that her roommate wanted to kill her and that her roommate was turning everyone against her. She said she feared for life. She started missing classes and stayed in her bed most the time. Sometimes she locked herself in her closet. Her parents took her home, and she was hospitalized and diagnosed with schizophrenia. She has since been maintained on psychotic medication while taking a few classes at the community college.

Sara tells the admitting nurse that she quit taking medication 4 weeks ago because the pharmacist who fills prescriptions is plotting to have her killed. She believes trying to poison her. She says she got this information from television message. As Sara speaks, the nurse notices that sometimes stops in midsentence and listens; sometimes cocks her head to the side and moves her lips as though is talking.

Answer the following questions related to Sara:

1. From the assessment data, what would be the most immediate nursing concern in working with Sara?
2. What is the nursing diagnosis related to this concern?
3. What interventions must be accomplished before the nurse can be successful in working with Sara?

---

me. During the last attempt to hospitalize me, I actually escaped and ran away, even though I was in pretty bad shape.

Karyn: So since you were knowledgeable about the laws, you could essentially be your own self-advocate and argue your case, so to speak?

Dr. Frese: Yes, and by that time, I was in grad school and had secured a job at what is now the Department of Mental Health and Addiction Services. I remember I was living in the hallway of some university housing, and one of the students, who saw me day after day just hanging around and not really doing anything, suggested that I might be eligible for a government job because of my military background. When I applied, the receptionist saw my history of mental health commitments and said I would never get the job, but I did. The last time I went to the hospital, I went voluntarily because I knew I needed more medication, but they thought I needed to be hospitalized and I didn't; so I ran away.

Karyn: Sounds like you were managing a lot of stuff—grad school, working—and, at the same time, episodically struggling with symptoms of illness. You were working in the field of mental health, too. Was the work environment supportive?

Dr. Frese: Not always. It seemed like even among my coworkers, when something strange happened, they thought it was something wrong with me.

Karyn: What do you mean by "something strange"?

Dr. Frese: Like one time when they perceived I was spending too much time interacting with patients, they assumed I was "going off again," and next thing I knew, they called a "blue alert" and wanted to hospitalize me. But that time, the medical director just told me to take some time off. I never did find out why they called that blue alert.

Karyn: So you haven't been hospitalized for a very long time, and you are internationally renowned for all of your work and advocacy in the field of mental health. What do you think has contributed most to your recovery?

Dr. Frese: No, I haven't been hospitalized since I got married. I think that has been central in my recovery: having a person who you trust to give you feedback and let me know when I need more medication.

Karyn: What role do medications play in recovery?

Dr. Frese: It's very individual. We need more research to identify who, among people with schizophrenia, will benefit most by continuous medication versus episodic, reduced doses, or no medication. Genetic research is hopeful, but we're not there yet. It's hard to advise any individual what to do without knowing their individual circumstances, and even knowing, it can be very hard.

...e to be disenfranchised, ... Even within healthcare, ... settings have been very ...ntal illnesses. One way ...h of people with mental ...ersonally. Dr. Fred Frese ...internationally renowned ...e field of mental illness.

...t about your history with

...my first episode. I was ...ad seen the movie *The* ...sly—and I began to think ...the same strategies from ...let my commanding of- ...hospitalized involuntarily, ...in and out of hospitals— ...ious medications, living ...employed.

Karyn: Were you getting any treatments or intervention that you thought were helpful to your recovery?

Dr. Frese: Well, at that time it was thought that schizophrenia was not an illness from which one could recover. Even recently, I've heard some folks who have a family member with schizophrenia say, "There's no way that anyone with this illness can get better." But that's starting to change, and now that the government, through SAMHSA (Substance Abuse and Mental Health Services Administration) is backing the recovery model approach, I think healthcare will improve. I remember being told that my brain was going to progressively deteriorate and that I would never be able to function on my own. All in all, I probably spent about a year of my life in hospitalizations. Once the laws changed and I knew I had to be of imminent harm to yourself or others in order to be hospitalized involuntarily, I talked some of the health professionals out of admitting

---

Real People, Real Stories features interviews with patients and provides a model for effective therapeutic communication.

CLINICAL JUDGMENT IN ACTION: CASE STUDY AND SAMPLE CARE PLAN

NURSING HISTORY AND ASSESSMENT

Recognizing cues: The nurse must demonstrate the ability to recognize what information is most important to making an assessment (National Council of State Boards of Nursing [NCSBN], 2021). This information is italicized in the following.

Frank is 22 years old. He joined the Marines just out of high school at age 18 for a 3-year enlistment. His final year was spent in Afghanistan. When his enlistment was up, he returned to his hometown and married a young woman with whom he had been a high school classmate. Frank has *always been quiet, somewhat withdrawn,* and *had very few friends.* He was the only child of a single mom who never married, and he does not know his father. His mother was killed in an automobile accident the spring before he enlisted in the Marines.

During the past year, he has become increasingly isolated and withdrawn. He is without regular employment but finds work as a day laborer when he can. His wife, Suzanne, works as a secretary and is the primary wage earner. Lately, *Frank has become very suspicious of Suzanne and sometimes follows her to work. He also drops in on her at work and*

Frank told the police that he *received a message over the radio from his Marine commanding officer telling him that he couldn't allow his wife to continue to commit adultery, and the only way he could stop it was to kill her.* The police took Frank to the emergency department of the VA Hospital, where he was *admitted to the psychiatric unit.* Suzanne is helping with the admission history.

Suzanne tells the nurse that she has never been unfaithful to Frank and she doesn't know why he believes that she has. Frank tells the nurse that he has been *"taking orders from my commanding officer through my car radio ever since I got back from Afghanistan."* He survived a helicopter crash in Afghanistan in which all were killed except Frank and one other man. Frank says, "I have to follow my CO's orders. *God saved me to annihilate the impure."*

After an evaluation, the psychiatrist diagnoses Frank with schizophrenia. He orders olanzapine 10 mg PO to be given daily and olanzapine 10 mg IM q6h prn for agitation.

Analyzing cues: The nurse must be able to interpret the information (NCSBN, 2021).

The nurse interprets that Frank's suspicious ideation

Chapters include case studies and review questions that challenge your **clinical judgment skills** to prepare you for the Next Generation NCLEX® and real-world practice.

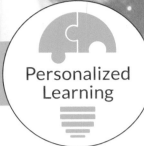

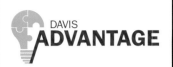
LEARN

STEP #2

Make the connections to key topics.

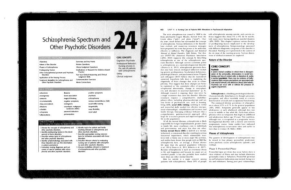

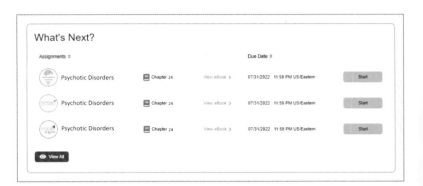

Assignments in Davis Advantage correspond to key topics in your book. Begin by reading from your printed text or click the eBook button to be taken to the **FREE, integrated eBook.**

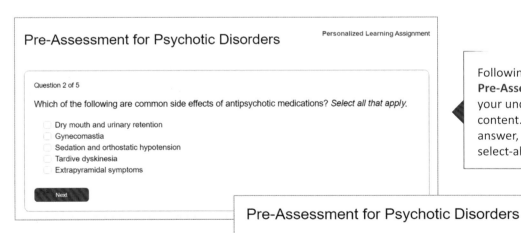

Following your reading, take the **Pre-Assessment** quiz to evaluate your understanding of the content. Questions feature single answer, multiple-choice, and select-all-that-apply formats.

Immediate feedback identifies your strengths and weaknesses using a thumbs up, thumbs down approach. *Thumbs up* indicates competency, while *thumbs down* signals an area of weakness that requires further study.

Content subject to change upon publication.

Psychotic Disorders

VIDEO

ACTIVITY

POST-ASSESSMENT

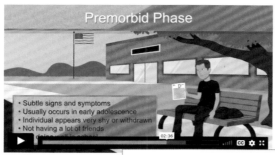

Premorbid Phase

- Subtle signs and symptoms
- Usually occurs in early adolescence
- Individual appears very shy or withdrawn
- Not having a lot of friends

02:36

Animated mini-lecture videos make key concepts easier to understand, while interactive learning activities allow you to expand your knowledge and make the connections to important topics.

Post-Assessment for Psychotic Disorders

Question 4 of 5

The RAISE approach stands for *Recovery After an Initial Schizophrenia Episode*. What are the approaches used in RAISE? *Select all that apply.*

- Personalized treatment plan
- Vocational support
- Case management
- Cognitive remediation
- Family education and support

Next

After working through the video and activity, a **Post-Assessment** quiz tests your mastery.

Personalized Learning at a Glance

Personalized Learning Assignments

Average

Performance	Time Spent	Participation
82% Average Score	18 min	15 / 36

Performance Summary

👍 Congratulations! You have demonstrated competency in 13 of the Personalized Learning topics.

👎 The following topics could use further study and review. Focus study time on:
- Depressive Disorders
- Bereaved Individual

Clinical Judgment Assignments

Average

Performance	Time Spent	Participation
75% Average Score	25 min	2 / 3

Quizzing Assignments

Average

Performance	Time Spent	Participation

Your **Dashboard** provides an at-a-glance snapshot of your performance as you work through your assignments.

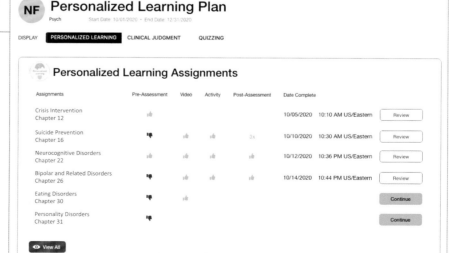

NF Personalized Learning Plan

Psych   Start Date: 10/01/2020 • End Date: 12/31/2020

DISPLAY   **PERSONALIZED LEARNING**   CLINICAL JUDGMENT   QUIZZING

Personalized Learning Assignments

Assignments	Pre-Assessment	Video	Activity	Post-Assessment	Date Complete		
Crisis Intervention Chapter 12	👍				10/05/2020	10:10 AM US/Eastern	Review
Suicide Prevention Chapter 16	👎	👍	👍	3x	10/10/2020	10:30 AM US/Eastern	Review
Neurocognitive Disorders Chapter 22	👍	👍	👍	👍	10/12/2020	10:36 PM US/Eastern	Review
Bipolar and Related Disorders Chapter 26	👎	👍	👍	👍	10/14/2020	10:44 PM US/Eastern	Review
Eating Disorders Chapter 30	👎	👍					Continue
Personality Disorders Chapter 31	👎						Continue

View All

KEY: 👍 80% – 100%   👍 70% – 79%   👎 ≤ 69%

Your **Personalized Learning Plan** is tailored to your individual needs and tracks your progress **across all your assignments**, helping you to identify the exact areas that require additional study.

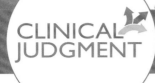
APPLY

STEP #3

Develop clinical judgment skills with Next Gen NCLEX® cases.

Psychotic Disorders

Clinical Judgment Assignment

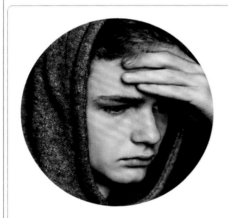

Psychotic Disorders

The nurse is caring for a 16-year-old boy presenting to the behavioral health provider's office with his mother for withdrawn behavior.

This case consists of six clinical judgment questions. Read each question carefully and select the best answer(s). Use the chart to help answer the question. The chart is dynamic and may change as the case progresses.

Real-world cases mirror the complex clinical challenges you will encounter in a variety of healthcare settings. Each **case study** begins with a patient photograph and a brief introduction to the scenario.

The **Patient Chart** displays tabs for History & Physical Assessment, Nurses' Notes, Vital Signs, and Laboratory Results. As you progress through the case, the chart expands and populates with additional data.

Scenario

The nurse is caring for a 16-year-old boy presenting to the behavioral health provider's office with his mother for withdrawn behavior. Use the chart to answer the questions. *The chart may update as the scenario progresses.*

| History and Physical Assessment | Nurses' Notes | Vital Signs | Laboratory Results |

to no interest in things that he used to like to do.

Family History: Paternal aunt with bipolar disorder. Maternal grandmother with depression.

Assessment: Client is a 16-year-old male who appears very withdrawn and disheveled. Only answers questions with one word and does not make eye contact. His movements are very slowed. He states that he feels like there is no hope for the future but denies suicidal ideation. Mother states that over the last 2 years, he has gotten progressively worse with hygiene, not completing schoolwork, and staying in his room all the time with the door locked. Mother states that more recently, he started to exhibit repetitive behaviors such as turning lights on and off seven times when entering the bathroom. Client states that "it's just something I need to do."

Medications: No current medications.

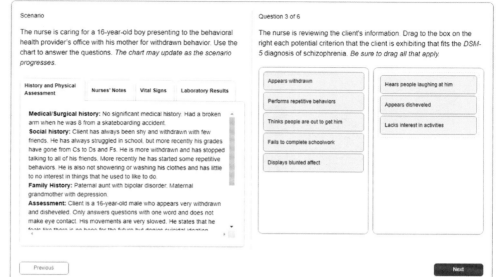

Psychotic Disorders

Scenario

The nurse is caring for a 16-year-old boy presenting to the behavioral health provider's office with his mother for withdrawn behavior. Use the chart to answer the questions. *The chart may update as the scenario progresses.*

| History and Physical Assessment | Nurses' Notes | Vital Signs | Laboratory Results |

Medical/Surgical history: No significant medical history. Had a broken arm when he was 8 from a skateboarding accident.
Social history: Client has always been shy and withdrawn with few friends. He has always struggled in school, but more recently his grades have gone from Cs to Ds and Fs. He is more withdrawn and has stopped talking to all of his friends. More recently he has started some repetitive behaviors. He is also not showering or washing his clothes and has little to no interest in things that he used to like to do.
Family History: Paternal aunt with bipolar disorder. Maternal grandmother with depression.
Assessment: Client is a 16-year-old male who appears very withdrawn and disheveled. Only answers questions with one word and does not make eye contact. His movements are very slowed. He states that he feels like there is no hope for the future but denies suicidal ideation.

Question 3 of 6

The nurse is reviewing the client's information. Drag to the box on the right each potential criterion that the client is exhibiting that fits the *DSM-5* diagnosis of schizophrenia. *Be sure to drag all that apply.*

| Appears withdrawn |
| Performs repetitive behaviors |
| Thinks people are out to get him |
| Fails to complete schoolwork |
| Displays blunted affect |

| Hears people laughing at him |
| Appears disheveled |
| Lacks interest in activities |

Previous | Next

NGN-format questions that align with the cognitive areas of the **NCSBN Clinical Judgment Measurement Model** require careful analysis, synthesis of the data, and multi-step thinking.

Psychotic Disorders

Results

You answered 2 out of 6 questions correctly.

Review the questions, answers and rationales below to improve your understanding. Identify which questions you answered correctly (indicated by a green check mark) and incorrectly (identified by a red x). Remember, you must choose all correct options and only the correct options to get a question correct. Expand the questions to review your individual answer choices, the correct answers (indicated by green shading), and complete rationales.

Hide All Details ▲ | Return to Assignments

❌ **Question 1 of 6** — Hide ▲

The nurse is reviewing the signs of schizophrenia. For each client finding below, specify whether it is consistent with the premorbid phase, prodromal phase, or both. *Select one option in each row.*

	Premorbid Phase	Prodromal Phase	Both Phases
Shy and withdrawn	●	○	○
Poor relationships with friends	●	○	○
Repetitive behaviors	○	●	○
Poor school performance	○	○	●
Not showering	○	○	●
Stays in room all day	○	●	○
No interest in activities	●	○	○

Rationale

The premorbid phase of schizophrenia is characterized by being shy and withdrawn and having poor peer relationships, poor school performance, and antisocial behavior. These signs occur before there is clear evidence to suggest a diagnosis of schizophrenia.

The prodromal phase of schizophrenia has more clearly manifested signs and symptoms and is a worsening of the premorbid phase. This phase can last from a few weeks to 5 years and the person shows significant deterioration in functioning. Half will have depressive symptoms and some will develop symptoms of OCD.

There is overlap in some of the signs and symptoms, but the prodromal phase is significantly worse than premorbid functioning.

Clinical Judgment Cognitive Skill: Analyze Cues   Page Reference: p. 341

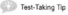 **Test-Taking Tip**   Make a chart for yourself to distinguish among the four phases of schizophrenia.

Immediate feedback with detailed rationales identifies the cognitive skills practiced according to the NCSBN Clinical Judgment Measurement Model and includes page references to the text for further remediation.

Test-taking tips provide important context and strategies for how to consider the structure of each question type when answering.

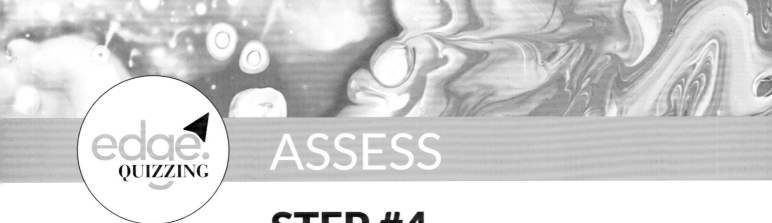

STEP #4

Improve scores and build confidence with NCLEX®-style questions.

High-quality questions, including **Next Gen NCLEX® bowtie and trend questions**, test your knowledge and challenge you to think critically.

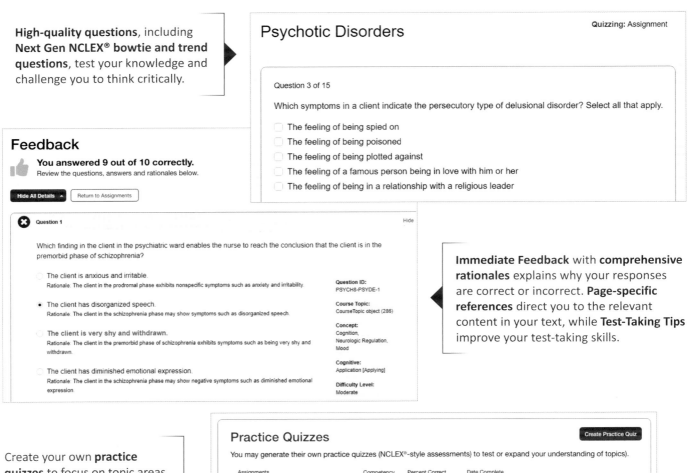

Psychotic Disorders

Quizzing: Assignment

Question 3 of 15

Which symptoms in a client indicate the persecutory type of delusional disorder? Select all that apply.

- ☐ The feeling of being spied on
- ☐ The feeling of being poisoned
- ☐ The feeling of being plotted against
- ☐ The feeling of a famous person being in love with him or her
- ☐ The feeling of being in a relationship with a religious leader

Feedback

👍 **You answered 9 out of 10 correctly.**
Review the questions, answers and rationales below.

[Hide All Details ▲] [Return to Assignments]

❌ **Question 1**   Hide

Which finding in the client in the psychiatric ward enables the nurse to reach the conclusion that the client is in the premorbid phase of schizophrenia?

○ The client is anxious and irritable.
  Rationale: The client in the prodromal phase exhibits nonspecific symptoms such as anxiety and irritability.

● The client has disorganized speech.
  Rationale: The client in the schizophrenia phase may show symptoms such as disorganized speech.

○ The client is very shy and withdrawn.
  Rationale: The client in the premorbid phase of schizophrenia exhibits symptoms such as being very shy and withdrawn.

○ The client has diminished emotional expression.
  Rationale: The client in the schizophrenia phase may show negative symptoms such as diminished emotional expression.

Question ID:
PSYCH8-PSYDE-1

Course Topic:
CourseTopic object (286)

Concept:
Cognition,
Neurologic Regulation,
Mood

Cognitive:
Application [Applying]

Difficulty Level:
Moderate

Immediate Feedback with **comprehensive rationales** explains why your responses are correct or incorrect. **Page-specific references** direct you to the relevant content in your text, while **Test-Taking Tips** improve your test-taking skills.

Create your own **practice quizzes** to focus on topic areas where you are struggling, or use as a study tool to review for an upcoming exam.

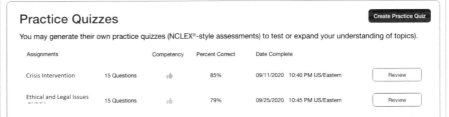

Practice Quizzes

[Create Practice Quiz]

You may generate their own practice quizzes (NCLEX®-style assessments) to test or expand your understanding of topics).

Assignments		Competency	Percent Correct	Date Complete	
Crisis Intervention	15 Questions	👍	85%	09/11/2020 10:40 PM US/Eastern	[Review]
Ethical and Legal Issues	15 Questions	👍	79%	09/25/2020 10:45 PM US/Eastern	[Review]

GET STARTED TODAY!

Use the access code on the inside front cover to unlock
Davis Advantage for **Townsend's Psychiatric Mental Health Nursing!**

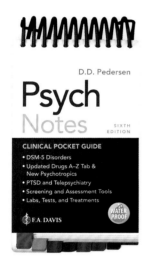
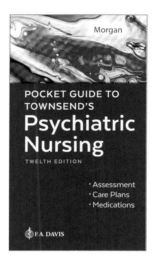
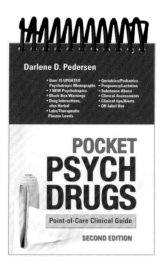

DAVIS ADVANTAGE for
Townsend's Psychiatric Mental Health Nursing

ELEVENTH EDITION

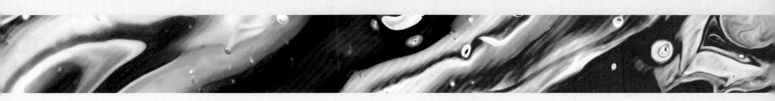

Karyn I. Morgan, RN, MSN, APRN-CNS

Psychiatric Clinical Nurse Specialist
Professor Emerita, Mental Health Nursing
The University of Akron
Akron, Ohio

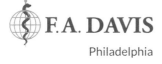 **F. A. DAVIS**

Philadelphia

F. A. Davis Company
1915 Arch Street
Philadelphia, PA 19103
www.fadavis.com

Copyright © 2024 by F. A. Davis Company

Printed in China

Last digit indicates print number: 10 9 8 7 6 5 4 3 2 1

Publisher, Nursing: Susan R. Rhyner
Content Project Manager 2: Amanda Minutola
Design and Illustrations Manager: Carolyn O'Brien

As new scientific information becomes available through basic and clinical research, recommended treatments and drug therapies undergo changes. The author(s) and publisher have done everything possible to make this book accurate, up to date, and in accord with accepted standards at the time of publication. The author(s), editors, and publisher are not responsible for errors or omissions or for consequences from application of the book, and make no warranty, expressed or implied, in regard to the contents of the book. Any practice described in this book should be applied by the reader in accordance with professional standards of care used in regard to the unique circumstances that may apply in each situation. The reader is advised always to check product information (package inserts) for changes and new information regarding dose and contraindications before administering any drug. Caution is especially urged when using new or infrequently ordered drugs.

Library of Congress Cataloging-in-Publication Data

Names: Morgan, Karyn I., author.
Title: Davis advantage for Townsend's psychiatric mental health nursing /
  Karyn I. Morgan.
Description: Eleventh edition. | Philadelphia, PA : F. A. Davis, [2024] |
  Includes bibliographical references and index.
Identifiers: LCCN 2023001186 (print) | LCCN 2023001187 (ebook) | ISBN
  9781719648240 (hardcover) | ISBN 9781719649872 (ebook)
Subjects: MESH: Psychiatric Nursing—methods | Evidence-Based
  Nursing—methods | Mental Disorders—nursing
Classification: LCC RC440 (print) | LCC RC440 (ebook) | NLM WY 160 | DDC
  616.89/0231—dc23/eng/20230417
LC record available at https://lccn.loc.gov/2023001186
LC ebook record available at https://lccn.loc.gov/2023001187

I dedicate this text to all of the nurses who have provided tireless and compassionate care during the recent, unprecedented, global challenges in our lifetime. Nurses continue to be trusted as a reliable source for evidence-based health care information and this is a critical role, especially in an environment where misinformation can be readily available.

—Karyn I. Morgan

Reviewers

Theresa Aldelman
Bradley University
Peoria, Illinois

Fredrick Astle
University of South Carolina
Columbia, South Carolina

Carol Backstedt
Baton Rouge Community College
Baton Rouge, Louisiana

Elizabeth Bailey
Clinton Community College
Pittsburgh, New York

Sheryl Banak
Baptist Health Schools—Little Rock
Little Rock, Arkansas

Joy A. Barham
Northwestern State University
Shreveport, Louisiana

Barbara Barry
Cape Fear Community College
Wilmington, North Carolina

Barbara B. Blozen
NJ City University
Jersey City, New Jersey

Carole Bomba
Harper College
Palatine, Illinois

Judy Bourrand
Samford University
Birmingham, Alabama

Susan Bowles
Barton Community College
Great Bend, Kansas

Wayne Boyer
College of the Desert
Palm Desert, California

Joyce Briggs
Ivy Tech Community College
Columbus, Indiana

Toni Bromley
Rogue Community College
Grants Pass, Oregon

Terrall Bryan
North Carolina A & T State University
Greensboro, North Carolina

Ruth Burkhart
New Mexico State University/Dona Ana Community
College
Las Cruces, New Mexico

Annette Cannon
Platt College
Aurora, Colorado

Deena Collins
Huron School of Nursing
Cleveland, Ohio

Martha Colvin
Georgia College & State University
Milledgeville, Georgia

Mary Jean Croft
St. Joseph School of Nursing
Providence, Rhode Island

Connie Cupples
Union University
Germantown, Tennessee

Karen Curlis
State University of New York Adirondack
Queensbury, New York

Nancy Cyr
North Georgia College and State Universitv
Dahlonega, Georgia

Carol Danner
Baptist Health Schools Little Rock—School
of Nursing
Little Rock, Arkansas

Carolyn DeCicco
Our Lady of Lourdes School of Nursing
Camden, New Jersey

Leona Dempsey
University of Wisconsin Oshkosh
Oshkosh, Wisconsin

Debra J. DeVoe
Our Lady of Lourdes School of Nursing
Camden, New Jersey

Victoria T. Durkee
University of Louisiana at Monroe
Monroe, Louisiana

J. Carol Elliott
St. Anselm College
Fairfield, California

Sandra Farmer
Capital University
Columbus, Ohio

Patricia Freed
Saint Louis University
St. Louis, Missouri

Diane Gardner
University of West Florida
Pensacola, Florida

Maureen Gaynor
Saint Anselm College
Manchester, New Hampshire

Denise Glenore
West Coast University
Riverside, California

Sheilia R. Goodwin
Winston Salem State University
Salem, North Carolina

Janine Graf-Kirk
Trinitas School of Nursing
Elizabeth, New Jersey

Susan B. Grubbs
Francis Marion University
Florence, South Carolina

Elizabeth Gulledge
Jacksonville State University
Jacksonville, Alabama

Kim Gurcan
Columbus Practical School of Nursing
Columbus, Ohio

Victoria Haynes
MidAmerica Nazarene University
Olathe, Kansas

Patricia Jean Hedrick Young
Washington Hospital School of Nursing
Washington, Pennsylvania

Melinda Hermanns
University of Texas at Tyler
Tyler, Texas

Alison Hewig
Victoria College
Victoria, Texas

Cheryl Hilgenberg
Millikin University
Decatur, Illinois

Lori Hill
Gadsden State Community College
Gadsden, Alabama

Ruby Houldson
Illinois Eastern Community College
Olney, Illinois

Eleanor J. Jefferson
Community College of Denver
Platt College
Metropolitan St. College
Denver, Colorado

Dana Johnson
Mesa State College/Grand Junction Regional Center
Grand Junction, Colorado

Janet Johnson
Fort Berthold Community College
New Town, North Dakota

Nancy Kostin
Madonna University
Livonia, Michigan

Linda Lamberson
University of Southern Maine
Portland, Maine

Irene Lang
Bristol Community College
Fall River, Massachusetts

Rhonda Lansdell
Northeast MS Community College
Baldwyn, Mississippi

Jacqueline Leonard
Franciscan University of Steubenville
Steubenville, Ohio

Debra Lett
Trenholm State Community College
Montgomery, Alabama

Judith Lynch-Sauer
University of Michigan
Ann Arbor, Michigan

Glenna Mahoney
University of Saint Mary
Leavenworth, Kansas

Jacqueline Mangnall
Jamestown College
Jamestown, North Dakota

Lori A. Manilla
Hagerstown Community College
Hagerstown, Maryland

Patricia Martin
West Kentucky Community and Technical College
Paducah, Kentucky

Christine Massey
Barton College
Wilson, North Carolina

Joanne Matthews
University of Kentucky
Lexington, Kentucky

Joanne McClave
Wayne Community College
Goldsboro, North Carolina

Mary McClay
Walla Walla University
Portland, Oregon

Susan McCormick
Brazosport College
Lake Jackson, Texas

Shawn McGill
Clovis Community College
Clovis, New Mexico

Margaret McIlwain
Gordon College
Barnesville, Georgia

Nancy Miller
Minneapolis Community and Technical College
Minneapolis, Minnesota

Vanessa Miller
California State University Fullerton
Fullerton, California

Mary Mitsui
Emporia State University
Emporia, Kansas

Cheryl Moreland
Western Nevada College
Carson City, Nevada

Daniel Nanguang
El Paso Community College
El Paso, Texas

Susan Newfield
West Virginia University
Morgantown, West Virginia

Dorothy Oakley
Jamestown Community College
Olean, New York

Christie Obritsch
University of Mary
Bismarck, North Dakota

Sharon Opsahl
Western Technical College
La Crosse, Wisconsin

Vicki Paris
Jackson State Community College
Jackson, Tennessee

Lillian Parker
Clayton State University
Morrow, Georgia

JoAnne M. Pearce
Idaho State University
Pocatello, Idaho

Karen Peterson
DeSales University
Center Valley, Pennsylvania

Kim Anne Pickett
Clemson University
Greenville, South Carolina

Carol Pool
South Texas College
McAllen, Texas

William S. Pope
Barton College
Wilson, North Carolina

Karen Pounds
Northeastern University
Boston, Massachusetts

Konnie Prince
Victoria College
Victoria, Texas

Cheryl Puntil
Hawaii Community College
Hilo, Hawaii

Larry Purnell
University of Delaware
Newark, Delaware

Melissa Reed
University of Alaska Anchorage
Anchorage, Alaska

Jeana Wilcox
Graceland University
Independence, Missouri

Jackie E. Williams
Georgia Perimeter College
Clarkston, Georgia

Rita L. Williams
Langston University School of Nursing & Health
Professions
Langston, Oklahoma

Rodney A. White
Lewis and Clark Community College
Godfrey, Illinois

Vita Wolinsky
Dominican College
Orangeburg, New York

Marguerite Wordell
Kentucky State University
Frankfort, Kentucky

Jan Zlotnick
City College of San Francisco
San Francisco, California

Acknowledgments

Sincere thanks to:

Susan Rhyner, for your skills, your integrity, and your gift of encouragement.

Amanda Minutola and Lynda Hatch, for all your support, accessibility, and assistance in preparing the manuscript.

The nursing educators, students, and clinicians, who provide critical information about the usability of the textbook and offer suggestions for improvements. Many changes have been made based on your input.

The individuals who critiqued the manuscript for this edition and shared your ideas, opinions, and suggestions for enhancement. I sincerely appreciate your contributions to the final product.

Special thanks also to Erin Barnard, Alan Brunner, Vic Farracane, Fred Frese, Bridget Hutchens, Myrle Weems, and the others who courageously allowed their stories to be told.

I appreciate each of you more than I can say.

Karyn I. Morgan

Contents

UNIT 5
Psychiatric-Mental Health Nursing of Special Populations 711

To the Instructor

The impact of the COVID-19 global pandemic put a spotlight on psychiatric and mental health concerns in ways we could not even imagine just a few short years ago. The need for confident nurses—well-versed in assessment and intervention across a broad spectrum of mental health disorders—remains higher than ever. As it has been with each new edition of *Psychiatric Mental Health Nursing*, the goal of this eleventh edition is to bring to practicing nurses and nursing students the most up-to-date information related to neurobiology, psychopharmacology, and evidence-based nursing interventions. This edition includes changes associated with the latest (fifth) edition, text revision of the American Psychiatric Association's *Diagnostic and Statistical Manual of Mental Disorders (DSM-5-TR)*.

Emphasis on Clinical Judgment and NCLEX Next Gen Preparation

As if the pressures of COVID-19 were not enough, the nursing community is simultaneously centered on the debut of the new Next Generation NCLEX exam. In anticipation of the heightened focus on clinical judgment skills, content in this edition of *Psychiatric Mental Health Nursing* has been augmented in several ways:

- *New Textbook Feature—Clinical Judgment in Action.* Case studies in most chapters have been redesigned to guide the student in the National Council of State Boards of Nursing's clinical judgment model that will include case studies as part of the updated licensure exam.
- *New NCLEX Next Gen style questions* have been added to the Instructor Test Bank and to Davis Edge Quizzing.
- *Textbook end of chapter review questions* are presented in two sections—general review of concepts or **Clinical Judgment Questions**—and are written to appear like **NCLEX test questions** for consistency with **The National Council of State Boards of Nursing**'s Next Gen test plan.

We hope this new content helps strengthen student readiness and preparation for their licensure exams as they are immersed in the coursework related to psychiatric-mental health nursing.

The Teaching and Learning Package: Davis Advantage

The past five years have also challenged faculty and students across the globe to migrate, almost overnight, from in-person, "brick-and-mortar" classroom settings to online and distance education. Recognizing those challenges, *Townsend's Psychiatric Mental Health Nursing* expanded the array of faculty and student resources to provide a complete teaching and learning package, including the online resource, *Davis Advantage for Psychiatric Mental Health Nursing*. Davis Advantage provides a wide variety of online activities, animations, and assessments, designed specifically to prepare students for the clinical judgment skills needed to successfully pass the NCLEX licensure exam, with a dashboard of metrics delivered seamlessly to faculty and students alike.

How students learn is constantly evolving, as they consume and process information in new ways. As instructors, we can be no less prepared, and must be ready to provide instruction in person and online, in ways that are engaging and dynamic. Classroom (traditional or online) time is valuable for active learning. This approach makes students responsible for the key concepts, allowing faculty to focus on clinical application. Relying on the textbook alone to support an active classroom leaves a gap. *Davis Advantage for Psychiatric Mental Health Nursing* fills that gap with the following resources:

- **A Strong Core Textbook** that provides the foundation of knowledge that today's nursing students need to pass the NCLEX and enter practice prepared for success.
- An **Online Solution** that provides resources for each step of the learning cycle: learn, apply, assess.
  - **Personalized Learning** assignments are the core of the product and are designed to prepare students for classroom (live or online) discussion. They provide directed learning based on needs. After completing text reading assignments, students take a pre-assessment for each *topic*. Their results feed into their *Personalized Learning Plan*. If students do not pass the pre-assessment, they are required to complete further work within the topic: watch an animated mini-lecture, work through an activity, and take the post-assessment.

The personalized learning content is designed to connect students with the foundational information about a given topic or concept. It provides the gateway to helping make the content accessible to all students and complements different learning styles.

- **Clinical Judgment** assignments are case-based and build off key Personalized Learning topics. These cases help students develop clinical judgment skills through exploratory learning. Students will link their knowledge base (developed through the text and personalized learning) to new data and patient situations. Cases include dynamic charts that expand as the case progresses and use complex question types that require students to analyze data, synthesize conclusions, and make judgments. Each case will end with comprehensive feedback, which provides detailed rationales for the correct and incorrect answers. **Davis Advantage Clinical Judgement Debriefing Guidelines** are also provided, which include reflection questions to enhance student understanding of the Clinical Judgment exercises.

- **Quizzing** assignments build off Personalized Learning topics (and are included for every topic) and help assess students' understanding of the broader scope and increased depth of that topic. The quizzes use NCLEX®-style questions to assess understanding and synthesis of content. Quiz results include comprehensive feedback for correct and incorrect answers to help students understand why their answer choices were right or wrong.

- **Online Instructor Resources** are aimed at creating a dynamic learning experience that relies heavily on interactive participation and is tailored to students' needs. Results from the post-assessments are available to faculty, in aggregate or by student, and inform a **Personalized Teaching Plan** that faculty can use to deliver a targeted classroom experience. Faculty will know students' strengths and weaknesses *before* they come to class and can spend class time focusing on where students are struggling. Suggested in-class activities are provided to help create an interactive, hands-on learning environment that helps students connect more deeply with the content. An accompanying **NCLEX-style test bank** and PowerPoint slides round out the teaching package, with slides that correspond to the textbook chapters referenced in the Personalized Teaching Plans. Finally, an Implementation Guide with a sample syllabus integrating the textbook and Davis Advantage can also be found on www.fadavis.com.

Updated or New Content in the Eleventh Edition Text

All content has been updated to reflect the current state of the discipline of nursing. This includes:

- All nursing diagnoses are current with the NANDA-I *2021–2023 Nursing Diagnoses Definitions and Classifications.*
- A new feature, **"Real Nurses, Real Advice",** has been added to selected chapters highlighting key nursing interventions as identified by practicing nurses.
- A new chapter, *Chapter 11, Psychosocial Interventions and Spiritual Care*, maintains content on milieu therapy while incorporating relaxation therapy and spiritual care from online chapters to a presence in the hardback text. Content on Cognitive Behavior Therapy and Assertiveness Training are mentioned in this chapter but continue to be expanded upon in distinct chapters throughout the text.
- Content on *forensic nursing* has been incorporated in Chapter 34, Survivors of Abuse or Neglect.
- **Updated and new psychotropic drugs** approved since the publication of the eleventh edition are included in the specific diagnostic chapters to which they apply.

Features that Have Been Retained in the Eleventh Edition

- The concept of **holistic nursing** is retained in the eleventh edition. An attempt has been made to ensure that the physical aspects of psychiatric-mental health nursing are not overlooked. In all relevant situations, the mind–body connection is addressed. The importance of trauma-informed care is integrated throughout the text with additional discussion in Chapter 34, Survivors of Abuse or Neglect.
- The term **patient** is used to refer to the recipient of nursing care and the term *client* is used to describe individuals in a broader concept of the individual who accesses a variety of mental health-related services. The purpose is to add consistency, particularly with concepts such as "patient-centered care," one of the six Quality and Safety Education for Nurses (QSEN) criteria.
- **Nursing process** is retained in the eleventh edition as the tool for delivery of care to the individual with a psychiatric disorder or to assist in the primary prevention or exacerbation of mental illness symptoms. The six steps of the nursing process, as described in the American Nurses Association's

Standards of Clinical Nursing Practice, are used to provide guidelines for the nurse. These standards of care are included for the *DSM-5-TR* diagnoses; as well as those on the aging individual, the bereaved individual, survivors of abuse or neglect, and military families; and as examples in several of the therapeutic approaches. The six steps are as follows:

- **Assessment:** Background assessment data, including a description of symptomatology, provides an extensive knowledge base from which the nurse may draw when performing an assessment. Several assessment tools are also included.
- **Diagnosis:** Nursing diagnoses common to specific psychiatric disorders are derived from analysis of assessment data.
- **Outcome Identification:** Outcomes are derived from the nursing diagnoses and stated as measurable goals.
- **Planning:** A plan of care is presented with selected nursing diagnoses for the *DSM-5-TR* diagnoses, as well as for the elderly client, the bereaved individual, victims of abuse or neglect, military veterans and their families, the elderly homebound client, and the primary caregiver of the client with a chronic mental illness. The planning standard also includes tables that list topics for educating clients and families about mental illness. Concept map care plans are included for all major psychiatric diagnoses.
- **Implementation:** The interventions that have been identified in the plan of care are included along with rationales for each. For each chapter in Unit 4, Nursing Care of Patients with Alterations in Psychosocial Adaptation, case studies are included to assist the student in the practical application of theoretical material. Unit 3, Therapeutic Approaches in Psychiatric Nursing Care, describes in detail nursing interventions for a variety of high-volume or high-risk patient problems. In addition, this section of the textbook speaks to the differentiation in scope of practice between the basic-level psychiatric nurse and the advanced practice-level psychiatric nurse.
- **Evaluation:** The evaluation standard includes a set of questions that the nurse may use to assess whether the nursing actions have been successful in achieving the objectives of care.

- **Chapter 4, Psychopharmacology,** describes each class of psychoactive substances. Lists of commonly used agents (along with generic and trade names, half-life, and dosage ranges) can be found in the chapters that discuss specific disorders.

For example, a list of commonly used antipsychotic agents appears in Chapter 24, Schizophrenia Spectrum and Other Psychotic Disorders. These lists also appear online at DavisPlus in the resource called Clinicals Toolkit.

- **Communication Exercises** are included in Chapters 12, Crisis Intervention; 16, Suicide Prevention; 20, The Recovery Model; 22, Neurocognitive Disorders; 23, Substance-Related and Addictive Disorders; 24, Schizophrenia Spectrum and Other Psychotic Disorders; 25, Depressive Disorders; 26, Bipolar and Related Disorders; 27, Anxiety, Obsessive-Compulsive, and Related Disorders; 30, Eating Disorders; 31, Personality Disorders; 34, Survivors of Abuse or Neglect; and 36, The Bereaved Individual; as well as online Chapter 42, Issues Related to Human Sexuality and Gender Dysphoria. These exercises portray clinical scenarios that allow the student to practice communication skills with patients. Examples of answers appear in an appendix at the back of the book.
- **Communication icons and clinical pearls** appear throughout the text and highlight tips for improving therapeutic communication.
- **"Real People, Real Stories" features** include interviews conducted by author Karyn I. Morgan, in which individuals discuss their experience of living with a mental illness and their thoughts on important information for nurses to know. These discussions can be used with students to explore communication issues and interventions to combat stigmatization and to build empathy through understanding individuals' unique experiences. "Real People, Real Stories" interviews are in Chapters 7, Therapeutic Communication; 16, Suicide Prevention; 23, Substance-Related and Addictive Disorders; 24, Schizophrenia Spectrum and Other Psychotic Disorders; 25, Depressive Disorders; 26, Bipolar and Related Disorders; 30, Eating Disorders; 32, Children and Adolescents; 37, Military Families; and 42, Issues Related to Human Sexuality and Gender Dysphoria.
- **QSEN icons** appear selectively throughout chapters to highlight content that reflects application of one or more of the six QSEN competencies (patient-centered care, evidence-based practice, teamwork and collaboration, maintaining safety, quality improvement, and informatics).

Other Features

- **Internet references** for each *DSM-5-TR* diagnosis, with website listings for information related to the disorder.

- **Tables that list topics for patient/family education** (in the clinical chapters).
- **Boxes that include current research studies** with implications for evidence-based nursing practice (in the clinical chapters).
- **Tables that assign nursing diagnoses to patient behaviors** (diagnostic chapters).
- **Taxonomy and diagnostic criteria from the *DSM-5-TR* (2022).** These criteria appear in selected chapters throughout the text.
- **Updated references throughout the text.** Classical references are distinguished from general references.
- **Boxes with definitions of core concepts** appear throughout the text.
- **Movie Connections** boxes at the end of selected chapters identify films relevant to the chapter topic.
- **Comprehensive glossary.**
- **Answers to end-of-chapter review questions** (Appendix A).
- **Answers to communication exercises** (Appendix B).
- **Additional chapters** on theories of personality development, cultural issues, complementary therapies and integrative health, and issues related to human sexuality and gender dysphoria.

Conclusion

Prior to COVID-19, as faculty we were already aware of dangerous trends related to suicide and addiction, especially opioids. Current federally endorsed initiatives, such as the Zero Suicide Initiative (2012) and HEAL (Helping to End Addiction Long-term) (2018), underscore the continuing magnitude of these two mental health issues and make clear that nurses practicing in any arena need a strong foundation in psychiatric mental health nursing care. Perhaps as never before, many nurse leaders see this period as an opportunity for nurses to expand their roles and assume key positions in education, prevention, assessment, and referral. Nurses are, and will continue to be, in key positions to assist individuals to attain, maintain, or regain optimal emotional wellness.

It is hoped that the revisions and additions to this eleventh edition continue to satisfy a need within psychiatric-mental health nursing practice. The mission of this textbook has been, and continues to be, to provide both students and clinicians with up-to-date information about psychiatric-mental health nursing. The user-friendly format and easy-to-understand language, for which we have received many positive comments, have been retained in this edition. We hope that this eleventh edition continues to promote and advance the commitment to psychiatric/mental health nursing.

Karyn I. Morgan

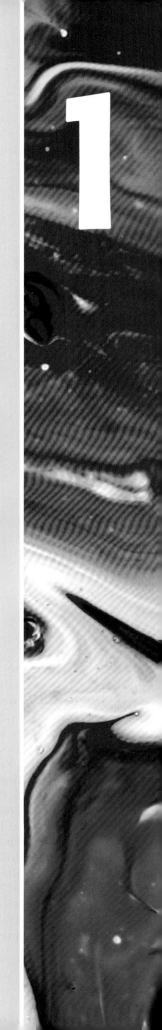

Basic Concepts in Psychiatric-Mental Health Nursing

1 The Concept of Stress Adaptation

KEY TERMS

adaptive responses
fight-or-flight syndrome
general adaptation syndrome
maladaptive responses

precipitating event
predisposing factors

OBJECTIVES
After reading this chapter, the student will be able to:

1. Define *adaptation* and *maladaptation*.
2. Identify physiological responses to stress.
3. Explain the relationship between stress and "diseases of adaptation."
4. Describe the concept of stress as an environmental event.
5. Explain the concept of stress as a transaction between the individual and the environment.
6. Discuss adaptive coping strategies in the management of stress.

Psychologists and others have struggled for many years to establish an effective definition of the term *stress*. This term is used loosely today and still lacks a definitive explanation. Stress may be viewed as an individual's reaction to any change that requires an adjustment or response, which can be physical, mental, or emotional. Responses directed at stabilizing internal biological processes and preserving self-esteem can be viewed as healthy adaptations to stress.

Roy (1976), a nursing theorist, defined **adaptive responses** as behaviors that maintain the integrity of the individual. Adaptation is viewed as positive and is correlated with a healthy response. When behavior disrupts the integrity of the individual, it is perceived as maladaptive. **Maladaptive responses** by the individual are considered to be harmful or unhealthy.

Various 20th-century researchers contributed to several different concepts of stress. Three of these concepts are stress as a biological response, stress as an environmental event, and stress as a transaction between the individual and the environment. This chapter includes an explanation of each of these concepts.

CORE CONCEPT
Stressor
A biological, psychological, social, or chemical factor that causes physical or emotional tension and may contribute to the development of certain illnesses.

Stress as a Biological Response

In 1956, Hans Selye published the results of his research on the physiological response of a biological system to an imposed change on the system.

2

Since his initial publication, his definition of stress has evolved to "the state manifested by a specific syndrome which consists of all the nonspecifically induced changes within a biological system" (Selye, 1976). This combination of symptoms has come to be known as the **fight-or-flight syndrome.** Schematics of these biological responses, both initially and with sustained stress, are presented in Figures 1–1 and 1–2. Selye called this phenomenon the **general adaptation syndrome.** He described three distinct stages of the reaction:

1. **Alarm reaction stage:** During this stage, the physiological responses of the fight-or-flight syndrome are initiated.
2. **Stage of resistance:** The individual uses the physiological responses of the first stage as a defense in the attempt to adapt to the stressor. If adaptation occurs, the third stage is prevented or delayed. Physiological symptoms may disappear.
3. **Stage of exhaustion:** This stage occurs when the body responds to prolonged exposure to a stressor. The adaptive energy becomes depleted, and the individual can no longer draw from the resources for adaptation described in the first two stages. Diseases of adaptation (e.g., headaches, mental disorders, coronary artery disease, ulcers, colitis) may occur. Without intervention for reversal, exhaustion, and in some cases even death, ensues (Selye, 1956, 1974).

The fight-or-flight response undoubtedly served our ancestors well. Those *Homo sapiens* who had to face giant grizzly bears or saber-toothed tigers as part of their struggle for survival must have used these adaptive resources to their advantage. The response was elicited in emergency situations, used in the preservation of life, and followed by restoration of the compensatory mechanisms to the preemergent condition (homeostasis).

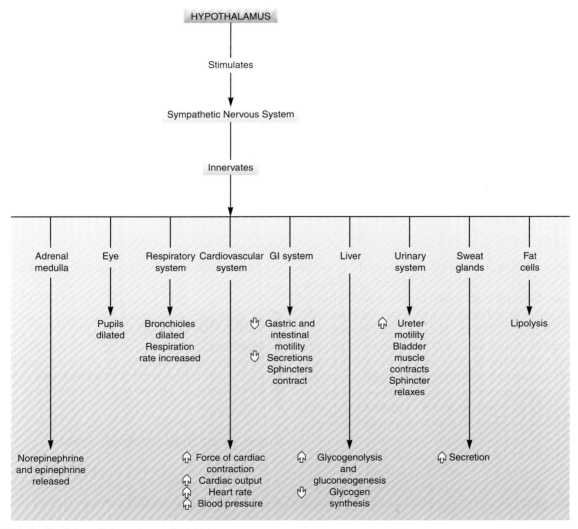

FIGURE 1–1   The fight-or-flight syndrome: The initial stress response.

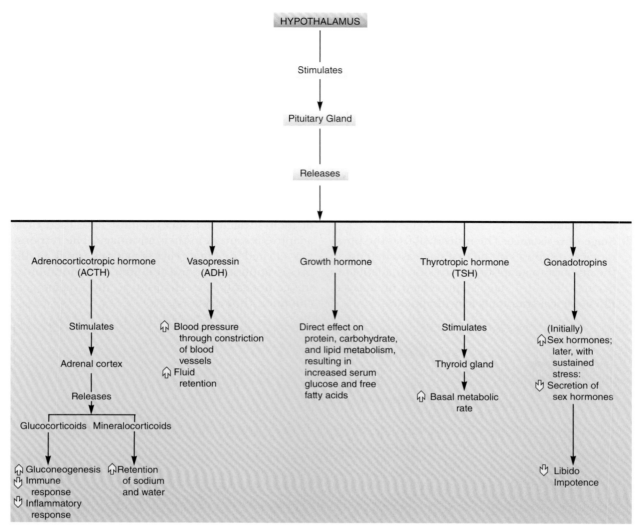

FIGURE 1–2   The fight-or-flight syndrome: The sustained stress response.

Selye performed his extensive research in a controlled setting with laboratory animals as subjects. He elicited the physiological responses with physical stimuli, such as exposure to heat or extreme cold, electric shock, injection of toxic agents, restraint, and surgical injury. Since the publication of his original research, it has become apparent that the fight-or-flight syndrome of symptoms occurs in response to psychological or emotional stimuli just as it does to physical stimuli. Psychological or emotional stressors are often not resolved as rapidly as physical stressors, so the body may be depleted of its adaptive energy more readily than it is from physical stressors. The fight-or-flight response may be inappropriate or even dangerous in our modern lifestyle in which stress has been described as a pervasive, chronic, and relentless psychosocial state. When the stress response becomes chronic, the body's persistent aroused condition for extended time periods increases an individual's risk for disease.

CORE CONCEPT
Adaptation
Adaptation is the process by which an individual's response to change results in the preservation of individual integrity or a timely return to equilibrium.

Stress as an Environmental Event

A second concept defines stress as an "event" that triggers an individual's adaptive physiological and psychological responses. The event creates change in the life pattern of the individual, requires significant adjustment in lifestyle, and taxes available personal resources. The change can be either positive, such as an outstanding personal achievement, or negative, such as being fired from a job. The emphasis here is on *change* from the existing steady state of the individual's life pattern.

Miller and Rahe (1997) have updated the original Social Readjustment Rating Scale devised in 1967 by Holmes and Rahe (1967) to reflect an increased number of modern stressors. Just as in the earlier version, numerical values are assigned to various common life events based on the stress these events create. In their research, Miller and Rahe (1997) found that women react to life stress events at higher levels than do men, and unmarried people gave higher scores than married people for most of the events. Younger participants rated more events at a higher stress level than did older participants. A high score on the Recent Life Changes Questionnaire (RLCQ) places the individual at greater susceptibility to physical or psychological illness. The questionnaire may be completed considering life stressors within a 6-month or 1-year period. Six-month totals equal to or greater than 300 life change units (LCUs) or 1-year totals equal to or greater than 500 LCUs are considered indicative of a high level of recent life stress, thereby increasing the individual's risk of illness. The RLCQ is presented in Table 1–1.

It is unknown whether stress overload merely predisposes a person to illness or actually precipitates it, but decades of research support that there is a link (Seiler et al., 2020). Individuals differ in their reactions to life events, and these variations are related to the degree to which the change is perceived as stressful.

Life changes questionnaires have been criticized because they do not consider the individual's perception of the event. These types of instruments also fail to consider cultural variations, the individual's coping strategies, and the available support systems

TABLE 1–1 The Recent Life Changes Questionnaire

LIFE CHANGE EVENT	LCU	LIFE CHANGE EVENT	LCU
HEALTH		Loss of job:	
An injury or illness which:	74	Laid off from work	68
Kept you in bed a week or more, or sent you to the hospital		Fired from work	79
Was less serious than above	44	Correspondence course to help you in your work	18
Major dental work	26	**PERSONAL AND SOCIAL**	
Major change in eating habits	27	Change in personal habits	26
Major change in sleeping habits	26	Beginning or ending school or college	38
Major change in your usual type/amount of recreation	28	Change of school or college	35
WORK		Change in political beliefs	24
Change to a new type of work	51	Change in religious beliefs	29
Change in your work hours or conditions	35	Change in social activities	27
Change in your responsibilities at work:		Vacation	24
More responsibilities	29	New, close, personal relationship	37
Fewer responsibilities	21	Engagement to marry	45
Promotion	31	Girlfriend or boyfriend problems	39
Demotion	42	Sexual difficulties	44
Transfer	32	"Falling out" of a close personal relationship	47
Troubles at work:		An accident	48
With your boss	29	Minor violation of the law	20
With coworkers	35	Being held in jail	75
With persons under your supervision	35	Death of a close friend	70
Other work troubles	28		
Major business adjustment	60		
Retirement	52		

Continued

TABLE 1–1 The Recent Life Changes Questionnaire–cont'd

LIFE CHANGE EVENT	LCU	LIFE CHANGE EVENT	LCU
Major decision regarding your immediate future	51	In-law problems	38
Major personal achievement	36	Change in the marital status of your parents:	
HOME AND FAMILY		Divorce	59
Major change in living conditions	42	Remarriage	50
Change in residence:		Separation from spouse:	
Move within the same town or city	25	Due to work	53
Move to a different town, city, or state	47	Due to marital problems	76
Change in family get-togethers	25	Divorce	96
Major change in health or behavior of family member	55	Birth of grandchild	43
		Death of spouse	119
Marriage	50	Death of other family member:	
Pregnancy	67	Child	123
Miscarriage or abortion	65	Brother or sister	102
		Parent	100
Gain of a new family member:		**FINANCIAL**	
Birth of a child	66	Major change in finances:	
Adoption of a child	65	Increased income	38
A relative moving in with you	59	Decreased income	60
		Investment and/or credit difficulties	56
Spouse beginning or ending work	46	Loss or damage of personal property	43
Child leaving home:		Moderate purchase	20
To attend college	41	Major purchase	37
Due to marriage	41		
For other reasons	45	Foreclosure on a mortgage or loan	58
Change in arguments with spouse	50		

LCU, life change unit.

Source: Miller, M.A., & Rahe, R.H. (1997). Life changes scaling for the 1990s. *Journal of Psychosomatic Research, 43*(3), 279–292, with permission.

at the time when the life change occurs. Amirkhan (2012) developed a tool to assess stress overload that attempts to correct for these limitations by asking a series of 30 questions that all begin with "In the past week have you felt..." followed by choices such as calm, inadequate, depressed, and others. The emphasis in this tool is on the individual's perception of events rather than on the events themselves. Artani et al. (2017) studied and subsequently adapted the RLCQ to better assess contextual stressors in a large urban community in Pakistan. One of the adaptations they made was to add a category assessing environmental stressors, noting that "stressful life events for adults living in Pakistan differ from developed countries because of poverty, lawlessness, and political instability" (p. 6). Although the approaches to assessing for stress and vulnerability vary, it is clear that positive coping mechanisms and strong social or familial support can reduce the intensity of stressful life changes and promote a more adaptive response.

Stress as a Transaction Between the Individual and the Environment

The concept of stress as a transaction between the individual and the environment emphasizes the *relationship* between internal variables (within an individual) and external variables (within the environment). This concept parallels the modern concept of disease etiology. No longer is causation viewed solely as an external entity; whether or not illness occurs depends also on the receiving organism's susceptibility. Similarly, to predict psychological stress as a reaction, the internal characteristics of the person in relation to the environment must be considered.

Precipitating Event

Lazarus and Folkman's seminal theory (1984) defined stress (and potentially illness) as a psychological phenomenon in which the relationship between the person and the environment is appraised by the person as taxing or exceeding their resources and endangering their well-being. A **precipitating event** is a stimulus arising from the internal or external environment and perceived by the individual in a specific manner. Determination of an event as stressful depends on the individual's cognitive appraisal of the situation. *Cognitive appraisal* is an individual's evaluation of the personal significance of the event or occurrence. The event "precipitates" a response on the part of the individual, and the response is influenced by the individual's perception of the event. The *cognitive response* consists of a primary appraisal and a secondary appraisal.

Individual's Perception of the Event
Primary Appraisal

Lazarus and Folkman (1984) identified three types of primary appraisal: irrelevant, benign-positive, and stressful. An event is judged *irrelevant* when the outcome holds no significance for the individual. A *benign-positive* outcome is one that is perceived as producing pleasure for the individual. *Stressful* appraisals include harm or loss, threat, and challenge. *Harm* or *loss* appraisals refer to damage or loss already experienced by the individual. Appraisals of a *threatening* nature are perceived as anticipated harms or losses. When an event is appraised as *challenging*, the individual focuses on potential for gain or growth rather than on risks associated with the event. Challenge produces stress even though the emotions associated with it (eagerness and excitement) are viewed as positive, and coping mechanisms must be called upon to face the new encounter. Challenge and threat may occur together when an individual experiences these positive emotions along with fear or anxiety over possible risks associated with the challenging event.

When stress is produced in response to harm or loss, threat, or challenge, a secondary appraisal is made by the individual.

Secondary Appraisal

The secondary appraisal is an assessment of skills, resources, and knowledge that the person possesses to deal with the situation. The individual appraises the situation by considering the following:

- Which coping strategies are available to me?
- Will the option I choose be effective in this situation?
- Do I have the ability to use that strategy in an effective manner?

The interaction between the primary appraisal of the event that has occurred and the secondary appraisal of available coping strategies determines the quality of the individual's adaptation response to stress.

Predisposing Factors

A variety of elements influence how an individual perceives and responds to a stressful event. These **predisposing factors** strongly influence whether the response is adaptive or maladaptive. Types of predisposing factors include genetic influences, past experiences, and existing conditions.

Genetic influences are those circumstances of an individual's life that are acquired through heredity. Examples include family history of physical and psychological conditions (strengths and weaknesses) and temperament (behavioral characteristics present at birth that evolve with development).

Past experiences are occurrences that result in learned patterns that can influence an individual's adaptation response. They include previous exposure to the stressor or other stressors, learned coping responses, and degree of adaptation to previous stressors.

Existing conditions incorporate vulnerabilities that influence the adequacy of the individual's physical, psychological, and social resources for dealing with adaptive demands. Examples include current health status, motivation, developmental maturity, severity and duration of the stressor, financial and educational resources, age, existing coping strategies, and a caring support system. Hobfoll's conservation of resources theory (Hobfoll, 1989; Hobfoll et al., 1998) adds that as existing conditions (loss or lack of resources) exceed the person's perception of adaptive capabilities, the person not only experiences stress in the present but also becomes more vulnerable to the effects of stress in the future due to a "weaker resource reservoir to call on to meet future demand" (Hobfoll et al., 1998, p. 191).

All of the preceding concepts and theories are foundational to the transactional model of stress and adaptation that serves as the framework for the process of nursing in this text. A graphic display of the model is presented in Figure 1–3.

CORE CONCEPT
Maladaptation
Maladaptation is the process by which an individual's response to change results in disruption of individual integrity or in persistent disequilibrium.

Stress Management

The growth of stress management into a multimillion-dollar-a-year industry attests to its importance in our society. Stress management involves the use of coping strategies in response to stressful situations. (Some stress management techniques are discussed

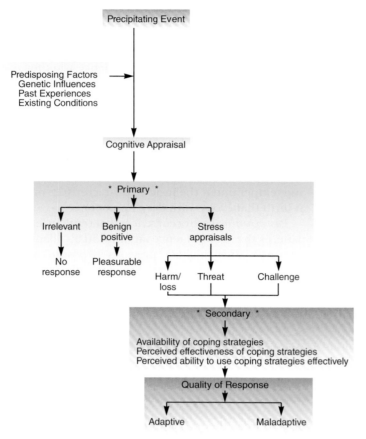

FIGURE 1-3 Transactional model of stress and adaptation.

at greater length in Chapter 11, "Psychosocial Interventions and Spiritual Care"). Coping strategies are adaptive when they protect the individual from harm (or additional harm) or strengthen the individual's ability to meet challenging situations. Adaptive responses help restore homeostasis to the body and impede the development of diseases of adaptation. Positive adaptation, particularly in response to adversity, has also been referred to as *resilience*.

Responses are considered maladaptive when the conflict goes unresolved or intensifies. Energy resources become depleted as the body struggles to compensate for the chronic physiological and psychological arousal experienced in response to the stressful event. The effect is a significant vulnerability to physical or psychological illness. One key to stress management is to identify factors and practices that contribute to adaptive coping and resilience.

Adaptive Coping Strategies

Awareness

The initial step in managing stress is awareness—to become aware of the factors that create stress and the feelings associated with a stressful response. Stress can be managed only when one recognizes the signs that it is occurring. As an individual becomes aware of stressors, they can choose to omit, avoid, or accept them.

Relaxation

Individuals experience relaxation in different ways. Some people relax by engaging in gross motor activities, such as sports, jogging, and physical exercise. Others use techniques such as breathing exercises and progressive relaxation. A discussion of relaxation therapy is described in more detail in Chapter 11, "Psychosocial Interventions and Spiritual Care."

Meditation

Meditation has been shown to produce a lasting reduction in blood pressure and other stress-related symptoms when practiced for 20 minutes once or twice a day (Scott, 2020). The practice of mindfulness meditation is foundational to many psychosocial interventions aimed at reducing anxiety and improving engagement in problem-solving. Meditation involves assuming a comfortable position, closing the eyes, casting off all other thoughts, and concentrating on a single word, sound, or phrase that has positive meaning to the individual. It may also involve concentrating on one's breathing or other mindfulness practices. Mindfulness meditation is described in more detail in Chapter 11, "Psychosocial Interventions and Spiritual Care."

Interpersonal Communication

As previously mentioned, the strength of an individual's available support system is an existing condition that significantly influences adaptation when coping with stress. Sometimes just "talking the problem out" with an empathetic individual can interrupt escalation of the stress response. Writing about one's feelings in a journal or diary can also be therapeutic.

Problem-Solving

Problem-solving is an adaptive coping strategy in which the individual is able to view the situation objectively (or to seek assistance from another individual to accomplish this if the anxiety level is too high to concentrate) and then apply a problem-solving and decision-making model such as the following:

- Assess the facts of the situation.
- Formulate goals for resolution of the stressful situation.
- Study the alternatives for dealing with the situation.
- Determine the risks and benefits of each alternative.
- Select an alternative.
- Implement the alternative selected.
- Evaluate the outcome of the alternative implemented.
- Select and implement a second option if the first choice is ineffective.

Pets

Studies show that those who care for pets, especially dogs and cats, are better able to cope with the stressors of life (Pendry & Vandagriff, 2019). The physical act of stroking a dog's or cat's fur can be therapeutic, giving the animal an intuitive sense of being cared for and providing the individual the calming feeling of warmth, affection, and interdependence with a reliable, trusting being. Studies have also shown that individuals with companion pets demonstrate improvements in heart health, allergies, anxiety, and mental illnesses such as depression (Casciotti & Zuckerman, 2022; Robinson, 2022).

Music

Studies have shown multiple benefits of listening to music, including relieving pain, improving motivation and performance, improving sleep, enhancing blood vessel function, reducing stress, relieving symptoms of depression, improving cognition, and easing recovery in stroke patients (Blocker, 2021; Traynor, 2021).

Summary and Key Points

- Stress has become a chronic and pervasive condition in the United States.
- Adaptive behavior is a stress response that maintains the integrity of the individual with a timely return to equilibrium. It is viewed as positive and is correlated with a healthy response.
- When behavior disrupts the integrity of the individual or results in persistent disequilibrium, it is perceived as maladaptive. Maladaptive responses by the individual are unhealthy.
- A stressor is defined as a biological, psychological, social, or chemical factor that causes physical or emotional tension and may be a factor in the etiology of certain illnesses.
- Hans Selye identified the biological changes associated with a stressful situation as the fight-or-flight syndrome. Selye called the general reaction of the body to stress the "general adaptation syndrome," which occurs in three stages: the alarm reaction stage, the stage of resistance, and the stage of exhaustion.
- When individuals remain in the aroused response to stress for an extended period of time, they become susceptible to diseases, including headaches, mental disorders, coronary artery disease, ulcers, and colitis.
- Stress may also be viewed as an environmental event, which results when a change from the existing steady state of the individual's life pattern occurs. When an individual experiences a high level of life change events, they become susceptible to physical or psychological illness.
- Limitations of the environmental concept of stress include failure to consider the individual's perception of the event, coping strategies, and available support systems at the time when the life change occurs.
- Stress is more appropriately expressed as a transaction between the individual and the environment that is appraised by the individual as taxing or exceeding their resources and endangering their well-being.
- The individual makes a cognitive appraisal of the precipitating event to determine the personal significance of the event or occurrence.
- Primary cognitive appraisals may conclude that an event is irrelevant, benign-positive, or stressful.
- Secondary cognitive appraisals include evaluation by the individual of skills, resources, and knowledge to deal with the stressful situation.
- Predisposing factors influence how an individual perceives and responds to a stressful event. They include genetic influences, past experiences, and existing conditions.

■ Stress management involves the use of adaptive coping strategies in response to stressful situations in an effort to impede the development of diseases of adaptation.

■ Examples of adaptive coping strategies include developing awareness, relaxation, meditation, interpersonal communication with caring other, problem-solving, pets, and music.

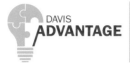 **DAVIS ADVANTAGE** | Go to **Davis Advantage** to complete your learning: strengthen understanding, apply your knowledge, and prepare for the Next Gen NCLEX®.

Review Questions

1. When assessing whether a client is exhibiting adaptive responses to stressors, the nurse must recognize which of the following?
   a. Adaptive responses are those that preserve the integrity of the individual.
   b. Adaptive responses eliminate all stressors.
   c. Adaptive responses can only be achieved through intensive therapy.
   d. Adaptive responses are whatever the client perceives them to be.

2. Why is stress management so important in one's overall health?
   a. Stress-related disorders strengthen the immune system.
   b. Sustained response to stress can increase vulnerability to a variety of diseases and maladaptive coping responses.
   c. Relaxation exercises are effective in preventing disorders such as depression and suicide.
   d. All of the above.

3. A client has just received a job promotion and, although excited about career advancement, has been experiencing anxiety since receiving the news. The nurse accurately assesses the client's primary appraisal of the situation as which of the following?
   a. Benign-positive
   b. Irrelevant
   c. Challenging
   d. Threatening

4. Which of the following statements by a client are examples of adaptive coping mechanisms?
   a. "I like to take the edge off by having a few drinks."
   b. "I need to pay more attention to my calorie intake because I gained 10 pounds in the last month."
   c. "When the stress gets to be too much, I feel better after I kick the dog."
   d. "I try to stay away from people because it's less stressful than arguing with everybody."

Clinical Judgment Questions

5. A client reports hearing on last night's evening news that 25 people were killed in a tornado in south Texas, but the individual appears to express no anxiety in response to this stressful situation. Which of these actions by the nurse is a priority?
   a. Ask where the client lives.
   b. Assess the client's perception about the relevance of this event.
   c. Encourage the client to use adaptive coping skills to help others through this tragedy.
   d. Ask where the client grew up.

6. A client regularly develops nausea and vomiting when faced with a stressful situation. Which of the following should be assessed when attempting to identify predisposing factors? (Select all that apply.)
   a. Identify what happened right before the most recent episode of nausea and vomiting.
   b. Consider genetic influences.
   c. Identify any existing physical conditions that might make the client more vulnerable to respond in this way.
   d. Explore past experiences that may have resulted in this becoming a learned response.

7. A client comes to the mental health clinic with reports of anxiety and depression. Using the transactional model of stress and adaptation, which of the following are important nursing actions when assessing these complaints? (Select all that apply.)
   a. Evaluate the client's perception of precipitating events.
   b. Ask the client about past stressors and degree of positive coping abilities.
   c. Assess the client's existing social supports.
   d. Evaluate the client's physical strength.
   e. Monitor the client's temperature.

8. A client says to the nurse, "I think that meditation might be a good thing for reducing my anxiety, but I've never learned how to do it." Which of these would be the most appropriate response by the nurse?
   a. Instruct the client that antianxiety medication must be taken before engaging in meditation.
   b. Ask why the client never learned this method of relaxation.
   c. Educate the client about the evidence supporting pet therapy as the most effective psychosocial coping mechanism.
   d. Educate the client about how to engage in mindfulness meditation.

9. A client tells the nurse, "My spouse and I got into a big fight, and I just stormed out because I didn't know what else to do." Which action by the nurse is a priority at this point?
   a. Encourage the client to seek legal advice from a divorce lawyer.
   b. Ask the client to describe the spouse's side of the story.
   c. Affirm the client's response as the most appropriate way to reduce anxiety in such situations.
   d. Assist the client to describe the event.

10. A new client tells the nurse at the mental health clinic, "I was so stressed out after work today and trying to get to my appointment here on time that I started having chest pain." Which action by the nurse is a priority at this point?
   a. Offer the client antianxiety medication as prescribed.
   b. Assess the client's physical status, including vital signs.
   c. Reinforce that since the client arrived on time there is nothing to worry about.
   d. Help the client to identify adaptive coping mechanisms for dealing with stress.

References

Amirkhan, J. H. (2012). Stress overload: A new approach to the assessment of stress. *American Journal of Community Psychology, 49*(1-2), 55–71. doi:10.1007/s10464-011-9438-x

Artani, A., Bhamani, S. S., Azam, I., AbdulSultan, M., Khoja, A., & Kama, A. K. (2017). Adaptation of the recent life changes questionnaire (RLCQ) to measure stressful life events in adults residing in an urban megapolis in Pakistan. *BMC Psychiatry 17*, 169, 1–12. https://doi.org/10.1186/s12888-017-1315-1

Blocker, K. (2021). *Benefits of music: 5 ways to use music to improve your daily life*. https://www.uchealth.org/today/benefits-of-music-5-ways-to-use-music-to-improve-your-daily life/

Casciotti, D., & Zuckerman, D. (2022). *The benefits of pets for human health*. http://www.center4research.org/benefits-pets-human-health/

Pendry, P., & Vandagriff, J. L. (2019). Animal visitation program (AVP) reduces cortisol levels of university students: A randomized controlled trial. *AERA Open, 5*(2). https://doi.org/10.1177/2332858419852592

Robinson, K. M. (2022). *How pets help manage depression*. https://www.webmd.com/depression/features/pets-depression

Scott, E. (2020). *The benefits of meditation for stress management*. https://www.verywell.com/meditation-research-and-benefits-3144996

Seiler, A., Fagundes, C. P., & Christian, L. M. (2020). The impact of everyday stressors on the immune system and health. In Choukèr, A. (Ed.), *Stress challenges and immunity in space*. Springer, Cham. https://doi.org/10.1007/978-3-030-16996-1_6

Traynor, C. (2021). What are the health benefits of music? *News Medical Life Sciences*. https://www.news-medical.net/health/What-Are-the-Health-Benefits-of-Music.aspx

Classical References

Hobfoll, S. (1989). Conservation of resources: A new attempt at conceptualizing stress. *American Psychologist, 44*(3), 513–524. doi: http://dx.doi.org/10.1037/0003-066X.44.3.513

Hobfoll, S., Schwarzer, R., & Chon, K. (1998). Disentangling the stress labyrinth: Interpreting the meaning of stress as it is studied in the health context. *Anxiety, Stress, and Coping, 11*(3), 181–212. doi:http://dx.doi.org/10.1080/10615809808248311

Holmes, T., & Rahe, R. (1967). The social readjustment rating scale. *Journal of Psychosomatic Research, 11*(2), 213–218. doi:http://dx.doi.org/10.1016/0022-3999(67)90010-4

Lazarus, R. S., & Folkman, S. (1984). *Stress, appraisal and coping*. Springer Publishing.

Miller, M. A., & Rahe, R. H. (1997). Life changes scaling for the 1990s. *Journal of Psychosomatic Research, 43*(3), 279–292. doi:10.1016/S0022-3999(97)00118-9

Roy, C. (1976). *Introduction to nursing: An adaptation model*. Prentice-Hall.

Selye, H. (1956). *The stress of life*. McGraw-Hill.

Selye, H. (1974). *Stress without distress*. Signet Books.

Selye, H. (1976). *The stress of life* (rev. ed.). McGraw Hill.

2 Mental Health and Mental Illness: Historical and Theoretical Concepts

KEY TERMS

anosognosia
coping skills
ego defense mechanisms
grief

mental health
mental illness
neurosis
psychosis

OBJECTIVES
After reading this chapter, the student will be able to:

1. Discuss the history of psychiatric care.
2. Define *mental health* and *mental illness.*
3. Discuss cultural elements that influence attitudes toward mental health and mental illness.
4. Describe psychological adaptation responses to stress.
5. Correlate adaptive and maladaptive responses to the mental health/mental illness continuum.

The consideration of mental health and mental illness has its basis in the cultural beliefs of the society in which the behavior takes place. What may be considered acceptable behavior in one culture may be considered abnormal in another.

A study of the history of psychiatric care reveals some shocking truths about past treatment of individuals with mental illness. Many were kept in control by means that today could be considered abuse.

This chapter deals with the evolution of psychiatric care from ancient times to the present. **Mental health** and **mental illness** are defined, and the psychological adaptation to stress is explained in terms of the two major responses: anxiety and grief. Behavioral responses are conceptualized along the mental health/mental illness continuum.

Historical Overview of Psychiatric Care

Primitive thoughts regarding mental disturbances varied and were often rooted in cultural and religious beliefs. Some cultures thought that an individual with mental illness had been dispossessed of their soul and wellness could be achieved only if the soul was returned. Others believed that evil spirits or supernatural or magical powers had entered the body. The "cure" for these individuals involved a ritualistic exorcism that often consisted of brutal beatings, starvation, or other harsh means to purge the body of these unwanted forces. Still other cultures considered that the mentally ill individual may have broken a taboo or sinned against another individual or God, for which ritualistic purification was required or various types of retribution were demanded.

The correlation of mental illness to demonology or witchcraft led to some mentally ill individuals being executed.

These ancient beliefs dwindled with increasing knowledge about mental illness and changes in cultural, religious, and sociopolitical attitudes. Around 400 BCE, the work of Hippocrates was the first to place mental illness in a physical rather than supernatural context. Hippocrates theorized that mental illness was caused by irregularity in the interaction of the four body fluids: blood, black bile, yellow bile, and phlegm. He called these body fluids *humors* and associated each with a particular disposition. Disequilibrium among these four humors was often treated by inducing vomiting and diarrhea with potent cathartic drugs.

During the Middle Ages (CE 500 to 1500), the association of mental illness with witchcraft and the supernatural continued to prevail in Europe. During this period, many people with mental illness were set to sea alone in sailing boats with little guidance to search for their lost rationality, a practice from which the expression "ship of fools" was derived. But in Middle Eastern countries, mental illness began to be perceived as a medical problem rather than a result of supernatural forces. This notion gave rise to the establishment of specialized hospital units and residential institutions specifically designed for clients with mental illness. They can likely be considered the first asylums for individuals with mental illness.

Colonial Americans tended to reflect the attitudes of the European communities from which they had emigrated. Particularly in the New England area, individuals were punished for behavior attributed to witchcraft. In the 16th and 17th centuries, institutions for people with mental illness did not exist in the United States, and care of these individuals was a family responsibility. Those without family or other resources became the responsibility of the communities in which they lived and were incarcerated in places where they could not harm themselves or others.

The first hospital in America to admit clients with mental illness was established in Philadelphia in the middle of the 18th century. Benjamin Rush, often called the father of American psychiatry, was a physician at the hospital. He initiated the provision of humanistic treatment and care for clients with mental illness. Although he included kindness, exercise, and socialization in his care, he also employed harsh methods such as bloodletting, purging, various types of physical restraints, and extremes of temperatures, reflecting the medical therapies of that era.

The 19th century brought the establishment of a system of state asylums, largely the result of the work of Dorothea Dix, a former New England schoolteacher who lobbied tirelessly on behalf of the mentally ill population. She was unwavering in her belief that mental illness was curable and that state hospitals should provide humanistic therapeutic care. This system of hospital care for individuals with mental illness grew, but the mentally ill population grew faster. The institutions became overcrowded and understaffed, and conditions deteriorated. Therapeutic care reverted to custodial care in state hospitals, which provided the largest resource for individuals with mental illness until the initiation of the community health movement of the 1960s (see Chapter 35, "Community Mental Health Nursing").

The emergence of psychiatric nursing began in 1873 with the graduation of Linda Richards from the nursing program at the New England Hospital for Women and Children in Boston. She has come to be known as the first American psychiatric nurse. During her career, Richards was instrumental in the establishment of a number of psychiatric hospitals and the first school of psychiatric nursing at the McLean Asylum in Waverly, Massachusetts, in 1882. This school and others like it provided training in custodial care for clients in psychiatric asylums—training that did not include the study of psychological concepts. Significant change in psychiatric nursing education did not occur until 1955, when incorporation of psychiatric nursing into the curricula became a requirement for all undergraduate schools of nursing. This new curriculum emphasized the importance of the nurse–patient relationship and therapeutic communication techniques. Nursing intervention in the somatic therapies (e.g., insulin and electroconvulsive therapy) provided impetus for the incorporation of these concepts into the profession's body of knowledge.

With the increasing need for psychiatric care in the aftermath of World War II, the government passed the National Mental Health Act of 1946. This legislation provided funds for the education of psychiatrists, psychologists, social workers, and psychiatric nurses. Graduate-level education in psychiatric nursing was established during this period. Around the same time, the introduction of antipsychotic medications made it possible for clients with psychoses to participate in their treatment more readily, including psychological therapies.

Knowledge of the history of psychiatric-mental health care contributes to the understanding of the concepts presented in this chapter and those in online Chapter 38, "Theoretical Models of Personality Development," which describe the theoretical models of personality development according to various 19th- and 20th-century leaders in the mental health movement. Modern American psychiatric care has its roots in ancient times. A great deal of opportunity exists for continued advancement of this specialty within the practice of nursing.

Mental Health

A number of theorists have attempted to define the concept of mental health. Many of these concepts focus on how well the individual is able to function. Maslow (1970) emphasized that mental health is associated with an individual's motivation toward self-actualization. He identified a "hierarchy of needs," with the most basic needs requiring fulfillment before those at higher levels can be achieved and with self-actualization defined as fulfillment of one's highest potential. An individual's position within the hierarchy may fluctuate on the basis of life circumstances. For example,

an individual facing major surgery who has been working to achieve self-actualization may become preoccupied, if only temporarily, with the need for physiological safety. A representation of the needs hierarchy is presented in Figure 2–1.

Maslow described self-actualization as being "psychologically healthy, fully human, highly evolved, and fully mature" (p. 149). He believed that self-actualized individuals possess the following characteristics:

■ An appropriate perception of reality
■ The ability to accept oneself, others, and human nature
■ The ability to manifest spontaneity
■ The capacity for focusing concentration on problem-solving
■ A need for detachment and desire for privacy
■ Independence, autonomy, and a resistance to enculturation
■ An intensity of emotional reaction

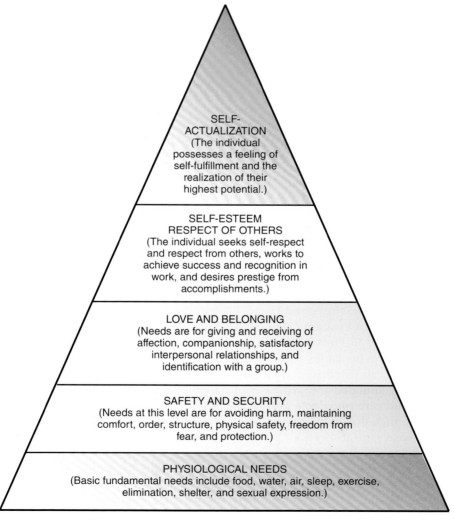

FIGURE 2–1   Maslow's hierarchy of needs.

- A frequency of "peak" experiences that validate the worthwhileness, richness, and beauty of life
- An identification with humankind
- The ability to achieve satisfactory interpersonal relationships
- A democratic character structure and strong sense of ethics
- Creativeness
- A degree of nonconformance

Jahoda (1958) identified a list of six indicators that are a reflection of mental health:

1. **A positive attitude toward self:** This indicator refers to an objective view of self, including knowledge and acceptance of strengths and limitations. The individual feels a strong sense of personal identity and security within their environment.

2. **Growth, development, and the ability to achieve self-actualization:** This indicator correlates with whether the individual successfully achieves the tasks associated with each level of development (see Chapter 31, "Personality Disorders," and online Chapter 38). With successful achievement in each level, the individual gains motivation for advancement to their highest potential.

3. **Integration:** The focus of this indicator is on maintaining equilibrium or balance among various life processes. Integration includes the ability to adaptively respond to the environment and the development of a philosophy of life, both of which help the individual maintain a manageable anxiety level in response to stressful situations.

4. **Autonomy:** This indicator refers to the individual's ability to perform in an independent, self-directed manner. The person makes choices and accepts responsibility for the outcomes.

5. **Perception of reality:** Accurate reality perception is a positive indicator of mental health. It includes perception of the environment without distortion as well as the capacity for empathy and social sensitivity—a respect and concern for the wants and needs of others.

6. **Environmental mastery:** This indicator suggests that the individual has achieved a satisfactory role within the group, society, or environment and is able to love and accept the love of others. When faced with life situations, the person is able to strategize, make decisions, change, adjust, and adapt. Life offers satisfaction to the individual who has achieved environmental mastery.

Robinson (1983) offered this definition of mental health: "A dynamic state in which thought, feeling, and behavior that is age-appropriate and congruent with the local and cultural norms is demonstrated" (p. 74).

Expanding on this model, mental health may be viewed as a relative state that occurs along a continuum of thoughts, feelings, and behaviors that are all part of the human psychological experience and are influenced by the perceived magnitude of stressors in interaction with adaptive capabilities.

In keeping with the framework of stress and adaptation, this text will use a modification of Robinson's definition of mental health. Thus, *mental health* will be defined as "the successful adaptation to stressors from the internal or external environment, evidenced by thoughts, feelings, and behaviors that are age-appropriate and congruent with local and cultural norms."

Mental Illness

Arriving at a universal concept of mental illness is difficult because of the many cultural factors that influence this concept. Horwitz (2010) attempted to define mental illness from a sociocultural perspective characterized by two elements: incomprehensibility and cultural relativity.

Incomprehensibility relates to the inability of the general population to understand the motivation behind an individual's behavior. When observers are unable to find meaning or comprehensibility in behavior, they are likely to label that behavior as mental illness. Horwitz stated, "Observers attribute labels of mental illness when the rules, conventions, and understandings they use to interpret behavior fail to find any intelligible motivation behind an action" (p. 17). The element of *cultural relativity* considers that these rules, conventions, and understandings are conceived within an individual's own particular culture. Behavior that is considered "normal" and "abnormal" is defined by one's cultural or societal norms. Therefore, a behavior that is recognized as evidence of mental illness in one society may be viewed as normal in another society, and vice versa.

The American Psychiatric Association (APA) (2022), in its *Diagnostic and Statistical Manual of Mental Disorders, Fifth Edition, Text Revision (DSM-5-TR)*, defined mental disorder as:

a syndrome characterized by clinically significant disturbance in an individual's cognitions, emotion regulation, or behavior that reflects a dysfunction in the psychological, biological, or developmental processes underlying mental functioning. Mental disorders are usually associated with significant distress or disability in social, occupational, or other important activities. An expected or culturally approved response to a common stressor or loss such as the death of a loved one is not a mental disorder (p. 14).

In this text, and in keeping with the transactional model of stress and adaptation, mental illness is characterized as "maladaptive responses to stressors from the internal or external environment, evidenced by thoughts, feelings, and behaviors that are incongruent with the local and cultural norms and that interfere with the individual's social, occupational, and/or physical functioning."

Psychological and Behavioral Adaptation to Stress

All individuals exhibit characteristics associated with both mental health and mental illness at any given point in time. Chapter 1, "The Concept of Stress Adaptation," described how an individual's response to stressful situations is influenced by physiological factors, their personal perception of the event, and a variety of predisposing factors such as heredity, temperament, learned response patterns, developmental maturity, existing coping strategies, and support systems of caring others.

Anxiety and grief have been described as two primary psychological response patterns to stress. A variety of thoughts, feelings, and behaviors are associated with each of these response patterns. Adaptation is determined by the degree to which the thoughts, feelings, and behaviors interfere with an individual's functioning.

CORE CONCEPT

Anxiety

Anxiety is a feeling of discomfort and apprehension related to fear of impending danger. Individuals may be unaware of the source of their anxiety, which is often accompanied by feelings of uncertainty and helplessness.

Anxiety

Feelings of anxiety are so common in our society that they are almost considered universal. Anxiety arises from the chaos and confusion that exists in the world. Fear of the unknown and conditions of ambiguity allow anxiety to take root and grow. Low levels of anxiety are adaptive and can provide the motivation required for survival. Anxiety becomes problematic when the individual is unable to prevent their response from escalating to a level that interferes with the ability to meet basic needs.

Peplau (1963) described four levels of anxiety: mild, moderate, severe, and panic. A synopsis of the characteristics associated with each of the four levels of anxiety is presented in Table 2–1. A variety of psychological and behavioral responses occur at each level of anxiety. Figure 2–2 depicts these responses on a continuum of anxiety ranging from mild to panic. Nurses must be able to recognize

TABLE 2–1	**Levels of Anxiety**			
LEVEL	**PERCEPTUAL FIELD**	**ABILITY TO LEARN**	**PHYSICAL CHARACTERISTICS**	**EMOTIONAL AND BEHAVIORAL CHARACTERISTICS**
Mild	Heightened perception (e.g., noises may seem louder; details within the environment are clearer) Increased awareness Increased alertness	Learning is enhanced	Restlessness Irritability	May remain superficial with others Rarely experienced as distressful Motivation is increased
Moderate	Reduction in perceptual field Reduced alertness to environmental events (e.g., someone talking may not be heard; part of the room may not be noticed)	Learning still occurs but not at optimal ability Decreased attention span Decreased ability to concentrate	Increased restlessness Increased heart and respiration rates Increased perspiration Gastric discomfort Increased muscular tension Increase in speech rate, volume, and pitch	A feeling of discontent May lead to a degree of impairment in interpersonal relationships as individual begins to focus on self and the need to relieve personal discomfort

TABLE 2–1	**Levels of Anxiety—cont'd**			
LEVEL	**PERCEPTUAL FIELD**	**ABILITY TO LEARN**	**PHYSICAL CHARACTERISTICS**	**EMOTIONAL AND BEHAVIORAL CHARACTERISTICS**
Severe	Greatly diminished; only extraneous details are perceived, or fixation on a single detail may occur May not take notice of an event even when attention is directed by another	Extremely limited attention span Unable to concentrate or problem-solve Effective learning cannot occur	Headaches Dizziness Nausea Trembling Insomnia Palpitations Tachycardia Hyperventilation Urinary frequency Diarrhea	Feelings of dread, loathing, horror Total focus on self and intense desire to relieve the anxiety
Panic	Unable to focus on even one detail within the environment Misperceptions of the environment common (e.g., a perceived detail may be elaborated and out of proportion)	Learning cannot occur Unable to concentrate Unable to comprehend even simple directions	Dilated pupils Labored breathing Severe trembling Sleeplessness Palpitations Diaphoresis and pallor Muscular incoordination Immobility or purposeless hyperactivity Incoherence or inability to verbalize	Sense of impending doom Terror Bizarre behavior, including shouting, screaming, running about wildly, clinging to anyone or anything from which a sense of safety and security is derived Hallucinations, delusions Extreme withdrawal into self

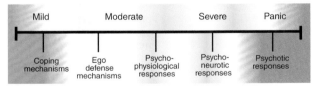

FIGURE 2–2   Adaptation responses on a continuum of anxiety.

the symptoms associated with each level to plan for appropriate intervention with anxious individuals.

Mild Anxiety

This level of anxiety is seldom a problem for the individual. It is associated with the tension experienced in response to the events of day-to-day living. Mild anxiety prepares people for action. It sharpens the senses, increases motivation for productivity, and results in a heightened awareness of the environment. Learning is enhanced, and the individual is able to function at an optimal level.

At the mild level, individuals employ any of a number of coping behaviors that satisfy their needs for comfort. Menninger (1963) described the following types of coping mechanisms that individuals use to relieve mild anxiety in stressful situations:

- Sleeping
- Yawning
- Eating
- Drinking
- Physical exercise
- Daydreaming
- Smoking
- Laughing
- Crying
- Cursing
- Pacing
- Nail biting
- Foot swinging
- Finger tapping
- Fidgeting
- Talking to someone with whom one feels comfortable

Undoubtedly, there are many more coping mechanisms, too numerous to mention here, considering that individuals develop their own unique ways to relieve anxiety at the mild level. Some of these behaviors are more adaptive than others. The term **coping skills** is used to describe those coping behaviors that enhance one's adaptation. These include enhancing knowledge, social affiliation with others, and problem-solving.

Moderate Anxiety

As the level of anxiety increases, the extent of the perceptual field diminishes. The moderately anxious individual is less alert to events occurring in the environment. The individual's attention span and ability to concentrate decrease, although they may still attend to needs with direction. Assistance with problem-solving may be required. Increased muscular tension and restlessness are evident.

Sigmund Freud (1961) identified the ego as the reality component of the personality, governing problem-solving and rational thinking. As the level of anxiety increases, the strength of the ego is tested, and energy is mobilized to confront the threat. Anna Freud (1953) identified a number of **ego defense mechanisms** employed by the ego in the face of threat to biological or psychological integrity. Some of these ego defense mechanisms are more adaptive than others, but all are used either consciously or unconsciously as protective devices by the ego to relieve moderate anxiety. They become maladaptive when an individual uses them to such a degree that the defense mechanism interferes with the ability to deal with reality, with interpersonal relations, or with occupational performance. Maladaptive use of defense mechanisms promotes disintegration of the ego. The major ego defense mechanisms identified by Anna Freud are summarized in Table 2–2.

Anxiety at the moderate-to-severe level that remains unresolved over an extended period can contribute to a number of physiological disorders. The *DSM-5-TR* (APA, 2022) described these disorders under the category "Psychological Factors Affecting Other Medical Conditions." The psychological factors may exacerbate symptoms of, delay recovery from, or interfere with treatment of the medical condition. The condition may be initiated or exacerbated by an environmental situation that the individual perceives as stressful. Measurable pathophysiology can be demonstrated. It is thought that psychological and behavioral factors may affect the course of almost every major category of disease, including cardiovascular, gastrointestinal, neoplastic, neurological, and pulmonary conditions.

Severe Anxiety

The perceptual field of the severely anxious individual is so greatly diminished that concentration may center on one particular detail only or on many extraneous details. Attention span is extremely limited, and the individual has difficulty completing even the simplest task. Physical symptoms (e.g., headaches, palpitations, insomnia) and emotional symptoms

TABLE 2–2 Ego Defense Mechanisms	
DEFENSE MECHANISM	**EXAMPLE**
COMPENSATION Covering up a real or perceived weakness by emphasizing a trait one considers more desirable	A physically disabled boy is unable to participate in football, so he compensates by becoming a great scholar.
DENIAL Refusing to acknowledge the existence of a real situation or the feelings associated with it	A woman drinks alcohol every day and cannot stop, failing to acknowledge that she has a problem.
DISPLACEMENT The transfer of feelings from one target to another that is considered less threatening or that is neutral	A patient is angry with his physician, does not express it, but becomes verbally abusive with the nurse.
IDENTIFICATION An attempt to increase self-worth by acquiring certain attributes and characteristics of an individual one admires	A teenager who required lengthy rehabilitation after an accident decides to become a physical therapist as a result of his experiences.
INTELLECTUALIZATION An attempt to avoid expressing actual emotions associated with a stressful situation by using the intellectual processes of logic, reasoning, and analysis	A woman's husband is being transferred by his job to a city far away from her parents. She hides anxiety by explaining to her parents the advantages associated with the move.
INTROJECTION Integrating the beliefs and values of another individual into one's own ego structure	A child integrates their parents' value system into the process of conscience formation. A child says to a friend, "Don't cheat. It's wrong."
ISOLATION Separating a thought or memory from the feeling, tone, or emotion associated with it	A young woman describes being attacked and raped without showing any emotion.
PROJECTION Attributing feelings or impulses unacceptable to one's self to another person	A man who is addicted to alcohol blames his wife for his excessive drinking.

TABLE 2–2 **Ego Defense Mechanisms—cont'd**	
DEFENSE MECHANISM	**EXAMPLE**
RATIONALIZATION	
Attempting to make excuses or formulate logical reasons to justify unacceptable feelings or behaviors	A patient tells the rehab nurse, "I drink because it's the only way I can deal with my bad marriage and my worse job."
REACTION FORMATION	
Preventing unacceptable or undesirable thoughts or behaviors from being expressed by exaggerating opposite thoughts or types of behaviors	A student who hates nursing and only attended nursing school to please her parents speaks to prospective students about the excellence of nursing as a career.
REGRESSION	
Retreating in response to stress to an earlier level of development and the comfort measures associated with that level of functioning	When a 2-year-old is hospitalized for tonsillitis, he will drink only from a bottle, even though his mother states he has been drinking from a cup for 6 months.
REPRESSION	
Involuntarily blocking unpleasant feelings and experiences from one's awareness	A trauma victim is unable to remember anything about the traumatic event.
SUBLIMATION	
Rechanneling of drives or impulses that are personally or socially unacceptable into activities that are constructive	A mother whose son was killed by a drunk driver channels her anger and energy into being the president of the local chapter of Mothers Against Drunk Driving.
SUPPRESSION	
The voluntary blocking of unpleasant feelings and experiences from one's awareness	"I don't want to think about that now. I'll think about that tomorrow."
UNDOING	
Symbolically negating or canceling out an experience that one finds intolerable	A man is nervous about his new job and yells at his wife. On his way home he stops and buys her some flowers.

(e.g., confusion, dread, horror) may be evident. Discomfort is experienced to the degree that virtually all overt behavior is aimed at relieving the anxiety.

Extended periods of repressed severe anxiety can result in neurotic patterns of behaving. Neurosis is

no longer considered a separate category of mental disorder. However, the term sometimes is still used in the literature to further describe the symptomatology of certain disorders and to differentiate them from behaviors that occur at the more serious level of psychosis.

A **neurosis** is a psychiatric disturbance characterized by excessive anxiety that is expressed directly or altered through defense mechanisms. Although there is no gross distortion of reality or severe personality disorganization, the symptoms are significant enough to impair a person's functioning. The following are common characteristics of people with neuroses:

- They are aware that they are experiencing distress.
- They are aware that their behaviors are maladaptive.
- They are unaware of any possible psychological causes of the distress.
- They feel helpless to change their situation.
- They experience no loss of contact with reality.

The following disorders are examples of psychoneurotic responses to severe anxiety as they appear in the *DSM-5-TR* (APA, 2022):

- *Anxiety disorders:* Disorders in which the characteristic features are symptoms of anxiety and avoidance behavior (e.g., phobias, panic disorder, generalized anxiety disorder, and separation anxiety disorder)
- *Somatic symptom and related disorders:* Disorders in which the characteristic feature is a preoccupation with distressing somatic symptoms for which there is no demonstrable organic pathology; psychological factors are judged to play a significant role in the onset, severity, exacerbation, or maintenance of the symptoms (e.g., somatic symptom disorder, illness anxiety disorder, conversion disorder, and factitious disorder)
- *Dissociative disorders:* Disorders in which the characteristic feature is a disruption in the usually integrated functions of consciousness, memory, identity, or perception of the environment (e.g., dissociative amnesia, dissociative identity disorder, and depersonalization-derealization disorder)

Panic Anxiety

In this most intense state of anxiety, the individual is unable to focus on even one detail in the environment. Misperceptions are common, and a loss of contact with reality may occur. The individual may experience hallucinations or delusions. Behavior may be characterized by wild and desperate actions or extreme withdrawal. Human functioning and communication with others is ineffective. Panic anxiety is associated with a feeling of terror, and individuals may be convinced that they have a life-threatening illness or fear that they are "going crazy," are losing control, or are emotionally weak. Prolonged panic anxiety can lead to physical and emotional exhaustion and can be a life-threatening situation.

At this extreme level of anxiety, an individual is not capable of processing what is happening in the environment and may lose contact with reality. **Psychosis** is defined as a significant thought disturbance in which reality testing is impaired, resulting in delusions, hallucinations, disorganized speech, or catatonic behavior. The following are common characteristics of people with psychoses:

■ They exhibit minimal distress (emotional tone is flat, bland, or inappropriate).
■ They are unaware that their behavior is maladaptive.
■ They are unaware of any psychological problems (**anosognosia**).
■ They are exhibiting a flight from reality into a less stressful world or one in which they are attempting to adapt.

Examples of psychotic responses to anxiety include delusions (fixed, false beliefs) and hallucinations (false sensory perceptions).

CORE CONCEPT
Grief
Grief is a subjective feeling of sorrow and sadness accompanied by emotional, physical, and social responses to the loss of a loved person or thing.

Grief

Most individuals experience intense emotional anguish in response to a significant personal loss. A loss is anything that is perceived as such by the individual. Losses may be real, in which case they can be substantiated by others (e.g., death of a loved one, loss of personal possessions), or they may be perceived by the individual alone, unable to be shared or identified by others (e.g., loss of the feeling of femininity after mastectomy). Any situation that

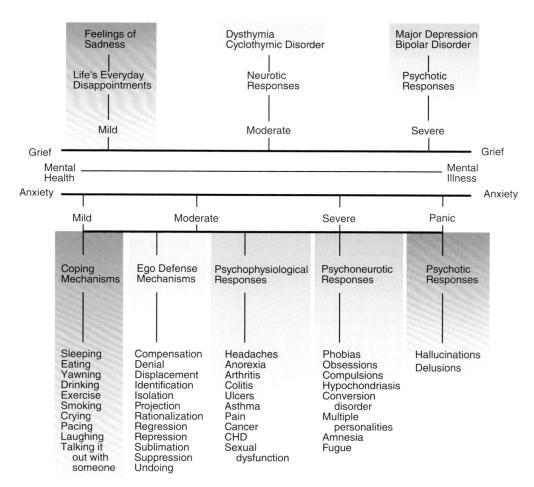

FIGURE 2–3 Conceptualization of anxiety and grief responses along the mental health/mental illness continuum.

creates change for an individual can be identified as a loss. Failure (either real or perceived) also can be viewed as a loss. Loss is typically a very stressful event and, like other stressors, an individual's response to loss may be adaptive or maladaptive.

The loss or anticipated loss of anything of value to an individual can trigger the grief response. This period of characteristic emotions and behaviors is called *mourning*. The "normal" mourning process, which may include feelings of sadness, guilt, anger, helplessness, hopelessness, and despair, is adaptive. Indeed, an absence of mourning after a loss may be considered maladaptive. Grief is not considered a mental illness, but maladaptive responses to grief may culminate in clinical depression or other symptoms of mental illness, including risk for suicide. In the latest edition of the *DSM-5-TR* (APA, 2022) a new diagnostic category, *prolonged grief disorder*, was added to the group of disorders identified as "Trauma and Stressor-Related" to clarify that intense distress and impaired functioning that endures beyond 12 months of the death of a loved one is beyond what is considered normal bereavement. Careful assessment to differentiate normal grief responses from those that require additional treatment is critical to maintaining patient safety. An in-depth discussion of the usual stages of grief and *maladaptive* grief responses can be found in Chapter 36, "The Bereaved Individual."

Anxiety and grief have been described as two primary responses to stress: the severity of symptoms and the ability to adapt effectively are influential along a continuum of one's experience of mental health or mental illness.

Mental Health/Mental Illness Continuum

Anxiety and grief have been described as two primary responses to stress. In Figure 2–3, both of these responses are presented on a continuum according to the degree of symptom severity. Disorders, as they appear in the *DSM-5-TR*, are identified at their appropriate placement along the continuum.

Summary and Key Points

■ Mental health is defined as "the successful adaptation to stressors from the internal or external environment evidenced by thoughts, feelings, and behaviors that are age appropriate and congruent with local and cultural norms."

■ Mental illness is defined as "maladaptive responses to stressors from the internal or external environment, evidenced by thoughts, feelings, and behaviors that are incongruent with the local and cultural norms, and interfere with the individual's social, occupational, and/or physical functioning."

■ From a sociocultural perspective, behavior may be labeled as mental illness on the basis of incomprehensibility and cultural relativity.

■ When observers are unable to find meaning or comprehensibility in behavior, they are likely to label that behavior as mental illness. The meaning of behaviors is determined within individual cultures.

■ Anxiety and grief have been identified as the two primary responses to stress.

■ Peplau (1963) defined anxiety by levels of symptom severity: mild, moderate, severe, and panic.

■ Behaviors associated with levels of anxiety include coping mechanisms, ego defense mechanisms, psychophysiological responses, psychoneurotic responses, and psychotic responses.

■ Grief is described as a response to loss of a valued entity. It can be an adaptive or a maladaptive experience.

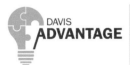

Go to **Davis Advantage** to complete your learning: strengthen understanding, apply your knowledge, and prepare for the Next Gen NCLEX®.

Review Questions

1. Which of the following is a true statement regarding Maslow's hierarchy of needs?
   a. Self-actualization cannot be effectively achieved if an individual is struggling with unmet safety and security needs.
   b. Self-actualized individuals have learned how to have no emotional reactions.
   c. Physiological health is the highest achievement in the hierarchy.
   d. All of the above.

2. A sociocultural perspective defines mental illness as:
   a. A disruption of brain chemicals in response to stress
   b. A *DSM-5-TR* diagnosis
   c. Behavior that is incomprehensible within one's culture
   d. Any illness that responds to psychotropic medication

3. When an individual remains under stress for a prolonged period, which of the following psychological and behavioral effects may occur? (Select all that apply.)
   a. Employment of ego defense mechanisms
   b. Inability to concentrate
   c. Psychosomatic symptoms
   d. All of the above

4. Which of the following are manifestations of mild anxiety?
   a. Less alertness to the environment and emotional numbness
   b. Sharp senses and motivation for productivity
   c. Ability to focus on only one detail
   d. Feeling out of control and exhibiting wild behavior

5. Extended periods of unmanaged or repressed severe anxiety may be associated with which of the following psychiatric disorders?
   a. Panic disorder
   b. Phobic disorders
   c. Somatic symptom disorders
   d. All of the above

Clinical Judgment Questions

6. A client with a history of substance use disorder is sent to the mental health clinic by their employer who expresses concern about their drinking alcohol on the job. The client denies having a problem and reports only drinking a little when the boss is "acting like a jerk." The nurse should document that the client is manifesting which defense mechanisms?
   a. Compensation and intellectualization
   b. Regression and reaction formation
   c. Denial and rationalization
   d. Undoing and projection

7. A client with a history of schizophrenia is brought to the emergency department by police who report that the individual was knocking down food displays at a grocery store and yelling that the food was all poisoned. The client reports to the nurse that they have no idea why they were brought to the emergency department because "there is nothing wrong with me." Which of these actions by the nurse demonstrates good clinical judgment?
   a. Instruct the police officer that this client should be incarcerated because there is nothing that can be done in an emergency department.
   b. Document that the client is manifesting psychotic symptoms and anosognosia.
   c. Ask the doctor to order gastric lavage because the client reports having been poisoned.
   d. Instruct the client that the food is not poisoned and there is something very wrong with them.

8. During a primary care physician appointment, a client who has been a widow for 7 years reports to the nurse not wanting to wake up in the morning and feeling like there is nothing left to live for. Which of these actions by the nurse is a priority?
   a. Listen empathically and encourage the client to find some activities to increase socialization.
   b. Encourage the client to discuss this with the physician.
   c. Assess the client for symptoms of depression and suicide risk.
   d. Instruct the client that grief takes a few months to resolve.

9. A client who has arrived at the health clinic for diabetic education is perspiring and states, "I'm so anxious about giving myself shots I can hardly breathe. I don't know what to do." Which of these actions by the nurse demonstrates good clinical judgment?
   a. Assist the client in relaxation exercises before commencing diabetes education.
   b. Instruct the client that it is not hard to give oneself a shot and commence teaching.
   c. Assess the client further for symptoms of anxiety.
   d. Cancel diabetic education and encourage the client to reschedule when they feel less anxious.

10. A client who was admitted to the psychiatric unit for major depressive disorder reports to the nurse, "Ever since my daughter died a year ago, I've been feeling depressed and thinking about suicide." Which of these actions by the nurse demonstrates prioritized, good clinical judgment?
    a. Encourage the client to attend group activities provided as part of the treatment program.
    b. Assess the client's grief response and risk for suicide.
    c. Educate the client about the stages of grief.
    d. Assess what caused the daughter's death.

References

American Psychiatric Association. (2022). *Diagnostic and statistical manual of mental disorders, fifth edition, text revision (DSM-5-TR).* American Psychiatric Association.

Horwitz, A.V. (2010). *The social control of mental illness.* Percheron Press.

Classical References

Freud, A. (1953). *The ego and mechanisms of defense.* International Universities Press.

Freud, S. (1961). The ego and the id. In *Standard edition of the complete psychological works of Freud* (Vol. XIX). Hogarth Press.

Jahoda, M. (1958). *Current concepts of positive mental health.* Basic Books.

Kübler-Ross, E. (1969). *On death and dying.* Macmillan.

Maslow, A. (1970). *Motivation and personality* (2nd ed.). Harper & Row.

Menninger, K. (1963). *The vital balance.* Viking Press.

Peplau, H. (1963). A working definition of anxiety. In S. Burd & M. Marshall (Eds.), *Some clinical approaches to psychiatric nursing.* Macmillan.

Robinson, L. (1983). *Psychiatric nursing as a human experience* (3rd ed.). WB Saunders.

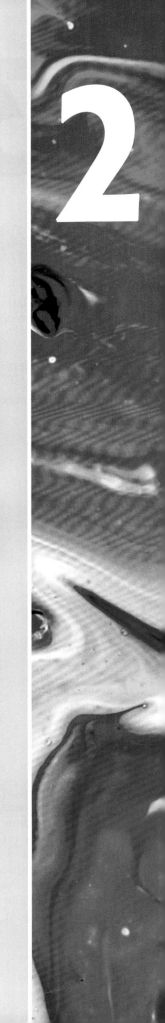

UNIT **2**

Foundations for Psychiatric-Mental Health Nursing

3 Concepts of Psychobiology

CORE CONCEPTS

Growth and
    Development:
    Genetics

Intracranial Regulation:
    Neuroendocrinology,
    Psychobiology,
    Nerve cells,
    Neurotransmitters

Immunity:
    Psychoneuroimmunology,
    Inflammation

Safety

CHAPTER OUTLINE

KEY TERMS

axon
cell body
circadian rhythms
dendrites

genotype
limbic system
neurons
neurotransmitters

phenotype
prefrontal cortex
receptor sites
synapse

OBJECTIVES
After reading this chapter, the student will be able to:

1. Identify gross anatomical structures of the brain and describe their functions.
2. Discuss the physiology of neurotransmission in the central nervous system.
3. Describe the role of neurotransmitters in human behavior.
4. Discuss the association of endocrine functioning to the development of psychiatric disorders.
5. Describe the role of genetics in the development of psychiatric disorders.
6. Discuss the correlation of altered brain function to various psychiatric disorders.
7. Identify diagnostic procedures used to detect alteration in biological functioning that may contribute to psychiatric disorders.
8. Discuss the influence of psychological factors on the immune system.
9. Describe the biological mechanisms of psychoactive drugs at neural synapses.
10. Recognize theorized influences in the development of psychiatric disorders, including brain physiology, genetics, endocrine function, immune system, and psychosocial and environmental factors.
11. Discuss the implications of psychobiological concepts for the practice of psychiatric-mental health nursing.

In recent years, increased emphasis has been placed on the organic basis for psychiatric illness. This "neuroscientific revolution" studies the biological basis of behavior, and several mental illnesses are now considered physical disorders resulting from malfunctions or malformations of the brain.

That some psychiatric illnesses and associated behaviors can be traced to biological factors does not imply that psychosocial and sociocultural influences are completely discounted. For example, there is evidence that *psychological* interventions influence brain activity in a way similar to that of psychopharmacological intervention (Collerton, 2013; Flor, 2014; Malhotra & Sahoo, 2017; Mason et al., 2017). Other evidence indicates that lifestyle choices, such as marijuana use, can precipitate mental illness (psychosis) in individuals with genetic vulnerability (National Institute on Drug Abuse, 2021). Ongoing research will build a better understanding of the complex interplay of neural activities within the brain and in interaction with one's environment.

The systems of biology, psychology, and sociology are not mutually exclusive—they are interacting systems. This interaction is clearly indicated by the fact that individuals experience biological changes in response to different environmental events. Indeed, one or several of these systems may, at various times, explain behavioral phenomena.

This chapter focuses on the role of neurophysiological, neurochemical, genetic, and endocrine influences on psychiatric illness. An introduction to psychopharmacology is included (discussed in more detail in Chapter 4, "Psychopharmacology"), and various diagnostic procedures used to detect alterations in biological function that may contribute to psychiatric illness are identified. The implications for psychiatric-mental health nursing are discussed.

The Nervous System: An Anatomical Review

The Brain

The brain has three major divisions, subdivided into six major parts:

1. Forebrain
   a. Cerebrum
   b. Diencephalon
2. Midbrain (Mesencephalon)
3. Hindbrain
   a. Pons
   b. Medulla
   c. Cerebellum

Each of these structures is discussed individually. A summary is presented in Table 3–1.

TABLE 3–1 Structure and Function of the Brain

STRUCTURE	PRIMARY FUNCTION
I. FOREBRAIN	
A. Cerebrum	Composed of two hemispheres connected by a band of nerve tissue that houses a band of 200 million axons called the *corpus callosum.* The outer layer is called the *cerebral cortex.* It is extensively folded and consists of billions of neurons. The left hemisphere appears to deal with logic and solving problems. The right hemisphere may be called the "creative" brain and is associated with affect, behavior, and spatial-perceptual functions. Each hemisphere is divided into four lobes.
1. Frontal lobes	Voluntary body movement, including movements that permit speaking, thinking and judgment formation, and expression of feelings
2. Parietal lobes	Perception and interpretation of most sensory information (including touch, pain, taste, and body position)
3. Temporal lobes	Hearing, short-term memory, and sense of smell; expression of emotions through connection with limbic system
4. Occipital lobes	Visual reception and interpretation
B. Diencephalon	Connects cerebrum with lower brain structures
1. Thalamus	Integrates all sensory input (except smell) on way to cortex; some involvement with emotions and mood
2. Hypothalamus	Regulates anterior and posterior lobes of pituitary gland; exerts control over actions of the autonomic nervous system; regulates appetite and temperature; regulates visceral responses to emotional situations and body rhythms such as mood changes and sleep–wakefulness cycles
3. Limbic system	The limbic system consists of medially placed cortical and subcortical structures and the fiber tracts connecting them with one another and with the hypothalamus. It is sometimes called the "emotional brain"—associated with feelings of fear and anxiety; anger and aggression; love, joy, and hope; and with sexuality and social behavior. As research has advanced our understanding of the connectivity in brain structures, it has become difficult to define the boundaries of the limbic system.

Continued

TABLE 3–1	Structure and Function of the Brain—cont'd
STRUCTURE	**PRIMARY FUNCTION**
II. MIDBRAIN (Mesencephalon)	Responsible for visual, auditory, and balance ("righting") reflexes
III. HINDBRAIN A. Pons	Regulation of respiration and skeletal muscle tone; ascending and descending tracts connect brainstem with cerebellum and cortex
B. Medulla	Pathway for all ascending and descending fiber tracts; contains vital centers that regulate heart rate, blood pressure, and respiration; reflex centers for swallowing, sneezing, coughing, and vomiting
C. Cerebellum	Regulates muscle tone and coordination and maintains posture and equilibrium

Cerebrum

The cerebrum consists of a right and left hemisphere and constitutes the largest part of the human brain. The two hemispheres are separated by a deep groove but remain connected to each other by a band of 200 million axons (nerve fibers) called the *corpus callosum*. Because each hemisphere controls different functions, information is processed through the corpus callosum so that each hemisphere is aware of the activity of the other.

The surface of the cerebrum consists of gray matter and is called the *cerebral cortex*. The gray matter is composed of neuron cell bodies that appear gray to the eye. These cell bodies are thought to be the actual "thinking" structures of the brain. The *basal ganglia,* four subcortical nuclei of gray matter (the striatum, the pallidum, the substantia nigra, and the subthalamic nucleus), are found deep within the cerebral hemispheres. They are responsible for certain subconscious aspects of voluntary movements, such as swinging the arms when walking, gesturing while speaking, and regulating muscle tone (Scanlon & Sanders, 2019).

The cerebral cortex is identified by numerous folds called *gyri* and deep grooves between the folds called *sulci.* This extensive folding extends the surface area of the cerebral cortex to permit the presence of millions more neurons than could be accommodated without the folds (as is the case in the brains of some animals, such as dogs and cats). Each hemisphere of the cerebral cortex is divided into the frontal lobe, parietal lobe, temporal lobe, and occipital lobe. These lobes, which are named for the overlying bones in the cranium, are identified in Figure 3–1.

The Frontal Lobes

Voluntary body movement is controlled by impulses through the frontal lobes. The right frontal lobe controls motor activity on the left side of the body, and the left frontal lobe controls motor activity on the right side of the body. The frontal lobe may also play a role in emotional experiences, as evidenced by changes in mood and character after damage to this area. Particularly, the **prefrontal cortex** (the front part of the frontal lobes) plays an essential role in the regulation and adaptation of our emotions to new situations. Morality, identified as one of the most sophisticated elements of human judgment, social cognition, decision making, and conflict resolution are affected by the function of the prefrontal cortex (Dashtestani et al., 2018; Lewis, 2017). Neuroimaging tests suggest there may be decreased activity in the frontal lobes (as well as temporal, parietal, and subcortical structures) in people with chronic schizophrenia (Boland et al., 2022).

The Parietal Lobes

The parietal lobes manage somatosensory input, including touch, pain, pressure, taste, temperature, perception of joint and body position, and visceral sensations. The parietal lobes also contain association fibers linked to the primary sensory areas through which interpretation of sensory-perceptual information is made. Language interpretation is associated with the left hemisphere of the parietal lobe.

The Temporal Lobes

The upper anterior temporal lobe is concerned with auditory functions, and the lower part is dedicated to short-term memory. The sense of smell has a connection to the temporal lobes, as the impulses carried by the olfactory nerves end in this area of the brain. The temporal lobes also play a role in the expression of emotions through an interconnection with the limbic system. The left temporal lobe (along with the left parietal lobe) is involved in language interpretation.

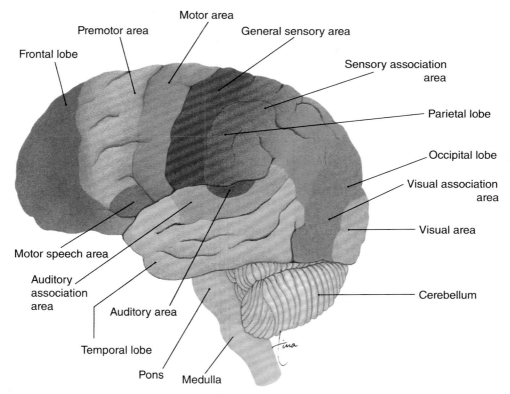

FIGURE 3–1 Left cerebral hemisphere showing some of the functional areas that have been mapped.

The Occipital Lobes

The occipital lobes are the primary area of visual reception and interpretation. Visual perception, the ability to judge spatial relationships such as distance and to see in three dimensions, is also processed in this area. Language interpretation is affected by the visual processing that occurs in the occipital lobes.

Diencephalon

The second part of the forebrain is the diencephalon, which connects the cerebrum with lower structures of the brain. The major components of the diencephalon include the thalamus and the hypothalamus, which are part of a neuroanatomical loop of structures known as the **limbic system** (sometimes called the emotional brain because these structures are associated with regulation of emotions). Commonly associated structures are identified in Figure 3–2.

Thalamus

The thalamus integrates all sensory input (except smell) on its way to the cortex. This integration allows for rapid interpretation of the whole rather than individual perception of each sensation. The thalamus is also involved in temporarily blocking minor sensations so that an individual can concentrate on one important event when necessary. For example, an individual who is studying for an examination may be unaware of the clock ticking in the room or another person entering because the thalamus has temporarily blocked these incoming sensations from the cortex. The effect of dopamine in the thalamus is associated with several neuropsychiatric disorders.

Hypothalamus

The hypothalamus is located just below the thalamus and just above the pituitary gland and has the following diverse functions:

1. **Regulation of the pituitary gland:** The pituitary gland consists of two lobes—the posterior lobe and the anterior lobe.

   a. The *posterior lobe* of the pituitary gland is actually extended tissue from the hypothalamus. The posterior lobe stores antidiuretic hormone (ADH), which helps to maintain blood pressure through regulation of water retention, and oxytocin, the hormone responsible for stimulation of the uterus during labor and the release of milk (along with prolactin) from the mammary glands. Both ADH and oxytocin are produced in the hypothalamus. When the hypothalamus detects the body's need for these hormones, it sends nerve impulses to the posterior pituitary for their release.

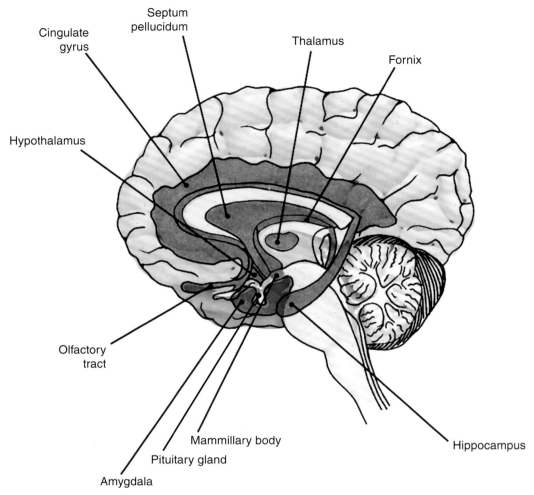

FIGURE 3–2 Structures of the limbic system.

b. The *anterior lobe* of the pituitary gland consists of glandular tissue that produces several hormones used by the body. These hormones are regulated by *releasing factors* from the hypothalamus. When the hormones are required by the body, the releasing factors stimulate the release of the hormone from the anterior pituitary, and the hormone in turn stimulates its target organ to carry out its specific functions.

2. **Direct neural control over the actions of the autonomic nervous system:** The hypothalamus regulates the appropriate visceral responses during various emotional states. The actions of the autonomic nervous system are described later in this chapter.

3. **Regulation of appetite, temperature, and thirst:** Appetite may be triggered or inhibited depending on which networks in the hypothalamus are stimulated. Temperature is regulated through the hypothalamus as it senses internal and external temperature changes on the skin and in the blood.

It then responds by triggering shivering or sweating to help maintain body temperature within the normal range. Thirst centers in the hypothalamus are stimulated by dry mouth or dehydration.

4. **Regulation of blood pressure:** The hypothalamus, which acts as an interface between the endocrine and nervous systems, coordinating signal transduction from central and peripheral stimuli, has been identified as a key component in the development of hypertension when activated. Inflammation in the hypothalamus has been found to disrupt signaling pathways affecting the control of blood pressure (Khor & Cai, 2017). Hypothalamic insufficiency leads to persistent increases in blood pressure (Goncharuk, 2021).

5. **Circadian rhythms (sleep and wakefulness cycles):** The output of the suprachiasmatic nucleus (SNC) of the hypothalamus promotes a state of arousal; as the output decreases, the onset of sleep is facilitated in a complex process that drives the homeostatic need for sleep. This process includes an

intrinsic 24-hour timing system and response to light or darkness. SNC neurons along with other peptides also produce gamma-aminobutyric acid (GABA) (Moore, 2019).

Limbic System

The limbic system is a group of structures typically identified as including the amygdala, mammillary body, olfactory tract, hypothalamus, cingulate gyrus, septum pellucidum, thalamus, hippocampus, and fornix, which, through communication with the hypothalamus, control several autonomic, endocrine, and somatic functions. This system has been called the "emotional brain" because of its association with feelings of fear and anxiety; anger, rage, and aggression; love, joy, and hope; and with sexuality and social behavior. However, as understanding of the complex connectivity within the brain has advanced, it has become increasingly difficult to define the boundaries of the limbic system, and research has demonstrated that some structures associated with the limbic system are involved in other complex brain processes such as memory (Melchitzky & Lewis, 2017). Nonetheless, the structures commonly associated with emotional regulation in the limbic system are identified in Figure 3–2.

Mesencephalon (Midbrain)

Structures of major importance in the mesencephalon, or midbrain, include nuclei and fiber tracts. The mesencephalon extends from the pons to the hypothalamus and is responsible for integration of various reflexes, including visual reflexes (e.g., automatically turning away from a dangerous object when it comes into view), auditory reflexes (e.g., automatically turning toward a sound that is heard), and righting reflexes (e.g., automatically keeping the head upright and maintaining balance).

Pons

The pons is a bulbous structure that lies between the midbrain and the medulla as part of the brainstem (see Fig. 3–1). It is composed of large bundles of fibers and forms a major connection between the cerebellum and the brainstem. The pons is a relay station that transmits messages between various parts of the nervous system, including the cerebrum and cerebellum. It contains the central connections of cranial nerves V through VIII and centers for respiration and skeletal muscle tone. The pons is also associated with sleep and dreaming.

Medulla

The medulla is the connecting structure between the spinal cord and the pons, and all of the ascending and descending fiber tracts pass through it. The vital centers are contained in the medulla, and its functions include regulation of heart rate, blood pressure, and respiration. The medulla contains reflex centers for swallowing, sneezing, coughing, and vomiting, as well as nuclei for cranial nerves IX through XII. The medulla, pons, and midbrain form the structure known as the *brainstem.*

Cerebellum

The cerebellum is separated from the brainstem by the fourth ventricle but is connected to it through bundles of fiber tracts (see Fig. 3–1). The cerebellum is associated with involuntary aspects of movement such as coordination, muscle tone, and the maintenance of posture and equilibrium.

Nerve Tissue

The tissue of the central nervous system (CNS) consists of nerve cells called **neurons** that generate and transmit electrochemical impulses. The structure of a neuron is composed of a cell body, an axon, and dendrites. The **cell body** contains the nucleus and is essential for the continued life of the neuron. The **dendrites** are processes that transmit impulses toward the cell body, and the **axon** transmits impulses away from the cell body. The axons and dendrites are covered by layers of cells called *neuroglia* that form a coating, or "sheath," of myelin. *Myelin* is a phospholipid that provides insulation against short-circuiting of the neurons during their electrical activity and increases the velocity of the impulse. The white matter of the brain and spinal cord is so called because of the whitish appearance of the myelin sheath covering the axons and dendrites. The gray matter is composed of cell bodies that contain no myelin.

Classes of Neurons

The three classes of neurons are afferent (sensory) neurons, efferent (motor) neurons, and interneurons:

- *Afferent neurons* carry impulses from receptors in the internal and external periphery to the CNS, where they are then interpreted into various sensations.
- *Efferent neurons* carry impulses from the CNS to *effectors* in the periphery, such as muscles (that respond by contracting) and glands (that respond by secreting).
- *Interneurons* exist entirely within the CNS, and 99% of all nerve cells belong to this group. They may carry only sensory or motor impulses, or they may serve as integrators in the pathways between afferent and efferent neurons. They account in large part for thinking, feelings, learning, language, and memory.

Synapses

Information is transmitted through the body from one neuron to another. Some messages may be processed through only a few neurons, whereas others may require thousands of neuronal connections. The neurons that transmit the impulses do not actually touch each other. The junction between two neurons is called a **synapse.** The small space between the axon terminals of one neuron and the cell body or dendrites of another is called the *synaptic cleft.* Neurons conducting impulses toward the synapse are called *presynaptic neurons,* and those conducting impulses away are called *postsynaptic neurons.*

Chemicals that act as **neurotransmitters** are stored in the axon terminals of the presynaptic neuron. An electrical impulse through the neuron causes the release of this neurotransmitter into the synaptic cleft. The neurotransmitter then diffuses across the synaptic cleft and combines with **receptor sites** that are situated on the cell membrane of the postsynaptic neuron. The type of combination determines whether or not another electrical impulse is generated. If an electrical impulse is generated, the result is called an *excitatory response,* and the electrical impulse moves on to the next synapse, where the same process recurs. If an electrical impulse is not generated by the neurotransmitter–receptor site combination, the result is called an *inhibitory response,* and synaptic transmission is terminated. Activity at the neural synapse is relevant in the study of psychiatric disorders because excessive or deficient activity of neurotransmitters influences a variety of cognitive and emotional symptoms. The synapse is also believed to be the primary site of activity for psychotropic drugs.

The cell body of the postsynaptic neuron also contains a chemical *inactivator* that is specific to the neurotransmitter released by the presynaptic neuron. When the synaptic transmission has been completed, the chemical inactivator quickly inactivates the neurotransmitter to prevent unwanted, continuous impulses until a new impulse from the presynaptic neuron releases more of the neurotransmitter. Continuous impulses can result in excessive activity of neurotransmitters such as dopamine, which is believed to be responsible for symptoms such as hallucinations and delusions seen in people with schizophrenia. A schematic representation of a synapse is presented in Figure 3–3.

Autonomic Nervous System

The autonomic nervous system (ANS) is considered part of the peripheral nervous system. Its regulation is modulated by the hypothalamus, and emotions exert a great deal of influence over its functioning. For this reason, the ANS has been implicated in the etiology of a number of psychophysiological disorders.

The ANS has two divisions: the sympathetic and the parasympathetic. The sympathetic division is

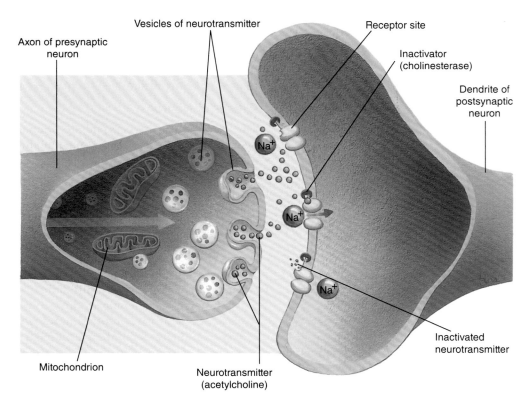

FIGURE 3–3 Impulse transmission at a synapse. The arrow indicates the direction of electrical impulses.

dominant in stressful situations and prepares the body for the fight-or-flight response (discussed in Chapter 1, "The Concept of Stress Adaptation"). The neuronal cell bodies of the sympathetic division originate in the thoracolumbar region of the spinal cord. Their axons extend to the chains of sympathetic ganglia where they synapse with other neurons that subsequently innervate the visceral effectors, resulting in an increase in heart rate and respiration and a decrease in digestive secretions and peristalsis. Blood is shunted to the vital organs and skeletal muscles to ensure adequate oxygenation.

The neuronal cell bodies of the parasympathetic division originate in the brainstem and the sacral segments of the spinal cord and extend to the parasympathetic ganglia where the synapse occurs either very close to or actually in the visceral organ being innervated. In this way, a localized response is possible. The parasympathetic division dominates when an individual is in a relaxed, nonstressful condition. The heart and respirations are maintained at a normal rate, and secretions and peristalsis increase for normal digestion. Elimination functions are promoted. A schematic representation of the ANS is presented in Figure 3–4.

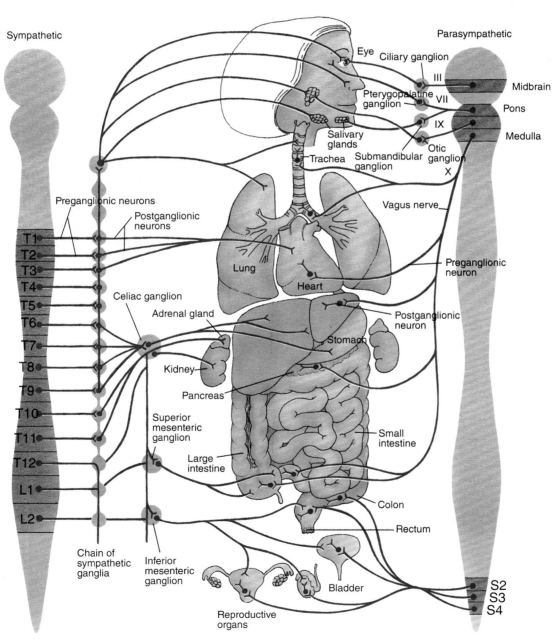

FIGURE 3–4 The autonomic nervous system. The sympathetic division is shown on the left, and the parasympathetic division is shown on the right (both divisions are bilateral).

Neurotransmitters

Although neurotransmitters were described during the explanation of synaptic activity, they are discussed here separately and in detail because of their essential roles in human emotion and behavior. Neurotransmitters are also central to the therapeutic action of many psychotropic medications.

Neurotransmitters are chemicals that convey information across synaptic clefts to neighboring target cells. They are stored in small vesicles in the axon terminals of neurons. When the action potential, or electrical impulse, reaches this point, the neurotransmitters are released from the vesicles. They cross the synaptic cleft and bind with receptor sites on the cell body or dendrites of the adjacent neuron to allow the impulse to continue its course or to prevent the impulse from continuing. After the neurotransmitter has performed its function in the synapse, it either returns to the vesicles to be stored and used again or is inactivated and dissolved by enzymes. The process of being stored for reuse is called *reuptake*, a function that holds significance for understanding the mechanism of action of certain psychotropic medications.

Many neurotransmitters exist in the central and peripheral nervous systems, but only a limited number have implications for psychiatry. Major categories include cholinergic neurotransmitters, monoamines, amino acids, and neuropeptides. Each of these is discussed separately and summarized in Table 3–2.

Cholinergic Neurotransmitters

Acetylcholine

Location: Acetylcholine was the first chemical to be identified as and proven to be a neurotransmitter. It is a major effector chemical in the ANS, producing

---

TABLE 3–2   Neurotransmitters in the Central Nervous System

NEUROTRANSMITTER	LOCATION AND FUNCTION	POSSIBLE IMPLICATIONS FOR MENTAL ILLNESS
I. CHOLINERGICS A. Acetylcholine	*ANS:* Sympathetic and parasympathetic pre-synaptic nerve terminals; parasympathetic postsynaptic nerve terminals *CNS:* Cerebral cortex, hippocampus, limbic structures, and basal ganglia *Functions:* Sleep, arousal, pain perception, movement, memory	*Decreased levels:* Alzheimer's disease, *Huntington's* disease, Parkinson's disease *Increased levels:* Depression
II. MONOAMINES A. Norepinephrine	*ANS:* Sympathetic postsynaptic nerve terminals *CNS:* Thalamus, hypothalamus, limbic system, hippocampus, cerebellum, cerebral cortex *Functions:* Mood, cognition, perception, locomotion, cardiovascular functioning, and sleep and arousal	*Decreased levels:* Depression *Increased levels:* Mania, anxiety states, schizophrenia
B. Dopamine	Frontal cortex, limbic system, basal ganglia, thalamus, posterior pituitary, spinal cord *Functions:* Movement and coordination, emotions, voluntary judgment, release of prolactin	*Decreased levels:* Parkinson's disease and depression *Increased levels:* Mania and schizophrenia
C. Serotonin	Hypothalamus, thalamus, limbic system, cerebral cortex, cerebellum, spinal cord *Functions:* Sleep and arousal, libido, appetite, mood, aggression, pain perception, coordination, judgment	*Decreased levels:* Depression *Increased levels:* Anxiety states (there are seven different types of serotonin receptors, increased levels of some serotonin subtypes [5HT1A] have an antianxiety effect, and increased levels of others [5HT3] may increase anxiety [Elsworth & Roth, 2017])
D. Histamine	Hypothalamus, hippocampus, cortex, cerebellum, basal ganglia, spinal cord, retina *Functions:* Wakefulness; pain sensation and inflammatory response	*Decreased levels:* Depression *Increased levels:* Sleep disorders, anxiety, Alzheimer's disease, psychosis

TABLE 3-2	Neurotransmitters in the Central Nervous System—cont'd	
NEUROTRANSMITTER	**LOCATION AND FUNCTION**	**POSSIBLE IMPLICATIONS FOR MENTAL ILLNESS**
III. AMINO ACIDS A. Gamma-aminobutyric acid	Hypothalamus *Functions:* Slowing of body activity	*Decreased levels:* Huntington's disease, anxiety disorders, schizophrenia, and various forms of epilepsy
B. Glycine	Spinal cord, brainstem *Functions:* Recurrent inhibition of motor neurons	*Toxic levels:* Glycine encephalopathy *Decreased levels:* Correlated with spastic motor movements
C. Glutamate and aspartate	Pyramidal cells of the cortex, cerebellum, and the primary sensory afferent systems; hippocampus, thalamus, hypothalamus, spinal cord *Functions:* Relay of sensory information and regulation of various motor and spinal reflexes; glutamate also has a role in memory and learning	*Decreased levels:* Schizophrenia *Increased levels:* Huntington's disease, temporal lobe epilepsy, spinal cerebellar degeneration, anxiety disorders, depressive disorders
D. d-Serine	Cerebral cortex, forebrain, hippocampus, cerebellum striatum, thalamus *Functions:* Binds at NMDA receptors and, with glutamate, is a co-agonist whose functions include mediating NMDA receptor transmission, synaptic plasticity, neurotoxicity	*Decreased levels:* Schizophrenia
IV. NEUROPEPTIDES A. Endorphins and enkephalins	Hypothalamus, thalamus, limbic structures, midbrain, brainstem; enkephalins are also found in the gastrointestinal tract *Functions:* Modulation of pain and reduced peristalsis (enkephalins)	*Modulation* of dopamine activity by opioid peptides may indicate some link to the symptoms of schizophrenia
B. Substance P	Hypothalamus, limbic structures, midbrain, brainstem, thalamus, basal ganglia, spinal cord; also found in gastrointestinal tract and salivary glands *Function:* Regulation of pain	*Decreased levels:* Huntington's disease, Alzheimer's disease *Increased levels:* Depression
C. Somatostatin	Cerebral cortex, hippocampus, thalamus, basal ganglia, brainstem, spinal cord *Function:* Depending on part of the brain affected, stimulates release of dopamine, serotonin, norepinephrine, and acetylcholine and inhibits release of norepinephrine, histamine, and glutamate; also acts as a neuromodulator for serotonin in the hypothalamus	*Decreased levels:* Alzheimer's disease *Increased levels:* Huntington's disease

ANS, autonomic nervous system; CNS, central nervous system; NMDA, *N*-methyl D-aspartate.

activity at all sympathetic and parasympathetic presynaptic nerve terminals and all parasympathetic postsynaptic nerve terminals. It is highly significant in the neurotransmission that occurs at the junctions of nerves and muscles. Acetylcholinesterase is the enzyme that destroys acetylcholine or inhibits its activity.

In the CNS, acetylcholine neurons innervate the cerebral cortex, hippocampus, and limbic structures. The pathways are especially dense through the area of the basal ganglia in the brain.

Functions: Functions of acetylcholine are manifold and include sleep, arousal, pain perception, the modulation and coordination of movement, and memory acquisition and retention.

Possible Implications in Mental Illness: Cholinergic mechanisms may have some role in certain disorders of motor behavior and memory, such as Parkinson's disease, Huntington's disease, and Alzheimer's disease.

Monoamine Neurotransmitters

Norepinephrine

Location: Norepinephrine is the neurotransmitter that produces activity at the sympathetic postsynaptic nerve terminals in the ANS, resulting in fight-or-flight responses in the effector organs. In the CNS, norepinephrine pathways originate in the pons and medulla and innervate the thalamus, dorsal hypothalamus, limbic system, hippocampus, cerebellum, and cerebral cortex. When norepinephrine is not returned for storage in the vesicles of the axon terminals, it is metabolized and inactivated by the enzymes monoamine oxidase (MAO) and catechol-*O*-methyltransferase (COMT).

Functions: The functions of norepinephrine include the regulation of mood, cognition, perception, locomotion, cardiovascular functioning, and sleep and arousal.

Possible Implications in Mental Illness: The activity of norepinephrine also has been implicated in certain mood disorders such as depression and mania, anxiety states, and schizophrenia.

Dopamine

Location: Dopamine pathways arise from the midbrain and hypothalamus and terminate in the frontal cortex, limbic system, basal ganglia, and thalamus. As with norepinephrine, the inactivating enzymes for dopamine are MAO and COMT.

Functions: Dopamine functions include regulation of movements and coordination, emotions, and voluntary decision-making ability, and because of its influence on the pituitary gland, it inhibits the release of prolactin.

Possible Implications in Mental Illness: Increased levels of dopamine are associated with mania and schizophrenia. Decreased levels of dopamine have been associated with Parkinson's disease and depression. Dopamine may also have a role in addictions.

Serotonin

Location: Serotonin pathways originate from cell bodies located in the pons and medulla and project to areas including the hypothalamus, thalamus, limbic system, cerebral cortex, cerebellum, and spinal cord. Serotonin that is not returned to be stored in the axon terminal vesicles is catabolized by the enzyme MAO.

Functions: Serotonin may play a role in sleep and arousal, libido, appetite, mood, aggression, and pain perception. The fact that both too much and too little serotonin have been associated with anxiety has led to the hypothesis that serotonin may modulate intense emotional states rather than influencing one kind of mood disruption. Further, there are seven different subgroups of serotonin receptors, which when activated result in different effects.

Possible Implications in Mental Illness: The serotoninergic (or serotonergic) system has been implicated in the etiology of certain psychopathological conditions including anxiety states, depression, and schizophrenia.

Histamine

Location: The role of histamine in mediating allergic and inflammatory reactions has been well documented. The source of histamine neurons in the brain is within the tuberomammillary nucleus, and they diffusely innervate the cortex, thalamus, and other wake-promoting regions in the brain (Scammell et al., 2019).

Functions: Brain histamine regulates many physiological functions: neuroendocrine, circadian rhythms, the sleep–wake cycle, psychomotor activity, mood, learning, cognition, appetite, and eating behavior. Although histamine is typically excitatory, it may also release GABA, an inhibitory neurotransmitter (Scammell et al., 2019). The enzyme that catabolizes histamine is MAO.

Possible Implications in Mental Illness: Alterations in brain histamine are associated with several pathological conditions, such as epilepsy, narcolepsy, stroke, anxiety, depression, psychosis, neurodegeneration, and neuroinflammatory processes (Scammell et al., 2019).

Amino Acids: Inhibitory Amino Acids

GABA

Location: GABA has a widespread distribution in the CNS, with high concentrations in the hypothalamus, hippocampus, cortex, cerebellum, and basal ganglia of the brain; in the gray matter of the dorsal horn of the spinal cord; and in the retina. GABA is catabolized by the enzyme GABA transaminase.

Functions: Inhibitory neurotransmitters such as GABA prevent postsynaptic excitation, interrupting the progression of the electrical impulse at the synaptic junction. This function is significant when slowdown of body activity is advantageous. Enhancement of the GABA system is the mechanism of action by which the benzodiazepines produce their calming effect.

Possible Implications in Mental Illness: Alterations in the GABA system have been implicated in the etiology of anxiety disorders, movement disorders (e.g., Huntington's disease), and various forms of epilepsy. GABA levels, in a complex interaction with other neurotransmitters such as dopamine, have also been implicated in substance use disorders and addiction.

Glycine

Location: The highest concentrations of glycine in the CNS are found in the spinal cord and brainstem.

Functions: Glycine appears to be the neurotransmitter of recurrent inhibition of motor neurons within the spinal cord and is possibly involved in the regulation of spinal and brainstem reflexes. It is also a co-agonist of the *N*-methyl-D-aspartate receptor (NMDAR) in excitatory glutamatergic neurotransmission. Evidence supports that glycine is a reciprocal modulator of both dopamine and glutamate (de Bartolomeis et al., 2020).

Possible Implications in Mental Illness: Novel human genetic findings and imaging genetics studies have linked glycine signaling to schizophrenia and may pave the way for novel treatment approaches (de Bartolomeis et al., 2020).

Amino Acids: Excitatory Amino Acids

Glutamate and Aspartate

Location: Glutamate and aspartate appear to be primary excitatory neurotransmitters in the pyramidal cells of the cortex, the cerebellum, and the primary sensory afferent systems. They are also found in the hippocampus, thalamus, hypothalamus, and spinal cord. Glutamate and aspartate are inactivated by uptake into the tissues and through assimilation in various metabolic pathways.

Functions: Glutamate and aspartate function in the relay of sensory information and regulation of various motor and spinal reflexes. Glutamate also plays a role in memory and learning.

Possible Implications in Mental Illness: Problems in making or using glutamate have been linked to many mental disorders, including autism, obsessive-compulsive disorder (OCD), schizophrenia, and depression (McGrath et al., 2022). Glutamatergic dysfunction has been implicated even in cases of schizophrenia that are not characterized by dopamine excess in subcortical regions and are not responsive to conventional antipsychotics, and recent research, using advanced magnetic resonance spectography, has identified high levels of both glutamate and glycine in first episodes of psychosis (de Bartolomeis et al., 2020). Alteration in glutamate and aspartate systems has been implicated in the etiology of certain neurodegenerative disorders, such as Huntington's disease, temporal lobe epilepsy, and spinal cerebellar degeneration.

Increases in glutamate have been associated with neuron degeneration in Alzheimer's disease (Liu et al., 2019).

Neuropeptides

Neuropeptides act as signaling molecules in the CNS. Their activities include regulating processes related to sex, sleep, stress and pain, emotion, and social cognition. They may contribute to symptoms and behaviors associated with psychosis, mood disorders, dementia, and autism spectrum disorders (ASDs). Opioid peptides, substance P, and somatostatin are discussed here. Hormonal neuropeptides are discussed later in the "Neuroendocrinology" section of this chapter.

Opioid Peptides

Location: Opioid peptides, which include the endorphins and enkephalins, have been widely studied. They are found in various concentrations in the hypothalamus, thalamus, limbic structures, midbrain, and brainstem. Enkephalins are also found in the gastrointestinal tract.

Functions: With their natural morphine-like properties, opioid peptides are thought to have a role in pain modulation. Released in response to painful stimuli, they may be responsible for producing the analgesic effect that results from acupuncture. Opioid peptides alter the release of dopamine and affect the spontaneous activity of the dopaminergic neurons.

Possible Implications in Mental Illness: Modulation of dopamine activity by opioid peptides may be associated with addiction and some symptoms of schizophrenia, and a growing body of research supports that opioid system dysregulation may contribute to depression (Peciña et al., 2019).

Substance P

Location: Substance P, the first neuropeptide to be discovered, is present in high concentrations in the hypothalamus, limbic structures, midbrain, and brainstem. It is also found in the thalamus, basal ganglia, and spinal cord.

Functions: Substance P plays a role in sensory transmission, particularly in the regulation of pain.

Possible Implications in Mental Illness: Substance P levels have been associated with depression and post-traumatic stress disorder (PTSD). Studies have demonstrated that people with depression and PTSD had elevated levels of substance P in their cerebral spinal fluid (Boland et al., 2022).

Somatostatin

Location: Somatostatin (also called *growth hormone–inhibiting hormone [GHIH]*) is found in the cerebral cortex, hippocampus, thalamus, basal ganglia, brainstem, and spinal cord.

Functions: In its function as a neurotransmitter, somatostatin exerts both stimulatory and inhibitory effects depending on the part of the brain affected. It has been shown to stimulate dopamine, serotonin, norepinephrine, and acetylcholine and to inhibit norepinephrine, histamine, and glutamate. It also acts as a neuromodulator for serotonin in the hypothalamus, thereby regulating its release (i.e., controlling whether it is stimulated or inhibited). Somatostatin may serve this function for other neurotransmitters as well.

Possible Implications in Mental Illness: High concentrations of somatostatin have been reported in brain specimens of clients with Huntington's disease, and low concentrations have been found in those with Alzheimer's disease.

CORE CONCEPTS

Neuroendocrinology
The study of the interaction between the nervous system and the endocrine system and the effects of various hormones on cognitive, emotional, and behavioral functioning.

Neuroendocrinology

Human endocrine functioning has a strong foundation in the CNS under the direction of the hypothalamus, which has direct control over the pituitary gland. The pituitary gland has two major lobes—the anterior lobe (also called the *adenohypophysis*) and the posterior lobe (also called the *neurohypophysis*). The pituitary gland is only about the size of a pea, but despite its size and because of the powerful control it exerts over endocrine functioning in humans, it is sometimes called the "master gland." Figure 3–5 shows the hormones of the pituitary gland and their target organs. Many of the hormones subject to hypothalamus-pituitary regulation may have implications for behavioral functioning. Discussion of these hormones is summarized in Table 3–3.

Pituitary Gland

The Posterior Pituitary (Neurohypophysis)

The hypothalamus has direct control over the posterior pituitary through efferent neural pathways. Two hormones are found in the posterior pituitary: vasopressin (ADH) and oxytocin. They are actually produced by the hypothalamus and stored in the posterior pituitary. Their release is mediated by neural impulses from the hypothalamus (Fig. 3–6).

Antidiuretic Hormone

The main function of ADH is to conserve body water and maintain normal blood pressure. The release of ADH is stimulated by pain, emotional stress, dehydration, increased plasma concentration, and decreases in blood volume. An alteration in the secretion of this hormone is related to the polydipsia seen in patients with diabetes. ADH alterations also may be one of many factors contributing to the polydipsia and water intoxication (a state of hyperhydration related to excessive consumption of water) observed in 10% to 20% of patients with severe mental illness, particularly those with schizophrenia. Other factors correlated with excessive thirst include adverse effects of psychotropic medications and features of the behavioral disorder itself. It is important to note that severe polydipsia can result in electrolyte imbalance and death. ADH also may play a role in learning and memory, alteration of the pain response, and modification of sleep patterns.

Oxytocin

Oxytocin causes contraction of the uterus during labor and stimulates release of milk from the mammary glands (Scanlon & Sanders, 2019). It is also released in response to stress and during sexual arousal. Oxytocin functions to promote mother–infant bonding and bonding between sexes and has been used experimentally with children with ASD to increase socialization.

Some research found that oxytocin may be more beneficial in treating core symptoms of ASD when baseline levels of oxytocin were already low (Parker et al., 2017). However, results are mixed. In a large, placebo-controlled trial, using intranasal oxytocin, the researchers found no significant improvements in cognitive or social functioning (Sikich et al., 2021).

Increases in oxytocin demonstrate antianxiety effects (in interaction with adrenocorticotrophic hormone [ACTH]) and may facilitate the development of substance use disorders, especially with "party drugs" (MDMA [Ecstasy, Molly] and GBH [Liquid X, Goop]) that are often used to decrease inhibitions in social interaction (Harris et al., 2017). Decreased levels of oxytocin have been reported both in patients with autism and anorexia.

The Anterior Pituitary (Adenohypophysis)

The hypothalamus produces releasing hormones that pass through capillaries and veins of the hypophyseal portal system to capillaries in the anterior pituitary, where they stimulate secretion of specialized hormones. The hormones of the anterior pituitary gland regulate multiple body functions and include growth hormone (GH),

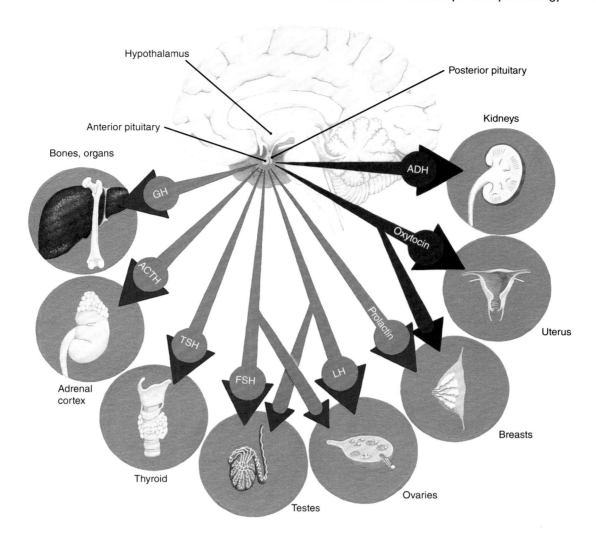

FIGURE 3-5 Hormones of the pituitary gland and their target organs.

TABLE 3-3	**Hormones of the Neuroendocrine System**			
HORMONE	**LOCATION AND STIMULATION OF RELEASE**	**TARGET ORGAN**	**FUNCTION**	**POSSIBLE BEHAVIORAL CORRELATION TO ALTERED SECRETION**
Antidiuretic hormone (ADH)	Posterior pituitary; release stimulated by dehydration, pain, stress	Kidney (causes increased reabsorption)	Conservation of body water; maintenance of blood pressure	Polydipsia; altered pain response; modified sleep pattern
Oxytocin	Posterior pituitary; release stimulated by end of pregnancy; stress; during sexual arousal	Uterus; breasts	Contraction of the uterus for labor; release of breast milk	May perform role in stress response by stimulation of adrenocorticotropic hormone (ACTH)

Continued

TABLE 3-3 Hormones of the Neuroendocrine System—cont'd

HORMONE	LOCATION AND STIMULATION OF RELEASE	TARGET ORGAN	FUNCTION	POSSIBLE BEHAVIORAL CORRELATION TO ALTERED SECRETION
Growth hormone (GH)	Anterior pituitary; release stimulated by growth hormone–releasing hormone from hypothalamus	Bones and tissues	Growth in children; protein synthesis in adults	Anorexia nervosa
Thyroid-stimulating hormone (TSH)	Anterior pituitary; release stimulated by thyrotropin-releasing hormone from hypothalamus	Thyroid gland	Stimulation of secretion of needed thyroid hormones for metabolism of food and regulation of temperature	*Increased levels of thyroid hormones (decreased secretion of TSH):* Insomnia, anxiety, emotional lability *Decreased levels of thyroid hormones (increased secretion of TSH):* Fatigue, depression
Adrenocortico-tropic hormone (ACTH)	Anterior pituitary; release stimulated by corticotropin-releasing hormone from hypothalamus	Adrenal cortex	Stimulation of secretion of cortisol, which performs a role in response to stress	*Increased levels:* Mood disorders, psychosis *Decreased levels:* Depression, apathy, fatigue
Prolactin	Anterior pituitary; release stimulated by prolactin-releasing hormone from hypothalamus	Breasts	Stimulation of milk production	*Increased levels:* Depression, anxiety, decreased libido, irritability
Gonadotropic hormones	Anterior pituitary; release stimulated by gonadotropin-releasing hormone from hypothalamus	Ovaries and testes	Stimulation of secretion of estrogen, progesterone, and testosterone; role in ovulation and sperm production	*Decreased levels:* Depression, anorexia nervosa *Increased testosterone:* Increased sexual behavior and aggressiveness
Melanocyte-stimulating hormone (MSH)	Anterior pituitary; release stimulated by onset of darkness	Pineal gland	Stimulation of secretion of melatonin	*Increased levels:* Depression

thyroid-stimulating hormone (TSH), ACTH, prolactin, gonadotropin-stimulating hormone, and melanocyte-stimulating hormone (MSH). Most of these hormones are regulated by a *negative feedback mechanism.* Once the hormone has exerted its effects, the information is "fed back" to the anterior pituitary, which inhibits the release and ultimately decreases the effects of the stimulating hormones.

Growth Hormone

The release of GH, also called *somatotropin,* is stimulated by growth hormone–releasing hormone (GHRH) from the hypothalamus. Its release is inhibited by GHIH, or somatostatin, also from the hypothalamus. It is responsible for growth in children and continued protein synthesis throughout life. During periods of fasting, it stimulates the release of

fat from the adipose tissue to increase energy. The release of GHIH is stimulated in response to periods of hyperglycemia. GHRH is stimulated in response to hypoglycemia and stressful situations. During prolonged stress, GH has a direct effect on protein, carbohydrate, and lipid metabolism, resulting in increased serum glucose and free fatty acids to be used for increased energy. GH deficiency has been noted in many patients with major depressive disorder, and several GH abnormalities have been noted in patients with anorexia nervosa.

Thyroid-Stimulating Hormone

Thyrotropin-releasing hormone (TRH) from the hypothalamus stimulates the release of TSH, or thyrotropin, from the anterior pituitary. TSH stimulates the thyroid gland to secrete triiodothyronine (T3)

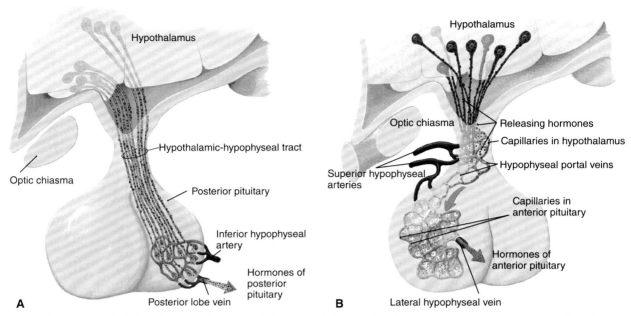

FIGURE 3-6 Structural relationships of hypothalamus and pituitary gland. (A) Posterior pituitary stores hormones produced in the hypothalamus. (B) Releasing hormones of the hypothalamus circulate directly to the anterior pituitary and influence its secretions. Notice the two networks of capillaries.

and thyroxine (T4). Thyroid hormones are integral to metabolism and the regulation of temperature.

A correlation between thyroid dysfunction and altered behavioral functioning has been well documented. Common symptoms of hyperthyroidism include irritability, insomnia, anxiety, restlessness, weight loss, and emotional lability, in some instances progressing to delirium or psychosis. Symptoms of fatigue, decreased libido, memory impairment, depression, and suicidal ideation have been associated with chronic hypothyroidism. Studies have correlated various forms of thyroid dysfunction with mood disorders, anxiety, eating disorders, psychosis, and dementia.

Adrenocorticotropic Hormone

Corticotropin-releasing hormone (CRH) from the hypothalamus stimulates the release of ACTH from the anterior pituitary. ACTH stimulates the adrenal cortex to secrete cortisol. CRH, ACTH, and cortisol levels all increase in response to stress. Disorders of the adrenal cortex have been associated with mood disorders, PTSD, Alzheimer's dementia, and substance use disorders.

Addison's disease is the result of hyposecretion of the hormones of the adrenal cortex. Behavioral symptoms of hyposecretion include mood changes with apathy, social withdrawal, impaired sleep, decreased concentration, and fatigue. Hypersecretion of cortisol results in Cushing's disease and is associated with

behaviors that include depression, mania, psychosis, and suicidal ideation. Cognitive impairments also have been observed.

Prolactin

Prolactin is mainly involved in reproductive functions and milk production in the mammary glands during and after pregnancy. First generation antipsychotic medications increase prolactin levels and may be responsible for the undesired side effect of lactation. High prolactin levels are also associated with depression, decreased libido, anxiety, irritability, and the negative symptoms of schizophrenia.

Gonadotropic Hormones

The gonadotropic hormones are so called because they produce an effect on the gonads—the ovaries and the testes. The gonadotropins include follicle-stimulating hormone (FSH) and luteinizing hormone (LH). In women, FSH initiates maturation of ovarian follicles into ova and stimulates secretion of estrogen from follicular granulosa cells. LH is responsible for ovulation and the secretion of progesterone from the corpus luteum. In men, FSH initiates sperm production in the testes, and LH increases secretion of testosterone by the interstitial cells of the testes (Scanlon & Sanders, 2019).

Limited evidence exists to correlate gonadotropins to behavioral functioning, although some observations warrant hypothetical consideration.

Increased sexual behavior and aggression have been linked to elevated testosterone levels in both men and women. Testosterone administration has also been associated with positive improvement in mood and energy (Boland et al., 2022). Decreased plasma levels of LH and FSH commonly occur in patients with anorexia nervosa. Supplemental estrogen therapy has resulted in improved mentation and mood in some women with depression.

Melanocyte-Stimulating Hormone

MSH from the hypothalamus stimulates the pineal gland to secrete melatonin. The release of melatonin appears to depend on the onset of darkness and is suppressed by light. Studies of this hormone have indicated that environmental light can affect neuronal activity and influence circadian rhythms (Boland, et al., 2022). Correlation between abnormal secretion of melatonin and symptoms of depression has led to the implication of melatonin as influential in seasonal affective disorder.

Circadian Rhythms

Human biological rhythms are largely determined by genetic coding, with input from the external environment influencing the cyclic effects. **Circadian rhythms** in humans follow a near-24-hour cycle and may influence a variety of regulatory functions, including the sleep–wakefulness cycle, body temperature regulation, patterns of activity such as eating and drinking, and hormone secretion. The 24-hour rhythms in humans are affected to a large degree by the cycles of lightness and darkness. These rhythms occur because of a "pacemaker" in the brain that sends messages to other systems in the body and maintains the 24-hour rhythm. This endogenous pacemaker appears to be the suprachiasmatic nuclei of the hypothalamus. These nuclei receive projections of light through the retina and in turn stimulate electrical impulses to various other systems in the body, mediating the release of neurotransmitters or hormones that regulate bodily functioning.

Most of the biological rhythms of the body operate for approximately 24 hours, but cycles of longer lengths have been studied. For example, women of menstruating age have monthly cycles of variable progesterone levels.

Some rhythms may last as long as a year. These circannual rhythms may influence the accuracy of some laboratory tests results and the effectiveness of some medications. Clinical studies have shown that administration of medications during the appropriate circadian phase and at the appropriate time of day can significantly increase the efficacy and decrease the toxic effects of some medications (Walton et al., 2021).

The Role of Circadian Rhythms in Psychopathology

Circadian rhythms may play a role in psychopathology. Abnormal circadian rhythms have been associated with a variety of mental illnesses including depression, bipolar disorder, and seasonal affective disorder. Because many hormones have been implicated in behavioral functioning, it is reasonable to believe that peak secretion times could be influential in predicting certain behaviors. The association of depression with increased secretion of melatonin during darkness hours has already been discussed. External manipulation of the light–dark cycle and removal of external time cues often have beneficial effects on mood disorders.

Symptoms that occur premenstrually have been linked to disruptions in biological rhythms. A number of the symptoms associated with premenstrual dysphoric disorder (PMDD) strongly resemble those attributed to depression, and hormonal changes have been implicated in the etiology. Some of these changes include progesterone–estrogen imbalance, increase in prolactin and mineralocorticoids, high level of prostaglandins, decrease in endogenous opiates, changes in metabolism of biogenic amines (serotonin, dopamine, norepinephrine, acetylcholine), and variations in secretion of glucocorticoids or melatonin.

The sleep–wakefulness cycle is probably the most fundamental of biological rhythms, and sleep disturbances are common in both mood disorders and PMDD. Neurochemicals such as serotonin and norepinephrine appear to be most active during non–rapid eye movement (NREM) sleep, whereas the neurotransmitter acetylcholine is activated during REM sleep (Skudaev, 2019). Several studies have revealed information about the sleep-inducing characteristics of serotonin. L-Tryptophan, the amino acid precursor to serotonin, has been used for many years as an effective sedative-hypnotic to induce sleep in individuals with sleep-onset disorder. A representation of bodily functions affected by 24-hour biological rhythms is presented in Figure 3–7.

Sleep

The sleep–wakefulness cycle is genetically determined rather than learned and is established after birth. Even when environmental cues, such as the

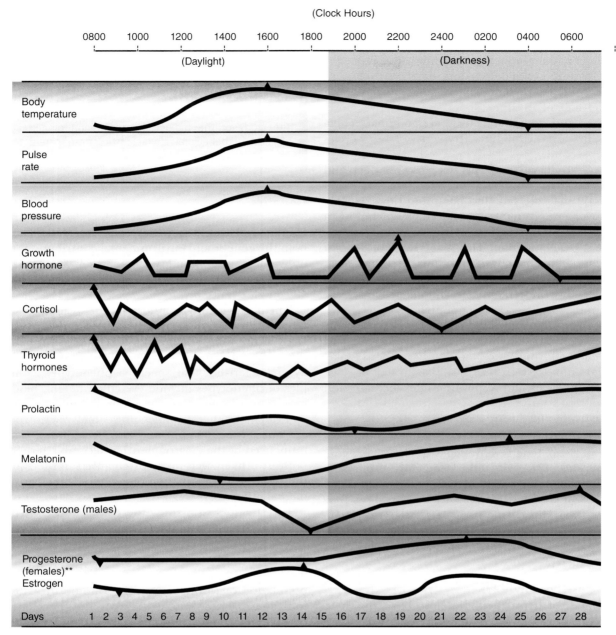

(Clock Hours)

FIGURE 3–7 Circadian biological rhythms.

▼ indicates low point and ▲ indicates peak time of these biological factors within a 24-hour circadian rhythm.
* The female hormones are presented on a monthly rhythm because of their influence on the reproductive cycle.
Daily rhythms of female gonadotropins are difficult to assay and are probably less significant than monthly.

ability to detect light and darkness, are removed, the human sleep–wakefulness cycle generally develops a periodicity of approximately 25 hours, which is close to the 24-hour normal circadian rhythm.

Sleep can be measured by the types of brain waves that occur during various stages of sleep activity. Dreaming episodes occur during REM sleep. The sleep–wakefulness cycle is represented by six distinct stages:

Stage 0—Alpha rhythm: This stage of the sleep–wakefulness cycle is characterized by a relaxed, waking state with eyes closed. The alpha brain wave rhythm has a frequency of 8 to 12 cycles per second.

Stage 1—Beta rhythm: Stage 1 characterizes the transition into sleep, a period of dozing in which thoughts wander and the person drifts in and out of sleep. Beta brain wave rhythm has a frequency of 18 to 25 cycles per second.

Stage 2—Theta rhythm: This stage comprises about one half of the time spent sleeping. Eye movement and muscular activity are minimal. Theta brain wave rhythm has a frequency of 4 to 7 cycles per second.

Stage 3—Delta rhythm: This is a period of deep and restful sleep. Muscles are relaxed, heart rate and blood pressure fall, and breathing slows. No eye movement occurs. Delta brain wave rhythm has a frequency of 1.5 to 3 cycles per second.

Stage 4—Delta rhythm: This is the stage of deepest sleep. Individuals with insomnia or other sleep disorders often do not experience this stage of sleep. Eye movement and muscular activity are minimal. Delta waves predominate.

REM sleep—Beta rhythm: The dream cycle occurs during REM sleep. Eyes dart about beneath closed eyelids, moving more rapidly than when awake. The brain wave pattern is similar to that of stage 1 sleep. Heart and respiration rates increase, and blood pressure may increase or decrease. Muscles are hypotonic during REM sleep.

Stages 2 through REM repeat throughout the cycle of sleep. One is more likely to experience longer periods of stages 3 and 4 sleep early in the cycle and longer periods of REM sleep later in the sleep cycle. Most people experience REM sleep about four to five times during the night. The amount of time spent in REM sleep and deep sleep decreases with age, and the time spent in drowsy wakefulness and dozing increases.

Neurochemical Influences

A number of neurochemicals have been shown to influence the sleep–wakefulness cycle. As noted previously, several studies have revealed information about the sleep-inducing characteristics of serotonin. L-Tryptophan, the amino acid precursor to serotonin, has been used for many years as an effective sedative-hypnotic to induce sleep in individuals with sleep-onset disorder. Serotonin and norepinephrine both appear to be most active during non-REM sleep, whereas the neurotransmitter acetylcholine is activated during REM sleep (Skudaev, 2019). The exact role of GABA in sleep facilitation is unclear, although the sedative effects of drugs that enhance GABA transmission, such as benzodiazepines, suggest that this neurotransmitter plays an important role in the regulation of sleep and arousal. Studies have suggested that acetylcholine induces and prolongs REM sleep, whereas histamine appears to have an inhibitory effect (Yamada & Ueda, 2020; Yu et al., 2018).

CORE CONCEPT

Genetics
The study of the biological transmission of certain physical or behavioral characteristics from parent to offspring.

Genetics

Human behavioral genetics seeks to understand both the genetic and environmental contributions to individual variations in human behavior. This type of study is complicated by the fact that behaviors, like all complex traits, involve *multiple genes.*

The term **genotype** refers to the complete set of genes present in an individual and coded in the DNA at the time of conception. The physical manifestations of a particular genotype are designated by characteristics that specify a **phenotype.** Examples of phenotypes include eye color, height, blood type, the characteristics of one's voice, and hair type. As evident by the examples presented, phenotypes are not *only* genetic but may also be acquired (i.e., influenced by the environment) or a combination of both. It is likely that many psychiatric disorders are the result of a combination of genetics and environmental influences.

Investigators who study the causes and contributing factors for psychiatric illness explore several risk factors. Studies to determine whether an illness is *familial* compare the percentage of family members with the illness to those in the general population or within a control group of unrelated individuals. These studies estimate the prevalence of psychopathology among relatives and predict predisposition to an illness based on familial risk factors. Schizophrenia, bipolar disorder, major depressive disorder, anorexia nervosa, panic disorder, somatic symptom disorder, antisocial personality disorder, and alcoholism are examples of psychiatric illnesses in which familial tendencies have been identified.

Studies that focus only on genetics search for a specific gene that causes a particular illness. A number of disorders exist in which the mutation of a specific gene or change in the number or structure of chromosomes are associated with the etiology. Examples include Huntington's disease, cystic fibrosis, phenylketonuria, Duchenne's muscular dystrophy, and Down's syndrome.

The search for genetic links to certain psychiatric disorders continues. Risk factors for early-onset Alzheimer's disease have been linked to mutations on chromosomes 21, 14, and 1 (National Institute on Aging, 2019). Other studies have linked a gene in the region of chromosome 19 that produces apolipoprotein E (ApoE) with late-onset Alzheimer's disease. One large study (Cross-Disorder Group of the Psychiatric Genomics Consortium, 2013) found similar genetic variations in patients with five mental disorders that were previously considered completely distinct. Autism, attention deficit-hyperactivity disorder (ADHD), bipolar disorder, major depression, and schizophrenia all showed some common gene variations, including differences in two genes that regulate the flow of calcium into cells. Although these findings are intriguing, they do not clearly explain all the genetic risks for mental illness, the nongenetic risks, or the interaction between the two. Future research will continue to search for answers with the ultimate goal of improving diagnosis and treatment and perhaps uncovering keys to prevention of mental illness.

In addition to familial and purely genetic investigations, other types of studies have been conducted to estimate the existence and degree of genetic and environmental contributions to the etiology of certain psychiatric disorders. Twin studies and adoption studies have been successfully employed for this purpose.

Twin studies examine the frequency of a disorder in monozygotic (genetically identical) and dizygotic (not genetically identical) twins. Twins are called *concordant* when both members have the disorder in question. Concordance in monozygotic twins is considered stronger evidence of genetic involvement than it is in dizygotic (fraternal) twins. Twin studies have supported genetic vulnerability in the etiology of several mental illnesses, including autism, PTSD, substance misuse (alcoholism), schizophrenia, bipolar disorder, major depression, OCD, risk for suicide, and others (Boland et al., 2022).

Adoption studies allow researchers to compare the influence of genetics versus environment on the development of a psychiatric disorder. Adoption studies include the following four types:

1. Adopted children whose biological parent(s) had a psychiatric disorder but whose adoptive parent(s) did not.
2. Adopted children whose adoptive parent(s) had a psychiatric disorder but whose biological parent(s) did not.
3. Adoptive and biological relatives of adopted children who developed a psychiatric disorder.
4. Monozygotic twins reared apart by different adoptive parents.

Disorders in which adoption studies have suggested a possible genetic link include alcoholism, schizophrenia, major depression, bipolar disorder, ADHD, and antisocial personality disorder (Boland et al., 2022).

Various psychiatric disorders and the possible biological influences discussed in this chapter are presented in Table 3–4. Diagnostic procedures used to detect alteration in biological functioning that may contribute to psychiatric disorders are presented in Table 3–5.

TABLE 3–4 Biological Implications of Psychiatric Disorders

ANATOMICAL BRAIN STRUCTURES INVOLVED	NEUROTRANSMITTER HYPOTHESIS	POSSIBLE ENDOCRINE CORRELATION	IMPLICATIONS OF CIRCADIAN RHYTHMS	POSSIBLE GENETIC LINK
SCHIZOPHRENIA				
Frontal cortex, temporal lobes, limbic system	Dopamine hyperactivity; decreased glutamate	Decreased prolactin levels	May correlate antipsychotic medication administration to times of lowest level	Twin, familial, and adoption studies suggest genetic link
DEPRESSIVE DISORDERS				
Frontal lobes, limbic system, temporal lobes	Decreased levels of norepinephrine, dopamine, and serotonin; increased glutamate	Increased cortisol levels; thyroid hormone hyposecretion; increased melatonin	DST* used to predict effectiveness of antidepressants; melatonin linked to depression during periods of darkness	Twin, familial, and adoption studies suggest a genetic link

Continued

TABLE 3-4   Biological Implications of Psychiatric Disorders—cont'd

ANATOMICAL BRAIN STRUCTURES INVOLVED	NEUROTRANSMITTER HYPOTHESIS	POSSIBLE ENDOCRINE CORRELATION	IMPLICATIONS OF CIRCADIAN RHYTHMS	POSSIBLE GENETIC LINK
BIPOLAR DISORDER				
Frontal lobes, limbic system, temporal lobes	Increased levels of norepinephrine and dopamine in acute mania	Some indication of elevated thyroid hormones in acute mania	Abnormal circadian rhythms have been associated with bipolar disorder	Twin, familial, and adoption studies suggest a genetic link
PANIC DISORDER				
Limbic system, midbrain	Increased levels of norepinephrine; decreased GABA activity	Elevated levels of thyroid hormones	May have some application for times of medication administration	Twin and familial studies suggest a genetic link
ANOREXIA NERVOSA				
Limbic system, particularly the hypothalamus	Decreased levels of norepinephrine, serotonin, and dopamine	Decreased levels of gonadotropins and growth hormone; increased cortisol levels	DST often shows same results as in depression	Twin and familial studies suggest a genetic link
OBSESSIVE-COMPULSIVE DISORDER				
Limbic system, basal ganglia (specifically caudate nucleus)	Decreased levels of serotonin	Increased cortisol levels	DST often shows same results as in depression	Twin studies suggest a possible genetic link
ALZHEIMER'S DISEASE				
Temporal, parietal, and occipital regions of cerebral cortex; hippocampus	Decreased levels of acetylcholine, norepinephrine, serotonin, and somatostatin	Decreased corticotropin-releasing hormone	Decreased levels of acetylcholine and serotonin may inhibit hypothalamic-pituitary axis and interfere with hormonal releasing factors	Familial studies suggest a genetic predisposition; late-onset disorder linked to marker on chromosome 19; early-onset disorder linked to chromosomes 21, 14, and 1

*DST, dexamethasone suppression test. Dexamethasone is a synthetic glucocorticoid that suppresses cortisol secretion via the feedback mechanism. In this test, 1 mg of dexamethasone is administered at 11:30 p.m., and blood samples are drawn at 8:00 a.m., 4:00 p.m., and 11:00 p.m. on the following day. A plasma value greater than 5 mcg/dL suggests that the individual is not suppressing cortisol in response to the dose of dexamethasone. This is a positive result for depression and may have implications for other disorders as well. GABA, gamma-aminobutyric acid.

TABLE 3-5   Diagnostic Procedures Used to Detect Altered Brain Functioning

EXAMINATION	TECHNIQUE USED	PURPOSE AND POSSIBLE FINDINGS
Electroencephalography (EEG)	Electrodes are placed on the scalp in a standardized position. Amplitude and frequency of beta, alpha, theta, and delta brain waves are graphically recorded on paper by ink markers for multiple areas of the brain surface.	Measures brain electrical activity; identifies dysrhythmias, asymmetries, or suppression of brain rhythms; used in the diagnosis of epilepsy, neoplasm, stroke, metabolic, or degenerative disease.
Computerized EEG mapping	EEG tracings are summarized by computer-assisted systems in which various regions of the brain are identified and functioning is interpreted by color coding or gray shading.	Measures brain electrical activity; used largely in research to represent statistical relationships between individuals and groups or between two populations of subjects (e.g., patients with schizophrenia vs. control subjects).

TABLE 3–5	**Diagnostic Procedures Used to Detect Altered Brain Functioning–cont'd**	
EXAMINATION	**TECHNIQUE USED**	**PURPOSE AND POSSIBLE FINDINGS**
Computed tomography (CT) scan	CT scan may be used with or without contrast medium. X-rays are taken of various transverse planes of the brain while a computerized analysis produces a precise reconstructed image of each segment.	Measures accuracy of brain structure to detect possible lesions, abscesses, areas of infarction, or aneurysm. CT has also identified various anatomical differences in patients with schizophrenia, organic mental disorders, and bipolar disorder.
Magnetic resonance imaging (MRI) (structural and functional [*f*MRI])	Within a strong magnetic field, the nuclei of hydrogen atoms absorb and reemit electromagnetic energy that is computerized and transformed into image information. No radiation or contrast medium is used.	Structural: Measures anatomical structures and biological status of various segments of the brain; detects brain edema, ischemia, infection, neoplasm, trauma, and other changes such as demyelination. Morphological differences have been noted in brains of patients with schizophrenia compared with control subjects. Functional: Measures metabolic functions in the brain. Can be used to locate brain areas and underlying brain processes that are associated with performing a particular cognitive or behavioral task.
Positron emission tomography (PET)	The patient receives an intravenous (IV) injection of a radioactive substance (type depends on brain activity to be visualized). The head is surrounded by detectors that relay data to a computer that interprets the signals and produces the image.	Measures specific brain functioning, such as glucose metabolism, oxygen utilization, blood flow, and, of particular interest in psychiatry, neurotransmitter-receptor interaction.
Single-photon emission computed tomography (SPECT)	The technique is similar to PET, but longer-acting radioactive substance must be used to allow time for a gamma-camera to rotate about the head and gather the data, which are then computer assembled into a brain image.	Measures various aspects of brain functioning, as with PET; has also been used to image activity of cerebrospinal fluid circulation.

CORE CONCEPT

Psychoneuroimmunology
The study of the relationship between the immune system, the nervous system, and psychological processes such as thinking and behavior is called **psychoneuroimmunology (PNI).**

Psychoneuroimmunology

The role of inflammation and disruptions in the function of the immune system have been implicated in many disease processes, including mental illnesses and substance use disorders. The role of prolonged, significant stress and trauma in immune system disruptions is central in this discussion.

Normal Immune Response

Cells responsible for *nonspecific* immune reactions include neutrophils, monocytes, and macrophages. They work to destroy invasive organisms and initiate and facilitate the healing of damaged tissue. If these cells do not accomplish a satisfactory healing response, *specific* immune mechanisms take over.

Cytokines are one such mechanism. These molecules, which regulate immune and inflammatory responses, are active when an individual is fighting an infection or any other condition that creates inflammation in the body. Research has demonstrated that cytokines are part of an essential and complex system of responses that are crucial for reducing inflammation and bolstering the immune response, and they are also active in mood disorders such as depression and bipolar disorder (Mao et al., 2018). Studies are also attempting to identify what happens when inflammation is not resolved and cytokines remain active or cross the blood–brain barrier.

The Role of the Immune System in Psychiatric Illness

Studies of the biological response to stress (Salleh, 2008) have hypothesized that individuals become more susceptible to physical illness after exposure to a stressful stimulus or life event (see Chapter 1, "The Concept of Stress Adaptation"). This response is thought to be caused by increased glucocorticoid release from the adrenal cortex after stimulation from the hypothalamic-pituitary-adrenal axis during stressful situations ("axis" refers to the complex interactions between these three glands). The result is suppression of lymphocyte proliferation and function.

Studies have shown that nerve endings exist in tissues of the immune system (Dantzer, 2018). The CNS has connections in both bone marrow and the thymus, where immune system cells are produced, and in the spleen and lymph nodes, where those cells are stored.

GH, which may be released in response to certain stressors, may enhance immune functioning, whereas testosterone is thought to inhibit immune functioning. Increased production of epinephrine and norepinephrine occurs in response to stress and may decrease immunity. Serotonin has been described as an immunomodulator because it has demonstrated both stimulatory and inhibitory effects on inflammation and immunity (Arreola et al., 2015).

Studies have correlated a decrease in lymphocyte function with periods of grief, bereavement, and depression, associating the degree of altered immunity with the severity of depression (Seiler et al., 2020). Several research studies have attempted to correlate the onset of schizophrenia with abnormalities of the immune system and these studies have implicated autoimmune responses, viral infections, and immunogenetics (Boland et al., 2022). A link has been identified between toxoplasmosis and psychiatric disorders such as schizophrenia, bipolar disorder, and particularly delusions and hallucinations (Torrey, 2022). *Toxoplasma gondii,* the parasite responsible for toxoplasmosis, has an affinity for brain tissue where it causes brain inflammation and may affect neurotransmitters such as dopamine. Immunological abnormalities have also been investigated in other psychiatric illnesses, including alcoholism, ASD, and neurocognitive disorder.

Although evidence exists to support a correlation between psychosocial stress and the onset of illness, more research is needed to determine the specific processes involved in stress-induced modulation of the immune system.

Psychopharmacology and the Brain

Understanding the brain and the biological processes involved in thoughts, feelings, and behavior has positive ramifications beyond better understanding of psychopharmacological treatment options.

As mentioned earlier, future research may continue to demonstrate the effect of psychological interventions on brain activity and neurotransmitters, which would open opportunities to hone psychological treatments and avoid the troubling side effects that accompany many medications. Furthermore, continued research in areas such as PNI may reveal causes of mental illness, which would provide the opportunity for primary prevention.

Despite these potential opportunities, psychopharmacology remains a primary treatment modality for mental disorders, and current evidence suggests that early medication treatment of schizophrenia at the first signs of psychosis may prevent the damaging effects of multiple psychotic episodes on the brain (Nasrallah, 2018). Understanding, as best we can with current evidence, the biological mechanisms at work in psychoactive drugs is essential to nursing practice. Figure 3–8 shows the biological mechanism of psychoactive drugs at the neural synapse. See Chapter 4, "Psychopharmacology," for further discussion of the influence of psychoactive drugs on neurosynaptic transmission.

Implications for Nursing

Psychiatric nurses must integrate knowledge of the biological sciences into their practices if they are to ensure safe and effective care to people with mental illness. Much progress has been made in understanding the biochemical, neuroanatomical, and genetic influences in mental illness, but much remains theoretical. Further, there is evidence that psychosocial influences, particularly a history of trauma such as abuse and neglect, interact significantly with an individual's biological vulnerabilities in the development of these illnesses (Substance Abuse and Mental Health Services Administration [SAMHSA], 2014).

To ensure a smooth transition from a strictly psychosocial focus to one of *bio*psychosocial emphasis, nurses must have a clear understanding of the following:

- **Neuroanatomy and neurophysiology:** The structure and functioning of the various parts of the brain and their correlation to human behavior and psychopathology
- **Neuronal processes:** The various functions of the nerve cells, including the role of neurotransmitters, receptors, synaptic activity, and information pathways
- **Neuroendocrinology:** The interaction of the endocrine and nervous systems and the role that the endocrine glands and their respective hormones play in behavioral functioning

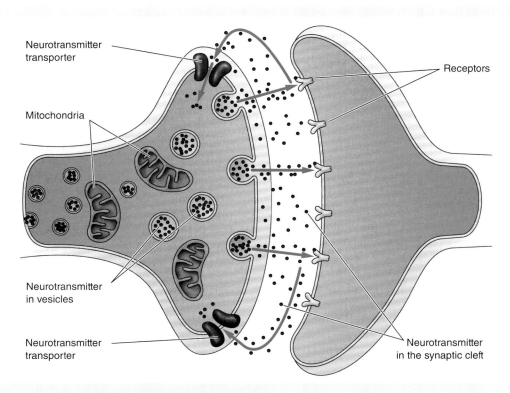

FIGURE 3-8 Area of synaptic transmission that is altered by drugs.
The transmission of electrical impulses from the axon terminal of one neuron to the dendrite of another is achieved by the controlled release of neurotransmitters into the synaptic cleft. Neurotransmitters include serotonin, norepinephrine, acetylcholine, dopamine, glutamate, gamma-aminobutyric acid (GABA), and histamine, among others. Before its release, the neurotransmitter is concentrated into specialized synaptic vesicles. Once fired, the neurotransmitter is released into the synaptic cleft where it encounters receptors on the postsynaptic membrane. Each neurotransmitter has receptors specific to it alone. Some neurotransmitters are considered to be *excitatory*, whereas others are *inhibitory*, a feature that determines whether another action potential will occur. In the synaptic cleft, the neurotransmitter rapidly diffuses, is catabolized by enzymatic action, or is taken up by the neurotransmitter transporters and returned to vesicles inside the axon terminal to await another action potential.

Psychotropic medications exert their effects in various ways in this area of synaptic transmission. Reuptake inhibitors block *reuptake* of the neurotransmitters by the transporter proteins, resulting in elevated levels of extracellular neurotransmitter. Drugs that inhibit catabolic enzymes promote excess buildup of the neurotransmitter at the synaptic site.

Some drugs cause *receptor blockade*, resulting in a reduction in transmission and decreased neurotransmitter activity. These drugs are called *antagonists*. Drugs that increase neurotransmitter activity by *direct stimulation* of the specific receptors are called *agonists*.

- **Circadian rhythms:** The regulation of biochemical functioning over periods of rhythmic cycles and its influence in predicting certain behaviors
- **Genetic influences:** The hereditary factors that predispose individuals to certain psychiatric disorders
- **PNI:** The influence of stress on the immune system and its role in the susceptibility to illness
- **The effect of trauma:** Both physical trauma (traumatic brain injury) and psychosocial trauma (especially early childhood trauma such as abuse, neglect, and abandonment) are influential in the development of several mental illnesses. (See Chapters 21, 28, 34, and 37 for further discussion of trauma and trauma-informed care.)

- **Psychopharmacology:** The increasing use of psychotropic drugs in the treatment of mental illness, demanding greater knowledge of psychopharmacological principles and nursing interventions necessary for safe and effective management
- **Diagnostic technology:** The imaging and other technological procedures for identifying alterations in brain structure and function associated with mental illness

Why are these concepts important to the practice of psychiatric-mental health nursing? The interrelationship between psychosocial adaptation and physical functioning has been established. Integrating biological and behavioral concepts into psychiatric nursing practice is essential for nurses to meet the complex needs of patients with mental illness. Psychobiological perspectives must be incorporated into nursing practice, education, and research to attain the evidence-based outcomes necessary for the delivery of competent care.

Summary and Key Points

- It is important for nurses to understand the interaction between biological and behavioral factors in the development and management of mental illness.
- Psychobiology is the study of the biological foundations of cognitive, emotional, and behavioral processes.
- The limbic system has been called the "emotional brain." Structures within this system are associated with feelings of fear and anxiety; anger, rage, and aggression; love, joy, and hope; and with sexuality and social behavior.
- The three classes of neurons are afferent (sensory) neurons, efferent (motor) neurons, and interneurons. The junction between two neurons is called a *synapse*.
- Neurotransmitters are chemicals that convey information across synaptic clefts to neighboring target cells. Many neurotransmitters have implications in the etiology of emotional disorders and in the pharmacological treatment of those disorders.
- Major categories of neurotransmitters include cholinergics, monoamines, amino acids, and neuropeptides.
- The endocrine system plays an important role in human behavior through the hypothalamic-pituitary axis.

- Hormones and their circadian rhythms of regulation significantly influence a number of physiological and psychological life cycle phenomena, such as moods, sleep and arousal, stress response, appetite, libido, and fertility.
- Research continues to validate the role of genetics in psychiatric illness.
- Familial, twin, and adoption studies suggest that genetics may be implicated in the etiology of schizophrenia, bipolar disorder, depressive disorder, panic disorder, anorexia nervosa, alcoholism, and OCD. Genetic studies, however, fail to entirely explain the complex factors involved in the development of these illnesses.
- PNI examines the relationship between psychological factors, the immune system, and the nervous system.
- Evidence exists to support a link between psychosocial stressors and suppression of the immune response.
- Technologies such as magnetic resonance imaging (structural and functional), computed tomography, positron emission tomography, and electroencephalography are used as diagnostic tools for detecting alterations in psychobiological functioning.
- Psychotropic medications act at the neural synapse to affect neurotransmitter activity and have been associated with improvement in symptoms of many mental disorders.
- Integrating knowledge of the expanding biological focus into psychiatric nursing is essential if nurses are to meet the changing needs of today's psychiatric clients.

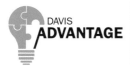 **DAVIS ADVANTAGE** | Go to **Davis Advantage** to complete your learning: strengthen understanding, apply your knowledge, and prepare for the Next Gen NCLEX®.

Review Questions

1. Which of the following parts of the brain is associated with multiple feelings and behaviors and is sometimes referred to as the "emotional brain"?
   a. Frontal lobe
   b. Pons
   c. Medulla
   d. Limbic system

2. Which of the following parts of the brain is concerned with visual reception and interpretation?
   a. Frontal lobe
   b. Parietal lobe
   c. Temporal lobe
   d. Occipital lobe

3. Which of the following parts of the brain is associated with voluntary body movement, thinking and judgment, and expression of feeling?
   a. Frontal lobe
   b. Parietal lobe
   c. Temporal lobe
   d. Occipital lobe

4. Which of the following parts of the brain integrates all sensory input (except smell) on the way to the cortex?
   a. Temporal lobe
   b. Thalamus
   c. Limbic system
   d. Hypothalamus

5. Which of the following parts of the brain deals with sensory perception and interpretation?
   a. Hypothalamus
   b. Cerebellum
   c. Parietal lobe
   d. Hippocampus

6. Which of the following parts of the brain is concerned with hearing, short-term memory, and sense of smell?
   a. Temporal lobe
   b. Parietal lobe
   c. Cerebellum
   d. Hypothalamus

7. Which of the following parts of the brain has control over the pituitary gland and autonomic nervous system, as well as regulation of appetite and temperature?
   a. Temporal lobe
   b. Parietal lobe
   c. Cerebellum
   d. Hypothalamus

8. At a synapse, the determination of further impulse transmission is accomplished by means of which of the following?
   a. Potassium ions
   b. Interneurons
   c. Neurotransmitters
   d. The myelin sheath

9. A decrease in which of the following neurotransmitters has been implicated in depression?
   a. GABA, acetylcholine, and aspartate
   b. Norepinephrine, serotonin, and dopamine
   c. Somatostatin, substance P, and glycine
   d. Glutamate, histamine, and opioid peptides

10. Which of the following hormones has been implicated as influential in seasonal affective disorder?
    a. Increased levels of melatonin
    b. Decreased levels of oxytocin
    c. Decreased levels of prolactin
    d. Increased levels of thyrotropin

11. Psychotropic medications may act at the neural synapse to accomplish which of the following? (Select all that apply.)
    a. Inhibit the reuptake of certain neurotransmitters, creating more availability
    b. Inhibit catabolic enzymes, promoting more availability of a neurotransmitter
    c. Block receptors, resulting in less neurotransmitter activity
    d. Add synthetic neurotransmitters found in the drug

12. Psychoneuroimmunology is a branch of science that involves which of the following? (Select all that apply.)
    a. The effect of psychoactive medications at the neural synapse
    b. The relationships between the immune system, the nervous system, and psychological processes including mental illness
    c. The correlation between psychosocial stress and the onset of illness
    d. The potential role of viruses in the onset of schizophrenia
    e. The genetic factors that influence the prevention of mental illness

References

Arreola, R., Becerril-Villanueva, E., Cruz-Fuentes, C., Velasco-Velázquez, M. A., Garcés-Alvarez, M. E., Hurtado-Alvarado, G., Hurtado-Alvarado, G., Quintero-Fabian, S., & Pavón, L. (2015). Immunomodulatory effects mediated by serotonin. *Journal of Immunology Research*. 2015:354957. http://doi.org/10.1155/2015/354957

Boland, R., Verduin, M. L., & P. Ruiz (Eds.). (2022). *Kaplan & Sadock's synopsis of psychiatry* (12th ed.). Wolters Kluwer.

Buckley, T., Sunari, D., Marshall, A., Bartrop, R., McKinley, S., & Tofler, G. (2012). Physiological correlates of bereavement and the impact of bereavement interventions. *Dialogues in Clinical Neuroscience, 14*(2), 129–139. https://doi.org/10.31887/DCNS.2012.14.2/tbuckley

Collerton, D. (2013). Psychotherapy and brain plasticity. *Frontiers in Psychology, 4*, 548. doi:10.3389/fpsyg.2013.00548

Cross-Disorder Group of the Psychiatric Genomics Consortium. (2013). Identification of risk loci with shared effects on five major psychiatric disorders: A genome-wide analysis. *Lancet, 381*(9875), 1371–1379. doi:10.1016/S0140-6736(12)62129-1

Dantzer, R. (2018). Neuroimmune interactions: From the brain to the immune system and vice versa. *Physiological Reviews, 98*(1), 477–504. https://doi.org/10.1152/physrev.00039.2016

Dashtestani, H., Zaragoza, R., Kermanian, R., Knutson, K. M., Halem, M., Casey, A., Shahni Karamzadeh, N., Anderson, A. A., Boccara, A.C., & Gandjbakhche, A. (2018). The role of prefrontal cortex in a moral judgment task using functional near-infrared spectroscopy. *Brain Behavior, 8*(11):e01116. doi: 10.1002/brb3.1116. Epub 2018 Sep 25. PMID: 30253084; PMCID: PMC6236239.

de Bartolomeis, A., Manchia, M., Marmo, F., Vellucci, L., Iasevoli, F., & Barone, A. (2020). Glycine signaling in the framework of dopamine-glutamate interaction and postsynaptic density: Implications for treatment-resistant schizophrenia. *Frontiers in Psychiatry, 11*, 369. doi: 10.3389/fpsyt.2020.00369

Elsworth, J. D., & Roth, R. H. (2017). Biogenic amine transmitters. In B. J. Sadock, V. A. Sadock, & P. Ruiz (Eds.), *Comprehensive textbook of psychiatry* (10th ed., pp. 61–75). Wolters Kluwer.

Flor, H. (2014). Psychological pain interventions and neurophysiology: Implications for a mechanism-based approach. *American Psychologist, 69*(2), 188–196. doi:http://dx.doi.org/10.1037/a0035254

Frick, A., Åhs, F., Palmquist, Å., Pissiota, A., Wallenquist, U., Fernandez, M., Jonasson, M., Appel, L., Frans, O., Lubberink, M., Furmark, T., von Knorring, L., & Fredrikson, M. (2016). Alterations in the serotonergic and substance P systems in posttraumatic stress disorder. *Molecular Psychiatry, 21*, 1323. https://doi.org/10.1038/mp.2016.159

Goncharuk, V. (2021). The hypothalamus and its role in hypertension. *Handbook of Clinical Neurology, 182*, 333–354. https://doi.org/10.1016/B978-0-12-819973-2.00023-X

Harris, D. S., Wolkowitz, M. D., & Reus, V. I. (2017). Psychoneuroendocrinology. In B. J. Sadock, V. A. Sadock, & P. Ruiz (Eds.), *Comprehensive textbook of psychiatry* (10th ed., pp. 164–178). Philadelphia, PA: Wolters Kluwer.

Jakka, N. R., & Ramesh, J. (2017). Role of depression, anxiety, testosterone and luteinizing hormone levels in disorders of sexual function. *International Journal of Advances in Medicine, 4*(4). https://doi.org/10.18203/2349-3933.ijam20173241

Khor, S., & Cai, D. (2017). Hypothalamic and inflammatory basis of hypertension. *Clinical Science, 131*(3), 211–223. https://doi.org/10.1042/CS20160001

Lewis, D. O. (2017). Adult antisocial behavior, criminality, and violence. In B. J. Sadock, V. A. Sadock, & P. Ruiz (Eds.), *Comprehensive textbook of psychiatry* (10th ed., pp. 2413–2430). Wolters Kluwer.

Liu, J., Chang, L., Song, Y., Li, H., & Wu, Y. (2019). The role of NMDA receptors in Alzheimer's disease. *Frontiers in Neuroscience, 13*,43. doi: 10.3389/fnins.2019.00043

Malhotra, S., & Sahoo, S. (2017). Rebuilding the brain with psychotherapy. *Indian Journal of Psychiatry. 59*(4), 411–419. doi: 10.4103/0019-5545.217299. PMID: 29497182; PMCID: PMC5806319.

Mao, R., Zhang, C., Chen, J., Zhao, G., Zhou, R., Wang, F., Xu, J., Yang, T., Su, Y., Huang, J., Wu, Z., Cao, L., Wang, Y., Hu, Y., Yuan, C., Yi, Z., Hong, W., Wang, Z., Peng, D., & Fang, Y. (2018). Different levels of pro- and anti-inflammatory cytokines in patients with unipolar and bipolar depression. *Journal of Affective Disorders, 237,* 65–72. https://doi.org/10.1016/j.jad.2018.04.115.

Mason, L., Peters, E., Williams, S.C., & Kumari, V. (2017). Brain connectivity changes occurring following cognitive behavioural therapy for psychosis predict long-term recovery. *Translational Psychiatry, 7*(1), e1001. doi:10.1038/tp.2016.263

McGrath, T., Baskerville, R., Rogero, M., & Castell, L. (2022). Emerging evidence for the widespread role of glutamatergic dysfunction in neuropsychiatric diseases. *Nutrients,14*(5), 917. doi: 10.3390/nu14050917.

Melchitzky, D. S., & Lewis, D. A. (2017). Functional neuroanatomy. In B. J. Sadock, V. A. Sadock, & P. Ruiz (Eds.), *Comprehensive textbook of psychiatry* (10th ed., pp. 3–39). Wolters Kluwer.

Moore, R. Y. (2019). *Clinical update—circadian rhythms, hypothalamus, and regulation of the sleep-wake cycle.* https://www.medscape.org/viewarticle/491041

Nasrallah, H.A. (2018). Preventing brain damage in psychosis. *Current Psychiatry, 17*(10), 9–10. https://www.mdedge.com/psychiatry/article/175767/schizophrenia-other-psychotic-disorders/page/0/1

National Institute on Aging. (2019). *Alzheimer's disease genetics fact sheet.* www.nia.nih.gov/alzheimers/publication/alzheimers-disease-genetics-fact-sheet

National Institute on Drug Abuse (NIDA). (2021). *Is there a link between marijuana use and psychiatric disorders?* https://nida.nih.gov/publications/research-reports/marijuana/there-link-between-marijuana-use-psychiatric-disorders

Peciña, M., Karp, J. F., Mathew, S., Todtenkopf, M. S., Ehrich, E.W., & Zubieta, J. K. (2019). Endogenous opioid system dysregulation in depression: Implications for new therapeutic approaches. *Molecular Psychiatry, 24,* 576–587. https://doi.org/10.1038/s41380-018-0117-2

Parker, K. J., Oztan, O., Libove, R. A., Sumiyoshi, R. D., Jackson, L. P., Karhson, D. S., Summers, J. E., Hinman, K. E., Motonaga, K. S., Phillips, J. M., Carson, D. S., Garner, J. P., & Hardan, A. Y. (2017). Intranasal oxytocin treatment for social deficits and biomarkers of response in children with autism. *Proceedings of the National Academy of Sciences of the United States of America, 114*(30), 8119–8124.

Pasco, J. A., Nicholson, G. C., Williams, L. J., Jacka, F. N., Henry, M. J., Kotowicz, M. A., Schneider, H. G., Leonard, B. E., & Berk, M. (2010). Association of high-sensitivity C-reactive protein with de novo major depression. *British Journal of Psychiatry, 197,* 372–377.

Ratnayake, U., Quinn, T., Walker, D. W., & Dickinson, H. (2013). Cytokines and the neurodevelopmental basis of mental illness. *Frontiers of Neuroscience, 7.* doi:10.3389/fnins.2013.00180

Salleh, M. R. (2008). Life event, stress and illness. *The Malaysian Journal of Medical Sciences, 15*(4), 9–18.

Scammell, T. E., Jackson, A. C., Franks, N. P., Wisden, W., & Dauvilliers, Y. (2019). Histamine: Neural circuits and new medications. *Sleep 42,* (1), 1–8. https://doi.org/10.1093/sleep/zsy183

Scanlon, V. C., & Sanders, T. (2019). *Essentials of anatomy and physiology* (8th ed., PE). F.A. Davis.

Seiler, A., von Känel, R., & Slavich, G. M. (2020). The psychobiology of bereavement and health: A conceptual review from the perspective of social signal transduction theory of depression. *Frontiers in Psychiatry 11,565239.* doi: 10.3389/fpsyt.2020.565239

Sikich, L., Kolevzon, A., King, B. H., McDougle, C. J., Sanders, K. B., Kim, S., Spanos, M., Chandrasekhar, T., Trelles, P., Rockhill, C. M., Palumbo, M. L., Cundiff, A. W., Montgomery, A., Siper, P., Minjarez, M., Nowinski, L. A., Marler, S., Shuffrey, L. C., Alderman, C., Weissman, J.... Veenstra-VanderWeele, J. (2021). Intranasal oxytocin in children and adolescents with autism spectrum disorder. *New England Journal of Medicine, 385,* 1462–1473. doi: 10.1056/NEJMoa2103583

Skudaev, S. (2019). *The neurophysiology and neurochemistry of sleep (review).* https://www.scribd.com/document/25882706/1022170-Neurophysiology-and-Neurochemistry-of-Sleep

Substance Abuse and Mental Health Services Administration (SAMHSA). (2014). *Trauma-informed care in behavioral health services. (Treatment Improvement Protocol (TIP) Series, No. 57)* https://www.ncbi.nlm.nih.gov/books/NBK207201/

Torrey, E. F. (2022). Cats, toxoplasmosis and psychosis: Understanding the risks. *Current Psychiatry, 21*(5), 15–19.

Walton, J. C., Walker, W. H., Bumgarner, J. R., Meléndez-Fernández, O. H., Liu, J. A., Hughes, H. L., Kaper, A. L., & Nelson, R. J. (2021). Circadian variation in efficacy of medications. *Clinical Pharmacology & Therapeutics, 109*(6), 1457–1488. doi: 10.1002/cpt.2073.

Yamada, R. G., & Ueda, H. R. (2020). Molecular mechanisms of REM sleep. *Frontiers in Neuroscience, 13,* 1402. doi: 10.3389/fnins.2019.01402

Yu, X., Franks, N. P., & Wisden, W. (2018). Sleep and sedative states induced by targeting the histamine and noradrenergic systems. *Frontiers in Neural Circuits 12,* 4. doi: 10.3389/fncir.2018.00004

4 Psychopharmacology

CORE CONCEPTS

Intracranial Regulation:
Neurotransmitters

Safety: Psychotropic
medication

Clinical Judgment

KEY TERMS

agonist

agranulocytosis

akathisia

akinesia

amenorrhea

antagonist

antianxiety agents

antidepressants

antiparkinsonian agents

antipsychotic agents

attention deficit-hyperactivity
disorder (ADHD) agents

boxed warning

dystonias

extrapyramidal symptoms
(EPS)

galactorrhea

gynecomastia

hypertensive crisis

mood stabilizing agents

neuroleptic malignant
syndrome

neurotransmitter

oculogyric crisis

photosensitivity

priapism

receptors

retrograde ejaculation

reuptake

sedative-hypnotic agents

serotonin syndrome

tardive dyskinesia

OBJECTIVES
After reading this chapter, the student will be able to:

1. Discuss historical perspectives related to
psychopharmacology.
2. Describe indications, actions, contraindications, precautions, side effects, and
nursing implications for the following
classifications of drugs:
   a. Antianxiety agents
   b. Antidepressants
   c. Mood-stabilizing agents

   d. Antipsychotics and agents for the treatment of tardive dyskinesia
   e. Antiparkinsonian agents
   f. Sedative-hypnotics
   g. Agents for attention deficit-hyperactivity
   disorder
3. Apply the steps of the nursing process
to the administration of psychotropic
medications.

The middle of the 20th century represents a pivotal
period in the treatment of individuals with mental
illness. It was during this time that the phenothiazine class of antipsychotics was introduced in the
United States. Before that time phenothiazines had
been used in France as preoperative medications.

As Dr. Henri Laborit (1914–1995) of the Hospital
Boucicaut in Paris stated:

> It was our aim to decrease the anxiety of the patients
> to prepare them in advance for their postoperative
> recovery. With these new drugs, the phenothiazines,
> we were seeing a profound psychic and physical

relaxation... a real indifference to the environment and to the upcoming operation. It seemed to me these drugs must have an application in psychiatry. (Sage, 1984)

Indeed, phenothiazines have had a significant application in psychiatry. Not only have they helped many individuals to function effectively, but they have also provided researchers and clinicians with information to study the origins, etiologies, and development of mental disorders. Dr. Arnold Scheibel, director of the UCLA Brain Research Institute, stated,

[When these drugs came out] there was a sense of disbelief that we could actually do something substantive for the patients... see them for the first time as sick individuals and not as something bizarre that we could literally not talk to. (Sage, 1984)

This chapter explores historical perspectives in the use of psychotropic medications in the treatment of mental illness. Seven classifications of medications are discussed, and their implications for psychiatric nursing are presented in the context of the steps of the nursing process.

CORE CONCEPT
Psychotropic Medication
Medication that affects psychic function, behavior, or experience.

Historical Perspectives

Historically, reaction to and treatment of individuals with mental illness have ranged from benign involvement to interventions that some would consider inhumane. Individuals with mental illness were feared because of common beliefs associating them with demons or the supernatural. They were looked upon as loathsome and often were mistreated.

Beginning in the late 18th century, a type of "moral reform" in the treatment of people with mental illness began to occur. Community and state hospitals concerned with the needs of individuals with mental illness were established. Considered a breakthrough in the humanization of care, these institutions, however well intentioned, fostered the concept of custodial care. Patients were ensured food and shelter but received little or no hope of change for the future. As they became increasingly dependent on the institution to fulfill their needs, the likelihood of their return to the family or community diminished.

The early part of the 20th century saw the advent of somatic therapies in psychiatry. Individuals with mental illness were treated with insulin-shock therapy, wet sheet packs, ice baths, electroconvulsive therapy, and psychosurgery. Before 1950, sedatives and amphetamines were the only significant psychotropic medications available. Even these drugs had limited use because of their potential for toxicity and physical dependence. Since the 1950s, the development of psychopharmacology has expanded to include widespread use of antipsychotic, antidepressant, antianxiety, and mood-stabilizer medications. Research into how these drugs work has provided an understanding of the biochemical influences in many psychiatric disorders.

Psychotropic medications are not a "cure" for mental illness. Most mental health practitioners who prescribe these medications for their clients use them as an adjunct to individual or group psychotherapy. Although their contribution to psychiatric care cannot be minimized, it must be emphasized that psychotropic medications relieve some physical and behavioral symptoms. They do not eliminate mental disorders.

The Role of the Nurse in Psychopharmacology

Ethical and Legal Implications

Nurses must understand the ethical and legal implications associated with the administration of psychotropic medications. Laws differ from state to state, but most adhere to the patient's right to refuse treatment. Exceptions exist in emergency situations when it has been determined that patients are likely to harm themselves or others. Many states have adopted laws that allow courts to order outpatient treatment, which may include medication, in circumstances where an individual is not seeking treatment and has a history of violent, aggressive behavior. The original law, called Kendra's law, was enacted after a young woman named Kendra Webdale was pushed in front of a New York City subway train by a man who lived in the community but was not seeking treatment for his mental illness (New York State Office of Mental Health, 2012). This law is perhaps more developed than those in other states. It includes a medication grant clause that provides uninterrupted medication for those transitioning from hospitals or correctional facilities. Some states do not have similar laws; it is important, then, for nurses to be informed about local, state, and federal laws when working in any health-care setting or correctional facility and providing care to patients with psychiatric disorders.

Assessment

A thorough baseline assessment must be conducted before a patient is placed on a regimen of psychopharmacological therapy. A nursing history and assessment (see Chapter 8, "The Nursing Process in Psychiatric-Mental Health Nursing"), an ethnocultural assessment, and a comprehensive medication assessment (Box 4–1) are all essential components of this database. The ethnocultural assessment is necessary because genetic variations in selected populations and cultural factors, including dietary preferences, may influence response to some medications; CYP450 isoenzyme variations,

---

BOX 4–1 Medication Assessment Tool

Date _____ Patient's Name _____ Age _____

Marital Status _____ Children _____ Occupation _____

Presenting Symptoms (subjective & objective) _____

Diagnosis (DSM-5-TR) _____

_____

Current Vital Signs: Blood Pressure: Sitting _____/_____; Standing _____/_____; Pulse _____;

Respirations _____ Height _____ Weight _____

CURRENT/PAST USE OF PRESCRIPTION DRUGS (Indicate with "c" or "p" beside name of drug whether current or past use):

Name	Dosage	How Long Used	Why Prescribed	By Whom	Side Effects/Results

CURRENT/PAST USE OF OVER-THE-COUNTER DRUGS (Indicate with "c" or "p" beside name of drug whether current or past use):

Name	Dosage	How Long Used	Why Prescribed	By Whom	Side Effects/Results

CURRENT/PAST USE OF STREET DRUGS, ALCOHOL, NICOTINE, OR CAFFEINE (Indicate with "c" or "p" beside name of drug):

Name	Amount Used	How Often Used	When Last Used	Effects Produced	Name

Any allergies to food or drugs? _____

Any special diet considerations? _____

Do you have (or have you ever had) any of the following? If yes, provide explanation on the back of this sheet.

	Yes	No		Yes	No		Yes	No
Difficulty swallowing	___	___	Chest pain	___	___	Shortness of breath	___	___
Delayed wound healing	___	___	Blood clots/pain in legs	___	___	Sexual dysfunction	___	___
Constipation problems	___	___	Fainting spells	___	___	Lumps in your breasts	___	___
Urination problems	___	___	Swollen ankles/			Blurred or double vision	___	___
Recent change in			legs/hands	___	___	Ringing in the ears	___	___
elimination patterns	___	___	Asthma	___	___	Insomnia	___	___
Weakness or tremors	___	___	Varicose veins	___	___	Skin rashes	___	___
Seizures	___	___	Numbness/tingling			Diabetes	___	___
Headaches	___	___	(location?)	___	___	Hepatitis (or other		
Dizziness	___	___	Ulcers	___	___	liver disease)	___	___
High blood pressure	___	___	Nausea/vomiting	___	___	Kidney disease	___	___
Palpitations	___	___	Problems with diarrhea	___	___	Glaucoma	___	___

Are you pregnant or breastfeeding? _____ Date of last menses _____ Type of contraception used _____

Describe any restrictions/limitations that might interfere with your use of medication for your current problem. _____

Prescription orders: Patient teaching related to medications prescribed:

Laboratory work or referrals prescribed:

Nurse's signature _____ Patient's signature _____

for example, influence metabolism of some medications and pharmacogenetic testing may be ordered to identify individuals at risk for being poor metabolizers (Table 4–1 shows degrees of risk for poor metabolism of selected medications). Individuals who metabolize drugs poorly are more vulnerable to adverse drug reactions including toxicity.

Medication Administration and Evaluation

The nurse is the key health-care professional in direct contact with individuals receiving psychotropic medication in inpatient settings, in partial hospitalization programs, day treatment centers, home health care, and other settings. Medication administration is followed by ongoing monitoring for side effects and adverse reactions. The nurse also evaluates the therapeutic effectiveness of the medication. It is essential for the nurse to have a thorough knowledge of psychotropic medications to be able to anticipate

potential problems and outcomes associated with their administration.

Patient Education

The information associated with psychotropic medications is copious and complex. An important role of the nurse is to translate this complex information into terms that can be easily understood by the patient. Patients must understand why the medication has been prescribed, when it should be taken, and what they may expect in terms of side effects and adverse reactions. They must know whom to contact when they have a question and when it is important to report to their physician. Medication education encourages patient collaboration and promotes accurate and effective management of the treatment regimen. For women of childbearing age, pregnancy risk information is an essential aspect of patient education. In 2015, a new U.S. Food and

TABLE 4–1	Variations in CYP450 Enzymes and Response to Selected Psychotropic Medications*		
CYP450 ISOENZYME	**% RISK FOR BEING POOR METABOLIZERS BY ETHNIC GROUP**	**SELECTED PSYCHOTROPIC MEDICATIONS AFFECTED**	**SELECTED POTENTIAL OUTCOMES**
2C19	Asian 12%–23% African, African American 18% Caucasian 3%–7%	Diazepam, tricyclics, citalopram	1. Higher blood levels and faster therapeutic response to tricyclic antidepressants. Experience more toxic side effects and more risk for tricyclic antidepressant delirium 2. Increased sensitivity to effects of alcohol
2D6	East Asian 0%–2% African, African American 0%–19% Caucasian 3%–9%	Tricyclics, fluoxetine, paroxetine, venlafaxine, sertraline, chlorpromazine, haloperidol, clozapine, risperidone	1. Higher incidence of extrapyramidal side effects with haloperidol 2. More sensitive to the effects of many psychotropic medications
3A4	Although results are inconsistent, poor metabolizers are rare (<1%) but drug–drug and drug–food interactions, such as interactions with grapefruit juice, may inhibit metabolism	Mirtazapine, sertraline, haloperidol, clozapine, quetiapine, risperidone, ziprasidone, gabapentin, lamotrigine, clonazepam, diazepam, zolpidem, buspirone, lurasidone, pimozide, ketamine, fentanyl, oxycodone, alfentanil, dextromethorphan, triazolam	1. Higher risk for respiratory depression with alfentanil, fentanyl, ketamine, and oxycodone 2. Higher risk for torsade de pointes with lurasidone, pimozide, and ziprasidone 3. Risk for hallucinations and somnolence with dextromethorphan 4. Increased sedation with buspirone and triazolam

*CYP450 enzymes are responsible for metabolizing many medications. Variations can occur due to genetic vulnerability or through drug–drug or drug–food interactions. CYP450 induction increases the metabolism of selected drugs thereby decreasing their effectiveness. Inhibition of CYP450 enzymes decreases the metabolism of selected drugs, which can result in severe toxicity and several adverse effects.
Sources: Anderson, L. (2018). *Drug interactions with grapefruit juice.* https://www.drugs.com/article/grapefruit-drug-interactions.html; Horn, J.R., & Hansten, P.D. (2008). Get to know an enzyme: CYP2C19. *Pharmacy Times.* https://www.pharmacytimes.com/publications/issue/2008/2008-05/2008-05-8538; Jones, D.S. (2006). Racial profiling in psychiatry: Does it help patients? *Psychiatric Times, 23*(14); Lynch, T., & Price, A. (2007). The effect of cytochrome P450 metabolism on drug response, interactions, and adverse effects. *American Family Physician, 76*(3): 391–396.

Drug Administration (FDA) rule went into effect that requires drug labeling to include specific narrative information on pregnancy-associated risks, lactation considerations, and reproductive potential (Drugs. com, 2022). This new system replaces the lettered risk categories that were criticized for being overly simplistic. Nurses should use the latest informatics resources to provide current and relevant education on this and other medication-related topics.

CORE CONCEPT

Neurotransmitters and Receptors

A **neurotransmitter** is a chemical that is stored in the axon terminals of the presynaptic neuron. An electrical impulse through the neuron stimulates the release of the neurotransmitter into the synaptic cleft, which in turn determines whether another electrical impulse is generated.

  Receptors are molecules situated on the cell membrane that are binding sites for neurotransmitters.

How Do Psychotropic Medications Work?

Most psychotropic medications affect the neuronal synapse, producing changes in neurotransmitter release and the receptors to which they bind

(Fig. 4–1). **Antagonist** drugs exert their effect by blocking a receptor and dampening the biological reaction. Conversely, **agonist** drugs activate receptors. Researchers hypothesize that most antidepressants work by blocking the reuptake of neurotransmitters, specifically, serotonin and norepinephrine. **Reuptake** is the process of neurotransmitter inactivation by which the neurotransmitter is reabsorbed into the presynaptic neuron from which it was released. Blocking the reuptake process allows more of the neurotransmitter to be available for neuronal transmission. This mechanism of action may also result in undesirable side effects (Table 4–2). Some antidepressants, for example, also block receptor sites that are unrelated to their mechanisms of action on mood and emotions. These include alpha-adrenergic, histaminergic, and muscarinic cholinergic receptors. Blocking these receptors is associated with certain side effects; for example, individuals treated with tricyclic antidepressants are at risk for developing postural hypotension. The specific type of receptor that a medication binds to is also relevant to the drug's level of antianxiety, antidepressant, and sedative properties (see Table 4–2).

Antipsychotic medications block dopamine receptors, and some affect muscarinic, cholinergic, histaminergic, and alpha-adrenergic receptors.

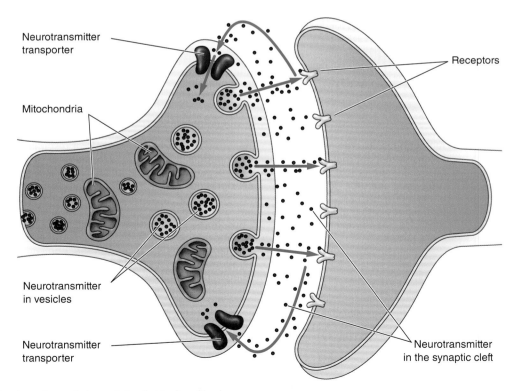

FIGURE 4–1 Area of synaptic transmission that is altered by drugs.

TABLE 4–2 Effects of Psychotropic Medications on Neurotransmitters

EXAMPLE OF MEDICATION	ACTION ON NEUROTRANSMITTER OR RECEPTOR	DESIRED EFFECTS	SIDE EFFECTS
Selective serotonin reuptake inhibitors (SSRIs)	Inhibit reuptake of serotonin (5-HT)	Reduce depression Control anxiety Control obsessions	Nausea, agitation, headache, sexual dysfunction
Tricyclic antidepressants	Inhibit reuptake of serotonin (5-HT) Inhibit reuptake of NE Block NE (α_1) receptor Block ACh receptor Block histamine (H_1) receptor	Reduce depression Relieve severe pain Prevent panic attacks	Sexual dysfunction (NE and 5-HT) Sedation, weight gain (H_1) Dry mouth, constipation, blurred vision, urinary retention (ACh) Postural hypotension and tachycardia (α_1)
Monoamine oxidase inhibitors (MAOIs)	Increase NE and 5-HT by inhibiting the enzyme that degrades them (MAO-A)	Reduce depression Control anxiety	Sedation, dizziness Sexual dysfunction Hypertensive crisis (interaction with tyramine and foods or beverages with high caffeine content)
Trazodone and nefazodone	5-HT reuptake block $5\text{-}HT_2$ receptor antagonism Adrenergic receptor blockade	Reduce depression Reduce anxiety	Nausea (5-HT) Sedation ($5\text{-}HT_2$) Orthostasis (α_1) Priapism (α_2)
Selective norepinephrine reuptake inhibitors (SNRIs): venlafaxine, desvenlafaxine, duloxetine, and levomilnacipran	Potent inhibitors of serotonin and norepinephrine reuptake Weak inhibitors of dopamine reuptake	Reduce depression Relieve pain of neuropathy (duloxetine) Relieve anxiety (venlafaxine)	Nausea (5-HT) ↑ Sweating (NE) Insomnia (NE) Tremors (NE) Sexual dysfunction (5-HT)
Bupropion	Inhibits reuptake of NE and D	Reduces depression Aids in smoking cessation Reduces symptoms of ADHD	Insomnia, dry mouth, tremor, seizures
Esketamine (nasal spray)	Nonselective, noncompetitive antagonist of the NMDA receptor (an ionotropic glutamate receptor)	Reduce depression in treatment-resistant depression (in conjunction with an oral antidepressant)	Dissociation, dizziness, nausea, sedation, vertigo, hypoesthesia, anxiety, lethargy, blood pressure increased, and vomiting
Antipsychotics: phenothiazines and haloperidol	Strong D_2 receptor blockades Weaker blockades of ACh, H_1, α_1-adrenergic, and $5\text{-}HT_2$ receptors	Relieve psychosis Relieve anxiety (Some) provide relief from nausea and vomiting and intractable hiccoughs	Blurred vision, dry mouth, ↓ sweating, constipation, urinary retention, tachycardia (ACh) EPS (D_2) ↑ Plasma prolactin (D_2) Sedation; weight gain (H_1) Ejaculatory difficulty ($5\text{-}HT_2$) Postural hypotension (α; H_1)

Continued

TABLE 4–2	**Effects of Psychotropic Medications on Neurotransmitters–cont'd**		
EXAMPLE OF MEDICATION	**ACTION ON NEUROTRANSMITTER OR RECEPTOR**	**DESIRED EFFECTS**	**SIDE EFFECTS**
Antipsychotics (second generation, atypical): aripiprazole, asenapine, brexpiprazole, cariprazine, clozapine, iloperidone, lurasidone, olanzapine, paliperidone, quetiapine, risperidone, ziprasidone	Receptor antagonism of 5-HT$_1$A and 5-HT$_2$A D$_1$–D$_5$ (varies with drug) H$_1$, α_1-adrenergic muscarinic (ACh)	Relieve psychosis (with minimal or no EPS) Relieve anxiety Relieve acute mania	Potential with some of the drugs for mild EPS (D$_2$) Sedation, weight gain (H$_1$) Orthostasis and dizziness (alpha-adrenergic) Blurred vision, dry mouth, ↓ sweating, constipation, urinary retention, tachycardia (ACh)
Antianxiety: benzodiazepines	Bind to BZ receptor sites on the GABAA receptor complex; increase receptor affinity for GABA	Relieve anxiety Produce sedation	Dependence (with long-term use) Confusion, memory impairment, motor incoordination
Antianxiety: buspirone	5-HT$_1$A agonist D$_2$ agonist D$_2$ antagonist	Relieves anxiety	Nausea, headache, dizziness Restlessness

5-HT, 5-hydroxytryptamine (serotonin); ACh, acetylcholine; ADHD, attention deficit-hyperactivity disorder; BZ, benzodiazepine; D, dopamine; EPS, extrapyramidal symptoms; GABA, gamma-aminobutyric acid; H, histamine; MAO, monoamine oxidase; MAO-A, monoamine oxidase A; NE, norepinephrine; NMDA, N-methyl-D-aspartate receptor.

Atypical (or second generation) antipsychotics focus primarily on blocking specific serotonin receptors. Benzodiazepines facilitate the transmission of the inhibitory neurotransmitter gamma-aminobutyric acid (GABA). Psychostimulants work by increasing norepinephrine, serotonin, and dopamine release.

Although each psychotropic medication affects neurotransmission, the specific drugs within each class have varying neuronal effects. Their exact mechanisms of action are unknown. Many neuronal effects occur rapidly; however, therapeutic effects of some medications, such as antidepressants and atypical antipsychotics, may take weeks to manifest full therapeutic benefits. Acute alterations in neuronal function do not fully explain how these medications work. Boland and Verduin (2022, p. 592) note that if merely raising or lowering levels of neurotransmitter activity is associated with the clinical effects of a drug, then all drugs that cause these changes should produce equivalent benefits [and] this predictability is not the case.

Long-term neuropharmacological reactions to increased norepinephrine and serotonin levels may better explain their mechanisms of action. Other researchers (Chaves et al., 2021; Yin & Yuan, 2015) suggest that the therapeutic effects are related to the nervous system's adaptation to increased levels of neurotransmitters. These adaptive changes result from a homeostatic mechanism, much like a thermostat, that regulates the cell and maintains equilibrium.

Applying the Nursing Process in Psychopharmacological Therapy

The Medication Assessment Tool, an assessment tool for obtaining a drug history (see Box 4–1), may be adapted for use by staff nurses admitting patients to the hospital or by nurse practitioners with prescriptive privileges. Some psychotropic medications (such as benzodiazepines, ketamine, and many sedative-hypnotic medications) are controlled substances because of their potential for misuse. Box 4–2 describes the different levels of controlled substance schedules.

One of the Quality and Safety Education for Nurses (QSEN) criteria culminating from the Institute of Medicine (IOM) (2003) report on essential competencies for health-care professionals stresses that the patient must be at the center of decisions about treatment (patient-centered care), and a type of assessment tool such as the Medication Assessment Tool provides an opportunity to actively engage the patient in describing what medications have been effective or ineffective and identifying side effects that may affect willingness to adhere to a medication regimen.

BOX 4–2 Controlled Substance Schedules

Schedule I: Substances in this schedule have no currently accepted medical use in the United States, a lack of accepted safety for use under medical supervision, and a high potential for abuse.

Schedule II: Substances in this schedule have a high potential for abuse which may lead to severe psychological or physical dependence.

Schedule III: Substances in this schedule have a potential for abuse less than substances in schedules I or II and abuse may lead to moderate or low physical dependence or high psychological dependence.

Schedule IV: Substances in this schedule have a low potential for abuse relative to substances in schedule III.

Schedule V: Substances in this schedule have a low potential for abuse relative to substances listed in schedule IV and consist primarily of preparations containing limited quantities of certain narcotics.

Source: *U.S. Department of Justice. (n.d.). Controlled substance schedules. https://www.deadiversion.usdoj.gov/schedules/#:~:text=Definition%*

Antianxiety Agents

Antianxiety agents are also called *anxiolytics* and historically were referred to as *minor tranquilizers*. Typically, this has included benzodiazepines, buspirone, and some selective serotonin reuptake inhibitors (SSRIs). Other medications that have been used off-label to treat anxiety disorders include anticonvulsants (such as divalproex, gabapentin, and pregabalin), beta blockers (such as atenolol, propranolol, and nadolol), antihistamines (hydroxyzine), and the antipsychotic medication quetiapine.

Background Assessment Data

Indications

Antianxiety agents are used in the treatment of anxiety disorders, anxiety symptoms, acute alcohol withdrawal, skeletal muscle spasms, convulsive disorders, status epilepticus, and preoperative sedation. They are most appropriate for the treatment of acute anxiety states rather than long-term treatment. Their use and efficacy for longer than 4 months have not been evaluated. For long-term management of anxiety disorders, antidepressants (such as SSRIs and selective norepinephrine reuptake inhibitors [SNRIs]) are often used as the first line of treatment because they are not addictive. (A table of current FDA-approved antianxiety agents' daily dosage ranges can be found in Chapter 27, "Anxiety, Obsessive-Compulsive, and Related Disorders.")

Action

Antianxiety drugs depress subcortical levels of the central nervous system (CNS), particularly the limbic system and reticular formation. They may potentiate the effects of the powerful inhibitory neurotransmitter GABA in the brain (inhibiting excitation), thereby producing a calmative effect. All levels of CNS depression can be affected from mild sedation to hypnosis to coma. The most commonly prescribed antianxiety agents are benzodiazepines (which are schedule IV controlled substances), including clonazepam (Klonopin), lorazepam (Ativan), diazepam (Valium), and alprazolam (Xanax). Benzodiazepines are similar to alcohol in their effects on GABA receptors, which explains why benzodiazepines may be used for the management of alcohol withdrawal.

The antianxiety agent buspirone (BuSpar) is not a benzodiazepine and does not depress the CNS. Although its action is unknown, the drug is believed to produce its effects through interactions with serotonin, dopamine, and other neurotransmitter receptors. Patients should be instructed that buspirone has a lag period of 7 to 10 days before full therapeutic benefits are achieved. It does not have the physical dependence potential of the other antianxiety agents; therefore it may be a better option for patients with anxiety disorders who also have substance use disorders.

One area of concern is the increased use of benzodiazepines in the older adult population despite known safety concerns, including psychomotor impairment, impaired cognitive function, and paradoxical increase in anxiety. Gerlach and associates (2018), in a systematic review, concluded that benzodiazepine prescribing to older adults "is significantly in excess of what the available evidence would suggest is appropriate" (p. 264). Other researchers (Gress et al., 2020) found that benzodiazepines are often prescribed for long-term use in older adults, a practice that has not been supported by scientific evidence and one that increases risks for side effects and dependence. Further, Maust and associates (2016) found that most older adults who were prescribed benzodiazepines did not receive a clinical mental health diagnosis and almost none were referred for psychotherapy. Nurses are in a position to assess safety risks and, in collaboration with the patient, physician, and other health-care team members, explore other options for treatment of anxiety and insomnia.

Despite the concerns about long-term use, side effects, and potential for dependence, benzodiazepines remain a mainstream treatment choice. In

2020 a new vehicle for diazepam administration came with the approval of diazepam nasal spray, but it should be noted that this is approved only for the rescue treatment of seizure clusters in patients with epilepsy age 6 years and older (Remaly, 2020).

Interactions

■ Increased effects of antianxiety agents can occur when they are taken concomitantly with alcohol, barbiturates, narcotics, antipsychotics, antidepressants, antihistamines, neuromuscular blocking agents, cimetidine, or disulfiram.

■ The FDA (2016c) added a boxed warning (its strongest warning, commonly called a *black box warning*) related to the serious risks and possible death associated with combining benzodiazepines with opioid pain or cough medicines.

■ Increased effects can also occur with herbal depressants (e.g., kava, valerian, lemon verbena, l-tryptophan, melatonin, and chamomile).

■ Decreased effects can be noted with cigarette smoking and caffeine consumption.

Diagnosis

The following nursing diagnoses may be considered for patients receiving therapy with antianxiety agents:

■ Risk for injury related to seizures, panic anxiety, acute agitation from alcohol withdrawal (indications), abrupt withdrawal from the medication after long-term use, or effects of medication intoxication or overdose

■ Anxiety related to threat to physical integrity or self-concept

■ Risk for activity intolerance related to side effects of sedation, confusion, and/or lethargy

■ Disturbed sleep pattern related to situational crises, physical condition, or severe level of anxiety

Safety Issues in Planning and Implementing Care

 The IOM (2003) identified *ensuring safety* as a core competency for health professions education. With that goal in mind, Table 4–3 notes some of the significant safety issues to be considered for clients taking antianxiety agents. Nursing interventions related to each side effect are noted in the right-hand column.

Outcome Criteria and Evaluation

The following criteria may be used for evaluating the effectiveness of therapy with antianxiety agents.
The patient:

■ Demonstrates a reduction in anxiety, tension, and restless activity

■ Experiences no seizure activity

■ Experiences no physical injury

■ Tolerates usual activities without excessive sedation

■ Exhibits no evidence of confusion

■ Tolerates the medication without gastrointestinal distress

■ Verbalizes understanding of the need for, side effects of, and regimen for self-administration

■ Verbalizes possible consequences of abrupt withdrawal from the medication

Antidepressants

There are several types of **antidepressants**, some of which are also prescribed to treat anxiety disorders. The first "antidepressant" drug was a monoamine oxidase inhibitor (MAOI), isoniazid, which was used to treat tuberculosis. When patients began describing their increased feelings of well-being on these drugs, MAOIs were developed specifically for the treatment of depression. Unfortunately, they were also potentially deadly for anyone who ate foods high in tyramine while taking these drugs, and several serious interactions occurred with other drugs. Because MAOIs increase the availability of norepinephrine, researchers focused on developing drugs that affected norepinephrine without the need for food restrictions, leading to the introduction of *tricyclic antidepressants (TCAs)*.

Tricyclics were the first line of treatment for depression for many years, but not everyone responded to them (it was generally identified that about 70% of people with depression improved with treatment, but that finding has been challenged in more recent studies). In addition, because all neurotransmitters bind to various receptor sites, increasing the availability of norepinephrine with tricyclics also causes anticholinergic effects (such as rapid heart rate) and increases the potential for postural hypotension. These side effects limit their use in the elderly and those with cardiovascular problems.

In the late 1980s, serotonin, an antianxiety hormone and neurotransmitter, became the latest biochemical believed to promote improvement in depression and anxiety without significant anticholinergic side effects. Consequently, a new group of drugs, SSRIs and SNRIs, became the preferred first-line treatment. Common SNRIs, which decrease reuptake of serotonin and norepinephrine, include desvenlafaxine (Pristiq), duloxetine (Cymbalta), levomilnacipran (Fetzima), and venlafaxine (Effexor). With these developments SSRIs and SNRIs became the preferred first line of treatment for depression.

Atypical antidepressants are a group of drugs that work differently and do not fit into the previously

TABLE 4–3 Safety Issues and Nursing Interventions for Patients Taking Antianxiety Agents

SAFETY ISSUES	NURSING INTERVENTIONS
Tolerance and physical dependence may develop. **Abrupt withdrawal can be life-threatening** (except with buspirone); signs include sweating, agitation, tremors, nausea and vomiting, delirium, seizures.	Instruct patient not to stop taking the drug abruptly. Assess the patient for signs of developing tolerance (requiring higher doses of medication to achieve effects). Educate the patient about symptoms of withdrawal. Contact the doctor immediately if symptoms of withdrawal are assessed.
Drowsiness, confusion, and lethargy are the most common side effects.	Instruct patient not to drive or operate dangerous machinery while taking this medication.
Effects of other CNS depressants are increased.	Instruct the patient not to drink alcohol or take other CNS depressants, antihistamines, cimetidine, antidepressants, neuromuscular blocking agents, or disulfiram while taking these drugs. The FDA (2016c) recently added a boxed warning (its strongest warning) related to the serious risks and possible death associated with combining benzodiazepines with opioid pain or cough medicines.
Antianxiety agents may **aggravate symptoms of depression.**	Assess the patient's mood and assess for suicide risk.
Orthostatic hypotension may occur.	Instruct the patient to rise slowly from a sitting to standing position to minimize risk for falls. Monitor lying and standing blood pressures to assess for orthostatic hypotension.
Paradoxical excitement (opposite from the desired effect) may occur. Especially the elderly may be at higher risk for agitation and increased anxiety. In general, safety risks associated with benzodiazepines may be greater for the older adult (especially with long-acting benzodiazepines and long-term use), including impaired cognitive function, reduced mobility, risk for falls, and chemical dependence (Gress et al., 2020).	Hold the medication and notify the doctor. Assess for other side effects and safety issues, including impaired cognition and impaired mobility. Use a patient-centered, collaborative team approach to explore options in safe management of anxiety and insomnia (lower dose, shorter-acting benzodiazepines; psychological interventions, etc.).
Blood dyscrasias, although rare, can be serious or life-threatening.	Assess for sore throat, fever, bruising, or unusual bleeding. Hold medication and report these symptoms immediately to the doctor.
Congenital malformations have been associated with use of these drugs during the first trimester of pregnancy.	Instruct the patient who is pregnant or anticipating pregnancy while on these drugs to explore alternative treatment options with their physician.

CNS, central nervous system.

mentioned classes. The following are FDA-approved atypical antidepressants:

■ Bupropion (Wellbutrin)—decreases reuptake of dopamine and, to a lesser extent, serotonin and norepinephrine
■ Mirtazapine (Remeron)—potentiates the effects of norepinephrine and serotonin
■ Nefazodone—inhibits reuptake of serotonin and norepinephrine by acting as an antagonist at the central 5-HT2 receptor
■ Vortioxetine (Trintellix)—action not well understood

■ Vilazodone (Viibryd)—partial agonist at serotonergic 5-HT1A receptors
■ Trazodone (Desyrel)—unknown but alters the effect of serotonin

One of the more recent additions to the pharmacological treatments for depression and anxiety are atypical antipsychotics that increase the availability of serotonin and dopamine. These medications are promoted as adjunctive to antidepressant therapy. The most popular example is aripiprazole (Abilify). In a large study sponsored by the National Institute of Mental Health, 44% of older adults who were not responding to a first-line antidepressant (venlafaxine) showed improvement in their symptoms when aripiprazole (Abilify) was added to treatment with venlafaxine. This finding has important implications for the treatment of older adult clients with depression because more than one-half of older adults with clinical depression do not respond to antidepressants alone (Lenze et al., 2015).

Despite these developments and client-subjective reports of improvement with antidepressant medications, our understanding of the exact mechanisms of action remains theoretical. Currently, the levels of neurotransmitters in the brain cannot be measured and in the STAR*D study (a large study funded by the National Institute of Mental Health), it was found that two-thirds of patients treated with an SSRI antidepressant medication did not experience full recovery (National Institute of Mental Health, 2006).

Research continues with the goal of identifying antidepressant therapies that are more effective and more rapid in achieving therapeutic benefits. All antidepressant therapies (TCA, SSRI, SNRI, and MAOI) may take up to 2 weeks before signs of improvement are noted and up to 4 weeks to achieve full therapeutic benefits. Several of the newest drugs on the market for treatment of depression are not significantly different from existing products. For example, a "new" antidepressant approved by the FDA in 2016, Oleptro, is a reformulation of trazodone. But new mechanisms are being explored in clinical trials. Glutamate receptors (*N*-methyl-D-aspartate [NMDA]) and a novel GABA modulator (Gunduz-Bruce et al., 2019) are being studied for potential antidepressant effects. Ketamine and midazolam (a benzodiazepine with transient effects similar to those of ketamine) are being explored as potentially faster-acting than traditional antidepressants.

In 2019, the FDA approved the nasal spray esketamine (Spravato) in conjunction with an oral antidepressant for individuals with treatment-resistant depression. In one of three short-term studies used to evaluate the drug's efficacy, Spravato demonstrated statistically significant benefit in reducing depressive symptoms, and some effect was seen within 2 days (FDA, 2019). Research into esketamine's mechanism of action, applications, and risks is ongoing. Because there are risks for serious adverse outcomes related to sedation, dissociation (difficulty with attention, judgment, and thinking), and the potential for substance misuse, this drug is classified as a schedule III controlled drug and is only available through a restricted distribution system. It must be administered in a certified medical office where the patient is under observation, and it requires a Risk Evaluation and Mitigation Strategy (REMS) (FDA, 2019).

Drugs that act on melatonin receptors are currently in clinical trials for use in depression (one is already approved for use in Europe). One study found a synergistic antidepressant effect when melatonin was combined with fluoxetine (Li et al., 2018), but more research is needed. There is concern that melatonin, although it may improve sleep disturbances in people with depression, may also worsen other symptoms of depression in some individuals (Tonon et al., 2021). A new group of antidepressants called *triple reuptake inhibitors* that simultaneously block reuptake of serotonin, norepinephrine, and dopamine have been studied but have demonstrated mixed results with regard to any superior benefits over highly selective serotonergic agents alone (Kose & Cetin, 2018).

The most current research is exploring the potential benefits of the psychedelic drugs ayahuasca, psilocybin, and lysergic acid diethylamide (LSD) for treatment-resistant depression. Studies thus far have found that when administered in a supportive setting, antidepressant and anxiolytic effects were immediate, consistent, and enduring for several months (Muttoni et al., 2019). In a recent study that incorporated two doses of psilocybin along with supportive therapy, researchers found substantial, enduring antidepressant effects at least through the follow-up period of 12 months (Gukasyan et al., 2022). The researchers caution, though, that at present the studies have been limited and small.

Pharmacogenetic research is ongoing to identify factors that may influence whether an individual is more likely to respond to one type of antidepressant than another. This type of research may provide a valuable resource for making decisions about which antidepressant to prescribe first.

The myriad searches for different treatment options speaks to the enormity of depression and suicide as public health concerns and the need for a more effective response. Nurses need to be informed of current, evidence-based pharmacological *and* nonpharmacological treatments to provide education and counseling to patients in and outside of psychiatric settings.

Background Assessment Data

Indications

In addition to the obvious indications for antidepressant medications in the treatment of major depressive and dysthymic disorders, some SSRIs, SNRIs, and atypical antidepressants have received FDA approval for the treatment of some anxiety disorders, bulimia nervosa and other eating disorders, premenstrual dysphoric disorder, borderline personality disorder, obesity, and smoking cessation.

A landmark review of the research on antidepressants (Fournier et al., 2010) found that the benefits of antidepressant therapy for clients with mild to moderate symptoms of depression may be minimal or nonexistent but that for clients with severe depression, the benefits, compared with placebo effects, are substantial. Therefore, these medications are particularly indicated when an individual is identified as having severe depression. (A table of current FDA-approved antidepressants can be found in Chapter 25, "Depressive Disorders.")

Action

Most antidepressants work to increase the concentration of norepinephrine, serotonin, and/or dopamine through a series of complex interactions in the body. For TCAs, SSRIs, SNRIs, and some atypical antidepressants this is believed to be accomplished by blocking the reuptake of neurotransmitters. MAOI antidepressants, on the other hand, act by inhibiting the enzyme monoamine oxidase (MAO), which is known to inactivate norepinephrine, serotonin, and dopamine.

Interactions

Tables 4–4 to 4–7 identify some of the significant, dangerous interactions between antidepressants and other drugs or foods. It is important to recognize that new information about drug interactions is discovered and published frequently. To fully understand safety issues related to medication administration, nurses need to access the most current, evidence-based informatics on drug interaction information.

TABLE 4–5 Selected Drug Interactions With Tricyclic Antidepressants (TCAs)

INTERACTING DRUGS	ADVERSE EFFECTS
Monoamine oxidase inhibitors	High fever, convulsions, death
St. John's wort, tramadol (Ultram)	Seizures, serotonin syndrome
Clonidine (Catapres), epinephrine	Severe hypertension
Acetylcholine blockers	Paralytic ileus
Alcohol and carbamazepine (Tegretol)	Blocks antidepressant action, increases sedation
Cimetidine (Tagamet), bupropion (Wellbutrin)	Increased TCA blood levels and increased side effects

TABLE 4–4 Selected Drug Interactions With Selective Serotonin Reuptake Inhibitors (SSRIs)

INTERACTING DRUGS	ADVERSE EFFECTS
Buspirone (BuSpar), tricyclic antidepressants (especially clomipramine), selegiline (Eldepryl), St. John's wort	Serotonin syndrome*
Monoamine oxidase inhibitors	Hypertensive crisis
Warfarin, NSAIDs	Increased risk of bleeding
Alcohol, benzodiazepines	Increased sedation
Antiepileptics	Lowered seizure threshold

*Serotonin syndrome is a potentially fatal syndrome of serotonin overstimulation with rapid onset that progresses from diarrhea, restlessness, agitation, hyperreflexia, fluctuations in vital signs to later symptoms of myoclonus, seizures, hyperthermia, uncontrolled shivering, muscle rigidity, and ultimately can lead to delirium, coma, status epilepticus, cardiovascular collapse, and death. Immediate cessation of offending drugs and comprehensive supportive intervention are essential (Boland & Verduin, 2022). NSAID, nonsteroidal anti-inflammatory drug.

TABLE 4–6 Selected Drug Interactions With Monoamine Oxidase Inhibitors (MAOIs)

INTERACTING DRUGS	ADVERSE EFFECTS
Selective serotonin reuptake inhibitor, tricyclic antidepressants, atomoxetine (Strattera), duloxetine (Cymbalta), dextromethorphan (an ingredient in many cough syrups), venlafaxine (Effexor), St. John's wort, ginkgo biloba	Serotonin syndrome
Morphine and other narcotic pain relievers, antihypertensives	Hypotension
All other antidepressants, pseudoephedrine, amphetamines, cocaine, cyclobenzaprine (Flexeril), dopamine, methyldopa, levodopa, epinephrine, buspirone (BuSpar)	Hypertensive crisis (these side effects can occur even if taken within 2 weeks of stopping MAOIs)
Buspirone	Psychosis, agitation, seizures
Antidiabetics	Hypoglycemia
Tegretol	Fever, hypertension, seizures

TABLE 4–7 Diet Restrictions for Clients on Monoamine Oxidase Inhibitor (MAOI) Therapy

FOODS CONTAINING TYRAMINE

HIGH TYRAMINE CONTENT (AVOID WHILE ON MAOI THERAPY)	MODERATE TYRAMINE CONTENT (MAY EAT OCCASIONALLY WHILE ON MAOI THERAPY)	LOW TYRAMINE CONTENT (LIMITED QUANTITIES PERMISSIBLE WHILE ON MAOI THERAPY)
Aged cheeses (cheddar, Swiss, Camembert, blue cheese, parmesan, provolone, Romano, brie)	Gouda cheese, processed American cheese, mozzarella	Pasteurized cheeses (cream cheese, cottage cheese, ricotta)
Raisins, fava beans, flat Italian beans, Chinese pea pods	Yogurt, sour cream	Figs
Red wines (chianti, burgundy, cabernet sauvignon)	Avocados, bananas	Distilled spirits (in moderation)
Liqueurs	Beer, white wine	
Smoked and processed meats (salami, bologna, pepperoni, summer sausage)	Coffee, colas, tea, hot chocolate (caffeinated beverages)	
Caviar, pickled herring, corned beef, chicken or beef liver	Meat extracts, such as bouillon	
Soy sauce, brewer's yeast, meat tenderizer (MSG)	Chocolate	
Sauerkraut		

Sources: Complied from Boland, R., & Verduin, M. L. (2022). *Kaplan & Sadock's synopsis of psychiatry* (P. Ruiz, Ed.). (12th ed.). Wolters Kluwer; Vallerand, A. H., & Sanoski, C. A. (2022). *Davis's drug guide for nurses* (18th ed.). F.A. Davis.

Drug interactions vary widely within these groups; the following are several examples:

- Concomitant use with MAOIs results in serious, sometimes fatal, effects resembling **neuroleptic malignant syndrome** (a rare but potentially life-threatening side effect characterized by muscle rigidity, severe hyperthermia, and cardiac effects that can progress rapidly over 24 to 72 hours). Coadministration is contraindicated.
- **Serotonin syndrome** (a potentially fatal syndrome associated with serotonin overstimulation) may occur when any of the following are used together: St. John's wort, sumatriptan, sibutramine, trazodone, nefazodone, venlafaxine, duloxetine, levomilnacipran, SSRIs, 5-HT-receptor agonists (triptans).
- Increased effects of haloperidol, clozapine, and desipramine may occur with concomitant use of venlafaxine.
- Increased effects of levomilnacipran may occur with concomitant use of CYP3A4 inhibitors.
- Increased effects of venlafaxine may occur with concomitant use of cimetidine.
- Increased effects of duloxetine may occur with concomitant use of CYP1A2 inhibitors (e.g., fluvoxamine, quinolone antibiotics) or CYP2D6 inhibitors (e.g., fluoxetine, quinidine, paroxetine).
- Risk of liver injury is increased with concomitant use of alcohol and duloxetine.

- Risk of toxicity or adverse effects from drugs extensively metabolized by CYP2D6 (e.g., flecainide, phenothiazines, propafenone, tricyclic antidepressants, thioridazine) is increased when these drugs are used concomitantly with duloxetine or bupropion.
- Decreased effects of bupropion and trazodone may occur with concomitant use of carbamazepine.
- The anticoagulant effect of warfarin may be altered with concomitant use of bupropion, venlafaxine, desvenlafaxine, duloxetine, levomilnacipran, or trazodone.
- Risk of seizures is increased when bupropion is coadministered with drugs that lower the seizure threshold (e.g., antidepressants, antipsychotics, systemic steroids, theophylline, tramadol).
- Effects of midazolam are decreased with concomitant use of desvenlafaxine.
- Effects of desvenlafaxine and levomilnacipran are increased with concomitant use of potent CYP3A4 inhibitors (e.g., ketoconazole).

Diagnosis

The following nursing diagnoses may be considered for patients receiving therapy with antidepressant medications:

- Risk for suicide related to depressed mood
- Risk for injury related to side effects of sedation, lowered seizure threshold, orthostatic hypotension,

priapism (painful penile erection enduring for hours in the absence of stimulation)**, photosensitivity** (increased sensitivity to ultraviolet [UV] rays such as sunlight), arrhythmias, **hypertensive crisis** (a severe increase in blood pressure to 180/120 or higher), or serotonin syndrome (a potentially fatal syndrome of serotonin overstimulation)

- Social isolation related to depressed mood
- Risk for constipation related to side effects of the medication
- Insomnia related to depressed mood and elevated level of anxiety

Safety Issues in Planning and Implementing Care

Some of the common but manageable side effects of antidepressant medications include dry mouth, sedation, and nausea. General nursing interventions such as offering hard candies, ice, and frequent sips of water are helpful in alleviating dry mouth. Patients may find that sedation is less bothersome if they take the daily dose of antidepressant at bedtime. They should be encouraged to discuss this side effect with the prescribing physician or nurse practitioner. Taking antidepressant medication with food may help minimize nausea.

Some patients taking SSRIs or SNRIs complain of sexual dysfunction. Men may report abnormal ejaculation or impotence, and women may report loss of orgasm. Because of these side effects, patients sometimes stop the medication abruptly, which may put them at risk for discontinuation syndrome and worsen symptoms of depression. Nurses must develop an open attitude regarding discussion and assessment of patient sexual concerns, and patients who are particularly troubled by this side effect can be encouraged to discuss their concerns with the prescribing physician or nurse practitioner to explore an alternative medication.

 Because there is so much information and new drug development is ongoing, practicing nurses should ensure that they are accessing evidence-based informatics to keep up to date on side effects as well. Many health-care organizations provide online medication resources to employees, and mobile device applications provide a readily available resource for updated drug information. Some important safety issues and nursing interventions are listed in Table 4–8.

> **CLINICAL PEARL** All antidepressants carry an FDA boxed warning for increased risk of suicidality in children, adolescents, and young adults up to 25 years of age.

> **CLINICAL PEARL** As antidepressant drugs take effect and mood begins to lift, the individual may have increased energy with which to implement a suicide plan. Suicide potential may increase as the level of depression decreases. The nurse should be particularly alert to sudden lifts or other dramatic changes in mood.

TABLE 4–8 Safety Issues and Nursing Interventions for Patients Taking Antidepressants

SAFETY ISSUES	NURSING INTERVENTIONS

Drug interactions (multiple, as discussed in the text)	Instruct patients to inform their physician or nurse practitioner of *all* medications they are taking, including herbal preparations, over-the-counter drugs, and any medications they have stopped taking within the previous 2 weeks.
	  Notify the physician immediately when any symptoms of serotonin syndrome are assessed. Do not administer the offending agent.
	■ Monitor vital signs.
	■ Protect from injury secondary to muscle rigidity or change in mental status.
	■ Provide cooling blankets for temperature regulation.
	■ Monitor intake and output.
	  The condition usually resolves when the offending agent is promptly discontinued but can be fatal without intervention (Cooper & Sejnowski, 2013).

Increased risk for suicide	Assess frequently for presence or worsening of suicide ideation.
	  Initiate suicide precautions as needed.
	  Monitor patients' use of medication as prescribed, because these medications can be lethal in overdose.

Sedation	Instruct patients not to drive or operate dangerous machinery when experiencing sedation.

Continued

TABLE 4–8 **Safety Issues and Nursing Interventions for Patients Taking Antidepressants—cont'd**	
SAFETY ISSUES	**NURSING INTERVENTIONS**
Discontinuation syndrome: SSRIs—dizziness, lethargy, headache, nausea TCAs—hypomania, akathisia, cardiac arrhythmias, gastrointestinal upset, panic attacks MAOIs—flu-like symptoms, confusion, hypomania	Instruct patients that all antidepressants have some potential for discontinuation syndrome and should not be stopped abruptly but rather tapered off. Paroxetine is associated with the highest risk for discontinuation syndrome (Janicak & Hussain, 2017).
Photosensitivity	Instruct patients of their vulnerability to severe sunburn and recommend sunscreen.
Orthostatic hypotension (TCAs)	Instruct patients to rise slowly from sitting to standing. Monitor blood pressure to assess for symptoms.
Tachycardia, arrhythmias (TCAs)	Monitor vital signs, especially in elderly with preexisting cardiovascular disorders.
Hyponatremia (SSRIs), especially among the elderly	Instruct patients to report any symptoms of nausea, malaise, lethargy, muscle cramps. Assess for disorientation or restlessness. Monitor sodium levels: ■ <120 mEq/L risk for seizure, coma, respiratory arrest ■ Withhold medication, contact physician, restrict water intake ■ Take a detailed history of antidepressant therapy, particularly the duration of new antidepressant use (Lien, 2018)
Blurred vision (TCAs and atypicals)	Instruct patients to avoid driving and reassure them that this side effect usually resolves within 3 weeks. Monitor blood pressure to rule out symptoms of hypertension.
Constipation	Recommend a high-fiber diet and regular exercise. Instruct patients to report any symptoms of ongoing difficulty with bowel movements.

MAOIs, monoamine oxidase inhibitors; SSRIs, selective serotonin reuptake inhibitors; TCAs, tricyclic antidepressants.

Outcome Criteria and Evaluation

The following criteria may be used for evaluating the effectiveness of therapy with antidepressant medications.

The patient:

■ Has not harmed self
■ Has not experienced injury caused by side effects
■ Exhibits vital signs within normal limits
■ Manifests symptoms of improvement in mood (presents brighter affect, interacts with others, demonstrates improved hygiene, expresses clear thought, conveys hopefulness, shows improved ability to make decisions)
■ Willingly participates in activities and interacts appropriately with others

Mood-Stabilizing Agents
Background Assessment Data

For many years, the drug of choice for treatment and management of bipolar mania was lithium carbonate.

In recent years, several other **mood-stabilizing agents** have demonstrated effectiveness either alone or in combination with lithium. Most notable are many drugs in the class of anticonvulsant medications, which are now FDA approved for mood stabilization. Some second generation atypical antipsychotics have also demonstrated benefits for management of this disorder.

Bipolar disorder is characterized by cycles of depression and manic episodes, which may manifest as grandiose thinking and behavior, rapid thoughts, hyperactivity, or impulsive agitation. The effective medication treatment for this disorder is one that reduces the rollercoaster of "ups and downs" often described by clients; thus the name "mood stabilizer" is an apt description of their purpose. Lithium was first identified as an antimanic but was later recognized as useful for stabilizing the mood *swings* of bipolar disorder as well.

Lithium is a salt present in mineral springs and added to spa baths. Although it was also used for other medicinal purposes, in 1949 Australian physician John Cade reported using lithium to treat manic excitement. It was so effective that some of his patients became symptom free and were able to be discharged after years of institutionalization (Shorter, 2009). It remains true that people who respond to lithium and remain on the medication may show no evidence of bipolar mood swings. Although it is not a cure, it is often described as "like insulin to a diabetic" in that proper use and response can reduce or eliminate symptoms. Unfortunately, not everyone responds with the same degree of success, and too much lithium can be fatal. Today, however, we are able to measure the blood levels of lithium and be confident of its safety when maintained within the specified therapeutic range (0.6 to 1.2 mEq/L). The exact mechanism of action remains unknown, but it is believed to have an effect on many of the same neurotransmitters (serotonin, norepinephrine, glutamate, GABA, and dopamine) as previously discussed.

In 1995 the FDA approved valproate (Depakote) as a mood stabilizer; since then, a significant shift toward this group of anticonvulsant mood stabilizers (including carbamazepine, clonazepam, topiramate, and lamotrigine) and away from lithium has occurred (Shorter, 2009). As with lithium, the mechanism of action for these drugs is unclear. The impact on cellular sodium transport, GABA modulation, and raising the seizure threshold have all been advanced as possible explanations for their effectiveness.

Both first and second generation antipsychotics have been used alone or as adjuncts to other medication treatment for bipolar mania. Because lithium has a lag period of 7 to 10 days, first generation antipsychotics, such as haloperidol, may be helpful in initial treatment because of their immediate sedative effects. They also increase the effects of lithium, so monitoring blood serum levels is especially important in the initial phase of treatment when these two drugs are used in combination. (A table of current FDA-approved mood-stabilizer medications can be found in Chapter 26, "Bipolar and Related Disorders.")

Several studies have explored dietary supplements and anti-inflammatory agents for their benefits as adjunct treatments in bipolar disorder (Aiken, 2020). Although studies have demonstrated benefits of N-acetylcysteine as an adjunctive treatment of subsyndromal depressive symptoms, the results for treatment of bipolar disorder have been mixed. Two anti-inflammatory agents, celecoxib and aspirin, have shown more promising results as adjunct treatments in major depressive disorder and depressive symptoms associated with bipolar disorder

(Köhler-Forsberg et al., 2019). A recent systematic review and meta-analysis also supported that skill-based psychosocial interventions, like cognitive behavior therapy (CBT; in combination with pharmacotherapy), reduced the recurrence of illness episodes better than medication treatment alone (Miklowitz et al., 2020).

Interactions

One of the interesting things about drug interactions with mood stabilizers is that many drugs either increase or decrease their effectiveness, as shown in Table 4–9. Understanding that lithium is a salt is relevant in explaining some of these interactions. Because lithium is an imperfect substitute for sodium, anything that depletes sodium will make more receptor sites available to lithium and increase the risk for lithium toxicity. This effect is why individuals taking lithium must maintain regular dietary sodium and fluid intake to avoid major fluctuations in their lithium levels and the resulting effects. For example, significant increases in dietary sodium intake may reduce the effectiveness of lithium because sodium will bind at more receptor sites and decrease the amount of lithium that can bind to these receptors. Other drugs that increase or decrease serum sodium levels also have an effect on lithium levels.

Diagnosis

The following nursing diagnoses may be considered for patients receiving therapy with mood-stabilizing agents:

■ Risk for injury related to manic hyperactivity
■ Risk for self-directed or other-directed violence related to unresolved anger turned inward on the self or outward on the environment
■ Risk for injury related to lithium toxicity
■ Risk for injury related to adverse effects of mood-stabilizing drugs
■ Risk for activity intolerance related to side effects of drowsiness and dizziness

Safety Issues in Planning and Implementing Care

One of the primary safety issues with lithium is its narrow therapeutic range. A description of lithium toxicity, other safety concerns with mood-stabilizing agents, and relevant nursing interventions are discussed in Table 4–10.

Lithium Maintenance

Patients who respond to lithium will typically remain on the medication indefinitely. To ensure safe maintenance and prevent lithium toxicity, patient education and regular monitoring are essential. An

TABLE 4-9 Selected Drug Interactions With Mood-Stabilizing Agents

THE EFFECTS OF:	ARE INCREASED BY:	ARE DECREASED BY:	CONCURRENT USE MAY RESULT IN:
ANTIMANIC AGENTS			
Lithium	Carbamazepine, fluoxetine, haloperidol, loop diuretics, methyldopa, NSAIDs, and thiazide diuretics	Acetazolamide, osmotic diuretics, theophylline, and urinary alkalinizers	Increased effects of neuromuscular blocking agents and tricyclic antidepressants; decreased pressor sensitivity of sympathomimetics; neurotoxicity may occur with phenothiazines or calcium channel blockers
ANTICONVULSANTS			
Clonazepam	CNS depressants, cimetidine, hormonal contraceptives, disulfiram, fluoxetine, isoniazid, ketoconazole, metoprolol, propranolol, valproic acid, probenecid	Rifampin, theophylline (↓ sedative effects), phenytoin	Increased phenytoin levels; decreased efficacy of levodopa
Carbamazepine	Verapamil, diltiazem, propoxyphene, erythromycin, clarithromycin, SSRIs, tricyclic antidepressants, cimetidine, isoniazid, danazol, lamotrigine, niacin, acetazolamide, dalfopristin, valproate, nefazodone	Cisplatin, doxorubicin, felbamate, rifampin, barbiturates, hydantoins, primidone, theophylline	Decreased levels of corticosteroids, doxycycline, quinidine, warfarin, estrogen-containing contraceptives, cyclosporine, benzodiazepines, theophylline, lamotrigine, valproic acid, bupropion, haloperidol, olanzapine, tiagabine, topiramate, voriconazole, ziprasidone, felbamate, levothyroxine, or antidepressants; increased levels of lithium; life-threatening hypertensive reaction with MAOIs
Valproic acid	Chlorpromazine, cimetidine, erythromycin, felbamate, salicylates	Rifampin, carbamazepine, cholestyramine, lamotrigine, phenobarbital, ethosuximide, hydantoins	Increased effects of tricyclic antidepressants, carbamazepine, CNS depressants, ethosuximide, lamotrigine, phenobarbital, warfarin, zidovudine, hydantoins
Lamotrigine	Valproic acid	Primidone, phenobarbital, phenytoin, rifamycin, succinimides, oral contraceptives, oxcarbazepine, carbamazepine, acetaminophen	Decreased levels of valproic acid; increased levels of carbamazepine and topiramate
Topiramate	Metformin, hydrochlorothiazide	Phenytoin, carbamazepine, valproic acid, lamotrigine	Increased risk of CNS depression with alcohol or other CNS depressants; increased risk of kidney stones with carbonic anhydrase inhibitors; increased effects of phenytoin, metformin, amitriptyline; decreased effects of oral contraceptives, digoxin, lithium, risperidone, and valproic acid
Oxcarbazepine		Carbamazepine, phenobarbital, phenytoin, valproic acid, verapamil	Increased concentrations of phenobarbital and phenytoin; decreased effects of oral contraceptives, felodipine, and lamotrigine
CALCIUM CHANNEL BLOCKER			
Verapamil	Amiodarone, beta blockers, cimetidine, ranitidine, and grapefruit juice	Barbiturates, calcium salts, hydantoins, rifampin, and antineoplastics	Increased effects of beta blockers, disopyramide, flecainide, doxorubicin, benzodiazepines, buspirone, carbamazepine, digoxin, dofetilide, ethanol, imipramine, nondepolarizing muscle relaxants, prazosin, quinidine, sirolimus, tacrolimus, and theophylline; altered serum lithium levels

TABLE 4–9 Selected Drug Interactions With Mood-Stabilizing Agents—cont'd

THE EFFECTS OF:	ARE INCREASED BY:	ARE DECREASED BY:	CONCURRENT USE MAY RESULT IN:
ANTIPSYCHOTIC AGENTS			
Olanzapine	Fluvoxamine and other CYP1A2 inhibitors, fluoxetine	Carbamazepine and other CYP1A2 inducers, omeprazole, rifampin	Decreased effects of levodopa and dopamine agonists; increased hypotension with antihypertensives; increased CNS depression with alcohol or other CNS depressants
Aripiprazole	Ketoconazole and other CYP3A4 inhibitors; quinidine, fluoxetine, paroxetine, or other potential CYP2D6 inhibitors	Carbamazepine, famotidine, valproate	Increased CNS depression with alcohol or other CNS depressants; increased hypotension with antihypertensives
Chlorpromazine	Beta blockers, paroxetine	Centrally acting anticholinergics	Increased effects of beta blockers; excessive sedation and hypotension with meperidine; decreased hypotensive effect of guanethidine; decreased effect of oral anticoagulants; decreased or increased phenytoin levels; increased orthostatic hypotension with thiazide diuretics; increased CNS depression with alcohol or other CNS depressants; increased hypotension with antihypertensives; increased anticholinergic effects with anticholinergic agents
Quetiapine	Cimetidine; ketoconazole, itraconazole, fluconazole, erythromycin, or other CYP3A4 inhibitors	Phenytoin, thioridazine	Decreased effects of levodopa and dopamine agonists; increased CNS depression with alcohol or other CNS depressants; increased hypotension with antihypertensives
Risperidone	Clozapine, fluoxetine, paroxetine, or ritonavir	Carbamazepine	Decreased effects of levodopa and dopamine agonists; increased effects of clozapine and valproate; increased CNS depression with alcohol or other CNS depressants; increased hypotension with antihypertensives
Ziprasidone	Ketoconazole and other CYP3A4 inhibitors	Carbamazepine	Life-threatening prolongation of QT interval with quinidine, dofetilide, other class Ia and III antiarrhythmics, pimozide, sotalol, thioridazine, chlorpromazine, pentamidine, arsenic trioxide, mefloquine, dolasetron, tacrolimus, droperidol, gatifloxacin, or moxifloxacin; decreased effects of levodopa and dopamine agonists; increased CNS depression with alcohol or other CNS depressants; increased hypotension with antihypertensives
Asenapine	Fluvoxamine, imipramine, valproate	Carbamazepine, cimetidine, paroxetine	Increased effects of paroxetine and dextromethorphan; increased CNS depression with alcohol or other CNS depressants; increased hypotension with antihypertensives; additive effects of QT interval prolongation with quinidine, dofetilide, other class Ia and III antiarrhythmics, pimozide, sotalol, thioridazine, chlorpromazine, pentamidine, arsenic trioxide, mefloquine, dolasetron, tacrolimus, droperidol, gatifloxacin, or moxifloxacin

CNS, central nervous system; MAOI, monoamine oxidase inhibitor; NSAID, nonsteroidal anti-inflammatory drug; SSRI, serotonin reuptake inhibitor.

TABLE 4–10 Safety Issues and Nursing Interventions for Patients Taking Mood Stabilizers	
SAFETY ISSUES	**NURSING INTERVENTIONS**
Lithium toxicity: ■ Blood levels >0.8 mmol (or mEq)/L are associated with increased risk for renal toxicity (N-acetylcysteine may prevent lithium-induced renal damage [Rege, 2020]). ■ At blood levels >1.2 mEq/L early signs of toxicity include vomiting and diarrhea. ■ At blood levels >1.5 mEq/L gastrointestinal (increasing nausea, anorexia, diarrhea) and CNS effects (muscle weakness, drowsiness, ataxia, coarse tremor and muscle twitching) occur (Rege, 2020). ■ At blood levels >2 mEq/L increasing disorientation and seizures can occur. ■ Blood levels ≥ 3.5 mEq/L are associated with coma, cardiovascular collapse, and death. ■ Chlorpromazine (Thorazine) may mask early signs of lithium toxicity (Vallerand & Sanoski, 2022).	Instruct patients to report all medications, herbals, and caffeine use to physician or nurse practitioner to evaluate for drug interactions. Encourage patients to maintain fluid intake at 2,000–3,000 mL/day and avoid activities in which excessive sweating and fluid loss are a risk because inadequate fluid intake can affect lithium levels. Instruct patients about the importance of regular monitoring of serum lithium levels. Blood levels should be drawn 12 hours after the last dose.
Increased risk of suicide for antiepileptics	Assess for suicide risk regularly and inform patients of risks associated with anticonvulsants.
Hyponatremia (lithium, carbamazepine)	Instruct patients to maintain usual dietary intake of sodium. Assess for and educate patients to report any episodes of nausea, vomiting, headache, muscle weakness, confusion, seizures, because these may be signs of hyponatremia.
Stevens-Johnson syndrome (especially with lamotrigine and carbamazepine) This toxic skin necrolysis can be life-threatening.	Assess for and educate patients to report any signs of rash or unusual skin breakdown.
Hypotension, arrhythmias (lithium)	Monitor vital signs and instruct patients to report any symptoms of dizziness or palpitations.
Blood dyscrasias (valproic acid, carbamazepine)	Educate patients to report infections or other illness while on these medications. Ensure that platelet counts and bleeding time are determined before initiation of therapy. Monitor for spontaneous bleeding or bruising.
Increased risk of birth defects (anticonvulsant mood stabilizers)	Inform female patients of the risks of birth defects and provide education about contraception as desired.
Drowsiness (lithium and all anticonvulsants)	Instruct patients to avoid driving or operating dangerous machinery when experiencing this side effect. Assess patients' mental status for level of alertness.

important component of monitoring is evaluation of serum lithium levels to ensure that they remain within the therapeutic range.

Although a typical therapeutic range for lithium is from 0.6 to 1.2 mEq/L, current American Psychiatric Association clinical practice guidelines recommend that when initiating treatment, the levels should be closer to 1.2 (the higher end of the range) and that in maintenance treatment the optimum levels should be closer to 0.6 (the lower end of the range)

(Rege, 2020). An international study group recently completed a systematic review and came to a consensus on a more conservative optimal range of 0.4 to 0.6 mEq/L if the patient is responding well to lithium therapy (Nolen et al., 2019).

Although higher levels (closer to 1.0) may be more efficacious for patients that are prone to more manic episodes (rather than more depressive episodes), higher levels are also associated with more adverse effects. At levels over 1.5 mEq/L, increasing nausea, anorexia, and diarrhea are common as well as CNS symptoms such as muscle weakness, drowsiness, ataxia, tremors, and muscle twitching. Even higher levels can lead to delirium, seizures, cardiovascular collapse, or death.

Serum lithium levels should be monitored once or twice a week after initial treatment until dosage and serum levels are stable and then monthly during maintenance therapy. Blood samples should be drawn 12 hours after the last dose.

Some individuals complain that they miss the "high" feeling of being in a manic or hypomanic state once they begin mood-stabilizer medications. They may be at risk for self-adjusting medication or discontinuing it altogether.

 Open discussion and exploring the benefits versus disadvantages of medication treatment promote patient-centered care and enable the nurse to troubleshoot with the patient ways to minimize risks.

One generally undesirable side effect of lithium is weight gain. Patients should be educated about this potential, and weight should be monitored at regular intervals. It may be helpful to discuss low-calorie diets while stressing the importance of not making significant changes in sodium intake because of its effect on serum blood levels of lithium.

> **CLINICAL PEARL** The FDA requires that all antiepileptic (anticonvulsant) drugs carry a warning label indicating that use of the drugs increases risk for suicidal thoughts and behaviors. Patients treated with these medications should be monitored for the emergence or worsening of depression, suicidal thoughts or behavior, or any unusual changes in mood or behavior.

Outcome Criteria and Evaluation

The following criteria may be used for evaluating the effectiveness of therapy with mood-stabilizing agents. The patient:

- Is maintaining stability of mood
- Has not harmed self or others
- Has experienced no injury from hyperactivity
- Is able to participate in activities without excessive sedation or dizziness
- Is maintaining appropriate weight
- Exhibits no signs of lithium toxicity
- Verbalizes importance of taking medication regularly and reporting for regular laboratory blood tests

Antipsychotic Agents

Antipsychotic agents are also called *neuroleptics*. Historically, they have been referred to as major tranquilizers and have clear sedative effects. The term *antipsychotic* is most descriptive because the primary benefit over time is the alleviation of psychotic symptoms, such as hallucinations and delusions.

Background Assessment Data

Antipsychotic agents were introduced in the United States in the 1950s with the phenothiazines. Other drugs in this classification soon followed, and these are called *typical* or *first generation antipsychotics*. Unfortunately, this group of medications has the potential for extrapyramidal side effects, also called **extrapyramidal symptoms (EPS)**, that interfere with normal movements, including acute **dystonias** (muscle spasms) that can be life-threatening, Parkinson-like symptoms, and **tardive dyskinesia** (later-onset involuntary movement disorders primarily in the tongue, lips, and jaw that may also involve other movement disturbances). Some of these side effects can be permanent, continuing even after the drug is discontinued. The first generation, typical antipsychotics include the phenothiazines, haloperidol, loxapine, pimozide, and thiothixene.

Second generation antipsychotic medications have since been developed with less potential for EPS. They have become the preferred first-line treatment. These are most often referred to as atypical antipsychotics, and they include aripiprazole, asenapine and asenapine transdermal (Secuado), clozapine, olanzapine, quetiapine, risperidone, paliperidone, iloperidone, lurasidone, ziprasidone, brexpiprazole (Rexulti), cariprazine (Vraylar), pimavanserin (Nuplazid), and lumateperone (Caplyta). Pimavanserin is indicated for hallucinations and delusions associated with Parkinson's disease psychosis. This group of drugs is used to alleviate positive symptoms hallucinations, delusions, and agitation and may be beneficial in treating some of the negative symptoms as well.

The atypical antipsychotic aripiprazole (Abilify) has sometimes been described as a third generation antipsychotic because of its unique functional profile with dopamine receptors, and it has been identified as having minimal risk for EPS. In 2017 the FDA approved a novel (and controversial) formulation of aripiprazole (called Abilify MyCite), which includes a sensor device embedded in the pill that enables the patient (and others) to track whether they are taking the medication. In 2020 the FDA approved a novel antipsychotic medication, lumateperone (Caplyta), which, although the action is unknown, reportedly demonstrates benefit in treating both positive and negative symptoms of schizophrenia.

Indications

Antipsychotics are used in the treatment of schizophrenia and other psychotic disorders. Selected agents are used in the treatment of bipolar mania (see previous section, "Mood-Stabilizing Agents"). Others are used as antiemetics (chlorpromazine, perphenazine, prochlorperazine), in the treatment of intractable hiccoughs (chlorpromazine), and for the control of tics and vocal utterances in Tourette's disorder (haloperidol, pimozide). Selected atypical antipsychotics, including aripiprazole (Abilify), are also being identified as adjuncts to the treatment of major depressive disorder. (A table of current FDA-approved antipsychotics as well as **antiparkinsonian agents**, which are used to treat EPS caused by antipsychotic medication, can be found in Chapter 24, "Schizophrenia Spectrum and Other Psychotic Disorders.")

Action

First generation, typical antipsychotics are antagonists that work by blocking postsynaptic dopamine receptors in the basal ganglia, hypothalamus, limbic system, brainstem, and medulla. They also demonstrate varying affinity for cholinergic, alpha1-adrenergic, and histaminic receptors.

Second generation, atypical antipsychotics are weaker dopamine receptor antagonists than conventional antipsychotics but are more potent antagonists of the serotonin type 2A (5-HT2A) receptors. They also exhibit antagonism for cholinergic, histaminic, and adrenergic receptors. As mentioned previously, aripiprazole (Abilify) is a dopamine receptor antagonist that seems to have a unique way of accomplishing its action and thus has a minimal risk of EPS.

Contraindications and Precautions

Certain individuals may be at greater risk for experiencing side effects associated with antipsychotic agents. Older adults have been identified as an at-risk population because of reports of stroke and sudden death while taking antipsychotic medication. Studies have indicated that older patients with psychosis related to neurocognitive disorder (NCD) who are treated with antipsychotic drugs are at increased risk of death, particularly from cerebrovascular events, and researchers have found a decrease in associated deaths since the FDA initiated boxed warnings about these risks for all antipsychotics (Rubino et al., 2020). All antipsychotic drugs now carry a boxed warning about these risks. A **boxed warning**, named for the black border around the warning text on a drug's package insert, is the highest level warning imposed by the FDA for prescription medications. Its purpose is to alert consumers about serious or life-threatening side effects the drug may have. Antipsychotic drugs are not approved for treatment of older patients with NCD-related psychosis. Rubino and associates (2020) also found that while prescriptions for antipsychotics declined in those with dementia-related psychosis since the initiation of boxed warnings, an increase in opioid and antiepileptic medication prescriptions (with other significant risks) ensued.

Both first and second generation antipsychotics are contraindicated in clients with known hypersensitivity. They should not be used in clients who are comatose or when CNS depression is evident; when blood dyscrasias exist; in clients with Parkinson's disease or narrow-angle glaucoma (first generation agents); for those with liver, renal, or cardiac insufficiency; in individuals with poorly controlled seizure disorders; or in elderly clients with dementia-related psychosis.

Ziprasidone, risperidone, paliperidone, asenapine, and iloperidone are contraindicated in patients with a history of QT prolongation or cardiac arrhythmias, recent myocardial infarction (MI), uncompensated heart failure, and concurrent use with other drugs that prolong the QT interval. Clozapine is contraindicated in patients with myeloproliferative disorders, a history of clozapine-induced agranulocytosis or severe granulocytopenia, or uncontrolled epilepsy. Lurasidone is contraindicated in individuals also using strong inhibitors of cytochrome P450 isozyme 3A4 (CYP3A4) (e.g., ketoconazole, an antifungal) and strong CYP3A4 inducers (e.g., rifampin, an antitubercular).

Caution is indicated when administering atypical antipsychotic medications to elderly or debilitated patients; patients with cardiac, hepatic, or renal insufficiency; those with a history of seizures; patients with diabetes or risk factors for diabetes; clients exposed to temperature extremes; under conditions that cause hypotension (dehydration, hypovolemia, treatment with antihypertensive medication); and to pregnant clients (several atypical antipsychotic medications, such as olanzapine, risperidone, and quetiapine, have been associated with congenital malformations) (Anderson et al., 2020).

Six atypical antipsychotic medications (aripiprazole, asenapine, olanzapine, paliperidone, quetiapine, and risperidone) have FDA approval for use in children and adolescents. Both aripiprazole and quetiapine (also approved for adjunctive treatment in depression) carry boxed warnings about increased risk for suicidal thinking in children, adolescents, and young adults.

Interactions

Table 4–11 highlights some drug interactions that warrant monitoring and assessment by nurses.

TABLE 4–11 Selected Drug Interactions With Antipsychotic Medications

DRUG INTERACTION	ADVERSE EFFECT
Antihypertensives, central nervous system depressants Epinephrine or dopamine in combination with haloperidol or phenothiazines	Additive and potentially severe hypotension
Oral anticoagulants with phenothiazines	Less effective anticoagulant effects
Drugs that prolong QT intervals	Additive effects
Drugs that trigger orthostatic hypotension	Additive hypotension
Drugs with anticholinergic effects, including prescription and over-the-counter drugs	Additive anticholinergic effects, including anticholinergic toxicity, signs of which are ■ Flushing ■ Dry mouth ■ Mydriasis ■ Altered mental status ■ Fever ■ Decreased bowel sounds ■ Ileus ■ Tachycardia ■ Urinary retention ■ Tremulousness ■ Myoclonic jerking ■ Hypertension (Ramnarine & Ahmed, 2022)

Diagnosis

The following nursing diagnoses may be considered for patients receiving antipsychotic therapy:

■ Risk for other-directed violence related to panic anxiety and mistrust of others
■ Risk for injury related to medication side effects of sedation, photosensitivity, reduction of seizure threshold, agranulocytosis, EPS, tardive dyskinesia, neuroleptic malignant syndrome, or QT prolongation
■ Risk for activity intolerance related to medication side effects of sedation, blurred vision, and weakness
■ Nonadherence with medication regimen related to suspiciousness and mistrust of others

Safety Issues in Planning and Implementing Care

Table 4–12 discusses some significant safety issues to consider and relevant nursing interventions for patients taking antipsychotic medication.

Additional Issues for Patient Education

Patients should be apprised of health risks when taking antipsychotic agents, including the following:

■ Smoking increases the metabolism of antipsychotics, requiring an adjustment in dosage to achieve a therapeutic effect. Patients should be encouraged to discuss this issue with the prescribing physician or nurse practitioner.
■ Body temperature is harder to maintain with antipsychotic medication, so patients should be encouraged to dress warmly in cold weather and

TABLE 4–12 Safety Issues and Nursing Interventions for Patients Taking Antipsychotic Medication

SAFETY ISSUES	NURSING INTERVENTIONS
Extrapyramidal side effects[a]	Instruct patient to report any signs of muscle stiffness or spasms. Hold the medication if this occurs. Administer antiparkinsonian agents as ordered and immediately when signs of acute dystonia are present. Assess the patient for abnormal involuntary movements (see Box 4–2). (See "Additional Issues for Patient Education" for further discussion.)
Hyperglycemia, weight gain, and diabetes (more common with atypical antipsychotic agents)	Assess for a history of diabetes. Evaluate blood sugars. Instruct the patient in these risks and the importance of diet and exercise. Assess for signs of hyperglycemia including polydipsia, polyphagia, polyuria, and weakness.
Hypotension	Educate the patient about the risk for hypotension. Monitor blood pressure.
Orthostatic hypotension	Instruct patient to rise slowly from sitting to standing. Monitor blood pressure lying and then standing to assess for postural changes.

Continued

TABLE 4–12 Safety Issues and Nursing Interventions for Patients Taking Antipsychotic Medication–cont'd	
SAFETY ISSUES	**NURSING INTERVENTIONS**
Lower seizure threshold (especially with clozapine)	Assess patient for history of seizure disorder. Monitor the patient for evidence of seizure activity and report to prescribing physician or nurse practitioner.
Prolonged QT interval,[b] especially ziprasidone, thioridazine, pimozide, haloperidol, paliperidone, iloperidone, asenapine, and clozapine.	Assess for history of arrhythmias, recent myocardial infarction, heart failure, and report to prescribing physician or nurse practitioner because these events are contraindications. Assess for other medications the patient is taking that prolong QT interval (there are many online resources), but note that erythromycin and clarithromycin are two that are commonly prescribed. Instruct patient to report any rapid heartbeat, dizziness, or fainting. Check baseline electrocardiogram (ECG) before beginning treatment.
Anticholinergic effects	Instruct patient about additive effects of other anticholinergic drugs in combination with antipsychotics, and to report any other medications taken including over-the-counter and herbal remedies. For minor symptoms such as dry mouth, recommend hard candies and sips of water. Instruct patient about the importance of good oral hygiene. Instruct patient to report and assess for any evidence of urinary retention, tachycardia, tremulousness, or hypertension, which may be signs of anticholinergic toxicity.
Sedation	Educate patient about this side effect and instruct patient not to drive or operate dangerous machinery if experiencing sedation.
Photosensitivity	Instruct patient to use sunblock and sunglasses and to wear protective clothing when in the sun because of the increased risk for severe sunburn while on these medications.
Agranulocytosis (more common with typical antipsychotics but especially with the atypical antipsychotic agent clozapine)	Instruct the patient receiving clozapine that regular monitoring of white blood cell and absolute neutrophil counts is essential. Instruct patient to report any signs of sore throat, fever, or malaise. (See additional guidelines in the section "Issues in Antipsychotic Maintenance Therapy.")
Neuroleptic malignant syndrome (NMS)[c]	Instruct patient to report immediately any fever, muscle rigidity, diaphoresis, tachycardia. Assess vital signs regularly, including temperature. Assess for deteriorating mental status or any other sign of NMS. Presence of any of these signs requires holding the medication and contacting the prescribing physician or nurse practitioner immediately, as well as monitoring vital signs and intake and output.
Drug reaction with eosinophilia and systemic symptoms (DRESS) (olanzapine)[d] (FDA, 2016b) New impulse control problems such as compulsive or uncontrollable urges to gamble, binge eat, shop, and have sex (aripiprazole) (FDA, 2016a)	Assess for symptoms of DRESS including fever, rash, swollen lymph glands, swelling in the face. Hold medication and contact physician immediately. Assess for newly developing impulse control problems for patients taking aripiprazole. Closely monitor patients who may be at increased risk for impulse control problems such as those with personal or family history of obsessive-compulsive disorder, bipolar disorder, impulsive personality, alcohol, drug, or other addictive behaviors.

[a]Acute dystonias can be life-threatening (more common with typical antipsychotic agents).
[b]Potentially life-threatening.
[c]Rare but potentially life-threatening side effect characterized by muscle rigidity, severe hyperthermia, and cardiac effects that can progress rapidly over 24–72 hours.
[d]Rare but serious; can lead to organ injury and even death.

avoid extended exposure to very high or low temperatures.

■ Antipsychotic medications increase photosensitivity to sunlight. Patients should be advised to wear sunscreen and protective clothing when exposed to the sun.

■ Alcohol and antipsychotic drugs potentiate each other's effects, so patients should be advised to avoid drinking alcohol while on antipsychotic therapy.

■ Many medications contain substances that interact with antipsychotics in a way that may be harmful. Patients should avoid taking other medications, including over-the-counter products, without first discussing it with the prescriber.

■ A significant number of patients on clozapine report excessive salivation. Sugar-free gum and medications (anticholinergic or alpha2-adrenoceptor agonists) may alleviate symptoms. Patients should be encouraged to discuss these options with the prescribing physician or nurse practitioner.

■ Safe use of antipsychotics during pregnancy has not been established. Antipsychotics are thought to readily cross the placental barrier; if so, a fetus could experience adverse effects of the drug. Patients should be aware of the possible risks and should inform the physician immediately if pregnancy occurs, is suspected, or is planned.

■ Clozapine carries a particular risk for agranulocytosis, which increases risk for severe infection. Patients should be instructed that regular measurement of neutrophils is essential (this is discussed in more detail later).

■ Clozapine also carries a risk for ileus (intestinal blockage) with a 15% to 28% fatality rate. Eighty percent of clozapine-treated patients have some hypomotility in their bowels, and in 2020 the FDA strengthened its warning on the risks of ileus (FDA, 2020). Patients should be instructed to report any change in bowel habits to their physician and to explore diet and medications to reduce constipation.

Issues in Antipsychotic Maintenance Therapy

The nurse must understand the management of side effects associated with antipsychotic medication to conduct a thorough assessment and minimize risks. In addition, some of these side effects can be difficult for patients to manage or understand, particularly when they are struggling with impaired mental status including psychosis and cognitive deficits. Three of these are discussed here.

Clozaril and the Risk for Agranulocytosis

The FDA requires close monitoring of patients on medications that increase the risk for life-threatening side effects. Clozaril is one such drug. Due to the risk of agranulocytosis, the FDA requires that clozapine be part of a REMS program to ensure that risk for agranulocytosis is monitored, managed, and reported. **Agranulocytosis** is a potentially fatal blood disorder in which the patient's absolute neutrophil count (ANC) drops to extremely low levels (less than or equal to 500 µL). This condition is called neutropenia. An ANC must be assessed before initiation of treatment with clozapine and weekly for the first 6 months of treatment. Initially, only a 1-week supply of medication is dispensed at a time. If the ANC remains within acceptable levels (i.e., ANC at least 1,500 µL) during the first 6 months, blood counts may be monitored biweekly for another 6 months and monthly thereafter. Some individuals with dark skin, particularly those of African and Middle Eastern descent, have normally lower ANC (benign ethnic neutropenia); in such cases the parameters for identifying clinically significant neutropenia are altered (Clozapine REMS, 2015).

Although the benefits of clozapine can be profound, this medication is typically used when patients fail to respond to other antipsychotics because of the strict protocols for adherence. If the patient agrees to this option, the nurse can be a vital resource in ensuring that support services, both professional and personal (such as family members or peers), are engaged to assist the patient with follow-through as needed.

Extrapyramidal Side Effects

To conduct a thorough assessment, the nurse must be familiar with several distinct types of extrapyramidal side effects of antipsychotic medications:

■ **Pseudoparkinsonism:** Symptoms of pseudoparkinsonism—tremor, shuffling gait, drooling, rigidity—may appear 1 to 5 days after initiation of antipsychotic medication. This side effect occurs most often in women, the elderly, and dehydrated individuals.

■ **Akinesia:** Absence or impairment in voluntary movement is termed **akinesia**.

■ **Akathisia:** Continuous restlessness and fidgeting, or **akathisia,** occurs most often in women and may manifest 50 to 60 days after therapy begins. Combining atypical antipsychotics and administration at doses greater than target ranges increases the incidence of akathisia (Chow et al., 2020)

■ **Dystonia:** This side effect—involuntary muscle spasms in the face, arms, legs, and neck—occurs most often in men and those younger than age 25. Dystonia should be treated as an emergency because laryngospasm follows these symptoms and can be fatal. The physician should be contacted, and intravenous or intramuscular benztropine mesylate (Cogentin) is commonly administered (see Chapter 24, "Schizophrenia Spectrum and Other Psychotic Disorders," for a list of antiparkinsonian agents used to treat EPS). Nurses should stay with the patient and offer reassurance.

■ **Oculogyric crisis:** Uncontrolled rolling back of the eyes, or **oculogyric crisis,** is a symptom of acute dystonia and can be mistaken for seizure activity. As with other symptoms of acute dystonia, this side effect should be treated as a medical emergency.

■ **Tardive dyskinesia:** This extrapyramidal side effect involves bizarre face and tongue movements, stiff neck, and difficulty swallowing. It may occur with all classifications but most commonly takes place with typical antipsychotics. All clients receiving antipsychotic therapy for months or years are at risk. Symptoms are potentially irreversible. Nurses should immediately report early signs of tardive dyskinesia (usually vermiform movements of the tongue) to the prescribing physician or nurse practitioner. Often, the drug is discontinued, changed to a different antipsychotic, or the dosage is altered. In 2017 the FDA approved the first drug for treating tardive dyskinesia, valbenazine (Ingrezza). It is hoped that this novel drug will effectively reduce this troubling condition and its sometimes stigmatizing effects (FDA, 2017). The involuntary movements associated with tardive dyskinesia can be measured by the Abnormal Involuntary Movement Scale (AIMS), developed in the 1970s by the National Institute of Mental Health. AIMS aids in early detection of movement disorders and provides means for ongoing surveillance. AIMS is featured in Box 4–3.

Some EPS can be life-threatening, and those that are not can sometimes be permanent. The abnormal movements in the tongue and lips are sometimes very visible and severe enough to interfere with a person's ability to speak or swallow.

 The nurse's empathic approach in listening to the patient's wishes regarding medication and advocating for exploring other options for management of symptoms is one way to promote patient-centered care, an essential nursing competency (IOM, 2003), and to promote a recovery model that empowers the patient to make decisions about management of the illness. There is evidence (Forma et al., 2020; Haddad et al., 2014) that remaining on antipsychotic medication can reduce the frequency of hospitalizations, and early treatment at the first psychotic episode may reduce some long-term consequences of illness. Educating patients about these risks and benefits is important in assisting them to make informed decisions about medication treatment.

Hormonal Side Effects

The following are sexual side effects that may accompany antipsychotic medications:

■ Decreased libido, **retrograde ejaculation** (the discharge of seminal fluid into the bladder rather than through the urethra); **gynecomastia** (breast enlargement in men)

■ **Amenorrhea** (absence of menses in women); **galactorrhea** (milky discharge from breasts of nonbreastfeeding women that may also occur in men)

These side effects can be troubling for anyone, but for a patient struggling with thought disturbances, they can become the foundation for delusions. A male patient with gynecomastia, for example, might begin to believe that external forces are taking over his body and turning him into a woman. An amenorrheic woman may begin to believe that she has been divinely impregnated. It is important for the nurse to clarify that these are side effects of the medication and offer reassurance that they are reversible. Women with amenorrhea should be instructed that this side effect does not indicate cessation of ovulation, so contraception use should continue as usual. Patients should be encouraged to explore alternative treatment if these side effects are deemed intolerable.

Current Developments in Psychopharmacological Treatment of Schizophrenia

One of the identified limitations of medication treatments available for schizophrenia is the cognitive deficits that are core symptoms of this illness, including deficits in working memory and long-term memory, reduced processing speed, limited verbal fluency, and impaired executive functions. Some atypical antipsychotics have demonstrated efficacy in lessening cognitive deficits but do not eliminate residual effects.

Cariprazine (Vraylar) has demonstrated some efficacy in treating the negative symptoms of schizophrenia, including flat affect, social withdrawal, and apathy (Correll et al., 2020). Although cariprazine is similar to other atypical antipsychotics, its particular affinity for certain dopamine receptors (D3) is believed to be associated with its superior effect on negative symptoms, particularly improving social behavior and self-care. In addition, cariprazine has demonstrated effectiveness in reducing substance misuse, a common comorbidity in patients with schizophrenia, and its long half-life enables maintenance of therapeutic levels even when a few doses are missed (Scarff, 2017). Negative symptoms can

BOX 4–3 Abnormal Involuntary Movement Scale (AIMS)

NAME _____ RATER NAME _____ DATE _____

Instructions: Complete the examination procedure before making ratings. For movement ratings, circle the highest severity observed. Rate movements that occur upon activation one less than those observed spontaneously. Circle movement as well as code number that applies.

Code: 0 = None
1 = Minimal, may be normal
2 = Mild
3 = Moderate
4 = Severe

Facial and Oral Movements	1. Muscles of facial expression (e.g., movements of forehead, eyebrows, periorbital area, cheeks, including frowning, blinking, smiling, grimacing)	0 1 2 3 4
	2. Lips and perioral area (e.g., puckering, pouting, smacking)	0 1 2 3 4
	3. Jaw (e.g., biting, clenching, chewing, mouth opening, lateral movement)	0 1 2 3 4
	4. Tongue (Rate only increases in movement both in and out of mouth. NOT inability to sustain movement. Darting in and out of mouth.)	0 1 2 3 4
Extremity Movements	5. Upper (arms, wrists, hands, fingers) Include choreic movements (i.e., rapid, objectively purposeless, irregular, spontaneous) and athetoid movements (i.e., slow, irregular, complex serpentine). *Do not include tremor* (i.e., repetitive, regular, rhythmic).	0 1 2 3 4
	6. Lower (legs, knees, ankles, toes) (e.g., lateral knee movement, foot tapping, heel dropping, foot squirming, inversion and eversion of foot)	0 1 2 3 4
Trunk Movements	7. Neck, shoulders, hips (e.g., rocking, twisting, squirming, pelvic gyrations)	0 1 2 3 4
Global Judgments	8. Severity of abnormal movements overall	0 1 2 3 4
	9. Incapacitation due to abnormal movements	0 1 2 3 4
	10. Patient's awareness of abnormal movements (Rate only the patient's report)	0 1 2 3 4

No awareness   0
Aware, no distress   1
Aware, mild distress   2
Aware, moderate distress   3
Aware, severe distress   4

Dental Status	11. Current problems with teeth and/or dentures?	No Yes
	12. Are dentures usually worn?	No Yes
	13. Edentia?	No Yes
	14. Do movements disappear in sleep?	No Yes

AIMS EXAMINATION PROCEDURE

Either before or after completing the examination procedure, observe the patient unobtrusively, at rest (e.g., in waiting room). The chair to be used in this examination should be a hard, firm one without arms.

1. Ask patient to remove shoes and socks.
2. Ask patient whether there is anything in his/her mouth (i.e., gum, candy, etc.), and if there is, to remove it.
3. Ask patient about the current condition of their teeth. Ask client if they wear dentures. Do teeth or dentures bother patient now?
4. Ask patient whether they notice any movements in mouth, face, hands, or feet. If yes, ask the patient to describe and to what extent they currently bother patient or interfere with their activities.
5. Have patient sit in chair with both hands on knees, legs slightly apart, and feet flat on floor. (Look at entire body for movements while in this position.)

Continued

BOX 4–3 Abnormal Involuntary Movement Scale (AIMS)—cont'd

6. Ask patient to sit with hands hanging unsupported. If male, between legs, if female and wearing a dress, hanging over knees. (Observe hands and other body areas.)
7. Ask patient to open mouth. (Observe tongue at rest within mouth.) Do this twice.
8. Ask patient to protrude tongue. (Observe abnormalities of tongue movement.) Do this twice.
9. Ask patient to tap thumb with each finger as rapidly as possible for 10 to 15 seconds; separately with right hand, then with left hand. (Observe facial and leg movements.)
10. Flex and extend patient's left and right arms (one at a time). (Note any rigidity.)
11. Ask patient to stand up. (Observe in profile. Observe all body areas again, hips included.)
12. Ask patient to extend both arms outstretched in front with palms down. (Observe trunk, legs, and mouth.)
13. Have patient walk a few paces, turn, and walk back to chair. (Observe hands and gait.) Do this twice.

INTERPRETATION OF AIMS SCORE

Add patient scores and note areas of difficulty.
Score of:

- 0 to 1 = Low risk
- 2 in only ONE of the areas assessed = borderline/observe closely
- 2 in TWO or more of the areas assessed or 3 to 4 in ONLY ONE area = indicative of TD

Source: *U.S. Department of Health and Human Services. Available for use in the public domain from Guy W. ECDEU Assessment Manual for Psychopharmacology:*
Revised (DHEW publication number ADM 76-338). Rockville, MD, US Department of Health, Education and Welfare, Public Health Service, Alcohol, Drug Abuse and Mental Health Administration, NIMH Psychopharmacology Research Branch, Division of Extramural Research Programs, 1976: 534–537.

complicate the prognosis in treatment of schizophrenia and as Scarff (2017) pointed out, the evidence supports "cautious optimism" that cariprazine may become the first-line treatment for patients with "disabling negative symptoms or impairment in self-care and interpersonal relationships" (p. 237). As mentioned previously, an even newer medication, lumateperone (Caplyta), is also being advanced as effective for treating both positive and negative symptoms of schizophrenia, although its action is unknown.

Outcome Criteria and Evaluation

The following criteria may be used for evaluating the effectiveness of therapy with antipsychotic medications.

The patient:

- Has not harmed self or others
- Has not experienced injury secondary to lowered seizure threshold or photosensitivity
- Maintains an ANC within normal limits
- Exhibits no symptoms of EPS, tardive dyskinesia, neuroleptic malignant syndrome, or hyperglycemia
- Maintains weight within normal limits
- Tolerates activity unaltered by the effects of sedation or weakness
- Adheres to medication schedule
- Verbalizes understanding of medication regimen and the importance of regular administration
- Demonstrates improvement in self-care and prosocial behavior

Sedative-Hypnotic Agents

Background Assessment Data

Indications

Sedative-hypnotic agents are used in the short-term management of various anxiety states and to treat insomnia. Selected agents are used as anticonvulsants (pentobarbital, phenobarbital) and preoperative sedatives (pentobarbital, secobarbital) and in the management of alcohol withdrawal. Examples of commonly used sedative-hypnotics are presented in Table 4–13.

Clinical guidelines typically recommend CBT as the first choice of treatment for insomnia, but there are currently four categories of medications approved by the FDA for this purpose (Neubauer, 2020):

- Benzodiazepines (estazolam, flurazepam, quazepam, temazepam, and triazolam) and alternative structured medications (eszopiclone, zaleplon, and zolpidem) with benzodiazepine-like properties
- Melatonin receptor agonists (ramelteon, tasimelteon)
- Histamine receptor antagonist (low-dose doxepin)
- Orexin receptor antagonists (suvorexant and lemborexant)

Action

Sedative-hypnotics cause generalized CNS depression. They may produce tolerance with chronic use and have the potential for psychological or physical dependence.

TABLE 4-13 Sedative-Hypnotic Agents

CHEMICAL CLASS	GENERIC (TRADE) NAME	CONTROLLED CATEGORIES	DAILY DOSAGE RANGE
Barbiturates	Amobarbital	CII	60–200 mg
	Butabarbital (Butisol)	CIII	45–120 mg
	Pentobarbital (Nembutal)	CII	150–200 mg
	Phenobarbital (Luminal; Solfoton)	CIV	30–200 mg
	Secobarbital (Seconal)	CII	100 mg (hypnotic); 200–300 mg (preoperative sedation)
Benzodiazepines	Estazolam	CIV	0.5–2 mg
	Flurazepam	CIV	15–30 mg
	Temazepam (Restoril)	CIV	7.5–30 mg
	Triazolam (Halcion)	CIV	0.125–0.5 mg
Miscellaneous	Eszopiclone (Lunesta)	CIV	1–3 mg
	Ramelteon (Rozerem)	N/A	8 mg
	Zaleplon (Sonata)	CIV	5–20 mg
	Zolpidem (Ambien)	CIV	5–10 mg (immediate release) 6.25–12.5 mg (extended release
	Lemborexant (Dayvigo)	(pending)	5–10 mg

Exception: Ramelteon (Rozerem) is not a controlled substance. It does not produce tolerance or physical dependence. Sleep-promoting properties are the result of ramelteon's agonist activity on selective melatonin receptors.

Contraindications and Precautions

Sedative-hypnotics are contraindicated in individuals with hypersensitivity to the drug or to any drug within the chemical class; in pregnancy (exceptions may be made in certain cases based on benefit-to-risk ratio); during lactation; in severe hepatic, cardiac, respiratory, or renal disease; and in children younger than age 15 years for flurazepam and those younger than age 18 years for estazolam, quazepam, temazepam, and triazolam. Triazolam is contraindicated with concurrent use of medications that impair the metabolism of triazolam by cytochrome P4503A (CYP3A), such as ketoconazole, itraconazole, and nefazodone. Ramelteon is contraindicated with concurrent use of fluvoxamine. Zolpidem, zaleplon, eszopiclone, and ramelteon are contraindicated in children.

Caution should be used in administering these drugs to patients with cardiac, hepatic, renal, or respiratory insufficiency. They should be used with caution in patients who may be suicidal or who previously may have been addicted to drugs. Hypnotic use should be short term. Elderly patients may be more sensitive to CNS depressant effects, and dosage reduction may be required.

Interactions

■ **Barbiturates:** The effects of barbiturates are increased with concomitant use of alcohol, other CNS depressants, MAOIs, or valproic acid. The effects of barbiturates may be decreased with rifampin. Possible decreased effects of the following drugs may occur when used concomitantly with barbiturates: anticoagulants, beta blockers, carbamazepine, clonazepam, oral contraceptives, corticosteroids, digitoxin, doxorubicin, doxycycline, felodipine, fenoprofen, griseofulvin, metronidazole, phenylbutazone, quinidine, theophylline, or verapamil. Concomitant use with methoxyflurane may enhance renal toxicity.

■ **Benzodiazepines:** The effects of the benzodiazepine hypnotics are increased with concomitant use of alcohol or other CNS depressants, cimetidine, oral contraceptives, disulfiram, isoniazid, or probenecid. Concomitant use with opioids increases the risk of respiratory depression, coma, and death. The effects of the benzodiazepine hypnotics are decreased with concomitant use of rifampin, theophylline, carbamazepine, or St. John's wort and with cigarette smoking. The effects of digoxin or phenytoin are increased when used concomitantly with benzodiazepines. Bioavailability of triazolam is increased with concurrent use of macrolides.

■ **Eszopiclone (Lunesta):** Additive effects of eszopiclone occur with alcohol or other CNS depressants. Decreased effects of eszopiclone occur with CYP3A4 inducers (e.g., rifampin, phenytoin, carbamazepine, phenobarbital), with lorazepam, or after a high-fat or heavy meal. Increased effects of eszopiclone occur with CYP3A4 inhibitors (e.g., ketoconazole, clarithromycin, nefazodone, ritonavir, and nelfinavir). The effects of lorazepam are decreased when used concomitantly with eszopiclone.

■ **Zaleplon (Sonata):** Additive effects of zaleplon occur with alcohol or other CNS depressants. Decreased effects of zaleplon occur with CYP3A4 inducers (e.g., rifampin, phenytoin, carbamazepine, phenobarbital) or after a high-fat or heavy meal. The effects of zaleplon are increased when used concomitantly with cimetidine.

■ **Zolpidem (Ambien, Ambien CR, Edluar, Intermezzo, Zolpimist):** Increased effects of zolpidem occur with alcohol or other CNS depressants, azole antifungals, ritonavir, or SSRIs. Decreased effects of zolpidem occur with flumazenil, rifampin, and with food. *There is a risk of life-threatening cardiac arrhythmias with concomitant use of amiodarone.*

■ **Ramelteon (Rozerem), tasimelteon (Hetlioz):** Increased effects occur with alcohol, ketoconazole (and other CYP3A4 inhibitors), and fluvoxamine (and other CYP1A2 inhibitors). Decreased effects occur with rifampin (and other CYP3A4 inducers) and after a heavy or high-fat meal.

Diagnosis

The following nursing diagnoses may be considered for patients receiving therapy with sedative-hypnotics:

■ Risk for injury related to abrupt withdrawal from long-term use or decreased mental alertness caused by residual sedation
■ Disturbed sleep pattern or insomnia related to situational crises, physical condition, or severe level of anxiety
■ Risk for activity intolerance related to side effects of lethargy, drowsiness, and dizziness

■ Risk for acute confusion related to action of the medication on the CNS

Safety Issues in Planning and Implementing Care

Refer to the earlier discussion of safety issues in the previous section "Antianxiety Agents." In addition to the side effects listed in that section, abnormal thinking and behavioral changes, including aggressiveness, hallucinations, and suicidal ideation, have also been noted in some individuals taking sedative-hypnotics. Certain complex behaviors, such as sleep-driving, preparing and eating food, and making phone calls, with amnesia for the behavior, have occurred. In 2019, the FDA added a boxed warning to prescribing information for eszopiclone, zaleplon, and zolpidem related to serious injuries and death associated with complex sleep behaviors that may occur with these medications. The emergence of any new behavioral sign or symptom of concern requires careful and immediate evaluation.

Outcome Criteria and Evaluation

The following criteria may be used for evaluating the effectiveness of therapy with sedative-hypnotic medications.

The patient:

■ Demonstrates reduced anxiety, tension, and restless activity
■ Falls asleep within 30 minutes of taking the medication and remains asleep for 6 to 8 hours without interruption
■ Is able to participate in usual activities without residual sedation
■ Experiences no physical injury
■ Exhibits no evidence of confusion
■ Verbalizes understanding of taking the medication on a short-term basis
■ Verbalizes understanding of potential for development of tolerance and dependence with long-term use

Attention Deficit-Hyperactivity Disorder Agents

Background Assessment Data

Indications

Attention deficit-hyperactivity disorder (ADHD) agents include CNS stimulants and nonstimulants. Amphetamines (which are CNS stimulants) are schedule II controlled substances indicating their high potential for misuse and dependence. They are also used in the treatment of narcolepsy and exogenous obesity. Nonstimulant medications include atomoxetine and bupropion (used off-label in ADHD treatment), which are also used in the treatment of major depression and for smoking cessation (Zyban only), and clonidine and guanfacine (also used to treat hypertension). (A table of current FDA-approved agents for ADHD can be found in Chapter 32, "Children and Adolescents.")

Action

CNS stimulants increase levels of neurotransmitters (probably norepinephrine, dopamine, and serotonin) in the CNS. They produce CNS and respiratory stimulation, vasoconstriction, dilated pupils, increased motor activity, mental alertness, decreased fatigue, and improved attention span in ADHD. The CNS stimulants discussed in this section include dextroamphetamine sulfate, methamphetamine, lisdexamfetamine, amphetamine mixtures, methylphenidate, and dexmethylphenidate. Their mechanism of action in the treatment of ADHD is unclear; however, it is believed that increasing dopamine and norepinephrine activity in the prefrontal cortex may explain the drugs' benefits because deficits in prefrontal functioning have been associated with ADHD, and dopamine and norepinephrine are key to enhancing prefrontal cortex functions (Guzman, 2021).

Atomoxetine inhibits the reuptake of norepinephrine, and bupropion blocks the neuronal uptake of serotonin, norepinephrine, and dopamine. Clonidine and guanfacine stimulate central alpha-adrenergic receptors in the brain, resulting in reduced sympathetic outflow from the CNS. The exact mechanism by which these nonstimulant drugs produce the therapeutic effect in ADHD is unclear.

One recent FDA approval in 2020 for the treatment of ADHD was not a drug but instead a novel interactive video game, EndeavorRx. Its developers identify that it directly targets neurological function, and studies support its effectiveness in improving attention (Tumolo, 2020). It requires a prescription and is currently advanced as a nondrug adjunctive treatment option. A second FDA-approved device is the Monarch external trigeminal nerve stimulation (eTNS) system, a trigeminal nerve stimulator. As Greenhill (2022) noted, FDA approvals for devices only require evidence of safety (unlike medications, which also require evidence of efficacy). More research is needed to evaluate the therapeutic benefits of these treatments.

Other advances in the treatment of ADHD include a delayed-release stimulant (methylphenidate hydrochloride) given at bedtime so that it reaches effectiveness levels in the morning; FDA approval of an SNRI, viloxazine (Qelbree), as another nonstimulant option; and a combination CNS stimulant drug (serdexmethylphenidate and dexmethylphenidate [Azstarys]) that is advanced as offering all-day relief in a single daily dose.

Contraindications and Precautions

CNS stimulants are contraindicated in individuals with hypersensitivity to sympathomimetic amines. They should not be used in clients with advanced arteriosclerosis, cardiovascular disease, hypertension, hyperthyroidism, glaucoma, or agitated or hyperexcitability states; in clients with a history of substance misuse; during or within 14 days of receiving therapy with MAOIs; in children younger than age 3; or during pregnancy and lactation. Atomoxetine and bupropion are contraindicated in clients with hypersensitivity to the drugs or their components, in lactation, and in concomitant use with or within 2 weeks of using MAOIs. Atomoxetine is contraindicated in clients with narrow-angle glaucoma. Bupropion is contraindicated in individuals with known or suspected seizure disorder, in the acute phase of MI, and in people with bulimia or anorexia nervosa. Because bupropion reduces the seizure threshold, doses should be given in equally spaced time increments during the day to minimize the risk of seizures. Risk of seizures increases fourfold in doses greater than 450 mg per day (Vallerand & Sanoski, 2022). Alpha-agonists are contraindicated in clients with known hypersensitivity to the drugs.

Caution is advised in using CNS stimulants in children with psychosis; in Tourette's disorder; in clients with anorexia or insomnia; in elderly, debilitated, or asthenic clients; and in clients with a history of suicidal or homicidal tendencies. Prolonged use may result in tolerance and physical or psychological dependence. Atomoxetine and bupropion should be used with caution in clients with urinary retention, hypertension, or hepatic, renal, or cardiovascular disease; in suicidal clients; during pregnancy; and in older and debilitated clients. Alpha-adrenergic agonists should be used with caution in clients with coronary insufficiency, recent MI, or cerebrovascular disease; in chronic renal or hepatic failure; in older adults; and in pregnancy and lactation.

Interactions

■ **CNS Stimulants (Amphetamines):** Effects of amphetamines are increased with furazolidone or urinary alkalinizers. Hypertensive crisis may occur with concomitant use of (and up to several weeks after discontinuing) MAOIs. Increased risk of serotonin syndrome occurs with coadministration of SSRIs. Decreased effects of amphetamines occur with urinary acidifiers, and decreased hypotensive effects of guanethidine occur with amphetamines.

■ *Dexmethylphenidate and Methylphenidate:* Effects of antihypertensive agents and pressor agents (e.g., dopamine, epinephrine, phenylephrine) are decreased with concomitant use of methylphenidates. Effects of coumarin anticoagulants, anticonvulsants (e.g., phenobarbital, phenytoin, primidone), TCAs, and SSRIs are increased with the methylphenidates. Hypertensive crisis may occur with coadministration of MAOIs.

■ *Atomoxetine and Viloxazine (SNRIs):* Effects are increased with concomitant use of CYP2D6 inhibitors (e.g., paroxetine, fluoxetine, quinidine). Potentially fatal reactions may occur with concurrent use of (or within 2 weeks of discontinuation of) MAOIs. Risk of cardiovascular effects is increased with concomitant use of albuterol or vasopressors.

■ *Bupropion (Nonstimulant, Antidepressant):* Effects of bupropion are increased with amantadine, levodopa, or ritonavir. Effects of bupropion are decreased with carbamazepine. There is an increased risk of acute toxicity with MAOIs. Increased risk of hypertension may occur with nicotine replacement agents, and adverse neuropsychiatric events may occur with alcohol. Increased anticoagulant effects of warfarin and increased effects of drugs metabolized by CYP2D6 (e.g., nortriptyline, imipramine, desipramine, paroxetine, fluoxetine, sertraline, haloperidol, risperidone, thioridazine, metoprolol, propafenone, and flecainide) occur with concomitant use.

■ *Alpha-adrenergic Agonists:* Synergistic pharmacological and toxic effects, possibly causing atrioventricular block, bradycardia, and severe hypotension, may occur with concomitant use of calcium channel blockers or beta blockers. Additive sedation occurs with CNS depressants, including alcohol, antihistamines, opioid analgesics, and sedative-hypnotics. Effects of clonidine may be decreased with concomitant use of TCAs and prazosin. Decreased effects of levodopa may occur with clonidine, and effects of guanfacine are decreased with barbiturates or phenytoin.

Diagnosis

The following nursing diagnoses may be considered for patients receiving therapy with agents for ADHD:

■ Risk for injury related to overstimulation and hyperactivity (CNS stimulants) or seizures (possible side effect of bupropion)

■ Risk for suicide secondary to major depression related to abrupt withdrawal after extended use (CNS stimulants)

■ Risk for suicide (children, adolescents, and young adults) as a side effect of atomoxetine and bupropion (boxed warning)

■ Imbalanced nutrition, less than body requirements, related to side effects of anorexia and weight loss (CNS stimulants)

■ Insomnia related to side effects of overstimulation

■ Nausea related to side effects of atomoxetine or bupropion

■ Pain related to side effect of abdominal pain (atomoxetine, bupropion) or headache (all agents)

■ Risk for activity intolerance related to side effects of sedation and dizziness with atomoxetine or bupropion

Safety Issues in Planning and Implementing Care

The plan of care should include monitoring for the following side effects from agents for ADHD. Nursing interventions related to each side effect are discussed in sub-bullets after each side effect.

■ *Overstimulation, restlessness, insomnia* (CNS stimulants)
  ■ Assess mental status for changes in mood, level of activity, degree of stimulation, and aggressiveness.
  ■ Ensure that the patient is protected from injury.
  ■ Keep stimuli low and environment as quiet as possible to discourage overstimulation.
  ■ Administer the last dose at least 6 hours before bedtime to prevent insomnia. Administer sustained-release forms in the morning.

■ *Palpitations, tachycardia* (CNS stimulants, atomoxetine, bupropion, clonidine), or bradycardia (clonidine, guanfacine)
  ■ Monitor and record vital signs at regular intervals (two or three times a day) throughout therapy. Report significant changes to the physician immediately.

Note: The FDA has issued warnings for CNS stimulants and atomoxetine about the risk for sudden death in patients who have cardiovascular disease. A careful personal and family history of heart disease, heart defects, or hypertension should be obtained before these medications are prescribed. Careful monitoring of cardiovascular function during administration must be ongoing.

■ *Anorexia, weight loss* (CNS stimulants, atomoxetine, bupropion)
  ■ Administer the medication immediately after meals to reduce anorexia.
  ■ Weigh the patient regularly (at least weekly) when receiving therapy with CNS stimulants, atomoxetine, or bupropion because of the potential for anorexia and weight loss and temporary interruption of growth and development.

- ***Tolerance, physical and psychological dependence*** (CNS stimulants)
  - Attempt a drug "holiday" periodically in children with ADHD, under the direction of the physician to determine the effectiveness of the medication and the need for continuation.
  - Do not abruptly withdraw CNS stimulants. To do so could initiate a syndrome of symptoms with nausea, vomiting, abdominal cramping, headache, fatigue, weakness, mental depression, *suicidal ideation*, increased dreaming, and psychotic behavior.
- ***Nausea and vomiting*** (atomoxetine and bupropion)
  - Recommend taking medication with food to minimize gastrointestinal upset.
- ***Constipation*** (atomoxetine, bupropion, clonidine, guanfacine)
  - Recommend increasing fiber and fluid in diet if not contraindicated.
- ***Dry mouth*** (clonidine and guanfacine)
  - Offer the patient sugarless candy, ice, and frequent sips of water.
  - Advise the patient that strict oral hygiene is very important.
- ***Sedation*** (clonidine and guanfacine)
  - Warn the patient that this effect is increased by concomitant use of alcohol and other CNS drugs.
  - Warn the patient to refrain from driving or performing hazardous tasks until response has been established.
- *Potential for seizures* (bupropion)
  - Protect the patient from injury if seizure should occur.
  - Instruct family and significant others of patients on bupropion therapy how to protect the patient during a seizure if one should occur.
  - Ensure that doses of the immediate-release medication are administered at least 4 to 6 hours apart and doses of the sustained-release medication at least 8 hours apart.
- ***Severe liver damage*** (with atomoxetine)
  - Monitor for the following side effects and report to the physician immediately: itching, dark urine, right upper quadrant pain, yellow skin or eyes, sore throat, fever, malaise.
- ***New or worsened psychiatric symptoms*** (with CNS stimulants and atomoxetine)
  - Monitor for psychotic symptoms (e.g., hearing voices, paranoid behaviors, delusions).
  - Monitor for manic symptoms, including aggressive and hostile behaviors.
- ***Rebound syndrome*** (with clonidine and guanfacine)
  - Instruct the patient not to discontinue therapy abruptly. To do so may result in symptoms of nervousness, agitation, headache, tremor, and a rapid rise in blood pressure. In addition, sudden withdrawal from stimulants may increase the risk of depression and suicide. Dosage should be tapered gradually under the supervision of the physician.
  - Assess the patient for signs of depression and risk for suicide because abrupt withdrawal increases these risks.

Patient and Family Education

Instruct the patient and family that the patient should:

- Use caution when driving or operating dangerous machinery. Drowsiness, dizziness, and blurred vision can occur.
- Not stop taking CNS stimulants abruptly. To do so could produce serious withdrawal symptoms.
- Avoid taking CNS stimulants late in the day to prevent insomnia. Take medication no later than 6 hours before bedtime.
- Not take other medications (including over-the-counter drugs) without the physician's approval. Many medications contain substances that, in combination with agents for ADHD, can be harmful.
- Monitor blood sugar two or three times a day or as instructed by the physician if the patient is diabetic. Be aware of the need for possible alteration in insulin requirements because of changes in food intake, weight, and activity.
- Avoid consumption of large amounts of caffeinated products (coffee, tea, colas, chocolate), as they may enhance the CNS stimulant effect.
- Notify physician if restlessness, insomnia, anorexia, or dry mouth becomes severe or if rapid, pounding heartbeat becomes evident.
- Report any of the following side effects to the physician immediately: shortness of breath, chest pain, jaw/left arm pain, fainting, seizures, sudden vision changes, weakness on one side of the body, slurred speech, confusion, itching, dark urine, right upper quadrant pain, yellow skin or eyes, sore throat, fever, malaise, increased hyperactivity, believing things that are not true, or hearing voices.
- Be aware of possible risks of taking agents for ADHD during pregnancy. Safe use during pregnancy and lactation has not been established. Inform the physician immediately if pregnancy is suspected or planned.
- Be aware of potential side effects of agents for ADHD. Refer to written materials furnished by health-care providers for safe self-administration.
- Carry a card or other identification at all times describing current medications.

Outcome Criteria and Evaluation

The following criteria may be used for evaluating the effectiveness of therapy with agents for ADHD.
  The patient:

■ Does not exhibit excessive hyperactivity
■ Has not experienced injury
■ Is maintaining expected parameters of growth and development
■ Verbalizes understanding of safe self-administration and the importance of not withdrawing medication abruptly

Summary and Key Points

■ Psychotropic medications are intended to be used as adjunctive therapy to individual or group psychotherapy.
■ *Antianxiety agents* are used in the treatment of anxiety disorders and to alleviate acute anxiety symptoms. Benzodiazepines are the most commonly used group of antianxiety agents. They are CNS depressants and have the potential for physical and psychological dependence. They should not be discontinued abruptly after long-term use because they can produce a life-threatening withdrawal syndrome. The most common side effects are drowsiness, confusion, and lethargy.
■ *Antidepressants* elevate mood and alleviate other symptoms associated with moderate-to-severe depression. These drugs work by increasing the concentration of norepinephrine, serotonin, or dopamine in the body.
■ The tricyclics and related drugs accomplish their effects by blocking the reuptake of norepinephrine at the neuron.
■ Another group of antidepressants inhibits MAO, an enzyme that is known to inactivate norepinephrine and serotonin. They are called MAOIs.
■ A third category of drugs, SSRIs, blocks neuronal reuptake of serotonin and has minimal or no effect on reuptake of norepinephrine or dopamine.
■ SNRIs are antidepressant medications that block reuptake of serotonin and norepinephrine.
■ Atypical antidepressants are a group of medications that act differently than other classes of antidepressants to decrease reuptake of serotonin, norepinephrine, and/or dopamine.
■ Esketamine nasal spray is a novel treatment for treatment-resistant depression that acts as an NMDA receptor antagonist. How it exerts antidepressant effects is unknown.
■ Antidepressant medications may take up to 2 weeks before desired effects are noticed and may take up to 4 weeks to produce full therapeutic

benefits. The most common side effects are anticholinergic effects, sedation, and orthostatic hypotension. They can also reduce the seizure threshold. MAOIs can cause a hypertensive crisis if food or other products containing tyramine are consumed while taking these medications.
■ Lithium carbonate is widely used as a *mood-stabilizing agent*. Its mechanism of action is not fully understood, but it is thought to enhance the reuptake of norepinephrine and serotonin in the brain, thereby lowering the levels in the body, resulting in decreased hyperactivity. The most common side effects are dry mouth, gastrointestinal upset, polyuria, and weight gain.
■ There is a narrow margin between the therapeutic and toxic levels of lithium. Serum levels must be drawn regularly to monitor for toxicity.
■ Symptoms of lithium toxicity are most noticeable at or greater than 1.5 mEq/L. If left untreated, lithium toxicity can be life-threatening.
■ Several other medications are used as mood-stabilizing agents. Two groups, anticonvulsants (carbamazepine, clonazepam, valproic acid, lamotrigine, oxcarbazepine, and topiramate) and the calcium channel blocker verapamil, have been used with some effectiveness. Their action in the treatment of bipolar mania is not well understood.
■ More recently, several atypical antipsychotic medications have been used with success in the treatment of bipolar mania. These include olanzapine, aripiprazole, quetiapine, risperidone, asenapine, and ziprasidone. The first generation phenothiazine, chlorpromazine, has also been used effectively. The action of antipsychotics in the treatment of bipolar mania is not well understood.
■ *Antipsychotic drugs* are primarily used in the treatment of acute and chronic psychoses. The action of typical antipsychotics is a result of blocking postsynaptic dopamine receptors in the basal ganglia. Their most common side effects include anticholinergic effects, sedation, weight gain, reduction in seizure threshold, photosensitivity, and EPS.
■ The newer generation of antipsychotic medications (atypical or second generation), which includes clozapine, risperidone, paliperidone, olanzapine, quetiapine, aripiprazole, asenapine, iloperidone, lurasidone, and ziprasidone, may have an effect on dopamine, serotonin, and other neurotransmitters. They show evidence of greater efficacy with less risk for EPS but have been associated with increased risk for metabolic disturbances and weight gain.

- *Antiparkinsonian agents* are used to counteract the EPS associated with antipsychotic medications. Antiparkinsonian drugs restore the natural balance of acetylcholine and dopamine in the brain. The most common side effects of these drugs are anticholinergic effects. They may also cause sedation and orthostatic hypotension.
- Agents for the treatment of tardive dyskinesia are used to reduce movement disturbances associated with antipsychotic medications. Their action is unknown but believed to be associated with inhibition of monoamine transport. Valbenazine (Ingrezza) and deutetrabenazine (Austeda) were both approved by the FDA for this indication in 2017.
- *Sedative-hypnotics* are used in the management of anxiety states and to treat insomnia. These CNS depressants (with the exception of ramelteon) have the potential for physical and psychological dependence. They are indicated for short-term use only. Many side effects and nursing implications are similar to those described for antianxiety medications.
- An FDA boxed warning is required in prescribing information for eszopiclone, zaleplon, and zolpidem related to serious injuries and death associated with complex sleep behaviors, which may occur with these medications.
- Several medications are used to treat ADHD. These include CNS stimulants, which have the potential for physical and psychological dependence. Tolerance develops quickly with CNS stimulants, and they should not be withdrawn abruptly because they can produce serious withdrawal symptoms. The most common side effects are restlessness, anorexia, and insomnia. Other nonstimulant medications that have demonstrated efficacy in treating ADHD include atomoxetine, viloxazine, bupropion, and the alpha-adrenergic agonists clonidine and guanfacine. Their mechanism of action in the treatment of ADHD is not clear.

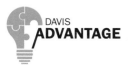 Go to **Davis Advantage** to complete your learning: strengthen understanding, apply your knowledge, and prepare for the Next Gen NCLEX®.

Review Questions

1. How do antianxiety medications, such as benzodiazepines, produce a calming effect?
   a. Depressing the CNS
   b. Decreasing levels of norepinephrine and serotonin in the brain
   c. Decreasing levels of dopamine in the brain
   d. Inhibiting production of the enzyme MAO

2. There is a narrow margin between the therapeutic and toxic levels of lithium carbonate. Symptoms of toxicity are most likely to appear when the serum levels exceed:
   a. 0.15 mEq/L
   b. 1.5 mEq/L
   c. 15.0 mEq/L
   d. 150 mEq/L

3. Initial symptoms of lithium toxicity include:
   a. Constipation, dry mouth
   b. Dizziness, thirst
   c. Vomiting, diarrhea
   d. Anuria, arrhythmias

4. Antipsychotic medications are thought to decrease psychotic symptoms by:
   a. Blocking reuptake of norepinephrine and serotonin
   b. Blocking the action of dopamine in the brain
   c. Inhibiting production of the enzyme MAO
   d. Depressing the CNS

5. Part of the nurse's ongoing assessment of the client taking antipsychotic medications is to observe for extrapyramidal symptoms. Which of the following are examples of extrapyramidal symptoms?
   a. Muscular weakness, rigidity, tremors, facial spasms
   b. Dry mouth, blurred vision, urinary retention, orthostatic hypotension
   c. Amenorrhea, gynecomastia, retrograde ejaculation
   d. Elevated blood pressure, severe occipital headache, stiff neck

Clinical Judgment Questions

6. A client who is prescribed haloperidol is observed to be staring at the ceiling and says they cannot move their eyes. The nurse notices that the client also appears to have muscle spasms in their legs and hands. What is the most appropriate action for the nurse to take at this point?
   a. Conduct an AIMS test.
   b. Administer prn benztropine (Cogentin).
   c. Withhold the next dose of antipsychotic medication.
   d. Contact the physician.

7. A client reports to the nurse that after having been on antidepressant medication (fluoxetine) for almost 2 weeks, they don't feel much better. Which of these actions by the nurse demonstrates the best clinical judgment?
   a. Educate the client that this medication may not be fully effective for up to 4 weeks.
   b. Hold the next dose and contact the physician to recommend an alternative antidepressant.
   c. Check the client's vital signs and check labs for therapeutic blood levels.
   d. Assess whether the client is aware of mood swings or history of bipolar disorder in their family.

8. A client who was recently prescribed an MAOI tells the nurse that they drink three to four cups of coffee with each meal. Which of these actions by the nurse demonstrates the best clinical judgment?
   a. Instruct the client that they only need to avoid foods high in tyramine; coffee consumption is not an issue with this medication.
   b. Inform the client that foods or beverages with high caffeine content increase the risk for serious hypertension and arrhythmias.
   c. Inform the client that caffeine interferes with the effectiveness of this medication.
   d. Instruct the client that red wines are a better beverage choice because they do not contain tyramine.

9. A young adult client has been prescribed an SSRI antidepressant, which they have been taking for 1 week. The client reports that they think they are getting worse and that nothing is going to help. Which of these actions by the nurse is a priority?
   a. Educate the client that SSRIs have a lag period before full therapeutic effectiveness is apparent.
   b. Ask the client to describe why they think they are depressed.
   c. Contact the physician to recommend a different medication.
   d. Conduct a suicide risk assessment.

10. A licensed practical nurse who is administering medications reports to the registered nurse (RN) in charge that they forgot to give the last scheduled dose of bupropion to a client. The licensed practical nurse (LPN) asks the RN if they should give the client two doses at the next scheduled time. Which of these responses by the RN demonstrates the best clinical judgment?
   a. "Yes, that would be fine. Just make sure the client stays in bed because this is a sedating medication."
   b. "No. Doses of this medication should not be doubled because that poses an increased risk for seizures."
   c. "Yes, as long as the client has not changed his sodium intake recently."
   d. "No, doses should not be doubled because there is an increased risk of tolerance and addiction."

References

Aiken, C. (2020). Novel approaches to bipolar: What worked, and what did not, in 2019. *Psychiatric Times*. https://www.psychiatrictimes.com/view/novel-approaches-bipolar-what-worked-and-what-did-not-2019

Anderson, K. N., Ailes, E. C., Lind, J. N., Broussard, C. S., Bitsko, R. H., Friedman, J. M., Bobo, W. V., Reefhuis, J., Tinker, S. C. (2020). Atypical antipsychotic use during pregnancy and birth defect risk: National Birth Defects Prevention Study, 1997–2011. *Schizophrenia Research, 215*, 81–88. doi: 10.1016/j.schres.2019.11.019

Anderson, L. (2018). *Drug interactions with grapefruit juice.* https://www.drugs.com/article/grapefruit-drug-interactions.html

Boland, R., & Verduin, M. L. (2022). *Kaplan & Sadock's synopsis of psychiatry* (P. Ruiz, Ed.). (12th ed.). Wolters Kluwer.

Chaves, T., Fazekas, C. L., Horváth, K., Correia, P., Szabó, A., Török, B., Bánrévi, K., & Zelena, D. (2021). Stress adaptation and the brainstem with focus on corticotropin-releasing hormone. *International Journal of Molecular Science, 22*(16), 9090. doi: 10.3390/ijms22169090. PMID: 34445795; PMCID: PMC8396605.

Chow, C. L., Kadouh, N. K., Bostwick, J. R., & VandenBerg, A. M. (2020). Akathisia and newer second generation antipsychotic drugs: A review of current evidence. *Pharmacotherapy, 40*(6), 565–574.

Clozapine REMS. (2015). *Clozapine and the risk of neutropenia: A guide for healthcare providers.* https://www.clozapinerems.com/CpmgClozapineUI/rems/pdf/resources/Clozapine_REMS_HCP_Guide.pdf

Cooper, B. E., & Sejnowski, C. A. (2013). Serotonin syndrome: Recognition and treatment. *AACN Advanced Critical Care, 24*(1), 15–20. doi: 10.1097/NCI.0b013e31827eecc6

Correll, C. U., Demyttenaere, K., Fagiolini, A., Hajak, G., Pallanti, S., Racagni, G., & Singh, S. (2020). Cariprazine in the management of negative symptoms of schizophrenia: State of the art and future perspectives. *Future Neurology, 15*(4). https://www.futuremedicine.com/doi/10.2217/fnl-2020-0012#:~:text=In%20patients%20with%20persistent%20predominant,prevent%20relapse%20in%20schizophrenic%20patients.

Drugs.com. (2022). *FDA pregnancy categories: FDA pregnancy risk information: An update.* https://www.drugs.com/pregnancy-categories.html

Food and Drug Administration (FDA). (2016a). *FDA Drug Safety Communication: FDA warns about new impulse-control problems associated with mental health drug aripiprazole (Abilify, Abilify Maintena, Aristada).* https://www.fda.gov/Drugs/DrugSafety/ucm498662.htm

Food and Drug Administration (FDA). (2016b). *FDA Drug Safety Communication: FDA warns about rare but serious skin reactions with mental health drug olanzapine (Zyprexa, Zyprexa Zydis, Zyprexa Relprevv, and Symbyax).* https://www.fda.gov/Drugs/DrugSafety/ucm499441.htm

Food and Drug Administration (FDA). (2016c). *FDA Drug Safety Communication: FDA warns about serious risks and death when combining opioid pain or cough medicines with benzodiazepines; requires its strongest warning.* http://www.fda.gov/Drugs/DrugSafety/ucm518473.htm

Food and Drug Administration (FDA). (2017). *FDA approves first drug to treat tardive dyskinesia.* https://www.fda.gov/NewsEvents/Newsroom/PressAnnouncements/ucm552418.htm

Food and Drug Administration (FDA). (2019). *FDA approves new nasal spray medication for treatment-resistant depression; available only at a certified doctor's office or clinic* [Press Release]. https://www.fda.gov/news-events/press-announcements/fda-approves-new-nasal-spray-medication-treatment-resistant-depression-available-only-certified

Food and Drug Administration (FDA). (2020). *FDA strengthens warning that untreated constipation caused by schizophrenia medicine clozapine (Clozaril) can lead to serious bowel problems.* https://www.fda.gov/drugs/fda-drug-safety-podcasts/fda-strengthens-warning-untreated-constipation-caused-schizophrenia-medicine-clozapine-clozaril-can#:~:text =

Forma, F., Green, T., Kim, S., & Teigland, C. (2020). Antipsychotic medication adherence and healthcare services utilization in two cohorts of patients with serious mental illness. *Clinicoeconomics and Outcomes Research, 12*, 123–132. doi: 10.2147/CEOR.S231000

Fournier, J. C., DeRubeis, R. J., Hollon, S. D., Dimidjian, S., Amsterdam, J. D., Shelton, R. C., & Fawcett, J. (2010). Antidepressant drug effects and depression severity: A patient-level meta-analysis. *Journal of the American Medical Association, 303*(1), 47–53. doi: 10.1001/jama.2009.1943

Gerlach, L. B., Wiechers, I. R., & Maust, D. T. (2018). Prescription benzodiazepine use among older adults: A critical review. *Harvard Review of Psychiatry, 26*(5), 264–273. https://doi.org/10.1097/HRP.0000000000000190

Greenhill, L. (2022). Advances in treatment for ADHD. *Psychiatric Times, 39*(1). https://www.psychiatrictimes.com/view/advances-in-treatments-for-adhd

Gress, T., Miller, M., Meadows, C., & Neitch, S. M. (2020). Benzodiazepine overuse in elders: Defining the problem and potential solutions. *Cureus, 2*(10), e11042. doi: 10.7759/cureus.11042

Gukasyan, N., Davis, A. K., Barrett, F. S., Cosimano, M. P., Sepeda, N. D., Johnson, M. W., & Griffiths, R. R. (2022). Efficacy and safety of psilocybin-assisted treatment for major depressive disorder: Prospective 12-month follow-up. *Journal of Psychopharmacology, 36*(2), 151–158. https://doi.org/10.1177/02698811211073759

Gunduz-Bruce, H., Silber, C., Kaul, I., Rothschild. A. J., Riesenberg, R., Sankoh, A.J., Li, H., Lasser, R., Zorumski, C. F., Rubinow, D. R., Paul, S. M., Jonas, J., Doherty, J. J., & Kanes, S. J. (2019). Trial of SAGE-217 in patients with major depressive disorder. *New England Journal of Medicine, 381*(10), 903–911. https://doi.org/10.1056/NEJMoa1815981

Guzman, F. (2021). Methylphenidate for ADHD: Mechanism of action and formulations. *Psychopharmacology Institute.* https://psychopharmacologyinstitute.com/publication/methylphenidate-for-adhd-mechanism-of-action-and-formulations-2194

Haddad, P. M., Brain, C., & Scott, J. (2014). Nonadherence with antipsychotic medication in schizophrenia: Challenges and management strategies. *Patient Related Outcome Measures, 5*, 43–62. http://www.ncbi.nlm.nih.gov/pmc/articles/PMC4085309/

Horn, J. R., & Hansten, P. D. (2008). Get to know an enzyme: CYP2C19. *Pharmacy Times.* https://www.pharmacytimes.com/publications/issue/2008/2008-05/2008-05-8538

Institute of Medicine. (2003). *Health professions education: A bridge to quality.* Washington, DC: Author.

Janicak, P. G., & Hussain, K. (2017). Medication induced movement disorders. In B. J. Sadock, V. A. Sadock, & P. Ruiz (Eds.), *Comprehensive textbook of psychiatry* (10th ed., pp. 2936–2944). Wolters Kluwer.

Jones, D. S. (2006). Racial profiling in psychiatry: Does it help patients? *Psychiatric Times, 23*(14).

Köhler-Forsberg, O., Lydholm, C.N., Hjorthøj, C., Nordentoft, M., Mors, O., Benros, M. E. (2019). Efficacy of anti-inflammatory treatment on major depressive disorder or depressive symptoms: Meta-analysis of clinical trials. *Acta Psychiatrica Scandinavica, 139*(5), 404–419. https://doi.org/10.1111/acps.13016

Kose, S., & Cetin, M. (2018). Triple reuptake inhibitors (TRIs): Do they promise us a rose garden? *Psychiatry and Clinical Pharmacology, 28*(2), 119–122. doi.org/10.1080/24750573. 2018.1443386

Lenze, E. J., Mulsant, B. H., Blumberger, D. M., Karp, J. F., Newcomer, J. W., Anderson, S. J., & Reynolds, C. F. (2015). Efficacy, safety, and tolerability of augmentation pharmacotherapy with aripiprazole for treatment resistant depression in late life: A randomized placebo-controlled study. *Lancet, 386*(10011), 2404–2412. doi:http://dx.doi.org/10.1016/So140-6736(15)00308-6

Li, K., Shen, S., Ji, Y. T., Li, X. Y., Zhang, L., &Wang, X. D. (2018). Melatonin BDNF-TrkB signaling. *Neuroscience Bulletin, 34*(2), 303–311. doi:10.1007/s12264-017-019-z

Lien, Y. H. H. (2018). Antidepressants and hyponatremia. *American Journal of Medicine, 131*(1), 7–8. doi.org/10.1016/j. amjmed.2017.09.002

Lynch, T., & Price, A. (2007). The effect of cytochrome P450 metabolism on drug response, interactions, and adverse effects. *American Family Physician, 76*(3), 391–396.

Maust, D. T., Kales, H. C., Weichers, I. R., Blow, F. C., & Olfson, M. (2016). No end in sight: Benzodiazepine use among older adults in the United States. *Journal of the American Geriatric Society, 64*(12), 2546–2553. https://doi.org/10.1111/jgs.14379

Miklowitz, D. J., Efthimiou, O., Furukawa, T. A., Scott, J., McLaren, R., Geddes, J. R., & Cipriani, A. (2020). Adjunctive psychotherapy for bipolar disorder: A systematic review and component network meta-analysis. *JAMA Psychiatry, 78*(2), 141–150. https://doi.org/10.1001/jamapsychiatry.2020.2993

Muttoni, S., Ardissino, M., & John, C. (2019). Classical psychedelics for the treatment of depression and anxiety: A systematic review. *Journal of Affective Disorders, 258*, 11–24. https://doi.org/10.1016/j.jad.2019.07.076

National Institute of Mental Health (NIMH). (2006). *Questions and answers about the NIMH sequenced treatment alternatives to relieve depression (STAR*D) study — All medication levels.* https:// www.nimh.nih.gov/funding/clinical-research/practical/stard/allmedicationlevelsNeubauer, D. N. (2020). Lemborexant for insomnia. *Current Psychiatry, 19*(11), 43–49.

New York State Office of Mental Health. (2012). An explanation of Kendra's law. https://www.omh.ny.gov/omhweb/kendra_web/ksummary.htm

Nolen, W. A., Licht, R. W., Young, A. H., Malhi, G. S., Tohen, M., Vieta, E., Kupka, R. W., Zarate, C., Nielsen, R. E., Baldessarini, R. J., Severus, E., & ISBD/IGSLI Task Force on the Treatment with Lithium. (2019). What is the optimal serum level for lithium in the maintenance treatment of bipolar disorder? A systematic review and recommendations from the ISBD/IGSLI Task Force on treatment with lithium. *Bipolar Disorders, 21*(5), 394–409. https://doi.org/10.1111/bdi.12805

Ramnarine, M., & Ahmed, D. (2022). *Anticholinergic toxicity.* http://emedicine.medscape.com/article/812644-overview

Rege, S. (2020). Lithium prescribing and monitoring in clinical practice—A practical guide. *Psychscenehub.* https://psychscenehub.com/psychinsights/lithium-prescribing-monitoring-clinical-practice/#:~:text = CLINICAL

Remaly, J. (2020). FDA approves diazepam nasal spray for seizure clusters. *Neurology Reviews.* https://www.mdedge.com/neurology/article/215442/epilepsy-seizures/fda-approves-diazepam-nasal-spray-seizure-clusters

Rubino, A., Sanon, M., Ganz, M. L., Simpson, A., Fenton, M. C., Sumit Verma, M. S., Hartry, A., Baker, R. A., Duffy, R. A., Gwin, K., & Fillit, H. (2020). Association of the US food and drug administration antipsychotic drug boxed warning with medication use and health outcomes in elderly patients with dementia. *JAMA Network Open, 3*(4), e203630. doi: 10.1001/jamanetworkopen.2020.3630

Scarff, J. R. (2017). The prospects of cariprazine in the treatment of schizophrenia. *Therapeutic Advances in Psychopharmacology, 7*(11), 237–239. doi: 10.1177/2045125317727260

Shorter, E. (2009). The history of lithium therapy. *Bipolar Disorders, 11*(Suppl. 2), 4–9. doi: 10.1111/j.1399-5618.2009.00706.x

Tonon, A. C., Pilz, L. K., Markus, R. P., Hidalgo, M. P., & Elisabetsky, E. (2021). Melatonin and depression: A translational perspective from animal models to clinical studies. *Frontiers in Psychiatry, 12*, 638981. doi: 10.3389/fpsyt.2021. 638981

Tumolo, J. (2020). FDA clears video game as treatment for ADHD. *Psych Congress Network.* https://www.psychcongress.com/article/fda-clears-video-game-treatment-adhd?hmpid =

U.S. Department of Health and Human Services. Available for use in the public domain from Guy W. *ECDEU Assessment Manual for Psychopharmacology:Revised (DHEW publication number ADM 76-338).* Rockville, MD, US Department of Health, Education and Welfare, Public Health Service, Alcohol, Drug Abuse and Mental Health Administration, NIMH Psychopharmacology Research Branch, Division of Extramural Research Programs, 1976: 534–537.

U.S. Department of Justice. (n.d.). *Controlled substance schedules.* https://www.deadiversion.usdoj.gov/schedules/#:~:text= Definition%

Vallerand, A. H., & Sanoski, C. A. (2022). *Davis's drug guide for nurses* (18th ed.). F.A. Davis.

Yin, J., & Yuan, Q. (2015). Structural homeostasis in the nervous system: A balancing act for wiring plasticity and stability. *Frontiers in Cellular Neuroscience, 8*, 439. doi: 10.3389/fncel.2014.00439

Classical References

Sage, D. L. (Producer). (1984). The brain: Madness [television broadcast]. Public Broadcasting Company.

Ethical and Legal Issues

5

CORE CONCEPTS

Professionalism: Ethics
Health Policy
Legal Aspects
Safety
Social Determinants
of Health
Clinical Judgment

KEY TERMS

advocacy	ethical dilemma	negligence
assault	ethical egoism	nonmaleficence
autonomy	ethics	privileged communication
battery	false imprisonment	rights
beneficence	informed consent	slander
bioethics	justice	statutory law
Christian ethics	Kantianism	tort
civil law	libel	utilitarianism
common law	malpractice	values
criminal law	moral behavior	values clarification
defamation of character	morals	veracity
divine command ethics	natural law theory	

OBJECTIVES
After reading this chapter, the student will be able to:

1. Differentiate between *ethics, morals, values,* and *rights.*
2. Discuss ethical theories, including *utilitarianism, Kantianism, Christian ethics, natural law theories,* and *ethical egoism.*
3. Define *ethical dilemma.*
4. Discuss the ethical principles of *autonomy, beneficence, nonmaleficence, justice,* and *veracity.*
5. Use an ethical decision-making model to make an ethical decision.
6. Describe ethical issues relevant to psychiatric-mental health nursing.
7. Define *statutory law and common law.*
8. Differentiate between *civil law* and *criminal law.*
9. Discuss legal issues relevant to psychiatric-mental health nursing.
10. Differentiate between *malpractice* and *negligence.*
11. Identify behaviors relevant to the psychiatric-mental health setting for which specific malpractice action could be taken.

Nurses are constantly faced with the challenge of making difficult decisions regarding good and evil or life and death. Complex situations frequently arise in caring for individuals with mental illness, and nurses are held to the highest level of legal and ethical accountability in their professional practice. This chapter presents basic ethical and legal concepts and their relationship to psychiatric-mental health nursing. A discussion of ethical theory is presented as a foundation on which ethical decisions may be made. The American Nurses Association (ANA) (2015) has established a code of ethics for nurses to use as a framework within which to make ethical choices and decisions. These revised provisions and interpretive guidelines have been expanded to address some of the complexities of the current health-care environment and include ethical principles regarding the nurse's duty not only to the patient but also to themselves and all people with whom they interact. According to the code, the nurse's primary responsibility is to the patient (whether that is an individual, family, group, community, or population), and all relationships should be conducted within a culture of respect and civility.

⬥ The ANA Code of Ethics interpretive guidelines include a discussion of the importance of teamwork and collaboration, which is consistent with one of the recommendations of the Institute of Medicine (IOM) (2003) (now renamed the National Academy of Medicine) for improving the future of health care and has become one of the Quality and Safety Education for Nurses (QSEN) competencies.

The ANA, in cooperation with the American Psychiatric Nurses Association and the International Society of Psychiatric-Mental Health Nurses (2022), has published a scope and standards of practice manual specifically for psychiatric-mental health nursing. It maintains consistency with the ANA code of ethics and applies those provisions to psychiatric-mental health nursing issues. Knowledge about the *Code of Ethics for Nurses* (ANA, 2015) and *Psychiatric-Mental Health Nursing: Scope and Standards of Practice* (ANA et al., 2022) is essential for guiding practice because they clarify the accepted expectations of the nurse in this field.

Because legislation determines what is *right* or *good* within a society, legal issues pertaining to psychiatric-mental health nursing are also discussed in this chapter. Definitions are presented along with a description of the generally accepted and legal rights of psychiatric clients. Nursing competency and client care accountability are compromised when the nurse has inadequate knowledge about the laws that regulate the practice of nursing.

Application of the legal and ethical concepts presented in this chapter promotes quality care in psychiatric-mental health nursing practice and promotes legal accountability. The right to practice nursing carries with it the responsibility to maintain a specific level of competency and to practice in accordance with certain ethical and legal standards of care.

CORE CONCEPTS

Ethics is a branch of philosophy that deals with systematic approaches to distinguishing right from wrong behavior (Butts & Rich, 2019). **Bioethics** is the term applied to these principles when they refer to concepts within the scope of medicine, nursing, and allied health.

Morals are fundamental standards of right and wrong that are learned and internalized (Catalano, 2020). **Moral behavior** is conduct that results from serious critical thinking about how individuals ought to treat others. Moral behavior reflects the way a person interprets basic respect for other people, such as the respect for autonomy, freedom, justice, honesty, and confidentiality. **Values** are personal beliefs about what is important and desirable (Butts & Rich, 2019). **Values clarification** is a process of self-exploration through which individuals identify and rank their personal values. This process increases awareness about why individuals behave in certain ways. Values clarification is important in nursing to increase understanding about why choices and decisions are made over others and how values affect nursing outcomes.

Rights are expectations to which an individual is entitled either by established laws, policies, or ethical principles. A right is *absolute* when there is no restriction whatsoever on the individual's entitlement. A *legal right* is one on which the society has agreed and formalized into law. Both the National League for Nursing (NLN) and the American Hospital Association (AHA) have established guidelines of patients' rights. Although these are not considered legal documents, nurses and hospitals are responsible for upholding these rights of patients.

Ethical Considerations

Theoretical Perspectives

An *ethical theory* is a set of philosophical principles that can be used to guide how an individual makes decisions on ethical questions and issues. Several ethical theories are described here.

Utilitarianism

The basis of **utilitarianism** is the "greatest-happiness principle." This principle holds that actions are right to the degree that they tend to promote happiness and are wrong as they tend to produce the reverse of happiness. Thus, the good is happiness and the right is that which promotes the good. Conversely, the wrongness of an action is determined by its tendency to bring about unhappiness. An ethical decision based on the utilitarian view looks at the end results of the decision. Action is taken on the basis of the end results that will produce the most good (happiness) for the most people.

Kantianism

Named for philosopher Immanuel Kant, **Kantianism** is directly opposed to utilitarianism. Kant argued that it is not the consequences or end results that make an action right or wrong; rather, it is the principle or motivation on which the action is based that is the morally decisive factor. Kantianism suggests that our actions are bound by a sense of duty. This theory is often called *deontology* (from the Greek word *deon,* which means "that which is binding; duty"). Kantian-directed ethical decisions are made out of respect for moral law. For example, "I make this choice because it is morally right and my duty to do so" (not because of consideration for a possible outcome).

Divine Command Ethics

The **divine command ethics** approach to decision making is focused on that which is commanded by God. Many contemporary religions, including Judaism, Islam, and Christianity and numerous polytheistic religions, incorporate the importance of divine commands in ethical decision making (Rae, 2009). In Christian ethics, ethical decisions are based in the way of life and teachings of Jesus Christ. This ethical theory advances the importance of virtues such as love, forgiveness, and honesty and is associated with the principle "Do unto others as you would have them do unto you." In Judaism, the Ten Commandments, which focus on loving God and loving others, are considered divine commands. In Islam, the focus is on the moral principles and virtues elaborated in Islamic religious texts, including good character, kindness, charity, and forgiveness.

Natural Law Theory

Natural law theory is based on the writings of St. Thomas Aquinas. It advances the idea that decisions about right versus wrong are self-evident and determined by human nature. The theory espouses that, as rational human beings, we inherently know the difference between good and evil (believed to be the knowledge that is given to man from God), and this knowledge directs our decision making.

Ethical Egoism

Ethical egoism espouses that what is right and good is what is best for the individual making the decision. An individual's actions are determined by what is to their advantage. The action may not be best for anyone else involved, but consideration is only for the individual making the decision.

 Providing patient-centered care, an important health professions education competency identified in the IOM report (2013), speaks to some elements of ethical egoism. This competency promotes listening to and respecting the patient's values, preferences, and expressed needs in care management decisions.

Ethical Dilemmas

An **ethical dilemma** in nursing is a situation that requires the nurse to make a choice between two equally balanced alternatives (Catalano, 2020). Evidence exists to support both moral "rightness" and moral "wrongness" related to a certain action. The individual who must make the choice experiences conscious conflict regarding the decision.

Not all ethical issues are dilemmas. An ethical dilemma arises when there is no clear reason to choose one action over another. Ethical dilemmas generally create a great deal of emotion. Often, the reasons supporting each side of the argument for action are logical and appropriate. The actions associated with both sides are desirable in some respects and undesirable in others. In most situations, taking no action is considered an action taken. For example, consider a patient who refuses to take a prescribed cardiac medication, claiming that they do not believe it is necessary. Although each patient has the right to refuse medication under ordinary circumstances, if the same patient is known to be depressed and suicidal, might they be intending self-harm by their refusal to take such a medication? And, if so, what is the best course of action?

Many health-care settings have established guidelines for how to proceed should an ethical question or dilemma arise. Hospitals typically have a formal committee to explore and analyze ethical issues from several vantage points. Nurses can improve their critical thinking and clinical judgment skills by identifying such issues and seeking clarification through collaborative exploration with others and through ethics committee involvement.

Ethical Principles

Ethical principles are fundamental guidelines that influence decision making. The ethical principles of autonomy, beneficence, nonmaleficence, veracity, and justice are examples that are used frequently by health-care workers to assist with ethical decision making.

Autonomy

The principle of **autonomy** arises from the Kantian view of people as autonomous moral agents whose right to determine their destinies should always be respected. This view presumes that individuals are always capable of making independent choices. Health-care workers know this is not always the case. Children, comatose individuals, and some people with serious mental illness are incapable of making informed choices. In these instances, a representative of the individual is usually asked to intervene and give consent. However, health-care workers must ensure that respect for an individual's autonomy is not disregarded in favor of what another person may view as best for the client.

Beneficence

Beneficence refers to one's duty to benefit or promote the good of others. Health-care workers who act in their clients' interests are beneficent, provided their actions serve the individuals' best interests. In fact, some duties do take preference over other duties. For example, the duty to respect the autonomy of an individual may be overridden when that individual has been deemed harmful to self or others. "Doing good" for the patient should not be confused with "doing whatever the patient wants" (Indiana State Nurses Association [ISNA] Bulletin, 2013). Good care must include a holistic focus that considers the patient's beliefs, feelings, and wishes; the wishes of the family and significant others; and considerations about competent nursing care (Catalano, 2020). Despite these guidelines, it is not always clear which action *is* in the best interest of the client. When such dilemmas occur, nurses should reach out to available resources, such as an ethics committee or a supervisor, to build confidence that their decisions have explored various vantage points.

Peplau (1991) recognized patient **advocacy** as an essential role for the psychiatric nurse. The term *advocacy* means acting in another's behalf as a supporter or defender. Being a patient advocate in psychiatric nursing means helping patients fulfill needs that, without assistance and because of their illness, may go unfulfilled. Individuals with mental illness are not always able to speak for themselves. Nurses serve in this manner to protect patients' rights and interests. Strategies include educating patients and their families about their legal rights, ensuring that patients have sufficient information to make informed decisions or to give informed consent, assisting patients to consider alternatives, and supporting them in the decisions they make. Additionally, nurses may act as advocates by speaking on behalf of individuals with mental illness to secure essential mental health services.

Nonmaleficence

Nonmaleficence is the requirement that health-care providers do no harm to their clients, either intentionally or unintentionally. Some philosophers suggest that this principle is more important than beneficence; that is, they support the notion that it is more important to avoid doing harm than it is to do good. In any event, ethical dilemmas arise when a conflict exists between an individual's rights and what is thought to best represent the welfare of the individual. An example of this conflict might occur when a psychiatric patient refuses antipsychotic medication (consistent with their rights), and the nurse must then decide how to maintain patient safety while psychotic symptoms continue.

Justice

The principle of **justice** has been referred to as the "justice as fairness" principle. It is sometimes called *distributive justice,* and its basic premise lies with the right of individuals to be treated equally and fairly regardless of race, gender, sexual orientation, marital status, medical diagnosis, social standing, economic level, or religious beliefs (Catalano, 2020). When applied to health care, the principle of justice suggests that all resources (including health-care services) ought to be distributed equally to all people. Thus, according to this principle, the vast disparity in the quality of care dispensed to the various socioeconomic classes within our society would be considered unjust. *Retribution* or *restorative justice* refers to the rules for responding when expectations for fairness are violated. *Social justice* assumes that rules for both distribution and rules for retribution should be fair and people should play by the rules (Maiese, 2017). It is important for nurses to recognize that in the latest revision of the *Code of Ethics for Nurses* (ANA, 2015), a new focus in one of the provisions states that nursing should integrate principles of social justice both in practice and in developing health policy.

Veracity

The principle of **veracity** refers to one's duty to always be truthful. Catalano (2020) stated that veracity "requires the health-care provider to tell the truth and not intentionally deceive or mislead clients" (p. 128). There are times when limitations must be placed on this principle, such as when the truth would knowingly produce harm or interfere with the recovery process. Being honest is not always easy, but rarely is lying justified. Clients have the right to know about their diagnosis, treatment, and prognosis.

A Model for Making Ethical Decisions

The following steps may be used in making an ethical decision. These steps are consistent with the steps of the nursing process.

1. **Assessment:** Gather the subjective and objective data about a situation. Consider personal values as well as values of others involved in the ethical dilemma.
2. **Problem identification:** Identify the conflict between two or more alternative actions.
3. **Planning:**
   a. Explore the benefits and consequences of each alternative.
   b. Consider principles of ethical theories.
   c. Select an alternative.
4. **Implementation:** Act on the decision made and communicate the decision to others.
5. **Evaluation:** Evaluate outcomes.

A schematic of this model is presented in Figure 5–1. A case study using this decision-making model is presented in Box 5–1. If the outcome is acceptable, action continues in the manner selected. If the outcome is unacceptable, benefits and consequences of the remaining alternatives are reexamined, and steps 3 through 7 in Box 5–1 are repeated.

Ethical and Legal Issues in Psychiatric-Mental Health Nursing

The Right to Treatment

Anyone who is admitted to the hospital has the right to treatment. For example, a psychiatric patient cannot legally be hospitalized and then denied appropriate treatment. The American Hospital Association (AHA) has also identified the rights of hospitalized patients. The AHA patient bill of rights was originally written with an emphasis on protecting the patient from a breach of reasonable standards while hospitalized. These guidelines were revised in 2003 to create an emphasis on the importance of the collaborative relationship between the patient and the hospital health-care team. Titled *The Patient Care Partnership,* this document informs patients of their rights to high-quality care while hospitalized, to a clean and safe environment, to be involved in their own care, to have their privacy protected, to get help when leaving the hospital, and to get help with their billing claims (AHA, 2003). In 2010 federal law expanded patient rights to include insurability despite preexisting conditions. However, federal health-care law continues to be a debated issue and will no doubt continue to change depending on the

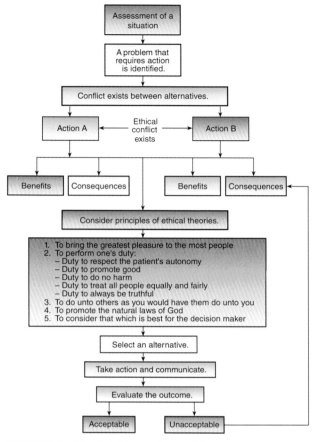

FIGURE 5–1   Ethical decision-making model.

prevailing political climate. Nurses practicing in hospital settings need to be aware of and adhere to legal statutes, accepted standards of practice, and organizational policies with regard to a patient's rights during hospital treatment.

The Right to Refuse Treatment (Including Medication)

Legally, patients have the right to refuse treatment unless immediate intervention is required to prevent death or serious harm to the patient or another person (Boland & Verduin, 2022). The U.S. Constitution and several of its amendments affirm this right (e.g., the First Amendment, which addresses the rights of speech, thought, and expression; the Eighth Amendment, which grants the right to freedom from cruel and unusual punishment; and the Fifth and Fourteenth Amendments, which grant due process of law and equal protection for all).

In psychiatry, however, both ethical and legal issues must be considered. Sometimes patients are involuntarily hospitalized because they are at risk of harm to themselves or others and do not recognize the severity of their symptoms. To protect the

BOX 5-1 Ethical Decision Making—A Case Study

STEP 1. ASSESSMENT

Tonja is a 17-year-old girl who is currently on the psychiatric unit with a diagnosis of conduct disorder. Tonja reports that she has been sexually active since she was 14. She had an abortion when she was 15 and a second one 6 weeks ago. She states that her mother told her she has "had her last abortion" and that she has to start taking birth control pills. She asks her nurse, Kimberly, to give her some information about the pills and to tell her how to go about getting some. Kimberly believes Tonja desperately needs information about birth control pills and other types of contraceptives, but the psychiatric unit is part of a Catholic hospital, and hospital policy prohibits distributing this type of information.

STEP 2. PROBLEM IDENTIFICATION

A conflict exists between the patient's need for information, the nurse's desire to provide that information, and the institution's policy prohibiting the provision of that information.

STEP 3. ALTERNATIVES—BENEFITS AND CONSEQUENCES

Alternative 1: Give the patient information and risk losing job.

Alternative 2: Do not give patient information and compromise own values of holistic nursing.

Alternative 3: Refer the patient to another source outside the hospital and risk reprimand from supervisor.

STEP 4. CONSIDER PRINCIPLES OF ETHICAL THEORIES

Alternative 1: Giving the patient information would certainly respect the patient's autonomy and would benefit her by decreasing her chances of becoming pregnant again. It would not be to the best advantage of Kimberly in that she would likely lose her job. According to the beliefs of the Catholic hospital, the natural laws of God would be violated.

Alternative 2: Withholding information restricts the patient's autonomy. It has the potential for doing harm in that without the use of contraceptives, the patient may become pregnant again (and she implies that this is not what she wants). Kimberly's Christian ethic is violated in that this action is not what she would want "done unto her."

Alternative 3: A referral would respect the patient's autonomy, would promote good, would do no harm (except perhaps to Kimberly's ego from the possible reprimand), and would comply with Kimberly's Christian ethic.

STEP 5. SELECT AN ALTERNATIVE

Alternative 3 is selected on the basis of the ethical theories of utilitarianism (does the most good for the greatest number of people), Christian ethics (Kimberly's belief of "Do unto others as you would have others do unto you"), and Kantianism (to perform one's duty) and on the basis of the ethical principles of autonomy, beneficence, and nonmaleficence. The success of this decision depends on the patient's follow-through with the referral and compliance with use of the contraceptives.

STEP 6. TAKE ACTION AND COMMUNICATE

Taking action involves providing information in writing for Tonja or perhaps making a phone call to set up an appointment for her with a health clinic. Communicating involves sharing the information with Tonja's mother. The referral should be documented in the patient's chart.

STEP 7. EVALUATE THE OUTCOME

An acceptable outcome might indicate that Tonja kept her appointment at the health clinic and is complying with the prescribed contraceptive regimen. It might also include Kimberly's input into the change process in her institution to implement these types of referrals to other patients who request them.

An unacceptable outcome might be indicated by Tonja's lack of follow-through with the appointment at the health clinic or lack of compliance in using the contraceptives, resulting in another pregnancy. Kimberly may also view a reprimand from her supervisor as an unacceptable outcome, particularly if she is told that she must select other alternatives should this situation arise in the future. Kimberly's disagreement with the institution's policy may motivate her to make another decision—that of seeking employment in an institution that supports a philosophy more consistent with her own.

patient's rights, specific legal criteria must be met to ensure that the involuntary hospitalization is justified. However, Saya and associates (2019) noted that the strictness of criteria for involuntarily hospitalization in the United States has made it harder to get treatment and has led to a criminalization of mental illness. Consequently, this population is detained in prisons in the United States more so than in any other country.

In emergency cases, sedative medication may be administered without the patient's consent in order to protect them from harming themselves or others. Unlike some other countries (such as Italy) where involuntary medication is automatically allowed for a hospitalized patient, in the United States there are, typically, specific criteria that must be met to justify medicating a patient without their consent (Saya et al., 2019). Because laws vary from state to state, nurses must know the laws that pertain in their local jurisdictions. Organizational policies in the nurse's practice setting should also guide decision making.

Although many courts support a client's right to refuse medications in the psychiatric area, exceptions do exist. Regarding decision making about forced medication, Weiss-Kaffie and Purtell (2001) stated:

> The treatment team must determine that three criteria be met to force medication without client consent. The client must exhibit behavior that is dangerous to self or others; the medication ordered by the physician must have a reasonable chance of providing help to the client; and clients who refuse medication must be judged incompetent to evaluate the benefits of the treatment in question. (p. 361)

Evidence supports the long-term benefits of involuntary medication, particularly for patients with schizophrenia and bipolar disorders (Mental Illness Policy Org., 2017). Current research (Dixon et al., 2018), demonstrating the particular benefits of treating a first episode of psychosis as important in decreasing long-term negative consequences, may increase acceptability of involuntary medication as an early intervention when needed.

More recently, some states have adopted laws that allow a court to mandate outpatient treatment for people with mental illness who have a history of violent behavior. In New York, this law, known as *Kendra's law* (see discussion later in this chapter), also includes a provision for ordering an individual to take medication as part of the treatment plan.

The Right to the Least Restrictive Treatment Alternative

The right to the least restrictive treatment alternative means that clients who can be adequately treated in an outpatient setting should not be hospitalized, and if they are hospitalized, they should not be sedated, restrained, or secluded unless less restrictive measures were unsuccessful. In other words, the client has a right to whatever level of treatment is effective and least restricts their freedom. The restrictiveness of psychiatric therapy can be described in the context of a continuum based on severity of illness. Clients may be treated on an outpatient basis, in day hospitals, or through voluntary or involuntary hospitalization. Symptoms may be treated with verbal rehabilitative techniques and move successively to behavioral techniques, chemical interventions, mechanical restraints, or electroconvulsive therapy. However, ethical issues arise in selecting the least restrictive means among involuntary chemical intervention, seclusion, and mechanical restraints. Boland and Verduin (2022) stated:

> Distinguishing among these interventions on the basis of restrictiveness proves to be a purely subjective exercise fraught with personal bias. Moreover, each of these three interventions is both more and less restrictive than each of the other two. Nevertheless, the effort should be made to think in terms of restrictiveness when deciding how to treat patients. (p. 841)

Although the right to the least restrictive treatment may seem reasonable and expected, it is important to recognize that clients with mental illness have historically been hospitalized against their will simply because they had a mental illness. In the case of *O'Connor v. Donaldson* (1976), the Supreme Court ruled that harmless mentally ill individuals cannot be confined against their will if they are able to remain safe outside of a hospital setting. They must be considered dangerous to themselves or others or be so unable to care for themselves that their safety and survival are at risk. In 1981 the case of *Roger v. Oken* culminated in the ruling that all patients, even those involuntarily hospitalized, are competent to refuse treatment, but a legal guardian may authorize treatment (Boland & Verduin, 2022). These laws and policies have better attempted to protect the rights of clients with mental illness while still recognizing that, at times, an individual with acute mental illness may be unable to make decisions in the interest of their safety and survival.

Ideally, it is hoped that a person recognizes their need for treatment and agrees voluntarily to be hospitalized if this measure is recommended by the health-care provider. The individual who is voluntarily hospitalized typically signs a consent to treatment upon admission, but it remains the person's right, as a voluntary patient, to revoke that consent and to be discharged from the hospital if they so choose.

Legal Considerations

The Patient Self-Determination Act, as part of the Omnibus Budget Reconciliation Act of 1990, went into effect on December 1, 1991. Cady (2010) stated:

> The Patient Self-determination Act requires health-care facilities to provide clear written information for every patient concerning his/her legal rights to make healthcare decisions, including the right to accept or refuse treatment. (p. 118)

Box 5–2 lists the rights of patients affirmed by this law.

Nurse Practice Acts

The legal parameters of professional and practical nursing are defined within each state by the state's nurse practice act. These documents are passed by

BOX 5–2 Patient Self-Determination Act–Patient Rights

A person admitted to a program or facility for the purpose of receiving mental health services should be accorded the following:

1. The right to appropriate treatment and related services in a setting and under conditions that are the most supportive of such person's personal liability and that restrict such liberty only to the extent necessary consistent with such person's treatment needs, applicable requirements of law, and applicable judicial orders.
2. The right to an individualized, written treatment or service plan (such plan to be developed promptly after admission of such person), the right to treatment based on such plan, the right to periodic review and reassessment of treatment and related service needs, and the right to appropriate revision of such plan, including any revision necessary to provide a description of mental health services that may be needed after such person is discharged from such program or facility.
3. The right to ongoing participation, in a manner appropriate to a person's capabilities, in the planning of mental health services to be provided (including the right to participate in the development and periodic revision of the plan).
4. The right to be provided, in terms and language appropriate to a person's condition and ability to understand, a reasonable explanation of the person's general mental and physical (if appropriate) condition, the objectives of treatment, the nature and significant possible adverse effects of recommended treatment, the reasons a particular treatment is considered appropriate, the reasons access to certain visitors may not be appropriate, and any appropriate and available alternative treatments,

services, and types of providers of mental health services.
5. The right not to receive a mode or course of treatment in the absence of informed, voluntary, written consent to treatment except during an emergency situation or as permitted by law when the person is being treated as a result of a court order.
6. The right not to participate in experimentation in the absence of informed, voluntary, written consent (includes human subject protection).
7. The right to freedom from restraint or seclusion, other than as a mode or course of treatment or restraint or seclusion during an emergency situation with a written order by a responsible mental health professional.
8. The right to a humane treatment environment that affords reasonable protection from harm and appropriate privacy with regard to personal needs.
9. The right to access, on request, to such person's mental health-care records.
10. The right, in the case of a person admitted on a residential or inpatient care basis, to converse with others privately, to have convenient and reasonable access to the telephone and mail, and to see visitors during regularly scheduled hours. (For treatment purposes, specific individuals may be excluded.)
11. The right to be informed promptly and in writing at the time of admission of these rights.
12. The right to assert grievances with respect to infringement of these rights.
13. The right to exercise these rights without reprisal.
14. The right of referral to other providers upon discharge.

Adapted from the U.S. Code, Title 42, Section 10841, The Public Health and Welfare, 1991.

the state legislature and are generally concerned with provisions such as the following:

■ The definition of important terms, including nursing itself and the various types of nurses
■ A statement of the education and other training or requirements for licensure and reciprocity
■ Broad statements that describe the scope of practice for various levels of nursing (advanced practice nurse [APN], registered nurse [RN], licensed practical nurse [LPN])
■ Conditions under which a nurse's license may be suspended or revoked and instructions for appeal
■ The general authority and powers of the state board of nursing

Most nurse practice acts are general in their terminology and do not provide specific guidelines for practice. Nurses must understand the scope of

practice protected by their license and should seek assistance from legal counsel if they are unsure about the proper interpretation of a nurse practice act.

Types of Law

The two general categories of law that are of most concern to nurses are statutory law and common law. These laws are identified by their source or origin.

Statutory Law

A **statutory law** is a law that has been enacted by a legislative body, such as a county or city council, state legislature, or the U.S. Congress. An example of statutory law is a nurse practice act.

Common Law

A **common law** is derived from decisions made in previous cases. These laws apply to a body of principles that evolve from court decisions resolving various controversies. Because common law in the United States has been developed by individual states, the law on specific subjects may differ from state to state. An example of a common law might be how different states deal with a nurse's refusal to provide care for a specific client.

Classifications Within Statutory and Common Law

Broadly speaking, there are two kinds of unlawful acts: civil and criminal. Both statutory law and common law have civil and criminal components.

Civil Law

Civil law protects the private and property rights of individuals and businesses. Private individuals or groups may bring a legal action to court for breach of civil law. These legal actions are of two basic types: torts and contracts.

Torts

A **tort** is a violation of a civil law in which an individual has been wronged. In a tort action, one party asserts that wrongful conduct on the part of the other has caused harm and seeks compensation. A tort may be *intentional* or *unintentional*. Examples of unintentional torts are malpractice and negligence actions. An example of an intentional tort is the touching of another person without that person's consent. Intentional touching (e.g., a medical treatment) without the client's consent can result in a charge of battery, an intentional tort.

Contracts

In a contract action, one party asserts that the other party, in failing to fulfill an obligation, has breached the contract, and either compensation or performance of the obligation is sought as remedy. An example is an action by a mental health professional whose clinical privileges have been reduced or terminated in violation of an implied contract between the professional and a hospital.

Criminal Law

Criminal law provides protection from conduct deemed injurious to the public welfare. It provides for punishment of those found to have engaged in such conduct, which can range from community service and fines to imprisonment and death depending on the scope of the crime (Aiken, 2020). An example of a violation of criminal law is the theft of supplies or drugs by a hospital employee. Catalano (2020) noted, "The most common violation by nurses of the criminal law is failure to renew nursing licenses. In this situation, the nurse is practicing nursing without a license, which is a crime in all states" (p. 184). He

adds that recent cases of intentional or unintentional death of clients and assisted suicide have also led to criminal charges against nurses.

Legal Issues in Psychiatric-Mental Health Nursing

Confidentiality and Right to Privacy

The Fourth, Fifth, and Fourteenth Amendments to the U.S. Constitution protect an individual's right to privacy. Most states have statutes protecting the confidentiality of client records and communications. Nurses must recognize that the only individuals who have a right to observe a client or have access to medical information are those involved in the client's medical care. The client must provide written consent for health-care information to be shared with anyone outside the current treatment team.

Health Insurance Portability and Accountability Act (HIPAA)

Until 1996 client confidentiality in medical records was not protected by federal law. In August 1996 President Clinton signed the Health Insurance Portability and Accountability Act (HIPAA) into law. This federal privacy rule pertains to data that is called *protected health information* (PHI) and applies to most individuals and institutions involved in health care. PHI is defined as individually identifiable health information indicators that "relate to past, present, or future physical or mental health or condition of the individual, or the past, present, or future payment for the provision of health care to an individual and (1) that identifies the individual; or (2) with respect to which there is a reasonable basis to believe the information can be used to identify the individual" (U.S. Department of Health and Human Services, 2003). These specific identifiers are listed in Box 5–3.

Under HIPAA, individuals have the rights to access their medical records, have corrections made to their medical records, and decide with whom their medical information may be shared. The actual document belongs to the facility or the therapist, but the information contained therein belongs to the client. The passage of HIPAA increased the level of control clients have over the information maintained in their medical records. Notice of privacy policies must be provided to clients upon entry into the health-care system.

In 2013 HIPAA privacy and security rules were again expanded to afford more rights to patients concerning their medical information and to ensure greater security of a person's health information. For example, when patients are paying out of pocket for their care, they can tell a provider that they do not want treatment information shared with their health insurance plan (U.S. Department of Health

BOX 5–3 Protected Health Information (PHI): Individually Identifiable Indicators

1. Names
2. Postal address information (except state), including street address, city, county, precinct, and zip code
3. All elements of dates (except year) for dates directly related to an individual, including birth date, admission date, discharge date, date of death; and all ages over 89 and all elements of dates (including year) indicative of such age, except that such ages and elements may be aggregated into a single category of age 90 or older
4. Telephone numbers
5. Fax numbers
6. Electronic mail addresses
7. Social Security numbers
8. Medical record numbers
9. Health plan beneficiary numbers
10. Account numbers
11. Certificate/license numbers
12. Vehicle identifiers and serial numbers, including license plate numbers
13. Device identifiers and serial numbers
14. Web Universal Resource Locators (URLs)
15. Internet protocol (IP) address numbers
16. Biometric identifiers, including finger and voice prints
17. Full face photographic images and any comparable images
18. Any other unique identifying number, characteristic, or code

From U.S. Department of Health and Human Services (HHS). (2003). Standards for privacy of individually identifiable health information. HHS.

& Human Services, 2013). Nurses in any practice setting need to be aware of HIPAA laws and any new legal provisions that will affect the conduct of their practice.

Pertinent medical information may be released without consent in a life-threatening situation. If information is released in an emergency, the following information must be recorded in the client's record: date of disclosure, person to whom information was disclosed, reason for disclosure, reason written consent could not be obtained, and the specific information disclosed.

Most states have statutes that pertain to the doctrine of **privileged communication.** Although the codes differ markedly from state to state, most grant certain professionals privileges under which they may refuse to reveal information about and communications with clients. In most states, the doctrine of privileged communication applies to psychiatrists and attorneys; in some instances, psychologists, clergy, and nurses are also included.

In certain instances, nurses may be called on to testify in cases in which the medical record is used as evidence. In most states, the right to privacy of these records is exempted in civil or criminal proceedings. Therefore, it is important that nurses document with these possibilities in mind. Strict record-keeping using objective and nonjudgmental statements, care plans that are specific in their prescriptive interventions, and documentation that describes those interventions and their subsequent evaluation all serve the best interests of the client, the nurse, and the institution, should questions regarding care arise. Documentation often weighs heavily in malpractice case decisions.

The right to confidentiality is a basic one, especially in psychiatry. Although societal attitudes are improving, individuals have experienced discrimination in the past for no other reason than having a history of mental illness. Nurses working in psychiatric-mental health nursing must guard the privacy of their patients with great diligence.

Exception: A Duty to Warn (Protection of a Third Party)

There are exceptions to the laws of privacy and confidentiality. One of these exceptions stems from the 1974 case of *Tarasoff v. Regents of the University of California.* The incident from which this case evolved occurred in the late 1960s. A young man from Bengal, India (Mr. P.), who was a graduate student at the University of California (UC), Berkeley, fell in love with another university student (Ms. Tarasoff). Because she was not interested in an exclusive relationship with Mr. P., he became resentful and angry. He began to stalk her and record some of their conversations in an effort to determine why she did not love him. He soon became very depressed and neglected his health, appearance, and studies.

Ms. Tarasoff spent the summer of 1969 in South America. During this time, Mr. P. entered therapy with a psychologist at UC. He confided in the psychologist that he intended to kill his former girlfriend (identifying Ms. Tarasoff by name) when she returned from vacation. The psychologist recommended civil commitment for Mr. P. and claimed that he had a diagnosis of acute and severe paranoid schizophrenia. Mr. P. was picked up by the campus police but released a short time later because he appeared rational and promised to stay away from Ms. Tarasoff. Neither Ms. Tarasoff nor her parents received any warning of Mr. P.'s stated intention to kill her.

When Ms. Tarasoff returned to campus in October 1969, Mr. P. resumed his stalking behavior and eventually stabbed her to death. Ms. Tarasoff's parents sued the psychologist, several psychiatrists, and the university for failure to warn the family of the danger. The case was referred to the California Supreme Court, which ruled that a mental health professional has a duty not only to a client but also to individuals who are being threatened by that client. The Court stated:

> Once a therapist does in fact determine, or under applicable professional standards should have determined, that a patient poses a serious danger of violence to others, he bears a duty to exercise reasonable care to protect the foreseeable victim of that danger. Although the discharge of this duty of due care will necessarily vary with the facts of each case, in each instance the adequacy of the therapist's conduct must be measured against the traditional negligence standard of reasonable care under the circumstances. (*Tarasoff v. Regents of University of California*, 1974a)

The defendants argued that warning the woman or her family would have breached professional ethics and violated the client's right to privacy. But the court ruled that "the confidential character of patient-psychotherapist communications must yield to the extent that disclosure is essential to avert danger to others. The protective privilege ends where the public peril begins" (*Tarasoff v. Regents of University of California*, 1974b).

In 1976 the California Supreme Court expanded the original case ruling (now referred to as *Tarasoff I*). The second ruling (known as *Tarasoff II*) broadened the ruling of "duty to warn" to include "duty to protect." It stated that under certain circumstances, a therapist might be required to warn an individual, notify police, or take whatever steps are necessary to protect the intended victim from harm. This duty to protect can also apply to health-care providers who are required to protect patients who are vulnerable due to their inability to identify harmful situations (Guido, 2014).

The *Tarasoff* rulings created a great deal of controversy in the psychiatric community regarding breach of confidentiality and the subsequent negative effect on the client-therapist relationship. However, most states now recognize that therapists have ethical and legal obligations to prevent their clients from harming themselves or others. Many states have passed their own variations on the original "protect and warn" legislation, but in most cases, courts have outlined the following guidelines for therapists to follow in determining their obligation to take protective measures:

1. Assessment of a threat of violence by a client toward another individual
2. Identification of the intended victim
3. Ability to intervene in a feasible, meaningful way to protect the intended victim

When these guidelines apply to a specific situation, it is reasonable for the therapist to notify the victim, law enforcement authorities, or relatives of the intended victim. They may also consider initiating voluntary or involuntary commitment of the client to prevent potential violence.

Implications for Nursing

Although the original decision in the Tarasoff ruling was directed toward psychotherapists, it has since been more broadly applied. Not all states identify RNs as having a duty to warn, but other statutes include a duty to warn for nurses at all levels, from LPNs to APNs. Four states currently have no duty to warn (Cottone, 2021). In 2018 New Jersey expanded its "duty to warn" law to require mental health professionals to notify local authorities whenever patients threaten harm to *themselves* or others (Sitrin, 2018). Although intended to promote greater gun safety by removing guns from people who are at risk of harming themselves or others with firearms, the law has far broader implications both professionally and politically.

Even in states that do not recognize a duty to warn, practitioners still must decide about warning a potential victim and others. Every nurse, not just those practicing in psychiatric nursing, should be informed about the laws in their state regarding duty to warn. As Henderson (2015) noted, emergency nurses are often the front-line health-care workers and thus are in a position to identify persons at risk for violence and to protect the safety of the patient and others. In psychiatric-mental health nursing practice, if a client confides in the nurse about the potential for harm to an intended victim, it is the nurse's duty to report this information to the psychiatrist and to other team members. Reporting this information is not a breach of confidentiality. In such situations, the nurse may be considered negligent for failure to report. All members of the treatment team must be made aware of the potential danger that the client poses to self or others. Detailed written documentation of the situation is also required.

Exception: Suspected Child or Elder Abuse

The Federal Child Abuse Prevention and Treatment Act (CAPTA) requires each state to have provisions or procedures for requiring certain individuals to report known or suspected instances of child abuse and neglect (Child Welfare Information Gateway, 2019a). Many jurisdictions also have statutes requiring that suspected elder abuse or neglect be reported. At times, health-care professionals are worried that they may be liable for false allegations and therefore may be reluctant to report, but reporting statutes generally grant immunity to anyone making a good faith report about a reasonable suspicion. In fact, nearly every state and U.S. territory imposes penalties, from imposing fines to possible imprisonment, for mandatory reporters who *fail to report* suspected child abuse or neglect as required by law; in some jurisdictions, failure to report is identified as a felony (Child Welfare Information Gateway, 2019b).

Implications for Nursing

There is often an element of clinical judgment about whether a patient's communication raises a reasonable suspicion of abuse. For example, when a person is experiencing hallucinations or delusions, their perception about events may be distorted. The nurse has a responsibility to explore all patient perceptions of abuse or mistreatment and discuss these with other health-care team members to identify the most appropriate decision with consideration of all legal, ethical, and clinical factors.

Informed Consent

According to law, all individuals have the right to decide whether to accept or reject medical treatment. A health-care provider can be charged with assault and battery for providing life-sustaining treatment to a patient when the patient has not agreed to the treatment. The rationale for the doctrine of **informed consent** is the preservation and protection of individual autonomy in determining what will and will not happen to a person's body (Guido, 2014).

Informed consent is permission granted by a patient to a physician to perform a therapeutic procedure. Before the procedure, the patient is presented with written information about the treatment and given adequate time to consider the benefits and risks of the procedure. Information should include treatment alternatives; why the physician believes this treatment is most appropriate; the possible outcomes, risks, and adverse effects; the possible outcome should the patient select another treatment alternative; and the possible outcome should the patient choose to decline all treatment. An example of a psychiatric treatment that requires informed consent is electroconvulsive therapy.

Under some conditions, treatment may be performed without obtaining informed consent from the patient. A patient's refusal to accept treatment may be challenged under the following circumstances (Guido, 2014):

1. When a patient is mentally incompetent to make a decision and treatment is necessary to preserve life or avoid serious harm

2. When refusing treatment endangers the life or health of another
3. During an emergency in which a patient is in no condition to exercise judgment
4. When the patient is a child (consent is obtained from parent or surrogate)
5. In the case of therapeutic privilege, information about a treatment may be withheld if the physician can show that full disclosure would
   a. hinder or complicate necessary treatment,
   b. cause severe psychological harm, or
   c. be so upsetting as to render a rational decision by the patient impossible.

Although most patients in psychiatric-mental health facilities are competent and capable of giving informed consent, those with severe psychiatric illness may not possess the cognitive ability to do so. If an individual has been legally determined to be mentally incompetent, consent is obtained from the legal guardian. Difficulty arises when no legal determination has been made, but the individual's current mental state prohibits informed decision making (e.g., a person who is psychotic, unconscious, or inebriated). In these instances, informed consent is usually obtained from the individual's nearest relative, or if none exist and time permits, the physician may ask the court to appoint a conservator or guardian. When time does not permit court intervention, permission may be sought from the hospital administrator.

A patient or guardian always has the right to withdraw consent after it has been given. When this occurs, the physician should inform (or reinform) the patient about the consequences of refusing treatment. If treatment has already been initiated, the physician should terminate treatment in a way least likely to cause injury to the patient and inform the patient or guardian of the risks associated with interrupted treatment (Guido, 2014).

The staff nurse's role in obtaining informed consent is usually defined by agency policy. A nurse may sign the consent form as a witness for the patient's signature. However, legal liability for informed consent lies with the physician. The nurse acts as a patient advocate, ensuring that the following three major elements of informed consent have been addressed:

1. **Knowledge:** The patient has received adequate information on which to base their decision.
2. **Competency:** The patient's cognition is not impaired to an extent that would interfere with decision making, or they have a legal representative.
3. **Free will:** The patient has given consent voluntarily without pressure or coercion from others.

Restraints and Seclusion

An individual's privacy and personal security are protected by the Patient Self-Determination Act of 1991. This legislation includes a set of patient rights, including an individual's right to freedom from restraint or seclusion except in an emergency. The use of seclusion and restraint as therapeutic interventions for psychiatric patients is controversial, and many efforts have been made through federal and state regulations and through standards set forth by accrediting bodies to minimize or eliminate their use.

In addition, there is an element of moral decision making when any kind of treatment is coerced, as is often the case with seclusion and restraint. Landeweer and associates (2011) pointed out that although coercion may sometimes be necessary, it can be detrimental to the patient, as it may produce trauma and mistrust. One advantage of using a forum such as a hospital-based ethics committee to guide moral decision making is that by exploring issues such as the use of seclusion and restraint with a diverse group of people who have different vantage points, alternative treatments can be identified and explored.

Because injuries and deaths have been associated with restraint and seclusion, this treatment requires careful attention whenever it is deemed necessary. Further, because laws, regulations, accreditation standards, and hospital policies are frequently revised, anyone practicing in inpatient psychiatric settings must remain well informed in each of these areas.

In psychiatry, the term *restraints* generally refers to a set of leather straps used to restrain the extremities of an individual whose behavior poses an immediate risk to the physical safety and psychological well-being of themselves and others. It is important to note that the currently accepted definition of restraint refers not only to leather restraints but also to any manual method or medication used to restrict a person's freedom of movement. Restraints are never to be used as punishment or for the convenience of staff. Other measures to decrease agitation, such as "talking down" (verbal intervention) and chemical restraints (tranquilizing medication), are usually tried first. If these interventions are ineffective, mechanical restraints may be instituted (although some controversy exists as to whether chemical restraints are indeed less restrictive than mechanical restraints). *Seclusion* is another type of physical restraint in which the client is confined alone in a room from which they are unable to leave. The room is usually minimally furnished with items to promote the client's comfort and safety.

Because seclusion and restraint are both considered high-risk interventions, institutions, health-care accrediting bodies (such as The Joint Commission), and state mental health departments define specific expectations for their use. These standards typically include requirements for staff training and competency in the use of seclusion or restraint; expectations that these interventions will be used only as a last resort and for the shortest amount of time necessary; and what kinds of assessment and intervention are required before, during, and after the individual is secluded or restrained.

The laws, regulations, accreditation standards, and hospital policies related to restraint and seclusion share a common priority of maintaining patient safety for a procedure that has the potential to incur injury or death. The importance of close and careful monitoring cannot be overstated.

False imprisonment is the deliberate and unauthorized confinement of a competent person with the intent to prevent them from leaving the hospital; this includes use of threats or medications that interfere with the patient's ability to leave the facility (Aiken, 2020). Health-care workers may be charged with false imprisonment for restraining or secluding—against the wishes of the client—anyone admitted to the hospital voluntarily. Should a voluntarily admitted client decompensate to a level that restraint or seclusion for protection of self or others is necessary, court intervention to determine competency and involuntary commitment is required to preserve the client's rights to privacy and freedom.

Hospitalization

Voluntary Admissions

Although the vast majority of mental health services are provided on a voluntary basis (Substance Abuse and Mental Health Services Administration [SAMHSA], 2019), much of voluntary treatment occurs in settings other than inpatient hospitalization. This has been influenced by the availability of a greater number of outpatient treatment options including partial hospitalization, intensive outpatient programs, and other specialized treatment programs.

To be admitted voluntarily, an individual makes direct application to the institution for services and may stay as long as treatment is deemed necessary. The person may sign out of the hospital at any time unless the health-care professional determines that they may be harmful to self or others after a mental status examination and recommends that admission status be changed from voluntary to involuntary. Even when admission is considered voluntary, it is important to ensure that the individual comprehends the meaning of their actions, has not been coerced in any manner, and is willing to proceed with admission.

Involuntary Commitment

Although the term *involuntary hospitalization* is preferred by some over the term *involuntary commitment* or *civil commitment*, this process needs to be conducted with respect to state and federal law. Because involuntary hospitalization results in substantial restrictions of the rights of an individual, the admission process is subject to the guarantee of the Fourteenth Amendment to the U.S. Constitution that provides citizens protection against loss of liberty and ensures due process rights. Involuntary hospitalizations may be made for various reasons. Most states commonly cite the following criteria:

- The person is imminently dangerous to themselves (i.e., suicidal intent).
- The person is a danger to others (i.e., physically aggressive, violent, or homicidal).
- The person is unable to take care of basic personal needs (the "gravely disabled").

Under the Fourth Amendment, individuals are protected from unlawful searches and seizures without probable cause. Therefore the person recommending involuntary hospitalization must show probable cause why the client should be hospitalized against their wishes; that is, the person must show that there is cause to believe that the client would be dangerous to self or others, is mentally ill and in need of treatment, or is gravely disabled.

Emergency Commitments

Emergency commitments are sought when an individual manifests behavior that is clearly and imminently dangerous to self or others. These admissions are usually instigated by relatives or friends of the individual or by police officers, the court, or healthcare professionals. Emergency commitments are time-limited, and a court hearing for the individual is scheduled, usually within 72 hours. At that time, the court may decide that the individual may be discharged or, if deemed necessary and voluntary admission is refused by the person, an additional period of involuntary hospitalization may be ordered. In most instances, another hearing is scheduled for a specified time (usually in 7 to 21 days).

The Mentally Ill Person in Need of Treatment

A second type of involuntary commitment is for the observation and treatment of mentally ill people in need of treatment. These commitments typically last longer than emergency commitments. Most states have established definitions of what constitutes "mentally ill" for purposes of state involuntary admission statutes. Some examples include individuals who, because of severe mental illness, are

- Unable to make informed decisions concerning treatment
- Likely to cause harm to self or others
- Unable to fulfill basic personal needs necessary for health and safety

In determining whether commitment is required, the court looks for substantial evidence of abnormal conduct—evidence that cannot be explained by a physical cause. There must be "clear and convincing evidence" as well as probable cause to substantiate the need for involuntary hospitalization to ensure that an individual's constitutional rights are protected. As mentioned earlier, the U.S. Supreme Court, in *O'Connor v. Donaldson,* held that the existence of mental illness alone does not justify involuntary hospitalization. State standards require a specific effect or consequence caused by mental illness that involves danger or an inability to care for one's own needs. These individuals are entitled to court hearings with representation, at which time determination of commitment and length of stay are considered. Legislative statutes governing involuntary commitments vary among states.

Involuntary Outpatient Commitment

Involuntary outpatient commitment (IOC) is a court-ordered mechanism used to compel a person with mental illness to submit to treatment on an outpatient basis. As these laws have evolved, they have taken a more "preventive approach." In this scenario a person with mental illness who is not currently dangerous, and therefore not legally committable to a hospital, could be ordered to community treatment on the basis of a complex clinical assessment and prediction about the future. Examples of eligibility criteria (SAMHSA, 2019) include those outlined in North Carolina's state statutes:

- The person must have a mental illness.
- The person is capable of surviving safely in the community with available supervision from family, friends, or others.
- Based on the person's psychiatric history, the person is in need of treatment in order to prevent further disability or deterioration that would predictably result in dangerousness.
- The person's current mental status or the nature of their illness limits or negates their ability to make an informed decision to seek voluntary admission or comply with recommended treatment.

Most states have already enacted IOC legislation or currently have agenda resolutions that pertain to this topic. Most commonly, clients who are committed into the IOC programs are those with severe and persistent mental illness such as schizophrenia. The rationale behind the legislation is to improve preventive care and reduce the number of readmissions and lengths of hospital stays for these clients. The need for this type of legislation arose after it was recognized that patients with schizophrenia who did not meet criteria for involuntary hospital treatment were, in some cases, ultimately dangerous to themselves or others. In New York, public attention to this need arose after a man with schizophrenia who had stopped taking his medication pushed a young woman into the path of a subway train. He would not have met the criteria for involuntary hospitalization until he was deemed dangerous to others, but advocates for this legislation argued that there should be provisions to prevent violence rather than waiting until it happens. The subsequent law governing IOC in New York became known as Kendra's law for the woman who was pushed to her death. Opponents of this legislation fear that it may violate the individual rights of psychiatric clients without significant improvement in outcomes. Although many states have enacted similar laws, New York's Kendra's law adds a stricter stipulation that the person must have been hospitalized at least twice within the prior 3 years as a result of noncompliance with treatment, or have committed, attempted, or threatened an act of violence or self-harm within the prior 2 years, and they would benefit from this type of treatment.

Research has attempted to evaluate whether IOC improves care, reduces lengths of stay in the hospital, and reduces episodes of violence. Some studies have shown positive outcomes with IOC, including a decrease in hospital readmissions (Swartz et al., 2017; Swartz & Swanson, 2008). However, a Cochrane literature review (Kisely et al., 2017) concluded that compulsory community treatment resulted in no significant differences in service use, social functioning, mental state, or quality of life, although those in mandated outpatient treatment were less likely to be victims of crimes. The issues around whether IOC will improve treatment compliance and enhance quality of life in the community for individuals with severe and persistent mental illness will continue to be a focus of study and debate.

The Gravely Disabled Client

Many states have statutes that specifically define the "gravely disabled" individual. For those that do not use this label, the description of the individual who is unable to take care of basic personal needs because of mental illness is very similar.

Gravely disabled is generally defined as a condition in which an individual, as a result of mental illness, is in danger of serious physical harm resulting from an inability to provide for basic needs such as food, clothing, shelter, medical care, and personal safety. Inability to care for oneself cannot be established by showing that an individual lacks the resources to provide the necessities of life; rather, it is the inability to make use of available resources.

Should it be determined that an individual is gravely disabled, a guardian, conservator, or committee will be appointed by the court to ensure the management of the person and their estate. Legal restoration of competency requires another court hearing to reverse the previous ruling. The individual whose competency is being determined has the right to be represented by an attorney.

It is an ethical and legal duty to ensure that whenever coercive treatments are used, including involuntary hospitalizations, seclusion and restraint, IOCs, mandated medication, and even prison commitments, the least restrictive intervention must first be considered. Sashadahran and Saraceno (2017) identified a current global shift toward more coercive care similar to that which existed before the community mental health movement. They cite increasing numbers of involuntary hospitalizations and note that in the United States there are currently three times as many individuals with mental illness in prisons as there are in hospitals. In addition, sexual predator laws in the United States allow indefinite hospital stays for serious sex offenders beyond their prison sentence completion. The authors posit that when risk management supersedes the most appropriate level of care for treatment, stigmatization of this population may increase (Sashadahran & Saraceno, 2017).

Nursing Liability

Mental health practitioners—psychiatrists, psychologists, psychiatric nurses, and social workers—have a duty to provide appropriate care based on the standards of their professions and the standards set by law. The standards of care for psychiatric-mental health nursing are presented in Chapter 8, "The Nursing Process in Psychiatric-Mental Health Nursing."

Malpractice and Negligence

The terms **malpractice** and **negligence** are often used interchangeably. Negligence has been defined as failure to exercise the care toward others that a reasonable or prudent person would do in the circumstances or taking action that a reasonable person would not. Negligence is accidental as distinguished from "intentional torts" (assault or trespass, for example) or from crimes, but a crime can also constitute negligence, such as reckless driving (Hill & Hill, 2022).

Any person may be negligent. In contrast, malpractice is a specialized form of negligence caused only by professionals. Malpractice may be defined as an act or continuing conduct of a professional that does not meet the standard of professional competence and results in provable damages to their patient. Such an error or omission may be through negligence, ignorance (when the professional should have known), or intentional wrongdoing (Hill & Hill, 2022).

In the absence of state statutes, common law is the basis of liability for injuries to patients caused by acts of malpractice and negligence by individual practitioners. In other words, most decisions of negligence in the professional setting are based on legal precedent (decisions that have been made previously about similar cases) rather than on any specific action taken by the legislature.

To summarize, when a breach of duty is characterized as malpractice, the action is weighed against the professional standard. When it is brought forth as negligence, the action is contrasted with what a reasonably prudent professional would have done in the same or similar circumstances.

Austin (2011) cited the following basic elements of a nursing malpractice lawsuit:

1. A duty to the patient existed, based on the recognized standard of care.
2. A breach of duty occurred, meaning that the care rendered was not consistent with the recognized standard of care.
3. The patient was injured.
4. The injury was directly caused by the breach of a standard of care.

For the client to prevail in a malpractice claim, each of these elements must be proven. Jury decisions are generally based on the testimony of expert witnesses because members of the jury are laypeople who cannot be expected to know what nursing interventions should have taken place. Without the testimony of expert witnesses, a favorable verdict usually goes to the defendant nurse.

Types of Lawsuits That Occur in Psychiatric Nursing

Most malpractice suits against nurses are civil actions, which means they are considered breach of conduct actions on the part of the professional from whom compensation is sought. The nurse in a psychiatric setting should be aware of the types of behavior that may result in malpractice charges.

The hospitalized psychiatric patient has a basic right to confidentiality and privacy. A nurse may be charged with *breach of confidentiality* for revealing aspects about a patient's case or even for revealing that an individual has been hospitalized if the patient can show that making this information known resulted in harm.

When shared information is detrimental to the client's or patient's reputation, the person sharing the information may be liable for **defamation of character.** When the information is in writing, the action is called **libel.** Oral defamation is called **slander.** Defamation of character involves communication that is malicious and false (Aiken, 2020). Occasionally, libel arises out of critical, judgmental statements written in a person's medical record. Nurses need to be very objective in their charting, backing up all statements with factual evidence.

Invasion of privacy is a charge that may result when an individual is searched without probable cause. Many institutions conduct body searches on patients with mental illness as a routine intervention. In these cases, there should be a physician's order and written rationale showing probable cause for the intervention. Many institutions are re-examining their policies regarding this procedure.

Assault is an act that results in a person's genuine fear and apprehension that they will be touched without consent. **Battery** is the nonconsensual touching of another person. These charges can result when a treatment is administered to an individual against their wishes and outside of an emergency situation. Harm or injury need not have occurred for these charges to be legitimate.

For confining a patient against their wishes outside of an emergency situation, the nurse may be charged with false imprisonment. Examples of actions that may invoke these charges include locking an individual in a room, taking a person's clothes for purposes of detainment against their will, and restraining a competent voluntary individual who demands to be released.

Avoiding Liability

Aiken (2020) suggested the following proactive nursing actions to avoid nursing malpractice and the risk of lawsuits:

1. *Effective communication* with patients and other caregivers. The SBAR (situation, background, assessment, and recommendations) model of reporting information has been identified as a useful tool for effective communication with caregivers. Establishing rapport with patients encourages open and honest communication.
2. *Accurate and complete documentation in the medical record.*

 The electronic health record (EHR) has been identified as the best way to document and share this information. The use of best informatics sources is identified as an essential nursing competency in the Quality and Safety Education for Nurses standards (QSEN Institute, 2013).

3. *Complying with standards of care,* including those established within the profession (such as ANA standards) and those identified by specific hospital policies.

4. *Rapport with and knowledge of the patient,* which includes helping the patient become involved in their care as well as understanding and responding to aspects of care in which the patient is dissatisfied.

5. *Practicing within the nurse's level of competence and scope of practice,* which includes not only adhering to professional standards (those of the ANA and state boards of nursing) but also keeping knowledge and nursing skills current through evidence-based literature, in-services, and continuing education.

Some patients appear to be more "suit prone" than others. Suit-prone patients are often very critical, complaining, uncooperative, and even hostile. A natural staff response to these patients is to become defensive or withdrawn. Aiken (2020) recommended instead that it is important to be direct and engage the patient in problem-solving. No matter how high the nurse's technical competence and skill, their insensitivity to a patient's complaints and failure to meet the patent's emotional needs often influence whether or not a lawsuit is generated. A great deal depends on the psychosocial skills of the health-care professional.

> **CLINICAL PEARL Always put the patient's rights and welfare first.**

Summary and Key Points

■ *Ethics* is a branch of philosophy that addresses methods for determining the rightness or wrongness of one's actions.

■ *Bioethics* is the term applied to these principles when they refer to concepts within the scope of medicine, nursing, and allied health.

■ *Moral behavior* is conduct that results from serious critical thinking about how individuals ought to treat others.

■ *Values* are personal beliefs about what is important or desirable.

■ *Rights* are expectations to which an individual is entitled either by established laws, policies, or ethical principles.

■ The ethical theory of utilitarianism is based on the premise that what is right and good is that which produces the most happiness for the most people.

■ The ethical theory of Kantianism suggests that actions are bound by a sense of duty and that ethical decisions are made out of respect for moral law.

■ Divine command ethics identifies ethical decisions as those that follow the divine commands of God.

■ The moral precept of the natural law theory is "do good and avoid evil." Good is viewed as that which is inscribed by God into the nature of things. Evil acts are never condoned, even if they are intended to advance the noblest of ends.

■ Ethical egoism espouses that what is right and good is what is best for the individual making the decision.

■ Ethical principles include autonomy, beneficence, nonmaleficence, veracity, and justice.

■ An ethical dilemma is a situation that requires an individual to decide between two equally unfavorable alternatives.

■ Ethical issues may arise in psychiatric-mental health nursing around a patient's right to refuse medication and right to the least restrictive treatment alternative.

■ Statutory laws are those that have been enacted by legislative bodies, and common laws are derived from decisions made in previous cases. Both types of laws have civil and criminal components.

■ Civil law protects the privacy and property rights of individuals and businesses, and criminal law provides protection from conduct deemed injurious to the public welfare.

■ Legal issues in psychiatric-mental health nursing center around confidentiality and the right to privacy, informed consent, restraints and seclusion, and commitment issues.

■ Nurses are accountable for their own actions in relation to legal issues, and violation can result in malpractice lawsuits against the physician, the hospital, and the nurse.

■ Developing and maintaining a good interpersonal relationship with the patient and their family appears to be a positive factor when the question of malpractice is being considered.

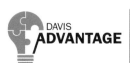 DAVIS **ADVANTAGE** | Go to **Davis Advantage** to complete your learning: strengthen understanding, apply your knowledge, and prepare for the Next Gen NCLEX®.

Review Questions

1. The nurse decides to go against family wishes and tell the client of their terminal status because that is what the nurse would want if they were the client. Which of the following ethical theories is considered in this decision?
   a. Kantianism
   b. Christian ethics
   c. Natural law theories
   d. Ethical egoism

2. The nurse decides to respect family wishes and not tell the client of their terminal status because that would bring the most happiness to the most people. Which of the following ethical theories is considered in this decision?
   a. Utilitarianism
   b. Kantianism
   c. Christian ethics
   d. Ethical egoism

3. The nurse decides to tell the client of their terminal status because the nurse believes it is their duty to do so. Which of the following ethical theories is considered in this decision?
   a. Natural law theories
   b. Ethical egoism
   c. Kantianism
   d. Utilitarianism

4. The nurse assists the physician with electroconvulsive therapy on a client who has refused to give consent. With which of the following legal actions might the nurse be charged because of this nursing action?
   a. Assault
   b. Battery
   c. False imprisonment
   d. Breach of confidentiality

5. A competent, voluntary client has stated they want to leave the hospital. The nurse hides the person's clothes to keep them from leaving. With which of the following legal actions might the nurse be charged because of this nursing action?
   a. Assault
   b. Battery
   c. False imprisonment
   d. Breach of confidentiality

6. A hospitalized client is very restless and is pacing a lot. The nurse says, "If you don't sit down in the chair and be still, I'm going to put you in restraints!" With which of the following legal actions might the nurse be charged because of this nursing action?
   a. Defamation of character
   b. Battery
   c. Breach of confidentiality
   d. Assault

Clinical Judgment Questions

7. A nurse reports to the supervisor that a depressed client is refusing medication to treat their heart condition and states the client "would rather just die." The nurse is not sure how to intervene because, although clients have a right to refuse medication, this client may be so depressed that their behavior represents risk for suicide. Which of these actions by the supervisor is a priority?
   a. Tell the nurse that medication will have to be given forcibly if the client continues to refuse medication.
   b. Instruct the nurse that, because the client is elderly, they are unable to make this decision and medication will need to be secretly mixed in the client's food.
   c. Educate the nurse that the physician has the final say so the nurse should ask the physician what to do.
   d. Activate appropriate hospital resources, such as an ethics committee, so this issue can be explored further.

8. A client on the psychiatric unit begins yelling out loud that no one is listening to them and that they are going to "blow up" soon. The orderly asks the nurse if they should go ahead and put the client in restraints for the safety of others. Which of these responses by the nurse is most appropriate?

   a. Educate the orderly that restraints may never be initiated without a physician's order.

   b. Instruct the orderly that it would be best to see if the client can be assisted to calm down by listening to their concerns.

   c. Instruct the orderly to put the client in restraints but make sure to assess the client every 15 minutes for issues regarding circulation, nutrition, respiration, hydration, and elimination.

   d. Instruct the orderly to get others to assist in restraining the client but be aware restraints should be discontinued at the earliest possible time regardless of when a physician's order is scheduled to expire.

9. The nurse collects the following information during the admission assessment. For which of these pieces of data should the nurse take additional action to ensure that "duty to warn" laws are followed?

   a. The client threatens violence toward another individual.

   b. The client states they want to kill everyone that has demons.

   c. The client is having command hallucinations.

   d. The client reveals paranoid delusions about another individual.

10. Which of these actions by the nurse demonstrates an application of the QSEN competency related to informatics?

   a. Learns how to effectively communicate information using EHRs

   b. Provides a verbal report of client behavioral issues at shift change

   c. Asks the supervisor for guidelines on how to prevent lawsuits

   d. Reads journals to learn information about new treatments and approaches to nursing care

References

Aiken, M. E. T. (2020). Nursing law and liability. In J. T. Catalano (Ed.), *Nursing now! Today's issues, tomorrow's trends* (8th ed., pp. 183–212). F.A. Davis.

American Hospital Association (AHA). (2003). *The patient care partnership: Understanding expectations, rights, and responsibilities.* www.aha.org/advocacy-issues/communicatingpts/pt-care-partnership.shtml

American Nurses Association (ANA). (2015). *Code of ethics for nurses with interpretive statements.* ANA.

American Nurses Association (ANA), American Psychiatric Nurses Association, & International Society of Psychiatric-Mental Health Nurses. (2022). *Psychiatric–mental health nursing: Scope and standards of practice* (3rd ed.). ANA.

Austin, S. (2011). Stay out of court with proper documentation. *Nursing2011, 41*(4), 25–29. doi:10.1097/01.NURSE.0000395202.86451.d4

Boland, R., & Verduin, M. L. (2022). *Kaplan & Sadock's synopsis of psychiatry* (P. Ruiz, Ed.). (12th ed.). Wolters Kluwer.

Butts, J., & Rich, K. (2019). *Nursing ethics: Across the curriculum and into practice* (5th ed.). Jones & Bartlett.

Cady, R. F. (2010). A review of basic patient rights in psychiatric care. *JONA's Healthcare Law, Ethics, and Regulation, 12*(4), 117–125. doi:10.1097/NHL.0b013e3181f4d357

Catalano, J. T. (2020). *Nursing now! Today's issues, tomorrow's trends* (8th ed.). F.A. Davis.

Child Welfare Information Gateway. (2019a). *Mandatory reporters of child abuse and neglect.* https://www.childwelfare.gov/pubPDFs/manda.pdf

Child Welfare Information Gateway. (2019b). *Penalties for failure to report and false reporting of child abuse and neglect.* https://www.childwelfare.gov/pubPDFs/report.pdf

Cottone, A. S. (2021). *Duty of mental health providers to warn and/or protect third party victims: The Tarasoff standard.* https://byrnecanaanlaw.com/news-post-5.html

Dixon, L. B., Goldman, H. H., Srihari, V. H., & Kane, J. M. (2018). Transforming the treatment of schizophrenia in the United States: The RAISE initiative. *Annual Review of Clinical Psychology, 7*(14), 237–258. https://doi.org/10.1146/annurev-clinpsy-050817-084934

Guido, G. W. (2014). *Legal and ethical issues in nursing* (6th ed.). Pearson.

Henderson, E. (2015). Potentially dangerous patients: A review of the duty to warn. *Journal of Emergency Nursing, 41*(3), 193–200. doi:http://dx.doi.org/10.1016/j.jen.2014.08.012

Hill, G., & Hill, K. (2022). *The people's law dictionary.* https://dictionary.law.com

Indiana State Nurses Association Bulletin. What do I do now? Ethical dilemmas in nursing and health care. (2013). *ISNA Bulletin, 13*(2), 5–12.

Institute of Medicine. (2003). *Health professions education: A bridge to quality.* Institute of Medicine.

Kisely, S. R., Campbell, L. A., & O'Reilly, R. (2017). *Compulsory community and involuntary outpatient treatment for people with severe mental disorders.* http://www.cochrane.org/CD004408/SCHIZ_compulsory-community-and involuntary-outpatient-treatment-people-severe-mental-disorders

Landeweer, E., Abma, T. A., & Widdershoven, G. (2011). Moral margins concerning the use of coercion in psychiatry. *Nursing Ethics, 18*(3), 304–316. doi:10.1177/0969733011400301

Maiese, M. (2017 [originally posted July 2003]). Principles of justice and fairness. *Beyond intractability.* G. Burgess & H. Burgess, Eds. Conflict Information Consortium, University of Colorado, Boulder. www.beyondintractability.org/essay/principles-of-justice

Mental Illness Policy Org. (2017). *The effects of involuntary medication on individuals with schizophrenia and manic-depressive disorder.* https://mentalillnesspolicy.org/medical/involuntary-medication.html

QSEN Institute. (2013). *Competencies.* http://qsen.org/competencies/

Rae, S. (2009). *Moral choices: An introduction to ethics.* Zondervan.

Sashadahran, S. P., & Saraceno, B. (2017). Is psychiatry becoming more coercive? *The British Medical Journal, 357.* doi:https://doi.org/10.1136/bmj.j2904

Saya, A., Brugnoli, C., Piazzi, G., Liberato, D., Di Ciaccia, G., Niolu, C., & Siracusano, A. (2019). Criteria, procedures, and future prospects of involuntary treatment in psychiatry around the world: A narrative review. *Frontiers in Psychiatry, 10,* 271. https://doi.org/10.3389/fpsyt.2019.00271

Sitrin, C. (2018). *Gov. Murphy signs New Jersey into new era of gun safety.* https://www.njspotlight.com/stories/18/06/13/gov-murphy-signs-new-jersey-into-new-era-of-gun-safety/

Substance Abuse and Mental Health Services Administration. (2019). *Civil commitment and the mental health care continuum: Historical trends and principles for law and practice.* https://www.samhsa.gov/sites/default/files/civil-commitment-continuum-of-care.pdf

Swartz, M. S., Bhattacharya, S., Robertson, A. G., & Swanson, J. W. (2017). Involuntary outpatient commitment and the elusive pursuit of violence prevention. *Canadian Journal of Psychiatry. 62*(2), 102–108. https://doi.org/10.1177/0706743716675857

Swartz, M. S., & Swanson, J. W. (2008). Outpatient commitment: When it improves patient outcomes. *Current Psychiatry, 7*(4), 25–35. doi:http://dx.doi.org/10.1176/appi.ps.52.3.325

Tarasoff v. Regents of University of California et al. (1974a), 551 P.d 345.

Tarasoff v. Regents of University of California et al. (1974b), 554 P.d 347.

U.S. Code, Title 42, Section 10841, The Public Health and Welfare, 1991.

U.S. Department of Health & Human Services (HHS). (2003). *Standards for privacy of individually identifiable health information.* HHS.

U.S. Department of Health & Human Services (HHS). (2013, Jan. 17). New rule protects patient privacy, secures health information [press release]. www.hhs.gov/news/press/2013pres/01/20130117b.html

Classical References

Patient Self-Determination Act—Patient Rights. (1991). U.S. Code, Title 42, Section 10841, The Public Health and Welfare.

Peplau, H. E. (1991). *Interpersonal relations in nursing: A conceptual frame of reference for psychodynamic nursing.* Springer.

Weiss-Kaffie, C. J., & Purtell, N. E. (2001). Psychiatric nursing. In M. E. O'Keefe (Ed.), *Nursing practice and the law: Avoiding malpractice and other legal risks* (pp. 352–371). F.A. Davis.

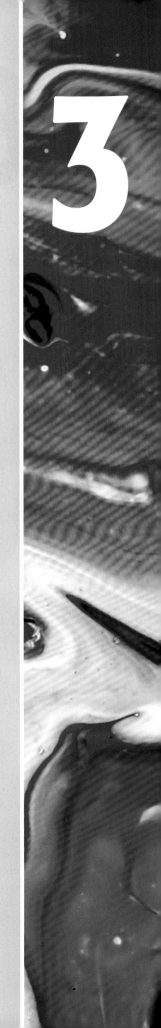

UNIT 3

Therapeutic Approaches in Psychiatric Nursing Care

6

Relationship Development

KEY TERMS

attitude	genuineness	sympathy
belief	material boundaries	transference
concrete thinking	personal boundaries	unconditional positive
confidentiality	professional boundaries	regard
countertransference	rapport	values
empathy	social boundaries	

OBJECTIVES
After reading this chapter, the student will be able to:

1. Describe the relevance of a therapeutic
   nurse–patient relationship.
2. Discuss the dynamics of a therapeutic
   nurse–patient relationship.
3. Discuss the importance of self-awareness
   in the nurse–patient relationship.
4. Identify goals of the nurse–patient
   relationship.
5. Identify and discuss essential conditions
   for a therapeutic relationship to occur.
6. Describe the phases of relationship
   development and the tasks associated
   with each phase.

The nurse–patient relationship is the foundation on which psychiatric nursing is established. It is a relationship in which both participants must recognize each other as unique and important human beings. It is also a relationship in which mutual learning occurs. In today's health-care environment, patient-centered care is promoted as central to quality and safety, and the therapeutic relationship remains at the foundation of this tenet. Concepts that were advanced over 60 years ago (by Hildegard Peplau in 1952) and have been the core of nursing practice to the present day

are now recognized by the larger medical community as not only still relevant but critical to improving quality and safety in health care. Peplau (1991) stated:

Shall a nurse do things *for* a patient or can participant relationships be emphasized so that a nurse comes to do things *with* a patient as her share of an agenda of work to be accomplished in reaching a goal—health. *It is likely that the nursing process is educative and therapeutic when nurse and patient can come to know and to respect each other, as persons who are alike, and yet, different, as persons who share in the solution of problems.* (p. 9, emphasis in original)

This chapter examines the role of the psychiatric nurse and the use of self as a therapeutic tool in the nursing care of patients with mental illness. Phases of the therapeutic relationship are explored, and conditions essential to the development of a therapeutic relationship are discussed. The importance of values clarification in the development of self-awareness is emphasized.

CORE CONCEPT
Therapeutic Relationship
An interaction between two people (usually a caregiver and a care receiver) in which input from both participants contributes to a climate of healing, growth promotion, and/or illness prevention.

Role of the Psychiatric Nurse

What is a nurse? Undoubtedly, this question would elicit as many different answers as the number of people to whom it was presented. Nursing as a *concept* has probably existed since the beginning of the civilized world, with the provision of "care" for the ill or infirm by anyone in the environment who took the time to administer to those in need. However, the emergence of nursing as a *profession* only began in the late 1800s with the graduation of Linda Richards from the New England Hospital for Women and Children in Boston upon achievement of the diploma in nursing. Since that time, the nurse's role has evolved from that of custodial caregiver and physician's handmaiden to recognition as a unique, independent member of the professional health-care team.

Peplau (1991) identified the following nursing roles:

1. **The stranger:** A nurse is at first a stranger to the patient. The patient is also a stranger to the nurse. Peplau (1991) stated:

   Respect and positive interest accorded a stranger is at first nonpersonal and includes the same ordinary courtesies that are accorded to a new guest who has been brought into any situation. This principle implies: (1) accepting the patient as he is; (2) treating the patient as an emotionally able stranger and relating to him on this basis until evidence shows him to be otherwise. (p. 44)

2. **The resource person:** According to Peplau, "A resource person provides specific answers to questions usually formulated with relation to a larger problem" (p. 47). In the role of resource person, the nurse explains, in language that the patient can understand, information related to the patient's health care.

3. **The teacher:** In this role, the nurse identifies learning needs and provides information required by the patient or family to improve the health situation.

4. **The leader:** According to Peplau, "Democratic leadership in nursing situations implies that the patient will be permitted to be an active participant in designing nursing plans for him" (p. 49). Autocratic leadership promotes overvaluation of the nurse and patients' substitution of the nurse's goals for their own. Laissez-faire leaders convey a lack of personal interest in the patient.

5. **The surrogate:** Outside of their awareness, patients often perceive nurses as symbols of other individuals. They may view the nurse as a mother figure, a sibling, a former teacher, or another nurse who has provided care in the past. This perception occurs when a patient is placed in a situation that generates feelings similar to ones they have experienced previously. Peplau (1991) explained that the nurse–patient relationship progresses along a continuum. When a patient is acutely ill they may incur the role of infant or child, while the nurse is perceived as the mother surrogate. Peplau (1991) stated, "Each nurse has the responsibility for exercising her professional skill in aiding the relationship to move forward on the continuum, so that person to person relations compatible with chronological age levels can develop" (p. 55).

6. **The technical expert:** The nurse understands various professional devices and possesses the clinical skills necessary to perform interventions that are in the best interest of the patient.

7. **The counselor:** The nurse uses "interpersonal techniques" to assist patients in adapting to difficulties or changes in life experiences. Peplau (1991) stated, "Counseling in nursing has to do with helping the patient to remember and to understand fully what is happening to him in the present situation, so that the experience can be integrated with, rather than dissociated from, other experiences in life" (p. 64).

Peplau (1952) believed that the counselor role is emphasized in psychiatric nursing. Many sources define the *nurse therapist* as a person with graduate preparation in psychiatric-mental health nursing. This person has developed skills through intensive, supervised educational experiences to provide helpful individual, group, or family therapy. Peplau suggested that it is essential for the *staff nurse working in psychiatry* to have a general knowledge of basic counseling techniques. A therapeutic or "helping" relationship is established through use of these interpersonal techniques and is based on a sound knowledge of theories of personality development and human behavior.

Sullivan (1953) believed that emotional problems stem from difficulties with interpersonal relationships. Interpersonal theorists, such as Peplau and Sullivan, emphasize the importance of relationship development in the provision of emotional care. Through the establishment of a satisfactory nurse–patient relationship, individuals learn to generalize the ability to achieve satisfactory interpersonal relationships to other aspects of their lives.

Dynamics of a Therapeutic Nurse–Patient Relationship

Travelbee (1971), who expanded on Peplau's theory of interpersonal relations in nursing, stated that only when each individual in the interaction perceives the other as a unique human being is a relationship possible. Travelbee referred not to a nurse–patient relationship but rather to a human-to-human relationship, which is described as a "mutually significant experience." That is, both the nurse and the recipient of care have needs met when each views the other as a unique human being, not as "an illness," as "a room number," or as "all nurses" in general.

Therapeutic relationships are goal oriented. Ideally, the nurse and patient decide together what the goal of the relationship will be. Most often, the goal is promotion of learning and growth to bring about change in the patient's life. In general, the goal of a therapeutic relationship may be based on a problem-solving model.

Example

Goal: The patient will demonstrate more adaptive coping strategies for dealing with (specific life situation).
Interventions:
■ Identify what is troubling the patient at the present time.
■ Encourage the patient to discuss changes they would like to make.
■ Discuss which changes are possible and which are not possible.
■ Explore feelings about aspects of their life that cannot be changed and alternative ways of coping more adaptively.
■ Discuss alternative strategies for creating changes the patient desires to make.
■ Weigh the benefits and consequences of each alternative.
■ Assist the patient to select an alternative.

■ Encourage the patient to implement the change.
■ Provide positive feedback for the patient's attempts to create change.
■ Assist the patient to evaluate outcomes of the change and make modifications as required.

Therapeutic Use of Self

Travelbee (1971) described the instrument for delivery of interpersonal nursing as the *therapeutic use of self*, which is defined as "the ability to use one's personality consciously and in full awareness in an attempt to establish relatedness and to structure nursing intervention" (p. 19). Use of the self in a therapeutic manner requires that the nurse possess self-awareness and self-understanding, which are achieved by developing a philosophical belief about life, death, and the overall human condition. The

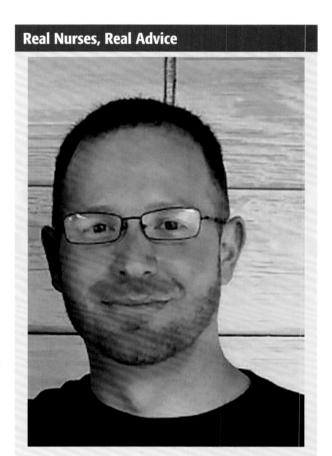

Real Nurses, Real Advice

"Many patients admitted to inpatient psychiatric settings are there involuntarily so establishing trust can sometimes be a challenge. Truthfulness, honesty, and genuineness are the best ways to earn a patient's trust. Trust is essential for earning the patient's respect and growing your nurse–patient relationship."

—Matt Mangus, RN, BSN

nurse must understand that the ability and the extent to which one can effectively help others in time of need is strongly influenced by this internal value system—a combination of intellect and emotions.

Gaining Self-Awareness

Values Clarification

Knowing and understanding oneself enhances the ability to form satisfactory interpersonal relationships. Self-awareness requires that an individual recognize and accept what they value and learn to accept the uniqueness of and differences in others. This concept is important in everyday life and in the nursing profession in general, but it is *essential* in psychiatric nursing.

An individual's value system is established very early in life and has its foundations in the value system held by one's primary caregivers. It is culturally oriented; consists of beliefs, attitudes, and values; and may change many times throughout one's lifetime. Values clarification is one process by which an individual may gain self-awareness.

Beliefs

A **belief** is an idea that one holds true, and it can take any of several forms:

- *Rational beliefs* are ideas for which objective evidence exists to substantiate their truth.
  - Example: Alcoholism is a disease.
- *Irrational beliefs* are ideas that an individual holds as true despite the existence of objective contradictory evidence. Delusions can be a form of irrational beliefs.
  - Example: Once an alcoholic has been through detoxification and rehabilitation, they can drink socially if desired.
- *Faith* (sometimes called *blind beliefs*) is a belief in something or someone that does not require proof.
  - Example: Belief in a higher power can help an alcoholic stop drinking.
- A *stereotype* is a socially shared belief that describes a concept in an oversimplified or undifferentiated matter.
  - Example: All alcoholics are skid-row bums.

Attitudes

An **attitude** is a frame of reference around which an individual organizes knowledge about their world. An attitude also has an emotional component. It can be a prejudgment and may be selective and biased. Attitudes fulfill the need to find meaning in life and to provide clarity and consistency for the individual. The prevailing stigma attached to mental illness is an example of a negative attitude. An associated stereotype might be that "all people with mental illness are dangerous."

Values

Values are abstract standards, positive or negative, that represent an individual's ideal mode of conduct and ideal goals. Examples of ideal modes of conduct include seeking truth and beauty; being clean and orderly; and behaving with sincerity, justice, reason, compassion, humility, respect, honor, and loyalty. Examples of ideal goals are security, happiness, freedom, equality, ecstasy, fame, and power.

Values differ from attitudes and beliefs in that they are action oriented or action producing. People may hold many attitudes and beliefs without behaving in a way that shows they hold those attitudes and beliefs. For example, a nurse may believe that all patients have the right to be told the truth about their diagnosis; however, they may not always act on the belief by telling all patients the complete truth about their conditions. Only when the belief is acted on does it become a value.

Attitudes and beliefs flow from one's set of values. An individual may have thousands of beliefs and hundreds of attitudes, but their values probably number only in the dozens. Values may be viewed as a kind of core concept or basic standard that determines one's attitudes, beliefs, and ultimately, behavior. Raths and associates (1978) identified a seven-step assessment process that can be used to help clarify personal values. This process is presented in Table 6–1. The process can be used by applying these seven steps to an attitude or belief that one holds. When an attitude or belief has met each of the seven criteria, it can be considered a personal value.

The Johari Window

The self arises out of self-appraisal and the appraisal of others. It represents each individual's unique pattern of values, attitudes, beliefs, behaviors, emotions, and needs. Self-awareness is the recognition of these aspects and understanding about their effect on the self and others. The Johari Window, presented in Figure 6–1, is a representation of the self and a tool that can be used to increase self-awareness (Luft, 1970). The Johari Window is divided into four quadrants (four aspects of the self): the open self, the unknowing self, the private self, and the unknown self.

The Open or Public Self

The upper-left quadrant of the window represents the part of the self that is public; that is, aspects of the self about which both the individual and others are aware.

TABLE 6–1 **The Process of Values Clarification**			
LEVEL OF OPERATIONS	**CATEGORY**	**CRITERIA**	**EXPLANATION**
Cognitive	Choosing	1. Freely 2. From alternatives 3. After careful consideration of the consequences	"This value is mine. No one forced me to choose it. I understand and accept the consequences of holding this value."
Emotional	Prizing	4. Satisfied; pleased with the choice 5. Making public affirmation of the choice, if necessary	"I am proud that I hold this value, and I am willing to tell others about it."
Behavioral	Acting	6. Taking action to demonstrate the value behaviorally 7. Demonstrating this pattern of behavior consistently and repeatedly	The value is reflected in the individual's behavior for as long as he or she holds it.

Adapted from: Raths, L., Harmin, M., & Simon, S. (1978). *Values and teaching: Working with values in the classroom* (2nd ed.). Merrill.

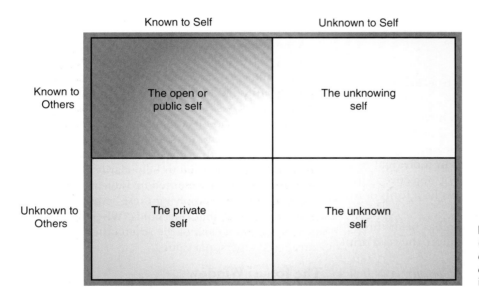

FIGURE 6–1 The Johari Window. (Source: Luft, J. (1970). *Group processes: An introduction to group dynamics* [3rd ed.]. Mayfield Publishing, 1984, with permission.)

Example

Susan, a nurse who is the adult child of an alcoholic, has strong feelings about helping alcoholics to achieve sobriety. She volunteers her time as a support person on call to help recovering alcoholics. She is aware of her feelings and her desire to help others. Members of the Alcoholics Anonymous group in which she volunteers her time are also aware of Susan's feelings, and they feel comfortable calling her when they need help with refraining from drinking.

The Unknowing Self

The upper-right quadrant of the window represents the part of the self that is known to others but remains hidden from the awareness of the individual.

Example

When Susan takes care of patients in detoxification, she does so without emotion, tending to the technical aspects of the task in a way that the patients perceive as cold and judgmental. She is unaware that she comes across to patients in this way.

The Private Self

The lower-left quadrant of the window represents the part of the self that is known to the individual but which the individual deliberately and consciously conceals from others.

Example

Susan would prefer not to take care of the patients in detoxification because doing so provokes painful memories from her childhood. However, because she does not want the other staff members to know about these feelings, she volunteers to take care of the detoxification patients whenever they are assigned to her unit.

The Unknown Self

The lower-right quadrant of the window represents the part of the self that is unknown to both the individual and to others.

Example

Susan felt very powerless as a child growing up with an alcoholic father. She seldom knew in what condition she would find her father or what his behavior would be. She learned over the years to find small ways to maintain control over her life situation, and she left home as soon as she graduated from high school. The need to stay in control has always been very important to Susan, and she is unaware that working with recovering alcoholics helps to fulfill this need. The people she is helping are also unaware that Susan is satisfying an unfulfilled personal need as she provides them with assistance.

The goal of increasing self-awareness by using the Johari Window is to increase the size of the quadrant that represents the open or public self. The individual who is open to self and others is able to be spontaneous and to share emotions and experiences with others. This individual also has a greater understanding of personal behavior and of others' responses to them. Increased self-awareness allows an individual to interact comfortably with others, to accept the differences in others, and to observe each person's right to respect and dignity.

Conditions Essential to Development of a Therapeutic Relationship

Several characteristics that enhance the achievement of a therapeutic relationship have been identified. These concepts are highly significant to the use of self as the therapeutic tool in interpersonal relationship development.

Rapport

Getting acquainted and establishing **rapport** is the primary task in relationship development. Rapport implies special feelings on the part of both the patient and the nurse based on acceptance, warmth, friendliness, common interest, a sense of trust, and a nonjudgmental attitude. Establishing rapport may be accomplished by discussing non–health-related topics. Travelbee (1971) stated:

> [To establish rapport] is to create a sense of harmony based on knowledge and appreciation of each

individual's uniqueness. It is the ability to be still and experience the other as a human being—to appreciate the unfolding of each personality one to the other. The ability to truly care for and about others is the core of rapport. (pp. 152, 155)

Trust

To trust another, one must feel confident in that person's presence, reliability, integrity, veracity, and sincere desire to provide assistance when requested. As summarized in Chapter 31, "Personality Disorders," and discussed in online Chapter 38, "Theoretical Models of Personality Development," trust is the initial developmental task described by Erikson (1963). If the task has not been achieved, this component of relationship development becomes more difficult. That is not to say that trust cannot be established, but only that additional time and patience may be required on the part of the nurse.

Trust cannot be presumed; it must be earned. Trustworthiness is demonstrated through nursing interventions that convey a sense of warmth and caring to the patient. These interventions are initiated simply and concretely and directed toward activities that address the patient's basic needs for physiological and psychological safety and security. Psychiatric patients with thought disorders, such as schizophrenia, may also have difficulty thinking abstractly (a symptom called **concrete thinking**) so it becomes even more important that the nurse communicate and behave in a simple, concrete manner to promote the development of trust. Examples of nursing interventions that promote trust in an individual who is thinking concretely include the following:

■ Providing a blanket when the patient is cold
■ Providing food when the patient is hungry
■ Keeping promises
■ Being honest (e.g., saying "I don't know the answer to your question, but I'll try to find out") and then following through
■ Providing reasons, simply and clearly, for certain policies, procedures, and rules
■ Providing a written, structured schedule of activities
■ Attending activities with the patient if they are reluctant to go alone
■ Being consistent in adhering to unit guidelines
■ Listening to the patient's preferences, requests, and opinions and making collaborative decisions concerning their care whenever possible
■ Ensuring **confidentiality;** providing reassurance that what is discussed will not be repeated outside the boundaries of the health-care team

Trust is the basis of a therapeutic relationship. The nurse working in psychiatry must perfect the skills that foster the development of trust. Trust must be established for the nurse–patient relationship to progress beyond the superficial level of tending to the patient's immediate needs.

Respect

To show respect is to believe in the dignity and worth of an individual regardless of their unacceptable behavior. Psychologist Carl Rogers called this **unconditional positive regard** (Rogers, 1951). The attitude is nonjudgmental, and the respect is unconditional in that it does not depend on the behavior of the patient to meet certain standards. The nurse, in fact, may not approve of the patient's lifestyle or behavior patterns. However, with unconditional positive regard, the patient is accepted and respected for no other reason than that they are considered to be a worthwhile and unique human being.

Many psychiatric patients have very little self-respect. Sometimes lack of self-respect is related to the low self-esteem that accompanies illnesses such as clinical depression, and sometimes it is related to rejection and stigmatization by others. Recognition that they are unconditionally accepted and respected as unique, valuable individuals can elevate feelings of self-worth and self-respect. The nurse can convey an attitude of respect by

- Calling the patient by name (and title, if they prefer).
- Spending time with the patient.
- Allowing sufficient time to answer the patient's questions and concerns.
- Promoting an atmosphere of privacy during therapeutic interactions with the patient and during physical examination or therapy.
- Always being open and honest with the patient, even when the truth may be difficult to discuss.
- Listening to the patient's ideas, preferences, and opinions and making collaborative decisions concerning their care whenever possible.
- Striving to understand the motivation behind the patient's behavior regardless of how unacceptable it may seem.

Genuineness

The concept of **genuineness** refers to the nurse's ability to be open, honest, and "real" in interactions with the patient. To be real is to be aware of what one is experiencing internally and to allow the quality of this inner experience to be apparent in the therapeutic relationship. When one is genuine, there is *congruence* between what is felt and what is expressed. The nurse who is genuine responds to the patient with truth and honesty rather than with responses they may consider more "professional" or ones that merely reflect the "nursing role."

Genuineness may call for a degree of *self-disclosure* on the part of the nurse. This is not to say that the nurse must disclose to the patient *everything* they are feeling or *all* personal experiences that relate to what the patient is going through. Indeed, care must be taken when using self-disclosure to avoid reversing the roles of nurse and patient. For example, when a patient tells the nurse, "I just get so upset when someone disrespects me; sometimes you have to smack someone to teach them a lesson," the nurse might respond, "I get upset by that, too. Let's talk about some different ways to respond to your anger rather than hitting someone." In this example, the nurse discloses a common feeling while maintaining a focus on the patient's need for problem-solving. When the nurse uses self-disclosure, a quality of "humanness" is revealed to the patient, creating a role for the patient to model in similar situations. The patient may then feel more comfortable revealing personal information to the nurse.

Most individuals have an uncanny ability to detect when others are artificial. When the nurse does not bring genuineness and respect to the relationship, a reality basis for trust cannot be established. These qualities are essential to helping the patient actualize their potential within the nurse–patient relationship and for change and growth to occur.

Empathy

Empathy is the ability to see beyond outward behavior and understand the situation from the patient's point of view. With empathy, the nurse can accurately perceive and comprehend the meaning and relevance of the patient's thoughts and feelings. The nurse must also be able to communicate this perception to the patient by attempting to translate words and behaviors into feelings.

It is not uncommon for the concept of empathy to be confused with that of **sympathy.** The major difference is that with *empathy* the nurse "accurately perceives or understands" what the patient is feeling and encourages the patient to explore these feelings. With *sympathy* the nurse actually "shares" what the patient is feeling and experiences a need to alleviate distress. Schuster (2000) stated:

> Empathy means that you remain emotionally separate from the other person, even though you can see the patient's viewpoint clearly. This is different from sympathy. Sympathy implies taking on the other's needs and problems as if they were your own and becoming emotionally involved to the point of losing your objectivity. To empathize rather than sympathize, you must show feelings but not get caught

up in feelings or overly identify with the patient's and family's concerns. (p. 102)

Empathy is considered to be one of the most important characteristics of a therapeutic relationship. Accurate empathetic perceptions on the part of the nurse assist the patient in identifying feelings that may have been suppressed or denied. Positive emotions are generated as the patient realizes that they are truly understood by another. As the feelings surface and are explored, the patient learns aspects about the self of which they may have been unaware. This exploration contributes to the process of personal identification and the promotion of positive self-concept.

With empathy, while understanding the patient's thoughts and feelings, the nurse is able to maintain sufficient objectivity to allow the patient to achieve problem resolution with minimal assistance. With sympathy, the nurse feels what the patient is feeling, objectivity is lost, and the nurse may become focused on relief of personal distress rather than on helping the patient resolve the problem at hand. The following example describes a sympathetic response and an empathetic response to the same situation.

Example

Situation: BJ is a patient on the psychiatric unit with a diagnosis of persistent depressive disorder (dysthymia). She is 5 feet 5 inches tall and weighs 295 pounds. BJ has been overweight all her life. She is single, has no close friends, and has never had an intimate relationship with another person. It is her first day on the unit, and she is refusing to come out of her room. When she appeared for lunch in the dining room after admission, she was embarrassed when several of the other patients laughed out loud and called her "fatso."
Sympathetic response: Nurse: "I can certainly identify with what you are feeling. I've been overweight most of my life, too. I just get so angry when people act like that. They are so insensitive! It's just so typical of skinny people to act that way. You have a right to want to stay away from them. We'll just see how loud they laugh when *you* get to choose what movie is shown on the unit after dinner tonight."
Empathetic response: Nurse: "You feel angry and embarrassed by what happened at lunch today." As tears fill BJ's eyes, the nurse encourages her to cry if she feels like it and to express her anger at the situation. She stays with BJ but does not dwell on her *own* feelings about what happened. Instead, she focuses on BJ and what the patient perceives are her most immediate needs at this time.

Rapport, trust, respect, genuineness, and empathy all are essential to forming therapeutic relationships,

and they can be assets in social relationships, too. The primary differences between social and therapeutic relationships are that therapeutic relationships always remain focused on the health-care needs of the patient, are never used to address the nurse's personal needs, and progress through identified phases of development to help the patient solve health-related problems.

Phases of a Therapeutic Nurse–Patient Relationship

Psychiatric nurses use interpersonal relationship development as the primary intervention with patients in psychiatric-mental health settings. This activity is congruent with Peplau's (1962) identification of *counseling* as the major role of nursing in psychiatry. Sullivan (1953), from whom Peplau patterned her interpersonal theory of nursing, strongly believed that many emotional problems are closely related to difficulties with interpersonal relationships. With this concept in mind, the counseling role of the nurse in psychiatry becomes especially meaningful and purposeful—an integral part of the total therapeutic regimen.

The therapeutic interpersonal relationship is the means by which the nursing process is implemented. Through the relationship, problems are identified and resolution is sought. Tasks of the relationship have been categorized into four phases: (1) the preinteraction phase, (2) the orientation (introductory) phase, (3) the working phase, and (4) the termination phase. Although each phase is presented as specific and distinct from the others, there may be some overlap of tasks, particularly when the interaction is limited. The major nursing goals during each phase of the nurse–patient relationship are listed in Table 6–2.

The Preinteraction Phase

The preinteraction phase involves preparation for the first encounter with the patient. Tasks include the following:

■ Obtaining available information about the patient from their chart, significant others, or other health-care team members. From this information, the initial assessment begins. The nurse may also become aware of personal responses to knowledge about the patient.

■ Examining one's feelings, fears, and anxieties about working with a particular patient. For example, the nurse may have been reared in an alcoholic family and have ambivalent feelings about caring for a patient who is dependent on alcohol. All individuals bring attitudes and feelings

TABLE 6–2	**Phases of Relationship Development and Major Nursing Goals**
PHASE	**GOALS**
1. Preinteraction	Explore self-perceptions
2. Orientation (introductory)	Establish trust Formulate contract for intervention
3. Working	Promote client change
4. Termination	Evaluate goal attainment Ensure therapeutic closure

from prior experiences to the clinical setting. The nurse needs to be aware of how these preconceptions may affect their ability to care for individual patients.

The Orientation (Introductory) Phase

During the orientation phase, the nurse and patient become acquainted. Tasks include the following:

■ Creating an environment for the establishment of trust and rapport.
■ Establishing a contract for intervention that details the expectations and responsibilities of both nurse and patient.
■ Gathering assessment information to build a strong patient database.
■ Identifying the patient's strengths and limitations.
■ Formulating nursing diagnoses.
■ Setting goals that are mutually agreeable to the nurse and patient.
■ Developing a plan of action that is realistic for meeting the established goals.
■ Exploring feelings of both the patient and nurse in terms of the introductory phase.

Introductions are often uncomfortable, and the participants may experience some anxiety until a degree of rapport has been established. Interactions may remain on a superficial level until anxiety subsides. Several interactions may be required to fulfill the tasks associated with this phase.

The Working Phase

The therapeutic work of the relationship is accomplished during this phase. Tasks include the following:

■ Maintaining the trust and rapport established during the orientation phase.
■ Promoting the patient's insight and perception of reality.

■ Problem-solving using the model presented earlier in this chapter.
■ Overcoming resistance behaviors on the part of the patient as the level of anxiety rises in response to discussion of painful issues.
■ Continuously evaluating progress toward goal attainment.

Transference and Countertransference

Transference and countertransference are common phenomena that often arise during a therapeutic relationship.

Transference

Transference occurs when the patient unconsciously displaces (or "transfers") to the nurse feelings formed toward a person from their past. These feelings may be triggered by something about the nurse's appearance or personality characteristics that remind the patient of another person. Transference can interfere with the therapeutic interaction when the feelings expressed include anger and hostility. Anger toward the nurse can be manifested by uncooperativeness and resistance to therapy.

Transference can also take the form of overwhelming affection for or excessive dependency on the nurse. The nurse is overvalued, and the patient forms unrealistic expectations of the nurse. When the nurse is unable to fulfill those expectations or meet the excessive dependency needs, the patient becomes angry and hostile.

Interventions for Transference

When the nurse suspects that transference may be affecting their relationship with the patient, it is helpful for the nurse to share with the patient their perceptions about patient behaviors and communication and help the patient to explore possible meanings in the context of the nurse–patient relationship. The goal is to assist the patient to develop more awareness of various influences on their behavior and communication and to develop more adaptive relationship skills.

Countertransference

Countertransference refers to the nurse's behavioral and emotional responses to the patient in which the nurse transfers feelings (often unconscious) about past experiences or people onto the patient. These responses may be related to unresolved feelings toward significant others from the nurse's past, or they may be generated in response to transference feelings on the part of the patient. It is not easy to refrain from becoming angry when the patient is consistently antagonistic, to feel flattered when showered with affection and attention by the patient, or even to feel quite powerful when the patient exhibits excessive dependency on the nurse. These feelings can interfere with the therapeutic relationship when they initiate the following types of behaviors:

■ The nurse overidentifies with the patient's feelings, as they remind the nurse of problems from their past or present.
■ The nurse and patient develop a social or personal relationship.
■ The nurse begins to give advice or attempts to "rescue" the patient.
■ The nurse encourages and promotes the patient's dependence.
■ The nurse's anger engenders feelings of disgust toward the patient.
■ The nurse feels anxious and uneasy in the presence of the patient.
■ The nurse is bored and apathetic in sessions with the patient.
■ The nurse has difficulty setting limits on the patient's behavior.
■ The nurse defends the patient's behavior to other staff members.

The nurse may be completely unaware or only minimally aware of the countertransference as it is occurring.

Interventions for Countertransference

The nurse's developing awareness of factors influencing their behavior and communication with patients is key to promoting more adaptive strategies. Peer or supervisory relationships are valuable resources for feedback. Consider the following example.

A coworker comments to a nursing peer, "I noticed when the patient said he started drinking again but it wasn't his fault, you seemed noticeably annoyed when you responded to him. What was going on there?" The nurse reflects on the coworker's feedback and notices "When he started saying it wasn't his fault, he reminded me of my ex-husband, who never took responsibility for his own behavior." The nurse's new awareness provides an opportunity to separate feelings associated with personal relationships and become more intentional in professional relationship with the patient.

The Termination Phase

Termination of the relationship may occur for a variety of reasons: the mutually agreed-on goals may have been reached, the patient may be discharged from the hospital, or, in the case of a student nurse, the clinical rotation ends. Termination can be difficult for both the patient and nurse. The main task involves bringing a therapeutic conclusion to the relationship. The relationship concludes when the following occur:

■ Progress has been made toward attainment of mutually set goals.
■ A plan for continuing care or for assistance during stressful life experiences is mutually established by the nurse and patient.
■ Feelings about termination of the relationship are recognized and explored. Both the nurse and patient may experience feelings of sadness and loss. The nurse should share their feelings with the patient. Through these interactions, the patient learns that it is acceptable to have these kinds of feelings at a time of separation. With this knowledge, the patient experiences growth during the process of termination. This is also a time when both nurse and patient may evaluate and summarize the learning that occurred as an outgrowth of their relationship.

CLINICAL PEARL When the patient feels sadness and loss, behaviors to delay termination may become evident. If the nurse experiences the same feelings, they may allow the patient's behaviors to delay termination. For therapeutic closure, the nurse must establish the reality of the separation and resist being manipulated into repeated delays by the patient.

Boundaries in the Nurse–Patient Relationship

A boundary indicates a border that determines the extent of acceptable limits. Many types of boundaries exist, such as the following.

■ **Material boundaries** can be seen, such as fences that border land.
■ **Social boundaries** are established within a culture and define how individuals are expected to behave in social situations.
■ **Personal boundaries** are boundaries that individuals define for themselves. They include *physical distance boundaries,* or how closely individuals will allow others to enter their physical space, and *emotional boundaries,* or how much individuals choose to disclose of their most private and intimate selves to others.
■ **Professional boundaries** limit and outline expectations for appropriate professional relationships with patients. "Professional boundaries are the spaces between a nurse's power and the patient's vulnerability" (National Council of State Boards of Nursing [NCSBN], 2018, p. 4). Nurses must recognize that they have an imbalance of power with

their patients because of their role and the patient information to which they have access. They must be consistently conscientious in avoiding any circumstance in which they might achieve personal gain within that relationship.

Concerns regarding professional boundaries are commonly related to the following issues:

- **Self-disclosure:** Self-disclosure on the part of the nurse may be appropriate when the information could therapeutically benefit the patient. It should never be undertaken to meet the nurse's needs.
- **Gift-giving:** Individuals who are receiving care often feel indebted toward health-care providers. The British Columbia College of Professional Nurses (BCCPN, 2023) clarifies in their practice standards that, although nurses do not generally exchange gifts with patients, when it is deemed to have therapeutic intent, groups of nurses may accept a token gift, but significant gifts should be returned or redirected. There is always a degree of clinical judgment necessary in deciding to accept or refuse a gift, including the appropriateness, the value, and the reason the gift is being offered. Cultural beliefs and values may also enter into the decision of whether to accept a gift from a patient. In some cultures, failure to do so would be interpreted as an insult (Choe, 2019). Accepting financial gifts is never appropriate, but in some instances, nurses may be permitted to instead suggest a donation to a charity of the patient's choice. If acceptance of a small gift of gratitude is deemed appropriate, the nurse may choose to share it with other staff members who have been involved in the patient's care. In all instances, nurses should exercise professional judgment when deciding whether to accept a gift from a patient, and refusal of a gift should be done with sensitivity for the patient's feelings. Attention should be given to what the gift-giving means to the patient, as well as to institutional policy, the American Nurses Association (ANA) *Code of Ethics for Nurses*, and the ANA *Scope and Standards of Practice*.
- **Touch:** Nursing, by its very nature, involves touching patients. Touching is required to perform the therapeutic procedures involved in providing physical care. Caring touch is the touching of patients when there is no physical need to do so. Touching or hugging can be beneficial when it is implemented with therapeutic intent and patient consent. When using caring touch, make sure it is appropriate, supportive, and welcomed (BCCPN, 2019). Caring touch may provide comfort or encouragement, but some vulnerable patients may misinterpret its meaning. In some cultures, touch is not considered acceptable unless the

parties know each other very well. The nurse must be sensitive to these cultural nuances and aware when touch is crossing a personal boundary. Additionally, patients who are experiencing high levels of anxiety, suspiciousness, or psychosis may interpret touch as aggressiveness. These are times when touch should be avoided or considered with extreme caution.

- **Friendship or romantic association:** When a nurse is previously acquainted with a patient, the relationship must move from a personal nature to professional. If the nurse is unable to accomplish this separation, they should withdraw from the nurse–patient relationship. Likewise, nurses must guard against personal relationships developing as a result of the nurse–patient relationship. Romantic, sexual, or otherwise intimate personal relationships are never appropriate between nurse and patient.

Certain warning signs indicate that professional boundaries of the nurse–patient relationship may be in jeopardy. These may include the following (Coltrane & Pugh, 1978):

- Favoring one patient's care over that of another
- Keeping secrets with a patient
- Changing dress style for working with a particular patient
- Swapping assignments to care for a particular patient
- Giving special attention or treatment to one patient over others
- Spending free time with a patient
- Frequently thinking about the patient when away from work
- Sharing personal information or work concerns with the patient
- Receiving gifts from or continuing contact or communication with the patient after discharge

Boundary crossing can threaten the integrity of the nurse–patient relationship. Nurses must gain self-awareness and insight to recognize when professional integrity is compromised. Although some variables, such as the care setting, community influences, patient needs, and the nature of therapy, affect how boundaries are delineated, "any actions that overstep the established boundaries to meet the needs of the nurse are boundary violations" (NCSBN, 2018, p. 6).

Summary and Key Points

- Nurses who work in the psychiatric-mental health field use special skills, or "interpersonal techniques," to assist patients in adapting to difficulties or changes in life experiences. Therapeutic nurse–patient relationships are goal oriented, and the problem-solving model is used to try to bring about some type of change in the patient's life.

■ The instrument for delivery of the process of interpersonal nursing is the therapeutic use of self, which requires that the nurse possess a strong sense of self-awareness and self-understanding.

■ Hildegard Peplau identified seven nursing roles within the therapeutic relationship: stranger, resource person, teacher, leader, surrogate, technical expert, and counselor.

■ Characteristics that enhance the achievement of a therapeutic relationship include rapport, trust, respect, genuineness, and empathy.

■ Phases of a therapeutic nurse–patient relationship include the preinteraction phase, orientation (introductory) phase, working phase, and termination phase.

■ Transference occurs when the patient unconsciously displaces (or "transfers") to the nurse feelings formed toward a person from the past.

■ Countertransference refers to the nurse's behavioral and emotional response to the patient in which the nurse transfers feelings (often unconscious) about past experiences or people onto the patient. These responses may be related to unresolved feelings toward significant others from the nurse's past, or they may be generated in response to transference feelings on the part of the patient.

■ Types of boundaries include material, social, personal, and professional.

■ Concerns associated with professional boundaries include self-disclosure, gift-giving, touch, and developing a friendship or romantic association.

■ Boundary crossings can threaten the integrity of the nurse–patient relationship.

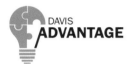

Go to **Davis Advantage** to complete your learning: strengthen understanding, apply your knowledge, and prepare for the Next Gen NCLEX®.

Review Questions

1. Which of the following behaviors suggest a possible breach of professional boundaries? (Select all that apply.)
   a. The nurse repeatedly requests to be assigned to a specific client.
   b. The nurse shares the details of her divorce with the client.
   c. The nurse makes arrangements to meet the client outside of the therapeutic environment.
   d. The nurse shares how she dealt with a similar difficult situation.

2. The nurse, who is an adult child of an alcoholic, is working with a client who abuses alcohol. The client has experienced a successful detoxification process and is beginning a rehabilitation program. The client says to the nurse, "I'm not going to go to those stupid AA meetings. They don't help anything." The nurse, whose father died of complications from alcoholism, responds with anger: "Don't you even care what happens to your children?" The nurse's response is an example of which of the following?
   a. Transference
   b. Countertransference
   c. Self-disclosure
   d. A breach of professional boundaries

3. Which of the following tasks are associated with the orientation phase of relationship development? (Select all that apply.)
   a. Promoting the patient's insight and perception of reality
   b. Creating an environment for the establishment of trust and rapport
   c. Using the problem-solving model toward goal fulfillment
   d. Obtaining available information about the patient from various sources
   e. Formulating nursing diagnoses and setting goals

4. Which of the following tasks are associated with the preinteraction phase of relationship development? (Select all that apply.)
   a. Promoting the client's insight and perception of reality
   b. Creating an environment for the establishment of trust and rapport
   c. Using the problem-solving model toward goal fulfillment
   d. Obtaining available information about the client from various sources
   e. Formulating nursing diagnoses and setting goals

5. The nurse is working with a client in the anger-management program. Which of the following identifies actions associated with the working phase of the therapeutic relationship?
   a. The nurse and the client work together to identify goals for developing more adaptive ways to handle anger.
   b. The client expresses a desire to continue in the anger management program after the goals have been met.
   c. The nurse reviews the client's medical record and assesses his or her personal feeling about working with a client who abused their spouse.
   d. The nurse assists the client in practicing various techniques to effectively manage anger and provides positive feedback when the client attempts to improve maladaptive behaviors.

6. When there is congruence between what is felt and what is expressed, the nurse is exhibiting which of the following characteristics?
   a. Trust
   b. Respect
   c. Genuineness
   d. Empathy

7. When the nurse shows unconditional acceptance of an individual as a worthwhile and unique human being, they are exhibiting which of the following characteristics?
   a. Trust
   b. Respect
   c. Genuineness
   d. Empathy

Clinical Judgment Questions

8. A client who is being discharged from an inpatient hospital stay has his wife bring a box of chocolates and a bouquet of flowers for his primary nurse. He presents these gifts to the nurse, saying, "Thank you for taking care of me." What is the most appropriate response by the nurse?
   a. "I don't accept gifts from patients."
   b. "Thank you so much! It is so nice to be appreciated."
   c. "Thank you. I will share these with the rest of the staff."
   d. "Hospital policy forbids me to accept gifts from patients."

9. A client states to the nurse, "I worked as a secretary to put my husband through college, and as soon as he graduated, he left me. I hate him! I hate all men!" Which of the following is an empathetic response by the nurse?
   a. "You are very angry now. This is a normal response to your loss."
   b. "I know what you mean. Men can be very insensitive."
   c. "I understand completely. My husband divorced me, too."
   d. "You are depressed now, but you will feel better in time."

10. A client with schizophrenia appears very watchful of others and tells the nurse, "There are infiltrators everywhere and I think they are trying to kill me." Which of these actions by the nurse would best promote development of trust with this client?
    a. Touch the client's shoulder and state, "I want you to feel safe here."
    b. State to the client, "I'm interested in hearing your thoughts. Would you like to talk more about this?"
    c. Ask the client, "Why would you think such a thing?"
    d. Tell the client, "It is an expectation that we will not talk about things that aren't real."

11. A client is being discharged from the inpatient psychiatric unit and states to their primary nurse, "Everyone abandons me and now you're probably going to abandon me, too." Which of these actions by the nurse best accomplishes termination of the therapeutic relationship?

a. Discuss the boundaries of this relationship and assist the client to explore their feelings.

b. Terminate the therapeutic relationship while exploring ways to remain connected as friends.

c. Provide discharge medication instructions and encourage the client to follow up with their physician.

d. Assure the client that they are not being abandoned and remind the individual that they can return to the unit in the future.

References

British Columbia College of Professional Nurses. (2023). *Boundaries in the nurse-client relationship: practice standard for registered nurses.* https://www.bccnm.ca/RN/PracticeStandards/Pages/boundaries.aspx

Choe, E. (2019). *Ethics in the language classroom: Gift giving culture.* https://multiolelo.com/2019/12/13/ethics-the-language-classroom-gift-giving-culture/

National Council of State Boards of Nursing (NCSBN). (2018). A nurse's guide to professional boundaries. https://www.ncsbn.org/public-files/ProfessionalBoundaries_Complete.pdf

Schuster, P. M. (2000). *Communication: The key to the therapeutic relationship.* F.A. Davis.

Classical References

Coltrane, F., & Pugh, C. (1978). Danger signals in staff/patient relationships. *Journal of Psychiatric Nursing & Mental Health Services, 16*(6): 34–36. doi:10.3928/0279-3695-19780601-06

Erikson, E. (1963). *Childhood and society* (2nd ed.). W.W. Norton.

Luft, J. (1970). *Group processes: An introduction to group dynamics* (3rd ed.). Mayfield Publishing.

Peplau, H.E. (1952) *Interpersonal relations in nursing.* Putnam.

Peplau, H. E. (1991). *Interpersonal relations in nursing.* Springer.

Raths, L., Harmin, M., & Simon, S. (1978). *Values and teaching: Working with values in the classroom* (2nd ed.). Merrill.

Rogers, C. (1951). *Client-centered therapy: Its current practice, implications and theory.* Constable.

Sullivan, H. S. (1953). *The interpersonal theory of psychiatry.* W.W. Norton.

Travelbee, J. (1971). *Interpersonal aspects of nursing* (2nd ed.). F.A. Davis.

7

Therapeutic Communication

KEY TERMS

density

distance

intimate distance

motivational interviewing

paralanguage

personal distance

public distance

social distance

territoriality

OBJECTIVES
After reading this chapter, the student will be able to:

1. Discuss the transactional model of communication.
2. Identify types of preexisting conditions that influence the outcome of the communication process.
3. Define *territoriality, density,* and *distance* as components of the environment.
4. Identify components of nonverbal expression.
5. Describe therapeutic and nontherapeutic verbal communication techniques.
6. Describe motivational interviewing as a communication strategy.
7. Describe active listening.
8. Discuss therapeutic feedback.

Development of the *therapeutic interpersonal relationship* is described in Chapter 6, "Relationship Development," as the process by which nurses provide care for patients in need of psychosocial intervention. *Therapeutic use of self* was identified as the instrument for delivery of care. The focus of this chapter is on *techniques* or, more specifically, *interpersonal communication techniques,* to facilitate delivery of that care.

In their classic work on therapeutic communication, Hays and Larson (1963) stated, "To relate therapeutically with a patient it is necessary for the nurse to understand his or her role and its relationship to the patient's illness" (p. 1). They describe the role of the nurse as providing the patient with the opportunity to accomplish the following:

1. Identify and explore problems in relating to others.
2. Discover healthy ways of meeting emotional needs.
3. Experience a satisfying interpersonal relationship.

These goals are achieved through the use of interpersonal communication techniques (both verbal and nonverbal). The nurse must be aware of the therapeutic or nontherapeutic value of the communication techniques used with the patient because they are the tools of psychosocial intervention.

CORE CONCEPT

Communication
An interactive process of transmitting information between two or more entities.

What Is Communication?

It has been said that individuals "cannot *not* communicate." Every word spoken, every movement made, and every action taken or not taken gives a message to someone. Interpersonal communication is a *transaction* between the sender and the receiver. In the transactional model of communication, both participants simultaneously perceive each other, listen to each other, and are mutually involved in creating meaning in a relationship. The transactional model is illustrated in Figure 7–1.

The Impact of Preexisting Conditions

In all interpersonal transactions, the sender and receiver each bring certain preexisting conditions to the exchange that influence both the intended message and how it is interpreted. Examples of these conditions include one's value system, internalized attitudes and beliefs, culture and religion, social status, gender, background knowledge and experience, and age or developmental level. The

type of environment in which the communication takes place may also influence the outcome of the transaction. Figure 7–2 shows how these influencing factors are positioned on the transactional model.

Values, Attitudes, and Beliefs

Values, attitudes, and beliefs are learned ways of thinking. Children generally adopt the value systems and internalize the attitudes and beliefs of their parents. Children may retain this way of thinking into adulthood or develop a different set of attitudes and values as they mature.

Values, attitudes, and beliefs can influence communication in numerous ways. For example, prejudice is expressed verbally through negative stereotyping. Attitudes may be communicated by use of certain words and through the volume and tone of voice. Values may be communicated directly through behaviors such as a person who expresses their value for religion by attending religious services.

One's value system may also be communicated with behaviors that are more symbolic in nature. For example, an individual who values youth may dress and behave in a manner that is characteristic of one who is much younger. People who value socioeconomic status may choose large homes, luxury cars, and other expensive personal possessions. In each of these situations, a message is being communicated.

Culture and Religion

Communication has its roots in culture. Cultural mores, norms, ideas, and customs provide the basis for our way of thinking. Cultural values are learned and differ from society to society. For example, in some European countries (e.g., Italy, Spain, France), men may greet each other with hugs and kisses; in the United States or Great Britain, shaking hands is a more culturally accepted style of greeting among men.

Religion also can influence communication. Priests and ministers who wear clerical collars

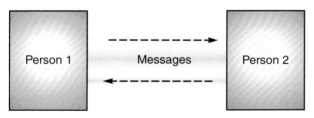

FIGURE 7–1 The transactional model of communication.

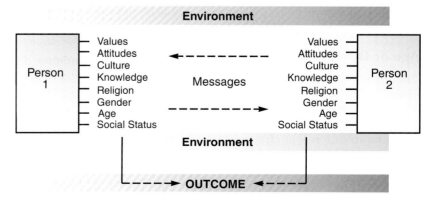

FIGURE 7–2 Factors influencing the transactional model of communication.

publicly communicate their mission in life. The collar may influence the way in which others relate to them, either positively or negatively. Other symbolic gestures, such as wearing a cross around the neck or wearing a hijab (a religious veil worn by some Muslim women in public), also communicate an individual's religious beliefs.

Social Status

Studies of nonverbal indicators of social status or power have suggested that individuals communicate status and power through body language such as eye contact and erect, open posture; louder voice pitch, and more frequent talking; approaching others and interacting with less interpersonal distance; as well as more covert cues such as formal dress and jewelry (Ali, 2021; Hall et al., 2005).

Gender

Gender may influence how individuals communicate. Within cultures and families, *gender signals* may be communicated as either masculine or feminine, and these are socially reinforced. Examples may include differences in posture and social distance.

Historically, many roles have been identified as either male or female. For example, in the United States traditional masculine roles included husband, father, breadwinner, doctor, lawyer, or engineer. Traditional female roles included those of wife, mother, homemaker, nurse, teacher, or secretary. Cultural beliefs about expected gender roles may also affect the communication process.

However, gender signals are changing in U.S. society as roles become less distinct. Behaviors once considered typically masculine or feminine may now be generally accepted in members of both genders. Words such as *nonbinary* communicate a desire by some individuals to diminish the distinction between genders and minimize the discrimination of either. Gender roles are changing as both women and men enter professions that were once dominated by members of the opposite gender. Thus, making *assumptions* about gender-based communication styles could negatively affect the communication process.

Age or Developmental Level

Age influences communication, which is especially evident during adolescence. In their struggle to separate from parental confines and establish their own identity, adolescents generate a unique pattern of communication that changes from generation to generation. Words such as *dude, dope, lit,* and *wasted* have had special meaning for different generations of adolescents. The technological age has produced a whole new language for today's adolescents.

Communication by text messaging includes such acronyms as BRB ("be right back"), BFF ("best friends forever"), and YOLO ("you only live once").

Developmental physiological alterations may also influence communication. One example is American Sign Language, the system of unique gestures used by many people who are deaf or hearing impaired. Individuals who are blind at birth never learn the subtle nonverbal gestures that accompany language, which can completely change the meaning of the spoken word.

Environment in Which the Transaction Takes Place

The place where communication occurs influences the outcome of the interaction. For example, some individuals who feel uncomfortable and refuse to speak during a group therapy session may be willing to discuss problems privately on a one-to-one basis with the nurse.

Territoriality, density, and distance are aspects of the environment that communicate messages. **Territoriality** is the innate tendency to own space. Individuals lay claim to areas around themselves as their own. When an interaction takes place in the territory "owned" by one or the other, it often influences communication. Interpersonal communication can be more successful if the interaction takes place in a "neutral" area. For example, with the concept of territoriality in mind, the nurse may choose to conduct the psychosocial assessment in an interview room rather than in their office or the patient's room.

Density refers to the number of people within a given environmental space. It has been shown to influence interpersonal interaction. Some animal studies indicate a correlation between prolonged high-density situations and certain behaviors, such as aggression or withdrawal (Dai et al., 2018).

Distance is the means by which various cultures use space to communicate. Hall (1966) identified four kinds of spatial interaction, or distances, that people maintain from each other in their interpersonal interactions and the kinds of activities in which people engage at these various distances.

1. **Intimate distance** is the closest distance that individuals will allow between themselves and others. In mainstream American culture, this distance, which is restricted to intimate interactions, is 0 to 18 inches.
2. **Personal distance** is approximately 18 to 40 inches and reserved for personal interactions, such as close conversations with friends or colleagues.
3. **Social distance** is about 4 to 12 feet away from the body. Interactions at this distance include

conversations with strangers or acquaintances, such as at a cocktail party or in a public building.

4. **Public distance** is one that exceeds 12 feet. Examples include speaking in public or yelling to someone some distance away. This distance is considered public space, and communicants are free to move about in it during the interaction.

Nonverbal Communication

Various studies have identified nonverbal communication as more reliable than verbal communication in expressing one's attitudes and feelings, and some describe it as the single most powerful way in which communication occurs (Heathfield, 2019). Some aspects of nonverbal expression were discussed in the previous section on preexisting conditions that influence communication. Other components of nonverbal communication include physical appearance and dress, body movement and posture, touch, facial expressions, eye behavior, and vocal cues or *paralanguage* (such as intonation, pitch, and speed; a more detailed description follows). These nonverbal messages vary from culture to culture.

Physical Appearance and Dress

Physical appearance and dress are part of the total nonverbal stimuli that influence interpersonal responses, and under some conditions, they are the primary determinants of such responses. Body coverings, both dress and hair, are manipulated by the wearer in a manner that conveys a distinct message to the receiver. Dress can be formal or casual, stylish or unkempt. Hair can be long or short, and even the presence or absence of hair conveys a message about the person. Other body adornments that are also considered potential communication messages include tattoos, masks, cosmetics, badges, jewelry, and eyeglasses. Some jewelry worn in specific ways can give special messages (e.g., a gold band or diamond ring worn on the third finger of the left hand, a pin bearing Greek letters worn on the lapel, or the wearing of a ring inscribed with the insignia of a college or university). Individuals may convey a specific message with the total absence of any body adornment.

Body Movement and Posture

The way in which an individual positions their body communicates messages regarding self-esteem, gender identity, status, and interpersonal warmth or coldness. The individual whose posture is slumped, with the head and eyes pointed downward, conveys a message of low self-esteem. Specific ways of standing or sitting are considered to be either feminine or masculine within a defined culture. In the United States, to stand straight and tall with head high and hands on hips indicates a superior status over the person being addressed.

Reece and Whitman (1962) identified response behaviors that were used to designate individuals as either a "warm" or "cold" person. Individuals who were perceived as warm responded to others with a shift of posture toward the other person, a smile, direct eye contact, and hands that remained still. Individuals who responded to others with a slumped posture, by looking around the room, drumming fingers on the desk, and not smiling were perceived as cold.

Touch

Touch is a powerful communication tool. It can elicit both negative and positive reactions, depending on the people involved and the circumstances of the interaction. It is a very basic and primitive form of communication, and the appropriateness of its use is culturally determined.

Touch can be categorized according to the message communicated (Knapp & Hall, 2014):

■ *Functional-professional:* This type of touch is impersonal and businesslike. It is used to accomplish a task.
  ■ EXAMPLE: A tailor measuring a customer for a suit or a physician examining a patient
■ *Social-polite:* This type of touch is still rather impersonal, but it conveys an affirmation or acceptance of the other person.
  ■ EXAMPLE: A handshake
■ *Friendship-warmth:* Touch at this level indicates a strong liking for the other person, a feeling that he or she is a friend.
  ■ EXAMPLE: Laying one's hand on the shoulder of another
■ *Love-intimacy:* This type of touch conveys an emotional attachment or attraction for another person.
  ■ EXAMPLE: Engaging in a strong, mutual embrace
■ *Sexual arousal:* Touch at this level is an expression of physical attraction only.
  ■ EXAMPLE: Caressing or touching another with intent to create sexual arousal

Some cultures encourage more touching of various types than do others. The nurse should understand the cultural meaning of touch before using this method of communication in specific situations. The best practice is to ask the patient's permission before using touch as an intervention.

Facial Expressions

Next to human speech, facial expression is the primary source of communication. Facial expressions reveal an individual's emotional state, such as happiness, sadness, anger, surprise, and fear. The face is a complex multimessage system. Facial expressions serve to complement and qualify other communication behaviors and at times even take the place of verbal messages. A summary of feelings associated with various facial expressions is presented in Table 7–1.

TABLE 7–1 **Summary of Facial Expressions**	
FACIAL EXPRESSION	**ASSOCIATED FEELINGS**
NOSE	
Nostril flare	Anger; arousal
Wrinkling up	Dislike; disgust
LIPS	
Grin; smile	Happiness; contentment
Grimace	Fear; pain
Compressed	Anger; frustration
Canine-type snarl	Disgust
Pouted; frown	Unhappiness; discontented; disapproval
Pursing	Disagreement
Sneer	Contempt; disdain
BROWS	
Frown	Anger; unhappiness; concentration
Raised	Surprise; enthusiasm
TONGUE	
Stick out	Dislike; disagree
EYES	
Widened	Surprise; excitement
Narrowed; lids squeezed shut	Threat; fear
Stare	Threat
Stare, blink, then look away	Dislike; disinterest
Eyes downcast; lack of eye contact	Submission; low self-esteem
Eye contact (generally intermittent as opposed to a stare)	Self-confidence; interest

Sources: Cherry, K. (2019). Understanding body language and facial expressions. https://www.verywellmind.com/understand-body-language-and-facial-expressions-4147228; Simon, M. (2005). *Facial expressions: A visual reference for artists.* Watson-Guptill.

Eye Behavior

Eyes have been called the "windows of the soul." It is through eye contact that individuals view and are viewed by others in a revealing way, creating an interpersonal connection. In American culture, eye contact conveys a personal interest in the other person. Eye contact indicates that the communication channel is open, and it is often the initiating factor in verbal interaction between two people.

Eye behavior is regulated by social rules. These rules dictate where, when, for how long, and at whom we can look. Staring is often used to register disapproval of the behavior of another. People are extremely sensitive to being looked at, and if the gazing or staring behavior violates social rules, they often assign meaning to it, such as the following statement implies: "He kept staring at me, and I began to wonder if I was dressed inappropriately or had mustard on my face!"

Vocal Cues or Paralanguage

Paralanguage is the gestural component of the spoken word. It consists of pitch, tone, and loudness of spoken messages; the rate of speaking; expressively placed pauses; and the emphasis assigned to certain words. These vocal cues greatly influence the way individuals interpret verbal messages. A normally soft-spoken individual whose pitch and rate of speaking increase may be perceived as being anxious or tense.

Different vocal emphases can alter the interpretation of the message. Three examples follow:

1. "I felt **SURE** you would notice the change."
   Interpretation: I was **SURE** you would, but you didn't.
2. "I felt sure **YOU** would notice the change."
   Interpretation: I thought **YOU** would, even if nobody else did.
3. "I felt sure you would notice the **CHANGE**."
   Interpretation: Even if you didn't notice anything else, I thought you would notice the **CHANGE**.

Verbal cues play a major role in determining responses in human communication situations. *How* a message is verbalized can be as important as *what* is verbalized.

CORE CONCEPT
Therapeutic Communication
Caregiver verbal and nonverbal techniques that focus on the care receiver's needs and advance the promotion of healing and change. Therapeutic communication encourages the exploration of feelings and fosters understanding of behavioral motivation. It is nonjudgmental, discourages defensiveness, and promotes trust.

Therapeutic Communication Techniques

Hays and Larson (1963) identified a number of techniques to assist the nurse in interacting more therapeutically with patients. These are important "technical procedures" carried out by the nurse working in psychiatry, and they should serve to enhance the development of a therapeutic nurse–patient relationship. Table 7–2 includes a list of these techniques, a short explanation of their usefulness, and examples of each.

Nontherapeutic Communication Techniques

Several approaches are considered to be barriers to open communication between the nurse and patient. Hays and Larson (1963) identified a number of these techniques, which are presented in Table 7–3. Nurses should recognize and eliminate the use of these patterns in their relationships with patients. Avoiding these communication barriers will maximize the effectiveness of communication and enhance the nurse–patient relationship.

TABLE 7–2 **Therapeutic Communication Techniques**		
TECHNIQUE	**EXPLANATION/RATIONALE**	**EXAMPLES**
Using silence	Silence encourages the patient to organize thoughts and put them into words and allows the patient time to think about the significance of events, thoughts, and feelings. Allowing the patient to break the silence often provides the nurse with important information about the patient's foremost concerns.	Patient: "My husband divorced me so I must be undesirable." Nurse: (silence) Patient: "You know, when I think about it, no matter what my husband does I always assume it's my fault or it's something wrong with me."
Accepting	Acceptance conveys an attitude of reception and regard.	"Yes, I understand what you said." Eye contact; nodding.
Giving recognition	Acknowledging and indicating awareness is better than complimenting; the former reflects an observation and the latter reflects the nurse's judgment.	"Hello, Mr. J. I notice that you made a ceramic ashtray in OT." "I see you made your bed."
Offering self	Willingness to spend time with the patient and show interest on an unconditional basis helps to increase the patient's feelings of self-worth.	"I'll stay with you a while." "How are you feeling today?" "I'm interested in hearing your thoughts about the group you just attended."
Giving broad openings	Broad openings allow the patient to direct the focus of the interaction and emphasize the importance of the patient's role in the communication process.	"What would you like to talk about today?" "Is there anything you want to discuss?"
General leads	General leads offer the patient encouragement to continue with minimal input from the nurse.	"Yes, I see." "Go on." "And after that?"
Placing the event in time or sequence	Encouraging the patient to identify the sequence of events and when they occurred in time facilitates organizing one's thoughts about their experiences.	"What happened first?" "What happened next?" "Was this before or after . . . ?" "When did this happen?"
Making observations	Verbalizing observations about a patient's behavior or appearance encourages the patient to develop awareness of how they are perceived by others and promotes exploration of issues that may be problematic.	"You appear sad today." "I notice you are pacing a lot." "I notice that when I ask you about whether you have thoughts of suicide you change the subject."

Continued

TABLE 7–2 Therapeutic Communication Techniques–cont'd

TECHNIQUE	EXPLANATION/RATIONALE	EXAMPLES
Encouraging description of perceptions	Asking the patient to verbalize their perceptions facilitates the patient's ability to develop awareness and understanding. For the patient experiencing hallucinations, it can facilitate both nurse's and patient's clarification about what the patient's perceptual experiences are communicating.	"Tell me more about the voices you said you are hearing." "What was it that increased your agitation during the group activity?" "Are these voices you hear directing you to take some action?"
Encouraging comparison	Asking the patient to compare similarities and differences in ideas, experiences, or interpersonal relationships helps the patient recognize life experiences that tend to recur and those aspects of life that are changeable.	"Was this episode similar to . . . ?" "How does this compare with the time when . . . ?" "What was your response the last time this situation occurred?"
Restating	Repeating the main idea of what the patient has said lets the patient know whether an expressed statement has been understood and gives them the chance to continue or to clarify if necessary.	Patient: "I can't study. My mind keeps wandering." Nurse: "You have trouble concentrating." Patient: "I can't take that new job. What if I can't do it?" Nurse: "You're afraid you will fail in this new position."
Reflecting	Questions and feelings are referred back to the patient so that the patient is empowered to actively engage in problem-solving rather than simply asking the nurse for advice.	Patient: "Don't you think I should tell my boss I'm not putting up with that?" Nurse: "What do you think you should do?" Patient: "She makes me so upset!" Nurse: "So you're feeling angry at your boss?"
Focusing	Taking notice of a single idea or even a single word works especially well with a patient who is moving rapidly from one thought to another. However, focusing is very difficult for a patient with severe anxiety, so in this case the nurse should not pursue focusing until the anxiety level decreases.	"Tell me more about this specific point."
Exploring	When the nurse hears the patient mention an issue or theme that seems relevant, the nurse asks the patient to explore this further. Exploring facilitates the patient's development of awareness and understanding about events, thoughts, and feelings. However, if the patient chooses not to disclose further information, the nurse should refrain from pushing or probing in an area that obviously creates discomfort.	"Please explain that situation in more detail." "Tell me more about that particular situation." "You mentioned feeling like no one cares about you. Tell me more about those feelings."
Seeking clarification and validation	Striving to explain vague or incomprehensible statements and searching for mutual understanding of what has been said facilitates and increases understanding for both patient and nurse.	"I'm not sure that I understand. Would you please explain?" "Tell me if my understanding agrees with yours." "Do I understand correctly that you said . . . ?"
Presenting reality	When the patient has a misperception of the environment, the nurse defines reality by expressing their perception of the situation without challenging the patient's perceptions.	"I understand that the voices seem real to you, but I do not hear any voices." "I don't see anyone else in the room but you and me."

TABLE 7–2	**Therapeutic Communication Techniques—cont'd**	
TECHNIQUE	**EXPLANATION/RATIONALE**	**EXAMPLES**
Voicing doubt	Expressing uncertainty as to the reality of the patient's perceptions is a technique often used with patients experiencing delusional thinking.	"It's difficult to believe that the president of the United States would be listening to all of your phone calls." "I find that hard to believe [or accept]." "That seems rather doubtful to me."
Verbalizing the implied	Putting into words what the patient has only implied or said indirectly is a technique that can be helpful with patients experiencing impaired verbal communication.	Patient: "I can't talk about this . . . you haven't been where I've been." Nurse: "Does it seem like no one could understand your thoughts and feelings unless they've had the same experiences you've had?" Patient: "I . . . I don't know where to begin." Nurse: "So it feels overwhelming to think about sharing the details of this experience."
Attempting to translate words into feelings	When the patient has difficulty identifying feelings or feelings are expressed indirectly, the nurse tries to "desymbolize" what has been said and to find clues to the underlying true feelings.	Patient: "I'm just an empty pit." Nurse: "It sounds like you are feeling hopeless, is that right?"
Formulating a plan of action	Encouraging the patient to identify a plan for behavior change promotes developing better coping skills.	"What could you do differently if you are faced with this situation in the future?" "What are some steps you could take to manage your anger without punching someone?" "What is one thing you might be willing to try to decrease your anxiety instead of using alcohol?"

Sources: Adapted from Hays, J. S., & Larson, K. H. (1963). *Interacting with patients.* Macmillan; Sullivan, H. S. (1954). *The psychiatric interview.* Norton.

TABLE 7–3	**Nontherapeutic Communication Techniques**	
TECHNIQUE	**EXPLANATION/RATIONALE**	**EXAMPLES**
Giving false reassurance	False reassurance conveys that the nurse already knows the outcome of a situation and minimizes the patient's expressed concerns. It may discourage the patient from further expression of feelings if they believe the feelings will be downplayed or ridiculed.	Patient: "My husband doesn't love me anymore. I think he wants a divorce." Nurse: "I'm sure he must still love you. Everything will be fine." **Better alternative:** "Tell me more about what's been happening in your relationship with your husband."
Rejecting	Refusing to consider or showing contempt for the patient's ideas or behavior may cause the patient to discontinue interaction with the nurse for fear of further rejection.	Patient: "Since I started taking this medication I can't be intimate with my girlfriend." Nurse: "Let's not talk about that right now." **Better alternative:** "Tell me more about what you mean by not being able 'to be intimate' with your girlfriend."
Approving or disapproving	Sanctioning or denouncing the patient's ideas or behavior implies that the nurse has the right to pass judgment on whether the patient's ideas or behaviors are "good" or "bad" and that the patient is expected to please the nurse. The nurse's acceptance of the patient is then seen as conditional depending on the patient's behavior.	"It's good that you confronted your wife about her behavior." "You shouldn't yell at your wife." **Better alternative:** "What happened after you confronted your wife in a loud voice?"

Continued

TABLE 7–3 **Nontherapeutic Communication Techniques–cont'd**		
TECHNIQUE	**EXPLANATION/RATIONALE**	**EXAMPLES**
Agreeing or disagreeing	Indicating accord with or opposition to the patient's ideas or opinions implies that the nurse has the right to pass judgment on whether the patient's ideas or opinions are "right" or "wrong." Agreement prevents the patient from later modifying their point of view without admitting error. Disagreement implies inaccuracy, provoking the need for defensiveness on the part of the patient.	Patient: "I think my doctor doesn't care about me." Nurse: "I disagree. You shouldn't think that way." Or "I can't believe that's true." **Better alternative:** "Tell me more about why you think your doctor doesn't care."
Giving advice	Telling the patient what to do or how to behave implies that the nurse knows what is best and nurtures the patient in the dependent role by discouraging independent thinking.	"You need to do deep breathing exercises when you become anxious." "You should stop drinking alcohol and start going to Alcoholics Anonymous meetings." **Better alternative:** "What do you think you should do?" or "Let's explore some options for solving this problem."
Probing	Persistent questioning of the patient and pushing for answers to issues the patient does not wish to discuss may contribute to the patient feeling used and valued only for what information the nurse is seeking and may place the patient on the defensive.	"Why was your family angry with you?" "How many times did you receive poor evaluations before you got fired?" "How many girlfriends were you lying to?" **Better alternative:** The nurse should actively listen to the patient's response and discontinue the interaction at the first sign of discomfort.
Defending	Defending someone or something the patient has criticized minimizes or completely ignores the patient's concerns. Defending may cause the patient to think the nurse is taking sides against them.	"None of the nurses here would lie to you." "You have a very capable physician." "Your children want only what's best for you." **Better alternative:** "Tell me more about these concerns you've expressed."
Requesting an explanation	This technique involves asking the patient why they have certain thoughts, feelings, and behaviors. Asking "why" a patient did something or feels a certain way can be very intimidating and implies that the patient must defend their behavior or feelings.	"Why do you think people are out to get you?" "Why do you feel depressed?" "Why were you taking drugs?" **Better alternative:** "Describe what you were feeling just before that happened."
Indicating the existence of an external source of power	Attributing the source of thoughts, feelings, and behavior to others or to outside influences encourages the patient to project blame for his or her thoughts or behaviors on others rather than accepting the responsibility personally.	"What made you go on a drinking binge?" "What made you say that you are a worthless person?" **Better alternative:** "What was happening just before you started binge drinking?" "What do you mean when you say you are 'a worthless person'?"
Belittling or minimizing feelings	When the nurse minimizes the degree of the patient's discomfort, a lack of empathy and understanding may be conveyed. When the nurse tells the patient to "cheer up" or "everybody feels that way," the patient may feel that their concerns are insignificant or unimportant.	Patient: "I don't even have the energy to go to work." Nurse: "We've all felt like that at times. You've just got to 'perk up' and get moving." **Better alternative:** "Tell me more about what you are feeling right now."

TABLE 7–3	Nontherapeutic Communication Techniques—cont'd	
TECHNIQUE	**EXPLANATION/RATIONALE**	**EXAMPLES**
Making stereotyped comments	Trite expressions are meaningless in a nurse–patient relationship. When the nurse uses meaningless expressions, it encourages a similar response from the patient.	"How are you?" "Hang in there." "It'll all work out." **Better alternative:** Choose words, sentences, and nonverbal language that convey a sincere interest in encouraging the patient to share more about their thoughts, feelings, and behaviors.
Using denial	Denying that a problem exists blocks discussion with the patient and avoids helping the patient identify and explore areas of difficulty.	Patient: "I have a problem interacting with people." Nurse: "You're doing fine." **Better alternative:** "Tell me more about that."
Interpreting	Interpreting attempts to tell the patient the meaning of their experience. Erroneous interpretations may leave the patient feeling that the nurse doesn't understand them, or that the nurse is being smug.	"What you really mean is. . . . " "Your continued drinking is your way of avoiding discussing your anger over the divorce. . . . " **Better alternative:** "Tell me more about what you're thinking (or feeling)."
Introducing an unrelated topic	When the nurse prematurely changes the subject, it conveys to the patient that the nurse does not want to discuss the original topic any further. This may occur in order to get to something that the nurse wants to discuss with the patient or to get away from a topic that the nurse would prefer not to discuss.	Patient: "I don't have anything to live for." Nurse: "How well did you sleep last night?" **Better alternative:** "Tell me more." Sometimes silence may be appropriate to convey that the nurse is willing to hear all of what the patient wants to say before moving on to a different topic.

Sources: Adapted from Hays, J. S., & Larson, K. H. (1963). *Interacting with patients.* Macmillan; Sullivan, H. S. (1954). *The psychiatric interview.* Norton.

Active Listening

To listen actively is to be attentive and demonstrate a desire to hear and understand what the patient is saying, both verbally and nonverbally. Attentive listening creates a climate in which the patient can communicate. With active listening, the nurse communicates acceptance and respect for the patient, and trust is enhanced. A climate is established within the relationship that promotes openness and honest expression.

Several nonverbal behaviors have been designated as facilitative skills for attentive listening. Those listed here can be identified by the acronym SOLER:

S: Sit squarely facing the patient. This nonverbal cue gives the message that the nurse is there to listen and is interested in what the patient has to say.

O: Present with an **open posture.** Posture is considered "open" when arms and legs remain uncrossed. This nonverbal cue suggests that the nurse is open to what the patient has to say. With a closed position, the nurse can convey a somewhat defensive

stance, possibly invoking a similar response in the patient.

L: Lean forward toward the patient. Leaning forward conveys to the patient that the nurse is involved in the interaction, interested in what is being said, and making a sincere effort to be attentive.

E: Establish **eye contact.** Eye contact, intermittently directed, is another behavior that conveys the nurse's involvement and willingness to listen to what the patient has to say. The absence of eye contact or the constant shifting of eye contact elsewhere in the environment gives the message that the nurse is not actually interested in what is being said.

> **CLINICAL PEARL** Ensure that eye contact conveys warmth and is accompanied by smiling and intermittent nodding of the head and does not come across as staring or glaring, which can create intense discomfort in the patient. Active observation and listening to discern an individual's comfort level with eye contact facilitates adapting one's level of eye contact if it appears to increase the patient's anxiety. For example, patients experiencing paranoia and some individuals with autism spectrum disorder may be very sensitive to levels of eye contact that in other situations would seem appropriate.

R: Relax. Whether sitting or standing during the interaction, the nurse should communicate a sense of being relaxed and comfortable with the patient. Restlessness and fidgetiness communicate a lack of interest and may convey a feeling of discomfort that is likely to be transferred to the patient.

Motivational Interviewing

Patient-centered care has been identified as an important focus in the quest to improve the quality of nurse communication and therapeutic relationships with patients (Institute of Medicine, 2003). **Motivational interviewing** is an evidence-based, patient-centered style of communicating that promotes behavior change by guiding patients to explore their motivation for change and the advantages and disadvantages of their decisions (Rubak et al., 2005). This style of communication incorporates active listening and verbal therapeutic communication techniques, but it is focused on what the patient wants (their current level of motivation) rather than on what the nurse thinks *should* be the next steps in behavior change. Motivational interviewing was originally developed for use with patients who have substance use disorders, primarily because this style of communication may decrease defensive responses. It has since gained widespread acceptance as a patient-centered communication strategy that promotes behavior change for patients with many different health-care issues. See the following "Real People, Real Stories" for an example of motivational interviewing described in a process recording format.

Process Recordings

Process recordings are written reports of verbal interactions with patients. They are verbatim accounts recorded by the nurse or student as a tool for improving interpersonal communication techniques. Process recording can take many forms but usually includes the verbal and nonverbal communication of both nurse and patient. The exercise provides a means for the nurse to analyze both the content and pattern of the interaction. Process recording, which is not considered documentation, is intended to be used as a learning tool for professional development. An example of one type of process recording is presented in Table 7–4.

Feedback

Feedback is a method of communication for helping the patient consider behavior modification by providing information about how they are perceived by others. Feedback can be useful to the patient if presented with objectivity by a trusted individual in a manner that discourages defensiveness.

Characteristics of useful feedback include the following:

■ *Feedback should be descriptive rather than evaluative and focus on the behavior rather than on the patient.* Avoiding evaluative language reduces the need for the patient to react defensively. Objective descriptions allow patients to use the information in whatever way they choose. When the focus is on the person, rather than the behavior, patients may perceive that they are being judged as "good" or "bad.

Example:

Descriptive and focused on behavior	"Jessica was very upset in group today when you called her 'a cow' and laughed at her in front of the others."
Evaluative	"You were very rude and inconsiderate to Jessica in group today."
Focus on patient	"You are a very insensitive person."

■ *Feedback should be specific rather than general.* Information that gives details about the patient's behavior is more effective than a generalized description in promoting behavior change.

Example:

Specific	"You were talking to Joe when we were deciding on the issue. Now you want to argue about the outcome."
General	"You just don't pay attention."

■ *Feedback should be directed toward behavior that the patient can modify.* To provide feedback about a characteristic or situation that the patient cannot change only provokes frustration.

Example:

Can modify	"I noticed that you did not want to hold your baby when the nurse brought her to you."
Cannot modify	"Your baby daughter is intellectually disabled because you took drugs when you were pregnant."

■ *Feedback should impart information rather than offer advice.* Giving advice fosters dependence and may convey the message to the patient that they are not capable of making decisions and solving problems independently. It is the patient's right and privilege to be as self-sufficient as possible.

Real People, Real Stories: A Sample of Motivational Interviewing in a Process Recording Format

The following is part of an interaction with Alan, incorporating motivational interviewing communication strategies in a process recording format. Learn more about Alan's story in Chapter 23, Substance-Related and Addictive Disorders

Interaction	Nurse's Thoughts and Feelings	Communication Technique/Evaluation
Karyn: You mentioned that you were at an event and you commented that you "needed a drink." Tell me more about what was happening. (SOLER) Alan: (nodding) I was perturbed. I felt like I was stuck at this event. There was supposed to be entertainment but it got canceled due to rain, and suddenly I noticed people were drinking and smoking. It brought back a lot of memories. (looks down)	I wasn't sure if Alan was willing to talk about this, but I thought it was important to facilitate his looking at his behavior in response to this experience. I was glad that Alan was open to discussing this experience, but he said so many things in this short statement that I had to be thoughtful about what to follow up on.	Technique: **Exploring** Evaluation: This approach was effective. Alan talked more about the event and was able to articulate some thoughts and feelings as well.
Karyn: So you felt perturbed and stuck. . . . (looking up, not making direct eye contact)	I was thinking that I don't usually explore feelings right off the bat because I believe it's better to help someone fully describe events and thoughts first (or at least it's less threatening). But I've interacted with Alan many times, he's been through rehab, sober for 7 years, and he's pretty comfortable talking about feelings. My immediate thought was that I want to tell him to go to an AA meeting or call his sponsor, but I was trying to incorporate a motivational interviewing strategy, and that meant it would be better to help him explore his motivation for how to respond to this experience. I didn't know what he meant by "blacked it out," but I felt uncomfortable when he said that. I thought this was an important statement to clarify because it might help him explore how he behaved in response to this event. Alan seemed to be thinking a lot about this and was responding with several different thoughts, so I felt like it was important to just use silence and facilitate his reflection. I thought Alan seemed to be genuinely considering a behavior change.	Technique: **Reflecting** Evaluation: This technique was effective. Alan began to process his thoughts about why he might be feeling perturbed and stuck. I think I may have been not making direct eye contact because of my perception that feelings can be a little more threatening for some people to talk about.
Alan: Yeah, but it didn't last long. Maybe it had something to do with the fact that there was nothing else going on and it seemed like the whole thing became about drinking. But then I just blacked it out.		
Karyn: What do you mean when you say you blacked it out? (SOLER) Alan: (silent for several seconds) I do need to go back to an AA meeting. I mean, am I different than other people? I know there are other people out there that have to be struggling with the same kind of things. When I was in rehab, my mom and her boyfriend were always there taking me to meetings. My sister went, too . . . (silent for several more seconds) I know it's important (silence) . . . about 75% of the people I went to rehab with are back out there using again.		Technique: **Clarifying** Evaluation: Asking this question was effective. Alan talked at length about his thoughts and feelings.

Continued

Real People, Real Stories: A Sample of Motivational Interviewing in a Process Recording Format–cont'd

Interaction	Nurse's Thoughts and Feelings	Communication Technique/Evaluation
Karyn: You said that you need to go back to a meeting and that they are important. Is it more helpful to go to meetings when you just start thinking about needing a drink, or do you think that meetings are only necessary after you actually take a drink? Alan: Oh no, you've got to go long before you take that first drink. (silence) People told me when I was in rehab that they could tell I was really listening in meetings . . . the meetings were helpful . . . (silence), and I just reconnected with my sponsor on Facebook, so I need to get back to a meeting to see him.	I knew that Alan had not been going to meetings regularly for the last couple of years, even though he acknowledges their importance, so I wanted to know more about whether he thought behavior change (such as going to AA meetings) was necessary at this point. Alan seemed like he was thinking about what is important to him, so I continued to remain silent to facilitate that process.	Technique: **Restating, focusing** Evaluation: Restatement was effective. The way I chose to focus was probably leading Alan to choose the "right" answer, and that makes it harder to evaluate whether he is just telling me what I want to hear or is really motivated. It might have been better to use the technique of formulating a plan of action.
Karyn: You've identified three reasons why you believe you need to go to a meeting: because they are helpful to you, because you want to find out if others are struggling with the same kinds of thoughts that you are, and because you need to reconnect with your sponsor. Do you have a plan in mind for how to follow through with that? Alan: Well, I haven't done it yet. I guess I'm still just thinking about it.	I was thinking that he talks about needing to go to AA, and *I* was feeling anxious about wanting him to commit to that, but at the same time, I recognized that the motivation for change and commitment to a plan of action has to come from him. I was appreciating his honesty and thinking that this is the challenge of motivational interviewing: accepting where the individual is at while continuing to explore and facilitate their motivations for behavior change.	Technique: **Summarizing, formulating a plan of action** Evaluation: I think the techniques were effective, although Alan may not be ready to formulate an action plan at present.

TABLE 7–4 Sample Process Recording

NURSE VERBAL (NONVERBAL)	PATIENT VERBAL (NONVERBAL)	NURSE'S THOUGHTS AND FEELINGS CONCERNING THE INTERACTION	ANALYSIS OF THE INTERACTION
Do you still have thoughts about harming yourself? (Sitting facing the patient; looking directly at patient.)	Not really. I still feel sad, but I don't want to die. (Looking at hands in lap.)	Felt a little uncomfortable. Always a hard question to ask.	Therapeutic. Asking a direct, closed-ended question about suicidal intent to elicit specific information.
Tell me what you were feeling before you took all the pills the other night. (Using SOLER techniques of active listening.)	I was just so angry! To think that my husband wants a divorce now that he has a good job. I worked hard to put him through college. (Fists clenched. Face and neck reddened.)	Beginning to feel more comfortable. Patient seems willing to talk, and I think she trusts me.	Therapeutic. Exploring. Delving further into the patient's feelings to help her better understand her experience.

TABLE 7–4 Sample Process Recording—cont'd

NURSE VERBAL (NONVERBAL)	PATIENT VERBAL (NONVERBAL)	NURSE'S THOUGHTS AND FEELINGS CONCERNING THE INTERACTION	ANALYSIS OF THE INTERACTION
You wanted to hurt him because you felt betrayed. (SOLER)	Yes! If I died, maybe he'd realize that he loved me more than that other woman. (Tears starting to well up in her eyes.)	Starting to feel sorry for her.	Therapeutic. Attempting to translate words into feelings to convey active listening.
Seems like a pretty drastic way to get your point across. (Small frown.)	I know. It was a stupid thing to do. (Wiping eyes.)	Trying hard to remain objective.	Nontherapeutic. Sounds disapproving. Better to have pursued patient's feelings.
How are you feeling about the situation now? (SOLER)	I don't know. I still love him. I want him to come home. I don't want him to marry her. (Starting to cry again.)	Wishing there was an easy way to help relieve some of her pain.	Therapeutic. Focusing on patient's current feelings to assess current mental status.
Yes, I can understand that you would like things to be the way they were before. (Offered patient a tissue.)	(Silence. Continues to cry softly.)	I'm starting to feel some anger toward her husband. Sometimes it's so hard to remain objective!	Therapeutic. Conveying empathy to support caring and connectedness.
What do you think are the chances of your getting back together? (SOLER)	None. He's refused marriage counseling. He's already moved in with her. He says it's over. (Wipes tears. Looks directly at nurse.)	Relieved to know that she isn't using denial about the reality of the situation.	Therapeutic. Reflecting on the patient's expressed feelings to encourage the patient to recognize and clarify their perceptions.
So how are you preparing to deal with this inevitable outcome? (SOLER)	I'm going to do the things we talked about: join a divorced women's support group, increase my job hours to full time, do some volunteer work, and call the suicide hotline if I feel like taking pills again. (Looks directly at nurse. Smiles.)	Positive feeling to know that she remembers what we discussed earlier and plans to follow through.	Therapeutic. Formulating a plan of action to set the foundation for problem-solving.
It won't be easy. But you have come a long way, and I feel you have gained strength in your ability to cope. (Standing. Looking at patient. Smiling.)	Yes, I know I will have hard times. But I also know I have support, and I want to go on with my life and be happy again. (Standing, smiling at nurse.)	Feeling confident that the session has gone well; hopeful that the patient will succeed in what she wants to do with her life.	Therapeutic. Presenting reality, making observations, and giving recognition to support patient's progress in problem-solving.

Example:

Imparting information	"There are various methods of assistance for people who want to lose weight, such as Overeaters Anonymous, Weight Watchers, regular visits to a dietitian, and the Physician's Weight Loss Program. You can decide what is best for you."
Giving advice	"You obviously need to lose a great deal of weight. I think the Physician's Weight Loss Program would be best for you."

■ *Feedback should be well timed.* Feedback is most useful when given at the earliest appropriate opportunity after the specific behavior.

Example:

Prompt response	"I saw you hit the wall with your fist just now when you hung up the phone after talking to your mother."
Delayed response	"You need to learn some more appropriate ways of dealing with your anger. Last week after group I saw you pounding your fist against the wall."

Summary and Key Points

- Interpersonal communication is a transaction between the sender and the receiver.
- In all interpersonal transactions, the sender and receiver each bring certain preexisting conditions to the exchange that influence both the intended message and how it is interpreted.
- Examples of these preexisting conditions include one's value system, internalized attitudes and beliefs, culture and religion, social status, gender, background knowledge and experience, age or developmental level, and the type of environment in which the communication takes place.
- Nonverbal expression is a primary communication system in which meaning is assigned to various gestures and patterns of behavior.
- Some components of nonverbal communication include physical appearance and dress, body movement and posture, touch, facial expressions, eye behavior, and vocal cues or paralanguage.
- The meaning of the nonverbal components of communication is culturally determined.
- Therapeutic communication is an intentional process that applies both verbal and nonverbal techniques to focus on the care *receiver's* needs and advance the promotion of healing and change.

- Motivational interviewing is an evidence-based, patient-centered style of therapeutic communication that facilitates patients' exploration of their motivations for behavior change and guides patients to explore the advantages and disadvantages of their decisions.
- Nurses must be aware of and avoid techniques that are considered barriers to effective communication.
- Active listening is described as attentiveness to what the patient is saying through both verbal and nonverbal cues. Skills associated with active listening include **SOLER**: **S**itting facing the patient, **O**pen posture, **L**eaning forward toward the patient, **E**stablishing eye contact, and being **R**elaxed.
- Process recordings are written reports of verbal interactions with patients. They are used as learning tools for professional development.
- Feedback is a method of communication for helping the patient consider a modification of behavior.
- The nurse must be aware of the therapeutic or nontherapeutic value of the communication techniques used with the patient because they are the tools of psychosocial intervention.

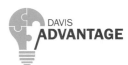

Go to **Davis Advantage** to complete your learning: strengthen understanding, apply your knowledge, and prepare for the Next Gen NCLEX®.

Review Questions

1. A client who is angry with their psychiatrist says to the nurse, "He doesn't know what he is doing. That medication isn't helping a thing!" The nurse responds, "He has been a doctor for many years and has helped many people." This is an example of what nontherapeutic technique?
   a. Rejecting
   b. Disapproving
   c. Probing
   d. Defending

2. A client says to the nurse, "I've been offered a promotion, but I don't know if I can handle it." The nurse replies, "You're afraid you may fail in the new position." This is an example of which therapeutic technique?
   a. Restating
   b. Making observations
   c. Focusing
   d. Verbalizing the implied

3. The environment in which communication takes place influences the outcome of the interaction. Which of the following are aspects of the environment that influence communication? (Select all that apply.)
   a. Territoriality
   b. Density
   c. Dimension
   d. Distance
   e. Intensity

4. The nurse says to a client, "You are being readmitted to the hospital. Why did you stop taking your medication?" What communication technique does this represent?
   a. Disapproving
   b. Requesting an explanation
   c. Disagreeing
   d. Probing

5. A client who has been in rehabilitation for alcohol dependence returns from a visit to their home and tells the nurse, "We were having a celebration and I did have one drink, but it really wasn't a problem." The nurse notices that their breath smells of alcohol. Which of the following responses by the nurse demonstrates a motivational interviewing style of communication?
   a. "You are obviously not motivated to change, so perhaps we should discuss your discharge from the treatment program."
   b. "You need to abstain from alcohol in order to recover, so let me talk to the doctor about the consequences of your behavior."
   c. "Why would you destroy everything you've worked so hard to achieve?"
   d. "What do you mean when you say, 'It really wasn't a problem'?"

6. A client who has been diagnosed with schizophrenia and has been on medication for several months states, "I'm not taking that stupid medication anymore." Which of the following responses by the nurse demonstrates a motivational interviewing style of communication?
   a. "Don't you know that if you don't take your medication you will never recover?"
   b. "Why won't you cooperate with the treatment your doctor prescribed?"
   c. "The medication is not stupid."
   d. "Tell me more about why you don't want to take the medication."

Clinical Judgment Questions

7. A client states, "I refuse to shower in this room. I must be very cautious. The FBI has placed a camera in here to monitor my every move." Which of the following is the most therapeutic response?
   a. "That's not true."
   b. "I have a hard time believing that is true."
   c. "Surely you don't really believe that."
   d. "I will help you search this room so that you can see there is no camera."

8. A depressed client who has been unkempt and untidy for weeks comes to group therapy today wearing makeup and a clean dress with hair washed and combed. Which of the following responses by the nurse is most appropriate?
   a. "I see you have put on a clean dress and combed your hair."
   b. "You look wonderful today!"
   c. "I'm sure everyone will appreciate that you have cleaned up for the group today."
   d. "Now that you see how important it is, I hope you will do this every day."

9. A client was involved in an automobile accident while under the influence of alcohol. They swerved the car into a tree and narrowly missed hitting a child on a bicycle. The client is in the hospital with multiple abrasions and contusions and is talking about the accident with the nurse. Which of the following statements by the nurse is most appropriate?
    a. "Now that you know what can happen when you drink and drive, I'm sure you won't let it happen again."
    b. "You know that was a terrible thing you did. That child could have been killed."
    c. "I'm sure everything is going to be okay now that you understand the possible consequences of such behavior."
    d. "How are you feeling about what happened?"

10. A client, who has been in the hospital for 3 weeks, has used Valium "to settle my nerves" for the past 15 years. The individual was admitted by their psychiatrist for safe withdrawal from the drug. The client has passed the physical symptoms of withdrawal at this time but states to the nurse, "I don't know if I will be able to make it without Valium after I go home. I'm already starting to feel nervous. I have so many personal problems." Which is the most appropriate response by the nurse?
    a. "Why do you think you need drugs to deal with your problems?"
    b. "Everybody has problems, but not everybody uses drugs to deal with them. You'll just have to do the best that you can."
    c. "Let's explore some things you can do to decrease your anxiety without resorting to drugs."
    d. "Just hang in there. I'm sure everything is going to be okay."

11. A client asks the nurse, "Do you think I should tell my spouse about my affair with my boss?" Which is the most appropriate response by the nurse?
    a. "What do you think would be best for you to do?"
    b. "Of course you should. Marriage has to be based on honesty."
    c. "Of course not. That would only make things worse."
    d. "I can't tell you what to do. You have to decide for yourself."

12. An adolescent who has just returned from group therapy is crying and says to the nurse, "All the other kids laughed at me! I try to fit in, but I always seem to say the wrong thing. I've never had a close friend. I guess I never will." Which is the most appropriate response by the nurse?
    a. "What makes you think you will never have any friends?"
    b. "You're feeling pretty down on yourself right now."
    c. "I'm sure they didn't mean to hurt your feelings."
    d. "Why do you feel this way about yourself?"

References

Ali, R. (2021). *The language of power and dominance.* https://sciencetranslated.org/the-language-of-nonverbal-dominance/

Cherry, K. (2019). *Understanding body language and facial expressions.* https://www.verywellmind.com/understand-body-language-and-facial-expressions-4147228

Dai, X., Zhou, L. Y., Cao, J. X., Zhang, Y. Q., Yang, F. P., Wang, A. Q., Wei, W. H., & Yang, S. M. (2018). Effect of group density on the physiology and aggressive behavior of male Brandt's voles *(Lasiopodomys brandtii). Zoological Studies, 18*(57), e35. doi: 10.6620/ZS.2018.57-35 PMID: 31966275; PMCID: PMC6517712.

Hall, J. A., Coats, E. J., & Smith LeBeau, L. (2005). Nonverbal behavior and the vertical dimension of social relations: A meta-analysis. *Psychological Bulletin, 131,* 898–924.

Heathfield, S. M. (2019). *How to understand your coworkers' nonverbal communication.* https://www.thebalancecareers.com/tips-for-understanding-nonverbal-communication-1918459

Institute of Medicine. (2003). *Health professions education: A bridge to quality.* Institute of Medicine.

Knapp, M. L., & Hall, J. A. (2014). *Nonverbal communication in human interaction* (8th ed.). Wadsworth.

Rubak, S., Sandbaek, A., Lauritzen, T., & Christensen, B. (2005). Motivational interviewing: A systematic review and meta-analysis. *The British Journal of General Practice: The Journal of the Royal College of General Practitioners, 55*(513), 305–312.

Simon, M. (2005). *Facial expressions: A visual reference for artists.* Watson-Guptill.

Classical References

Hall, E. T. (1966). *The hidden dimension.* Doubleday.

Hays, J. S., & Larson, K. H. (1963). *Interacting with patients.* Macmillan.

Reece, M., & Whitman, R. (1962). Expressive movements, warmth, and verbal reinforcement. *Journal of Abnormal and Social Psychology, 64,* 234–236. doi:http://dx.doi.org/10.1037/h0039792

Sullivan, H. S. (1954). *The psychiatric interview.* Norton.

The Nursing Process in Psychiatric-Mental Health Nursing

8

CORE CONCEPTS

Professional Behavior: Nursing Process

Assessment

Nursing Diagnosis

Outcomes

Planning

Implementation

Evaluation

Clinical Judgment

KEY TERMS

case management

case manager

concept mapping

critical pathways of care (CPCs)

Focus Charting

interdisciplinary

managed care

Nursing Interventions Classification (NIC)

Nursing Outcomes Classification (NOC)

nursing process

PIE charting

problem-oriented recording

OBJECTIVES
After reading this chapter, the student will be able to:

1. Define *nursing process.*
2. Identify six steps of the nursing process and describe nursing actions associated with each.
3. Describe the benefits of using nursing diagnosis.
4. Discuss the list of nursing diagnoses approved by NANDA International (NANDA-I) for clinical use and testing.
5. Define and discuss the use of case management and critical pathways of care in the clinical setting.
6. Apply the six steps of the nursing process in caring for a client in the psychiatric setting.
7. Describe the six areas of focus identified by The Institute of Medicine (IOM) (and Quality and Safety Education for Nurses [QSEN] competencies) as critical to the improvement of health care.
8. Document patient care that validates use of the nursing process.

For many years, the **nursing process** has provided a systematic framework for the delivery of nursing care. This framework fulfills the requirement for a *scientific methodology* in order for nursing to be considered a profession.

This chapter examines several essential models that guide the implementation of the nursing process. The first of these is the steps of the nursing process as they are set forth by the American Nurses Association (ANA), in *Nursing: Scope and Standards of Practice* (ANA, 2021). The second is the *Psychiatric-Mental Health Nursing: Scope and Standards of Practice* established specifically for psychiatric mental health nursing (ANA, American Psychiatric Nurses Association [APNA], International Society of Psychiatric-Mental Health Nurses [ISPN], 2022). Third, the landmark IOM (now called the National Academy of Medicine) report (2003) identified six critical areas of focus (patient-centered care, safety, teamwork and collaboration, evidence-based practice, informatics, and quality improvement) that are needed to shape the future and improve quality of health care. These six critical areas are incorporated as an important model for implementing nursing care. These areas have become known as QSEN competencies (Cronenwett et al., 2007). An explanation is provided for the implementation of case management and the critical pathways of care (CPC) tool used with this methodology. A description of concept mapping is included, and documentation that validates the use of the nursing process is discussed.

The Nursing Process

Definition

The nursing process consists of six steps (Figure 8–1) and uses a problem-solving approach that is now accepted as nursing's scientific methodology. It is goal directed with the objective of quality patient care delivery.

The nursing process is dynamic, not static. It is an ongoing process that continues for as long as the nurse and patient have interactions directed toward change in the patient's physical or behavioral responses.

Standards of Practice

The ANA, in collaboration with the APNA and the ISPN (2022), has delineated a set of standards that psychiatric-mental health nurses (PMHNs) are expected to follow as they provide care for their patients. The ANA (2021) describes a *standard of practice* as an authoritative statement that is defined and promoted by the profession and that provides the foundation for evaluating quality of nursing practice. The nursing process is a critical thinking model that integrates professional standards of practice to assess, diagnose, identify outcomes, plan, implement, and evaluate nursing care. Although the nursing process is often written as a detailed care plan in educational settings, it is rarely documented this way in practice. It is important for the nursing student to recognize that although they will not likely document care plans with the same measure of detail in practice, learning and using this critical thinking methodology is fundamental to nursing practice in any setting.

The following is a discussion of the standards of practice for PMHNs as set forth by the ANA, APNA, and ISPN (2022). Many of these standards outline the registered nurse's role in each step of the nursing process and apply them to the PMHN. The *PMHN Scope and Standards of Practice* evolve and change with current trends in health care and society and with the evolution of the science of nursing practice. For example, national frameworks such as Healthy People 2030 (n.d.) advance that health-care providers must focus on health-care needs of individuals, families, and populations to improve health-care outcomes. This framework also informs the scope and standards of practice for PMHNs. The latest iteration of the scope and standards clarifies that the term "patient" is used to describe recipients of PMH nursing care in acute care and "client" is used to describe those in community and private practice settings (ANA et al., 2022).

The psychiatric-mental health advanced practice registered nurse (PMH-APRN) education and practice roles are evolving toward a life span approach to meet the needs of individuals, families, and communities throughout life (ANA et al., 2022). Current research on the effect of childhood and prior trauma in mental and physical health outcomes informs PMH nursing standards with regard to trauma-informed care. The trend toward recovery-focused models of care, patient-centered care, and the recognition of the need for housing and early intervention in first episodes of psychosis are all relevant to the evolution of PMH nursing standards of practice. As the roles of advanced practice nurses have evolved, counseling interventions (performed by psychiatric-mental health registered nurses) are now differentiated from psychotherapy (performed by psychiatric-mental health *advanced practice* registered nurses). In addition, Standard 5H. "Counseling and Psychotherapy" (ANA et al., 2022) incorporates language in the nursing competencies

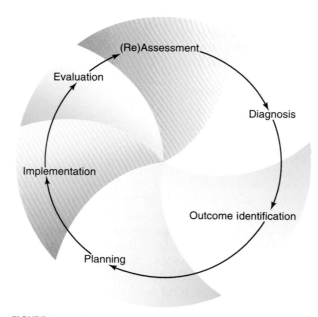

FIGURE 8–1 The ongoing nursing process.

such as "promoting...personal recovery goals" and "empowers patients/clients to be active participants," which highlight principles associated with recovery models of practice. (See Chapter 20, "The Recovery Model," for more information.)

CORE CONCEPT

Assessment

Assessment is a systematic, dynamic process by which the registered nurse, through interaction with the patient, family, groups, communities, populations, and health-care providers, collects and analyzes data. Assessment may include the following dimensions: physical, psychological, sociocultural, spiritual, cognitive, functional abilities, developmental, economic, and lifestyle (ANA et al., 2022, p. 93).

Standard 1. Assessment

"The psychiatric-mental health registered nurse [PMH-RN] collects and synthesizes comprehensive health data that are pertinent to the patient/client's health and/or situation" (ANA et al., 2022. p. 59).

In this first step, a database to determine the best possible patient care is established. Information for this database is gathered from a variety of sources, including interviews with the patient and family, observation of the patient and their environment, consultation with other health team members, review of the patient's records, and a nursing physical examination.

Many tools are available to assist the nurse in gathering this information. For example, a biopsychosocial assessment tool based on the stress-adaptation framework is included in Box 8–1. The primary focus
Text continued on page 151

BOX 8–1 Nursing History and Assessment Tool

I. GENERAL INFORMATION

Patient name: _____

Room number: _____

Doctor: _____

Age: _____

Sex: _____ Name and phone no. of significant other: _____

Race: _____

Dominant language: _____

Marital status: _____

Chief complaint: _____

Allergies: _____

Diet: _____

Height/weight: _____

Vital signs: TPR/BP _____

City of residence: _____

Diagnosis (admitting & current): _____

Conditions of admission: _____

Date: _____   Time: _____

Accompanied by: _____

Route of admission (wheelchair; ambulatory; cart): _____

Admitted from: _____

II. PREDISPOSING FACTORS

A. Genetic Influences

1. Family configuration (use genograms):

   Family of origin: Present family:

   Family dynamics (describe significant relationships between family members): _____
   _____
   _____
   _____
   _____

2. Medical/psychiatric history: _____
   a. Patient: _____
      _____
      _____

   b. Family members: _____
      _____
      _____

BOX 8–1 **Nursing History and Assessment Tool–cont'd**

3. Other genetic influences affecting present adaptation. This might include effects specific to gender, race, appearance, such as genetic physical defects, or any other factor related to genetics that is affecting the patient's adaptation that has not been mentioned elsewhere in this assessment.
_____
_____

B. Past Experiences
1. Cultural and social history:
   a. Environmental factors (family living arrangements, type of neighborhood, special working conditions):
   _____
   _____
   _____

   b. Health beliefs and practices (personal responsibility for health; special self-care practices):
   _____
   _____

   c. Religious beliefs and practices: _____
   _____

   d. Educational background: _____
   _____

   e. Significant losses/changes (include dates): _____
   _____

   f. Peer/friendship relationships: _____
   _____

   g. Occupational history: _____
   _____

   h. Previous pattern of coping with stress: _____
   _____
   _____

   i. Other lifestyle factors contributing to present adaptation: _____
   _____
   _____

C. Existing Conditions
1. Stage of development (Erikson):
   a. Theoretically: _____
   b. Behaviorally: _____
   c. Rationale: _____
   _____
   _____
   _____

2. Support systems: _____
   _____

3. Economic security: _____
   _____

4. Avenues of productivity/contribution:
   a. Current job status: _____
   _____

   b. Role contributions and responsibility for others: _____
   _____

BOX 8–1 **Nursing History and Assessment Tool—cont'd**

III. PRECIPITATING EVENT

Describe the situation or events that precipitated this illness/hospitalization: _____
_____
_____

IV. PATIENT'S PERCEPTION OF THE STRESSOR

Patient's or family member's understanding or description of stressor/illness and expectations of hospitalization:
_____
_____
_____

V. ADAPTATION RESPONSES

A. Psychosocial

1. Anxiety level (circle one of the 4 levels and check the behaviors that apply): Mild Moderate Severe Panic
   calm ____ friendly ____ passive ____ alert ____ perceives environment correctly ____ cooperative ____ impaired attention ____ "jittery" ____ unable to concentrate ____ hypervigilant ____ tremors ____ rapid speech ____ withdrawn ____ confused ____ disoriented ____ fearful ____ hyperventilating ____ misinterpreting The environment (hallucinations or delusions) ____ depersonalization ____ obsessions ____ compulsions ____ somatic complaints ____ excessive hyperactivity ____ other _____
   Judgment: Intact ____ Impaired ____
   Associated behaviors: _____
   Insight: Intact: ____ Impaired ____
   Associated patient statements: _____

2. Mood/affect (check as many as apply): happiness ____ sadness ____ dejection ____ despair ____ elation ____ euphoria ____ suspiciousness ____ apathy (little emotional tone) ____ anger/hostility ____

3. Level of self-esteem (check one): low ____ moderate ____ high ____
   Things patient likes about self _____
   Things patient would like to change about self _____
   Objective assessment of self-esteem: _____
   Eye contact _____
   General appearance _____
   Personal hygiene _____
   Participation in group activities and interactions with others _____

4. Stage and manifestations of grief (check one):
   Denial ____ Anger ____ Bargaining ____ Depression ____ Acceptance ____
   Describe the patient's behaviors and communication that are associated with this stage of grieving in response to loss or change.
   _____
   _____
   _____

5. Thought processes (check as many as apply): clear ____ logical ____ easy to follow ____ relevant ____ confused ____ blocking ____ delusional ____ rapid flow of thoughts ____ slowness in thought ____ suspicious ____

6. Memory
   Recent memory (check one): loss ____ intact ____ Remote memory (check one): loss ____ intact ____
   Other: _____

Continued

BOX 8–1 **Nursing History and Assessment Tool–cont'd**

7. Communication patterns (check as many as apply): clear _____ coherent _____ slurred speech _____ incoherent _____ neologisms _____ loose associations _____ flight of ideas _____ aphasic _____ perseveration _____ rumination _____ tangential speech _____ loquaciousness _____ slow, impoverished speech _____ speech impediment (describe) _____
   Other _____
   _____

8. Interaction patterns (describe patient's pattern of interpersonal interactions with staff and peers on the unit, e.g., manipulative, withdrawn, isolated, verbally or physically hostile, argumentative, passive, assertive, aggressive, passive-aggressive, other): _____
   _____
   _____
   _____

9. Reality orientation (check those that apply):
   Oriented to: Time _____ Person _____
                 Place _____ Situation _____

10. Ideas of destruction to self/others (circle one)?   Yes   No
    If yes, consider plan; available means _____

11. Nonsuicidal intent to self-injury (circle one)?   Yes   No

12. Intent to die (circle one)?   Yes   No
    If yes, consider plan; available means: _____

13. Previous history of ideation and/or attempts (describe) _____

14. Intensity of current ideation (if present) _____

15. Other risk factors _____

16. Other warning signs

B. Physiological
1. Psychosomatic manifestations (describe any somatic complaints that may be stress-related):
   _____
   _____
   _____

2. Drug history and assessment:
   Use of prescribed drugs:

Name	Dosage	Prescribed for	Results

   Use of over-the-counter drugs:

Name	Dosage	Used for	Results

BOX 8–1 **Nursing History and Assessment Tool–cont'd**

Medication Side Effects:
What symptoms is the patient experiencing that may be attributed to current medication usage? _____

Use of street drugs or alcohol:

Name	Amount Used	How Often Used	When Last Used	Effects Produced

3. Pertinent physical assessments:
   a. Respirations: normal _____ labored _____
      Rate _____ Rhythm _____

   b. Skin: warm _____ dry _____ moist _____ cool _____ clammy _____ pink _____
      cyanotic _____ poor turgor _____ edematous _____
      Evidence of: rash _____ bruising _____ needle tracks _____ hirsutism _____
      loss of hair _____ other _____

   c. Musculoskeletal status: _____ weakness _____ tremors
      Degree of range of motion (describe limitations) _____

      Pain (describe) _____

      Skeletal deformities (describe) _____
      Coordination (describe limitations) _____

   d. Neurological status:
      History of (check all that apply): seizures _____ (describe method of control) _____

      headaches (describe location and frequency) _____
      fainting spells _____ dizziness _____
      tingling/numbness (describe location) _____

   e. Cardiovascular: B/P _____ Pulse _____
      History of (check all that apply):
      hypertension _____ palpitations _____
      heart murmur _____ chest pain _____
      shortness of breath _____ pain in legs _____
      phlebitis _____ ankle/leg edema _____
      numbness/tingling in extremities _____
      varicose veins _____

   f. Gastrointestinal:
      Usual diet pattern: _____
      Food allergies: _____
      Dentures? Upper _____ Lower _____
      Any problems with chewing or swallowing? _____
      Any recent change in weight? _____
      Any problems with:
      Indigestion/heartburn? _____
         Relieved by _____
      Nausea/vomiting? _____
         Relieved by _____

Continued

BOX 8–1 Nursing History and Assessment Tool—cont'd

History of ulcers? _____
Usual bowel pattern _____
   Constipation? _____ Diarrhea? _____
   Type of self-care assistance provided for either of the above problems _____

_____

g. Genitourinary/Reproductive:
Usual voiding pattern _____
Urinary hesitancy? _____ Frequency? _____
Nocturia? _____ Pain/burning? _____
Incontinence? _____
Any genital lesions? _____
   Discharge?_____Odor?_____
History of sexually transmitted disease? _____
   If yes, please explain: _____

Any concerns about sexuality/sexual activity? _____

Method of birth control used _____
Females:
   Date of last menstrual cycle _____
   Length of cycle _____
   Problems associated with menstruation? _____

Breasts: Pain/tenderness? _____
   Swelling? _____ Discharge? _____
   Lumps? _____ Dimpling? _____
Practice breast self-examination? _____
   Frequency? _____
Males:
   Penile discharge? _____
   Prostate problems? _____

h. Eyes:	Yes	No	Explain
Glasses?	_____	_____	_____
Contacts?	_____	_____	_____
Swelling?	_____	_____	_____
Discharge?	_____	_____	_____
Itching?	_____	_____	_____
Blurring?	_____	_____	_____
Double vision?	_____	_____	_____

i. Ears:	Yes	No	Explain
Pain?	_____	_____	_____
Drainage?	_____	_____	_____
Difficulty hearing?	_____	_____	_____
Hearing aid?	_____	_____	_____
Tinnitus?	_____	_____	_____

_____

j. Altered laboratory values and possible significance:

_____
_____

BOX 8–1 **Nursing History and Assessment Tool–cont'd**

k. Activity/rest patterns:
Exercise (amount, type, frequency) ⎯⎯⎯⎯⎯⎯⎯⎯⎯⎯⎯⎯⎯⎯⎯⎯⎯⎯⎯⎯⎯⎯⎯⎯⎯⎯⎯⎯⎯⎯⎯⎯

Leisure time activities: ⎯⎯⎯⎯⎯⎯⎯⎯⎯⎯⎯⎯⎯⎯⎯⎯⎯⎯⎯⎯⎯⎯⎯⎯⎯⎯⎯⎯⎯⎯⎯⎯⎯⎯⎯⎯⎯

Patterns of sleep: Number of hours per night ⎯⎯⎯⎯⎯⎯⎯⎯⎯⎯⎯⎯⎯⎯⎯⎯⎯⎯⎯⎯⎯⎯⎯⎯⎯
Use of sleep aids? ⎯⎯⎯⎯⎯⎯⎯⎯⎯⎯⎯⎯⎯⎯⎯⎯⎯⎯⎯⎯⎯⎯⎯⎯⎯⎯⎯⎯⎯⎯⎯⎯⎯⎯⎯⎯⎯⎯⎯
Pattern of awakening during the night? ⎯⎯⎯⎯⎯⎯⎯⎯⎯⎯⎯⎯⎯⎯⎯⎯⎯⎯⎯⎯⎯⎯⎯⎯⎯⎯⎯

Feel rested upon awakening? ⎯⎯⎯⎯⎯⎯⎯⎯⎯⎯⎯⎯⎯⎯⎯⎯⎯⎯⎯⎯⎯⎯⎯⎯⎯⎯⎯⎯⎯⎯⎯⎯

l. Personal hygiene/activities of daily living:
Patterns of self-care: independent ⎯⎯⎯⎯⎯⎯⎯⎯⎯⎯⎯⎯⎯⎯⎯⎯⎯⎯⎯⎯⎯⎯⎯⎯⎯⎯⎯⎯⎯⎯
Requires assistance with: mobility ⎯⎯⎯⎯⎯⎯⎯⎯⎯⎯⎯⎯⎯⎯⎯⎯⎯⎯⎯⎯⎯⎯⎯⎯⎯⎯⎯⎯⎯⎯
hygiene ⎯⎯⎯
toileting ⎯⎯
feeding ⎯⎯⎯
dressing ⎯⎯
other ⎯⎯⎯
Statement describing personal hygiene and general appearance ⎯⎯⎯⎯⎯⎯⎯⎯⎯⎯⎯⎯⎯⎯

m. Other pertinent physical assessments: ⎯⎯⎯⎯⎯⎯⎯⎯⎯⎯⎯⎯⎯⎯⎯⎯⎯⎯⎯⎯⎯⎯⎯⎯⎯⎯⎯⎯

VI. SUMMARY OF INITIAL PSYCHOSOCIAL/PHYSICAL ASSESSMENT:
Knowledge Deficits Identified:

Nursing Diagnoses Indicated:

---

of this assessment is to evaluate the patient's mental status and identify its effect on their safety and ability to function. Mental status evaluation can be either brief or extensive. An example of a simple and quick mental status evaluation is presented in Table 8–1. Sometimes the term *mental status assessment* is used to describe an assessment of the cognitive aspects of functioning, as is the case with tools such as Folstein's Mini-Mental State Evaluation (Folstein et al., 1975). Likewise, the tool in Table 8–1 focuses strictly on a brief assessment of the cognitive aspects of mental functioning. In psychiatry and psychiatric-mental health nursing, mental status assessment assumes a much broader definition and includes assessment of mood, affect, behavior, relationships, speech, perceptual disturbances, insight, and judgment in addition to cognitive function. A comprehensive mental status assessment guide, with explanations and selected sample interview questions, is provided in Appendix C, "Mental Status Assessment."

CORE CONCEPT

Nursing Diagnosis

A nursing diagnosis is a clinical judgment concerning a human response to health conditions/life processes, or a susceptibility to that response, that is recognized in an individual, caregiver, family, group, or community. A nursing diagnosis provides the basis for selection of nursing interventions to achieve outcomes for which the nurse has accountability (Herdman et al., 2021).

Standard 2. Diagnosis

"*The psychiatric-mental health registered nurse analyzes the assessment data to determine diagnoses, problems, and areas of focus for care and treatment, including level of risk*" (ANA et al., 2022, p. 61).

In the second step, data gathered during the assessment are analyzed. Diagnoses and potential problem statements are formulated and prioritized.

TABLE 8–1 Brief Mental Status Evaluation

AREA OF MENTAL FUNCTION EVALUATED	EVALUATION ACTIVITY
Orientation to time	"What year is it?" "What month is it?" "What day is it?" (3 points)
Orientation to place	"Where are you now?" (1 point)
Attention and immediate recall	"Repeat these words now: bell, book, and candle." (3 points) "Remember these words, and I will ask you to repeat them in a few minutes."
Abstract thinking	"What does this mean: No use crying over spilled milk." (3 points)
Recent memory	"Say the 3 words I asked you to remember earlier." (3 points)
Naming objects	Point to eyeglasses and ask, "What is this?" Repeat with 1 other item (e.g., calendar, watch, pencil). (2 points possible)
Ability to follow simple verbal command	"Tear this piece of paper in half and put it in the trash container." (2 points)
Ability to follow simple written command	Write a command on a piece of paper (e.g., TOUCH YOUR NOSE), give the paper to the patient, and say, "Do what it says on this paper." (1 point for correct action)
Ability to use language correctly	Ask the patient to write a sentence. (3 points if sentence has a subject, a verb, and valid meaning)
Ability to concentrate	"Say the months of the year in reverse, starting with December." (1 point each for correct answers from November through August; 4 points possible)
Understanding spatial relationships	Instruct patient to draw a clock, put in all the numbers, and set the hands on 3 o'clock. (clock circle = 1 pt; numbers in correct sequence = 1 pt; numbers placed on clock correctly = 1 pt; two hands on the clock = 1 pt; hands set at correct time = 1 pt; 5 points possible)

Scoring: 30–21 = normal; 20–11 = mild cognitive impairment; 10–0 = severe cognitive impairment (scores are not absolute and must be considered within the comprehensive diagnostic assessment).
Sources: Folstein, M. F., Folstein, S. E., & McHugh, P. R. (1975). Mini-mental state: A practical method for grading the cognitive state of patients for the clinician. *Journal of Psychiatric Research, 12*(3), 189–198; Kaufman, D. M., & Zun, L. (1995). A quantifiable, brief mental status examination for emergency patients. *Journal of Emergency Medicine, 13*(4), 440–456; Kokman, E., Smith, G. E., Petersen, R. C., Tangalos, E., & Ivnik, R. C. (1991). The short test of mental status: Correlations with standardized psychometric testing. *Archives of Neurology, 48*(7), 725–728; Pfeiffer, E. (1975). A short portable mental status questionnaire for the assessment of organic brain deficit in elderly patients. *Journal of the American Geriatric Society, 23*(10), 433–441.

Diagnoses are congruent with available and accepted classification systems (e.g., *NANDA International Nursing Diagnoses: Definitions and Classification*).

CORE CONCEPT

Outcomes
Patient behaviors and responses that are collaboratively agreed upon, measurable, desired results of nursing interventions.

Standard 3. Outcomes Identification

"*The psychiatric-mental health registered nurse identifies expected outcomes based on the patient's/client's goals and their individual circumstances*" (ANA et al., 2022, p. 63).

Expected outcomes are derived from the diagnosis. They must be measurable and include a time estimate for attainment. They must be realistic for the patient's capabilities, and they are most effective when formulated cooperatively by the interdisciplinary team members, the patient, and significant others.

Nursing Outcomes Classification

The **Nursing Outcomes Classification (NOC)** is a comprehensive, standardized classification of patient outcomes developed to evaluate the effects of nursing interventions (Moorhead et al., 2018). The outcomes have been linked to NANDA International (NANDA-I) diagnoses and the **Nursing Interventions Classification (NIC)**. NANDA-I, NIC, and NOC represent all domains of nursing and can be used together or separately (Moorhead & Dochterman, 2012). Each of the NOC outcomes has a label name, a definition, a list of indicators to evaluate patient status in relation to the outcome, and a five-point Likert scale to measure patient status (Moorhead et al., 2018).

Standard 4. Planning

"The psychiatric-mental health registered nurse develops a patient/client-centered plan that prescribes strategies and alternatives to attain expected outcomes" (ANA et al., 2022, p. 64).

The care plan is individualized to the patient's mental health problems, condition, or needs and is developed in collaboration with the patient, significant others, and interdisciplinary team members if possible. For each diagnosis identified, the most appropriate interventions based on current psychiatric-mental health nursing practice, standards, relevant statutes, and research evidence are selected. Patient education and necessary referrals are included. Priorities for delivery of nursing care are determined based on safety needs and the patient's risk for harm to self or others. Elements of the plan should be prioritized with input from the patient/client, support system, health-care providers, and others as appropriate (ANA et al., 2022).

Nursing Interventions Classification

NIC is a comprehensive, standardized language describing treatments that nurses perform in all settings and specialties (Butcher et al., 2018). NIC includes both physiological and psychosocial interventions as well as those for illness treatment, illness prevention, and health promotion. NIC interventions are comprehensive, supported by research, and reflect current clinical practice. They were developed inductively based on existing practice.

Each NIC intervention has a definition and a detailed set of activities that describe what a nurse does to implement the intervention. The use of standardized language is thought to enhance continuity of care and facilitate communication among nurses and between nurses and other providers.

Standard 5. Implementation

The psychiatric-mental health registered nurse implements the patient/client-centered plan (ANA et al., 2022, p. 66).

Interventions selected during the planning stage are executed, taking into consideration the nurse's level of practice, education, and certification. This standard incorporates, among others, competencies in principles of recovery and trauma-sensitive care, integrative health practices (a coordination of traditional and complementary practices), and cultural humility. Cultural humility, a new addition to terminology in the latest PMHN *Scope and Standards of Practice,* is described as "a lifelong commitment to self-evaluation and personal critique, to acknowledging and addressing power imbalances, and to developing mutually beneficial and nonpaternalistic partnerships with communities on

behalf of individuals, groups, and populations" (ANA et al., 2022, p. 95). The care plan serves as a blueprint for delivery of safe, ethical, and appropriate interventions. Documentation of interventions also occurs at this step in the nursing process. Several specific interventions, discussed later, are included among the standards of psychiatric-mental health clinical nursing practice (ANA et al., 2022).

Standard 5A. Coordination of Care

"The psychiatric-mental health registered nurse coordinates care delivery" (ANA et al., 2022, p. 68).

 One of the QSEN competencies, teamwork and collaboration, is consistent with this ANA standard of practice. For the nurse to coordinate care it is critical that they understand the roles of other health-care team members and develop strategies for effectively collaborating to meet the patient's needs.

Standard 5B. Health Teaching, Health Literacy, and Health Promotion

"The psychiatric-mental health registered nurse employs strategies to promote health and a safe environment" (ANA et al., 2022, p. 69).

Standard 5C. Consultation

"The psychiatric-mental health advanced practice registered nurse provides consultation to maximize outcomes from the identified plan, collaborate with other clinicians to provide services for patients/clients, and contribute to system" (ANA et al., 2022, p. 71).

Standard 5D. Pharmacological/Biological Therapies and Prescriptive Authority

"The psychiatric mental health registered nurse incorporates knowledge of pharmacological and biological interventions with applied skills to restore the patient's/client's health and prevent further disability.

"The psychiatric-mental health advanced practice registered nurse uses prescriptive authority, procedures, referrals, treatments, and therapies in accordance with state and federal laws and regulations" (ANA et al., 2022, p. 71).

Standard 5E. Complementary/Integrative Therapies

"The psychiatric-mental health registered nurse incorporates knowledge of complementary/integrative interventions (e.g., meditation, yoga, acupuncture, Reiki, Healing Touch, nutrition, physical exercises, dietary supplements, aromatherapy, herbology, art, and music) with applied clinical skills to restore the patient's/client's health and prevent further disability" (ANA et al., 2022, p. 73).

(See online Chapter 40, "Complementary Therapies and Integrative Health for further discussion of this topic.)

Standard 5F. Milieu Therapy

"The psychiatric-mental health registered nurse (including the graduate-level prepared PMH-RN and PMH-APRN) provides a safe, therapeutic, recovery-oriented environment in collaboration with patients/clients, families, and other clinicians/ancillary staff/care partners" (ANA et al., 2022, p. 74).

Several models have been developed to identify what constitutes a therapeutic environment. These models are discussed in greater detail in Chapter 11, "Psychosocial Interventions and Spiritual Care." Incorporation of the health-care environment and the community of patients, their families, and health-care providers is a unique aspect of treatment for patients in psychiatric care settings.

Standard 5G. Therapeutic Relationship

"The psychiatric-mental health registered nurse (including the graduate-level prepared PMH-RN and PMH-APRN) uses the therapeutic relationship as the basis for interactions and the provision of care" (ANA et al., 2022, p. 75).

As mentioned previously, therapeutic relationship and counseling interventions are part of the role of registered nurses practicing in psychiatric-mental health settings. These are basic psychoeducational and problem discussion interventions and are differentiated from psychotherapy that requires advanced practice education and competency.

Standard 5H. Counseling and Psychotherapy

"The psychiatric-mental health registered nurse (PMH-RN) uses counseling interventions to assist patients/clients in their individual recovery journeys.

"The psychiatric-mental health advanced practice registered nurse conducts individual, couples, group, and family psychotherapy using evidence-based psychotherapeutic frameworks within the nurse-client therapeutic relationship" (ANA et al., 2022, p. 76).

CORE CONCEPT

Evaluation

Evaluation involves measuring the patient's progress toward achieving expected outcomes as established in the nursing care plan. This includes identifying whether the patient has improved, has made no change, or has gotten worse.

Standard 6. Evaluation

"The psychiatric-mental health registered nurse evaluates progress toward attainment of expected outcomes" (ANA et al., 2022, p. 77).

During the evaluation step, the nurse measures the success of the interventions in meeting the outcome criteria. The patient's response to treatment is documented, validating use of the nursing process in the delivery of care. The diagnoses, outcomes, and plan of care are reviewed and revised as determined by the evaluation.

Why Nursing Diagnosis?

The concept of nursing diagnosis is not new. For centuries, nurses have identified specific patient responses for which nursing interventions were used to improve quality of life. However, because of the limitations imposed by their licensure, nurses have lacked autonomy in provision of care. Nurses assisted physicians as required and performed a group of specific tasks that were considered within their scope of responsibility. Formal identification of nursing diagnoses, however, affirms those aspects of nursing practice that are within their scope of practice *and* independently directed or implemented.

The term *diagnosis* in relation to nursing first began to appear in the literature in the early 1950s. The formalized organization of the concept, however, was initiated in 1973 with the convening of the First Task Force to Name and Classify Nursing Diagnoses. The Task Force of the National Conference Group on the Classification of Nursing Diagnoses formed during this conference was charged with the task of identifying and classifying nursing diagnoses.

Also in the 1970s, the ANA began to write standards of practice around the steps of the nursing process, of which nursing diagnosis is an inherent part. This format encompassed both the general and specialty standards outlined by the ANA.

From this progression, a policy statement that includes a definition of nursing was published in 1980. The ANA defined nursing as "the diagnosis and treatment of human responses to actual or potential health problems" (ANA, 2010). This definition has been expanded to describe more appropriately nursing's commitment to society and the profession. The ANA (no date) currently describes nursing as follows:

> Beyond the time-honored reputation for compassion and dedication lies a highly specialized profession, which is constantly evolving to address the needs of society. From ensuring the most accurate diagnoses to the ongoing education of the public about critical health issues; nurses are indispensable in safeguarding public health.... Through the critical thinking exemplified in the nursing process, nurses use their judgment to integrate objective data with subjective experience of a patient's biological, physical and behavioral needs. This ensures that every patient, from city hospital to community health center;

state prison to summer camp, receives the best possible care regardless of who they are, or where they may be.

Decisions regarding professional negligence are made based on the standards of practice defined by the ANA and the individual state nurse practice acts. Many states have incorporated the steps of the nursing process, including nursing diagnosis, into the scope of nursing practice described in their nurse practice acts. When this is the case, it is the legal duty of the nurse to show that the nursing process and nursing diagnosis were accurately implemented in the delivery of nursing care. The National Council of State Boards of Nursing (2023), in the most recent iteration of the NCLEX framework (Next Generation NCLEX [NGN]), reinforces the importance of every nurse's competence in this critical thinking process by incorporating case studies in the testing format that evaluate the nurse's ability to problem solve using each of the steps of the nursing process. Several chapters in this text include case studies to guide the student in developing these critical thinking skills.

NANDA-I evolved from the original 1973 task force to name and classify nursing diagnoses. The major purpose of NANDA-I is "to develop, refine and promote terminology that accurately reflects nurses' clinical judgments … NANDA-I will be a global force for the development and use of nursing's standardized terminology to ensure patient safety through evidence-based care, thereby improving the health care of all people" (NANDA-I, 2021). The list of NANDA-I-approved diagnoses is by no means all inclusive. In an effort to maintain a common language within nursing and encourage clinical testing, most of the nursing diagnoses used in this text are taken from the 2021–2023 list approved by NANDA-I. However, in one instance, a nursing diagnosis (disturbed sensory perceptions) that has been retired by NANDA-I for various reasons will continue to be used because of its appropriateness and suitability in describing specific behaviors.

The use of nursing diagnosis affords a degree of autonomy that historically has been lacking in the practice of nursing. Nursing diagnosis describes the patient's unhealthy or potentially unhealthy responses, facilitating the prescription of interventions and establishment of parameters for outcome criteria based on aspects of practice that are unique to nursing. The ultimate benefit is to the patient, who receives effective and consistent nursing care based on knowledge of the problems that they are experiencing and of the most beneficial nursing interventions to resolve them.

Nursing Case Management

The concept of case management evolved with the advent of diagnosis-related groups (DRGs) and shorter hospital stays. Case management is a model of care delivery that can result in improved client care. In this model, clients are assigned a manager who negotiates with multiple providers to obtain diverse services. This type of health-care delivery process serves to decrease fragmentation of care while striving to contain cost of services.

Case management in the acute care setting aims to organize patient care through an episode of illness so that specific clinical and financial outcomes are achieved within an allotted time frame. Commonly, the allotted time frame is determined by the established protocols for length of stay as defined by the DRGs.

Case management has been shown to be an effective method of treatment for individuals with severe and persistent mental illness. This type of care strives to improve functioning by assisting the individual in solving problems, improving work and socialization skills, promoting leisure-time activities, and enhancing overall independence.

Ideally, case management incorporates concepts of care at the primary, secondary, and tertiary levels of prevention (see Chapter 35, "Community Mental Health Nursing," for further discussion of the different levels of prevention). Various terms that are used in the arena of case management are clarified, as follows.

Managed care refers to a strategy employed by purchasers of health services who make determinations about various services to maintain quality and control costs. In a managed care program, individuals receive health care based on need as assessed by coordinators of the providership. Managed care exists in many settings, including (but not limited to):

- Insurance-based programs
- Employer-based medical providerships
- Social service programs
- The public health sector

Managed care may exist in virtually any setting in which a private or government-based organization is responsible for payment of health-care services for a group of people. Examples of managed care are health maintenance organizations (HMOs) and preferred provider organizations (PPOs).

Case management, the method used to achieve managed care, is the actual coordination of services required to meet the needs of a client within the fragmented health-care system. Case management strives to help at-risk clients prevent avoidable episodes of illness while controlling health-care costs for the consumer and third-party payers. Types of clients who benefit from case management include (but are not limited to):

■ The frail elderly
■ Individuals with developmental disabilities
■ Individuals with physical disabilities
■ Individuals with mental disabilities
■ Individuals with long-term, medically complex problems who require multifaceted, costly care (e.g., high-risk infants, those who are HIV positive or who have AIDS, and transplant clients)
■ Individuals who are severely compromised by an acute episode of illness or an acute exacerbation of a severe and persistent illness (e.g., schizophrenia)

The **case manager** is responsible for negotiating with multiple health-care providers to obtain a variety of services for the client. Nurses are exceptionally qualified to serve as case managers. The very nature of nursing, which incorporates knowledge about the biological, psychological, and sociocultural aspects related to human functioning, makes nurses highly appropriate for this role. Several years of experience as a registered nurse are usually required for employment as a case manager. Some case management programs prefer advanced practice registered nurses who have experience working with the specific populations for whom the service will be rendered. The American Nurses Credentialing Center (ANCC) offers an examination for nurses to become board certified in nursing case management.

Critical Pathways of Care

CPCs (also called *clinical pathways*) may be used as the tools for provision of care in a case management system. A critical pathway is an abbreviated care plan that provides guidelines for goal achievement within a designated length of stay. A sample CPC is presented in Table 8–2. Only one nursing diagnosis is used in this sample, but a comprehensive CPC may have nursing diagnoses for several individual problems and incorporates the responsibilities of other team members as well.

CPCs are intended to be used by the entire interdisciplinary team, which may include a nurse, case manager, clinical nurse specialist, social worker, psychiatrist, psychologist, dietitian, occupational therapist, recreational therapist, chaplain, and others. The team decides what categories of care are to be performed, by what date, and by whom. Each member of the team is then expected to carry out their functions according to the timeline designated on the CPC.

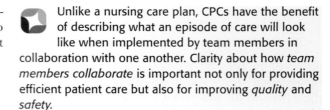 Unlike a nursing care plan, CPCs have the benefit of describing what an episode of care will look like when implemented by team members in collaboration with one another. Clarity about how *team members collaborate* is important not only for providing efficient patient care but also for improving *quality* and *safety.*

As a case manager, the nurse is ultimately responsible for ensuring that each assignment is carried out. If variations occur in any of the categories of care, the rationale must be documented in the progress notes. For example, with the sample CPC presented in Table 8–2, the nurse case manager may admit the client into the detoxification center. The nurse contacts the psychiatrist to inform them of the admission. The psychiatrist performs additional assessments to determine whether other consultations are required and writes the orders for the initial diagnostic work-up and medication regimen.

Within 24 hours, the interdisciplinary team meets to decide on other categories of care, complete the CPC, and make individual care assignments from the CPC. This particular sample CPC relies heavily on nursing care of the patient through the critical withdrawal period. However, other problems for the same patient, such as imbalanced nutrition, impaired physical mobility, or spiritual distress, may involve other members of the team to a greater degree. Each member of the team stays in contact with the case manager regarding individual assignments. Ideally, team meetings are held daily or every other day to review progress and modify the plan as required.

CPCs can be standardized, as they are intended to be used with uncomplicated cases. A CPC can be viewed as protocol for clients who have specific problems for which a designated outcome can be predicted.

Applying the Nursing Process in the Psychiatric Setting

Based on the definition of *mental health* stated in Chapter 2, "Mental Health and Mental Illness: Historical and Theoretical Concepts," the nurse's role in psychiatry is to help the patient successfully adapt to stressors in the environment. Goals are directed toward changes in thoughts, feelings, and behaviors that are age appropriate and congruent with local and cultural norms.

Therapy in the psychiatric setting is most often team oriented, or **interdisciplinary.** Therefore, it is important to delineate nursing's involvement in the treatment regimen. Nurses are valuable members of the team and they provide defined services within the scope of nursing practice. Nursing diagnosis is

TABLE 8–2 Sample Critical Pathway of Care for Patient in Alcohol Withdrawal

Estimated Length of Stay: 7 Days—Variations from designated pathway should be documented in progress notes

NURSING DIAGNOSES AND CATEGORIES OF CARE	TIME DIMENSION	GOALS AND/OR ACTIONS	TIME DIMENSION	GOALS AND/OR ACTIONS	TIME DIMENSION	DISCHARGE OUTCOME
Risk for injury related to CNS agitation					Day 7	Patient shows no evidence of injury obtained during ETOH withdrawal
Referrals	Day 1	Psychiatrist Assess need for: Neurologist Cardiologist Internist			Day 7	Discharge with follow-up appointments as required
Diagnostic studies	Day 1	Blood alcohol level Drug screen (urine and blood) Chemistry profile Urinalysis Chest x-ray ECG	Day 4	Repeat selected diagnostic studies as necessary		
Additional assessments	Day 1 Day 1–5 Ongoing Ongoing	VS q4h I&O Assess withdrawal symptoms: tremors, nausea/vomiting, tachycardia, sweating, high blood pressure, seizures, insomnia, hallucinations	Day 2–3 Day 6 Day 4	VS q8h if stable DC I&O Marked decrease in objective withdrawal symptoms	Day 4–7 Day 7	VS bid; remain stable Discharge; absence of objective withdrawal symptoms
Medications	Day 1 Day 2 Day 1–6 Day 1–7	*Librium 200 mg in divided doses Librium 160 mg in divided doses Librium prn Maalox pc & hs *Note: Some physicians may elect to use alternative medications in the detoxification process	Day 3 Day 4	Librium 120 mg in divided doses Librium 80 mg in divided doses	Day 5 Day 6 Day 7	Librium 40 mg Discontinue Librium Discharge; no withdrawal symptoms
Patient education			Day 5	Discuss goals of AA and need for outpatient therapy	Day 7	Discharge with information regarding AA attendance or outpatient treatment

AA, Alcoholics Anonymous; bid, twice a day; CNS, central nervous system; DC, discontinue; ECG, electrocardiogram; ETOH, alcohol; hs, bedtime; I&O, intake and output; pc, after meals; prn, as needed; q4h, every 4 hours; q8h, every 8 hours; VS, vital signs.

helping to define these nursing boundaries and provides a degree of autonomy and professionalism.

For example, a newly admitted patient with the medical diagnosis of schizophrenia may be demonstrating the following behaviors:

■ Inability to trust others
■ Hearing voices
■ Refusal to interact with staff and peers
■ Fear of failure
■ Poor personal hygiene

From these assessments, the treatment team may determine that the patient has the following problems:

■ Paranoid delusions
■ Auditory hallucinations
■ Social withdrawal
■ Developmental regression

Team goals would be directed toward the following:

■ Reducing suspiciousness
■ Terminating auditory hallucinations
■ Increasing feelings of self-worth

From this team treatment plan, nursing may identify the following nursing diagnoses:

■ Disturbed sensory perception, auditory (evidenced by hearing voices)
■ Disturbed thought processes (evidenced by delusions)
■ Low self-esteem (evidenced by fear of failure and social withdrawal)
■ Self-care deficit (evidenced by poor personal hygiene)
■ Social isolation

Nursing diagnoses are prioritized according to life-threatening potential. Maslow's hierarchy of needs is an appropriate model to follow when prioritizing nursing diagnoses. In this instance, Disturbed sensory perception (auditory) is identified as the priority nursing diagnosis because the patient may be hearing voices that command them to harm themselves or others. Psychiatric nursing, regardless of the setting—hospital (inpatient or outpatient), office, home, community—is goal-directed care. The goals (or expected outcomes) are patient oriented, measurable, and focused on problem resolution (if this is realistic) or on a more short-term outcome (if resolution is unrealistic). For example, in the previous situation, expected outcomes for the identified nursing diagnoses might be as follows:

The patient:

■ Demonstrates trust in one staff member within 3 days
■ Verbalizes understanding that the voices are not real (not heard by others) within 5 days
■ Completes one simple craft project within 5 days
■ Takes responsibility for self-care and performs activities of daily living independently by time of discharge

Nursing's contribution to the interdisciplinary treatment regimen will focus on establishing trust on a one-to-one basis (thus reducing the level of anxiety that may be promoting hallucinations), giving positive feedback for small day-to-day accomplishments to build self-esteem, and assisting with and encouraging independent self-care. These interventions describe *independent nursing* actions and goals that are evaluated apart from, while also being directed toward the achievement of, the *team's* treatment goals.

In this manner of collaboration with other team members, nursing provides a unique service based on sound knowledge of psychopathology, scope of practice, and legal implications of the role. Although implementing physician's orders is acknowledged as an important aspect of nursing care, nursing interventions that enhance the achievement of the overall goals of treatment are important contributions as well. The nurse who administers a medication prescribed by the physician to decrease anxiety may also choose to stay with the anxious patient and offer reassurance of safety and security, thereby providing an independent nursing action that is distinct from, yet complementary to, the medical treatment.

Concept Mapping*

Concept mapping is a diagrammatic teaching and learning strategy that allows students and faculty to visualize interrelationships between medical diagnoses, nursing diagnoses, assessment data, and treatments. The concept map is a diagram of patient problems and interventions. Compared with the commonly used column format care plans, concept map care plans are more succinct. They primarily serve to enhance critical-thinking skills and clinical reasoning ability by creating a holistic picture of various patient problems and their interconnectedness to one another.

The nursing process is foundational to developing and using the concept map care plan, just as with all types of nursing care plans. Patient data are collected and analyzed, nursing diagnoses are formulated, outcome criteria are identified, nursing actions are planned and implemented, and the success of the interventions in meeting the outcome criteria is evaluated.

The concept map care plan may be presented in its entirety on one page, or the assessment data

---

*Content in this section is adapted from Doenges et al. (2022) and Schuster (2020).

and nursing diagnoses may appear in diagram format on one page, with outcomes, interventions, and evaluation written on a second page. Alternatively, the diagram may appear in circular format, with nursing diagnoses and interventions branching off the "patient" in the center of the diagram. Or, it may begin with the "patient" at the top of the diagram, with branches emanating downward in a linear fashion.

Whatever format is chosen to visualize the concept map, the diagram should reflect the nursing process in a stepwise fashion, beginning with the patient and their reason for needing care, nursing diagnoses with subjective and objective clinical evidence for each, nursing interventions, and outcome criteria for evaluation.

Figure 8–2 presents one example of a concept map care plan. It is assembled for the hypothetical

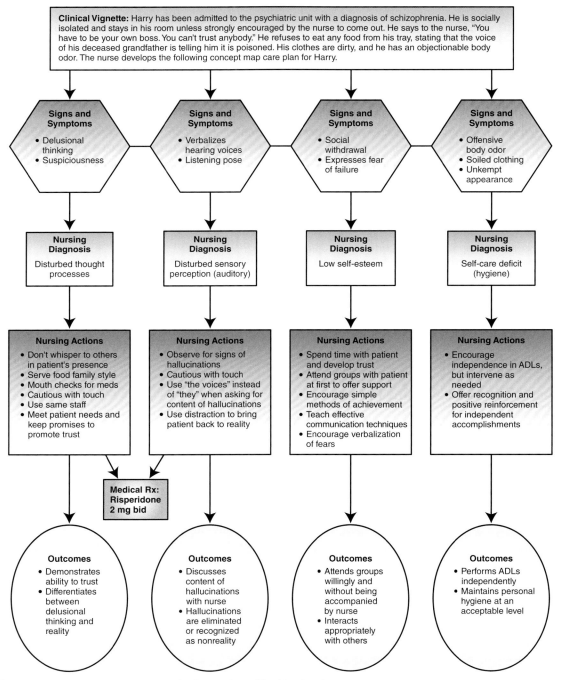

Clinical Vignette: Harry has been admitted to the psychiatric unit with a diagnosis of schizophrenia. He is socially isolated and stays in his room unless strongly encouraged by the nurse to come out. He says to the nurse, "You have to be your own boss. You can't trust anybody." He refuses to eat any food from his tray, stating that the voice of his deceased grandfather is telling him it is poisoned. His clothes are dirty, and he has an objectionable body odor. The nurse develops the following concept map care plan for Harry.

Signs and Symptoms
- Delusional thinking
- Suspiciousness

Signs and Symptoms
- Verbalizes hearing voices
- Listening pose

Signs and Symptoms
- Social withdrawal
- Expresses fear of failure

Signs and Symptoms
- Offensive body odor
- Soiled clothing
- Unkempt appearance

Nursing Diagnosis
Disturbed thought processes

Nursing Diagnosis
Disturbed sensory perception (auditory)

Nursing Diagnosis
Low self-esteem

Nursing Diagnosis
Self-care deficit (hygiene)

Nursing Actions
- Don't whisper to others in patient's presence
- Serve food family style
- Mouth checks for meds
- Cautious with touch
- Use same staff
- Meet patient needs and keep promises to promote trust

Nursing Actions
- Observe for signs of hallucinations
- Cautious with touch
- Use "the voices" instead of "they" when asking for content of hallucinations
- Use distraction to bring patient back to reality

Nursing Actions
- Spend time with patient and develop trust
- Attend groups with patient at first to offer support
- Encourage simple methods of achievement
- Teach effective communication techniques
- Encourage verbalization of fears

Nursing Actions
- Encourage independence in ADLs, but intervene as needed
- Offer recognition and positive reinforcement for independent accomplishments

Medical Rx: Risperidone 2 mg bid

Outcomes
- Demonstrates ability to trust
- Differentiates between delusional thinking and reality

Outcomes
- Discusses content of hallucinations with nurse
- Hallucinations are eliminated or recognized as nonreality

Outcomes
- Attends groups willingly and without being accompanied by nurse
- Interacts appropriately with others

Outcomes
- Performs ADLs independently
- Maintains personal hygiene at an acceptable level

FIGURE 8–2 Example of a concept map care plan for a patient with schizophrenia.

patient with schizophrenia discussed in the previous section, "Applying the Nursing Process in the Psychiatric Setting." Different colors may be used in the diagram to designate various components of the care plan. Connecting lines are drawn between components to indicate relationships. For example, there may be a relationship between two nursing diagnoses (e.g., between the nursing diagnoses of Pain or Anxiety and Disturbed sleep pattern). A line between these nursing diagnoses should be drawn to show the relationship.

Concept map care plans permit viewing the "whole picture" without generating a great deal of paperwork. Because they reflect the steps of the nursing process, concept map care plans also are valuable guides for documentation of patient care. Doenges and associates (2019) noted that traditional care plans fail to clarify how all the patient's identified needs are related, so the user may not develop a holistic view. The concept map clarifies those linkages. Whether these care-planning strategies are used for learning or in actual practice, both the concept map and traditional care plan are useful tools for developing and visualizing the critical-thinking process that goes into planning patient care.

 The concept map can be expanded to visualize an episode of care that not only includes various patient needs and associated nursing care but also visualizes how other disciplines within the treatment team are collaborating to address those needs. In this format, the concept map informs about *teamwork and collaboration,* one of the six QSEN competencies.

Documentation of the Nursing Process

Equally as important as using the nursing process in the delivery of care is documenting its use in writing. Some contemporary nursing leaders advocate that with solid standards of practice and procedures in place within the institution, nurses need only chart when there has been a deviation in the care as outlined by that standard. This method of documentation, known as *charting by exception,* is not widely accepted, as many legal decisions are still based on the precept that "if it was not charted, it was not done."

Because nursing process and diagnosis are mandated by nurse practice acts in some states, documentation of their use is considered evidence in those states when determining certain cases of negligence by nurses. Some health-care organization accrediting agencies also require that the nursing process be reflected in the delivery of care.

A variety of documentation methods can be used to reflect use of the nursing process in the delivery of nursing care. Three examples are presented here: problem-oriented recording (POR); Focus Charting; and the problem, intervention, evaluation (PIE) system of documentation.

Electronic health records (EHRs) have become a primary vehicle for documentation of patient care, and many rely heavily on preset menus and checklists. However, the various methods of documentation described next remain an important model for critical thinking about the essential aspects to be included in communicating and documenting patient care. These methods can be incorporated in electronic nurses' notes when there is an opportunity or need to provide additional documentation in the EHR.

Problem-Oriented Recording

POR, based on a list of problems, follows the subjective, objective, assessment, plan, implementation, and evaluation (SOAPIE) format. When used in nursing, the problems (nursing diagnoses) are identified on a written plan of care, with appropriate nursing interventions described for each. Documentation written in the SOAPIE format includes the following:

S = Subjective data: Information gathered from what the patient, family, or other source has said or reported

O = Objective data: Information gathered through direct observation by the person performing the assessment; may include a physiological measurement such as blood pressure or a behavioral response such as affect

A = Assessment: The nurse's interpretation of the subjective and objective data

P = Plan: The actions or treatments to be carried out (may be omitted in daily charting if the plan is clearly explained in the written nursing care plan and no changes are expected)

I = Intervention: Those nursing actions that were actually carried out

E = Evaluation: Evaluation of the problem after nursing intervention (some nursing interventions cannot be evaluated immediately, so this section may be optional)

Table 8–3 shows how POR corresponds to the steps of the nursing process. The following is an example of a three-column documentation in the POR format.

Example

DATE/TIME	PROBLEM	PROGRESS NOTES
9-12-2024 1000	SOCIAL ISOLATION	**S:** States he does not want to sit with or talk to others; "they frighten me."
		O: Stays in room alone unless strongly encouraged to come out; no group involvement; at times listens to group conversations from a distance but does not interact; some hypervigilance and scanning noted
		A: Inability to trust; panic level of anxiety; delusional thinking
		P: Facilitate patient's ability to attend group activities with manageable level of anxiety
		I: Initiated trusting relationship by spending time alone with the patient; discussed his feelings regarding interactions with others; discussed strategies for decreasing anxiety; accompanied patient to group activities; provided positive feedback for voluntarily participating in assertiveness training
		E: Patient stayed throughout the group activity; reported using deep breathing exercises to decrease anxiety and felt "a little less anxious"; identified that the assertive communication techniques he learned are something he needs to use more often

TABLE 8–3 Validation of the Nursing Process With Problem-Oriented Recording

PROBLEM-ORIENTED RECORDING	WHAT IS RECORDED	NURSING PROCESS
S and O (Subjective and Objective data)	Verbal reports to, and direct observation and examination by, the nurse	Assessment
A (Assessment)	Nurse's interpretation of S and O	Diagnosis and outcome identification
P (Plan) (Omitted in charting if written plan describes care to be given)	Description of appropriate nursing actions to resolve the identified problem	Planning
I (Intervention)	Description of nursing actions actually carried out	Implementation
E (Evaluation)	A reassessment of the situation to determine results of nursing actions implemented	Evaluation

Focus Charting

Another type of documentation that reflects use of the nursing process is **Focus Charting.** Focus Charting differs from POR in that the main perspective has been changed from "problem" to "focus," and a data, action, and response (DAR) format has replaced SOAPIE.

Lampe (1985) suggested that a focus for documentation can be any of the following:

■ Nursing diagnosis
■ Current patient concern or behavior
■ Significant change in the patient status or behavior
■ Significant event in the patient's therapy

The focus cannot be a medical diagnosis. The documentation is organized in the format of DAR. These categories are defined as follows:

D = Data: Information that supports the stated focus or describes pertinent observations about the patient

A = Action: Immediate or future nursing actions that address the focus, and evaluation of the present care plan along with any changes required

R = Response: Description of patient's responses to any part of the medical or nursing care

Table 8–4 shows how Focus Charting corresponds to the steps of the nursing process.

The following is an example of a three-column documentation in the DAR format.

Example

DATE/TIME	FOCUS	PROGRESS NOTES
9-12-2024 1000	Social isolation related to mistrust, panic anxiety, delusions	**D:** States he does not want to sit with or talk to others; they "frighten" him; stays in room alone unless strongly encouraged to come out; no group involvement; at times listens to group conversations from a distance, but does not interact; some hypervigilance and scanning noted **A:** Initiated trusting relationship by spending time alone with patient; discussed his feelings regarding interactions with others; accompanied patient to group activities; provided positive feedback for voluntarily participating in assertiveness training **R:** Cooperative with therapy; still acts uncomfortable in the presence of a group of people; accepted positive feedback from nurse

TABLE 8–4 Validation of the Nursing Process With Focus Charting

FOCUS CHARTING	WHAT IS RECORDED	NURSING PROCESS
D (Data)	Information that supports the stated focus or describes pertinent observations about the patient	Assessment
Focus	A nursing diagnosis; current patient concern or behavior; significant change in patient status; significant event in the patient's therapy (*Note:* If outcome appears on written care plan, does not need to be repeated in daily documentation unless a change occurs.)	Diagnosis and outcome identification
A (Action)	Immediate or future nursing actions that address the focus; appraisal of the care plan along with any changes required	Plan and implementation
R (Response)	Description of patient responses to any part of the medical or nursing care	Evaluation

The PIE Method

The PIE method, or more specifically, "APIE" (assessment, problem, intervention, evaluation), is a systematic approach of documenting to nursing process and nursing diagnosis. A problem-oriented system, **PIE charting** uses accompanying flow sheets that are individualized by each institution. Criteria for documentation are organized in the following manner:

A = Assessment: A complete patient assessment is conducted at the beginning of each shift. Results are documented under this section in the progress notes. Some institutions elect instead to use a daily patient assessment sheet designed to meet specific needs of the unit. Explanation of any deviation from the norm is included in the progress notes.

P = Problem: A problem list, or list of nursing diagnoses, is an important part of the APIE method of charting. The name or number of the problem being addressed is documented in this section.

I = Intervention: Nursing actions are performed, directed at resolution of the problem.

E = Evaluation: Outcomes of the implemented interventions are documented, including an evaluation of patient responses to determine the effectiveness of nursing interventions and the presence or absence of progress toward resolution of a problem.

Table 8–5 shows how APIE charting corresponds to the steps of the nursing process. The following is an example of a three-column documentation in the APIE format.

Example

DATE/TIME	PROBLEM	PROGRESS NOTES
9-12-2024 1000	Social isolation	**A:** States he does not want to sit with or talk to others; they "frighten" him; stays in room alone unless strongly encouraged to come out; no group involvement; at times listens to group conversations from a distance but does not interact; some hypervigilance and scanning noted **P:** Social isolation related to inability to trust, panic level of anxiety, and delusional thinking **I:** Initiated trusting relationship by spending time alone with patient; discussed his feelings regarding interactions with others; accompanied patient to group activities; provided positive feedback for voluntarily participating in assertiveness training **E:** Cooperative with therapy; still uncomfortable in the presence of a group of people; accepted positive feedback from nurse

TABLE 8–5 Validation of the Nursing Process With APIE Method

APIE CHARTING	WHAT IS RECORDED	NURSING PROCESS
A (Assessment)	Subjective and objective data about the patient that are gathered at the beginning of each shift	Assessment
P (Problem)	Name (or number) of nursing diagnosis being addressed from written problem list, and identified outcome for that problem (*Note:* If outcome appears on written care plan, it does not need to be repeated in daily documentation unless a change occurs.)	Diagnosis and outcome identification
I (Intervention)	Nursing actions performed, directed at problem resolution	Plan and implementation
E (Evaluation)	Appraisal of patient responses to determine effectiveness of nursing interventions	Evaluation

Electronic Documentation

Most health-care facilities have implemented an EHR or electronic documentation system. Federal regulations and programs have incentivized the move to EHR systems by requiring health-care organizations to use them to receive Medicare and Medicaid reimbursement; as of 2015, progressive reductions in reimbursement have been initiated for health-care providers who are not demonstrating meaningful use of EHRs.

 The rationale for this move is that EHR systems have been shown to improve both the quality of patient care and the efficiency of the health-care system (U.S. Government Accountability Office, 2010). *Quality improvement and informatics* are both QSEN competencies. Further, as the IOM (2003) noted, EHRs can improve communication among team members thus facilitating *teamwork and collaboration,* another QSEN competency.

In 2003, the U.S. Department of Health and Human Services commissioned the IOM to study the capabilities of an EHR system. The IOM identified a set of eight core functions that EHR systems should perform in the delivery of safer, higher quality, and more efficient health care (IOM, 2003):

1. **Health information and data:** EHRs provide more rapid access to important patient information (e.g., allergies, laboratory test results, a medication list, demographic information, and clinical narratives), thereby improving care providers' abilities to make sound clinical decisions in a timely manner.

2. **Results management:** Computerized results of all types (e.g., laboratory test results, radiology procedure result reports) can be accessed more easily by the provider at the time and place they are needed.

3. **Order entry and order management:** Computer-based order entries improve workflow processes

by eliminating lost orders and ambiguities caused by illegible handwriting, generating related orders automatically, monitoring for duplicate orders, and improving the speed with which orders are executed.

4. **Decision support:** Computerized decision support systems enhance clinical performance for many aspects of health care. Reminders and prompts help improve adherence to regular screenings and other preventive practices. Other aspects of health-care support include identifying possible drug interactions and facilitating diagnosis and treatment.

5. **Electronic communication and connectivity:** Improved communication among care associates, such as medicine, nursing, laboratory, pharmacy, and radiology team members, can enhance patient safety and quality of care. Efficient communication among providers improves continuity of care, allows for more timely interventions, and reduces the risk of adverse events.

6. **Patient support:** Computer-based interactive patient education, self-testing, and self-monitoring have been shown to improve control of chronic illnesses.

7. **Administrative processes:** Electronic scheduling systems (e.g., for hospital admissions and outpatient procedures) increase the efficiency of health-care organizations and provide more timely service to patients.

8. **Reporting and population health management:** Health-care organizations are required to report health-care data to government and private sectors for patient safety and public health. Uniform electronic data standards facilitate this process at the provider level, reduce the associated costs, and increase the speed and accuracy of the data reported.

Summary and Key Points

■ The nursing process provides a methodology for critical thinking by which nurses may deliver care using a systematic, scientific approach.

■ The focus of the nursing process is goal directed and based on a decision-making or problem-solving model consisting of six steps: assessment, diagnosis, outcome identification, planning, implementation, and evaluation.

■ Assessment is a systematic, dynamic process by which the nurse, through interaction with the

patient, significant others, and health-care providers, collects and analyzes data about the patient.

■ Nursing diagnoses are clinical judgments about individual, family, or community responses to actual or potential health problems and life processes.

■ Outcomes are measurable, expected, patient-focused goals that translate into observable behaviors.

■ Evaluation is the process of determining both the patient's progress toward the attainment of expected outcomes and the effectiveness of nursing care.

■ The psychiatric nurse uses the nursing process to assist patients to adapt successfully to stressors within the environment.

■ Standards of practice for PMHNs, set forth by the ANA, APNA, and ISPN, outline the nurse's role in each step of the nursing process when caring for the patient within psychiatric services.

■ The nurse serves as a valuable member of the interdisciplinary treatment team, working both independently and cooperatively with other team members.

■ Case management is a model of care delivery that serves to provide quality patient care while controlling health-care costs. CPCs serve as the tools for provision of care in a case management system.

■ Nurses may serve as case managers who are responsible for negotiating with multiple health-care providers to obtain a variety of services for the patient.

■ Concept mapping is a diagrammatic teaching and learning strategy that allows students and faculty to visualize interrelationships between medical diagnoses, nursing diagnoses, assessment data, and treatments. It can be expanded to include a visual picture of how other disciplines are collaborating with nursing to meet specific patient needs. Nurses must document that the nursing process has been used in the delivery of care.

■ Nurses must document that the nursing process has been used in the delivery of care. Three methods of documentation that reflect use of the nursing process are POR, Focus Charting, and the PIE method.

■ Many health-care facilities have implemented the use of EHRs or electronic documentation systems. EHRs have been shown to improve both the quality of patient care and the efficiency of the health-care system.

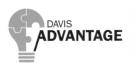

DAVIS **ADVANTAGE** | Go to **Davis Advantage** to complete your learning: strengthen understanding, apply your knowledge, and prepare for the Next Gen NCLEX®.

Review Questions

1. The nurse is using the nursing process to care for a client who is suicidal. Which of the following nursing actions is a part of the *assessment* step of the nursing process?
   a. Identifies nursing diagnosis: Risk for suicide.
   b. Notes that client's family reports recent suicide attempt.
   c. Prioritizes the necessity of maintaining a safe client environment.
   d. Obtains a commitment from the patient to work collaboratively to identify adaptive coping skills.

2. The nurse is using the nursing process to care for a client who is suicidal. Which of the following nursing actions is a part of *the diagnosis* step of the nursing process?
   a. Identifies the client as "At risk for suicide."
   b. Notes that client's family reports recent suicide attempt.
   c. Prioritizes the necessity for maintaining a safe environment for the client.
   d. Obtains a commitment from the patient to work collaboratively to identify adaptive coping skills.

3. The nurse is using the nursing process to care for a client who is suicidal. Which of the following nursing actions is a part of the *outcome identification* step of the nursing process?
   a. Prioritizes the necessity for maintaining a safe environment for the client.
   b. Determines whether nursing interventions have been appropriate to achieve desired results.
   c. Obtains a commitment from the patient to work collaboratively to identify adaptive coping skills.
   d. Identifies that the "Client will not harm self during hospitalization."

4. The nurse is using the nursing process to care for a client who is suicidal. Which of the following nursing actions is a part of the *planning* step of the nursing process?
   a. Prioritizes the necessity for maintaining a safe environment for the client.
   b. Determines whether nursing interventions have been appropriate to achieve desired results.
   c. Obtains a commitment from the patient to work collaboratively to identify adaptive coping skill.
   d. Identifies that the "Client will not harm self during hospitalization."

5. The nurse is using the nursing process to care for a client who is suicidal. Which of the following nursing actions is a part of the *implementation* step of the nursing process?
   a. Prioritizes the necessity for maintaining a safe environment for the client.
   b. Determines whether nursing interventions have been appropriate to achieve desired results.
   c. Collaborates with the client to develop a plan for ongoing safety and suicide prevention.
   d. Identifies that the "Client will not harm self during hospitalization."

6. The nurse is using the nursing process to care for a client who is suicidal. Which of the following nursing actions is a part of the *evaluation* step of the nursing process?
   a. Prioritizes the necessity for maintaining a safe environment for the client.
   b. Determines whether nursing interventions have been appropriate to achieve desired goals.
   c. Collaborates with the client to develop a plan for ongoing safety and suicide prevention.
   d. Identifies that the "Client will not harm self during hospitalization."

Clinical Judgment Questions

7. A 15-year-old female client is admitted to the adolescent psychiatric unit with a diagnosis of anorexia nervosa. She is 5 feet 5 inches tall and weighs 82 pounds. She was selected to join the cheerleading squad for the fall but states that she is not as good as the others on the squad. The treatment team has identified the following problems: refusal to eat, occasional purging, refusing to interact with staff and peers, and fear of failure. Which of the following nursing diagnoses would be appropriate for this client? (Select all that apply.)
   a. Social isolation
   b. Disturbed body image
   c. Low self-esteem
   d. Imbalanced nutrition: Less than body requirements

8. Which of the following nursing diagnoses would be the *priority* diagnosis for the client described in question 7?
   a. Social isolation
   b. Disturbed body image
   c. Low self-esteem
   d. Imbalanced nutrition: Less than body requirements

9. The nurse is transferring a client to a different unit and is providing a transfer report to the nurse that will be receiving this client. The receiving nurse asks what medications this individual received within the last 2 hours. Which source should the nurse use to convey this information?
   a. Handwritten notes from a shift change report.
   b. Memory of what was given to the client earlier.
   c. The electronic health record.
   d. All of the above.

10. A client is admitted to the psychiatric unit with depression. Which of these activities by the nurse is a priority?
    a. Assess the client's risk for suicide.
    b. Establish a care plan that includes suicide precautions.
    c. Contact the physician for orders.
    d. Orient the client to unit activities.

References

American Nurses Association (no date). *What is nursing?* https://www.nursingworld.org/practice-policy/workforce/what-is-nursing/

American Nurses Association (ANA). (2010). *Nursing's social policy statement: The essence of the profession* (3rd ed.). ANA.

American Nurses Association (ANA). (2021). *Nursing: Scope and standards of practice* (4th ed.). ANA.

American Nurses Association (ANA), American Psychiatric Nurses Association (APNA), & International Society of Psychiatric-Mental Health Nurses (ISPN). (2022). *Psychiatric-mental health nursing: Scope and standards of practice* (3rd ed.). ANA.

Butcher, H. K., Bulechek, G. M., Dochterman, J. M., & Wagner, C. M. (Eds.). (2018). *Nursing interventions classification (NIC)* (7th ed.). Elsevier.

Cronenwett, L., Sherwood, G., Barnsteiner, J., Disch, J., Johnson, J., Mitchell, P., Sullivan, D. T., & Warren, D. J. (2007). Quality and safety education for nurses. *Nursing Outlook, 55*(3), 122–131. doi:10.1016/j.outlook.2007.02.006

Doenges, M. E., Moorhouse, M. F., & Murr, A. C. (2022). *Nursing diagnosis manual: Planning, individualizing, and documenting client care* (7th ed.). F.A. Davis.

Healthy People 2030, U.S. Department of Health and Human Services, Office of Disease Prevention and Health Promotion. (n.d.). *Healthy people 2030 framework.* https://health.gov/healthypeople/about/healthy-people-2030-framework

Herdman, T. H., Kamitsuru, S., & Lopes, C. T. (Eds.). (2021). *NANDA-International, Inc. Nursing diagnoses: Definitions and classification, 2021–2023* (12th ed.). Thieme.

Institute of Medicine (IOM). (2003). *Key capabilities of an electronic health record system: Letter report.* The National Academies Press. doi:https://doi.org/10.17226/10781.

Moorhead, S., & Dochterman, J. M. (2012). Languages and development of the linkages. In M. Johnson, S. Moorhead, G. Bulechek, H. Butcher, M. Maas, & E. Swanson, *NOC and NIC linkages to NANDA-I and clinical conditions: Supporting critical reasoning and quality care* (3rd ed., pp. 1–10). Mosby.

Moorhead, S., Swanson, E., Johnson, M., & Maas, M. (2018). *Nursing Outcomes Classification (NOC): Measurement of health outcomes* (6th ed.). Elsevier.

NANDA International. (2021). *About NANDA International.* https://nanda.org/who-we-are/our-story/

National Council of State Boards of Nursing. (2023). *Next generation NCLEX: An enhanced NCLEX.* https://www.nclex.com/next-generation-nclex.page

Schuster, P. M. (2020). *Concept mapping: A clinical judgment approach to care planning* (5th ed.). F.A. Davis.

U.S. Government Accountability Office (GAO). (2010). *Features of integrated systems support patient care strategies and access to care, but systems face challenges.* GAO-11-49. GAO.

Classical References

Folstein, M. F., Folstein, S. E., & McHugh, P. R. (1975). Mini-mental state: A practical method for grading the cognitive state of patients for the clinician. *Journal of Psychiatric Research, 12*(3), 189–198. doi:http://dx.doi.org/10.1016/0022-3956(75)90026-6

Kaufman, D. M., & Zun, L. (1995). A quantifiable, brief mental status examination for emergency patients. *Journal of Emergency Medicine, 13*(4), 440–456. doi:10.1016/0736-4679(95)80000-X

Kokman, E., Smith, G. E., Petersen, R. C., Tangalos, E., & Ivnik, R. C. (1991). The short test of mental status: Correlations with standardized psychometric testing. *Archives of Neurology, 48*(7), 725–728. doi:10.1001/archneur.1991.00530190071018

Lampe, S. S. (1985). Focus charting: Streamlining documentation. *Nursing Management, 16*(7), 43–46.

Pfeiffer, E. (1975). A short portable mental status questionnaire for the assessment of organic brain deficit in elderly patients. *Journal of the American Geriatric Society, 23*(10), 433–441. doi:10.1111/j.1532-5415.1975.tb00927.x

Therapeutic Groups 9

CORE CONCEPTS

Professional Behavior: Intervention in groups

Family: Family therapy

Clinical Judgment

KEY TERMS

altruism

autocratic leaders

catharsis

democratic leaders

group

laissez-faire leaders

psychodrama

universality

OBJECTIVES

After reading this chapter, the student will be able to:

1. Define a group.
2. Discuss eight functions of a group.
3. Identify various types of groups.
4. Describe physical conditions that influence groups.
5. Discuss therapeutic factors that occur in groups.
6. Describe the phases of group development.
7. Identify various leadership styles in groups.
8. Identify various roles that members assume within a group.
9. Discuss psychodrama as a specialized form of group therapy.
10. Describe the role of the nurse in group therapy.

Human beings are complex creatures who share their activities of daily living with various *groups* of people. As Forsyth (2019) stated, "The tendency to join with others in groups is perhaps the single most important characteristic of humans and the processes that unfold within these groups leave an indelible imprint on their members and on society" (p. 1). Groups provide a sense of belonging, establish norms for accepted behavior, provide support, and facilitate problem-solving.

Health-care professionals share their personal lives with groups of people and encounter multiple group situations in their professional operations. Team conferences, committee meetings, grand rounds, and in-service sessions are but a few instances in which this occurs. In psychiatry, work with patients and families often takes the form of groups. With group work, not only does the nurse have the opportunity to reach out to a greater number of people at one time, but those individuals also assist each other by sharing their feelings, opinions, ideas, and behaviors with the group. Patients learn from each other in a group setting.

This chapter explores various types and methods of therapeutic groups that can be used with psychiatric patients and the role of the nurse in group intervention.

CORE CONCEPT

Group

A **group** is a collection of individuals whose association is founded on commonalities of interest, values, norms, or purpose. Membership in a group is generally by chance (born into the group), by choice (voluntary affiliation), or by circumstance (the result of life cycle events over which an individual may or may not have control).

Functions of a Group

Sampson and Marthas (1990) outlined the following eight functions that groups serve for their members. They contend that groups may serve more than one function and usually serve different functions for different members of the group.

1. **Socialization:** The cultural group into which individuals are born begins the process of teaching social norms. This process is continued throughout their lives by members of other groups with which they become affiliated.

2. **Support:** One's fellow group members are available in times of need. Individuals derive a feeling of security from group involvement.

3. **Task completion:** Group members provide assistance in endeavors that are beyond the capacity of one individual alone or when results can be achieved more effectively as a team.

4. **Camaraderie:** Members of a group provide the joy and pleasure that individuals seek from interactions with significant others.

5. **Information sharing:** Learning takes place within groups. Knowledge is gained when individual members learn how others in the group have resolved situations similar to those with which they are currently experiencing.

6. **Normative influence:** This function relates to the ways in which groups enforce the established norms. As group members interact, they influence each other about expected norms for communication and behavior.

7. **Empowerment:** Groups help to bring about improvement in existing conditions by providing support to individual members who seek to bring about change. Groups have power that individuals alone do not.

8. **Governance:** Groups provide oversight functions and direction of activities (such as strategic planning or quality assurance) often within the context of a larger group organization.

Types of Groups

The functions of a group vary depending on the reason the group was formed. Clark (2009) identified three types of groups in which nurses most often participate: task, teaching, and supportive/therapeutic groups.

Task Groups

The function of a task group is to accomplish a specific outcome or task. The focus is on solving problems and making decisions to achieve this outcome. Often, a deadline is placed on completion of the task. Because a satisfactory outcome is so important to these types of groups, conflicts may be smoothed over or ignored to focus on the priority at hand.

Teaching Groups

Teaching, or educational, groups convey knowledge and information to a number of individuals. Nurses can be involved in many types of teaching groups, such as medication education, childbirth education, breast self-examination, and effective parenting classes. These groups usually have a set time frame or a specific number of meetings. Members learn from each other as well as from the designated instructor. The objective of teaching groups is for the learner to verbalize or demonstrate mastery of the material presented by the end of the designated period.

Supportive/Therapeutic Groups

Supportive or therapeutic groups are primarily concerned with participants sharing thoughts, feelings, events, and coping strategies to help them learn effective ways to deal with emotional stress arising from situational or developmental crises.

CORE CONCEPT

Group Therapy

A form of psychosocial treatment in which several clients meet together with a therapist for purposes of sharing, gaining personal insight, and improving interpersonal coping strategies.

For the purposes of this text, it is important to differentiate between *therapeutic groups* and *group therapy*. Leaders of group therapy generally have advanced degrees in psychology, social work, nursing, or medicine. They often have additional training or experience under the supervision of a professional accomplished in conducting group psychotherapy based on various theoretical frameworks such as cognitive, behavioral, psychodynamic, interpersonal, and family dynamics. Approaches based on these theories are used by the group therapy leaders to promote improvement in group members' abilities to function on an interpersonal level. Supportive/therapeutic groups, on the other hand, are not designed to conduct psychotherapy. They focus instead on group relations, interactions among group members, and the consideration of selected issues. Like group therapists, individuals who lead therapeutic groups must be knowledgeable in *group process;* that is, the *way* in which group members interact with each other. Interruptions, silences, judgments, nonverbal communication, and scapegoating are examples of group processes. These interactions may occur whether or not there is a designated group leader, but nurses acting as group leaders can guide the ways in which members interact to facilitate accomplishing the group's goals or tasks. This guidance is one reason why group leaders are often referred to as *group facilitators.* They must also have a thorough knowledge of *group content,* the topic or issue being discussed by the group, and the ability to present the topic in language that can be understood by all members. Many nurses who work in psychiatry lead supportive/therapeutic groups.

Self-Help Groups

Nurses may also be involved in self-help groups, a type of group that has grown in number and credibility in recent years. Self-help groups allow individuals to talk about their fears and relieve feelings of isolation while receiving comfort and advice from others undergoing similar experiences. Examples of self-help groups include WW (formerly Weight Watchers), Alcoholics Anonymous, Reach to Recovery, Parents Without Partners, Overeaters Anonymous, Adult Children of Alcoholics, and many others related to specific needs or illnesses. These groups may or may not have a professional leader or consultant. They are run by the members, and leadership often rotates from member to member.

Nurses may become involved with self-help groups either voluntarily or because members have their advice or participation. The nurse may function as a referral agent, resource person, member of an advisory board, or leader of the group. When nurses refer patients to self-help groups they must be knowledgeable about the purposes of the group, membership, leadership, benefits, and the appropriateness of this group for the specific patient before making a referral. Many self-help groups will allow nurses, student nurses, or other health professionals to attend group meetings for the purpose of better understanding the functions of the group.

Physical Conditions That Influence Group Dynamics

The physical aspects, including arrangement of seating, the number of group members, and whether the membership is consistent or variable, has an effect on the dynamics of interaction within the group.

Seating

When preparing the setting for a group, there should be no barrier between members. For example, a circle of chairs is better than chairs set around a table. Members should be encouraged to sit in different chairs at each meeting. This openness and change create a feeling of discomfort that encourages anxious and unsettled behaviors that can then be explored within the group.

Size

Various authors have suggested different ranges of size as ideal for group interaction: 5 to 10 (Yalom & Leszcz, 2020), 8 to 12 (Ezhumalai et al., 2018), and 4 to 12 (Clark, 2009). Group size does make a difference in the interaction among members. The larger the group, the less time is available to devote to individual members. In larger groups, more aggressive individuals are most likely to be heard, whereas quieter members may be left out of the discussions altogether. Understanding this dynamic alerts nurse group leaders to this possibility and allows them to facilitate interaction that promotes greater involvement for all members. However, larger groups provide more opportunities for individuals to learn from other members. The wider range of life experiences and knowledge provides a greater potential for effective group problem-solving. Ultimately, there is no single right answer in identifying optimal group size because it is influenced by several variables including the group's purpose, group members' functional abilities, and expected outcomes.

Membership

Whether the group is open or closed is another condition that influences the dynamics of group process. Open groups are those in which members leave and others join at any time while the group is active. The continuous movement of members in and out of the group creates a type of discomfort that may foster exploration of feelings, and it allows new members to observe benefits of group therapy that longer-term members have already begun to achieve. Open groups are the most common types of groups held on short-term inpatient units, although they are used in outpatient and long-term care facilities as well. Closed groups usually have a predetermined, fixed time frame. All members join at the time the group is organized and terminate at the end of the designated time period. Closed groups are often composed of individuals with common issues or problems they wish to address.

Therapeutic Factors

Why are therapeutic groups helpful? Yalom and Leszcz (2020) described seven therapeutic factors that individuals can achieve through interpersonal interactions within the group, some of which are present in most groups in varying degrees:

1. **Instillation of hope:** By observing the progress of others in the group with similar problems, a group member garners hope that his or her problems can also be resolved.
2. **Universality:** Through **universality,** individuals come to realize that they are not alone in the problems, thoughts, and feelings they are experiencing. Anxiety is relieved by the support and understanding of others in the group who share similar (universal) experiences.
3. **Imparting of information:** Knowledge is gained through formal instruction as well as sharing of advice and suggestions among group members.
4. **Altruism:** Mutual sharing and concern for each other is called **altruism.** Providing assistance and support to others creates a positive self-image and promotes self-growth.
5. **Corrective recapitulation of the primary family group:** Group members are able to reexperience unresolved conflicts that originated in the primary family. Attempts at resolution are promoted through feedback and exploration.
6. **Development of socializing techniques:** Through interaction with and feedback from other members within the group, individuals are able to correct maladaptive social behaviors and learn and develop new social skills.
7. **Imitative behavior:** In a group setting, one who has mastered a particular psychosocial skill or developmental task can be a valuable role model for others. Individuals may imitate selected behaviors that they wish to develop in themselves.

Two additional aspects important in the effectiveness of a therapeutic group include the development of group cohesiveness (members develop an alliance within the group and the feeling emerges that individuals and the total group are of value to each other) and the opportunity for interpersonal learning.

Phases of Group Development

Groups, like individuals, move through phases of therapeutic relationship development. Ideally, groups progress from the phase of getting oriented to one another and advance to trusted working relationships that promote fulfillment of the group members' goals. As with individuals, some groups become fixed in superficial relationships and never progress, or they experience periods of regression in the developmental process. Three phases of group development are discussed here.

Phase I. Initial or Orientation Phase
Group Activities

Leader and members work together to establish the rules that will govern the group (e.g., when and where meetings will occur, the importance of confidentiality, how meetings will be structured). Goals of the group are established. Members are introduced to each other.

Leader Expectations

The leader is expected to orient members to specific group processes, encourage members to participate without disclosing too much too soon, promote an environment of trust, and ensure that rules established by the group do not interfere with fulfillment of the goals.

Member Behaviors

In phase I, members have not yet established trust and will respond to this lack of trust by being overly polite. There is a fear of not being accepted by the group. They may try to "get on the good side" of the leader with compliments and conforming behaviors. A power struggle may ensue as members compete for their position in the "pecking order" of the group.

Phase II. Middle or Working Phase
Group Activities

Ideally, during the working phase, cohesiveness has been established within the group. This phase is when productive work toward completion of the task is undertaken. Problem-solving and decision making occur within the group. In the mature group, cooperation prevails, and differences and disagreements are confronted and resolved.

Leader Expectations

The leader becomes less of a leader and more of a facilitator during the working phase. Some leadership functions are shared by certain members of the group as they progress toward resolution. The leader helps to resolve conflict and continues to foster cohesiveness among the members while ensuring that they do not deviate from the intended task or purpose for which the group was organized.

Member Behaviors

At this point, trust has been established among the members. They turn more often to each other and less often to the leader for guidance. They accept criticism from each other, using it constructively to create change. Occasionally, subgroups form in which two or more members conspire with each other to the exclusion of the rest of the group. These subgroups must be confronted and discussed by the entire membership to maintain group cohesion. Conflict is managed by the group with minimal assistance from the leader.

Phase III. Final or Termination Phase

Group Activities

The longer a group has existed, the more difficult termination is likely to be for the members. Termination should be mentioned from the outset of group formation and be discussed in depth for several meetings before the final session. A sense of loss that precipitates the grief process may be evident, particularly in groups that have been successful in their stated purpose.

Leader Expectations

In the termination phase, the leader encourages the group members to reminisce about what has occurred within the group, review the goals and discuss the actual outcomes, and provide feedback to each other about individual progress within the group. The leader encourages members to discuss feelings of loss associated with termination of the group.

Member Behaviors

Members may express surprise when the group actually ends. They may experience grief responses as they come to grips with the impending loss of the group relationships. Anger toward other group members or the leader may reflect feelings of abandonment (Sampson & Marthas, 1990). These feelings may lead to individual members' discussions of previous losses for which similar emotions were experienced.

Successful termination of the group may help members develop the skills needed when losses occur in other dimensions of their lives.

Leadership Styles

Lippitt and White's classic work (1958) identified three of the most common group leadership styles: autocratic, democratic, and laissez-faire. Table 9–1 outlines various similarities and differences between the three leadership styles.

Autocratic

Autocratic leaders have personal goals for the group. They withhold information from group members, particularly issues that may interfere with the achievement of their own objectives. The message that is conveyed to the group is: "We will do it my way. My way is best." The focus in this style of leadership is on the leader. Members are dependent on the leader for problem-solving, decision making, and permission to perform. The approach of the autocratic leader is one of persuasion, striving to convince others in the group that his or her ideas and methods are superior. Productivity is high with this type of leadership, but often morale within the group is low because of the lack of member input and creativity.

Democratic

Democratic leaders focus on including input from the members of the group. Information is shared with members to allow them to make decisions regarding group goals. Members are encouraged to participate fully in solving problems that affect the

TABLE 9–1 **Leadership Styles–Similarities and Differences**			
CHARACTERISTICS	**AUTOCRATIC**	**DEMOCRATIC**	**LAISSEZ-FAIRE**
Focus	Leader	Members	Undetermined
Task strategy	Members are persuaded to adopt leader's ideas	Members engage in group problem-solving	No defined strategy exists
Member participation	Limited	Unlimited	Inconsistent
Individual creativity	Stifled	Encouraged	Not addressed
Member enthusiasm and morale	Low	High	Low
Group cohesiveness	Low	High	Low
Productivity	High	High (may not be as high as autocratic)	Low
Individual motivation and commitment	Low (tend to work only when leader is present to urge them to do so)	High (satisfaction derived from personal input and participation)	Low (feelings of frustration from lack of direction or guidance)

group, including taking action to effect change. The message that is conveyed to the group is: "Decide what must be done, consider the alternatives, make a selection, and proceed with the actions required to complete the task." The leader provides guidance and expertise as needed. Productivity is lower than it is with autocratic leadership, but morale is much higher because of the extent of input allowed all members of the group and the potential for individual creativity.

Laissez-Faire

This leadership style allows people to do as they please. There is no direction from the leader. In fact, the approach of **laissez-faire leaders** is noninvolvement. Goals for the group are undefined. No decisions are made, no problems are solved, and no action is taken. Members become frustrated and confused, and productivity and morale are low.

Member Roles

Benne and Sheats' classic work (1948) identified three major types of roles that individuals play within the membership of the group. These are roles that serve to

1. Complete the task of the group.
2. Maintain or enhance group processes.
3. Fulfill personal or individual needs.

Task roles and maintenance roles contribute to the success or effectiveness of the group. Personal roles satisfy the needs of the individual members, sometimes to the extent of interfering with the effectiveness of the group. Table 9–2 outlines specific roles within these three major types and the behaviors associated with each.

Psychodrama

A specialized type of therapeutic group, called **psychodrama,** was introduced in 1921 by Jacob L. Moreno, a Viennese psychiatrist. Moreno's method employs a dramatic approach in which clients become "actors" in life-situation scenarios. Cruz and associates (2018), in a systematic review of the literature, identified and defined 11 distinct techniques that are core techniques of Morenian psychodrama, all of which are directed toward offering the client, in a group format, an opportunity to "act out" roles and situations in which the client has unresolved conflicts.

The group leader is called the *director,* group members are the *audience,* and the *set* or *stage* may be specially designed or just a room or area selected for this purpose. Actors are members from the audience who agree to take part in the "drama" by role-playing a situation about which the director has informed

TABLE 9–2 Member Roles Within Groups	
ROLE	**BEHAVIORS**
TASK ROLES	
Coordinator	Clarifies ideas and suggestions that have been made within the group; fosters relationships between members to facilitate pursuit of common goals
Evaluator	Examines group plans and performance, measuring against group standards and goals
Elaborator	Explains and expands on group plans and ideas
Energizer	Encourages and motivates group to perform at its maximum potential
Initiator	Outlines the task at hand for the group and proposes methods for solution
Orienter	Maintains direction within the group
MAINTENANCE ROLES	
Compromiser	Relieves conflict within the group by assisting members to reach a compromise agreeable to all
Encourager	Offers recognition and acceptance of others' ideas and contributions
Follower	Listens attentively to group interaction; is a passive participant
Gatekeeper	Encourages acceptance of and participation by all members of the group
Harmonizer	Minimizes tension within the group by intervening when disagreements produce conflict

TABLE 9–2 **Member Roles Within Groups—cont'd**	
ROLE	**BEHAVIORS**
INDIVIDUAL (PERSONAL) ROLES	
Aggressor	Expresses negativism and hostility toward other members; may use sarcasm to degrade the status of others
Blocker	Resists group efforts; demonstrates rigid and sometimes irrational behaviors that impede group progress
Dominator	Manipulates others to gain control; behaves in an authoritarian manner
Help-seeker	Uses the group to gain sympathy from others; seeks to increase self-confidence from group feedback; lacks concern for others or the group as a whole
Monopolizer	Maintains control of the group by dominating the conversation
Mute or silent member	Does not participate verbally; remains silent for a variety of reasons—may feel uncomfortable with self-disclosure or may be seeking attention through silence
Recognition seeker	Talks about personal accomplishments to gain attention for self
Seducer	Shares intimate details about self with group; is the least reluctant of the group to do so; may frighten others in the group and inhibit group progress with excessive premature self-disclosure

Source: Compiled from Benne, K. D., & Sheats, P. (1948, Spring). Functional roles of group members. *Journal of Social Issues, 4*(2), 41–49; Hobbs, D. J., & Powers, R. C. (1981). *Group member roles: For group effectiveness.* Iowa State University, Cooperative Extension Service.

them. Usually, the situation is an issue with which an individual client has been struggling. The client plays the role of themself and is called the *protagonist.* In this role, the client is able to express true feelings toward individuals (represented by group members) with whom unresolved conflicts exist.

In some instances, the group leader may ask for a client to volunteer as the protagonist for that session. The client may choose a situation they wish to enact and select the audience members to portray the roles of others in the life situation. The psychodrama setting provides the client with a safer and less threatening atmosphere than the real situation, facilitating the expression of true feelings and resolution of interpersonal conflicts.

When the drama has been completed, group members from the audience discuss the situation they have observed, offer feedback, express their feelings, and relate their own similar experiences. In this way, all group members benefit from the session, either directly or indirectly. Role-playing is often incorporated in other therapy groups (not specifically identified as psychodrama groups) to accomplish similar objectives.

Nurses often serve as actors or role players in psychodrama sessions. Leaders of psychodrama groups typically have graduate degrees in psychology, social work, nursing, or medicine with additional training in group therapy and specialty preparation to become a psychodramatist.

The Role of the Nurse in Therapeutic Groups

Nurses participate in group situations on a daily basis. In health-care settings, nurses serve on or lead task groups that create policy, describe procedures, and plan patient care. They are also involved in a variety of other groups aimed at the institutional effort of serving the consumer. Nurses are encouraged to use the steps of the nursing process as a framework for task group leadership.

In psychiatry, nurses may lead various types of therapeutic groups, such as patient education, assertiveness training, grief support, parenting, and transition to discharge groups, among others. To function effectively in the leadership capacity for these groups, nurses must recognize the various processes that occur in groups, such as the phases of group development, the roles that people play within groups, and the motivation behind these behaviors. They also need to be able to select the most appropriate leadership style for the type of group. Generalist nurses may develop these skills as part of their undergraduate education, or they may pursue additional study while serving and learning as the co-leader of a group with a more experienced nurse leader.

Generalist nurses in psychiatry should not serve as leaders of psychotherapy groups. The *Psychiatric-Mental Health Nursing Scope and Standards of Practice* (American Nurses Association [ANA], American Psychiatric Nurses Association [APNA], & International Society of Psychiatric Nurses [ISPN], 2022) specifies that nurses who serve as group psychotherapists should have a minimum of a master's degree in psychiatric nursing. Educational preparation in group theory, extended practice as a group co-leader or leader under the supervision of an experienced psychotherapist, and participation in group therapy on an experiential level are also recommended. Additional specialist training is required beyond the master's level to prepare nurses to become family therapists, psychodramatists, or specialists in other models of group therapy.

Leading therapeutic groups is within the realm of nursing practice. Because group work is such a common therapeutic approach in the discipline of psychiatry, nurses working in this field must continually strive to expand their knowledge and use of group process as a significant psychiatric nursing intervention.

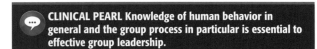

💬 **CLINICAL PEARL Knowledge of human behavior in general and the group process in particular is essential to effective group leadership.**

Summary and Key Points

- A group has been defined as a collection of individuals whose association is founded on shared commonalities of interest, values, norms, or purpose.
- Eight group functions have been identified: socialization, support, task completion, camaraderie, informational, normative, empowerment, and governance.
- The three major types of groups are task groups, teaching groups, and supportive/therapeutic groups.
- The function of task groups is to solve problems, make decisions, and achieve a specific outcome.
- In teaching groups, knowledge and information are conveyed to several individuals.
- The function of supportive/therapeutic groups is to educate people to deal effectively with emotional stress in their lives.

- In self-help groups, members share the same type of problem and help each other to prevent decompensation related to that problem.
- Therapeutic groups differ from group therapy in that the focus is not on psychotherapy but rather on interaction and relationships among group members about a selected issue. Group therapy is more focused on specific models of psychotherapy, and the leaders generally have advanced degrees in psychology, social work, nursing, or medicine. Placement of the seating and size of the group can influence group interaction.
- Groups can be open (when members leave and others join at any time while the group is active) or closed (when groups have a predetermined, fixed time frame and all members join at the same time and leave when the group disbands).
- Yalom and Leszcz (2020) described the following therapeutic factors that individuals derive from participation in therapeutic groups: instillation of hope, universality, imparting of information, altruism, corrective recapitulation of the primary family group, development of socializing techniques, and imitative behavior. General aspects of a therapeutic group that are important to its effectiveness include opportunities for interpersonal learning and the development of group cohesiveness.
- Groups progress through three phases: initial (orientation), working, and termination.
- Group leadership styles include autocratic, democratic, and laissez-faire.
- Members play various roles within groups. These roles are categorized as task, maintenance, and personal roles.
- Psychodrama is a specialized type of group therapy that uses a dramatic approach in which clients become "actors" in life-situation scenarios.
- The psychodrama setting provides the client with a safer and less-threatening atmosphere than the real situation in which to express and work through unresolved conflicts.
- Nurses lead various types of therapeutic groups in the psychiatric setting. Knowledge of human behavior in general and the group process in particular is essential to effective group leadership.
- Specialized training, in addition to a master's degree, is required for nurses to serve as group psychotherapists or psychodramatists.

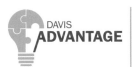

DAVIS **ADVANTAGE** | Go to **Davis Advantage** to complete your learning: strengthen understanding, apply your knowledge, and prepare for the Next Gen NCLEX®.

Review Questions

1. A nurse who is leading a childbirth preparation group shows a film each week and sets out reading materials. She expects the participants to utilize their time on a topic of their choice or practice skills they have observed in the films. Which type of group and style of leadership is described in this situation?
   a. Task group, democratic leadership
   b. Teaching group, laissez-faire leadership
   c. Self-help group, democratic leadership
   d. Supportive-therapeutic group, autocratic leadership

2. A psychiatric nurse is leading a group for people who desire to lose weight. The criterion for membership is that members must be at least 20 pounds overweight. All have tried to lose weight on their own many times in the past without success. At their first meeting, the nurse provides suggestions as the members determine what their goals will be and how they plan to go about achieving those goals. They decide how often they want to meet and what they plan to do at each meeting. Which type of group and style of leadership is described in this situation?
   a. Task group, autocratic leadership
   b. Teaching group, democratic leadership
   c. Self-help group, laissez-faire leadership
   d. Supportive-therapeutic group, democratic leadership

3. A staff nurse on a surgical unit is the leader of a newly established group of staff nurses organized to determine ways to decrease the number of medication errors occurring on the unit. The group leader has definite ideas about how to bring this about and believes that if they are successful in leading the group toward achievement of its goals, it will facilitate their own chances for promotion. At each meeting, the nurse addresses the group to convince the members to adopt the nurse's ideas. Which type of group and style of leadership is described in this situation?
   a. Task group, autocratic leadership
   b. Teaching group, autocratic leadership
   c. Self-help group, democratic leadership
   d. Supportive-therapeutic group, laissez-faire leadership

4. A nurse leader who is explaining about group "therapeutic factors" tells the group members that group situations are beneficial because members can see that they are not alone in their experiences. Which of the following therapeutic factors is the nurse describing?
   a. Altruism
   b. Imitative behavior
   c. Universality
   d. Imparting of information

5. In a bereavement group for the recently widowed, one of the new members hears a longer-term member describe that the group support has helped them adjust to the loss of their spouse. The new member states, "Well, maybe I can get through this, too." This statement is evidence of which of the following therapeutic factors?
   a. Universality
   b. Imitative behavior
   c. Installation of hope
   d. Imparting of information

Clinical Judgment Questions

6. A nurse has been asked to facilitate a group in the outpatient mental health clinic that is focused on helping clients problem solve issues with adherence to medications. Which of these decisions about group size is most appropriate?
  a. The group should be open to all clients who express interest.
  b. The optimal size for this type of group is around 7 to 8 clients.
  c. Clients should democratically decide on the size of the group.
  d. The group should be limited to the first 35 clients who sign up.

7. A psychiatric nurse has been asked to lead an educational group on anger management for clients admitted to the psychiatric unit. Which of these actions by the nurse is the most important priority?
  a. Provide information and handouts on anger management.
  b. Ask clients how long they would like the group to last.
  c. Restrict the group to only those who have been complying with unit rules and expectations.
  d. Ask clients if they would rather have a group on something else.

8. A generalist nurse in the outpatient mental health clinic is approached by the medical director who requests that the nurse initiate a cognitive behavior therapy group. Which of these is the most appropriate action by the nurse?
  a. Establish a self-help group for any clients who are interested.
  b. Conduct cognitive behavior therapy for a small group of 7 to 10 clients.
  c. Educate the medical director that according to nursing practice standards, therapy groups should be conducted by nurses who have a minimum of a master's degree in psychiatric nursing.
  d. Ask the nursing supervisor for approval to initiate the medical director's request.

9. The nursing supervisor asks one of the staff nurses to initiate a group with other staff nurses to identify new ways to prevent client falls. Which of these would be the most appropriate style of leadership for the nurse to implement?
  a. Autocratic
  b. Democratic
  c. Laissez-faire
  d. Militaristic

10. A nurse is conducting a diabetic medication education group for clients on a medical unit. Which of these actions by the nurse is the most important priority during the first meeting of this group?
  a. Ask the clients where they would like to begin.
  b. Try to identify what role each of the members is assuming.
  c. Conduct fingerstick blood sugars on each attendee.
  d. Explain how the meetings will be structured.

References

American Nurses Association (ANA), American Psychiatric Nurses Association (APNA), & International Society of Psychiatric Nurses (ISPN). (2022). *Psychiatric-mental health nursing: Scope and standards of practice* (3rd ed.). ANA.

Clark, C. C. (2009). *Group leadership skills for nurses and health professionals* (5th ed.). Springer.

Cruz, A., Sales, C., Alves, P., & Moita, G. (2018). The core techniques of Morenian psychodrama: A systematic review of literature. *Frontiers in Psychology, 9*, 1263. https://doi.org/10.3389/fpsyg.2018.01263

Ezhumalai, S., Muralidhar, D., Dhanasekarapandian, R., & Nikketha, B. S. (2018). Group interventions. *Indian Journal of Psychiatry, 60*(Suppl 4), S514–S521. doi: 10.4103/psychiatry.IndianJPsychiatry_42_18

Forsyth, D. R. (2019). *Group dynamics* (7th ed.). Cengage Learning.

Yalom, I. D., & Leszcz, M. (2020). *The theory and practice of group psychotherapy* (6th ed.). Basic Books.

Classical References

Benne, K. D., & Sheats, P. (1948, Spring). Functional roles of group members. *Journal of Social Issues, 4*(2), 41–49. doi:10.1111/j.1540-4560.1948.tb01783.x

Hobbs, D. J., & Powers, R. C. (1981). *Group member roles: For group effectiveness.* Iowa State University, Cooperative Extension Service.

Lippitt, R., & White, R. K. (1958). An experimental study of leadership and group life. In Maccoby, E. E., Newcomb, T. M., & Hartley, E. L. (Eds.), *Readings in social psychology* (3rd ed.). Holt, Rinehart, & Winston.

Sampson, E. E., & Marthas, M. (1990). *Group process for the health professions* (3rd ed.). Delmar Publishers.

Intervention With Families

10

CHAPTER OUTLINE

Objectives

Stages of Family Development

Major Variations

Family Functioning

Therapeutic Modalities With Families

The Nursing Process—A Case Study

Summary and Key Points

Review Questions

Clinical Judgment Questions

CORE CONCEPTS

Family

Professional behavior: Nursing process in the care of families

KEY TERMS

boundaries

disengagement

double-bind communication

enmeshment

family structure

family system

genograms

marital schism

marital skew

paradoxical intervention

pseudohostility

pseudomutuality

reframing

scapegoating

subsystems

triangles

OBJECTIVES

After reading this chapter, the student will be able to:

1. Define the term *family.*
2. Identify stages of family development.
3. Describe major variations in the American middle-class family life cycle.
4. Discuss characteristics of adaptive family functioning.
5. Describe behaviors that interfere with adaptive family functioning.
6. Discuss the essential components of family systems, structural, and strategic therapies.
7. Construct a family genogram.
8. Apply the steps of the nursing process in therapeutic intervention with families.

What is a family? Robinson (2022, p. 5) proposes the following definition: "Family refers to two or more individuals who depend on one another for emotional, physical, and economic support. The members of the family are self-defined." This definition allows for the broad diversity seen in American families today and respects the idea that families tell us who their members are, not the other way around.

Many nurses have daily interactions with family members. An individual's illness or hospitalization affects all members of the family, and nurses must understand how to work with the family as a unit, knowing that family members can have a profound effect on the client's healing process.

Nurse generalists should be familiar with the tasks associated with adaptive family functioning. With this knowledge, they can assess family interaction and recognize problems when they arise. They can provide support to families with ill members and make referrals to other professionals when assistance is required to restore adaptive functioning.

Nurse specialists usually possess an advanced degree in nursing. Some nurse specialists have education or experience that qualifies them to perform family therapy. Family therapy is an approach that incorporates theories and models designed to explore family dynamics, dysfunctional patterns, and methods for adaptive change within the context of the family. This

177

chapter explores the stages of family development and compares the "typical" family within various subcultures. Characteristics of adaptive family functioning and behaviors that interfere with this adaptation are discussed. Theoretical components of selected therapeutic approaches are described. Instructions for construction of a family genogram are included. Nursing process provides the framework for nursing intervention with families.

CORE CONCEPT

Family

Two or more individuals who depend on one another for emotional, physical, and economical support. The members of the family are self-defined (Robinson, 2022, p. 5).

Stages of Family Development

McGoldrick and associate (2015) discussed the stages and developmental tasks that describe the traditional family life cycle while acknowledging that it is only one of many trajectories for family development in today's society. The accomplishment of these tasks can vary among diverse cultural groups and the various forms of family structure. These stages, however, provide a valuable framework from which the nurse may study families, emphasizing expansion (the addition of members), contraction (the loss of members), and realignment of relationships as members experience developmental changes. These stages of family development are described in the following paragraphs and summarized in Table 10–1.

The Single Young Adult

This model begins with the launching of the young adult from the family of origin. This stage is challenging because young adults must decide what social standards they will preserve from the family of origin and eventually incorporate into a new family. Tasks of this stage include forming an identity separate from the parents, establishing intimate peer relationships, and advancing toward financial independence. Problems can arise when either the young adults or the parents encounter difficulty terminating the interdependent relationship that has existed in the family of origin.

The Family Joined Through Marriage or Other Union

Uniting as a couple is a difficult transition that must include the integration of contrasting issues that each partner brings to the relationship and issues they may have redefined for themselves as a couple. The new couple must also renegotiate relationships with parents, siblings, and other relatives in view of the new partnership. Tasks of this stage include establishing a new identity as a couple, realigning relationships

TABLE 10–1 **Stages of the Traditional Family Life Cycle**		
FAMILY LIFE CYCLE STAGES	**EMOTIONAL PROCESS OF TRANSITION: KEY PRINCIPLES**	**CHANGES REQUIRED IN FAMILY STATUS TO PROCEED DEVELOPMENTALLY**
The single young adult	Accepting separation from parents and emotional and financial responsibility for self	■ Differentiation of self in relation to family of origin ■ Development of intimate peer relationships ■ Establishment of self with respect to work and financial independence ■ Establishment of self in community and larger society
The family joined through marriage or other union	Commitment to new system	■ Formation of partner systems ■ Realignment of relationships with extended family, friends, and larger community and social system to include new partners
The family with young children	Accepting new members into the system	■ Adjustment of couple system to make space for children ■ Collaboration in child-rearing, financial and housekeeping tasks ■ Realignment of relationships with extended family to include parenting and grandparenting roles ■ Realignment of relationships with community and larger social system to include new family structure and relationships

TABLE 10–1	**Stages of the Traditional Family Life Cycle–cont'd**	
FAMILY LIFE CYCLE STAGES	**EMOTIONAL PROCESS OF TRANSITION: KEY PRINCIPLES**	**CHANGES REQUIRED IN FAMILY STATUS TO PROCEED DEVELOPMENTALLY**
The family with adolescents	Increasing flexibility of family boundaries to permit children's independence and grandparents' frailties	■ Shifting of parent-child relationships to permit adolescents to move in and out of system ■ Refocus on midlife couple and career issues ■ Beginning shift toward caring for older generation ■ Realignment with community and larger social system to include shifting family of emerging adolescent and parents in new formation patterns of relating
The family launching children and moving on in midlife	Accepting a multitude of exits from and entries into the family system	■ Renegotiation of couple system as a dyad ■ Development of adult-to-adult relationships between parents and grown children ■ Realignment of relationships to include in-laws and grandchildren ■ Realignment of relationships with community and larger social system to include new structure and constellation of family relationships ■ Exploration of new interests/career given the freedom from child-care responsibilities ■ Dealing with care needs, disabilities and death of parents (grandparents)
The family in later life (late middle age to end of life)	Accepting the shifting of generational roles Accepting the realities of limitations and death	■ Maintaining personal and/or couple functioning and interests in the face of physiological decline; exploration of new familial and social role options ■ Supporting a more central role of middle generations ■ Realignment of the system in relation to community and larger social system to acknowledge changed pattern of family relationships of this stage ■ Making room in the system for the wisdom and experience of the elders; supporting the older generation without overfunctioning for them ■ Dealing with loss of spouse, siblings, and other peers and preparation for own death; life review and integration ■ Managing reversed roles in caretaking between middle and older generations

Adapted from McGoldrick, M., Garcia-Preto, N., & Carter, B. (2015). Overview: The life cycle in its changing context. In McGoldrick, M., Garcia-Preto, N., & Carter, B. (Eds.), *The expanding family life cycle: Individual, family, and social perspectives* (5th ed., pp. 1–19). Allyn & Bacon. Reprinted by permission.

with extended family members, and making decisions about having children. Problems can arise if either partner remains too enmeshed with their family of origin or when the couple chooses to cut themselves off completely from extended family.

The Family With Young Children

Adjustments in relationships must occur with the arrival of children. The entire family system is affected, and role realignments are necessary for both new parents and new grandparents. Tasks of this stage include making adjustments to meet the responsibilities associated with parenthood while maintaining the integrity of the couple relationship, sharing equally in the tasks of child-rearing, and integrating the roles of extended family members into the newly expanded family organization. Problems can arise when parents lack knowledge about normal childhood development and how to allow children to express themselves through behavior.

The Family With Adolescents

This stage of family development may be characterized by turmoil and transition. Parents may be approaching a midlife stage, and adolescents are undergoing biological, emotional, and sociocultural changes that place demands on each individual and the family unit. Grandparents, too, may require assistance with the tasks of later life. These developments can create a "sandwich" effect for the parents, who must deal with issues confronting three generations. Tasks of this stage include redefining the level of dependence so that adolescents are provided with greater autonomy while parents remain responsive to the teenager's dependency needs. Midlife issues related to marriage, career, and aging parents must also be resolved during this period. Problems can arise when parents are unable to relinquish control and allow the adolescent greater autonomy and freedom to make independent decisions or when parents are unable to agree and support each other in this effort.

The Family With Children Leaving Home

Realignment of family roles occurs during this stage, characterized by the intermittent exiting and entering of various family members. Children leave home for further education and careers; marriages occur, and new spouses, in-laws, and children enter the system; and new grandparent roles are established. Adult-to-adult relationships among grown children and their parents are renegotiated. Tasks associated with this stage include reestablishing the bond of the dyadic marital relationship; realigning relationships to include grown children, in-laws, and new grandchildren; and accepting the additional caretaking responsibilities and eventual death of elderly parents. Problems can arise when feelings of loss and depression become overwhelming in response to the departure of children from home, when parents are unable to accept their children as adults or cope with the disability or death of their own parents, and when the marital bond has deteriorated.

The Family in Later Life (Late Middle Age to End of Life)

This stage can begin with retirement and last until the death of both spouses. However, some older people who have the opportunity to do so are choosing to retire early, and large numbers of those over age 65 are remaining in the workforce and delaying retirement. Thus, the beginning of this stage varies widely. Most adults in their later years are still a prominent part of the family system, and many are able to offer support to their grown children in the middle generation. Tasks traditionally associated with this stage include exploring new social roles related to retirement and possible change in socioeconomic status; accepting some decline in physiological functioning; dealing with the deaths of spouse, siblings, and friends; and confronting and preparing for one's own death. When older adults have failed to fulfill the tasks associated with earlier levels of development and are dissatisfied with the way their lives have gone, they may be unable to find happiness in retirement or emotional satisfaction with children and grandchildren. They may also have difficulty accepting the deaths of loved ones or preparing for their own impending deaths.

A growing trend is an increasing number of older adults living with and in many cases assuming primary responsibility for their grandchildren. Henig (2018) reported that this number has doubled since the 1970s and has increased by 7% in the last 5 years alone. The U.S. Census Bureau reports that currently 2.7 million children are being raised in the home of grandparents (Administration for Community Living [ACL], 2021); Native American, Alaska Native, Black, and African American children are overrepresented in this group.

For many older adults, caring for grandchildren introduces financial and social burdens that may be difficult to manage. According to the American Community Survey (ACL, 2021), 43% of the children who lived with a "grandmother-only" in 2012 lived in poverty. The opioid epidemic has contributed (but not exclusively) to growing numbers of children in this population who have been orphaned or require caregivers other than the parent. In 2018 *The Supporting Grandparents Raising Grandchildren (SGRG) Act* was enacted to explore the complex needs of this growing sector.

Major Variations

Divorce

McGoldrick and associates (2020) also discussed stages and tasks of families experiencing divorce and remarriage. Stages in the family life cycle of divorce include deciding to divorce, planning the breakup of the system, separation, and divorce. Tasks include accepting one's part in the failure of the marriage, working cooperatively on problems related to finances and child custody and visitation, realigning relationships with extended family, and mourning the loss of the marriage relationship and the intact family.

After the divorce, the custodial parent must adjust to functioning as the single leader of an ongoing family while working to rebuild a new social network. The noncustodial parent must find ways to continue to be an effective parent in a different kind of parenting role.

Remarriage

Approximately 75% of people who divorce eventually remarry and about 50% of the 60 million children younger than age 13 are living with one biological parent and that parent's current partner (The Stepfamily Foundation, 2021). The challenges that face the joining of two established families are immense, and statistics reveal that the rate of divorce for remarried couples is even higher than the divorce rate after first marriages (Gaspard, 2022). Stages in the remarried family life cycle include entering the new relationship, planning the new marriage and family, and remarriage and reestablishment of family. Tasks include making a firm commitment to confronting the complexities of combining two families, maintaining open communication, facing fears, realigning relationships with extended family to include new spouse and children, and encouraging healthy relationships with biological (noncustodial) parents and grandparents.

Problems can arise when there is a blurring of boundaries between the custodial and noncustodial families. Common issues that children may face include the following:

- Who is the boss now?
- Who is most important, the child or the new spouse?
- Mom loves her new husband more than she loves me.

- Dad lets me do more than my new stepdad does.
- I don't have to mind him; he's not my real dad.

Confusion and distress for both the children and the parents can be minimized with the establishment of clear boundaries and open communication.

Cultural Variations

It is difficult to generalize about variations in family life cycle development according to culture. Although many families in the United States progress through the life cycle stages previously described, cultural variations exist, and nurses must assess for differences in family expectations related to sociocultural beliefs. Cultural and religious values may influence beliefs about marriage, divorce, children, and the importance of extended family.

Family Functioning

Boyer and Jeffrey (1994) described six elements on which families are assessed to be either functional or dysfunctional. Each can be viewed on a continuum, although families rarely fall at extreme ends of the continuum. Rather, they tend to be dynamic and fluctuate from one point to another within the different areas. These six elements of assessment are described in the following sections and summarized in Table 10–2.

TABLE 10–2 Family Functioning: Elements of Assessment

ELEMENTS OF ASSESSMENT	CONTINUUM	
	FUNCTIONAL	**DYSFUNCTIONAL**
Communication	Clear, direct, open, honest, with congruence between verbal and nonverbal; members listen to one another	Indirect, vague, controlled, with many double-bind messages; ignoring one another
Self-concept reinforcement	Supportive, loving, praising, approving, with behaviors that instill confidence	Unsupportive, blaming, put-downs, refusing to allow self-responsibility
Family members' expectations	Flexible, realistic, individualized, respects the privacy of each member; exhibits a sense of shared responsibility	Judgmental, rigid, controlling, ignoring individuality
Handling differences	Tolerant, dynamic, negotiating; admits to problems and seeks help	Attacking, avoiding, surrendering, denying
Family interactional patterns	Workable, constructive, flexible; promoting the needs of all members; shares leisure time; balance of interaction among members	Contradictory, rigid, self-defeating, destructive, disengaged; imbalance of interaction (such as monopolizing)
Family climate	Trusting, growth-promoting, caring; general feeling of well-being; teaches a sense of right and wrong	Distrusting, emotionally painful, with absence of hope for improvement

Sources: Adapted from Boyer, P. A., & Jeffrey, R. J. (1994). *A guide for the family therapist.* Jason Aronson; Robinson, M. (2022). Family health care nursing: An introduction. In M. Robinson, D. Padgett Coehlo, & P. S. Smith (Eds.), *Family health care nursing* (7th ed., pp. 3–24). F.A. Davis.

Communication

Functional communication patterns are those in which verbal and nonverbal messages are clear, direct, and congruent between the sender and the intended receiver. Family members are encouraged to express honest feelings and opinions, and all members participate in decisions that affect the family system. Each member is an active listener to the other members of the family.

Behaviors that interfere with functional communication include the following:

Making Assumptions

With this behavior, one assumes that others will know what is meant by an action or an expression (or sometimes even what one is thinking), or, conversely, assumes to know what another member is thinking or feeling without checking to make certain.

> **Example**
>
> A father says to his teenaged daughter, "You should have known that I expected you to clean up the kitchen while I was gone!"

Belittling Feelings

This behavior involves ignoring or minimizing another's feelings when they are expressed. Belittling a person's feelings encourages the individual to withhold honest feelings to avoid being hurt by the negative response.

> **Example**
>
> When the young woman confides to her mother that she is angry because the grandfather has touched her breast, the mother responds, "Oh, don't be angry. He doesn't mean anything by that."

Failing to Listen

With this behavior, one does not hear what the other individual is saying. Failing to listen can mean not hearing the words by "tuning out" the message, or it can be "selective" listening, in which a person hears only a selective part of the message or interprets it selectively.

> **Example**
>
> The father explains to Johnny, "If the contract comes through and I get this new job, we'll have a little extra money, and we will consider sending you to State U." Johnny relays the message to his friend, "Dad says I can go to State U!"

Communicating Indirectly

Indirect communication usually means that an individual does not or cannot present a message to a receiver directly, so the individual seeks to communicate through a third person.

> **Example**
>
> A father does not want his teenage daughter to see a certain boyfriend but wants to avoid the angry response he expects from his daughter if he tells her so. He expresses his feelings to his wife, hoping she will share them with their daughter.

Presenting Double-Bind Messages

Double-bind communication conveys a confusing message about expected behavior. A family member may respond to a direct request by another family member, only to be rebuked when the request is fulfilled. This concept appears again in the section on the strategic model of family therapy later in this chapter.

> **Example**
>
> The father tells his son he is spending too much time playing football, and as a result, his grades are falling. The son is expected to bring his grades up over the next 9 weeks or his car will be taken away. When the son tells the father he has quit the football team so he can study more, Dad responds angrily, "I won't allow any son of mine to be a quitter!"

Self-Concept Reinforcement

Functional families strive to reinforce and strengthen each member's self-concept, with the positive result that family members feel loved and valued. Boyer and Jeffrey (1994) stated:

> The manner in which children see and value themselves is influenced most significantly by the messages they receive concerning their value to other members of the family. Messages that convey praise, approval, appreciation, trust, and confidence in decisions and that allow family members to pursue individual needs and ultimately to become independent are the foundation blocks of a child's feelings of self-worth. Adults also need and depend heavily on this kind of reinforcement for their own emotional well-being. (p. 27)

Behaviors that interfere with self-concept reinforcement include the following:

Expressing Denigrating Remarks

These remarks are commonly called "put-downs." Individuals receive messages that they are worthless or unloved.

> **Example**
>
> A child spills a glass of milk at the table. The mother responds, "You are hopeless! How could anybody be so clumsy?!"

Withholding Supportive Messages

Some family members find it very difficult to provide others with reinforcing and supportive messages.

This difficulty may occur because they themselves have not been the recipients of reinforcement from significant others and have not learned how to provide support to others.

Example

A 10-year-old boy playing Little League baseball retrieves the ball and throws it to second base for an out. After the game, he says to his dad, "Did you see my play on second base?" Dad responds, "Yes, I did, son, but if you had been paying better attention, you could have caught the ball for a direct and immediate out."

Taking Over

Taking over occurs when one family member fails to permit another member to develop a sense of responsibility and self-worth. Instead, the person who takes over does things for the individual preventing him or her from managing the situation independently.

Example

Twelve-year-old Eric has a job delivering the evening paper, which he usually begins right after school. Today he must serve a 1-hour detention after school for being late to class yesterday. He tells his mom, "Tommy said he would throw my papers for me today if I help him wash his dad's car on Saturday." Mom responds, "Never mind. Tell Tommy to forget it. I'll take care of your paper route today."

Family Members' Expectations

All individuals have some expectations about the outcomes of the life situations they experience. These expectations are related to and significantly influenced by earlier life experiences. In functional families, expectations are realistic, thereby avoiding setting up members for failure. In functional families, expectations are also flexible. Life situations are full of extraneous and unexpected interferences. Flexibility allows for changes and interruptions to occur without creating conflict. Finally, in functional families, expectations are individualized. Each family member is different, with different strengths and limitations. The outcome of a life situation for one family member may not be realistic for another. Each member must be valued independently, and comparison among members must be avoided.

Behaviors that interfere with adaptive functioning in terms of member expectations include the following:

Ignoring Individuality

When family members are expected to perform or behave in ways that undermine their individuality or do not suit their current life situation, their individuality is being ignored. This sometimes happens when parents expect their children to fulfill the hopes and dreams the parents have failed to achieve, yet the children have different hopes and dreams.

Example

Bob, an only child, leaves for college next year. Bob's father, Robert, inherited a hardware store that was founded by Bob's great-grandfather and has been in the family for three generations. Robert expects Bob to major in business, work in the store after college, and take over the business when Robert retires. Bob, however, has a talent for writing, wants to major in communication, and wants to work in television news when he graduates. Robert sees this plan as a betrayal of the family.

Demanding Proof of Love

Boyer and Jeffrey (1994) stated:

> Family members place expectations on others' behavior that are used as standards by which the expecting member determines how much the other members care for him or her. The message attached to these expectations is: "If you will not be as I wish you to be, you don't love me." (p. 32)

Example

"If you don't take over the hardware store, you don't love me" is the message that Bob receives from his father in the previous example.

Handling Differences

It is difficult to conceive of two or more individuals living together who agree on everything all of the time. Serious problems in a family's functioning appear when differences become equated with disapproval or when disagreement is perceived as offensive. Members of a functional family understand that it is acceptable to disagree and deal with differences in an open, nonattacking manner. Members are willing to hear the other person's position, respect the other person's right to hold an opposing position, and work to modify the expectations on both sides of the issue to negotiate a workable solution.

Behaviors that interfere with successful family negotiations include the following:

Attacking

Personal attacks can occur when differences of opinion culminate in blaming and verbal or physical aggression and the situation intensifies with destructive expressions of anger and hurt.

Example

When Nadya's husband, Denis, buys an expensive set of golf clubs, Nadya responds, "How could you do such a thing? You know we can't afford those! No wonder we don't have a nice house like all our friends. You spend all our money before we can save for a down payment. You're so selfish! We'll never have anything nice, and it's all your fault!"

Avoiding

Avoiding refers to differences that are never acknowledged openly. Rather than resolving conflicts, the individuals resist discussing issues for fear that the other person will withdraw love or approval or become angry in response to the disagreement. Avoidance also occurs when an individual fears loss of control of their temper if the disagreement is brought out into the open.

Example

Vicki and Clint have been married for 6 months. This is Vicki's second marriage, and she has a 4-year-old son, Derek, from her first marriage who now lives with them. Both Vicki and Clint work, and Derek goes to day care. Since the marriage 6 months ago, Derek cries every night continuously unless Vicki spends all her time with him, which she does to keep him quiet. Clint resents this but says nothing for fear he will come across as interfering. He has started returning to work in his office in the evenings to avoid the family situation.

Surrendering

The person who surrenders in the face of disagreement does so at the expense of denying their own needs or rights. The individual avoids expressing a difference of opinion for fear of angering another person or of losing approval and support.

Example

Elaine is the only child of wealthy parents. She attends an exclusive private college in a small New England town, where she met Andrew, the son of a farming couple from the area. Andrew attended the local community college for 2 years but chose to work on his parents' farm rather than continue college. Elaine and Andrew love each other and want to be married, but Elaine's parents say they will disown her if she marries Andrew, who they believe is beneath her social status. Elaine breaks off her relationship with Andrew rather than challenge her parents' wishes.

Family Interactional Patterns

Interactional patterns have to do with the ways in which families "behave." All families develop recurring, predictable patterns of interaction over time. These are often thought of as family rules. The mentality conveys, "This is the way we have always done it," and provides a sense of security and stability for family members that comes from predictability. These interactions may involve communication, self-concept reinforcement, expressing expectations, and handling differences (all of the behaviors that were discussed previously), but because they are repetitive and recur over time, they become the rules that govern patterns of interaction among family members.

Family rules are functional when they are workable, constructive, and promote the needs of all family members. They are dysfunctional when they become contradictory, self-defeating, and destructive. Family therapists often find that individuals are unaware that dysfunctional family rules exist and may vehemently deny their existence even when confronted with a specific behavioral interaction. The development of dysfunctional interactional patterns occurs through a habituation process and out of fear of change or reprisal or through a lack of knowledge as to how a given situation might be handled differently. Many are derived from the parents' childhood experiences.

Patterns of interaction that interfere with adaptive family functioning include the following:

Patterns That Cause Emotional Discomfort

Interactions can promote hurt and anger in family members, especially when individuals are uncomfortable expressing their feelings or when family rules do not permit them to do so. These interactional patterns include behaviors such as never apologizing or never admitting that one has made a mistake, forbidding flexibility in life situations ("You must do it my way, or you will not do it at all"), making statements that devalue the worth of others, or withholding statements that promote increased self-worth.

Example

Priscilla and Bill had been discussing buying a new car but could not agree on the make or model to buy. One day, Bill appeared at Priscilla's office over the lunch hour and said, "Come outside and see our new car." In front of the building, Bill had parked a brand-new sports car that he explained he had purchased with their combined savings. Priscilla was furious but kept quiet and proceeded to finish her workday. At home, she expressed her anger to Bill for making the purchase without consulting her. Bill refused to apologize or admit to making a mistake. They both remained cool and hardly spoke to each other for weeks.

Patterns That Perpetuate or Intensify Problems

When problems go unresolved over a long period of time, it sometimes appears to be easier to ignore them. If problems of the same nature occur, the tendency to ignore them then becomes the safe and predictable pattern of interaction for dealing with this type of situation. The problem may intensify to a point where it can no longer be ignored.

Example

Dan works hard in the automobile factory and demands peace and quiet from his family when he comes home from work. His children have learned over the years not to share their problems with him because they fear his explosive temper. Their mother attempts to handle unpleasant situations alone as best she can. When son Ron was expelled from school for being caught smoking pot for the third time, Dan yelled, "Why wasn't I told about this before?"

Patterns That Are in Conflict With Each Other

Some family rules may appear to be functional—very workable and constructive—on the surface, but in practice they may serve to destroy healthy interactional patterns. Boyer and Jeffrey (1994) described the following scenario as an example.

Example

Dad insists that all members of the family eat dinner together every evening. No one may leave the table until everyone is finished because dinnertime is one of the few times when the family can be together. Yet Dad frequently uses the time to reprimand Bobby about his poor grades in math, to scold Ann for her sloppy room, or to make not-so-subtle gibes at Mom for not being able to finding a "better paying job."

Family Climate

The atmosphere or climate of a family is composed of a blend of the feelings and experiences that result from family members' verbal and nonverbal sharing and interacting. A positive family climate is founded on trust and reflected in open communication, joyfulness and laughter, expressions of caring and mutual respect, the valuing of each individual as unique, and a general feeling of security and well-being. In a dysfunctional family, the climate is evidenced by tension, frustration, guilt, anger and resentment, depression, and despair.

CORE CONCEPT

Family Therapy
A type of therapeutic modality in which the focus of treatment is on the family as a unit. In this type of intervention, family members are assisted to identify and change maladaptive behaviors and relationship patterns to facilitate improvement in family functioning.

Therapeutic Modalities With Families

Although family therapy is reserved for the advanced practice psychiatric nurse, the theoretical foundations for family therapy are useful to the generalist nurse for understanding and assessing family dynamics and making appropriate referrals when family dysfunction is identified.

The Family as a System

General systems theory is a way of organizing thought according to the holistic perspective. A system is considered greater than the sum of its parts. A system is considered dynamic and ever changing. A change in one part of the system causes a change in the other parts of the system and in the system as a whole. When studying families, it is helpful to conceptualize a hierarchy of systems.

The family can be viewed as a system composed of various subsystems, such as the marital subsystem, parent-child subsystems, and sibling subsystems. Each of these subsystems is further divided into subsystems of individuals. The family system is also a subsystem of a larger supersystem, such as the neighborhood or community. A schematic of a hierarchy of systems is presented in Figure 10–1.

Major Concepts

Bowen (1978) did a great deal of work with families using a systems approach. Bowen's theoretical approach to family therapy is composed of eight major concepts: (1) differentiation of self, (2) triangles, (3) nuclear family emotional process, (4) family projection process, (5) multigenerational transmission process, (6) sibling position, (7) emotional cutoff, and (8) societal emotional process.

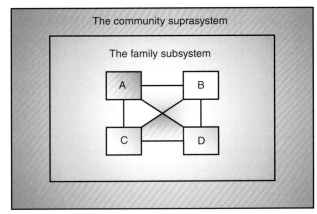

Key:
A = Father subsystem   CD = Sibling subsystem
B = Mother subsystem   AD = Parent-child subsystem
C = Child subsystem   BC = Parent-child subsystem
D = Child subsystem   AC = Parent-child subsystem
AB = Marital subsystem   BD = Parent-child subsystem

FIGURE 10–1 A hierarchy of systems.

Differentiation of Self

Differentiation of self is the ability to define oneself as a separate being. The Bowen theory suggests that "a person with a well-differentiated self recognizes his [or her] realistic dependence on others, but can stay calm and clear headed enough in the face of conflict, criticism, and rejection to distinguish thinking rooted in a careful assessment of the facts from thinking clouded by emotionality" (Bowen Center, 2021).

The degree of differentiation of self can be viewed on a continuum from high levels, in which an individual manifests a clearly defined sense of self, to low or undifferentiated levels, in which emotional fusion exists and the individual is unable to function separately from a relationship system. Healthy families encourage differentiation, and the process of separation from the family ego mass is most pronounced between the ages of 2 and 5 and again between the ages of 13 and 15. Families that do not understand the child's need to be different during these times may perceive the child's behavior as objectionable.

Bowen (1971) used the term *stuck-togetherness* to describe the family with a fused ego mass. When family fusion occurs, none of the members have a true sense of self as an independent individual. Boundaries between members are blurred, and the family becomes enmeshed without individual distinguishing characteristics. In this situation, family members can neither gain true intimacy nor separate and become individuals.

Triangles

The concept of **triangles** refers to a three-person emotional configuration that is considered a significant element in evaluating the communication, behavior, and relationships within the family system. Bowen (1978) offered the following description of triangles:

> The basic building block of any emotional system is the triangle. When emotional tension in a two-person system exceeds a certain level, it triangles in a third person, permitting the tension to shift about within the triangle. Any two in the original triangle can add a new triangle. An emotional system is composed of a series of interlocking triangles. (p. 306)

Triangles are dysfunctional in that they offer relief from anxiety through diversion rather than through resolution of the issue. To diffuse stress and conflict in a two-person relationship, one or both individuals may draw a third person into the mix either for sympathy or to deflect from the issues that are creating the stress between them. When the dynamics within a triangle stabilize, a fourth person may be brought in to form additional triangles to reduce tension. This triangulation can continue almost indefinitely as extended family and people outside the family, including the family therapist, may become entangled in the process. The therapist working with families must strive to remain "de-triangled" from this emotional system.

Nuclear Family Emotional Process

The nuclear family emotional process describes the patterns of emotional functioning in a single generation. The nuclear family begins with a relationship between two people who form a couple. The most open relationship usually occurs during courtship, when most individuals choose partners with similar levels of differentiation. The lower the level of differentiation, the greater the possibility of problems in the future. A degree of fusion occurs with permanent commitment. This fusion results in anxiety and must be dealt with by each partner to maintain a healthy degree of differentiation.

Family Projection Process

Spouses who are unable to work through the undifferentiation or fusion that occurs with permanent commitment may project the resulting anxiety onto the children when they become parents. This occurrence is manifested as a father-mother-child triangle. These triangles are common and exist in various gradations of intensity in most families with children.

The child who becomes the target of the projection may be selected for various reasons:

- A particular child reminds one of the parents of an unresolved childhood issue.
- The child is of a particular gender or position in the family.
- The child is born with special needs.
- The parent has a negative attitude about the pregnancy.

This behavior is called **scapegoating.** It is harmful to both the child's emotional stability and their ability to function outside the family. A child who is scapegoated may become identified as "the problem child" and is vulnerable to accepting this label as their identity. The potential outcomes are poor self-esteem, difficulty developing healthy relationships, and other emotional problems.

Multigenerational Transmission Process

Bowen (1978) described the multigenerational transmission process as the manner in which interactional patterns are transferred from one generation to another. Attitudes, values, beliefs, behaviors, and patterns of interaction are passed from parents to children over many lifetimes. It therefore becomes possible to show in a family assessment that a certain behavior has existed within a family through multiple generations.

Genograms

Pictorial representations of family members and relationships are called **genograms**. They are a convenient way to plot a multigenerational assessment and offer the convenience of summarizing a great deal of information in a small amount of space. They can also be used as teaching tools with the family itself. An overall picture of the life of the family over several generations can be conveyed, including roles that various family members play as well as emotional distance between specific individuals. Areas for change can be easily identified. A sample genogram is presented in Figure 10–2.

Sibling Position

This concept in Bowen's theory suggests that birth order in a family influences the development of predictable personality characteristics. For example, firstborn children have been thought to be perfectionistic, reliable, and conscientious; middle children have been described as independent, loyal, and intolerant of conflict; and youngest children are often characterized as charming, precocious, and gregarious. Bowen used this thesis to help determine levels of differentiation within a family and the possible direction of the family projection process. For example, if the oldest child exhibits characteristics more representative of the youngest child, there is evidence that this child may be the product of triangulation. Sibling position profiles are also used when studying multigenerational transmission processes and verifiable data are missing for certain family members.

Is there evidence to support profiled sibling personality traits based on birth order? The answer is complex. Hartshorne (2010) stated that the majority of the 65,000 research studies on this topic are flawed, and the remainder show no significant effect. Eckstein and Kaufman's work (2012) suggested that perceptions about roles and personality characteristics may be influenced by parents' expectations and stereotypes about birth-order related roles. In a large, multinational study, Rohrer and associates

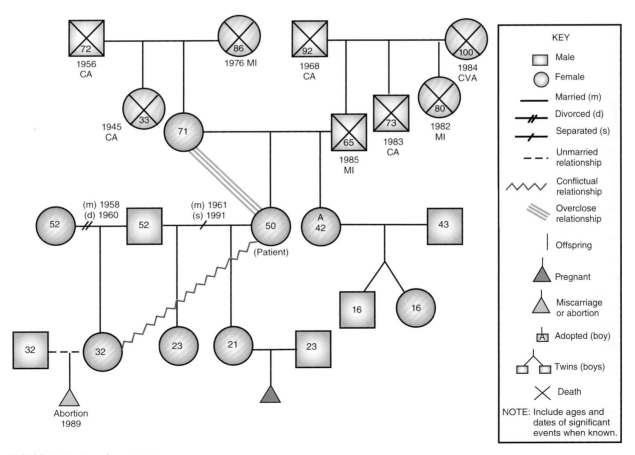

FIGURE 10–2   Sample genogram.

(2015) found that firstborn children objectively and subjectively scored higher on intelligence, but birth order did not affect personality traits such as extroversion, emotional stability, agreeability, conscientiousness, or imagination. When assessing the effect of birth order among siblings in family roles and functions, the nurse needs to consider many variables to make the best clinical judgment.

Emotional Cutoff

"The concept of emotional cutoff describes how people manage their unresolved emotional issues with parents, siblings, and other family members by reducing or totally cutting off emotional contact with them" (Bowen Center, 2021). Bowen (1976) suggested that emotional cutoff is the result of dysfunction within the family of origin and that it promotes the same type of dysfunction in the new nuclear family. He contends that maintaining some emotional contact with the family of origin promotes healthy differentiation.

Societal Emotional Process

The Bowen theory views society as an emotional system. The concept of societal emotional process suggests that societal responses to stress influence similar responses in individuals and families: stress creates uncomfortable levels of anxiety that lead to hasty solutions, which add to the problems, and the cycle continues. This concept of Bowen's theory is explained as follows (Bowen Center, 2021):

> Human societies undergo periods of regression and progression in their history. The current regression seems related to factors such as the population explosion, a sense of diminishing frontiers, and the depletion of natural resources... The "symptoms" of societal regression include a growth of crime and violence, an increasing divorce rate, a more litigious attitude, a greater polarization between racial groups, less principled decision-making by leaders, the drug abuse epidemic, an increase in bankruptcy, and a focus on rights over responsibilities.

One outcome is that during periods of societal regression, families have a more difficult time raising children, perhaps because societal stressors are greater and expectations for how the family should respond to stressors become blurred.

Goals and Techniques of Therapy

The goal of Bowen's systems approach to family therapy is to increase the level of differentiation of self while remaining in touch with the family system. The premise is that intense emotional problems within the nuclear family can be resolved only by resolving undifferentiated relationships with the family of origin. Emphasis is given to the understanding of past relationships.

The therapeutic role is that of "coach" or supervisor, and emotional involvement with the family is minimized. Therapist techniques include the following:

1. Defining and clarifying the relationship between the family members
2. Helping family members develop one-to-one relationships with each other and minimizing triangles within the system
3. Teaching family members about the functioning of emotional systems
4. Promoting differentiation by encouraging members to speak as individuals rather than as a family unit

The Structural Model

Structural family therapy is associated with a model developed by Minuchin (1974). In this model, the family is viewed as a social system within which the individual lives and to which the individual must adapt. The individual both contributes and responds to stresses within the family.

Major Concepts

Systems

The structural model views the family as a system. The structure of the **family system** is founded on a set of invisible principles that influence the interaction among family members. These principles concern how, when, and with whom to relate, and are established over time and through repeated transactions until they become rules that govern the conduct of various family members.

Transactional Patterns

Transactional patterns are the rules established over time that organize the ways in which family members relate to one another. A hierarchy of authority is one example of a transactional pattern. Usually, parents have a higher level of authority in a family than the children, so parental behavior reflects this role. A balance of authority may exist between the two parents, or one may reflect a higher level than the other. These patterns of behavioral expectations differ from family to family and may trace their origin over generations of family negotiations.

Subsystems

Minuchin (1974) described **subsystems** as smaller elements that make up the larger family system. Subsystems can be individuals or can consist of two or more people united by gender, relationship, generation, interest, or purpose. A family member may belong to several subsystems at the same time, in which the individual may experience different levels of power and require different types of skills. For example, a young man has a different level of power and a different set of expectations in his father-son subsystem than in a subsystem with his younger brother.

Boundaries

Boundaries define the level of participation and interaction among subsystems. Boundaries are appropriate when they permit appropriate contact with others while preventing excessive interference. Clearly defined boundaries promote adaptive functioning. Maladaptive functioning can occur when boundaries are *rigid* or *diffuse.*

A rigid boundary is characterized by decreased communication and lack of support and responsiveness. Rigid boundaries prevent a subsystem (family member or subgroup) from achieving appropriate closeness or interaction with others in the system. Rigid boundaries promote **disengagement,** or extreme separateness, among family members.

A diffuse boundary is characterized by dependency and overinvolvement. Diffuse boundaries interfere with adaptive functioning because of the overinvestment, overinvolvement, and lack of differentiation between certain subsystems. Diffuse boundaries promote **enmeshment,** or exaggerated connectedness, among family members.

Example

Sally and Jim have been married for 12 years, during which time they have tried without success to have children. Six months ago they were thrilled to have the opportunity to adopt a 5-year-old girl, Annie. Because both Sally and Jim have full-time teaching jobs, Annie stays with her maternal grandmother, Krista, during the day after she gets home from half-day kindergarten. At first, Annie was a polite and obedient child. However, in the last few months, she has become insolent and oppositional and has temper tantrums when she cannot have her way. Sally and Krista agree that Annie should have whatever she desires and should not be punished for her behavior. Jim believes that discipline is necessary, but Sally and Krista refuse to enforce any guidelines he tries to establish. Annie is aware of this discordance and manipulates it to her full advantage.

In this situation, diffuse boundaries exist among the Sally-Krista-Annie subsystems. They have become enmeshed. They have also established a rigid boundary against Jim, disengaging him from the system.

Goal and Techniques of Therapy

The goal of structural family therapy is to facilitate change in the family structure. **Family structure** is changed with modification of the family principles, or transactional patterns, that are contributing to dysfunction within the family. The family is viewed as the unit of therapy, and all members are counseled together. Little, if any, time is spent exploring past experiences. The focus of structural therapy is on the present. Therapist techniques include the following:

- **Joining the family:** The therapist must become a part of the family if restructuring is to occur. The therapist joins the family but maintains a leadership position. At different times the therapist may join various subsystems within the family but ultimately includes the entire family system as the target of intervention.
- **Evaluating the family structure:** Even though a family may come for therapy because of the behavior of one family member (the identified patient), the family as a unit is considered problematic. The family structure is evaluated by assessing transactional patterns, system flexibility and potential for change, boundaries, family developmental stage, and role of the identified patient within the system.
- **Restructuring the family:** An alliance or contract for therapy is established with the family. By becoming an actual part of the family, the therapist is able to manipulate the system and facilitate the circumstances and experiences that can lead to structural change.

The Strategic Model

The strategic model of family therapy uses the interactional or communications approach. Communication theory is viewed as the foundation for this model. Communication is the actual transmission of information among individuals. All behavior sends a message, so all behavior in the presence of two or more individuals is communication. In this model, families considered to be functional are open systems where clear and precise messages, congruent with the situation, are sent and received. Healthy communication patterns promote nurturance and individual self-worth. Dysfunctional families are viewed as partially closed systems in which communication is vague and messages are often inconsistent and incongruent with the situation. Destructive patterns of communication tend to inhibit healthful nurturing and decrease individual feelings of self-worth.

Major Concepts

Double-Bind Communication

Double-bind communication occurs when a statement is made and succeeded by a contradictory statement. It also occurs when a statement is made accompanied by a nonverbal expression that is inconsistent with the verbal communication. These incompatible communications can interfere with ego development in an individual and promote mistrust of all communications. Double-bind communication often results in a confusing message about the appropriate or expected response.

Example

A mother freely gives and receives hugs and kisses from her 6-year-old son some of the time, while at other times she pushes him away saying, "Big boys don't act like that." The little boy receives a conflicting message and is presented with an impossible dilemma: "To please my mother I must not show her that I love her, but if I do not show her that I love her, I'm afraid I will lose her."

Pseudomutuality and Pseudohostility

A healthy, functioning individual is able to relate to other people while still maintaining a sense of separate identity. In a dysfunctional family, patterns of interaction may be reflected in the remoteness or closeness of relationships. These relationships may reflect erratic interaction (i.e., sometimes remote and sometimes close) or inappropriate interaction (i.e., excessive closeness or remoteness).

Pseudomutuality and pseudohostility are seen as collective defenses against the reality of the underlying meaning of the relationships in a dysfunctional family system. **Pseudomutuality** is characterized by a facade of mutual regard. Emotional investment is directed at maintaining the outward representation of reciprocal fulfillment rather than in the relationship itself. The style of relating is fixed and rigid and allows family members to deny underlying fears of separation and hostility.

Example

A couple, early in their relationship, discuss their hopes for the future. When one person says they hope to have a large family, the other person agrees (although that person doesn't really wish to have any children). In an effort to "help" the relationship grow by appearing to have similar values, the communication is not a true reflection of values or beliefs and creates a foundation for conflict later on when dissimilarities in values or beliefs emerge.

Pseudohostility is also a fixed and rigid style of relating, but the facade being maintained is that of a state of chronic conflict and alienation among family members. This relationship pattern allows family members to deny underlying fears of tenderness and intimacy.

Example

Jack, 14, and his sister Jill, 15, have nothing to do with each other. When they are together, they can agree on nothing, and the barrage of put-downs is constant. This behavior reflects pseudohostility used by individuals who are afraid to reveal feelings of intimacy.

Schism and Skew

Lidz and associates (1957) observed two patterns within dysfunctional marital relationships. **Marital schism** is defined as "a state of severe chronic disequilibrium and discord, with recurrent threats of separation." Each partner undermines the other, mutual trust is absent, and competition exists for closeness with the children. Often a partner establishes an alliance with their parent against the spouse. Children lack appropriate role models. **Marital skew** describes a relationship in which there is a lack of equal partnership. One partner dominates both the relationship and the other partner. The marriage remains intact as long as the passive partner allows the domination to continue. Children also lack role models when a marital skew exists.

Goal and Techniques of Therapy

The goal of strategic family therapy is to create change in destructive behavior and communication patterns among family members. The identified family *problem* is the unit of therapy, and all family members need not be counseled together. In fact, strategic therapists may prefer to see subgroups or individuals separately to achieve problem resolution. Therapy is oriented in the present, and the therapist assumes full responsibility for devising an effective strategy for family change. Therapeutic techniques include the following:

■ **Paradoxical intervention:** A paradox can be called a contradiction in therapy, or "prescribing the symptom." With **paradoxical intervention,** the therapist requests that the family continue to engage in the behavior that they are trying to change. Alternatively, specific directions may be given for continuing the defeating behavior. This intervention requires an established, trusting relationship between a skilled therapist and family. For example, a couple that regularly engages in insulting shouting matches is instructed to have one of these encounters on Tuesdays and Thursdays from 8:30 to 9 p.m. Boyer and Jeffrey (1994) explained this technique in the following manner:

A family using its maladaptive behavior to control or punish other people loses control of the situation when it finds itself continuing the behavior under a therapist's direction and being praised for following instructions. If the family disobeys the therapist's instruction, the price it pays is sacrificing the old behavior pattern and experiencing more satisfying ways of interacting with one another. A family that maintains it has no control over its behavior, or whose members contend that others must change before they can themselves suddenly finds itself unable to defend such statements. (p. 125)

■ **Reframing:** Reframing involves restating an issue with a different, more positive interpretation that encourages the client to consider alternative interpretations. This technique facilitates exploring different responses to a behavior or event because of a change in the meaning attached to the behavior. This technique is sometimes referred to as *positive reframing*.

Example

A wife tells the family therapist that her husband obviously doesn't care about her because he works so many hours and "thinks it's all about making money." The therapist reframes this comment by responding "So your husband places a lot of value in providing for his family."

The Evolution of Family Therapy

Bowen's family theory and the structural and strategic models are sometimes referred to as basic models of family therapy. Although some family therapists adhere to a specific theoretical framework, Nichols and Davis (2021) suggested that contemporary family therapists "borrow from each other's arsenal of techniques." The basic models described here have provided a foundation for the progression and growth of the discipline of family therapy. Examples of newer models include the following:

■ **Narrative therapy:** Narrative therapy is an approach to treatment that emphasizes the role of the stories people construct about their experience.

■ **Feminist family therapy:** This form of family therapy employs a collaborative, egalitarian, nonsexist intervention, applicable to both men and women, addressing family gender roles, patriarchal attitudes, and social and economic inequalities in male-female relationships.

■ **Social constructionist therapy:** Social constructionist therapy shifts attention away from an inspection of the origin or the exact nature of a family's presenting problems to an examination of the stories (interpretations, explanations, theories about relationships) family members have told themselves that account for how they have lived their lives. This approach facilitates clients' reevaluation of their views of the world.

■ **Psychoeducational family therapy:** This type of family therapy emphasizes educating family members to help them understand and cope with a seriously disturbed family member. Although family therapists may use a psychoeducational approach in treatment, psychiatric-mental health registered nurses also use psychotherapeutic education strategies with individual patients and with families (American Nurses Association [ANA], American Psychiatric Nurses Association, & International Society of Psychiatric-Mental Health Nurses, 2022). When provided with supportive education about mental illness and management strategies, families can have an important and positive affect on patient recovery. In one 14-year follow-up study (Ran et al., 2015), researchers found that in families where psychoeducational family interventions were used for patients with schizophrenia, patient adherence to treatment and social functioning maintained enduring improvement over the course of the study.

CLINICAL JUDGMENT IN ACTION: CASE STUDY AND SAMPLE CARE PLAN

ASSESSMENT

The Calgary Family Assessment Model (CFAM), created by Shajani and Snell (2019), is a multidimensional model originally adapted from a framework developed by Tomm and Sanders (1983). The CFAM consists of three major categories: structural, developmental, and functional. Shajani and Snell (2019) stated:

Each category contains several subcategories. It is important for each nurse to decide which subcategories are relevant and appropriate to explore and assess with each family at each point in time—that is, not all subcategories need

to be assessed at a first meeting with a family, and some subcategories need never be assessed. If the nurse uses too many subcategories, he or she may become overwhelmed by all the data. If the nurse and the family discuss too few subcategories, each may have a distorted view of the family's strengths or problems and the family situation. (pp. 51–52)

A diagram of the CFAM is presented in Figure 10–3. The three major categories are listed, along with the subcategories for assessment under each. This diagram is used to assess the Marino family, a case study presented in Box 10–1.

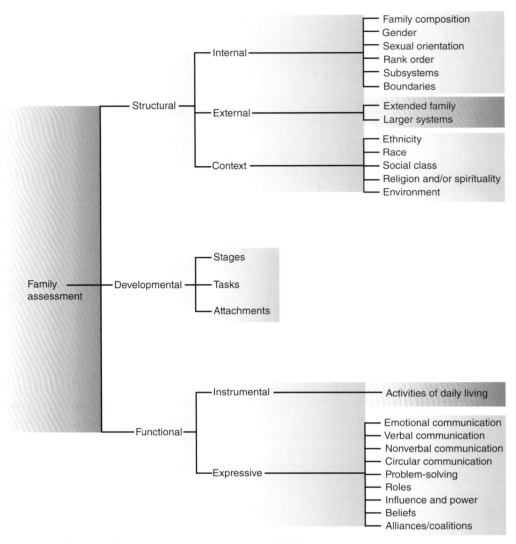

FIGURE 10–3 Branching diagram of the Calgary Family Assessment Model (CFAM).

BOX 10–1 The Marino Family—A Case Study

John and Nancy Marino have been married for 19 years. They have a 17-year-old son, Peter, and a 15-year-old daughter, Anna. Anna was recently hospitalized for taking an overdose of fluoxetine, her mother's prescription antidepressant. The family is attending family therapy sessions while Anna is in the hospital. Anna states, "I just couldn't take the fighting anymore! Our house is an awful place to be. Everyone hates each other, and everyone is unhappy. Dad drinks too much, and Mom is always sick! Peter stays away as much as he can, and I don't blame him. I would too if I had some place to stay. I just thought I'd be better off dead."

John Marino, age 44, is the oldest of five children. His father, Paulo, age 66, is a first generation Italian American whose parents emigrated from Italy in the early 1900s. Paulo retired last year after 32 years as a cutter in a meatpacking plant. His wife, Carla, age 64, has never worked outside the home. John and his siblings all worked at minimum-wage jobs during high school, and John and his two brothers worked their way through college. His two sisters married young, and both are housewives and mothers. John was able to go to law school with the help of loans, grants, and scholarships. He has held several positions since graduation and is currently employed as a corporate attorney for a large aircraft company.

Nancy, age 43, is the only child of Sam and Ethel Jones. Sam, age 67, inherited a great deal of money from his family who had been in the shipping business. He is currently the chief executive officer of this business. Ethel, also 67, was an aspiring concert pianist when she met Sam. She chose to give up her career for marriage and family, although Nancy believes her mother always resented

BOX 10–1 **The Marino Family—A Case Study—cont'd**

doing so. Nancy was reared in an affluent lifestyle. She attended private boarding schools as she was growing up and chose an exclusive college in the East to pursue her interest in art. She studied in Paris during her junior year. Nancy states that she was never emotionally close to her parents. They traveled a great deal, and she spent much of her time under the supervision of a nanny.

Nancy's parents were opposed to her marrying John. They perceived John's family to be beneath their social status. Nancy, on the other hand, loved John's family. She felt them to be very warm and loving, so unlike what she was used to in her own family. Her family is Protestant and also disapproved of her marrying in the Roman Catholic Church.

FAMILY DYNAMICS

As their marriage progressed, Nancy's health became very fragile. She had continued her artistic pursuits but seemed to achieve little satisfaction from it. She tried to keep in touch with her parents but often felt spurned by them. They traveled a great deal and often did not even inform her of their whereabouts. They were not present at the birth of her children. She experiences many aches and pains and spends many days in bed. She sees several physicians, who have prescribed various pain medications, antianxiety agents, and antidepressants but can find nothing organically wrong. Five years ago, she learned that John had been having an affair with his secretary. He promised to break it off and fired the secretary, but Nancy has had

difficulty trusting him since that time. She brings up his infidelity whenever they have an argument, which is increasingly often lately. When he is home, John drinks, usually until he falls asleep. Peter frequently comes home smelling of alcohol, and several times has been clearly intoxicated.

When Nancy called her parents to tell them that Anna was in the hospital, Ethel replied, "I'm sorry to hear that, dear. We certainly never had any of those kinds of problems on our side of the family. But I'm sure everything will be okay now that you are getting help. Please give our love to your family. Your father and I are leaving for Europe on Saturday and will be gone for 6 weeks."

Although more supportive, John's parents view this situation as somewhat shameful for the family. John's dad responded, "We had hard times when you were growing up, but never like this. We always took care of our own problems. We never had to tell a bunch of strangers about them. It's not right to air your dirty laundry in public. Bring Anna home. Give her your love, and she will be okay."

In therapy, Nancy blames John's drinking and his admitted affair for all their problems. John states that he drinks because it is the only way he can tolerate his wife's complaining about his behavior and her many illnesses. Peter is very quiet most of the time but says he will be glad when he graduates in 4 months and can leave "this looney bunch of people." Anna cries as she listens to her family in therapy and says, "Nothing's ever going to change."

The goal of family therapy, in general, is to promote change and improve adaptive functioning within the context of the family. Because nurses interact with families in most health-care settings, understanding these frameworks for assessing and intervening with families is an important aspect of every nurse's knowledge base.

Structural Assessment

A graphic representation of the Marino family structure is presented in the genogram in Figure 10–4.

Internal Structure

The Marino family consists of a husband, wife, and their teenage biological son and daughter who live together in the same home. They conform to traditional gender roles. John is the eldest child from a rather large family, and Nancy has no siblings. In this family, their son, Peter, is the firstborn, and his sister, Anna, is 2 years younger. Neither spousal, sibling, nor spousal-sibling subsystems appear to be close in this family, and some are clearly conflictual. Problematic subsystems include John-Nancy, John-Nancy-children, and Nancy-Ethel (Nancy's mother).

The subsystem boundaries are quite rigid, and the family members appear to be emotionally disengaged from one another. One of the overt issues affecting the family is Anna's recent hospitalization after taking an overdose of her mother's prescription antidepressant.

External Structure

This family has ties to extended family, although the availability of support is questionable. Nancy's parents offered little emotional support to her as a developing child. They never approved of her marriage to John and remain distant and cold. John's family consists of a father, mother, two brothers, and two sisters. They are warm and supportive most of the time, but cultural influences interfere with their understanding of the current situation. At this time, the Marino family is probably receiving the most support from health-care professionals who have intervened during Anna's hospitalization.

Context

John is a second generation Italian American. His family of origin is large, warm, and supportive.

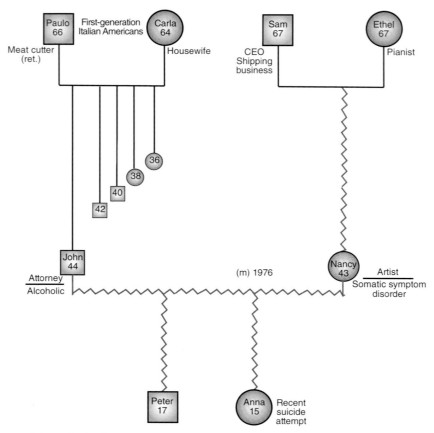

FIGURE 10–4 Genogram of the Marino family.

However, John's parents believe that family problems should be dealt with in the family, and they disapprove of bringing "strangers" in to hear what they consider to be private information. They believe that Anna's physical condition should be stabilized, and then she should be discharged to deal with family problems at home.

John and Nancy were reared in different social classes. In John's family, money was not available to seek professional help for every problem that arose. Instead, it was expected that help would be provided within the nuclear and extended family network. If outside counseling is sought, it is often with the family priest. John and Nancy did not seek this type of counseling because they no longer attend church regularly.

In Nancy's family, money was available to obtain the very best professional help at the first sign of trouble. However, Nancy's parents refused to acknowledge, both then and now, that any difficulty ever existed in their family situation.

The Marino family lives comfortably on John's salary as a corporate attorney. They have health insurance and access to any referrals that are deemed necessary. They are well educated but have been

attempting to deny the dysfunctional dynamics that exist in their family.

Developmental Assessment

The Marino family falls within the "family with adolescents" stage of McGoldrick and associates' (2020) family life cycle. In this stage, parents are expected to respond to adolescents' requests for increasing independence while being available to continue to fulfill dependency needs. They may also be required to provide additional support to aging grandparents. This is a time when parents may also begin to reexamine their own marital and career issues.

The Marino family is not fulfilling the dependency needs of its adolescents; in fact, they may be establishing premature independence. The parents are absorbed in their personal problems to the exclusion of their children. Peter responds to this neglect by staying away as much as possible, drinking with his friends, and planning to leave home at the first opportunity. Anna's attempted suicide is a cry for help. She has needs that are unfulfilled by her parents, and this crisis situation may be required for them to recognize that a problem exists. This may be the time when they begin to reexamine their unresolved marital issues. Extended family are still self-supporting and do not require assistance from John and Nancy at this time.

Functional Assessment

Instrumental Functioning

This family has managed to adjust to the maladaptive functioning to meet the physical activities of daily living. They subsist on fast food, or sometimes Nancy or Anna will prepare a meal. Seldom do they sit down at a table to eat together. Nancy must take pain medication or sedatives to sleep. John usually drinks himself to sleep. Anna and Peter take care of their own needs independently. Often they do not even see their parents in the evenings. Each manages to do fairly well in school. Peter says, "I don't intend to ruin my chances of getting out of this hell hole as soon as I can!"

Expressive Functioning

John and Nancy Marino argue a great deal about many topics. This family seldom shows affection to one another. Nancy and Anna express sadness with tears, whereas John and Peter tend to withdraw or turn to alcohol when experiencing unhappiness. Nancy somaticizes her internal pain and numbs this pain with medication. Anna internalized her emotional pain until it became unbearable. A notable lack of constructive communication is evident.

This family is unable to solve its problems effectively. In fact, it is unlikely that it has even identified its problems, which undoubtedly have been in existence for a long while. These problems have only recently been revealed in light of Anna's suicide attempt.

Diagnosis

The following nursing diagnoses were identified for the Marino family:

■ **Interrupted family processes** related to unsuccessful achievement of family developmental tasks and dysfunctional coping strategies evidenced by inability of family members to relate to each other in an adaptive manner, adolescents' unmet dependency needs, and inability of family members to express a wide range of feelings and to send and receive clear messages.

■ **Disabled family coping** related to highly ambivalent family relationships and lack of support evidenced by inability to problem solve; each member copes in response to dysfunctional family processes with destructive behavior (John drinks, Nancy somaticizes, Peter drinks and withdraws, and Anna attempts suicide).

Outcome Identification

The following criteria were identified as measurement of outcomes in counseling of the Marino family:

■ Family members will demonstrate effective communication patterns.
■ Family members will express feelings openly and honestly.
■ Family members will establish more adaptive coping strategies.
■ Family members will be able to identify destructive patterns of functioning and problem solve them effectively.
■ Boundaries between spousal subsystems and spousal-children subsystems will become more clearly defined.
■ Family members will establish stronger bonds with extended family.

Planning and Implementation

The Marino family will undoubtedly require many months of outpatient therapy. It is even likely that each member will need individual psychotherapy in addition to family therapy. Once Anna has been stabilized physiologically and is discharged from the hospital, family and individual therapy will begin.

Several strategies for family therapy have been discussed in this chapter. As mentioned previously, family therapy has a strong theoretical framework and is performed by individuals with specialized education in family theory and process. Some advanced practice nurses possess the credentials required to perform family therapy. It is important, however, for all nurses to have some knowledge about working with families, to be able to assess family interaction, and to recognize when problems exist.

Some interventions with the Marino family might include the following:

1. Create a therapeutic environment that fosters trust in which the family members can feel safe and comfortable. Promote this type of environment by being empathetic, listening actively (see Chapter 7, "Therapeutic Communication"), accepting feelings and attitudes, and being nonjudgmental.
2. Promote effective communication by doing the following:
   a. Seek clarification when vague and generalized statements are made (e.g., Anna states, "I just want my family to be like my friends' families." Ask Anna, "Would you please explain to the group exactly what you mean by that?").
   b. Set clear limits (e.g., "Peter, it is okay to state when you are angry about something that has been said. It is not okay to throw the chair against the wall.")

c. Be consistent and fair (e.g., "I encourage each of you to contribute to the group process and to respect one another's opportunity to contribute equally").

d. Address each individual clearly and directly and encouraging family members to do the same (e.g., "Nancy, I think it would be more appropriate if you directed that statement to John instead of to me").

3. Identify patterns of interaction that interfere with successful problem resolution. For example, John asks Nancy many "Why?" questions that keep her on the defensive. He criticizes her for "always being sick." Nancy responds by frequently reminding John of his infidelity. Peter and Anna interrupt each other and their parents when the level of conflict reaches a certain point. Provide examples of more appropriate ways to communicate that can improve interpersonal relations and lead to more effective patterns of interaction.

4. Help the Marino family identify problems that may necessitate change. Encourage each member to discuss a family process that they would like to change. As a group, promote discussion of what must take place for change to occur and allow each member to explore whether they could realistically cooperate with the necessary requirements for change.

5. As the problem-solving process progresses, encourage all family members to express honest feelings. Address each one directly: "John (Nancy, Peter, Anna), how do you feel about what the others are suggesting?" Ensure that all participants understand that each member may express honest feelings (e.g., anger, sadness, fear, anxiety, guilt, disgust, helplessness) without criticism, judgment, or fear of personal reprisal.

6. Avoid becoming triangled in the family emotional system. Remain neutral and objective. Do not take sides in family disagreements; instead, provide alternative explanations and suggestions (e.g., "Perhaps we can look at that situation in a different light...").

7. Reframe vague problem descriptions into ones for which resolution is more realistic. For example, rather than defining the problem as "We don't love each other anymore," the problem could be defined as "We do not spend time together in family activities anymore." This definition evolves from the family members' description of what they mean by the more general problem description.

8. Discuss present coping strategies. Encourage each family member to describe how they cope with stress and with the adversity within the family. Explore each member's possible contribution to the family's problems. Encourage family members to discuss possible solutions among themselves.

9. Identify community resources that may assist individual family members and provide support for establishing more adaptive coping mechanisms. For example, Alcoholics Anonymous for John, Al-Anon for Nancy, and Alateen for Peter and Anna. Other groups that may be of assistance to this family include Emotions Anonymous, Parents Support Group, Families Helping Families, Marriage Enrichment, Parents of Teenagers, and We Saved Our Marriage (WESOM). Local self-help networks often provide a directory of resources within specific communities.

10. Discuss with the family the possible need for psychotherapy for individual members. Provide names of therapists who can perform assessments to determine individual needs. Encourage follow-through with appointments.

11. Assist family members in planning leisure time activities together. These could include time to play together, exercise together, or engage in a shared project.

Evaluation

Evaluation is the final step in the nursing process. In this step, progress toward attainment of outcomes is measured.

1. Do family members demonstrate effective patterns of communication?
2. Can family members express feelings openly and honestly without fear of reprisal?
3. Can family members accept their personal contributions to the family's problems?
4. Can individual members identify maladaptive coping methods and express a desire to improve?
5. Do family members work together to solve problems?
6. Can family members identify resources in the community from which they can seek assistance and support?
7. Do family members express a desire to form stronger bonds with the extended family?
8. Are family members willing to seek individual psychotherapy?
9. Are family members pursuing shared activities?

Summary and Key Points

■ Family may be defined as two or more individuals who depend on one another for emotional, physical, and economic support. The members of the family are self-defined.

- Nurses must have sufficient knowledge of family functioning to assess family interaction and recognize when problems exist.
- McGoldrick and associates (2020) identified the following stages and associated tasks that describe the traditional family life cycle:
  - The single young adult
  - The family joined through marriage/union
  - The family with young children
  - The family with adolescents
  - The family launching children and moving on in midlife
  - The family in later life (late middle age to end of life)
- Tasks of families experiencing divorce and remarriage, as well as those that vary according to cultural norms, are also important to understand as the demographics of family life continue to change in society.
- Families are assessed as functional or dysfunctional based on the following six elements: communication, self-concept reinforcement, family members' expectations, handling differences, family interactional patterns, and family climate.
- Bowen viewed the family as a system that was composed of various subsystems. His theoretical approach to family therapy includes eight major concepts: differentiation of self, triangles, nuclear family emotional process, family projection process, multigenerational transmission process, sibling position, emotional cutoff, and societal emotional process.
- In the structural model of family therapy, the family is viewed as a social system within which the individual lives and to which the individual must adapt.
- In the strategic model of family therapy, communication is viewed as the foundation of functioning. Functional families are open systems where clear and precise messages are sent and received. Dysfunctional families are viewed as partially closed systems in which communication is vague, and messages are often inconsistent and incongruent with the situation.
- Many family therapists today follow an eclectic approach and incorporate concepts from several models into their practices.
- The nursing process is used as a framework for assessing, diagnosing, planning, implementing, and evaluating care to families who require assistance to maintain or regain adaptive functioning.

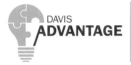 DAVIS ADVANTAGE | Go to **Davis Advantage** to complete your learning: strengthen understanding, apply your knowledge, and prepare for the Next Gen NCLEX®.

Review Questions

1. The nurse-therapist is counseling the Smith family: Mr. and Mrs. Smith, 10-year-old Rob, and 8-year-old Lisa. When Mr. and Mrs. Smith start to argue, Rob hits Lisa and Lisa starts to cry. The Smiths then turn their attention to comforting Lisa and scolding Rob, complaining that he is "out of control" and "we don't know what to do about his behavior." These dynamics are an example of which of the following?
   a. Double-bind messages
   b. Triangulation
   c. Pseudohostility
   d. Multigenerational transmission

2. Using Bowen's systems approach with a family in therapy, the therapist would:
   a. Try to change family principles that may be promoting dysfunctional behavior patterns.
   b. Strive to create change in destructive behavior through improvement in communication and interaction patterns.
   c. Encourage differentiation of individual family members.
   d. Promote change in dysfunctional behavior by encouraging the formation of more diffuse boundaries between family members.

3. Using the structural approach with a family in therapy, the therapist would:
   a. Try to change family transactions that may be promoting dysfunctional behavior patterns.
   b. Strive to create change in destructive behavior through improvement in communications and inter-action patterns.
   c. Encourage differentiation of individual family members.
   d. Promote change in dysfunctional behavior by encouraging the formation of more diffuse boundaries between family members.

4. Using the strategic approach with a family in therapy, the therapist would:
   a. Try to change family principles that may be promoting dysfunctional behavior patterns.
   b. Strive to create change in destructive behavior through improvement in communication and inter-action patterns.
   c. Encourage differentiation of individual family members.
   d. Promote change in dysfunctional behavior by encouraging the formation of more diffuse boundaries between family members.

5. During a family meeting, the parents, who are in the process of getting a divorce, report to the nurse that their teenage son with his "depression and attention-seeking behavior" is the root of all of their problems. Using concepts from Bowen's theory, which of these is the most accurate interpretation of this parental communication?
   a. The parents are scapegoating.
   b. Parental boundaries are diffuse.
   c. The parents are assuming healthy roles.
   d. The parents are disengaged.

Clinical Judgment Questions

6. A couple reports to the generalist staff nurse at the mental health clinic that they are having trouble in their marriage and want to enter therapy. Which of these is the most appropriate next action by the nurse?
   a. Offer to begin meeting with them as a couple.
   b. Recommend referral to a marriage and family therapist.
   c. Assess how many times each partner has been married before.
   d. Assess which of the partners is responsible for the marital discord.

7. The staff nurse on a psychiatric unit is approached by the client's husband, who reports, "I know my wife has bipolar disorder, but I can't tolerate the lying and the infidelity when she has manic episodes. I don't want a divorce, but I don't know what to do next." Which of these would be the most appropriate response by the nurse?
   a. "I can't discuss this with you, but I can refer you to a family therapist."
   b. "These are illness symptoms that are permanent. You will have to learn to cope with them."
   c. "Let's sit down and explore some options for next steps."
   d. "I'm sure you and your family will get through this. It will just take some time."

8. A client, who expresses interest in family therapy, says that he and his two roommates with whom he has lived for the past 20 years are unable to stop fighting about how to manage finances. Which of these is the most appropriate response by the nurse?
   a. Instruct the client that family therapy can only be conducted with blood relatives.
   b. Discuss and explore available resources that he and his roommates might access for family therapy.
   c. Assess which family members the client would like to invite in addition to the roommates.
   d. Instruct the client to discuss this with his family doctor.

9. A client reports to the nurse that her children are threatening to break up her second marriage because they don't like their stepfather. She admits that he is a disciplinarian and that he broke her son's arm when they got into an argument about her son's report card. Which of these is the most important priority action by the nurse?
   a. Make a referral to a family therapist.
   b. Encourage the client to consider divorce as an acceptable option.
   c. Suggest that her husband consider anger management classes.
   d. Report suspicions of child abuse to child protective services.

References

Administration for Community Living. (2021). *Advisory council to support grandparents raising grandchildren delivers report and recommendations for improving support to kin and grandparent caregivers*. https://acl.gov/news-and-events/announcements/advisory-council-support-grandparents-raising-grandchildren-delivers

American Nurses Association (ANA), American Psychiatric Nurses Association, & International Society of Psychiatric-Mental Health Nurses. (2022). *Psychiatric-mental health nursing: Scope and standards of practice* (3rd ed.). ANA.

Bowen Center. (2021). *Learn about Bowen theory*. https://www.thebowencenter.org/core-concepts-diagrams

Eckstein, D., & Kaufman, J. A. (2012). The role of birth order in personality: An enduring intellectual legacy of Alfred Adler. *Journal of Individual Psychology, 68*(1), 60–74. doi:10.1037/gpr0000013

Gaspard, T. (2022). *10 rules for a successful second marriage*. https://www.gottman.com/blog/10-rules-successful-second-marriage/#:~:text = While%20many%20couples%20see%20remarriage,around%2050%25%20for%20first%20marriages

Hartshorne, J. K. (2010). How birth order affects your personality. *Scientific American*. www.scientificamerican.com/article/ruled-by-birth-order

Henig, R. (2018). The age of grandparents is made of many tragedies. *The Atlantic*. https://www.theatlantic.com/family/archive/2018/06/this-is-the-age-of-grandparents/561527/

McGoldrick, M., Garcia-Preto, N., & Carter, B. (2020). *The expanding family life cycle: Individual, family, and social perspectives* (5th ed.). Pearson.

Nichols, M. P., & Davis, S. D. (2021). *Family therapy: Concepts and methods* (12th ed.). Pearson.

Ran, M. S., Chan, C.L.-W., Ng, S.-M., Guo, L.-T., & Xiang, M.-Z. (2015). The effectiveness of psychoeducational family intervention for patients with schizophrenia in a 14 year follow-up study in a Chinese rural area. *Psychological Medicine, 45*(10), 2197–2204. doi:10.1017/S0033291715000197

Robinson, M. (2022). Family health care nursing: An introduction. In Robinson, M., Padgett Coehlo, D., & Smith, P. S. (Eds.), *Family health care nursing* (7th ed., pp. 3–24). F.A. Davis.

Rohrer, J. M., Egloff, B., & Schmukle, S. C. (2015). Examining the effects of birth order on personality. *Proceedings of the National Academy of Sciences, 112*(46), 14224–14229. https://doi.org/10.1073/pnas.1506451112

Shajani, Z., & Snell, D. (2019). *Wright and Leahey's nurses and families: A guide to family assessment and intervention* (7th ed.). F.A. Davis.

The Stepfamily Foundation. (2021). *Stepfamily statistics*. www.stepfamily.org/stepfamily-statistics.html

Classical References

Bowen, M. (1971). The use of family theory in clinical practice. In Haley, J. (Ed.), *Changing families*. Grune & Stratton.

Bowen, M. (1976). Theory in the practice of psychotherapy. In Guerin, P. (Ed.), *Family therapy: Theory and practice*. Gardner Press.

Bowen, M. (1978). *Family therapy in clinical practice*. Jason Aronson.

Boyer, P. A., & Jeffrey, R. J. (1994). *A guide for the family therapist*. Jason Aronson.

Lidz, T., Cornelison, A., Fleck, S., & Terry, D. (1957). The intrafamilial environment of schizophrenic patients: II. Marital schism and marital skew. *American Journal of Psychiatry, 114*, 241–248. doi:http://dx.doi.org/10.1176/ajp.114.3.241

Minuchin, S. (1974). *Families and family therapy*. Harvard University Press.

Tomm, K., & Sanders, G. (1983). Family assessment in a problem oriented record. In Hansen, J. C., & Keeney, B. F. (Eds.), *Diagnosis and assessment in family therapy*. Aspen Systems.

11 Psychosocial Interventions and Spiritual Care

KEY TERMS

cognitive behavior therapy (CBT)

dialectical behavior therapy (DBT)

interpersonal psychotherapy (IPT)

milieu therapy

psychoanalysis

reality therapy

relaxation therapy

religion

spirituality

therapeutic community

OBJECTIVES
After reading this chapter, the student will be able to:

1. Discuss objectives and therapeutic strategies of selected psychosocial therapies, including individual psychotherapy, dialectical behavior therapy, and cognitive behavior therapy.
2. Discuss objectives and therapeutic strategies for various psychosocial interventions including assertiveness training, relaxation therapy, and milieu therapy.
3. Differentiate formal therapy from psychosocial interventions that are

conducted by generalist and psychiatric nurses.
4. Define and differentiate between spirituality and religion.
5. Conduct an assessment of a patient's spiritual needs.
6. Apply the six steps of the nursing process to individuals with spiritual and religious needs.

Conventional interventions for patients with a mental illness include psychopharmacological, psychosocial, spiritual, and physical interventions such as electroconvulsive therapy, transcranial magnetic stimulation, and light therapy. Complementary care comprises a variety of adjunctive interventions that may include over-the-counter supplements, exercise and diet interventions, acupuncture, and chiropractic services, among others. The term *integrative health* has been used to describe a holistic approach that incorporates complementary and conventional interventions in a coordinated, comprehensive treatment plan.

Psychopharmacological interventions (see Chapter 4, "Psychopharmacology"), physical interventions (see Chapter 25, "Depressive Disorders"), and complementary care (see online Chapter 40, "Complementary Therapies and Integrative Health") are covered elsewhere in the text. The focus of this chapter is on introducing selected psychosocial therapies, exploring psychosocial interventions that are often incorporated in nursing practice, and discussing spiritual care. Psychosocial *therapy*, in the formal sense, refers to a variety of specialized treatment strategies that require advanced education, licensure, or certification. Other psychosocial interventions, such as milieu therapy, relaxation therapy, and assertiveness training, are not therapies in a formal sense but rather a series of interventions that are well within the scope of practice for generalist and psychiatric nurses with basic education.

Individual Psychosocial Therapies

Individual psychotherapy takes place on a one-to-one basis between a client and a therapist. Mental health professionals who usually perform individual psychotherapy include advanced practice registered nurses, psychiatric social workers, psychiatrists, psychologists, and licensed mental health counselors. An agreement is established, and, within a therapeutic environment, the therapist assists the client to overcome behavioral symptoms or resolve interpersonal problems. Several models of individual psychotherapy are discussed in this section.

Psychoanalysis and Psychoanalytic Psychotherapy

Psychoanalysis is a theoretical approach that focuses on the unconscious mind and its influence on one's thoughts, feelings, and behaviors; it was originated by Freud in the early 20th century. It is considered by many to be the historical foundation for individual psychotherapy. Psychoanalytic psychotherapy uses in-depth talk therapy to assist the client to gain insight and understanding about current relationships and behavior patterns by confronting unconscious conflicts that surface in therapy with the analyst. Psychoanalytic psychotherapy is a lengthy and costly treatment, often lasting years, although more recently brief psychoanalytic psychotherapy models have been developed that are completed in 10 to 20 sessions. Some of the techniques used in psychoanalysis are described in the following subsections.

Free Association

Free association is a technique in which the therapist is largely nonverbal, perhaps simply introducing words or phrases. The client then verbalizes whatever thoughts come to mind. Proponents of this form of therapy believe that through freely associating, a conflict or issue may surface. Psychoanalytic psychotherapy rarely uses free association because it is more focused on already-identified conflicts.

Dream Analysis

In psychoanalysis, dreams are considered a symbolic window to unconscious conflict, so interpreting dreams is an important tool in this type of therapy.

Freud even believed that some symbols that occur in dreams are universal symbols. Analyzing dreams may include free association as well as exploring the meaning of symbols expressed in dream content.

Hypnosis

Hypnotherapy is sometimes used in psychoanalysis as a tool for unlocking the unconscious. Hypnosis is very deep relaxation during which the therapist, who has been trained in techniques of trance formation, asks certain questions of the client. Guided imagery also may be used to help the client envision a specific situation to explore aspects of a problem that were not available in the client's conscious memory. At the close of the session, while the individual is still in the trance state, the therapist may offer some posthypnotic suggestions.

Catharsis

Catharsis is defined as a releasing of unconscious conflicts into conscious awareness, generally through individual or group psychotherapy, accompanied by emotional release. Psychoanalysis proposes that maladaptive symptoms may be resolved by bringing unconscious thoughts and feelings into consciousness. Sometimes the individual not only may recall the painful experience but also may actually relive it, experiencing the feelings and emotions associated with the event. This process is called *abreaction*.

Interpersonal Psychotherapy

Interpersonal psychotherapy (IPT) is a time-limited therapy that was originally developed for the treatment of major depression. Time-limited psychotherapies (also called *brief psychotherapy*) have a specific focus, identified goals, and a limited number of sessions. Theoretical approaches include psychoanalytic, psychodynamic, interpersonal, and integrative. IPT is based on the concepts of Harry Stack Sullivan (1953) and assumes that the symptoms and social dysfunction associated with depression (and other psychiatric disorders) are correlated with difficulties in interpersonal relations. The overall goal of IPT is improvement in current interpersonal skills. Sessions generally occur weekly for about 12 to 16 weeks.

In the initial sessions, the therapist gathers information by taking a psychiatric history, identifying the major problem, establishing a diagnosis, and, together with the client, outlining the goals of therapy. A plan of action for the remaining therapy sessions defines specific interventions targeted at resolving the identified problem. The therapist's role is to guide the client to meet specifically identified treatment goals that are focused on change in interpersonal behaviors and responses. Guynn (2017, p. 2779) identified phrases such as "moving forward on your goals" and "making important changes" that are used to encourage clients to be responsible for their treatment while reminding them that altering interpersonal patterns requires attention and persistence.

Outcome studies have demonstrated IPT's efficacy in treating various types of depression, including nonpsychotic major depression, recurrent depression, bipolar disorder, postpartum depression, and dysthymic disorder as well as bulimia nervosa and binge eating disorder (Guynn, 2017). Some evidence suggests that IPT may also be effective for treating substance use disorders with dual diagnoses (a co-occurring mental disorder, such as depression, with an addiction) (Crane, 2023). In this context, motivational interviewing is often incorporated, and the focus is on interpersonal patterns that are detrimental to recovery.

Reality Therapy

Reality therapy was developed in the mid-1960s by the American psychiatrist William Glasser (1965). In **reality therapy**, psychopathology is viewed in terms of ineffective behaviors rather than mental illnesses. Diagnoses and labels (e.g., neurotic or dysfunctional) are perceived as not particularly useful. As such, it is not entirely compatible with a medical model of psychiatric treatment. The concept of responsibility is emphasized. Accepting responsibility for one's own behavior is equated with mental health. An individual who behaves responsibly is able to fulfill their basic needs without interfering with others' attempts at need fulfillment.

The tenets of reality therapy are rooted in personality development. Personality is defined as an individual's characteristic patterns of thinking, feeling, and behaving, and personality development may be viewed as an attempt to fulfill five basic needs: power, belonging, freedom, fun, and survival. Individuals choose behaviors that will either be effective or ineffective in satisfying those needs. In the course of reality therapy, the therapist helps the client identify needs that are not being met, correlate the unmet needs to current ineffective behaviors, and make conscious choices to change to more effective patterns of behavior in an effort to satisfy basic needs. In reality therapy, emphasis is on the present: the here and now. The past is addressed only as it affects present choices or future behavior. A primary function of the therapist is to assist the client in dealing with getting needs met in the present.

Cognitive Behavior Therapy

Cognitive behavior therapy (CBT), developed by Aaron Beck (1976) and originally identified as simply cognitive therapy, was initially developed for the treatment of mood disorders, but evidence supports its benefits in the treatment of many other disorders including schizophrenia, eating disorders, posttraumatic stress disorders, substance use disorders, and personality disorders. In the cognitive model, irrational thoughts (also referred to as *thought distortions*) are considered a factor in the development and maintenance of mental and emotional disorders. Teaching and guiding the client to challenge and reframe dysfunctional patterns of thinking is believed to contribute to more positive mood and behavior and relief of symptoms. Developing skill in mindfulness is considered foundational to achieving these outcomes. A more in-depth discussion on CBT can be found in Chapter 18, "Cognitive Behavior Therapy."

Dialectical Behavior Therapy

Dialectical behavior therapy (DBT) was originally developed by Marsha Linehan (1993) as a treatment approach for people with borderline personality disorder (BPD) and suicidal ideation. Originally conceptualized as a CBT, it shares several features with CBT including mindfulness as a foundational skill. Like CBT, DBT focuses on the therapist working with the client to develop a series of skills. Where the central focus in CBT is learning how to reframe troubling thoughts, DBT focuses more on learning how to regulate troubling emotions. Some of the skills that are unique to DBT include learning nonjudgmental self-acceptance, structuring the environment to positively reinforce progress, developing skills in distress tolerance, and interpersonal effectiveness. Evidence supports the effectiveness of DBT for individuals with several psychiatric disorders including BPD, eating disorders, mood disorders, and substance use disorders.

Psychosocial Interventions in Nursing Practice

Psychiatric nurses, while not prepared to conduct formal therapy, are often involved in education and counseling on psychosocial issues. Three psychosocial interventions within the scope of nursing practice include milieu therapy, relaxation therapy, and assertiveness training. Assertiveness Training is explored in more detail in Chapter 13, "Assertiveness Training."

Milieu Therapy: The Therapeutic Community

Standard 5F of the *Psychiatric–Mental Health Nursing: Scope and Standards of Practice* (American Nurses

Association [ANA], American Psychiatric Nurses Association, & International Society of Psychiatric Nurses, 2022) states, "The psychiatric-mental health nurse (including the graduate-level prepared PMH-RN and PMH-APRN) provides a safe, therapeutic, recovery-oriented environment in collaboration with patients/clients, families, and other clinicians/ancillary staff/care partners" (p. 74).

Milieu, Defined

The word *milieu,* French for "middle," is translated in English as "surroundings, or environment." In psychiatry, therapy involving the milieu, or environment, may be called **milieu therapy,** the **therapeutic community,** the therapeutic environment, or the therapeutic milieu. The goal of milieu therapy is to manipulate the environment so that all aspects of the patient's hospital experience are considered therapeutic. Within this therapeutic community setting, the patient is expected to learn adaptive coping, interaction, and relationship skills that can be adapted to other aspects of their life.

> ## CORE CONCEPT
> ### Milieu Therapy
> A scientific structuring of the environment in order to effect behavioral changes and improve the psychological health and functioning of the individual (Skinner, 1979).

Milieu therapy came into its own from the 1960s through the early 1980s. The milieu was the inpatient hospital setting. During this period, psychiatric inpatient treatment provided sufficient time to implement programs of therapy aimed at social rehabilitation. Lengths of stay averaged from 28 to 30 days for acute care hospitalizations and several months or years for long-term hospitalizations. Nursing's focus on establishing interpersonal relationships with patients fit well within this concept of therapy. Patients were encouraged to be active participants in their therapy, and individual autonomy was emphasized. Because acute care hospital lengths of stay now average 2 to 3 days, the focus of inpatient psychiatric care has changed to primarily biologically based stabilization of acute symptoms, but patients still interact within a community environment that can be used to promote their recovery.

Although some of the original strategies for milieu therapy are still used, they have been modified to conform to the short-term approach to care or to outpatient treatment programs. Some programs (e.g., those for children and adolescents, people with substance use disorders, and geriatric clients) have successfully adapted the concepts of milieu treatment to their specialty needs (Menninger Clinic, 2022; O-School, 2022; Valley View, 2022).

Evidence supports the benefits of therapeutic communities in prison settings for individuals with substance use disorders (National Institutes of Health [NIH], 2015). In this context, work assignments, peer support, formal treatment, and accepting responsibility for one's actions are key elements, and the therapeutic community treatment may last 12 months or more. Evidence also supports milieu therapy for longer-term treatment of patients with schizophrenia. For these patients, milieu therapy has demonstrated positive benefits at lower doses of antipsychotic medications, leading researchers to conclude that the positive emotional experience of milieu therapy is not only an important aspect of treatment but also one that may enable lower doses of medication (Ciompi & Hoffman, 2004; Kvarnstrom, 2017). Even in acute care hospital settings, evidence supports that milieu therapy is effective in decreasing aggressive behavior, self-harm behavior, and general rule-breaking behavior among patients with schizophrenia (Bhat et al., 2020).

Whether the inpatient treatment setting is short term or longer term, some basic principles of milieu therapy are applicable. In a therapeutic community, the setting is the foundation, and everything that happens to the patient or within the patient's environment is considered part of the treatment program. Unlike a medical or surgical hospital setting, patients in an inpatient psychiatric setting are exposed to a tremendous amount of interaction and activity with one another. Community factors, such as social interactions, the physical structure of the treatment setting, and schedule of activities, may generate negative responses from some patients. These stressful experiences are used as opportunities to help the patient learn how to manage stress more adaptively in real-life situations.

Under what conditions, then, is a hospital environment considered therapeutic? Gunderson (1978) identified five elements of a community environment that are necessary for therapeutic outcomes:

1. *Containment:* The environment is contained to create a sense of safety and security. Patients who are struggling with strong suicidal intentions, for example, often find that locked doors and lack of access to easy methods of self-harm provide the containment they need to resist self-destructive impulses.
2. *Structure:* The environment needs to have a structure that promotes the goals of treatment. This includes a schedule of activities so that patients

know what, when, and where activities are taking place. Group therapies, for example, are scheduled at specific times so patients can structure their day to attend. Knowing to whom they should go (perhaps a primary nurse or team leader) to express concerns, ask for medication, or contact other team members is another aspect of unit structure that promotes therapeutic outcomes.

3. *Involvement:* The environment must encourage involvement so that patients develop a sense of social community. Common dining areas, small group seating arrangements, and community meetings to discuss aspects of community living are examples of elements that promote involvement.

4. *Support:* The environment must be supportive and affirming rather than rigid or punitive. The nurse plays an active role in offering emotional support, reinforcing the expectations within the community environment by promoting supportive interaction, and redirecting patients who are struggling to accomplish therapeutic interaction with others. Support also includes creating a sense that patients are not only involved in treatment but empowered in decision making and direction about their care.

5. *Validation:* The environment must support and affirm the needs of the individual both within and separate from the community. Active, empathic listening to the patient's perceptions and concerns and promoting autonomy are examples of validation.

The Role of the Nurse in Milieu Therapy

Several professional health-care disciplines contribute to the function of the therapeutic milieu and collaborate with one another through interdisciplinary team treatment planning and intervention. Table 11–1 describes some of the roles and functions of these team members. Nursing, however, is the only discipline that provides in-person care for patients 24 hours a day and, as such, plays a crucial role in establishing and maintaining the therapeutic milieu.

One of the most important initial nursing interventions in establishing a therapeutic milieu and a foundation for trust is orienting the new patient to the environment, including their rights and responsibilities within the unit milieu, the structured activities designed for personal growth, and any limits or restrictions necessary to maintain safety. Availability to provide support and validation to patients throughout their treatment is also an essential nursing competency in milieu therapy (ANA et al., 2022), and this, too, is rooted in a trusting relationship. Active listening and inquiring about the patient's expectations for treatment are key communication skills in providing support and validation and in establishing a foundation for patient-centered care.

In acute care hospitalizations, the ability to establish trust quickly and to assess and collaborate with

TABLE 11–1 **The Interdisciplinary Treatment Team in Psychiatry**		
TEAM MEMBER	**RESPONSIBILITIES**	**CREDENTIALS**
Psychiatrist	Serves as the leader of the team. Responsible for diagnosis and treatment of mental disorders. Prescribes medication and other somatic therapies. May perform psychotherapy.	Medical degree with residency in psychiatry and license to practice medicine.
Clinical psychologist	Conducts individual, group, and family therapy. Administers, interprets, and evaluates psychological tests that assist in the diagnostic process.	Doctorate in clinical psychology with 2- to 3-year internship supervised by a licensed clinical psychologist. State license is required to practice.
Psychiatric clinical nurse specialist or psychiatric nurse practitioner	Conducts individual, group, and family therapy. Presents educational programs for nursing staff. Provides consultation services to nurses who require assistance in the planning and implementation of care for individual patients. May also prescribe and manage the medication regimen.	Registered nurse with a minimum of a master's degree in psychiatric nursing. Some institutions and most states require certification by national credentialing association.
Psychiatric nurse	Provides ongoing mental and physical assessment of the patient's condition. Manages the therapeutic milieu on a 24-hour basis. Administers medications. Assists patients with all therapeutic activities as required. Focus is on one-to-one relationship development.	Registered nurse with hospital diploma, associate degree, or baccalaureate degree. Some psychiatric nurses have national certification.

TABLE 11–1	**The Interdisciplinary Treatment Team in Psychiatry—cont'd**	
TEAM MEMBER	**RESPONSIBILITIES**	**CREDENTIALS**
Mental health technician (also called psychiatric aide or assistant or psychiatric technician)	Functions under the supervision of the psychiatric nurse. Provides assistance to patients in the fulfillment of their activities of daily living. Assists activity therapists as required in conducting their groups. May also participate in one-to-one relationship development.	Varies by state. Requirements include high school education, with additional vocational education or on-the-job training. Some hospitals hire individuals with a baccalaureate degree in psychology in this capacity. Some states require a licensure examination to practice.
Psychiatric social worker	Conducts individual, group, and family therapy. Is concerned with patient's social needs, such as placement, financial support, and community requirements. Conducts in-depth psychosocial history on which the needs assessment is based. Works with patient and family to ensure that requirements for discharge are fulfilled and needs can be met by appropriate community resources.	Minimum of a master's degree in social work. Some states require additional supervision and subsequent licensure by examination.
Occupational therapist	Works with patients to help develop (or redevelop) independence in performance of activities of daily living. Focus is on rehabilitation and vocational training in which clients learn to be productive, thereby enhancing self-esteem. Creative activities and therapeutic relationship skills are used.	Baccalaureate or master's degree in occupational therapy.
Recreation therapist	Uses recreational activities to promote patients to redirect their thinking or to rechannel destructive energy in an appropriate manner. Patients learn skills (e.g., bowling, volleyball, exercises, jogging) that can be used during leisure time and during times of stress after discharge from treatment. Some longer-term settings include activities such as picnics, swimming, and group attendance at certain events (e.g., the state fair).	Baccalaureate or master's degree in recreational therapy.
Music therapist	Encourages patients in self-expression through music. Patients listen to music, play instruments, sing, dance, and compose songs that help them get in touch with feelings and emotions that they may not be able to experience in any other way.	Graduate degree with a specialty in music therapy.
Art therapist	Uses the patient's creative abilities to encourage the expression of emotions and feelings through artwork. Helps patients to analyze their own work in an effort to recognize and resolve underlying conflict.	Graduate degree with a specialty in art therapy.
Dietitian	Plans nutritious meals for all patients. Consults with patients with specific eating disorders, such as anorexia nervosa, bulimia nervosa, obesity, and pica.	Baccalaureate or master's degree with a specialty in dietetics.
Chaplain	Assesses, identifies, and attends to the spiritual needs of patients and their family members. Provides spiritual support and comfort as requested by the patient or family. May provide counseling if educational background includes this type of preparation.	College degree with advanced education in theology, seminary, or rabbinical studies.

patients about their post-discharge needs has become an essential role for nurses because many aspects of the recovery treatment plan will occur in treatment settings other than inpatient hospitalization. Do not underestimate the importance of these short-term relationships. Patients in outpatient treatment often identify that something a nurse said or something they learned within the hospital milieu planted the seeds for their ongoing recovery plan.

> **CLINICAL PEARL** Developing trust entails being reliable and transparent. It requires acceptance of the individual as a person, separate from behaviors that are unacceptable. It means responding to the patient with concrete actions that are easy to understand (e.g., "If you are frightened, I will stay with you"; "If you are cold, I will bring you a blanket"; "If you are thirsty, I will bring you a drink of water").

Reorienting patients who are confused, redirecting and setting limits when patient behavior is disruptive within the community, patient education, and role modeling communication and social skills are all activities in which nurses contribute to promoting a therapeutic milieu.

In the therapeutic milieu, nurses are also responsible for ensuring that patients' physiological needs are met. Patients must be encouraged to perform as independently as possible in fulfilling activities of daily living. However, the nurse must make ongoing assessments and provide assistance for those who require it. Assessing physical status is an important nursing responsibility that must not be overlooked in a psychiatric setting.

Therapeutic Milieu as a Professional Nursing Practice Model

Meehan (2020) reimagined the idea of therapeutic milieu as a model for professional practice that involves six principles and can be adopted in any practice setting. Some of these principles are patient centered, others pertain to the nurses, and some are the responsibility of the health-care team. These principles are listed as follows:

1. *Contagious calmness:* This principle refers to the nurse's ability to maintain composure, even during stressful events. Nurses encounter patients' anxiety on a daily basis, and the nurse's ability to respond with calm composure creates the foundation for a healing environment for the patient.
2. *Respect for inherent human dignity:* Widely recognized as a core value in nursing, this principle can be overlooked in practice if not given careful thought. Patients with mental illness have been victims of stigmatizing attitudes and behaviors.

Referring to patients with derogatory language such as "those crazies" or "nuts," even when doing so with other health-care professionals, devalues the inherent dignity of the patient.
3. *Nurse's care for self and one another:* Caring for self implies attending to one's own needs to achieve inner and outer wellness. Caring for others implies attending to relational wellness. Nurses sometimes express that their relationships with patients and their relationships with other team members are two mutually exclusive entities. However, patients who see inconsistencies in how health-care professionals relate to one another and their patients may have more difficulty trusting that the milieu is safe and therapeutic.
4. *Intellectual engagement:* The therapeutic milieu is developed and enhanced by the nurse's active engagement in critical thinking, creativity, and problem-solving around relevant practice issues. Examples may include exploring the best ways to maintain a safe environment or studying a patient care intervention to improve its effectiveness. Intellectual engagement is the essence of quality improvement, which has been identified as an essential Quality and Safety Education for Nurses (QSEN) competency.
5. *Caritas:* Caritas refers to the nurse's ability to experience and express benevolent affection for patients regardless of their characteristics. Patients with mental illness may say things that are reflections of disrupted thought processes; they may be anxious and angry and they may behave in ways that are not socially acceptable. The ability to relate to patients with caritas, or what Carl Rogers (1951; the founder of client-centered psychology) described as "unconditional positive regard," is foundational to establishing a healing, therapeutic environment.
6. *Safe and restorative physical surroundings:* In the inpatient psychiatric unit, safety of the physical environment is paramount. Many adjustments are made to doors, windows, and furniture to minimize risks for suicide or violence toward others. Standards and unit policies dictate the manner and frequency with which patients are observed and assessed to ensure their safety. All of these efforts communicate to the patient a concern for a safe, therapeutic milieu and begin to lay the foundation for establishing trust. Whether the therapeutic milieu is adopted as a treatment strategy within psychiatric treatment settings or broadened in scope to be viewed as a professional practice model for nurses in any setting, evidence supports that establishing a therapeutic environment of care is essential to the development of

trust, relationship building, and therapeutic outcomes in patient care.

Relaxation Therapy

Stress is a part of our everyday lives. It can be positive or negative, but it cannot be eliminated. Keeping stress at a manageable level is a lifelong process. Individuals under stress respond with a physiological arousal that can be dangerous over long periods. Indeed, the stress response has been shown to be a major contributor, either directly or indirectly, to coronary heart disease, cancer, lung ailments, accidental injuries, cirrhosis of the liver, and suicide—six of the leading causes of death in the United States.

Relaxation therapy is an effective means of reducing the stress response in some individuals. The degree of anxiety that an individual experiences in response to stress is related to certain predisposing factors, such as innate temperament, past experiences resulting in learned patterns of responding, and existing conditions, such as health status, coping strategies, and adequacy of support systems. Nurses can play an active role in educating patients about the stress response and various methods to achieve relaxation. Deep relaxation can counteract the physiological and behavioral manifestations of stress. Various methods of relaxation are described in the following subsections.

Deep-Breathing Exercises

Tension is released when the lungs are allowed to breathe in as much oxygen as possible. Deep-breathing exercises involve inhaling slowly and deeply through the nose, holding the breath for a few seconds, and then exhaling slowly through the mouth, pursing the lips as if trying to whistle.

Progressive Relaxation

Progressive relaxation is a method of deep-muscle relaxation that is based on the premise that the body responds to anxiety-provoking thoughts and events with muscle tension. Each muscle group is tensed for 5 to 7 seconds and then relaxed for 20 to 30 seconds, during which time the individual concentrates on the difference in sensations between the two conditions. Soft, slow background music may facilitate relaxation. A modified version of this technique, called *passive progressive relaxation,* involves relaxation of the muscles by concentrating on the feeling of relaxation within the muscle, rather than on the actual tensing and relaxing of the muscle.

Meditation

The goal of meditation is to gain mastery over attention. It brings on a special state of consciousness as attention is concentrated solely on one thought or object. During meditation, as the individual becomes completely preoccupied with the selected focus, respiration rate, heart rate, and blood pressure decrease.

Mindfulness meditation, a practice rooted in Buddhist traditions, has gained popularity as a foundational skill in several psychological therapies. The practice of mindfulness is a form of meditation focused on nonjudgmental awareness of the present moment. For example, focusing on one's breathing (the sounds, the depth of each breath, the sensations in the body as one is breathing) and nonjudgmentally returning one's attention to breathing when they notice their mind wandering, is associated with relaxation and improved ability to focus on the present. Developing the skill of "being present in the moment" facilitates problem-solving and behavior change.

Mental Imagery

Mental imagery uses the imagination of a relaxing environment to reduce the body's response to stress. The frame of reference is very personal, based on what each individual considers to be a relaxing environment. Imagining the relaxing environment by engaging multiple sensory experiences (imagining the sights, the smells, the sounds, etc.) enhances the mental imagery. For example, one might find it relaxing to imagine a warm beach, the sound of the water ebbing and flowing at the shoreline, the smell of the sea air, and the feel of a warm breeze. Combining this practice with muscle relaxation and deep breathing often facilitates one's ability to experience the relaxing environment. The relaxing scenario may be taped and played back at a time when the individual wishes to achieve relaxation.

Biofeedback

Biofeedback is the use of instrumentation to become aware of processes in the body that usually go unnoticed and to help bring them under voluntary control. Biological conditions, such as muscle tension, skin surface temperature, blood pressure, and heart rate, are monitored by the biofeedback equipment. As biofeedback training progresses, the individual learns to use relaxation and voluntary control to modify the biological condition, in turn indicating a modification of the autonomic function it represents. Biofeedback is often used together with other relaxation techniques such as deep breathing, progressive relaxation, and mental imagery. Nurses may be involved in providing biofeedback services after completing specialized training and/or certification.

Assertiveness Training

Assertive behavior and communication promote positive self-esteem by encouraging open and honest expression of one's needs and respecting one's basic human rights as well as the rights of others. Assertive communication is an important skill for nurses to develop in professional relationships with peers and supervisors in any practice setting. In psychiatric nursing, assertive communication and behavior are important tools that can be taught and role modeled in interaction with patients to promote their development of effective communication skills in interpersonal relationships.

The basic goal in assertive communication training is to teach individuals to express what they feel and need without becoming defensive and without violating the rights of others. Some people who are beginning to learn these skills wrongly believe that assertive communication will get people to respond in certain ways or will allow them to get what they want from another person. Manipulation is not the goal of assertive communication. Further, no one can control another person's behaviors or responses, and if individuals do not understand these limitations at the outset, they may be setting themselves up for failure. It is important to educate people that assertive communication skills are designed to empower them to express themselves and their needs more effectively. The skills associated with assertiveness training are discussed in detail in Chapter 13, "Assertiveness Training."

Spiritual Care

Assessing a patient's spiritual needs is recognized as an important aspect of holistic nursing care, but definitions and activities to accomplish this have not always been well understood. Historically, spiritual care has had distinctly religious connections, with a spiritual person being described as "someone with whom the Spirit of God dwelt." Koenig (2012) described **spirituality** as distinguished by its connection to that which is considered sacred and transcendent. He identifies spirituality as connected to the supernatural, the mystical, and organized religion but extending beyond and beginning before organized religion. In other words, spirituality may be considered a quest for the transcendent that might lead to staunch belief or nonbelief.

> ## CORE CONCEPT
> ### Spirituality
> The human quality that gives meaning and sense of purpose to an individual's existence. Spirituality exists within each individual regardless of belief system and serves as a force for interconnectedness between the self and others, the environment, and a higher power.

Contemporary research supports the value of addressing spirituality for both medical and psychiatric patients (Clark & Emerson, 2021; Lichter, 2013; Liefbroer et al., 2019; Reeves & Reynolds, 2009). Within nursing, focus on spirituality is identified as a nursing responsibility in the International Council of Nurses *Code of Ethics* (2021) and the American Holistic Nurses Association (in collaboration with the American Nurses Association) *Holistic Nursing: Scope and Standards of Practice* (2019). Spiritual care is recognized as an important aspect of care in two *NANDA International* nursing diagnoses: Spiritual distress and spiritual well-being (Herdman et al., 2021). Although spiritual care has been identified as an important aspect of recovery, a recent study (Neathery et al., 2020) found that nurses who had a spiritual perspective with a religious affiliation and more years of experience as a psychiatric-mental health nurse were more likely to provide spiritual care. The authors suggest that more development for nurses in their understanding of spiritual care is necessary to enhance the frequency with which this aspect of nursing care is provided.

Specifically in psychiatric nursing, issues related to spiritual distress and spiritual well-being are common. The sense of hopelessness that is symptomatic in major depressive disorders raises spiritual questions for many patients with this condition. The thought disruptions that are characteristic in schizophrenia lead some to misinterpret their experience as induced by evil forces. Patients with grandiose delusions may falsely believe they are a prophet, the messiah, or other person of great religious or spiritual significance. How should the nurse respond to these issues and questions around spirituality with respect for the patient's needs, values, and beliefs? A prerequisite to conducting a meaningful spiritual assessment is exploration of concepts related to meaning and purpose in life, connectedness, faith, hope, love, and forgiveness.

Spiritual Needs
Meaning and Purpose in Life

Humans by nature strive for order and structure in their lives. Having a purpose in life gives one a sense of control and the feeling that life is worth living. Each individual's exploration of what is most important in their lives is foundational to their awareness of their spirituality and provides a platform for spiritual growth. Further, each nurse's exploration of their own spirituality and efforts to grow spiritually are foundational to being responsive to those needs in others. Walsh (1999) described seven perennial practices that he believes promote enlightenment, aid in transformation, and encourage spiritual growth:

1. ***Transform your motivation:*** Reduce craving and find your soul's desire.
2. ***Cultivate emotional wisdom:*** Heal your heart and learn to love.
3. ***Live ethically:*** Feel good by doing good.
4. ***Concentrate and calm your mind:*** Accept the challenge of mastering attention and mindfulness.
5. ***Awaken your spiritual vision:*** See clearly and recognize the sacred in all things.
6. ***Cultivate spiritual intelligence:*** Develop wisdom and understand the purpose of life.
7. ***Express spirit in action:*** Embrace generosity and the joy of service. (p. 14)

In the final analysis, individuals must determine their own perception of what is important and what gives meaning to life. Throughout one's existence, the meaning of life will undoubtedly be challenged many times. A solid spiritual foundation may help an individual confront the challenges that result from life's experiences.

Erik Erikson, who elaborated a classic model of developmental tasks throughout the life span (1950), recognized that as people continue to live into older adulthood, his identified tasks did not address what he referred to as the older, older adult (those adults age 80 years and older). His widow compiled his notes and subsequently published his work on an additional developmental stage. This stage is *transcendence*, in which adults 80 years and older focus more on clarifying meaning in their life as well as those things that transcend beyond themselves. Erikson suggests that as individuals continue to grow older, spirituality becomes a more important part of their development.

Connectedness

Clark and Emerson, in their concept analysis of spirituality in psychiatric nursing (2021), found that connectedness was one of the top two key attributes of spirituality (along with life meaning and purpose). Connectedness may include "transcendental connections with the sacred, with the deep [inner] being … and with ordinary everyday life" (Lavorato-Neto et al., 2018, p. 281). Patients during acute episodes of a psychiatric disorder are often in a crisis of disconnectedness. Symptoms such as hopelessness, disrupted thought processes, anxiety, and anger are contributing factors. The experience of stigmatization and disenfranchisement confounds the risk for a sense of isolation.

The importance of connectedness in suicide prevention has been identified in research. Klonsky and May (2015) found that connectedness prevents suicide ideation from escalating in those at risk and when pain and hopelessness exceed one's sense of connectedness, suicide ideation becomes active. Patient-centered care and collaboration in the context of a trusting relationship are nursing skills that promote connectedness.

Faith

Faith is often thought of as the acceptance of a belief in the absence of physical or empirical evidence. Smucker (2001) stated:

> For all people, faith is an important concept. From childhood on, our psychological health depends on having faith or trust in something or someone to help meet our needs. (p. 7)

Having faith requires that individuals rise above that which they can experience only through the five senses. Faith transcends the appearance of the physical world. An increasing amount of medical and scientific research is showing that what individuals believe exists can have as powerful an effect as what actually exists (Bogousslavsky & Inglin, 2007; Harvard Health, 2021; Sathyanarayana Rao et al., 2009; Tétreault et al., 2016). Karren and associates (2010) added that there is a growing appreciation of the healing power of faith among members of the medical community.

Hope

Hope is defined as a positive, optimistic outlook. With hope, individuals look at a situation, and no matter how negative, find something positive on which to focus. Hope functions as an energizing force. In addition, research indicates that hope may promote healing, facilitate coping, and enhance the quality of life (Enayati, 2013; Nekolaichuk et al., 1999).

Kübler-Ross (1969), in her classic study of dying patients, stressed the importance of hope. She suggested that even though these patients could not hope for a cure, they could hope for additional time to live, to be with loved ones, for freedom from pain, or for a peaceful death with dignity. She found hope to be a satisfaction unto itself, whether or not it was fulfilled. She stated, "If a patient stops expressing hope, it is usually a sign of imminent death" (p. 140).

Researchers in the field of psychoneuroimmunology have found that the attitudes we have and the emotions we experience have a definite effect on inflammation in the body (Jones, 2019; Jones & Graham-Engeland, 2021). An optimistic feeling of hope is not just a mental state. Hope and optimism produce positive physical changes in the body that can influence the immune system and the functioning of specific body organs. Medical literature abounds with countless examples of individuals with terminal conditions who suddenly improve when they find hope. Conversely, there are many accounts of patients whose conditions deteriorate when they lose hope.

Love

Love may be identified as a projection of one's own good feelings onto others. To love others, one must first experience love of self and then be able and willing to project that warmth and affectionate concern for others (Karren et al., 2013). Smucker (2001) stated:

> Love, in its purest unconditional form, is probably life's most powerful force and our greatest spiritual need. Not only is it important to receive love, but equally important to give love to others. Thinking about and caring for the needs of others keeps us from being too absorbed with ourselves and our needs to the exclusion of others. We all have experienced the good feelings that come from caring for and loving others. (p. 10)

Love may be an important component of the healing process. Thaik, a cardiologist, stated that love, as one of many strong human emotions, releases a cascade of hundreds or thousands of neuropeptides and hormones that can affect physical and mental health (2013). Among the beneficial effects, Thaik reported that:

1. Love counteracts the fight-or-flight syndrome and decreases production of the stress hormone cortisol.
2. Love encourages the production of oxytocin, the "feel-good" hormone, which can reduce cardiovascular stress and improve the immune system.
3. Love increases the production of norepinephrine and dopamine and may stave off depression.
4. Love decreases inflammation, which affects immune function and pain relief.

Some researchers present evidence that love has a positive effect on the immune system in adults, children, and animals (Murray et al., 2019; Ornish, 1998; Pace et al., 2009). The giving and receiving of love may also result in higher levels of endorphins, thereby contributing to a sense of euphoria and helping to reduce pain.

In a classic long-term study, researchers Werner and Smith (1992) studied children who were reared in impoverished environments. Their homes were troubled by discord, desertion, or divorce or were marred by parental alcoholism or mental illness. The participants were studied at birth, childhood, adolescence, and adulthood. Two of three of these high-risk children had developed serious learning and/or behavioral problems by age 10 or had a record of delinquencies, mental health problems, or pregnancies by age 18. One-fourth of them had developed "very serious" physical and psychosocial problems. By the time they reached adulthood, more than three-fourths had profound psychological and behavioral problems, and even more were in poor physical health. But of particular interest to the researchers were the 15% to 20% who remained resilient and well despite their impoverished and difficult existence. These children had experienced a warm and loving relationship with another person during their first year of life, whereas the children who developed serious psychological and physical problems did not. This research indicates that the earlier people have the benefit of a strong, loving relationship, the better they seem able to resist the effects of a deleterious lifestyle.

Forgiveness

Forgiveness has been defined as the letting go of resentments and thoughts of revenge (Mayo Clinic, 2022). Feelings of bitterness and resentment take a physical toll on an individual by generating stress hormones. When maintained for long periods, these feelings can have a detrimental effect on health. Forgiveness enables a person to cast off resentment and begin the pathway to healing. Owen, as cited by Harrison (2011), conducted research with patients who were HIV positive to study the effects of forgiveness on the immune system and found that forgiveness was correlated with improvements in immune function.

Forgiveness is not easy. Individuals often have great difficulty when called upon to forgive others, and even greater difficulty in attempting to forgive themselves. To forgive is not necessarily to condone or excuse one's own or someone else's inappropriate behavior. Karren and associates (2013) suggested that forgiveness is an attitude of owning responsibility for one's own perceptions and moving beyond the perception of being a helpless victim to the perception of being empowered in choosing one's own responses to hurts and offenses.

It is important for nurses to be able to assess the spiritual needs of their patients. The aforementioned aspects are relevant to one's spiritual well-being as well as their physical well-being. Nurses need not serve the role of a professional counselor or spiritual guide, but because of the ongoing contact with patients and the trust that is developed within a therapeutic nurse–patient relationship, nurses may be the part of the health-care team to whom patients reveal the most intimate details of their lives. As Balboni and Balboni (2019) noted, "spiritual care should be patient-centered and appropriate to the professional role and training of the clinician. A simple minimal standard is that clinicians should be expected to ask each patient if and how spirituality or religion might be important to their illness" (para 17). Smucker (2001) stated:

> Just as answering a patient's question honestly and with accurate information and responding to his needs in a timely and sensitive manner communicates caring, so also does high-quality professional nursing care reach beyond the physical body or the illness to that part of the person where identity, self-worth, and spirit lie. In this sense, good nursing care is also good spiritual care. (pp. 11–12)

Religion

> ### CORE CONCEPT
> **Religion**
> **Religion** is a set of beliefs, values, rites, and rituals adopted by a group of people. The practices are usually grounded in the teachings of a spiritual leader.

Religion is one way an individual's spirituality may be expressed. There are more than 6,500 religions in the world (Bronson, 2005). Globally, Christianity remains the largest religious group (31.2%), followed by Islam (24.1%), and unaffiliated individuals (16%) (Pew Research Center, 2017). Some individuals seek out various religions in an attempt to find answers to fundamental questions that they have about life and, indeed, about their very existence. Others, although they may regard themselves as spiritual, choose not to affiliate with an organized religious group. In either situation, however, it is inevitable that questions related to life and the human condition arise during the progression of spiritual maturation.

Evidence supports that affiliation with a religious group is a health-enhancing endeavor (Karren et al., 2013). Defining what constitutes unhealthy religious adaptation is difficult and multilayered. Certainly, an individual's general psychological adaptation is influential. Healthy religious adaptation may generally be defined as participation in religious activities that promote well-being and spiritual growth. Several studies indicate a correlation between religious faith, church attendance, increased chance of survival after serious illness, fewer instances of depression and mental illness, longer life, and overall better physical and mental health. In an extensive review of the literature, Levin (2010) concluded that the weight of the evidence across studies suggests that religious involvement is a general protective factor for mental illness and psychological distress.

Despite these findings, confidence in organized religion and church attendance have been declining in American society. Over the past four decades, there has been a steady decline in Americans' confidence in religion. In 2018, church membership reached an all-time low, with 50% of Americans reporting belonging to a church, synagogue, or mosque (Jones, 2019). The trend toward declining membership has been particularly pronounced over the last two decades. Church attendance has shown similar declines.

Despite declining church membership, a recent Gallup poll (Jones, 2019) identified that 77% of Americans report identifying with some organized religion. Although the majority of Americans still identify as affiliated with some branch of Christianity, the number of Americans identifying as having no religious affiliation has more than doubled (from 8% to 19%) since the turn of the century (Jones, 2019). These findings suggest that although a majority of Americans may still value faith and worship, their mechanisms for expressing those values are undergoing cultural change.

Addressing Spiritual and Religious Needs Through the Nursing Process

Assessment

It is important for nurses to consider spiritual and religious needs when planning care for their patients. The Joint Commission, as part of its accreditation standards, identifies that nurses should address the psychosocial, spiritual, and cultural variables that influence their perception of illness. Dossey (1998) developed a spiritual assessment tool about which she stated:

> The Spiritual Assessment Tool provides reflective questions for assessing, evaluating, and increasing awareness of spirituality in patients and their significant others. The tool's reflective questions can facilitate healing because they stimulate spontaneous, independent, meaningful initiatives to improve the patient's capacity for recovery and healing. (p. 45)

An adapted version of this spiritual assessment tool can be found in Box 11–1.

Assessing the spiritual needs of a patient with a psychotic disorder can pose some additional challenges. Approximately 25% of people with schizophrenia and 15% to 22% of people with bipolar disorder have religious delusions (Koenig, 2012). Sometimes these delusions can be difficult to differentiate from general religious or cultural beliefs, but nonpsychotic religious activity may actually improve long-term prognosis in patients with psychotic disorders (Koenig, 2012). Engaging family members

BOX 11–1 Spiritual Assessment Tool

The following reflective questions may assist you in assessing, evaluating, and increasing awareness of spirituality in yourself and others.

MEANING AND PURPOSE

These questions assess a person's ability to seek meaning and fulfillment in life, manifest hope, and accept ambiguity and uncertainty.

- What gives your life meaning?
- Describe your sense of purpose in life.
- How does your illness affect your life goals?
- How hopeful are you about obtaining a better degree of health?
- How would you describe your role in maintaining your health?
- What kind of changes will you be able to make in your life to maintain your health?
- Describe your level of motivation to get well.
- What is the most important or powerful thing your life?

INNER STRENGTHS

These questions assess a person's ability to manifest joy and recognize strengths, choices, goals, and faith.

- What brings you joy and peace in your life?
- What can you do to feel alive and full of spirit?
- What traits do you like about yourself?
- What are your personal strengths?
- What choices are available to you to enhance your healing?
- What life goals have you set for yourself?
- What do you think is the role of stress, if any, in your illness?
- How aware were you of your body before you became sick?
- What do you believe in?
- How has your illness influenced your faith?
- How important is faith in your overall health and sense of well-being?

INTERCONNECTIONS

These questions assess a person's positive self-concept, self-esteem, and sense of self; sense of belonging in the world with others; capacity to pursue personal interests; and ability to demonstrate love of self and self-forgiveness.

- How do you feel about yourself right now?
- How do you feel when you have a true sense of yourself?
- Describe any activities of personal interest that you pursue.
- What do you do to show love for yourself?
- Can you forgive yourself?
- What do you do to heal your spirit?

RELATIONSHIPS

These questions assess a person's ability to connect in life-giving ways with family, friends, and social groups and to engage in the forgiveness of others.

- Who are the significant people in your life?
- Who are your readily available, nearby, support people?
- Who are the people to whom you are closest?
- Describe any groups in which you are an active participant.
- How comfortable are you with asking people for help when you need it?
- How comfortable are you with sharing your feelings with others?
- What are some of the most loving things that others have done for you?
- What are the loving things that you do for other people?
- What are your thoughts about forgiving others?

BEHAVIOR AND ACTIVITIES

These questions assess a person's capacity for finding meaning in worship or religious activities and a connectedness with a divinity.

- How important is worship to you?
- What do you consider the most significant act of worship in your life?
- Describe any religious activities in which you are an active participant.
- Describe any spiritual activities, if any, that you find meaningful.
- Do you find prayer meaningful?
- To whom do you turn for support?
- Describe any activities in which you engage for coping and support.
- Describe any activities in which you have previously engaged and have not found helpful.

ENVIRONMENT

These questions assess a person's ability to experience a sense of connection with life and nature, an awareness of the effects of the environment on life and well-being, and a capacity or concern for the health of the environment.

- How does your environment effect your state of well-being?
- What are your environmental stressors at work and at home?
- What strategies reduce your environmental stressors?
- Do you have any concerns for the state of your immediate environment?
- Are you involved with environmental issues such as recycling environmental resources at home, work, or in your community?
- Are you concerned about the survival of the planet?

Source: Compiled from Burkhardt, M. A. (1989). Spirituality: The analysis of the concept. *Holistic Nursing Practice, 3*(3), 69–77; Dossey, B. M., & American Holistic Nurses' Association. (1995). *Holistic nursing: A handbook for practice* (2nd ed.). Aspen; and Dossey, B. M. (1998). Holistic modalities and healing moments. *American Journal of Nursing, 98*(6), 44–47.

and significant others in the assessment process can be a great help in determining which religious beliefs and activities have been beneficial to the patient and which have been detrimental to their progress.

Diagnoses/Outcome Identification

Nursing diagnoses that may be used when addressing spiritual and religious needs of patients include the following:

■ Risk for spiritual distress
■ Spiritual distress
■ Readiness for enhanced spiritual well-being
■ Risk for impaired religiosity
■ Impaired religiosity
■ Readiness for enhanced religiosity

The following outcomes may be used as guidelines for care and to evaluate effectiveness of the nursing interventions. The patient:

■ Identifies meaning and purpose in life that reinforce hope, peace, and contentment.

■ Verbalizes acceptance of self as a worthwhile human being.
■ Accepts and incorporates change into life in a healthy manner.
■ Expresses understanding of the relationship between difficulties in current life situation and interruption in previous religious beliefs and activities.
■ Discusses beliefs and values about spiritual and religious issues.
■ Expresses desire and ability to participate in beliefs and activities of desired religion.

Planning and Implementation

Sample care plans using nursing diagnoses for spiritual distress and impaired religiosity are presented in Table 11–2.

Evaluation

Evaluation of nursing actions is directed at achievement of the established outcomes. Part of the

Table 11–2 | CARE PLAN FOR THE PATIENT WITH SPIRITUAL AND RELIGIOUS NEEDS

NURSING DIAGNOSIS: RISK FOR SPIRITUAL DISTRESS

RELATED TO: Life changes; environmental changes; stress; anxiety; depression

OUTCOME CRITERIA	NURSING INTERVENTIONS	RATIONALE
Patient identifies meaning and purpose in life that reinforce hope, peace, contentment, and self-satisfaction.	1. Assess current situation. 2. Listen to the patient's expressions of anger, concern, self-blame. 3. Note the patient's perceptions about reason for living and whether it is directly related to situation. 4. Determine the patient's religious and/or spiritual orientation, current involvement, and presence of conflicts, especially in current circumstances. 5. Assess sense of self-concept, worth, ability to enter into loving relationships. 6. Observe behavior indicative of poor relationships with others. 7. Determine support systems available to and used by the patient and significant others. 8. Assess substance use/misuse.	1–8. Thorough assessment is necessary to develop an accurate care plan.

Continued

Table 11–2 | CARE PLAN FOR THE PATIENT WITH SPIRITUAL AND RELIGIOUS NEEDS–cont'd

OUTCOME CRITERIA	NURSING INTERVENTIONS	RATIONALE
	9. Establish an environment that promotes free expression of feelings and concerns.	9. Trust is the basis of a therapeutic nurse–patient relationship.
	10. Have the patient identify and prioritize current/immediate spiritual needs.	10. Helps patients focus on what needs to be done and identify manageable steps to take.
	11. Discuss philosophical issues related to the effect of current situation on spiritual beliefs and values.	11. Helps patients to understand that certain life experiences can cause individuals to question personal values and that this response is not uncommon.
	12. Use therapeutic communication skills of reflection and active listening.	12. Helps patients explore and identify solutions to concerns.
	13. Review coping skills used and their effectiveness in current situation.	13. Identifies strengths to incorporate into plan and techniques that need revision.
	14. Provide a role model for open discussion of spiritual concerns.	14. Sharing of experiences and hope assists patients to deal with reality.
	15. Suggest use of journaling.	15. Journaling can assist in clarifying beliefs and values and in recognizing and resolving feelings about current life situation.
	16. Discuss the patient's interest in the arts, music, and literature.	16. Provides insight into meaning of these issues and how they are integrated into an individual's life.
	17. Role-play new coping techniques. Discuss possibilities of taking classes, becoming involved in discussion groups, cultural activities of the patient's choice.	17. These activities will help to enhance integration of new skills and necessary changes in the patient's lifestyle.
	18. Refer the patient to appropriate resources for spiritual support and guidance.	18. Patients may require additional assistance with an individual who specializes in these types of concerns.

NURSING DIAGNOSIS: RISK FOR IMPAIRED RELIGIOSITY
RELATED TO: Suffering; depression; illness; life transitions

OUTCOME CRITERIA	NURSING INTERVENTIONS	RATIONALE
Patient expresses achievement of support and personal satisfaction from spiritual and/or religious practices.	1. Assess current situation (e.g., illness, hospitalization, prognosis of death, presence of support systems, financial concerns).	1. This information identifies problems the patient is dealing with in the moment that is affecting desire to be involved with religious activities.

Table 11–2 | CARE PLAN FOR THE PATIENT WITH SPIRITUAL AND RELIGIOUS NEEDS—cont'd

OUTCOME CRITERIA	NURSING INTERVENTIONS	RATIONALE
	2. Listen nonjudgmentally to the patient's expressions of anger and possible belief that illness or condition may be a result of lack of faith.	2. Individuals often blame themselves for what has happened and reject previous religious beliefs and/or God.
	3. Determine the patient's usual religious and/or spiritual beliefs, current involvement in specific church activities.	3. This information is important background for establishing a database about the patient's impaired religiosity.
	4. Note quality of relationships with significant others and friends.	4. Individuals may withdraw from others in relation to the stress of illness, pain, and suffering.
	5. Assess substance use/misuse.	5. When in distress, individuals may turn to use of various substances, which can affect the ability to deal with problems in a positive manner.
	6. Develop nurse–patient relationship in which the individual can express feelings and concerns freely.	6. Trust is the basis for a therapeutic nurse–patient relationship.
	7. Use therapeutic communication skills of active listening, reflection, and "I" messages.	7. Helps patients explore and identify solutions to problems and concerns and promotes sense of control.
	8. Be accepting and nonjudgmental when the patient expresses anger and bitterness toward God. Stay with the patient.	8. The nurse's presence and nonjudgmental attitude increase the patient's feelings of self-worth and promote trust in the relationship.
	9. Encourage the patient to discuss previous religious practices and how these practices provided support in the past.	9. A nonjudgmental discussion of previous sources of support may help the patient work through current rejection of them as potential sources of support.
	10. Allow the patient to take the lead in initiating participation in religious activities, such as prayer.	10. Patients may be vulnerable in current situation and need to be allowed to decide own resumption of these actions.
	11. Contact spiritual leader of patient's choice, if they request one.	11. These individuals serve to provide relief from spiritual distress and often can do so when other support persons cannot.

Source: The interventions for this care plan were adapted from Doenges, M. E., Moorhouse, M. F., & Murr, A. C. (2022). *Nursing diagnosis manual: Planning, individualizing, and documenting client care* (7th ed.). F.A. Davis.

evaluation process is continuous reassessment to ensure that the selected actions are appropriate and the goals and outcomes are realistic. Including the family and extended support systems in the evaluation process is essential if spiritual and religious implications of nursing care are to be measured. Modifications to the plan of care are made as the need is determined.

Summary and Key Points

■ Selected psychosocial therapies include psychoanalysis, interpersonal psychotherapy, reality therapy, cognitive behavior therapy, and dialectical behavior therapy. Advanced practice psychiatric nurses may use some of these therapies in their practices.

■ Generalist psychiatric nurses play active roles in milieu therapy and educating patients about relaxation and assertiveness skills.

■ In psychiatry, milieu therapy (or the therapeutic community) constitutes a manipulation of the environment to create behavioral changes and to improve the psychological health and functioning of the individual.

■ The goal of a therapeutic community is for the patient to learn adaptive coping, interaction, and relationship skills that can be generalized to other aspects of their life.

■ Six principles for establishing therapeutic milieu as a practice model for nurses in any health-care setting are contagious calmness, respect for inherent human dignity, nurse's care for self and others, intellectual engagement, caritas, and maintaining safe and restorative physical surroundings (Meehan, 2020).

■ Spirituality is the human quality that gives meaning and sense of purpose to an individual's existence.

■ Individuals possess a number of spiritual needs that include meaning and purpose in life, faith or trust in someone or something beyond themselves, hope, love, and forgiveness.

■ Religion is a set of beliefs, values, rites, and rituals adopted by a group of people.

■ Religion is one way in which an individual's spirituality may be expressed.

■ Affiliation with a religious group has been shown to be a health-enhancing endeavor.

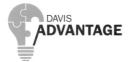

DAVIS ADVANTAGE | Go to **Davis Advantage** to complete your learning: strengthen understanding, apply your knowledge, and prepare for the Next Gen NCLEX®.

Review Questions

1. Interpersonal psychotherapy assumes that a client's psychiatric disorder is related to:
   a. Irrational, automatic thought patterns
   b. Emotional dysregulation
   c. Difficulties in relationships
   d. Negative reinforcement

2. Which of the following are basic assumptions of milieu therapy? (Select all that apply.)
   a. Individuals own their own environment.
   b. Individuals own their own behavior.
   c. Peer pressure is a useful and powerful tool.
   d. Inappropriate behaviors are punished immediately.

3. Within the therapeutic milieu of an inpatient psychiatric unit, duties of the staff psychiatric nurse include which of the following? (Select all that apply.)
   a. Medication administration
   b. Client teaching
   c. Medical diagnosis
   d. Reality orientation
   e. Relationship development
   f. Group therapy

4. Relaxation therapy is composed of a variety of interventions designed to:
   a. Educate the client to reframe automatic thought distortions
   b. Reduce the stress response
   c. Decrease oxygen intake
   d. Treat epilepsy

Clinical Judgment Questions

5. In a medication education group, which of the following actions is most important for reinforcing the therapeutic milieu?
   a. Allowing each person a specific and equal amount of time to talk
   b. Reviewing group rules and behavioral limits that apply to all clients
   c. Reading the medication information
   d. Restricting the group to only those clients who are currently adhering to medication schedules

6. One of the goals of therapeutic milieu is for clients to become more independent and accept self-responsibility. Which of the following approaches by staff best encourages the fulfillment of this goal?
   a. Including client input and decisions into the treatment plan
   b. Insisting that each client take a turn leading a group activity
   c. Making decisions for the client regarding plans for treatment
   d. Requiring that the client bathe, dress, and attend breakfast on time each morning

7. A client admitted to the inpatient psychiatric unit appears anxious and states, "I've never been on a unit like this before." Which action by the nurse is a priority for beginning to establish a therapeutic milieu?
   a. Instruct the client to remain in their room until they feel less anxious.
   b. Orient the client to the physical surroundings, milieu rules, and activities.
   c. Offer to medicate the client with antianxiety medication.
   d. Instruct the client not to worry because they will only be on the unit for a few days.

8. A client approaches the nurse and says, "I'm sick of the rules on this unit about not touching each other. I'm an adult and if I want to give one of the ladies a massage, it's my own business." Which of these responses best incorporates milieu therapy principles?
   a. "If you don't follow the established rules, you will be put in seclusion."
   b. "You don't make the rules, so just do as you're told."
   c. "Why are you on this unit?"
   d. "Let me try to explain why these rules are important for everyone's safety."

9. A client reports feeling "anxious all the time" but doesn't want to take the benzodiazepine medication prescribed by their family physician. Which of these is the most appropriate action for the nurse to take next?
   a. Instruct the client to continue to take the prescribed medication for several weeks in order to begin to feel relaxed.
   b. Recommend that the client begin using melatonin nightly.
   c. Assess whether the client has tried relaxation exercises or meditation.
   d. Provide medical massage therapy.

10. A fellow nurse approaches you and states, "Since you knew I was swamped you could have offered to pass my medications. You are so lazy!" Which response by the nurse is most assertive?
    a. "I'm sorry you're feeling overwhelmed. I'll try to be more sensitive next time."
    b. "You're the lazy one. I've got my own work to do."
    c. "I will go ahead and pass your medications this time, but in the future, you need to stop talking to me that way."
    d. "I deserve to be treated with respect and I will not be bullied into doing your work."

11. A client who has come to the mental health clinic with symptoms of depression says to the nurse, "My father is dying. I have always hated my father. He physically abused me when I was a child. We haven't spoken for many years. He wants to see me now, but I don't know if I want to see him." Which nursing diagnoses is a priority?
    a. Spiritual distress
    b. Risk for physical injury
    c. Altered mental status
    d. Risk for self-harm

12. As a child, a client was physically abused by their father. The father is now dying and has expressed a desire to see his child before he dies. The patient is depressed and says to the mental health nurse, "I'm so angry! Why did God have to give me a father like this? I feel cheated of a father! I've always been a good person. I deserved better. I hate God!" Which nursing intervention is a priority?
    a. Ask the client why they think God gave him such an abusive father.
    b. Instruct the client to set aside their feelings temporarily to meet the needs of their dying father.
    c. Ask the client to describe in detail how they were physically abused.
    d. Ask the client if they would be willing to talk with a chaplain.

References

American Holistic Nurses Association & American Nurses Association. (2019). *Holistic nursing: Scope and standards of practice.* (3rd ed.).

American Nurses Association, American Psychiatric Nurses Association, & International Society of Psychiatric Nurses. (2022). *Psychiatric-mental health nursing: Scope and standards of practice.* (3rd ed.). Nursesbooks.org

Balboni, M., & Balboni, T. (2019). *Do spirituality and medicine go together? When exploring the indelible connection between medicine and spirituality, follow the evidence.* https://bioethics.hms.harvard.edu/journal/spirituality-medicine

Bhat, S., Rentala, S., Nanjegowda, R. B., & Chellappan, X. B. (2020). Effectiveness of milieu therapy in reducing conflicts and containment rates among schizophrenia patients. *Investigacion y Educacion en Enfermeria, 38*(1), e06. doi: 10.17533/udea.iee.v38n1e06

Bogousslavsky, J., & Inglin, M. (2007). Beliefs and the brain. *European Neurology, 58,* 129–132.

Bronson, M. (2005). *Why are there so many religions?* http://www.biblehelp.org/relig.htm

Ciompi, L., & Hoffman, H. (2004). Soteria Berne: An innovative milieu therapeutic approach to acute schizophrenia based on the concept of affect-logic. *World Psychiatry, 3*(3), 140–146.

Clark, M., & Emerson, A. (2021). Spirituality in psychiatric nursing: A concept analysis. *Journal of the American Psychiatric Nurses Association, 27*(1), p. 22–32.

Crane, M. (2023). *Interpersonal therapy for mood disorders and substance abuse.* https://recovery.org/treatment-therapy/interpersonal/

Doenges, M. E., Moorhouse, M. F., & Murr, A. C. (2022). *Nursing diagnosis manual: Planning, individualizing, and documenting client care* (7th ed.). F.A. Davis.

Enayati, A. (2013). *How hope can help you heal.* https://www.cnn.com/2013/04/11/health/hope-healing-enayati/index.html

Guynn, R. W. (2017). Interpersonal psychotherapy. In Sadock, B. J., Sadock, V. A., & Ruiz, P. (Eds.), *Comprehensive textbook of psychiatry* (10th ed., pp. 2775–2784). Wolters Kluwer.

Harrison, P. (2011). *Forgiveness can improve immune function.* http://www.medscape.com/viewarticle/742198

Harvard Health. (2021). *The power of the placebo effect.* https://www.health.harvard.edu/mental-health/the-power-of-the-placebo-effect

Herdman, T. H., Kamitsuru, S., & Lopes, C. T. (Eds.). (2021). *NANDA-I, Inc. nursing diagnoses: Definitions and classification, 2021–2023* (12th ed.). Thieme.

International Council of Nurses. (2021). *The ICN code of ethics for nurses.* https://www.icn.ch/system/files/2021-10/ICN_Code-of-Ethics_EN_Web_0.pdf

Jones, D. R., & Graham-Engeland, J. E. (2021). Positive affect and peripheral inflammatory markers among adults: A narrative review. *Psychoneuroendocrinology,123.* https://doi.org/10.1016/j.psyneuen.2020.104892

Jones, J. (2019). *U.S. church membership down sharply in past two decades.* Gallup. https://news.gallup.com/poll/248837/church-membership-down-sharply-past-two-decades.aspx?g

Karren, K. J., Hafen, B. Q., Smith, N. L., & Jenkins, K. J. (2010). *Mind/body health: The effects of attitudes, emotions, and relationships* (4th ed.). Benjamin Cummings.

Karren, K. J., Smith, N. L., Gordon, K., & Frandsen, K. J. (2013). *Mind/body health: The effects of attitudes, emotions, and relationships* (5th ed.). Pearson.

Klonsky, D. E., & May, A. M., (2015). The three-step theory (3ST): A new theory of suicide rooted in the "ideation to action" framework. *International Journal of Cognitive Therapy, 8*(2), 114–129. https://doi.org/10.1521/ijct.2015.8.2.114

Koenig, H. G. (2012). Religion, spirituality, and health: The research and clinical implications. *International Scholarly Research Notices, 2012.* https://doi.org/10.5402/2012/278730

Kvarnstrom, E. (2017). *A social treatment: Mental health benefits of milieu therapy for people living with schizophrenia.* https://www.brightquest.com/blog/a-social-treatment-mental-health-benefits-of-milieu-therapy-for-people-living-with-schizophrenia/

Lavorato-Neto, G., Rodrigues, L., Turato, E. R., & Campos, C. J. G. (2018). The free spirit: Spiritualism meanings by a nursing team on psychiatry. *Revista Brasileira Enfermagem, 71*(2), 280–288. doi: http://dx.doi.org/10.1590/0034-7167-2016-0428

Levin, J. (2010). Religion and mental health: Theory and research. *International Journal of Applied Psychoanalytic Studies, 7*(2), 102–115. https://doi.org/10.1002/aps.240

Lichter, D. A. (2013, March-April). Studies show spiritual care linked to better health outcomes. *Health Progress.* https://www.chausa.org/publications/health-progress/article/march-april-2013/studies-show-spiritual-care-linked-to-better-health-outcomes

Liefbroer, A. I., Ganzevoort, R. R., & Olsman, E. (2019). Addressing the spiritual domain in a plural society: What is the best mode of integrating spiritual care into healthcare? *Mental Health, Religion & Culture, 22*(3), 244–260. https://doi.org/10.1080/13674676.2019.1590806

Mayo Clinic. (2022). *Forgiveness: Letting go of grudges and bitterness.* http://www.mayoclinic.org/healthy-lifestyle/adult-health/in-depth/forgiveness/art-20047692

Meehan, T. C. (2020). *The therapeutic milieu.* https://www.carefulnursing.ie/go/overview/professional_practice_model/therapeutic_milieu

Menninger Clinic. (2022). *Adolescent treatment program.* https://www.menningerclinic.org/treatment/treatment-for-children-adolescents/inpatient-programs/adolescent-treatment-program

Murray, D. R., Haselton, M. G., Fales, M., & Cole, S. W. (2019). Falling in love is associated with immune system gene regulation. *Psychoneuroendocrinology 100,* 120–126. https://doi.org/10.1016/j.psyneuen.2018.09.043

National Institutes of Health. (2015). *How are therapeutic communities integrated into the criminal justice system?* https://www.drugabuse.gov/publications/research-reports/therapeutic-communities/how-are-therapeutic-communities-integrated-criminal-justice-system

Neathery, M., He, Z., Johnston Taylor, E., & Deal, B. (2020). Spiritual perspectives, spiritual care, and knowledge of recovery among psychiatric mental health nurses. *Journal of the American Psychiatric Nurses Association 26*(1), 364–372. https://doi.org/10.1177/1078390319846548

O-School. (2022). *The six components of modern milieu therapy.* https://www.oschool.org/about/blog/haven-and-hope/~board/haven-and-hope/post/the-six-components-of-modern-milieu-therapy

Pace, T. W., Negi, T. L., Adame, D. D., Cole, S. P., Sivilli, T. I., Brown, T. D., Issa, M. J., & Raison, C. L. (2009). Effect of compassion meditation on neuroendocrine, innate immune and behavioral responses to psychosocial stress. *Psychoneuroendocrinology, 34*(1), 87–98. https://doi.org/10.1016/j.psyneuen.2008.08.011

Pew Research Center. (2017). *The changing global religious landscape.* https://www.pewresearch.org/religion/2017/04/05/the-changing-global-religious-landscape/

Reeves, R., & Reynolds, M. (2009). What is the role of spirituality in mental health treatment? *Journal of Psychosocial Nursing, 54*(5), 8–9. https://doi.org/10.3928/02793695-20090301-05

Sathyanarayana Rao, T. S., Asha, M. R., Jagannatha Rao, K. S., & Vasudevaraju, P. (2009). The biochemistry of belief. *Indian Journal of Psychiatry, 51*(4), 239–241. https://doi.org/10.4103/0019-5545.58285

Tétreault, P., Mansour, A., Vachon-Presseau, E., Schnitzer, T. J., Apkarian, A. V., & Baliki, M. N. (2016). Brain connectivity predicts placebo response across chronic pain clinical trials. *PLoS Biology 14*(10), e1002570. https://doi.org/10.1371/journal.pbio.1002570

Thaik, C. (2013). *Love heals!* http://www.huffingtonpost.com/dr-cynthia-thaik/love-health-benefits_b_3131370.html

Valley View. (2022). *Therapeutic milieu.* https://www.valleyviewschool.org/Therapeutic-Milieu

CLASSICAL REFERENCES

Beck, A. (1976). *Cognitive therapy and the emotional disorders.* Penguin Books.

Burkhardt, M. A. (1989). Spirituality: The analysis of the concept. *Holistic Nursing Practice, 3*(3), 69–77.

Dossey, B. M. (1998). Holistic modalities and healing moments. *American Journal of Nursing, 98*(6), 44–47.

Dossey, B. M., & American Holistic Nurses' Association. (1995). *Holistic nursing: A handbook for practice* (2nd ed.). Aspen.

Erikson, E. H. (1950). *Childhood and society.* Norton.

Glasser, W. (1965). *Reality therapy: A new approach to psychiatry.* Harper & Row.

Gunderson, J. G. (1978). Defining the therapeutic processes in psychiatric milieus. *Psychiatry: Interpersonal and Biological Processes, 41*(4), 327–335.

Kübler-Ross, E. (1969). *On death and dying.* Macmillan.

Linehan, M. M. (1993). *Cognitive-behavioral treatment of borderline personality disorder.* Guilford Press.

Nekolaichuk, C. L., Jevne, R. F., & Maguire, T. O. (1999). Structuring the meaning of hope in health and illness. *Social Science and Medicine, 48*(5), 591–605. http://doi.org/10.1016/S0277-9536(98)00348-7

Ornish, D. (1998). *Love and survival: Eight pathways to intimacy and health.* Harper Perennial.

Rogers, C. (1951). *Client-centered therapy: Its current practice, implications and theory.* Constable.

Skinner, B. F. (1979). *Beyond freedom and dignity.* Knopf.

Smucker, C. J. (2001). Overview of nursing the spirit. In Wilt D. L., & Smucker, C. J. (Eds.), *Nursing the spirit: The art and science of applying spiritual care* (pp. 1–18). American Nurses.

Sullivan, H. S. (1953). *The interpersonal theory of psychiatry.* W.W. Norton and Company.

Walsh, R. (1999). *Essential spirituality.* Wiley.

Werner, E. E., & Smith, R. S. (1992). *Overcoming the odds: High risk children from birth to adulthood.* Cornell University Press.

12 Crisis Intervention

KEY TERMS

crisis intervention

disaster

OBJECTIVES

After reading this chapter, the student will be able to:

1. Define *crisis.*
2. Describe four phases in the development of a crisis.
3. Identify types of crises that occur in people's lives.
4. Discuss the goal of crisis intervention.
5. Describe the steps in crisis intervention.
6. Identify the role of the nurse in crisis intervention.
7. Apply the nursing process to care for victims of disasters.

Stressful situations are part of everyday life. Any stressful situation can precipitate a crisis. Crises result in a disequilibrium from which many individuals require assistance to recover. **Crisis intervention** is a short-term approach focused on managing the immediate needs of the client and minimizing the negative consequences that often follow unmanaged or unresolved crises. Assistance with problem-solving during the crisis period preserves self-esteem and promotes growth with resolution.

In recent years, individuals in the United States have been faced with a number of catastrophic events, including a worldwide pandemic, and natural disasters such as tornados, earthquakes, hurricanes, and floods. Man-made disasters, such as the Oklahoma City and Boston Marathon bombings, the attacks on the World Trade Center and the Pentagon, and mass shootings have created considerable psychological stress in populations around the world.

This chapter examines the phases in the development of a crisis and the types of crises that occur in people's lives. The methodology of crisis intervention, including the role of the nurse, is explored. A discussion of disaster nursing is also presented.

CORE CONCEPT

Crisis

An acute event perceived by the individual as distressing and in which coping mechanisms and support systems are inadequate to manage associated anxiety.

Characteristics of a Crisis

The concept of crisis has several defining characteristics (Aguilera, 1998; Caplan, 1964):

1. Crisis occurs in all individuals at one time or another and is not necessarily equated with psychopathology.
2. Crises are precipitated by specific, identifiable events.
3. Crises are personal by nature. What may be considered a crisis situation by one individual may not be so for another.
4. Crises are acute, not chronic, and will be resolved in one way or another within a brief period.
5. A crisis situation contains the potential for psychological growth or deterioration.

Individuals who are in crisis feel helpless to change. They do not believe they have the resources to cope with the precipitating stressor. Levels of anxiety rise to the point that the individual becomes nonfunctional, thoughts become obsessional, and all behavior is aimed at relief of the anxiety being experienced. The feeling is overwhelming and may affect the individual physically as well as psychologically.

Bateman and Peternelj-Taylor (1998) stated:

Outside Western culture, a crisis is often viewed as a time for movement and growth. The Chinese symbol for crisis consists of the characters for *danger* and *opportunity* [Fig. 12–1]. When a crisis is viewed as an opportunity for growth, those involved are much more capable of resolving related issues and more able to move toward positive changes. When the crisis experience is overwhelming because of its scope and nature or when there has not been adequate preparation for the necessary changes, the dangers seem paramount and overshadow any potential growth. The results are maladaptive coping and dysfunctional behavior. (pp. 144–145)

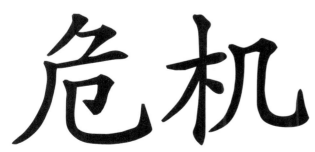

FIGURE 12–1   Chinese symbol for crisis.

Phases in the Development of a Crisis

The development of a crisis follows a relatively predictable course. Caplan (1964) outlined four phases through which individuals progress in response to a precipitating stressor and that culminate in the state of acute crisis.

Phase 1: *The individual is exposed to a precipitating stressor.* Anxiety increases; previous problem-solving techniques are employed.

Phase 2: *When previous problem-solving techniques do not relieve the stressor, anxiety increases further.* The individual begins to feel a great deal of discomfort at this point. Coping techniques that have worked in the past are attempted, only to create feelings of helplessness when they are not successful. Feelings of confusion and disorganization prevail.

Phase 3: *All possible resources, both internal and external, are called on to resolve the problem and relieve the discomfort.* The individual may try to view the problem from a different perspective or even to overlook certain aspects of it. New problem-solving techniques may be used, and, if effective, resolution may occur at this phase, with the individual returning to a higher, a lower, or the previous level of precrisis functioning.

Phase 4: *If resolution does not occur in previous phases, Caplan states that "the tension mounts beyond a further threshold or its burden increases over time to a breaking point. Major disorganization of the individual with drastic results often occurs"* (p. 41). Anxiety may reach panic levels. Cognitive functions are disordered, emotions are labile, and behavior may reflect the presence of psychotic thinking.

These phases are congruent with the transactional model of stress adaptation outlined in Chapter 1, "The Concept of Stress Adaptation." The relationship between the two perspectives is presented in Figure 12–2. When an individual perceives a stressor as a threat to their well-being and lacks adaptive coping strategies or employs maladaptive strategies, crisis ensues. Similarly, Aguilera (1998) spoke of "balancing factors" that affect how an individual perceives and responds to a precipitating stressor. A schematic of these balancing factors is illustrated in Figure 12–3.

The paradigm set forth by Aguilera suggests that whether or not an individual experiences a crisis in response to a stressful situation depends on the following three factors:

1. **The individual's perception of the event:** If the event is perceived realistically, the individual is

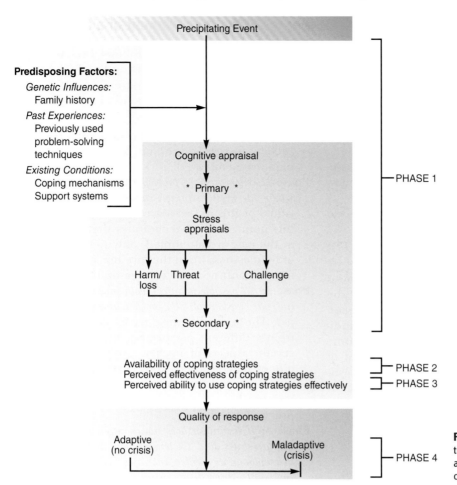

FIGURE 12–2 Relationship between transactional model of stress/adaptation and Caplan's phases in the development of a crisis.

more likely to draw upon adequate resources to restore equilibrium. If the perception of the event is distorted, attempts at problem-solving are likely to be ineffective, and equilibrium is not restored.

2. **The availability of situational supports:** Aguilera stated, "Situational supports are those persons who are available in the environment and who can be depended on to help solve the problem" (p. 37). Without adequate situational supports during a stressful situation, an individual is most likely to feel overwhelmed and alone.

3. **The availability of adequate coping mechanisms:** When a stressful situation occurs, individuals draw upon behavioral strategies that have been successful for them in the past. If these coping strategies work, a crisis may be diverted. If not, disequilibrium may continue and tension and anxiety increase.

Crises are acute, time-limited situations that will be resolved in one way or another within 1 to 3 months. Crises can become growth opportunities when individuals learn new methods of coping that can be preserved and used when similar stressors recur. However, when new coping mechanisms or balancing factors are not identified and incorporated, the crisis can evolve into longer-term problems and sometimes symptoms of emotional or mental illness, including depression, anxiety, and trauma/stressor-related disorders.

Types of Crises

Baldwin (1978) identified six classes of emotional crises, which progress by degree of severity. As the measure of psychopathology increases, the source of the stressor changes from external to internal. The type of crisis determines the method of intervention selected.

Class 1: Dispositional Crises

Definition An acute response to an external situational stressor.

Example

Brittany and Ethan have been married for 3 years and have a 1-year-old daughter. Ethan has been having difficulty with his boss at work. Twice during the past

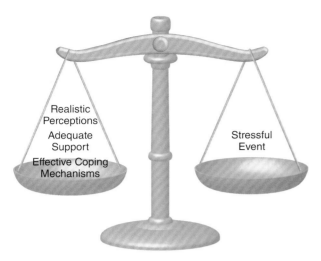

Stressful event is balanced by realistic perceptions, adequate support, effective coping mechanisms ➡ Equilibrium ➡ **No crisis**

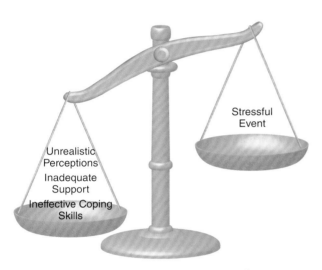

Problem unresolved ➡ Disequilibrium ➡ **Crisis**

FIGURE 12–3 The effect of balancing factors in a stressful event.

6 months, he has exploded in anger at home and become abusive with Brittany. Last night he became angry that dinner was not ready when he expected. He grabbed the baby from Brittany and tossed her, screaming, into her crib. He hit and punched Brittany until she feared for her life. This morning when he left for work, she took the baby and went to the emergency department of the city hospital, not knowing what else to do.

Intervention Physical care of wounds and screening for domestic violence issues should be conducted in the emergency department. The mental health counselor can provide support and guidance in terms of presenting alternatives for managing the health and safety of Brittany and her child. The emergency department nurse should encourage and empower Brittany to clarify her needs and issues so referrals for agency assistance can be made.

Class 2: Crises of Anticipated Life Transitions

Definition Normal life cycle transitions that are anticipated but over which the individual may feel a lack of control.

Example

College student J.T. is placed on probationary status because of low grades this semester. His wife had a baby and had to quit her job. He had increased his working hours from part time to full time to compensate and therefore had little time for studies. He presents himself to the student-health nurse practitioner complaining of numerous vague physical complaints.

Intervention Physical examination should be performed (physical symptoms could be caused by depression) and expression of feelings encouraged. Reassurance and support should be provided as needed. J.T. should be referred to services that can provide financial and other types of assistance. Problematic areas should be identified and approaches to change discussed.

Class 3: Crises Resulting from Traumatic Stress

Definition Crisis precipitated by an unexpected external stressor over which the individual has little or no control and as a result of which they feel emotionally overwhelmed and defeated.

Example

Ava is a doctor whose last shift ended at midnight 2 weeks ago. At that point, while walking to her car, she was abducted by two men with guns, taken to an abandoned building, and raped and beaten. Since that time, her physical wounds have nearly healed. However, Ava cannot be alone; is constantly fearful; relives the experience in flashbacks and dreams; and is unable to eat, sleep, or work at her job in the hospital. Her friend offers to accompany her to the mental health clinic.

Intervention The nurse should offer Ava the opportunity to talk about the experience and express her feelings about the trauma when she demonstrates readiness. The nurse should offer reassurance and support and discuss how rape may precipitate feelings of loss, including loss of control, power, and sense of self-worth, that trigger the grief response. After a discussion of the stages of grief, the nurse should identify support systems that can help Ava to resume her normal activities and explore new methods of coping with emotions arising from a situation with which she has had no previous experience. These interventions should be conducted in an environment that is sensitive to the effect of trauma on a person's sense of self, and all interventions should convey dignity, respect, and hopefulness and promote the patient's empowerment to make choices in their care (Substance Abuse and Mental Health Services Administration [SAMHSA], 2014). See Chapter 28, "Trauma- and Stressor-Related Disorders," for more information on trauma-informed care.

Class 4: Maturational/Developmental Crises

Definition Crises that occur in response to failed attempts to master developmental tasks associated with transitions in the life cycle.

Example

Jada and Caleb have been married for 2 years, and their firstborn child is 4 months old. Jada's mother was recently diagnosed with cancer, and the prognosis is unclear. Over the past 3 weeks, Jada has become increasingly anxious and disorganized, calling the nurse practitioner 10 to 15 times each day with new fears that she is not addressing her child's health needs. Jada has been screaming at Caleb that he is never there when she needs help with the baby and states she is thinking of dropping their child off at the Children's Service Agency because she believes they are both unable to be good parents. She agrees to see a counselor at Caleb's insistence.

Intervention The primary intervention is to help Jada with anxiety reduction. When individuals have intense anxiety, their ability to gain insight about contributing factors and explore options for behavior change is impaired. The safety of their child should also be carefully assessed. Referrals and guidance in parenting skills may lessen the anxiety associated with this new developmental phase. Anxiety and grief related to Jada's mother's illness could also be explored as a possible factor contributing to the current crisis.

Class 5: Crises Reflecting Psychopathology

Definition A crisis that is influenced or triggered by preexisting psychopathology. Examples of psychopathology that may precipitate crises include personality disorders, anxiety disorders, bipolar disorder, and schizophrenia.

Example

Sonja, age 29, was diagnosed with borderline personality disorder at age 18. This disorder is believed to be rooted in a deep fear of abandonment. She has been in weekly therapy for 10 years, with several hospitalizations for suicide attempts during that time. She has had the same therapist for the past 6 years. This therapist told Sonja today that she is to be married in 1 month and will be moving across the country with her new husband. Sonja is distraught, stating that no one cares about her and that she would be better off dead. She is found wandering in and out of traffic on a busy expressway, oblivious to her surroundings. Police bring her to the emergency department of the hospital.

Intervention The initial intervention is aimed at helping Sonja to reduce her anxiety. She requires that someone stay with her and reassure her of her safety and security. After the feelings of panic and anxiety have subsided, she should be encouraged to verbalize her feelings of abandonment. Regressive behaviors should be discouraged. Positive reinforcement should be given for independent activities and accomplishments. The primary therapist will need to pursue this issue of termination with Sonja and facilitate transfer of services to another therapist or treatment program. Hospitalization may be necessary to maintain patient safety.

Class 6: Psychiatric Emergencies

Definition Crisis situations in which general functioning has been severely impaired and the individual is rendered incompetent or unable to assume personal responsibility for their behavior. Examples include acute suicide risk, drug overdose, reactions to hallucinogenic drugs, acute psychoses, uncontrollable anger, and alcohol intoxication.

Example

Olivia, age 14, had been dating Liam, the star high school football player, for 6 months. After the game on Friday night, Olivia and Liam went to Alexandra's house, where several high school students had gathered for an after-game party. No adults were present. About midnight, Liam told Olivia that he did not want to date her anymore. Olivia became hysterical, and Alexandra was frightened by her behavior. She took Olivia to her parent's bedroom and gave her a Valium from a bottle in her mother's medicine cabinet. She left Olivia lying on her parent's bed and returned to the party downstairs. About an hour later, she returned to her parent's bedroom and found that Olivia had removed the bottle of Valium from the cabinet and swallowed all of the tablets. Olivia was unconscious, and Alexandra could not awaken her. An ambulance was called, and Olivia was transported to the local hospital.

Intervention Emergency medical care, including monitoring vital signs, ensuring maintenance of adequate airway, and initiating gastric lavage or activated charcoal, is the priority in this case. Olivia is a minor, so notifying the parents is essential as well. Inpatient hospitalization is justifiable to ensure patient safety. Discussing feelings about self-esteem, rejection, and loss will help Olivia explore more adaptive methods of dealing with stressful situations.

Crisis Intervention

Individuals experiencing crises have an urgent need for assistance. In crisis intervention, the therapist or other intervener becomes part of the individual's life situation. Because of the individual's emotional state, they are unable to problem solve and consequently require guidance and support from another to help mobilize the resources needed to resolve the crisis.

Lengthy psychological interpretations are not appropriate for crisis intervention. It is a time for doing what is needed to help the individual get relief and for calling into action all the people and resources required to do so. Aguilera (1998) stated:

> The goal of crisis intervention is the resolution of an immediate crisis. Its focus is on the supportive, with the restoration of the individual to his precrisis level of functioning or possibly to a higher level of functioning. The therapist's role is direct, supportive, and that of an active participant. (p. 24)

Crisis intervention takes place in inpatient settings, outpatient settings, and the community. In the past few decades, people with mental illness have been increasingly involved with criminal justice personnel as first responders to manage mental health crisis situations. In 1988, the fatal shooting by police officers of a man with mental illness prompted the development of the *crisis intervention team (CIT) model* to ensure that a subset of police officers are trained to identify mental illness and substance abuse, use de-escalation techniques, and divert individuals from criminal justice systems to mental health professionals (Watson & Fulambarker, 2012). Not all states have CIT training programs, but several studies have demonstrated improved safety outcomes for patients with mental illness where CIT-trained officers are available (National Alliance on Mental Illness, 2022). Other resources that may be available for patients with mental illness who are experiencing an acute crisis include 24-hour crisis phone lines, walk-in crisis centers, mobile crisis teams, respite and residential services, and hospital services, including emergency departments and 23-hour observation beds. Nurses have a responsibility to know what resources exist in their community of practice. They can then become advocates for crisis intervention training in communities and provide support to families by encouraging them to ask for CIT-trained police officers (where available) when faced with a family member's psychiatric crisis.

A more recent development in some states, counties, and mental health facilities is to use *peer support specialists*. These individuals have personal experience with mental illness and are trained or credentialed to help clients navigate everyday challenges of living with a mental illness. Evidence has demonstrated their effectiveness in several aspects of mental health care and treatment including diffusing psychiatric crises, reducing hospitalizations, empowering the client, and enhancing social network support (Bouchery et al., 2018; Puschner et al., 2019; Shalaby & Agyapong, 2020; White et al., 2020), all of which may be beneficial in crisis intervention.

The basic methodology for crisis intervention by health-care professionals relies on orderly problem-solving techniques and structured activities focused on change. Through adaptive change, crises are resolved, and growth occurs. Because of the time limit of crisis intervention, the individual must experience some degree of relief almost from the first interaction. Crisis intervention, then, is not aimed at major personality change or reconstruction (as may be the case in long-term psychotherapy), but rather at using a given crisis to restore functioning and at most to enhance personal growth.

Phases of Crisis Intervention: The Role of the Nurse

Nurses respond to crisis situations on a daily basis. Crises can occur in every unit in the general hospital, home setting, community health-care setting, schools and offices, and private practice. Nurses may be called on to function as crisis helpers in virtually any setting committed to the practice of nursing.

Aguilera (1998) described four phases in the technique of crisis intervention that are clearly comparable to the steps of the nursing process. These phases are discussed in the following paragraphs.

Phase 1. Assessment

In this phase, the nurse gathers information regarding the precipitating stressor and the resulting crisis that prompted the individual to seek professional help. In crisis intervention the nurse might perform some of the following assessments:

■ Ask the individual to describe the event that precipitated this crisis.
■ Determine when it occurred.
■ Assess the individual's mental *and* physical status.
■ Determine whether the individual has experienced this stressor before. If so, what method of

coping was used? Have these methods been tried this time?
- If previous coping methods were tried, what was the result?
- If new coping methods were tried, what was the result?
- Assess suicide or homicide potential, plan, and means.
- Assess the adequacy of support systems.
- Determine the level of the individual's precrisis functioning. Assess the usual coping methods, available support systems, and ability to problem solve.
- Assess the individual's perception of personal strengths and limitations.
- Assess the individual's use of substances.

Next, information from the comprehensive assessment is analyzed, and appropriate nursing diagnoses reflecting the immediacy of the crisis situation are identified. Some nursing diagnoses that may be relevant include the following:

- Ineffective coping
- Anxiety (severe to panic)
- Disturbed thought processes
- Risk for self- or other-directed violence
- Rape-trauma syndrome
- Post-trauma syndrome
- Fear

Phase 2. Planning of Therapeutic Intervention

In the planning phase of crisis intervention, the nurse selects the appropriate nursing actions for the identified nursing diagnoses. In planning the interventions, the type of crisis, as well as the individual's strengths, desired choices, and available resources for support, are considered. Goals are established for crisis resolution and a return to or increase in the precrisis level of functioning.

Phase 3. Intervention

During phase 3, the actions identified in phase 2 are implemented. The following interventions are the focus of nursing in crisis intervention:

- Use a reality-oriented approach. The focus of the problem is on the here and now.
- Remain with the individual experiencing panic anxiety.
- Establish a rapid working relationship by showing unconditional acceptance, active listening, and attending to immediate needs.
- Discourage lengthy explanations or rationalizations of the situation; promote an atmosphere for verbalization of true feelings.

- Set firm limits on aggressive, destructive behaviors. At high levels of anxiety, behavior is likely to be impulsive and regressive. Establish at the outset what is acceptable and what is not and maintain consistency.
- Clarify the problem the individual is facing by describing the problem and comparing it with the individual's perception of the problem.
- Help the individual determine what they believe precipitated the crisis.
- Acknowledge feelings of anger, guilt, helplessness, and powerlessness without judgment.
- Guide the individual through a problem-solving process by which they may move in the direction of positive life change:
  - Help the individual confront the factors that are contributing to the experience of crisis.
  - Encourage the individual to discuss changes they would like to make. Jointly determine whether or not desired changes are realistic.
  - Encourage exploration of feelings about aspects of the situation that cannot be changed and explore alternative ways of coping more adaptively in these situations.
  - Discuss alternative strategies for creating changes that are realistically possible.
  - Weigh the benefits and consequences of each alternative.
  - Assist the individual in selecting alternative coping strategies that will help alleviate future crisis situations.
- Identify external support systems and new social networks from which the individual may seek assistance in times of stress.

> **CLINICAL PEARL** Coping mechanisms are highly individual, and the choice ultimately must be made by the patient. The nurse may offer suggestions and provide guidance to help the patient identify realistic coping mechanisms that can promote positive outcomes in a crisis situation.

Phase 4. Evaluation of Crisis Resolution and Anticipatory Planning

To evaluate the outcome of crisis intervention, the nurse should reassess the individual to determine whether the following objectives have been achieved:

- Have positive behavioral changes occurred?
- Has the individual developed more adaptive coping strategies? Have they been effective?
- Has the individual grown from the experience by gaining insight into their responses to crisis situations?

■ Does the individual believe that they could respond with healthy adaptation in future stressful situations to prevent crisis development?

■ Can the individual describe a plan of action for dealing with stressors similar to the one that precipitated this crisis?

During the evaluation period, the nurse and patient summarize what has occurred during the intervention. They review what the individual has learned and anticipate how they will respond in the future. A determination is made regarding follow-up therapy; if needed, the nurse provides referral information.

Disaster Nursing

Although there are many definitions of a **disaster,** a common feature is that the event overwhelms local resources and threatens the function and safety of the community. A violent disaster, whether natural or man-made, may cause devastation to property or life. These crises leave victims with a damaged sense of safety and well-being and varying degrees of emotional trauma. Spiritual distress often occurs as victims ask, "How could this have happened?" and "What is most important in life?" A care plan for responding to spiritual distress is included in Table 12–1. Children, who lack life experiences and coping skills, are particularly vulnerable. Their sense of order and security has been seriously disrupted, and they are unable to understand that the disruption is time-limited and that their world will eventually return to normal.

Application of the Nursing Process to Disaster Nursing

Background Assessment Data

Individuals respond to traumatic events in many ways. Grieving is a natural response after any loss, and it may be more extreme if the disaster is directly experienced or witnessed. The emotional effects of loss and disruption may occur immediately or appear weeks or months later.

Psychological and behavioral responses common in adults after trauma and disaster include anger; disbelief; sadness; anxiety; fear; irritability; arousal; numbing; sleep disturbance; and increases in alcohol, caffeine, and tobacco use. Preschool children commonly experience separation anxiety, regressive behaviors, nightmares, and hyperactive or withdrawn behaviors. Older children may have difficulty concentrating, somatic complaints, sleep disturbances, and concerns about safety. Adolescents' responses are often similar to those of adults.

Traumatic bereavement is a term used to describe the grief process that accompanies unexpected losses resulting from traumatic events such as disasters. In these circumstances the survivor must come to grips not only with the loss but also the manner in which the loss occurred, and this can include powerful emotions ranging from guilt (at having survived when others lost their lives) to overwhelming fear of additional traumas (catastrophic thinking) and anger. Barlé et al. (2017) reported that, most often, the symptoms associated with traumatic loss are more intense and more prolonged than those after a natural death. These authors propose that three critical elements for intervention include building resources, processing trauma, and facilitating mourning. Ongoing assessment includes looking for signs of post-traumatic stress disorder (PTSD) and major depression or anxiety disorders that require additional intervention and treatment.

Nursing Diagnoses and Outcome Identification

Information from the assessment is analyzed, and appropriate nursing diagnoses reflecting the immediacy of the situation are identified. Some nursing diagnoses that may be relevant include the following:

■ Risk for injury (trauma, suffocation, poisoning)
■ Risk for infection
■ Anxiety (panic)
■ Fear
■ Spiritual distress
■ Risk for post-trauma syndrome
■ Ineffective community coping

The following criteria may be used for measurement of outcomes in the care of the patient having experienced a traumatic event. Timelines are individually determined.

The patient:

■ Demonstrates behaviors necessary to protect self from further injury
■ Identifies interventions to prevent/reduce risk of infection
■ Does not have an infection or physical injury
■ Maintains anxiety at a manageable level
■ Expresses beliefs and values about spiritual issues
■ Demonstrates ability to cope with emotional reactions in an individually appropriate manner
■ Demonstrates an increase in activities to improve community functioning

Planning and Implementation

Table 12–1 provides a plan of care for the patient who has experienced a traumatic event. Selected nursing diagnoses are presented, along with *Text continued on page 234*

Table 12–1 | CARE PLAN FOR THE PATIENT WHO HAS EXPERIENCED A TRAUMATIC EVENT

NURSING DIAGNOSIS: ANXIETY (PANIC)/FEAR

RELATED TO: Real or perceived threat to physical well-being; threat of death; situational crisis; exposure to toxins; unmet needs

EVIDENCED BY: Persistent feelings of apprehension and uneasiness; sense of impending doom; impaired functioning; verbal expressions of having no control or influence over situation, outcome, or self-care; sympathetic stimulation; extraneous physical movements

OUTCOME CRITERIA	NURSING INTERVENTIONS	RATIONALE
Patient demonstrates that anxiety is at a manageable level. Patient demonstrates use of positive coping mechanisms to manage anxiety.	1. Determine degree of anxiety/fear present, associated behaviors (e.g., laughter, crying, calm or agitation, excited or hysterical behavior, expressions of disbelief or self-blame), and reality of perceived threat.	1. Clearly understanding the patient's perception is pivotal to providing appropriate assistance in overcoming the fear. Individual may be agitated or completely overwhelmed. Panic state anxiety increases risk for the patient's safety and the safety of others in the environment to be compromised.
	2. Note degree of disorganization.	2. The patient may be unable to handle activities of daily living or work requirements and need more intensive intervention.
	3. Create as quiet an area as possible. Maintain a calm, confident manner. Speak in even tone using short, simple sentences.	3. Decreases sense of confusion or overstimulation; enhances sense of safety. Helps the patient focus on what is said and reduces transmission of anxiety.
	4. Develop trusting relationship with patient.	4. Trust is the basis of a therapeutic nurse–patient relationship and enables effective collaboration.
	5. Identify whether incident has reactivated preexisting or coexisting situations (physical or psychological trauma).	5. Concerns and psychological issues may be recycled each time trauma is reexperienced and affect how patient views the current situation.
	6. Determine presence of physical symptoms (e.g., numbness, headache, tightness in chest, nausea, and pounding heart).	6. Physical problems need to be differentiated from anxiety symptoms so that appropriate treatment can be given.
	7. Identify psychological responses (e.g., anger, shock, acute anxiety, panic, confusion, denial). Record emotional changes.	7. Although these are normal responses at the time of the trauma, they will repeatedly recycle until they are dealt with adequately.
	8. Discuss with patient the perception of what is causing the anxiety.	8. Increases the ability to connect symptoms to subjective feeling of anxiety, providing opportunity to gain insight/control and make desired changes.

Table 12–1 | CARE PLAN FOR THE PATIENT WHO HAS EXPERIENCED A TRAUMATIC EVENT—cont'd

OUTCOME CRITERIA	NURSING INTERVENTIONS	RATIONALE
	9. Assist the patient in correcting any distortions in thinking. Share perceptions with patient.	9. Perceptions based on reality will help to decrease fearfulness. How the nurse views the situation may help the patient to see it differently.
	10. Explore with the patient or significant other the manner in which patient has previously coped with anxiety-producing events.	10. May help the patient regain sense of control and recognize significance of trauma.
	11. Engage the patient in learning new coping behaviors (e.g., progressive muscle relaxation, thought-stopping).	11. Replacing maladaptive behaviors can enhance ability to manage and cope with stress. Interrupting obsessive thinking allows the patient to use energy to address underlying anxiety, whereas continued rumination about the incident can retard recovery.
	12. Encourage use of techniques to manage stress and vent emotions such as anger and hostility.	12. Reduces the likelihood of eruptions that can result in abusive behavior.
	13. Give positive feedback when the patient demonstrates better ways to manage anxiety and is able to appraise the situation calmly and realistically.	13. Provides acknowledgment and reinforcement, encouraging use of new coping strategies. Enhances ability to manage fearful feelings and gain control over situation, promoting future successes.
	14. Administer medications as indicated, such as antianxiety (diazepam, alprazolam, oxazepam) or antidepressants (fluoxetine, paroxetine, bupropion).	14. Antianxiety medication provides temporary relief of anxiety symptoms, enhancing ability to cope with situation. Antidepressants lift mood and help suppress intrusive thoughts and explosive anger.

NURSING DIAGNOSIS: SPIRITUAL DISTRESS

RELATED TO: Physical or psychological stress; energy-consuming anxiety; loss(es), intense suffering; separation from religious or cultural ties; challenged belief and value system

EVIDENCED BY: Expressions of concern about disaster and the meaning of life and death or belief systems; inner conflict about current loss of normality and effects of the disaster; anger directed at deity; engaging in self-blame; seeking spiritual assistance

OUTCOME CRITERIA	NURSING INTERVENTIONS	RATIONALE
Patient expresses beliefs and values about spiritual issues.	1. Determine the patient's religious/spiritual orientation, current involvement, and presence of conflicts.	1. Provides baseline for planning care and accessing appropriate resources.

Continued

Table 12–1 | CARE PLAN FOR THE PATIENT WHO HAS EXPERIENCED A TRAUMATIC EVENT–cont'd

OUTCOME CRITERIA	NURSING INTERVENTIONS	RATIONALE
	2. Establish environment that promotes free expression of feelings and concerns. Provide calm, peaceful setting when possible.	2. Promotes awareness and identification of feelings so they can be processed.
	3. Listen to the patient's and significant others' expressions of anger, concern, alienation from God, belief that situation is a punishment for wrongdoing, and so on.	3. It is helpful to understand the patient's and significant others' points of view and how their faith is affected in the face of tragedy.
	4. Note sense of futility, feelings of hopelessness and helplessness, lack of motivation to help self.	4. These thoughts and feelings can result in the patient feeling paralyzed and unable to move forward to resolve the situation.
	5. Listen to expressions of inability to find meaning in life and reason for living. Evaluate for suicidal ideation.	5. May indicate need for further intervention to prevent suicide attempt.
	6. Determine support systems available to the patient.	6. Presence or lack of support systems can affect the patient's recovery.
	7. Ask how you can be most helpful. Convey acceptance of the patient's spiritual beliefs and concerns.	7. Promotes trust and comfort, encouraging the patient to be open about sensitive matters.
	8. Make time for nonjudgmental discussion of philosophical issues and questions about spiritual effect of current situation.	8. Helps the patient to begin to look at basis for spiritual confusion. *Note:* There is a potential for the care provider's belief system to influence the patient's thoughts. Therefore, it is most beneficial for caregivers to remain neutral and not express their individual beliefs.
	9. Discuss difference between grief and guilt and help the patient to identify and explore each, assuming responsibility for own actions, expressing awareness of the consequences of acting out of false guilt.	9. Blaming self for what has happened impedes dealing with the grief process.
	10. Use therapeutic communication skills of reflection and active listening.	10. Helps the patient find solutions to concerns.

Table 12-1 | CARE PLAN FOR THE PATIENT WHO HAS EXPERIENCED A TRAUMATIC EVENT—cont'd

OUTCOME CRITERIA	NURSING INTERVENTIONS	RATIONALE
	11. Encourage the patient to experience meditation, prayer, and forgiveness according to their wishes. Provide information that anger with God is a normal part of the grieving process.	11. These actions can help the patient to reconnect with spiritual supports and coping mechanisms to heal past and present pain.
	12. Assist the patient in developing goals for coping with life situation.	12. Enhances commitment to goal, optimizing outcomes and promoting sense of hope.
	13. Identify and refer to resources that can be helpful (e.g., pastoral/parish nurse or religious counselor, crisis counselor, psychotherapy, Alcoholics/Narcotics Anonymous).	13. Specific assistance may be helpful to recovery (e.g., relationship problems, substance abuse, suicidal ideation).
	14. Encourage participation in support groups.	14. Discussing concerns and questions with others can help the patient gain support and identify new coping strategies.

NURSING DIAGNOSIS: RISK FOR POST-TRAUMA SYNDROME

RELATED TO: Events outside the range of usual human experience; serious threat or injury to self or loved ones; witnessing violent or tragic events; exaggerated sense of responsibility; survivor's guilt or role in the event; inadequate social support

OUTCOME CRITERIA	NURSING INTERVENTIONS	RATIONALE
Community demonstrates ability to deal with emotional reactions in an individually appropriate manner.	1. Determine involvement in event (e.g., survivor, significant other, rescue/aid worker, health-care provider, family member).	1. All those concerned with a traumatic event are at risk for emotional trauma and have needs related to their involvement in the event. *Note:* Close involvement with victims affects individual responses and may prolong emotional suffering.
	2. Evaluate current factors associated with the event, such as displacement from home due to illness or injury, natural disaster, or terrorist attack. Identify how the patient's past experiences may affect current situation.	2. Affects the patient's reaction to the current event and is the basis for planning care and identifying appropriate support systems and resources.
	3. Listen for comments of taking on responsibility (e.g., "I should have been more careful or gone back to get her").	3. Statements such as these are indicators of "survivor's guilt" and blaming self for actions.

Continued

Table 12-1 | CARE PLAN FOR THE PATIENT WHO HAS EXPERIENCED A TRAUMATIC EVENT—cont'd

OUTCOME CRITERIA	NURSING INTERVENTIONS	RATIONALE
	4. Identify the patient's current coping mechanisms.	4. Noting positive or negative coping skills provides direction for care.
	5. Determine availability and usefulness of the patient's support systems, family, social contacts, and community resources.	5. Family and others close to the patient may also be at risk and require assistance to cope with the trauma.
	6. Provide information about signs and symptoms of post-trauma response, especially if individual is involved in a high-risk occupation.	6. Awareness of these factors helps individual identify need for assistance when signs and symptoms occur.
	7. Identify and discuss the patient's strengths as well as vulnerabilities.	7. Provides information to build on for coping with the traumatic experience.
	8. Evaluate individual's perceptions of events and personal significance (e.g., rescue worker trained to provide lifesaving assistance but recovering only dead bodies).	8. Events that trigger feelings of despair and hopelessness may be more difficult to cope with and require long-term interventions.
	9. Provide emotional and physical presence by sitting with patient/significant other and offering solace.	9. Offering oneself promotes the establishment of trust and the potential to provide emotional and physical comfort measures.
	10. Encourage expression of feelings. Note whether feelings expressed appear congruent with events experienced.	10. It is important to talk about the incident repeatedly. Incongruencies may indicate deeper conflict and can impede resolution.
	11. Note presence of nightmares, reliving the incident, loss of appetite, irritability, numbness and crying, and family or relationship disruption.	11. These responses are normal in the early post-incident time frame. If prolonged and persistent, they may indicate a need for more intensive therapy.
	12. Provide a calm, safe environment.	12. Promotes the patient's ability to regain a sense of balance and control.
	13. Encourage and assist the patient in learning stress-management techniques.	13. Promotes relaxation and helps individual exercise control over self and what has happened.
	14. Recommend participation in debriefing sessions that may be provided after major disaster events.	14. Exploring stress and identifying coping strategies promptly may facilitate recovery from the event or prevent exacerbation.

Table 12–1 | CARE PLAN FOR THE PATIENT WHO HAS EXPERIENCED A TRAUMATIC EVENT–cont'd

OUTCOME CRITERIA	NURSING INTERVENTIONS	RATIONALE
	15. Identify employment, community resource groups.	15. Provides opportunity for ongoing support to cope with recurrent feelings related to the trauma.
	16. Administer prescribed medications as indicated, such as antipsychotic medications (e.g., chlorpromazine, haloperidol, olanzapine, or quetiapine) or carbamazepine (Tegretol).	16. Low doses of antipsychotic medications may be used for reduction of psychotic symptoms when loss of contact with reality occurs, usually for patients with especially disturbing flashbacks. Carbamazepine may be used to alleviate intrusive recollections or flashbacks, impulsivity, and violent behavior.

NURSING DIAGNOSIS: INEFFECTIVE COMMUNITY COPING

RELATED TO: History of exposure to disasters (earthquakes, tornados, floods, reemerging infectious agents, terrorist activity); ineffective or nonexistent community resources (e.g., lack of or inadequate emergency medical system, transportation system, or disaster planning systems), inadequate resources for problem-solving

EVIDENCED BY: Deficits of community participation; community does not meet expectations of its members; expressed perception of vulnerability and powerlessness; stressors perceived as excessive; excessive community conflicts or problems (vandalism, robbery, unemployment, homicides, terrorism, poverty); high illness rates

OUTCOME CRITERIA	NURSING INTERVENTIONS	RATIONALE
Community demonstrates an increase in activities to improve community functioning.	1. Evaluate community activities that are related to meeting collective needs within the community and between the community and the larger society. Note immediate needs, such as health care, food, shelter, funds.	1. Provides a baseline to determine community needs in relation to current concerns or threats.
	2. Note community reports of functioning, including areas of weakness or conflict.	2. Provides a view of how the community sees these areas.
	3. Identify effects of related factors on community activities.	3. In the face of a current threat, local or national, community resources need to be evaluated, updated, and given priority to meet the identified need.
	4. Determine availability and use of resources. Identify unmet demands or needs of the community.	4. This information is necessary to identify additional resources that are needed to meet the current situation.
	5. Determine community strengths.	5. Promotes understanding of the ways in which the community is already meeting the identified needs.

Continued

Table 12–1 | CARE PLAN FOR THE PATIENT WHO HAS EXPERIENCED A TRAUMATIC EVENT—cont'd

OUTCOME CRITERIA	NURSING INTERVENTIONS	RATIONALE
	6. Encourage community members/groups to engage in problem-solving activities.	6. Promotes a sense of working together to meet the needs.
	7. Develop a plan jointly with the members of the community to address immediate needs.	7. Provides insight into potential deficits in community response to crisis.
	8. Create plans managing interactions within the community and between the community and the larger society.	8. Meets collective needs when the concerns/threats are shared beyond a local community.
	9. Make information accessible to the public. Provide channels for dissemination of information to the community as a whole (e.g., print media, radio/television reports and community bulletin boards; Internet sites; speaker's bureau; reports to committees, councils, advisory boards).	9. Readily available accurate information can help citizens cope with the situation.
	10. Make information available in different modalities and geared to differing educational levels and cultures of the community.	10. Using languages other than English and making written materials accessible to all members of the community promotes understanding.
	11. Seek out and evaluate needs of underserved populations.	11. Homeless individuals and those residing in lower-income areas may have special requirements that need to be addressed with additional resources.

Source: Doenges, M. E., Moorhouse, M. F., & Murr, A. C. (2022). *Nurse's pocket guide: Diagnoses, prioritized interventions, and rationales* (16th ed.). F.A. Davis. With permission.

outcome criteria, appropriate nursing interventions, and rationales for each.

Evaluation

In the final step of the nursing process, a reassessment is conducted to determine whether the nursing actions have been successful in achieving the objectives of care. Evaluation of the nursing actions for the patient who has experienced a traumatic event may be facilitated by gathering information using the following types of questions:

Has the patient:

■ Been assessed and treated for serious injury or infections, or have they been resolved?

■ Been able to maintain anxiety at a manageable level?

■ Demonstrated appropriate problem-solving skills?

■ Discussed their beliefs about spiritual issues?

■ Demonstrated the ability to cope with emotional reactions in an individually appropriate manner?

■ Verbalized a subsiding of the physical manifestations (e.g., pain, nightmares, flashbacks, fatigue) associated with the traumatic event?

■ Recognized factors affecting the community's ability to meet its own demands or needs?

■ Demonstrated increased activities to improve community functioning?

■ Established and put in place a plan to deal with future contingencies?

When acute crises are not resolved, an individual may be vulnerable to acute stress disorders and trauma-related disorders. See Chapter 28, "Trauma- and Stressor-Related Disorders," for more information on these topics.

Summary and Key Points

■ A *crisis* is defined as an acute event in one's life, perceived by the individual as distressing and in which coping mechanisms and support systems are inadequate to manage associated anxiety.

■ All individuals experience crises at one time or another. A crisis does not necessarily indicate psychopathology. However, individuals with psychopathology are also vulnerable to crisis and may experience an exacerbation of psychiatric symptoms when in crisis.

■ Crises are precipitated by specific identifiable events and are determined by an individual's perception of the situation.

■ Crises are acute rather than chronic and generally last no more than a few weeks to a few months.

■ Crises occur when an individual is exposed to a stressor, and previous problem-solving techniques are ineffective, causing an increase in the level of anxiety. Panic may ensue when new techniques are tried, but resolution fails to occur.

■ Six types of crises have been identified: dispositional crises, crises of anticipated life transitions, crises resulting from traumatic stress, maturation/developmental crises, crises reflecting psychopathology, and psychiatric emergencies. The type of crisis determines the method of intervention selected.

■ Crisis intervention is designed to provide rapid assistance for individuals who have an urgent need.

■ The minimum therapeutic goal of crisis intervention is the psychological resolution of the individual's immediate crisis and restoration to at least the level of functioning that existed before the crisis period. A maximum goal is improvement in functioning above the precrisis level.

■ Nurses regularly respond to individuals in crisis in all types of settings. The nursing process is the vehicle by which nurses assist individuals in crisis with a short-term problem-solving approach to change.

■ A four-phase technique of crisis intervention includes assessment/analysis, planning of therapeutic intervention, intervention, and evaluation of crisis resolution and anticipatory planning.

■ Through this structured method of assistance, nurses help individuals in crisis develop more adaptive coping strategies for dealing with stressful situations in the future.

■ Nurses have many important skills that can assist individuals and communities in the wake of traumatic events. Nursing interventions presented in this chapter were developed for the nursing diagnoses of panic anxiety/fear, spiritual distress, risk for post-trauma syndrome, and ineffective community coping.

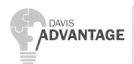

Go to **Davis Advantage** to complete your learning: strengthen understanding, apply your knowledge, and prepare for the Next Gen NCLEX®.

Review Questions

1. Which of the following is a correct assumption regarding the concept of crisis?
   a. Crises occur only in individuals with psychopathology.
   b. The stressful event that precipitates crisis is seldom identifiable.
   c. A crisis situation contains the potential for psychological growth or deterioration.
   d. Crises are chronic situations that recur many times during an individual's life.

2. Crises occur when an individual:
   a. Is exposed to a precipitating stressor.
   b. Perceives a stressor to be threatening.
   c. Has no support systems.
   d. Experiences a stressor and perceives coping strategies to be ineffective.

3. Which of the following events would likely precipitate a crisis? (Select all that apply)
   a. First-time parenthood when the parents perceive they have inadequate support and education
   b. Receiving a pay raise when the worker perceived they had to work very hard to accomplish their financial goals
   c. A natural disaster such as a forest fire in which lives and property were lost
   d. A peer or family member dies by suicide

4. Which of the following is a desired outcome of working with an individual who has witnessed a traumatic event and is now experiencing panic anxiety?
   a. The individual will experience no anxiety.
   b. The individual will demonstrate hope for the future.
   c. The individual will identify that anxiety is at a manageable level.
   d. The individual will verbalize the acceptance of self as worthy.

5. The client, a firefighter who responded to an industrial explosion, lost a coworker and close friend when they entered a building that collapsed. The client reports that since this event, they have had frequent nightmares and anxiety attacks and says to the mental health worker, "I should have died, but instead I lost my best friend!" This statement suggests that the client is experiencing:
   a. Spiritual distress.
   b. Night terrors.
   c. Survivor's guilt.
   d. Suicidal ideation.

Clinical Judgment Questions

6. A client whose home was destroyed during a tornado expresses to the nurse that they have been having disabling anxiety and nightmares for the last 2 weeks after this disaster. The most appropriate crisis intervention would be to:
   a. Encourage them to recognize how lucky they are to be alive.
   b. Discuss stages of grief and feelings associated with each.
   c. Identify helpful community resources.
   d. Suggest that they find a place to live that provides a storm shelter.

7. A teenager tells the high school nurse that their parents are drinking alcohol every day and they don't know what to do. The student's grades are starting to drop, and they complain of feeling anxious and overwhelmed. The most appropriate nursing action in response to the client's complaint would be to:
   a. Facilitate arrangements for the student to start attending Alateen meetings.
   b. Help the teenager identify the positive things in their life and recognize that the situation could be a lot worse than it is.
   c. Teach the student about the effects of alcohol on the body and that it can be hereditary.
   d. Refer the teenager to a psychiatrist for private therapy to learn to cope with their home situation.

8. A college student, who is an only child and attending school 500 miles away from their parents, reports to the nurse practitioner at the student health center that they have been having difficulty making decisions and will not undertake anything new without first consulting their mother. The student has recently started having anxiety attacks. Which nursing action is most appropriate in response to this client's maturational crisis?
   a. Suggest that they move to a college closer to home.
   b. Help the client to explore factors contributing to this crisis.
   c. Help the client find someone in the college town from whom they could seek assistance rather than calling their mother regularly.
   d. Recommend that the college physician prescribe an antianxiety medication for the client.

9. A client is brought to the emergency department by her college roommate and appears to be emotionless. The client reports that she was raped at a party earlier that evening. Which of these actions by the nurse is a priority?
   a. Ask the client if she would like to shower before she is examined.
   b. Confront the client about her apparent lack of emotion and ask if this was consensual sex.
   c. Affirm the client for seeking help and ask her to describe what happened.
   d. Ask the roommate if the client is typically so emotionless.

10. A client is admitted to the inpatient psychiatric unit after a suicide attempt. They report having become acutely suicidal after a recent job loss. Which of these nursing actions is a priority in response to this client's psychiatric crisis?
    a. Assess why the client lost their job.
    b. Ensure that the client remains safe and free from further self-injury.
    c. Explore career interests and other job opportunities.
    d. Assess for substance use disorder.

Communication Exercises

1. A patient you have been working with for several days approaches you with apparent signs of agitation and yells in a loud voice, "I want out of this hospital right now! You don't listen to a thing I say, and my doctor just wants my money." How will you respond?

2. Shelley enters the emergency department accompanied by a friend who reports that Shelley was raped after leaving a college campus party the night before. Shelley is staring off into space, exhibits a closed posture, and is mumbling inaudibly. How will you introduce yourself and begin to intervene in this situation?

3. Thomas was secluded and restrained after punching another patient on the inpatient psychiatric unit. The next day, Thomas asks you what happened last night, stating they do not remember, and says they want to know why they were arrested and tied up like an animal. What will you communicate to Thomas about the prior events and the crisis intervention process?

References

Barlé, N., Wortman, C. B., & Latack, J. A. (2017). Traumatic bereavement: Basic research and clinical implications. *Journal of Psychotherapy Integration, 27*(2), 127–139. https://doi.org/10.1037/int0000013

Bouchery, E. E., Barna, M., Babalola, E., Friend, D., Brown, J. D., Blyler, C., & Ireys, H. T. (2018). The effectiveness of a peer-staffed crisis respite program as an alternative to hospitalization. *Psychiatric Services.* https://doi.org/10.1176/appi.ps.201700451

Doenges, M. E., Moorhouse, M. F., & Murr, A. C. (2022). *Nurse's pocket guide: Diagnoses, prioritized interventions, and rationales* (16th ed.). F.A. Davis.

National Alliance on Mental Illness. (2022). *Crisis intervention team (CIT) programs.* https://www.nami.org/Advocacy/Crisis-Intervention/Crisis-Intervention-Team-(CIT)-Programs

Puschner, B., Repper, J., Mahlke, C., Nixdorf, R., Basangwa, D., Nakku, J., Ryan, G., Baillie, D., Shamba, D., Ramesh, M., Moran, G., Lachmann, M., Kalha, J., Pathare, S., Müller-Stierlin, A., & Slade, M. (2019). Using peer support in developing empowering mental health services (UPSIDES): Background, rationale and methodology. *Annals of Global Health, 85*(1): 53. https://doi.org/10.5334/aogh.2435

Shalaby, R., & Agyapong, V. (2020). Peer support in mental health: Literature review. *JMIR Mental Health, 7*(6), e15572. https://doi.org/10.2196/15572

Substance Abuse and Mental Health Services Administration (SAMHSA). (2014). *SAMHSA's concept of trauma and guidance for a trauma-informed approach.* https://s3.amazonaws.com/static.nicic.gov/Library/028436.pdf

Watson, A. C., & Fulambarker, A. J. (2012). The crisis intervention team model of police response to mental health crisis: A primer for mental health practitioners. *Best Practices in Mental Health, 8*(2), 71–81.

White, S., Foster, R., Marks, J., Morshead, R., Goldsmith, L., Barlow, S., Sin, J., & Gillard, S. (2020). The effectiveness of one-to-one peer support in mental health services: A systematic review and meta-analysis. *BMC Psychiatry 20,* 534. https://doi.org/10.1186/s12888-020-02923-3

Classical References

Aguilera, D. C. (1998). *Crisis intervention: Theory and methodology* (8th ed.). Mosby.

Baldwin, B. A. (1978, July). A paradigm for the classification of emotional crises: Implications for crisis intervention. *American Journal of Orthopsychiatry, 48*(3), 538–551. doi:10.1111/j.1939-0025.1978.tb01342.x

Bateman, A., & Peternelj-Taylor, C. (1998). Crisis intervention. In Glod, C. A. (Ed.), *Contemporary psychiatric-mental health nursing: The brain-behavior connection.* F.A. Davis.

Caplan, G. (1964). *Principles of preventive psychiatry.* Basic Books.

13

Assertiveness Training

KEY TERMS

aggressive	emotional intelligence (EI)	passive-aggressive
assertive	nonassertive	thought-stopping

OBJECTIVES
After reading this chapter, the student will be able to:

1. Define assertive behavior.
2. Discuss basic human rights.
3. Differentiate among nonassertive, assertive, aggressive, and passive-aggressive behaviors.
4. Describe techniques that promote assertive behavior.
5. Demonstrate thought-stopping techniques.
6. Discuss the role of the nurse in assertiveness training.

Alberti and Emmons (2017) have proposed the following questions:

> Are you able to express warm, positive feelings to another person? Are you comfortable starting a conversation with strangers at a party? Do you sometimes feel ineffective in making your desires clear to others? Do you have difficulty saying no to persuasive people? Are you often at the bottom of the "pecking order," pushed around by others? Or maybe you're the one who pushes others around to get your way? (p. 14)

Assertive behavior promotes a feeling of personal power and self-confidence. These two components are commonly lacking in clients with emotional disorders. Becoming more assertive empowers individuals by promoting self-esteem without diminishing the esteem of others.

This chapter describes several rights that are considered basic to human beings. Various kinds of behaviors are explored, including assertive, nonassertive, aggressive, and passive-aggressive. Techniques that promote assertive behavior and the nurse's role in assertiveness training are presented.

CORE CONCEPT
Assertive Behavior
Assertive behavior is a style of relating to other people that promotes clear and direct expression of one's needs and rights without impinging on the rights of others.

Assertive Communication

Assertive behavior helps us feel good about ourselves and increases our self-esteem. It helps us feel good about other people and increases our ability to develop satisfying relationships. Assertive communication is characterized by honesty, directness, appropriateness, and respect for one's basic rights as well as the rights of others.

Honesty is basic to assertive behavior. Assertive honesty is not an outspoken declaration of everything that is on one's mind. It is instead an accurate representation of feelings, opinions, or preferences expressed in a manner that promotes self-respect and respect for others. Direct communication is stating what one wants to convey with clarity and candor. Hinting and "beating around the bush" are indirect forms of communication.

Communication must occur in an appropriate context to be considered assertive. The location and timing, as well as the manner (tone of voice, nonverbal gestures) in which the communication is presented, must be correct for the situation.

Basic Human Rights

Many authors have identified "assertive rights" (Alberti & Emmons, 2017; Bishop, 2013; Davis et al., 2008; Grosaru, 2020; Lloyd, 2002). The following list is a composite of 10 basic assertive human rights adapted from an aggregation of sources:

1. The right to be treated with respect
2. The right to express feelings, opinions, and beliefs
3. The right to say "no" without feeling guilty or needing to justify your feelings or behavior
4. The right to make and accept responsibility for mistakes
5. The right to be listened to and taken seriously
6. The right to change your mind
7. The right to ask for what you want
8. The right to put yourself first, sometimes
9. The right to set your own priorities
10. The right to be assertive

In accepting these rights, an individual also accepts the responsibilities that accompany them. Rights and responsibilities are reciprocal entities. To experience one without the other is inherently destructive to an individual. Some responsibilities associated with basic assertive human rights are presented in Table 13–1.

Response Patterns

Individuals develop patterns of responding to others. Some of these patterns have developed through

■ Watching other people (role modeling).
■ Being positively reinforced or punished for a certain response.
■ Inventing an individual response style.
■ Not being able to think of different or better ways to respond.
■ Not developing the proper skills for a better response.
■ Consciously and intentionally choosing a response style.

The nurse should be able to recognize their individual pattern of responding as well as that of others. Four common response patterns are discussed here: nonassertive, assertive, aggressive, and passive-aggressive.

TABLE 13–1 **Assertive Rights and Responsibilities**	
RIGHTS	**RESPONSIBILITIES**
1. To be treated with respect	To treat others in a way that recognizes their human dignity
2. To express feelings, opinions, and beliefs	To accept ownership of our feelings and show respect for those that differ from our own
3. To say "no"	To analyze each situation individually, recognizing all human rights as equal (others have the right to say "no," too)
4. To make mistakes	To accept responsibility for own mistakes and try to correct them
5. To be listened to	To listen to others
6. To change your mind	To accept the possible consequences that the change may incur; to accept the same flexibility in others
7. To ask for what you want	To accept others' right to refuse your request
8. To put yourself first, sometimes	To put others first, sometimes
9. To set your own priorities	To consider one's limitations as well as strengths in directing independent activities, to be a dependable person
10. To refuse to justify feelings or behavior	To accept ownership of own feelings and behavior, to accept others without requiring justification for their feelings and behavior

Nonassertive Behavior

Individuals who behave in a **nonassertive** (sometimes called *passive*) manner seek to please others at the expense of their basic human rights. They seldom let their true feelings show and often feel hurt and anxious because they allow others to choose for them. They seldom achieve their desired goals. They come across as apologetic and tend to be self-deprecating. They use actions instead of words and hope someone will "guess" what they want. Their voices are hesitant, weak, and expressed in a monotone. Their eyes are usually downcast. They feel uncomfortable in interpersonal interactions. All they want is to please and to be liked by others. Their behavior helps them avoid unpleasant situations and confrontations with others; however, they often harbor anger and resentment.

Assertive Behavior

Individuals who demonstrate **assertive** behavior stand up for their own rights while protecting the rights of others. Feelings are expressed openly and honestly. These individuals assume responsibility for their own choices and allow others to choose for themselves. They maintain self-respect and respect for others by treating everyone equally and with human dignity. They communicate tactfully, using lots of "I" statements. Their voices are warm and expressive, and eye contact is intermittent but direct. These individuals desire to communicate effectively with and be respected by others. They are self-confident and experience satisfactory and pleasurable relationships with others.

Aggressive Behavior

Individuals who use **aggressive** response patterns defend their own basic rights by violating the basic rights of others. Feelings are often expressed dishonestly and inappropriately. They say what is on their mind, often at the expense of others. Aggressive behavior commonly results in *put-downs,* leaving the receiver feeling hurt, defensive, and humiliated. Individuals responding aggressively devalue the self-worth of those on whom they impose their choices. They typically express an air of superiority, and their voices are often loud, demanding, angry, or cold and emotionless. Eye contact may be an attempt to intimidate others by "staring them down." They want to increase their feelings of power by dominating or humiliating others. Aggressive behavior hinders interpersonal relationships.

Passive-Aggressive Behavior

Individuals using **passive-aggressive** behavior *respond* to others by appearing passive and accepting of others' demands while *behaving* in ways that suggest anger and resentment are their true feelings. This kind of behavior is sometimes referred to as *indirect* or *covert aggression* and takes the form of passive, nonconfrontational action. This pattern of communication is dishonest, manipulative, and sly, and it undermines others with behavior that expresses the opposite of what these individuals are feeling. It is critical and sometimes sarcastic. Individuals employing passive-aggressive behavior allow others to make choices for them, then resist by using passive behaviors such as procrastination, dawdling, stubbornness, and "forgetfulness." They use actions instead of words to convey their messages, and the actions express covert aggression. They become sulky, irritable, or argumentative when asked to do something they do not want to do. They may protest to others about the demand but will not confront the person who has made the demand. The goal is domination through retaliation. This behavior offers a feeling of control and power, although the individual actually feels resentment. This style of communication is associated with extremely low self-confidence.

A comparison of these four behavior patterns is presented in Table 13–2.

Behavioral Components of Assertive Behavior

Alberti and Emmons (2017) have identified several defining characteristics of assertive behavior:

- **Eye contact:** Eye contact is considered appropriate when intermittent (i.e., looking directly at the person to whom one is speaking but looking away now and then). Individuals feel uncomfortable when someone stares at them continuously and intently. Intermittent eye contact conveys the message that one is interested in what is being said.
- **Body posture:** Sitting and leaning slightly toward the other person in a conversation suggests an active interest in what is being said. Emphasis on an assertive stance can be achieved by standing with an erect posture squarely facing the other person. A slumped posture conveys passivity or nonassertiveness.
- **Distance/physical contact:** The distance between two individuals in an interaction or the physical contact between them has a strong cultural influence. For example, the predominant culture of the United States considers intimate distance as approximately 18 inches from the body. Some individuals may interpret invasion of this space as very aggressive.
- **Gestures:** Nonverbal gestures also are variable among different cultures. In assertive communication, gestures add emphasis, warmth, depth, or

TABLE 13-2 **Comparison of Behavioral Response Patterns**			
	NONASSERTIVE	**ASSERTIVE**	**AGGRESSIVE**	**PASSIVE-AGGRESSIVE**
BEHAVIORAL CHARACTERISTICS	■ Passive ■ Does not express true feelings ■ Self-deprecating ■ Denies own rights	■ Stands up for own rights ■ Protects rights of others ■ Honest, direct, appropriate	■ Violates rights of others ■ Expresses feelings dishonestly and inappropriately	■ Defends own rights with passive resistance ■ Is critical and sarcastic ■ Often expresses opposite of true feelings
EXAMPLES	"Uh, well, uh, sure, I'll be glad to stay and work an extra shift."	"I don't want to stay and work an extra shift today. I stayed over yesterday. It's someone else's turn today."	"You've got to be kidding!"	"Okay, I'll stay and work an extra shift." (Then to peer: "How dare she ask me to work over again! Well, we'll just see how much work she gets out of me!")
GOALS	To please others; to be liked by others	To communicate effectively; to be respected by others	To dominate or humiliate others	To dominate through retaliation
FEELINGS	Anxious, hurt, disappointed with self, angry, resentful	Confident, successful, proud, self-respecting	Self-righteous, controlling, superior	Anger, resentment, manipulated, controlled
COMPENSATION	Is able to avoid unpleasant situations and confrontations with others	Increased self-confidence, self-respect, respect for others, satisfying interpersonal relationships	Anger is released, increasing feeling of power and superiority	Feels self-righteous and in control
OUTCOMES	Goals not met; others meet *their* goals at nonassertive person's expense; anger and resentment grow; feels violated and manipulated	Goals met; desires most often fulfilled while defending own rights as well as rights of others	Goals may be met but at the expense of others; they feel hurt and vengeful	Goals not met, nor are the goals of others met due to retaliatory nature of the interaction

Sources: Alberti, R. E., & Emmons, M. L. (2017). *Your perfect right* (10th ed.). Impact Publishers; Bishop, S. (2013). *Develop your assertiveness*. Kogan Page; Davis, M., Eshelman, E. R., & McKay, M. (2008). *The relaxation and stress reduction workbook* (6th ed.). New Harbinger Publications; Lloyd, S. R. (2002). *Developing positive assertiveness* (3rd ed.). Crisp Publications; and Powell, T. J., & Enright, S. J. (1990). *Anxiety and stress management*. Routledge.

power to the spoken word with awareness of and sensitivity to the effect on the receiver.

■ **Facial expression:** Various facial expressions convey different messages (e.g., surprise, anger, fear). It is difficult to "fake" these messages. In assertive communication, the facial expression is congruent with the verbal message.

■ **Voice:** The voice conveys a message by its loudness, softness, degree and placement of emphasis, and evidence of emotional tone. In assertive communication, the voice conveys an acceptable volume to communicate confidence without being too loud or forceful.

■ **Fluency:** The ability to discuss a subject with ease and obvious knowledge conveys assertiveness and self-confidence. This message is impeded by numerous pauses or filler words such as "and, uh …" or "you know …"

■ **Timing:** Assertive responses are most effective when they are spontaneous and immediate. However, most people have experienced times when it was inappropriate to respond (e.g., in front of a group of people) or times when an appropriate response is generated only after the fact ("If only I had said …"). It is correct and worthwhile to seek out the individual at a later time and express the assertive response if an immediate response seems ill-timed.

■ **Listening:** Assertive listening means giving the other individual full attention by making eye contact, nodding to indicate acceptance of what is said, and taking time to understand the message before responding.

■ **Thoughts:** Cognitive processes affect one's assertive behavior. Two such processes are an individual's attitudes about the appropriateness of assertive behavior in general and the appropriateness of assertive behavior for oneself specifically. Assertive communication is supported by a belief that being assertive is a reasonable, appropriate, and healthy way to communicate.

■ **Content:** The content of assertive communication includes "I" statements to describe one's feelings and needs. "You" statements, such as "You never listen to me" or "You don't respect my parenting decisions," tend to put others on the defensive. Instead, "I" statements, such as "I'm upset because I don't feel like you're hearing me" or "I need you to respect my decision on this parenting issue," tend to lessen defensiveness and increase the likelihood that the message will be received and heard.

■ **Persistence:** This element of assertive behavior involves maintaining confidence in and commitment to one's needs and feelings even when someone is pressuring the individual to cave into demands. It often means repeating a stated feeling or need in an effort to be heard and respected. Persistence, as with other aspects of assertive behavior, employs "I" communication statements. For example, when someone is trying to pressure another person to drink alcohol, a persistent response might be "As I already told you, I am not interested in drinking alcohol, and I need for you to stop pressuring me."

Techniques That Promote Assertive Behavior

The following techniques have been shown to be effective in responding to criticism and avoiding manipulation by others:

1. **Standing up for one's basic human rights.**

Example

"I have the right to express my opinion."

2. **Assuming responsibility for one's own statements.**

Example

"I don't want to go out with you tonight," instead of "I can't go out with you tonight." The latter implies a lack of power or ability.

3. **Responding as a broken record;** that is, persistently repeating in a calm voice what is wanted.

Example

Telephone salesperson: I want to help you save money by changing long-distance services.
Assertive response: I don't want to change my long-distance service.
Telephone salesperson: I can't believe you don't want to save money!
Assertive response: I don't want to change my long-distance service.

4. **Agreeing assertively;** that is, assertively accepting negative aspects about oneself and admitting when an error has been made.

Example

Ms. Jones: You sure let that meeting get out of hand. What a waste of time.
Ms. Smith: Yes, I didn't do a very good job of conducting the meeting today.

5. **Inquiring assertively;** that is, seeking additional information about critical statements.

Example

Staff nurse #1: You made a real fool of yourself at the staff meeting this afternoon.
Staff nurse #2: Oh, really? Just what about my behavior offended you?
Staff nurse #1: You were so damned pushy!
Staff nurse #2: Were you offended that I spoke up for my beliefs, or was it because my beliefs are in direct opposition to yours?

6. **Shifting from content to process;** that is, changing the focus of the communication from discussing the topic at hand to analyzing what is actually going on in the interaction.

Example

Wife: Would you please call me if you will be late for dinner?
Husband: Why don't you just get off my back! I always have to account for every minute of my time with you!
Wife: Sounds to me like we need to discuss some other things here. What are you *really* angry about?

7. **Clouding or fogging;** that is, concurring with the critic's argument without becoming defensive and without agreeing to change.

Example

Nurse 1: You never come to the Nurses Association meetings. I don't know why you even belong!
Nurse 2: You're right. I haven't attended very many of the meetings.

8. **Defusing;** that is, putting off further discussion with an angry individual until they are calmer.

Example

"You are very angry right now. I don't want to discuss this matter with you while you are so upset. I will discuss it with you in my office at 3 o'clock this afternoon."

9. **Delaying assertively;** that is, putting off further discussion with another individual until one is calmer.

Example

"That's a very challenging position you have taken, Mr. Brown. I'll need time to give it some thought. I'll call you later this afternoon."

10. **Responding assertively with irony.**

Example

Confronter: You think you're so smart!
Assertive responder: Why, yes, I do try to stay well informed. Thank you for noticing.

11. **Using "I" statements,** which allow an individual to take ownership for their feelings rather than saying they are caused by another person.

"I" statements are sometimes called "feeling" statements. They express directly what an individual is feeling. "You" statements are accusatory and put the receiver on the defensive. "I" statements have four parts:

1. How I feel: These are my feelings and I accept ownership of them.
2. When: Describe in a neutral manner the behavior that is the problem.
3. Why: Describe what it is about the behavior that is objectionable.
4. What I need (suggesting change): Offer a preferred alternative to the behavior using "I" statements.

Example

John has just returned from a hunting trip and walked into the living room in his muddy boots, leaving a trail of mud on the carpet. His wife, Mary, may respond as follows:

With a "you" statement: "You are such a jerk! Can't you see the trail of mud you are leaving on the carpet? I just cleaned this carpet. You make me so angry!"
With an "I" statement: "I feel so angry when you walk on the carpet in your muddy boots. I just cleaned it, and now I will have to clean it again. I would appreciate it if you would remove your boots on the porch before you come in the house."

"You" statements are negative and focus on what the person has done wrong. They do not explain what is being requested of the person. "I" statements are more positive. They explain *how* one is feeling, *why* they are feeling that way, and *what* the individual wants instead. Hopkins (2022) stated the following about the importance of "I" statements:

Part of being assertive involves the ability to appropriately express your needs and feelings. You can accomplish this by using "I" statements. These [statements] indicate ownership, do not attribute blame, focus on behavior, identify the effect of the behavior, are direct and honest, and contribute to the growth of your relationship with each other. (p. 2)

Thought-Stopping Techniques

Assertive thinking is sometimes inhibited by repetitive, negative thoughts of which the mind refuses to let go. Individuals with low self-worth may be obsessed with thoughts such as, "I know he'd never want to go out with me. I'm too ugly (or plain, or fat, or dumb)" or "I just know I'll never be able to do this job well" or "I just can't seem to do anything right." This type of thinking fosters the belief that one's individual rights do not deserve the same consideration as those of others and reflects nonassertive communication and behavioral response patterns.

Thought-stopping techniques, as described here, were developed by psychiatrist Joseph Wolpe (1990), and are intended to eliminate intrusive, unwanted thoughts.

Method

In a practice setting, with eyes closed, the individual concentrates on an unwanted recurring thought. Once the thought is clearly established in the mind, the person shouts aloud: "STOP!" This action interrupts the thought, and it is actually removed from one's awareness. The individual then immediately shifts their thoughts to one that is considered pleasant and desirable.

It is possible that the unwanted thought may soon recur, but with practice, the length of time between recurrences will increase until the unwanted thought is no longer intrusive. Obviously, one cannot go about their daily life shouting, "STOP!" in public places. After several practice sessions, the technique is equally effective if "stop!" is used silently in the mind.

Role of the Nurse in Assertiveness Training

It is important for nurses to become aware of and recognize their own behavioral responses. Common questions used to assess and develop self-awareness include the following: Are my behaviors mostly non-assertive? Assertive? Aggressive? Passive-aggressive? Do I consider my behavioral responses effective? Do I wish to change? Remember, all individuals have the right to choose whether or not they want to be assertive. A self-assessment of assertiveness is found in Box 13–1.

Assertive communication is part of a larger set of competencies referred to as **emotional intelligence (EI).** This concept, first developed by Salovey and Mayer (1990) and elaborated by Goleman (2006), includes four sets of competencies:

- Self-awareness (of emotions and behavior)
- Social awareness (awareness of others' feelings, or empathy)
- Self-management (which includes self-control)
- Relationship management (which includes skills in teamwork and collaboration).

Each of these competencies is relevant to developing assertive communication skills. To communicate assertively, individuals must be aware of their own feelings and the feelings of others; they must be aware of and develop skill in their ability to control their emotions and behavior; and they must respond in ways that effectively manage relationships, including skills that resolve conflicts rather than escalate them. In professional roles, assertive communication and EI are important competencies for effective teamwork and collaboration. The ability to respond assertively is especially important to nurses who are committed to the further development of the profession. Assertiveness skills facilitate the implementation of change that is required if the image of nursing is to be elevated to the level of professionalism that most nurses desire. Assertive communication is useful in the political arena for nurses who choose to become involved at the state and national levels in striving to influence legislation and ultimately improve our country's system of health-care provision.

Nurses who understand and use assertiveness skills themselves can, in turn, assist patients who wish to effect behavioral change to increase self-esteem and improve interpersonal relationships. When

---

BOX 13–1 An Assertiveness Quiz

Assign a number to each item using the following scale: 1 = Never; 3 = Sometimes; 5 = Always

_____ 1. I ask others to do things without feeling guilty or anxious.
_____ 2. When someone asks me to do something I don't want to do, I say no without feeling guilty or anxious.
_____ 3. I am comfortable when speaking to a large group of people.
_____ 4. I confidently express my honest opinions to authority figures (such as my boss).
_____ 5. When I experience powerful feelings (anger, frustration, disappointment, and so on), I verbalize them easily.
_____ 6. When I express anger, I do so without blaming others for "making me mad."
_____ 7. I am comfortable speaking up in a group situation.
_____ 8. If I disagree with the majority opinion in a meeting, I can "stick to my guns" without feeling uncomfortable or being abrasive.
_____ 9. When I make a mistake, I acknowledge it.
_____ 10. I tell others when their behavior creates a problem for me.
_____ 11. Meeting new people in social situations is something I do with ease and comfort.
_____ 12. When discussing my beliefs, I do so without labeling the opinions of others as "crazy," "stupid," "ridiculous," or "irrational."
_____ 13. I assume that most people are competent and trustworthy, and I do not have difficulty delegating tasks to others.
_____ 14. When considering doing something I have never done, I feel confident I can learn to do it.
_____ 15. I believe that my needs are as important as those of others, and I am entitled to have my needs satisfied.
_____ TOTAL SCORE

SCORING:
1. If your total score is 60 or higher, you have a consistently assertive philosophy and probably handle most situations well.
2. If your total score is 45 to 59, you have a fairly assertive outlook but may benefit from some assertiveness training.
3. If your total score is 30 to 44, you may be assertive in some situations, but your natural response is either nonassertive or aggressive. Assertiveness training is suggested.
4. If your total score is 15 to 29, you have considerable difficulty being assertive. Assertiveness training is recommended.

Source: Lloyd, S. R. (2002). *Developing positive assertiveness* (3rd ed.). Crisp Publications. With permission.

using assertive communication and teaching patients about assertiveness, it is important to be clear that assertive communication does not necessarily ensure a particular response. For example, a spouse may assertively communicate that they feel overwhelmed and need more help with the housework, but the other spouse still has control over whether or not to respect those wishes. Instead, assertive communication is a way to communicate one's feelings and needs in a manner that is less likely to generate defensiveness from the receiver and more likely to allow the message to be heard. Evidence supports that assertiveness skills training is beneficial in reducing symptoms of depression, anxiety, and interpersonal difficulties and for improving one's self-esteem and help-seeking skills even among individuals with severe mental illness such as schizophrenia (Ayhan & Öz, 2021; Cantero-Sánchez et al., 2021; Maaly et al., 2016; Shean, 2013; Speed et al., 2017; Tavakoli et al., 2014).

The nursing process is a useful tool for nurses who are involved in helping patients increase their assertiveness. The following sections detail how to achieve this objective in each phase of the nursing process.

Assessment

Nurses can help patients become more aware of their behavioral responses. Many tools exist for assessing the level of assertiveness, but it is difficult to *generalize* when attempting to measure assertive behaviors.

Box 13–2 and Figure 13–1 represent examples of assertiveness inventories that can be personalized to explore life situations of individual patients more specifically. Obviously, the everyday situations that require assertiveness are not the same for all individuals.

Diagnosis

Possible nursing diagnoses for individuals needing assistance with assertiveness include the following:

■ Coping, defensive
■ Coping, ineffective
■ Decisional conflict
■ Denial
■ Personal identity, disturbed
■ Powerlessness
■ Rape-trauma syndrome
■ Self-esteem, low
■ Social interaction, impaired
■ Social isolation

Outcome Identification and Implementation

The goal for nurses working with individuals needing assistance with assertiveness is to help them develop satisfying interpersonal relationships. Individuals who do not feel good about themselves either allow others to violate their rights or cover up their low self-esteem by being overtly or covertly aggressive. Individuals should be given information regarding

---

BOX 13–2 Everyday Situations That May Require Assertiveness

AT WORK
How do you respond when:

1. You receive a compliment on your appearance or someone praises your work?
2. You are criticized unfairly?
3. You are criticized legitimately by a superior?
4. You have to confront a subordinate for continual lateness or sloppy work?
5. Your boss makes a sexual innuendo or makes a pass at you?

IN PUBLIC
How do you respond when:

1. In a restaurant, the food you ordered arrives cold or overcooked?
2. A fellow passenger in a no-smoking compartment lights a cigarette?
3. You are faced with an unhelpful shop assistant?
4. Somebody barges in front of you in a waiting line?
5. You take an inferior article back to a shop?

AMONG FRIENDS
How do you respond when:

1. You feel angry with the way a friend has treated you?
2. A friend makes what you consider to be an unreasonable request?
3. You want to ask a friend for a favor?
4. You ask a friend for repayment of a loan of money?
5. You have to negotiate with a friend on which film to see or where to meet?

AT HOME
How do you respond when:

1. One of your parents criticizes you?
2. You are irritated by a persistent habit in someone you love?
3. Everybody leaves the cleaning-up chores to you?
4. You want to say "no" to a proposed visit to a relative?
5. Your partner feels amorous but you are not in the mood?

Source: Powell, T. J., & Enright, S. J. (1990). *Anxiety and stress management.* Routledge. With permission.

DIRECTIONS: Fill in each block with a rating of your assertiveness on a 5-point scale. A rating of 0 means you have no difficulty asserting yourself. A rating of 5 means that you are completely unable to assert yourself. Evaluation can be made by analyzing the scores:

1. Totally by activity, including all of the different people categories
2. Totally by people, including all of the different activity categories
3. On an individual basis, considering specific people and specific activities

PEOPLE / ACTIVITY	Friends of the same sex	Friends of the opposite sex	Intimate relations or spouse	Authority figures	Relatives/ family members	Colleagues and sub-ordinates	Strangers	Service workers: waiters, shop assistants, etc.
Giving and receiving compliments								
Asking for favors/help								
Initiating and maintaining conversation								
Refusing requests								
Expressing personal opinions								
Expressing anger/dis-pleasure								
Expressing liking, love, affection								
Stating your rights and needs								

FIGURE 13–1 Rating your assertiveness. (From Powell, T. J., & Enright, S. J. [1990]. *Anxiety and stress management*. Routledge. With permission.)

their individual human rights. They must know these rights before they can assert them.

Outcome criteria are derived from specific nursing diagnoses. Timelines are individually determined. Examples include the following:

The patient:

■ Verbalizes and accepts responsibility for their own behavior.
■ Expresses opinions and disagrees with the opinions of others in a socially acceptable manner without feeling guilty.
■ Verbalizes positive aspects about self.
■ Verbalizes choices made in a plan to maintain control over their life situation.
■ Approaches others in an appropriate manner for one-to-one interaction.

In a clinical setting, nurses can teach patients techniques to increase their assertive responses. This education can be done on a one-to-one basis or in group situations. Once these techniques have been discussed, nurses can assist patients in practicing them through role-playing. Each patient should compose a list of specific personal examples of situations that create difficulties for them. These situations will then be simulated in a role-play so that the patient may practice assertive responses in a nonthreatening environment. In a group situation, feedback from peers can provide valuable insight into the effectiveness of the response. The nurse's ability to role model assertive communication in relationships with patients, peers, and other health-care team members can be a powerful teaching tool.

CLINICAL PEARL An important part of this type of intervention is to ensure that patients are aware of the differences among assertive, nonassertive, aggressive, and passive-aggressive behaviors in the same situation. When a discussion is held about what the best (assertive) response would be, it is also important to discuss the other types of responses as well so that patients can begin to recognize their pattern of response and make changes accordingly.

Evaluation

Evaluation requires that the nurse and patient assess whether or not these techniques are achieving the desired outcomes. Reassessment might include the following questions:

- Is the patient able to accept criticism without becoming defensive?
- Can the patient express true feelings (to spouse, friend, boss, and others) when their basic human rights are violated?
- Is the patient able to decline a request without feeling guilty?
- Can the patient verbalize positive qualities themselves?
- Does the patient verbalize improvement in interpersonal relationships?

Assertiveness training serves to extend and create more flexibility in an individual's communication style so that they have a greater choice of responses in various situations. Although change does not come easily, assertiveness training can be an effective way of changing behavior. Nurses can assist individuals to become more assertive, thereby encouraging them to become what they want to be, promoting an improvement in self-esteem, and fostering a respect for their own rights and the rights of others.

Summary and Key Points

- Assertive behavior helps individuals feel better about themselves by encouraging them to communicate their own needs clearly and directly.
- Basic human rights have equal representation for all individuals.
- Along with rights comes an equal number of responsibilities. Part of being assertive includes living up to these responsibilities.
- Assertive behavior increases self-esteem and the ability to develop satisfying interpersonal relationships. This behavior is accomplished through honesty, directness, appropriateness, and respecting one's rights and the rights of others.

CASE STUDY

Alessa comes to the day hospital once a week to attend group therapy and assertiveness training. She has had problems with depression and low self-esteem and is married to a man who is verbally abusive. He is highly critical, is seldom satisfied with anything Alessa does, and blames her for negative consequences that occur in their lives whether or not she is involved.

Since the beginning of the assertiveness training group, the nurse who leads the group has taught the participants about basic human rights and the various types of response patterns. When the nurse asks for patient situations to be presented in group, Alessa volunteers to discuss an incident that occurred in her home this week. She related that she had just put some chicken on the stove to cook for supper when her 7-year-old son came running in the house yelling that he had been hurt. Alessa went to him and observed that he had blood dripping down the side of his head from his forehead. He said he and some friends had been playing on the jungle gym in the schoolyard down the street and he had fallen and hit his head. Alessa went with him to the bathroom to clean the wound and apply some medication. Her husband, Joe, was reading the newspaper in the living room. By the time she got back to the chicken on the stove, it was burned and inedible. Her husband shouted, "You stupid woman! You can't do anything right!" Alessa did not respond but burst into tears.

The nurse asked the other members in the group to present some ideas about how Alessa could have responded to Joe's criticism. After some discussion, they agreed that Alessa might have stated, "I made a mistake. I am not stupid, and I do lots of things right." They also discussed other types of responses and why they were less acceptable. They recognized that Alessa's lack of verbal response and bursting into tears was a nonassertive response. They also identified other examples, such as the following:

1. An aggressive response might be, "Cook your own supper!" and toss the skillet out the back door.
2. A passive-aggressive response might be to fix sandwiches for supper and not speak to Joe for 3 days.

Practice on the assertive response began, with the nurse and various members of the group playing the role of Joe so that Alessa could practice until she felt comfortable with the response. She participated in the group for 6 months, regularly submitting situations with which she needed help. She also learned from the situations presented by other members of the group. These weekly sessions gave Alessa the self-confidence that she needed to respond assertively to Joe's criticism. She became aware of her basic human rights and, with practice, was able to protect her rights by communicating them assertively. She was happy to report to the group after a few months that Joe seemed to be less critical and that their relationship was improving.

■ Individuals develop patterns of responding in various ways, such as role modeling, by receiving positive or negative reinforcement, or by conscious choice.

■ Patterns of communication and behavior can take the form of nonassertive, assertive, aggressive, or passive-aggressive responses.

■ Individuals who communicate in a *nonassertive* manner seek to please others at the expense of denying their basic human rights.

■ Individuals who communicate in an *assertive* manner stand up for their rights while protecting the rights of others.

■ Those who respond *aggressively* defend their rights by violating the basic rights of others.

■ Individuals who respond in a *passive-aggressive* manner defend their rights by expressing resistance to social and occupational demands.

■ Some important behavioral considerations of assertive behavior include eye contact, body posture, distance/physical contact, gestures, facial expression, voice, fluency, timing, listening, thoughts, content, and persistence.

■ Using "I" statements is an important technique of assertive communication.

■ Competency in the skills of emotional intelligence is foundational to effective assertive communication and behavior.

■ Negative thinking can sometimes interfere with one's ability to respond assertively. Thought-stopping techniques help individuals remove negative, unwanted thoughts from awareness and promote the development of a more assertive attitude.

■ Nurses can assist individuals to learn and practice assertiveness techniques.

■ The nursing process is an effective vehicle for providing the information and support to patients as they strive to create positive change in their lives.

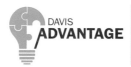 **DAVIS ADVANTAGE**

Go to **Davis Advantage** to complete your learning: strengthen understanding, apply your knowledge, and prepare for the Next Gen NCLEX®.

Review Questions

1. Your spouse says, "You're crazy to think about going to college! You're not smart enough to handle the studies along with everything else." Which of the following is an example of an ***assertive*** response?
   a. "I will do what I can and the best that I can."
   b. (Thinking to yourself): "I'll just go anyway and keep it a secret."
   c. "You're probably right. Maybe I should reconsider."
   d. "I'm going to do what I want to do, when I want to do it, and you can't stop me!"

2. You are having company for dinner, and they are due to arrive in 20 minutes. You are about to finish cooking and still have to shower and dress. The doorbell rings, and it is a man selling a new product for cleaning windows. Which of the following is an example of an ***aggressive*** response?
   a. "I don't do windows!" and slam the door in his face.
   b. "I'll take a case," and write him a check.
   c. "Sure, I'll take three bottles." Then to yourself you think: "I'm calling this company tomorrow and complaining to the manager about their salespeople coming around at dinnertime!"
   d. "I'm very busy at the moment. I don't wish to purchase any of your product. Thank you."

3. A nurse who is giving a change-of-shift report to the oncoming nurse reports having been unable to obtain an ordered urine specimen because the patient was sleeping the entire shift. The oncoming nurse retorts "Well thanks a lot for making more work for me! Do I have to do everything for you?" Which of these is an ***assertive*** response?
   a. Say nothing and continue reporting on the next patient.
   b. "This was a circumstance beyond my control, and I don't appreciate the implication that I'm not doing my work."
   c. "I'll make sure to wake up patients in the middle of the night and tell them *you'd* rather not have to wait until they are up and about."
   d. "You're the worst nurse I've ever met!"

4. A spouse comes home from work and angrily shouts, "Why the heck isn't dinner ready?" Which of the following is an example of a ***passive-aggressive*** response?
   a. "I'm sorry. I'll have it done in no time, honey." But then intentionally takes a long time to cook the meal.
   b. "I'm tired, too. Make your own dinner, you bum! I'm tired of being your slave!"
   c. "I haven't started dinner yet. I'd like some help from you."
   d. "I'm so sorry. I know you're tired and hungry. It's all my fault!"

5. You and your best friend have had plans for 6 months to go on vacation together to Hawaii. You have saved your money and have plane tickets to leave in 3 weeks. Your friend just called and said they have to cancel the trip because another friend has offered some free tickets to a concert during the same time period. Which of the following is an example of an ***assertive*** response?
   a. "I'm very disappointed and very angry. I'd like to talk to you about this later. I'll call you."
   b. "I'm very happy for you. It sounds like it will be a great concert."
   c. Tell your friend that you understand and privately vow to never speak again.
   d. "What? You can't do that to me! We've had plans! You're acting like a real selfish brat!"

Clinical Judgment Questions

6. A client on the psychiatric unit approaches the nurse, strokes the nurse's arm, and says, "Why don't you be a sweetie and get me some pain medication." Which of these actions by the nurse demonstrates the best clinical judgment?
   a. Ignore the client's behavior and assess pain level.
   b. Inform the client that patronizing attitudes are not the best way to get more pain medication.
   c. Tell the client that this behavior is not appropriate and clarify unit rules and policies regarding touching others.
   d. Tell the client, "If you call me sweetie or touch me one more time, I will call security and have you restrained."

7. A client tells the nurse, "I know I need to communicate more assertively, but I don't really know how." Which of these is the best response by the nurse?
   a. Inform the client that you will make a referral to an advanced practice nurse because generalist nurses are not within their scope of practice to teach assertiveness skills.
   b. Affirm that the client must know how to communicate assertively because they just did communicate their needs.
   c. Instruct the client that as long as they use "I" statements their communication will be assertive.
   d. Ask the client to further describe their concerns and offer to provide education in assertiveness skills.

8. During a client education group on assertiveness skills, a client asks a question while some other group members are carrying on a separate conversation, appearing not to listen. The client states, "When you appear not to be listening, I feel disrespected. I need for the group to listen to my question." How should the nurse respond to this event?
   a. Reinforce that the client used assertive communication to express their needs and affirm that respect for other group members includes not having private conversations during the group.
   b. Tell the client to ask the question again and speak louder.
   c. Instruct the client that no one is being disrespectful but their low self-esteem may be influencing their perception.
   d. Terminate the group and offer to talk with the client privately about their questions.

9. A nurse is approached by a mental health technician who states, "I need for you to do 15-minute checks on my clients because I've got too many other things to do." This has been a regular occurrence with the mental health technician, and other staff members have complained that this worker is "just being lazy." Which of these is the best response by the nurse?
   a. Commend the technician for using good "I" communication.
   b. Instruct the technician that his peers think he is just being lazy.
   c. Reinforce to the technician that everyone is busy.
   d. State to the technician the expectation that they will complete their assigned duties.

10. A physician approaches the nurse, yelling loudly and stating, "You must be the stupidest person to ever get out of nursing school. I said I wanted vital signs on this client every 4 hours and there are no recordings of temperatures. Do I need to teach you what vital signs are?" Which of these is the best response by the nurse?

    a. "Yes, doctor, I know what vital signs are."

    b. "I will try to find the information you are looking for, but I don't appreciate your belittling comments. I need for you to treat me with respect."

    c. "If *you* weren't so stupid you would know that the temperatures are recorded on a separate graph in the electronic health record."

    d. "I'm not doing a thing for you until you treat me with respect."

References

Alberti, R. E., & Emmons, M. L. (2017). *Your perfect right* (10th ed.). Impact Publishers.

Ayhan, D., & Öz, H. S. (2021). Effect of assertiveness training on the nursing students' assertiveness and self-esteem levels: Application of hybrid education in COVID-19 pandemic. *Nursing Forum, 56*(4), 807–815. doi: 10.1111/nuf.12610

Bishop, S. (2013). *Develop your assertiveness.* Kogan Page.

Cantero-Sánchez, F. J., León-Rubio, J. M., Vázquez-Morejón, R., & León-Pérez, J. M. (2021). Evaluation of an assertiveness training based on the social learning theory for occupational health, safety and environment practitioners. *Sustainability, 13*, 11504. https://doi.org/10.3390/su132011504

Davis, M., Eshelman, E. R., & McKay, M. (2008). *The relaxation and stress reduction workbook* (6th ed.). New Harbinger Publications.

Goleman, D. (2006). *Working with emotional intelligence.* Bantam.

Grosaru, L. (2020). *Assertive rights and principles explained.* https://psychologycorner.com/assertive-rights-and-principles-explained/

Hopkins, L. (2022). Assertive communication: Six tips for effective use. *EzineArticles.* http://ezinearticles.com/?Assertive-Communication-6-Tips-For-Effective-Use&id=10259

Lloyd, S. R. (2002). *Developing positive assertiveness* (3rd ed.). Crisp Publications.

Maaly, I. E. M., Merfat, A. M., & Faten, A. H. (2016). The effectiveness of social skill training on depressive symptoms, self-esteem, and interpersonal difficulties among schizophrenic patients. *International Journal of Advanced Nursing Studies, 5*(1), 43–50. doi:10.14419/ijans.v5i1.5386

Shean, G. D. (2013). Empirically based psychosocial therapies for schizophrenia: The disconnection between science and practice. *Schizophrenia Research and Treatment.* https://www.hindawi.com/journals/schizort/2013/792769

Speed, B. C., Goldstein, B. L., & Goldfried, M. R. (2017). Assertiveness training: A forgotten evidence-based treatment. *Clinical Psychology: Science and Practice, 25*, 1–20. doi:10.1111/cpsp.12216

Tavakoli, P., Setoodeh, G., Dashtbozorgi, B., Komili-Sani, H., & Pakseresht, S. (2014). The influence of assertiveness training on self-esteem in female students of government high schools of Shiraz, Iran: A randomized controlled trial. *Nursing Practice Today 2014, 1*(1), 17–23.

Classical References

Powell, T. J., & Enright, S. J. (1990). *Anxiety and stress management.* Routledge.

Salovey, P., & Mayer, J. D. (1990). Emotional intelligence. *Imagination, Cognition, and Personality, 9*, 185–211. doi:0.2190/DUGG-P24E-52WK-6CDG

Wolpe, J. (1990). *The practice of behavior therapy* (4th ed.) Pergamon Press.

Promoting Self-Esteem

14

CORE CONCEPTS

Self: Self-Esteem
Teaching and Learning
Professional Behavior: Nursing process in the care of patients with low self-esteem
Clinical Judgment

KEY TERMS

body image
boundaries
contextual stimuli
enmeshed boundaries

flexible boundaries
focal stimulus
ideal self
moral-ethical self

residual stimuli
rigid boundaries
self-consistency

OBJECTIVES
After reading this chapter, the student will be able to:

1. Identify and define components of the self-concept.
2. Discuss influencing factors in the development of self-esteem and its progression through the life span.
3. Describe the verbal and nonverbal manifestations of low self-esteem.
4. Discuss the concept of boundaries and its relationship to self-esteem.
5. Apply the nursing process with patients who are experiencing disturbances in self-esteem.

Whereas self-concept describes individuals' *thoughts and beliefs* about themselves, self-esteem describes how individuals *feel* about themselves. Hosogi and associates (2012) described self-esteem as a feeling of self-appreciation that is indispensable for adaptation in society. The awareness of self (i.e., the ability to form an identity and then attach a value to it) is an important differentiating factor between humans and other animals. The capacity for judgment becomes a contributing factor in disturbances of self-esteem.

The promotion of self-esteem is about stopping irrational self-judgments. It is about helping individuals change how they perceive and feel about themselves. Cognitive behavior therapy, which focuses on helping the client correct irrational thoughts about themselves, is an evidence-based strategy for improving self-esteem. A healthy self-esteem means having a balanced, accurate view of oneself, which includes being able to recognize one's flaws while maintaining a good opinion of one's abilities (Mayo Clinic, 2022). This chapter describes the developmental progression and the verbal and behavioral manifestations of self-esteem. The concept of boundaries and its relationship to self-esteem is explored. Nursing care of patients with disturbances in self-esteem is described in the context of the nursing process.

CORE CONCEPT
Self-Concept
Self-concept is one's overall idea about oneself, including beliefs about oneself physically, emotionally, socially, and functionally.

Components of Self-Concept

Body Image

An individual's **body image** is a subjective perception of their physical appearance based on self-evaluation and reactions and feedback from others. This perception may be realistic or distorted; in either case, it is intimately linked to one's self-concept and self-esteem.

■ An individual's body image may not necessarily coincide with their actual appearance. For example, individuals who have been overweight for many years and then lose weight often have difficulty perceiving of themselves as thin. They may even continue to choose clothing in the size they were before they lost weight.

■ A disturbance in one's body image may occur with changes in structure or function. Examples of changes in body structure include amputations, mastectomy, and facial disfigurements. Functional alterations are conditions such as colostomy, paralysis, and impotence. Alterations in body image are often experienced as losses.

Personal Identity

This component of self-concept is composed of the moral-ethical self, self-consistency, and the ideal self.

■ **Moral-ethical self** is that aspect of the personal identity that evaluates who the individual says they are. This component of the self observes, compares, sets standards, and makes judgments that influence an individual's self-evaluation.

■ **Self-consistency** is the component of the personal identity that strives to maintain a stable self-image. Even if the self-image is negative, because of this need for stability and self-consistency, the individual resists letting go of the image from which they have achieved a measure of constancy.

■ **Ideal self** relates to an individual's perception of what they want to be, do, or become. The ideal self is borne out of societal expectations, admired qualities in others, and personal perceptions about what or who one should strive to become. Disturbances in self-concept can occur when individuals are unable to achieve their ideals and self-expectations.

> ## CORE CONCEPT
> ### Self-Esteem
> Self-esteem is the degree of regard or respect that individuals have for themselves and is a measure of worth that they place on their abilities and judgments.

Self-Esteem

Warren (1991) stated:

> Self-esteem breaks down into two components: (1) the ability to say that "I am important," "I matter," and (2) the ability to say "I am competent," "I have something to offer to others and the world." (p. 1)

Maslow (1970) postulated that individuals must achieve positive self-esteem before they can achieve self-actualization (see Chapter 2, "Mental Health and Mental Illness: Historical and Theoretical Concepts"). One's self-value is challenged daily by changes within the environment. With a positive self-worth, individuals are able to adapt successfully to the demands associated with situational and maturational stressors that occur. The ability to adapt to these environmental changes is impaired when individuals hold themselves in low esteem. Self-esteem is closely related to the other components of the self-concept. Just as with body image and personal identity, the development of self-esteem is largely influenced by perceptions about how one is viewed by significant others. It begins in early childhood and vacillates throughout the life span.

Development of Self-Esteem

How self-esteem is established has been the topic of investigation for many theorists and clinicians. In a longitudinal study of self-esteem development (Erol & Orth, 2011), several factors were consistently correlated with higher self-esteem:

■ **Emotional stability:** At each age, individuals who had emotional stability had higher self-esteem than those who had unstable emotions.

■ **Extroversion:** The personality trait of extroversion, which includes a social, outgoing personality, was consistently associated with higher self-esteem than was the trait of introversion.

■ **Conscientiousness:** At each age, the personality trait of conscientiousness, which includes a desire to be thoughtful, careful, and to do the right thing, was associated with higher self-esteem.

■ **A high sense of mastery:** The sense that one has control over the forces affecting one's life or that one is able to be effective was consistently associated with higher self-esteem. Part of developing a sense of mastery involves clear differentiation of those things over which a person has control and those things that are beyond a person's ability to control. For example, individuals can choose how they communicate with another person, but they do not have control over how the other person responds. Clarity about these differences supports a person's sense of mastery. In contrast, becoming overly concerned with what someone else's responses and opinions (something one has no control over) say about their worth may contribute to a person devaluing themselves, which is the foundation for low self-esteem.

- **Low risk taking:** At any age, a tendency to engage in risky behavior was associated with lower self-esteem, and low risk-taking was correlated with higher self-esteem.
- **Being healthy:** At any age, the perception of being healthy was associated with higher self-esteem.

Warren (1991) outlined the following focus areas to be emphasized by parents and others who work with children when encouraging the growth and development of positive self-esteem:

- **A sense of competence:** Everyone needs to feel skilled at something. Warren (1991) stated, "Children do not necessarily need to be THE best at a skill in order to have positive self-esteem; what they need to feel is that they have accomplished their PERSONAL best effort" (p. 1).
- **Unconditional love:** Children need to know that they are loved and accepted by family and friends regardless of success or failure. Unconditional love is demonstrated by expressive touch, realistic praise, and separation of criticism of the person from criticism of the behavior.
- **A sense of survival:** Everyone fails at something from time to time. Self-esteem is enhanced when individuals learn from failure and grow in the knowledge that they are stronger for having experienced it.
- **Realistic goals:** Low self-esteem can be the result of not being able to achieve established goals. Individuals may set themselves up for failure by setting unattainable goals. Goals can be unrealistic when they are beyond a child's capability to achieve, require an inordinate amount of effort to accomplish, and are based on exaggerated fantasy.
- **A sense of responsibility:** Children gain positive self-worth when they are assigned areas of responsibility or are expected to complete tasks that they perceive are valued by others.
- **Reality orientation:** Personal limitations abound within our world, and it is important for children to recognize and achieve a healthy balance between what they can possess and achieve and what is beyond their capability or control.

Other factors have been found to be influential in the development of self-esteem:

- **The responses of others:** The development of self-esteem can be positively or negatively influenced by the responses of others, particularly significant others, and by how individuals perceive those responses. Role modeling and teaching children strategies for evaluating and keeping in perspective the responses of others contributes to their ability to develop self-esteem.
- **Hereditary factors:** Factors that are genetically determined, such as physical appearance, size, or inherited infirmity, can affect the development of self-esteem. Reinforcing a child's strengths and helping the child to differentiate factors over which they have control or the ability to change contributes to a sense of mastery and self-esteem.
- **Environmental conditions:** The development of self-esteem can be influenced by demands from the environment. For example, intellectual prowess may be incorporated into the self-worth of an individual who is reared in an academic environment.

Developmental Progression of Self-Esteem Through the Life Span

The development of self-esteem progresses throughout the life span. Erikson's (1963) theory of personality development provides a useful framework for illustration. Erikson described eight transitional or maturational crises, the resolution of which can have a profound influence on self-esteem. If a crisis is successfully resolved at one stage, the individual develops healthy coping strategies that they can draw on to help fulfill tasks of subsequent stages. When an individual fails to achieve the tasks associated with a developmental stage, emotional growth is inhibited, and they are less able to cope with subsequent maturational or situational crises.

Trust versus Mistrust (Birth to 18 Months)

The development of trust results in a feeling of confidence in the predictability of the environment. Achievement of trust results in positive self-esteem through the instillation of self-confidence, optimism, and faith in the gratification of needs. Unsuccessful resolution results in the individual experiencing emotional dissatisfaction with the self and suspiciousness of others, thereby promoting negative self-esteem.

Autonomy versus Shame and Doubt (18 Months to 3 Years)

With motor and mental development come greater movement and independence within the environment. The child begins active exploration and experimentation. Achievement of the task results in a sense of self-control and the ability to delay gratification, as well as a feeling of self-confidence in one's ability to perform.

This task remains unresolved when the child's independent behaviors are restricted or when the child fails because of unrealistic expectations. Negative self-esteem is promoted by a lack of self-confidence, a lack of pride in the ability to perform, and a sense of being controlled by others.

Initiative versus Guilt (3 to 6 Years)

Positive self-esteem is gained through initiative when creativity is encouraged and performance is recognized and positively reinforced. In this stage, children strive to develop a sense of purpose and the ability to initiate and direct their own activities.

This is the stage during which the child begins to develop a conscience. They become vulnerable to the labeling of behaviors as "good" or "bad." Guidance and discipline that rely heavily on shaming the child create guilt and result in a decrease in self-esteem.

Industry versus Inferiority (6 to 12 Years)

Self-confidence is gained at this stage through learning, competing, performing successfully, and receiving recognition from significant others, peers, and acquaintances. Negative self-esteem is the result of nonachievement, unrealistic expectations, or when accomplishments are consistently met with negative feedback. The child develops a sense of personal inadequacy.

Identity versus Role Confusion (12 to 20 Years)

During adolescence, the individual is striving to redefine the sense of self. Positive self-esteem occurs when individuals are allowed to experience independence by making decisions that influence their lives.

Failure to develop a new self-definition results in a sense of self-consciousness, doubt, and confusion about one's role in life. This can occur when adolescents are encouraged to remain in a dependent position; when discipline in the home has been overly harsh, inconsistent, or absent; and when parental support has been lacking. These conditions are influential in the development of low self-esteem.

Intimacy versus Isolation (20 to 30 Years)

Intimacy is achieved when one is able to form a lasting relationship or a commitment to another person, a cause, an institution, or a creative effort. Positive self-esteem is promoted through this capacity for giving of oneself to another.

Failure to achieve intimacy results in behaviors such as withdrawal, social isolation, aloneness, and the inability to form lasting, intimate relationships. Isolation occurs when love in the home has been deprived or distorted throughout the younger years, causing severe impairment in self-esteem.

Generativity versus Stagnation (30 to 65 Years)

Generativity promotes positive self-esteem through gratification from personal and professional achievements and from meaningful contributions to others. Failure to achieve generativity occurs when earlier developmental tasks are not fulfilled, and the individual does not achieve the degree of maturity required to derive gratification out of personal concern for the welfare of others. The person lacks self-worth and becomes withdrawn and isolated.

Ego Integrity versus Despair (65 Years and Older)

Ego integrity results in a sense of self-worth and self-acceptance as one reviews life goals, accepting that some were achieved and some were not. The individual has little desire to make major changes in how their life has progressed. Positive self-esteem is evident.

Individuals in despair possess a sense of self-contempt and disgust with how life has progressed. They feel worthless and helpless and would like to have a second chance at life. Earlier developmental tasks of self-confidence, self-identity, and concern for others remain unfulfilled. Negative self-esteem prevails.

In the late 1990s, Erikson advanced the concept of transcendence as an additional stage that occurs after the stage of integrity versus despair (Erikson & Erikson, 1997). This stage incorporates the tasks of broadening personal boundaries and developing an increased sense of meaning in life. Accomplishment of these tasks in the life span of 80 years and beyond contributes to one's sense of self-worth and satisfaction with life.

Manifestations of Low Self-Esteem

Individuals with low self-esteem perceive themselves to be incompetent, unlovable, insecure, and unworthy and manifest behaviors that demonstrate their feelings about themselves. The number of manifestations exhibited is influenced by the degree to which an individual experiences low self-esteem. Nursing theorist Roy (1976, 2009) categorized these behaviors according to the type of stimuli that give rise to manifestations of low self-esteem and affirmed the importance of collecting this type of information in the nursing assessment. Stimulus categories are identified as *focal, contextual,* and *residual.*

Focal Stimuli

A **focal stimulus** is the *immediate* concern that is causing the threat to self-esteem and the stimulus that is engendering the current behavior. Examples of focal stimuli include termination of a significant relationship or loss of employment.

Contextual Stimuli

Contextual stimuli are all of the other stimuli present in the person's environment that *contribute* to the behavior being caused by the focal stimulus. Examples of contextual stimuli (related to the previously mentioned focal stimuli) might be preoccupation with guilt about the effects a divorce may have on one's children or the perception that advanced age will interfere with obtaining employment.

Residual Stimuli

Residual stimuli are previous experiences that influence one's maladaptive behavior in response to focal and contextual stimuli. For example, being reared in an atmosphere of ridicule and deprecation may affect one's current adaptation to divorce. Previous experiences with multiple job losses may affect one's current perceptions about self-efficacy in acquiring a new job.

Symptoms of Low Self-Esteem

Driever (1976) identified several behaviors manifested by the individual with low self-esteem. It is clear that low self-esteem and depression share many of the same symptoms. Indeed, low self-esteem is an underlying feature in many types of depressive disorders. These behaviors are presented in Box 14–1.

Boundaries

The term **boundaries** is used to denote the personal space, both physical and psychological, that individuals identify as their own. Boundaries are sometimes referred to as *limits:* the limit or degree to which individuals feel comfortable in a relationship. Boundaries define and differentiate an individual's physical and psychological space from the physical and psychological space of others.

Boundaries help individuals define the self and are part of the individuation process. More importantly, boundaries are a measure of self-esteem; healthy boundaries communicate self-respect and an expectation to be treated well in interpersonal relationships (Collingwood, 2022). Types of physical boundaries include physical closeness, touching, sexual behavior, eye contact, privacy (e.g., mail, diary, doors, nudity, bathroom, telephone), and pollution (e.g., noise and smoke), among others. Examples of invasions of physical boundaries are reading someone else's diary, smoking in a nonsmoking public area, and touching someone who does not wish to be touched.

Types of psychological boundaries include beliefs, feelings, choices, needs, time alone, interests, confidences, individual differences, and spirituality, among others. Examples of invasions of psychological boundaries are being criticized for doing something differently than others; having personal information shared in confidence told to others; and being told one "should" believe, feel, decide, choose, or think in a certain way.

BOX 14–1 Manifestations of Low Self-Esteem

1. Loss of appetite/weight loss
2. Overeating
3. Constipation or diarrhea
4. Sleep disturbances (insomnia or difficulty falling or staying asleep)
5. Hypersomnia
6. Complaints of fatigue
7. Poor posture
8. Withdrawal from activities
9. Difficulty initiating new activities
10. Decreased libido
11. Decrease in spontaneous behavior
12. Expression of sadness, anxiety, or discouragement
13. Expression of feeling of isolation, being unlovable, unable to express or defend oneself, and too weak to confront or overcome difficulties
14. Fearful of angering others
15. Avoidance of situations of self-disclosure or public exposure
16. Tendency to stay in background, be a listener rather than a participant
17. Sensitivity to criticism; self-conscious
18. Expression of feelings of helplessness
19. Various complaints of aches and pains
20. Expression of being unable to do anything "good" or productive; expression of feelings of worthlessness and inadequacy
21. Expressions of self-deprecation, self-dislike, and unhappiness with self
22. Denial of past successes and accomplishments and of possibility for success with current activities
23. Feeling that anything one does will fail or be meaningless
24. Ruminating about problems
25. Seeking reinforcement from others; making efforts to gain favors but failing to reciprocate such behavior
26. Seeing self as a burden to others
27. Alienation from others by clinging and self-preoccupation
28. Self-accusatory
29. Demanding reassurance but not accepting it
30. Hostile behavior
31. Angry at self and others but unable to express these feelings directly
32. Decreased ability to meet responsibilities
33. Decreased interest, motivation, concentration
34. Decrease in self-care, hygiene

Adapted from Lloyd, S. R. (2002). *Developing positive assertiveness* (3rd ed.). Crisp Learning.

Boundary Pliancy

Boundaries can be rigid, flexible, or enmeshed. The behavior of dogs and cats can be a good illustration of rigid boundaries and flexible boundaries. Most dogs want to be as close to people as possible. When "their people" walk into the room, the dog is likely to be all over them. They want to be where their people are and do what they are doing. Dogs have very flexible boundaries.

Cats, on the other hand, have very distinct boundaries. They do what they want, when they want. They decide how close they will be to their people, and when. Cats take notice when their people enter a room but may not even acknowledge their presence (until the cat decides the time is right). Their boundaries are less flexible than those of dogs.

Rigid Boundaries

Individuals who have **rigid boundaries** often have a hard time trusting others and are unable to alter a boundary even when it is appropriate and healthy. They keep others at a distance and are difficult to communicate with. They reject new ideas or experiences and often withdraw, both emotionally and physically.

Example

Brent and Meghan were seeing a marriage counselor because they were unable to agree on many aspects of raising their children, and it was beginning to interfere with their relationship. Meghan runs a day-care service out of their home, and Brent is an accountant. Meghan states, "He never once changed a diaper or got up at night with a child. Now that they are older, he refuses to discipline them in any way." Brent responds, "In my family, my Mom took care of the house and kids and my Dad kept us clothed and fed. That's the way it should be. It's Meghan's job to raise the kids. It's my job to make the money." Brent's boundaries are considered rigid because he refuses to consider the ideas of others or to experience alternative ways of doing things.

Flexible Boundaries

Healthy boundaries are flexible. That is, individuals with **flexible boundaries** are able to let go of their boundaries and limits *when appropriate*. In order to have flexible boundaries, individuals must be aware of who is considered safe and when it is safe to let others invade their personal space.

Example

Kristen always takes the hour from 4 to 5 p.m. for her own. She takes no phone calls and tells the children that she is not to be disturbed during that hour. Today her private time was interrupted when her 15-year-old daughter came home from school crying because she had not made the cheerleading squad. Kristen used her private time to comfort her daughter, who was grieving the failure.

Sometimes boundaries can be too flexible. Individuals with boundaries that are too loose are like chameleons. They take their "colors" from whomever they happen to be with at the time. That is, they allow others to make their choices and direct their behavior.

Example

At a cocktail party, Diane agreed with one person that she didn't like hugging people when they approach you. Later, at the same party, she approached others and greeted them with hugs.

Enmeshed Boundaries

Enmeshed boundaries occur when two people's boundaries are so blended together that neither can be sure where one stops and the other begins, or one individual's boundaries may be blurred with another's. The individual with enmeshed boundaries may be unable to differentiate their feelings, wants, and needs from the other person's.

Examples

1. Leila's parents are in town for a visit. They say to Leila, "Dear, we want to take you and Josh out to dinner tonight. What is *your* favorite restaurant?" Leila automatically responds, "Villa Roma," knowing that the Italian restaurant is Josh's favorite.
2. Aileen got her hair cut without her mother's knowledge. It was styled with spikes across the top of her head. When her mother saw it, she said, "How dare you go around looking like that! What will people think of me?"

Establishing Boundaries

Boundaries are established in childhood. Unhealthy boundaries are the products of unhealthy, troubled, or dysfunctional families. The boundaries enclose painful feelings that have their origin in the dysfunctional family and that have not been dealt with. McKay and Fanning (2000) explained the correlation between unhealthy boundaries and self-esteem disturbances and how they can arise out of negative role models:

> Modeling self-esteem means valuing oneself enough to take care of one's own basic needs. When parents put themselves last or chronically sacrifice for their kids, they teach them that a person is only worthy insofar as he or she is of service to others. When parents set consistent, supportive limits and protect themselves from overbearing demands, they send a

message to their children that both are important and both have legitimate needs. (p. 312)

In addition to the lack of positive role models, unhealthy boundaries may also be the result of abuse or neglect. These circumstances can cause a delay in psychosocial development. Individuals must then resume the grief process as an adult to continue the developmental progression. They learn to recognize feelings, work through core issues, and tolerate emotional pain as their own. They complete the individuation process, go on to develop healthy boundaries, and learn to appreciate their self-worth.

The Nursing Process in Promoting Positive Self-Esteem

Assessment

Patients with self-esteem problems may manifest any of the symptoms presented in Box 14–1. Some patients with disturbances in self-esteem make direct statements that reflect guilt, shame, or negative self-appraisal, but often it is necessary for the nurse to ask specific questions to obtain this type of information. In particular, patients who have experienced abuse or other severe trauma often have kept feelings and fears buried for years, and behavioral manifestations of low self-esteem may not be readily evident.

Various tools for measuring self-esteem exist. One is presented in Box 14–2. This particular tool can be used as a self-inventory by the patient, or it can be adapted and used by the nurse to format questions for assessing the level of self-esteem in the patient.

Diagnosis and Outcome Identification

NANDA International has accepted for use and testing four nursing diagnoses that relate to self-esteem. These diagnoses are chronic low self-esteem, situational low self-esteem, risk for chronic low self-esteem, and risk for situational low self-esteem (Herdman et al., 2021). Each is described here with its definitions and defining characteristics.

BOX 14–2 Self-Esteem Inventory

Place a checkmark in the column that most closely describes your answer to each statement. Each check is worth the number of points listed above each column.

	3 Often or a Great Deal	2 Sometimes	1 Seldom or Occasionally	0 Never or Not at All
1. I become angry or hurt when criticized.				
2. I am afraid to try new things.				
3. I feel stupid when I make a mistake.				
4. I have difficulty looking people in the eye.				
5. I have difficulty making small talk.				
6. I feel uncomfortable in the presence of strangers.				
7. I am embarrassed when people compliment me.				
8. I am dissatisfied with the way I look.				
9. I am afraid to express my opinions in a group.				
10. I prefer staying home alone to participating in group social situations.				
11. I have trouble accepting teasing.				
12. I feel guilty when I say "no" to people.				
13. I am afraid to make a commitment to a relationship for fear of rejection.				
14. I believe that most people are more competent than I.				
15. I feel resentment toward people who are attractive and successful.				
16. I have trouble thinking of any positive aspects about my life.				
17. I feel inadequate in the presence of authority figures.				
18. I have trouble making decisions.				
19. I fear the disapproval of others.				
20. I feel tense, stressed out, or uptight.				

Problems with low self-esteem are indicated by items scored with a 3 or by a total score higher than 46.

Chronic Low Self-Esteem

Definition "Long-standing negative perception of self-worth, self-acceptance, self-respect, competence, and attitude toward self" (Herdman et al., 2021, p. 348).

Defining characteristics

■ Dependent on others' opinions
■ Underestimates ability to deal with situations
■ Hesitant to try new things
■ Indecisive behavior
■ Exaggerates negative feedback about self
■ Guilt
■ Nonassertive behavior
■ Excessively seeks reassurance
■ Overly conforming
■ Shame
■ Passive
■ Frequent lack of success in life events
■ Rejection of positive feedback

Situational Low Self-Esteem

Definition "Change from positive to negative perception of self-worth, self-acceptance, self-respect, competence, and attitude toward self in response to a current situation" (Herdman et al., 2021, p. 351).

Defining characteristics

■ Helplessness
■ Indecisive behavior
■ Nonassertive behavior
■ Purposelessness
■ Self-negating verbalizations
■ Situational challenges to self-worth
■ Underestimates ability to deal with the situation

Risk for Chronic Low Self-Esteem

Definition "Susceptible to long-standing negative perception of self-worth, self-acceptance, self-respect, competence, and attitude toward self, which may compromise health" (Herdman et al., 2021, p. 350).

Risk factors

■ Cultural incongruence
■ Exposure to a traumatic situation
■ Inadequate affection received
■ Inadequate group membership
■ Inadequate respect from others
■ Ineffective coping with loss
■ Insufficient feeling of belonging
■ Psychiatric disorder
■ Spiritual incongruence
■ Repeated failures
■ Repeated negative reinforcement

Risk for Situational Low Self-Esteem

Definition "Susceptible to change from positive to negative perception of self-worth, self-acceptance, self-respect, competence, and attitude toward self in response to a current situation, which may compromise health" (Herdman et al., 2021, p. 353).

Risk factors

■ Alterations in body image
■ Alteration in social role
■ Behavior inconsistent with values
■ Decrease in control over environment
■ Developmental transition
■ Functional impairment
■ History of abandonment
■ History of abuse
■ History of loss
■ History of neglect
■ History of rejection
■ Inadequate recognition
■ Pattern of failure
■ Pattern of helplessness
■ Physical illness
■ Unrealistic self-expectations

Outcome Criteria

Outcome criteria include short- and long-term goals. Timelines for achievement are individually determined. The following criteria may be used for measurement of outcomes in the care of the patient with disturbances of self-esteem.

The patient:

■ Expresses positive aspects about self and life situation
■ Accepts positive feedback from others
■ Attempts new experiences
■ Accepts personal responsibility for own problems
■ Accepts constructive criticism without becoming defensive
■ Makes independent decisions about life situation
■ Uses intermittent, appropriate eye contact
■ Develops positive interpersonal relationships
■ Communicates needs and wants to others assertively

Planning and Implementation

In Table 14–1, a plan of care using selected self-esteem diagnoses accepted by NANDA International is presented. Outcome criteria, appropriate nursing interventions, and rationales are included for each diagnosis.

> **CLINICAL PEARL** Ensure that patient goals are realistic. Unrealistic goals set up the patient for failure. Provide encouragement and positive reinforcement for attempts at change. Give recognition of accomplishments, however small.

Evaluation

Reassessment is conducted to determine whether the nursing actions have been successful in achieving the

Table 14–1 | CARE PLAN FOR THE PATIENT WITH PROBLEMS RELATED TO SELF-ESTEEM

NURSING DIAGNOSIS: CHRONIC LOW SELF-ESTEEM

RELATED TO: Lack of affection/approval; repeated failures; repeated negative reinforcement

EVIDENCED BY: Exaggerates negative feedback about self and expressions of shame and guilt

OUTCOME CRITERIA	NURSING INTERVENTIONS	RATIONALE
Patient verbalizes positive aspects of self and abandons irrational, negative self-judgments.	1. Be supportive, accepting, and respectful without invading the patient's personal space.	1. Individuals who have had long-standing feelings of low self-worth may be uncomfortable with personal attentiveness.
	2. Explore inaccuracies in self-perception with the patient.	2. Patients may not see positive aspects of self that others see and bringing it to awareness may help change perception.
	3. Have the patient list successes and strengths. Provide positive feedback.	3. Helps patients to develop internal self-worth and new coping behaviors.
	4. Assess content of negative self-talk and educate the patient about the effect of cognitive distortions (irrational thinking) on self-esteem.	4. Self-blame, shame, and guilt promote feelings of low self-worth. Depending on chronicity and severity of the problem, this is likely to be the focus of long-term psychotherapy with the patient. Assisting patients to recognize the effect of negative cognition on self-esteem lays the foundation for referral to longer-term treatment such as cognitive therapies (see Chapter 18, "Cognitive Behavior Therapy").

NURSING DIAGNOSIS: SITUATIONAL LOW SELF-ESTEEM

RELATED TO: Failure (either real or perceived) in a situation of importance to the individual or loss (either real or perceived) of a concept of value to the individual

EVIDENCED BY: Indecisive behavior and expressions of helplessness and uselessness

OUTCOME CRITERIA	NURSING INTERVENTIONS	RATIONALE
Patient identifies source of threat to self-esteem and works through the stages of the grief process to resolve the loss or failure.	1. Convey an accepting attitude; encourage the patient to express self openly.	1. An accepting attitude enhances trust and communicates that the nurse believes they are a worthwhile person, regardless of what is expressed.
	2. Encourage the patient to express anger. Do not become defensive if initial expression of anger is displaced on nurse/therapist. Assist the patient in exploring angry feelings and direct them toward the intended object/person or other loss.	2. Verbalization of feelings in a nonthreatening environment may help patients come to terms with unresolved issues related to the loss.

Continued

Table 14–1 | CARE PLAN FOR THE PATIENT WITH PROBLEMS RELATED TO SELF-ESTEEM—cont'd

OUTCOME CRITERIA	NURSING INTERVENTIONS	RATIONALE
	3. Help the patient avoid ruminating about past failures. Withdraw attention if the patient persists.	3. Lack of attention to these undesirable behaviors may discourage their repetition.
	4. Educate the patient about the importance of focusing on positive attributes if self-esteem is to be enhanced. Encourage discussion of past accomplishments and offer support in undertaking new tasks. Offer recognition of successful endeavors and positive reinforcement of attempts made.	4. Recognition and positive reinforcement enhance self-esteem and encourage repetition of desirable behaviors.

NURSING DIAGNOSIS: RISK FOR SITUATIONAL LOW SELF-ESTEEM

RISK FACTORS: Developmental changes; functional impairment; disturbed body image; loss; history of abuse or neglect; unrealistic self-expectations; physical illness; failures/rejections

OUTCOME CRITERIA	NURSING INTERVENTIONS	RATIONALE
Patient's self-esteem is preserved.	1. Provide an open environment and trusting relationship.	1. Facilitates the patient's ability to deal with current situation.
	2. Determine the patient's perception of the loss or failure and its personal meaning.	2. Assessment of the cause or contributing factor is necessary to provide assistance to the patient.
	3. Identify response of family or significant others to the patient's current situation.	3. Provides additional background assessment data with which to plan the patient's care.
	4. Permit appropriate expressions of anger.	4. Anger is a stage in the normal grieving process and must be dealt with for progression to occur.
	5. Provide information about normalcy of individual grief reaction.	5. Individuals who are unaware of normal feelings associated with grief may feel guilty and try to deny certain feelings.
	6. Discuss and assist with planning for the future. Communicate hope but avoid giving false reassurance.	6. In a state of anxiety and grief, individuals need assistance with decision making and problem-solving. They may find it difficult or impossible to envision any hope for the future.

objectives of care. Evaluation of the nursing actions for the patient with self-esteem disturbances may be facilitated by gathering information using the following types of questions:

Does the patient:

■ Discuss past accomplishments and other positive aspects about their life?
■ Accept praise and recognition from others in a gracious manner?
■ Try new experiences without extreme fear of failure?
■ Accept constructive criticism now without becoming overly defensive and shifting the blame to others?
■ Accept personal responsibility for problems rather than attributing feelings and behaviors to others?
■ Participate in decisions that affect their life?
■ Make rational decisions independently?
■ Behave more assertively in interpersonal relations?
■ Manifest the physical presentation of self-esteem, such as eye contact, posture, changes in eating and sleeping, fatigue, libido, elimination patterns, self-care, and complaints of aches and pains?

Summary and Key Points

■ Emotional wellness requires that an individual have some degree of self-worth—a perception that they possess a measure of value to self and others.
■ Self-concept is a cognitive component of the self that includes a set of beliefs about oneself.
■ Body image encompasses one's appraisal of physical attributes, functioning, sexuality, wellness-illness state, and appearance.
■ The personal identity component of self-concept is composed of the moral-ethical self, self-consistency, and the ideal self.
■ Self-consistency is the component of the personal identity that strives to maintain a stable self-image.
■ Ideal self relates to an individual's perception of what they want to be, do, or become.
■ Self-esteem refers to the degree of regard or respect that individuals have for themselves and is

a measure of worth that they place on their abilities and judgments. It is largely influenced by the perceptions of how one is viewed by significant others.

■ Irrational self-judgments negatively influence one's self-esteem, and cognitive behavior therapy is an evidence-based strategy for correcting one's irrational thinking, thereby improving one's self-esteem.
■ High self-esteem is associated with emotional stability, extroversion, conscientiousness, a sense of mastery, low risk-taking, and better health. Genetics and environmental conditions may also be influencing factors.
■ The development of self-esteem progresses throughout the life span. Erikson's theory of personality development elaborates on the importance of accomplishing developmental tasks in self-esteem. The behaviors associated with low self-esteem are numerous and correlated with signs and symptoms of depression.
■ Maslow identified positive self-esteem as a prerequisite to self-actualization.
■ Stimuli that trigger behaviors associated with low self-esteem may include focal, contextual, and residual stimuli.
■ Boundaries, or personal limits, help individuals define the self and are part of the individuation process.
■ Boundaries are a measure of self-esteem.
■ Boundaries are physical and psychological and may be rigid, flexible, or enmeshed.
■ Unhealthy boundaries are often the result of dysfunctional family systems.
■ The nursing process is the vehicle for delivery of care to patients needing assistance with self-esteem disturbances.
■ The four nursing diagnoses relating to self-esteem accepted by NANDA International include chronic low self-esteem, situational low self-esteem, risk for chronic low self-esteem, and risk for situational low self-esteem.

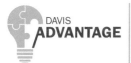
DAVIS
ADVANTAGE   Go to **Davis Advantage** to complete your learning: strengthen understanding, apply your knowledge, and prepare for the Next Gen NCLEX®.

Review Questions

1. A law school graduate failing the bar examination and a 15-year-old high school girl not being selected for the cheerleading squad are examples of which of the following?
   a. Focal stimuli
   b. Contextual stimuli
   c. Residual stimuli
   d. Spatial stimuli

2. The husband says to his wife, "What do you want to do tonight?" and his wife responds, "Whatever you want to do." This is an example of which of the following?
   a. Extremely rigid boundaries
   b. A boundary violation
   c. Extremely flexible boundaries
   d. Showing respect for the boundary of another

3. Twins Jan and Jean still dress alike even though they are grown and married. This is an example of which of the following?
   a. Rigid boundaries
   b. Enmeshed boundaries
   c. A boundary violation
   d. Boundary pliancy

4. A counselor asks the client if they would like a hug. This is an example of which of the following?
   a. Rigid boundary
   b. A boundary violation
   c. Enmeshed boundary
   d. Showing respect for the boundary of another

5. Jessica told Andrea a secret that Eva had told her. This is an example of which of the following?
   a. Too flexible a boundary
   b. A boundary violation
   c. Too rigid a boundary
   d. An enmeshed boundary

6. Tommy says to his friend, "I can't ever talk to my Daddy until after he has read his newspaper." This is an example of which of the following?
   a. A rigid boundary
   b. A boundary violation
   c. An enmeshed boundary
   d. A flexible boundary

Clinical Judgment Questions

7. A nurse is engaging in psychoeducation about improving self-esteem with a client who has depression and low self-esteem. Which of the following are important for the nurse to assess? (Select all that apply.)
   a. Focal, contextual, and residual stimuli
   b. The client's abilities with regard to establishment of boundaries
   c. The client's age and whether or not they are married
   d. The nurse's awareness of their own ability to establish appropriate boundaries
   e. The client's predominant communication style and their understanding of assertiveness

8. A teenage client is brought to the mental health clinic by her mother, who reports that her child has been very depressed since they were not accepted into the high school National Honor Society. The client states, "What's the use? I'm not good at anything." Which of these is the best action by the nurse at this point?
   a. Reinforce to the client that they have many strengths.
   b. Assist the client in determining why they weren't accepted into the Honor Society.
   c. Assess whether the client was raised in a punitive environment.
   d. Explore with the client their past accomplishments and successes.

9. A client who is hospitalized for depression tells the nurse, "I feel like nobody loves me. I must be the most unattractive person on the planet." Which of the following is the best nursing action at this point?

   a. Give the client a hug and reassure them that *you* love them.

   b. Spend time with the client exploring their thoughts and feelings about themselves.

   c. Assess the client's failed relationships to identify opportunities for change.

   d. Offer to help the client with a makeover to improve their self-esteem.

10. Which of these actions by the nurse is the best approach for promoting positive self-esteem in a depressed client who is expressing helplessness?

    a. Facilitate the client's accomplishment of realistic goals and give positive feedback when goals are accomplished.

    b. Teach the client about the negative health effects of chronic helplessness and depression.

    c. Assess why the client is feeling depressed.

    d. Reinforce the importance of medication adherence.

References

Collingwood, J. (2022). The importance of personal boundaries. *PsychCentral.* http://psychcentral.com/lib/the-importance-of-personal-boundaries

Erol, R. Y., & Orth, U. (2011). Self-esteem development from age 14 to 30 years: A longitudinal study. *Journal of Personality and Social Psychology, 101*(3), 607–619. doi:http://dx.doi.org/10.1037/a0024299

Herdman, T. H., Kamitsuru, S., & Lopes, C. T. (Eds.). (2021). *NANDA-I, Inc. nursing diagnoses: Definitions and classification, 2021–2023.* Thieme.

Hosogi, M., Okada, A., Fujii, C., Noguchi, K., & Watanabe, K. (2012). Importance and usefulness of evaluating self-esteem in children. *Biopsychosocial Medicine, 6*(9). doi:10.1186/1751-0759-6-9

Lloyd, S. R. (2002). *Developing positive assertiveness* (3rd ed.). Crisp Learning.

Mayo Clinic. (2022). *Self-esteem check: Too low or just right?* www.mayoclinic.org/healthy-lifestyle/adult-health/in-depth/self-esteem/art-20047976

McKay, M., & Fanning, P. (2000). *Self-esteem: A proven program of cognitive techniques for assessing, improving, and maintaining your self-esteem* (3rd ed.). New Harbinger Publications.

Roy, C. (2009). *The Roy adaptation model* (3rd ed.). Pearson Education.

Classical References

Driever, M. J. (1976). Problem of low self-esteem. In Roy, C. (Ed.), *Introduction to nursing: An adaptation model* (pp. 232–242). Prentice-Hall.

Erikson, E. H. (1963). *Childhood and society* (2nd ed.). W.W. Norton.

Erikson, E.H. & Erikson, J. M. (1997). *The life cycle completed: Extended version with new chapters on the ninth stage of development.* W.W. Norton.

Maslow, A. (1970). *Motivation and personality* (2nd ed.). Harper & Row.

Roy, C. (1976). *Introduction to nursing: An adaptation model.* Prentice Hall.

Warren, J. (1991). Your child and self-esteem. *The Prairie View, 30*(2), 1.

15 Anger and Aggression Management

KEY TERMS

modeling   operant conditioning   prodromal syndrome

OBJECTIVES
After reading this chapter, the student will be able to:

1. Define and differentiate between *anger* and *aggression.*
2. Identify when the expression of anger becomes a problem.
3. Discuss predisposing factors to the maladaptive expression of anger.
4. Apply the nursing process to patients expressing anger or aggression.
   a. Assessment: Describe physical and psychological responses to anger.
   b. Diagnosis/Outcome Identification: Formulate nursing diagnoses and outcome criteria for patients expressing anger and aggression.
   c. Planning/Intervention: Describe nursing interventions for patients demonstrating maladaptive expressions of anger.
   d. Evaluation: Evaluate achievement of the projected outcomes in the intervention with patients demonstrating maladaptive expression of anger.

Anger is not always a negative expression. It is a normal human emotion that, when handled appropriately and expressed assertively, can provide an individual with a positive force to solve problems and make decisions concerning life situations. Anger becomes a problem when it is not expressed or when it is expressed aggressively. Violence occurs when individuals lose control of their anger. The rate of violent crimes in the United States in 2020 was 398.5 per 100,000 inhabitants and aggravated assault accounted for around two-thirds of all violent crimes (Statistica, 2021). Although the rate of violent crimes (reported by the Federal Bureau of Investigation) has seen a downward trend since the 1990s, 2020 saw an increase in violent crimes, particularly in murder and nonnegligent manslaughter rates. Violent crimes are reported daily by the news media, and health-care workers see the results each day in the emergency departments of general hospitals.

This chapter addresses the concepts of anger and aggression. Predisposing factors to the maladaptive expression of anger are discussed, and the nursing process as a vehicle for delivery of care to assist clients in the management of anger and aggression is described.

Anger and Aggression, Defined

CORE CONCEPT
Anger
Anger is "an emotional state that varies in intensity from mild irritation to intense fury and rage," according to Charles Spielberger, a clinical psychologist best

known for developing the State/Trait Anxiety Inventory. Anger is accompanied by physiological and biological changes, such as increases in heart rate, blood pressure, and levels of the energy hormones adrenaline and noradrenaline (American Psychological Association [APA], 2022).

Anger is a normal, healthy emotion that serves as a warning signal and alerts us to potential threat or trauma. It triggers energy that sets us up for a good fight or quick flight and can range from mild irritation to rage. Warren (1993) outlined some fundamental points about anger:

- Anger is not a primary emotion, but it is typically experienced as an almost automatic inner response to hurt, frustration, or fear.
- Anger is physiological arousal. It instills feelings of power and generates preparedness.
- Anger and aggression are significantly different.
- The expression of anger is learned.
- The expression of anger can come under personal control.

Anger is a very powerful emotion. When it is denied or buried, it can precipitate a number of physical problems such as migraine headaches, ulcers, colitis, and even coronary heart disease. When turned inward on oneself, anger can result in depression and low self-esteem. When it is expressed inappropriately, it commonly interferes with relationships. When suppressed, anger may turn into resentment, which often manifests in negative, passive-aggressive behavior.

Anger creates a state of preparedness by arousing the sympathetic nervous system. The activation of this system results in increased heart rate and blood pressure, increased secretion of epinephrine (resulting in additional physiological arousal), and increased levels of serum glucose, among others. Anger prepares the body, physiologically, to fight. When anger is unresolved, this physiological arousal can be the predisposing factor to several health problems. Even if the situation that created the anger is removed by miles or years, it can be replayed through the memory, reactivating the sympathetic arousal when this occurs. Table 15–1 lists positive and negative functions of anger.

CORE CONCEPT

Aggression

Aggression has many different definitions depending on the context in which it is described. When describing aggression as a behavioral response to anger, aggression has been defined as a behavior intended to threaten or injure the victim's security or self-esteem. It means "to go against," "to assault," or "to attack." It is a response that aims at inflicting pain or injury on objects or persons (Warren, 1993, pp. 119–120). Aggression may include verbal and physical attacks that intend harm to another and often reflect a desire for dominance and control (Kassinove, 2023). Aggression, in general, may range from a self-protective response to a destructive, violent act.

The term *anger* often takes on a negative connotation because of its link with aggression. Aggression is one way individuals express anger. It is sometimes used to try to force someone into compliance with

TABLE 15–1 **The Functions of Anger**	
POSITIVE FUNCTIONS OR CONSTRUCTIVE USES	**NEGATIVE FUNCTIONS OR DESTRUCTIVE USES**
Anger energizes and mobilizes the body for self-defense.	Without cognitive input, anger may result in impulsive behavior, disregarding possible negative consequences.
Communicated assertively, anger can promote conflict resolution.	Communicated passive-aggressively or aggressively, conflict escalates, and the problem that created the conflict goes unresolved.
Anger arousal is a personal signal of threat or injustice against the self. The signal elicits coping responses to deal with the distress.	Anger can lead to aggression when the coping response is displacement. Anger can be destructive if it is discharged against an object or person unrelated to the true target of the anger.
Anger is constructive when it provides a feeling of control over a situation and the individual is able to assertively take charge of a situation.	Anger can be destructive when the feeling of control is exaggerated and the individual uses the power to intimidate others.
Anger is constructive when it is expressed assertively, serves to increase self-esteem, and leads to mutual understanding and forgiveness.	Anger can be destructive when it masks honest feelings, weakens self-esteem, and leads to hostility and rage.

the aggressor's wishes, but at other times, the only objective seems to be the infliction of punishment and pain. In virtually all instances, aggression is a negative function or destructive use of anger.

Predisposing Factors to Anger and Aggression

A number of factors have been implicated in the way an individual expresses anger. Some theorists view aggression as purely biological, and some suggest that it results from individuals' interactions with their environments. It is likely a combination of both.

Modeling

Role **modeling** is one of the strongest forms of learning. Children model their behavior at a very early age after their primary caregivers, usually parents. How parents or significant others express anger becomes the child's method of anger expression.

Whether role modeling is positive or negative depends on the behavior of the models. Much has been written about the abused child becoming physically abusive as an adult, which may be connected to a learned response.

Role models are not always related to home life relationships, however. Evidence supports the role of television and video violence as a predisposing factor to later aggressive behavior (APA, 2013). Zhang and associates (2021) found that even brief exposure to violent video games increased aggressive cognition and behavior and that the effect was stronger in boys than in girls. Whether modeling occurs in the home, community, or popular media, its role in the development of aggression has been well supported.

Operant Conditioning

Operant conditioning occurs when a specific behavior is reinforced. Positive reinforcement is a response to a specific behavior that is pleasurable or offers a reward. Negative reinforcement is a response to a specific behavior that prevents an undesirable result from occurring.

Anger responses can be learned through operant conditioning. For example, when a child wants something and has been told no by a parent, the child might have a temper tantrum. If the parent then gives the child an ice cream cone, the anger displayed during the temper tantrum has been positively reinforced (or rewarded).

An example of learning by negative reinforcement follows: A mother asks the child to pick up their toys, and the child becomes angry and has a temper tantrum. If, when the temper tantrum begins, the mother thinks, "Oh, it's not worth all this!" and picks up the toys herself, the anger has been negatively reinforced (the child was rewarded by not having to pick up their toys).

Neurophysiological Factors

The neurophysiology of aggression is extremely complex and only partially understood despite years of research. Perry (2016) described the findings as such: "Any factors which increase the activity or reactivity of the brainstem (e.g., chronic traumatic stress, testosterone, dysregulated serotonin or norepinephrine systems) or decrease the moderating capacity of the limbic or cortical areas (e.g., neglect) will increase an individual's aggressivity, impulsivity, and capacity to display violence." Loss of function in the frontal cortex (and subsequently decreased moderating capacity) can also occur as a result of many pathological processes, including stroke, dementia, alcohol intoxication, and traumatic brain injuries, and has been associated with increased aggression. Tumors in the brain, particularly in the areas of the limbic system and the temporal lobes; trauma to the brain resulting in cerebral changes; and diseases such as encephalitis (or medications that may effect this syndrome) have all been implicated in the predisposition to aggression and violent behavior.

Individuals may be genetically predisposed to aggression related to genetic variants that control levels of serotonin in the central and peripheral nervous systems. Consequently, administration of selective serotonin reuptake inhibitors (SSRIs) has been associated with increased frontal cortex activity and decreased aggression (Merritt, 2017; Pavlov et al., 2012).

Biochemical Factors

The effect of hormones, particularly testosterone, in aggression has been the focus of animal research, and although it has been associated with increased aggression in animals and correlation studies in humans, the effects of testosterone administration have yielded mixed results (Boland & Verduin, 2022). For example, in one controlled study where anabolic-androgenic steroids were given to normal subjects, the participants reported both positive and negative mood symptoms; the latter included anger, hostility, and violent feelings (Boland & Verduin, 2022). Although aggression is modulated by several hormonal systems, testosterone is identified as playing a key role, and deficits in serotonin have been associated with an increase in impulsivity (Vetulani, 2013). Oxytocin administration has been associated with decreasing activation in the amygdala and decreasing aggression in men (Merritt, 2017).

Socioeconomic Factors

High rates of violence exist within the subculture of poverty in the United States. Exposure to violence has been identified as having an effect on future tendencies toward aggression. An ongoing controversy exists as to whether economic inequality or absolute poverty is most responsible for aggressive and violent behavior within this subculture. That is, does violence occur because individuals perceive themselves as disadvantaged relative to other persons, or does violence occur because of the deprivation itself? These concepts are not easily understood and are still under investigation.

Environmental Factors

Three environmental factors that have been shown to increase risks for aggression are crowding, temperature, and noise (Archer, 2012). All three of these environmental factors increase stress, which has a multitude of effects on mood and behavior. Past experiences and current behavior also influence aggressive expression. The three most common predictors of violent behavior in this context are a history of childhood abuse, a history of violent acts with criminal activity or arrests, and alcohol intake (Boland & Verduin, 2022). Numerous other substances of abuse have been associated with aggression, including methamphetamines and amphetamines, bath salts, anabolic steroids, synthetic marijuana, PCP, and alpha PVP (also known as *flakka*).

The Nursing Process in Anger Management

> ## CORE CONCEPT
> ### Anger Management
> The use of various techniques and strategies to control responses to anger-provoking situations. The goal of anger management is to reduce both the emotional feelings and the physiological arousal that anger engenders.

Assessment

Sometimes crises occur for hospitalized psychiatric patients when they become unable to manage personal responsibility for their behaviors in response to anger. Nurses must be aware of the risk factors and symptoms associated with anger and aggression to make an accurate assessment. In a meta-analysis of prevalence and risk factors for violence by psychiatric acute inpatients (Iozzino et al., 2015), the researchers found that close to 1 in 5 patients may commit an act of violence. The highest risk factors were male sex, a diagnosis of schizophrenia, substance use, and a history of violence. Assessing for violence potential is an important aspect of nursing care in efforts to prevent violence in psychiatric settings. Strategies to accomplish this are presented in the following section.

Anger

Anger is often manifested in the following ways:
- Frowning facial expression
- Clenched fists
- Low-pitched verbalizations forced through clenched teeth
- Yelling and shouting
- Intense eye contact or avoidance of eye contact
- Hypersensitivity, easily offended
- Defensive response to criticism
- Passive-aggressive behaviors
- Lack of control or overcontrolled emotions
- Intense discomfort; continuous state of tension
- Flushed face
- Anxious, tense, angry facial expression (affect)

Anger is often described as a secondary emotion. For example, it may be a response to unresolved grief, depression, fear, anxiety, or unresolved post-traumatic stress. Anger is also one of the stages of the normal grief process and thus is an expected emotion. Because of the negative connotation of the word *anger,* some people will not acknowledge that they are feeling angry. These individuals need assistance to recognize their true feelings and understand that anger is a perfectly acceptable emotion; it is one's *behavior* in response to anger that may be unacceptable, such as when it results in aggression.

Aggression

Aggression can arise from a number of feeling states, including anger, anxiety, guilt, frustration, or suspiciousness. Kassinove (2023) stated that aggression may include verbal and physical attacks that intend harm to another and often reflect a desire for dominance and control. Aggressive behaviors can be classified as mild (e.g., sarcasm), moderate (e.g., slamming doors), severe (e.g., threats of physical violence against others), or extreme (e.g., physical acts of violence against others). Aggression may be associated with (but not limited to) the following defining characteristics:

- Pacing, restlessness
- Threatening body language
- Verbal or physical threats
- Loud voice, shouting, use of obscenities, argumentative

■ Threats of homicide or suicide
■ Increase in agitation, with overreaction to environmental stimuli
■ Panic anxiety, leading to misinterpretation of the environment
■ Suspiciousness and defensive posturing
■ Angry mood, often disproportionate to the situation
■ Destruction of property
■ Acts of physical harm toward another person

Aggression may be differentiated as reactive versus proactive. Reactive aggression is defined as fear based and impulsive; proactive aggression is described as predatory and calculated. In both cases, there is intent to harm another, but the motives differ. *Intent* is a requisite in the definition of aggression. It refers to behavior that is *intended* to inflict harm or destruction. Accidents that lead to *unintentional* harm or destruction are not considered aggression.

Assessing Risk Factors

Prevention is a key issue in managing aggressive or violent behavior. The individual who becomes violent usually feels an underlying helplessness. The following three factors have been identified as important considerations in assessing for potential violence:

1. Past history of violence
2. Patient diagnosis
3. Current behavior

Past history of violence is widely recognized as a major risk factor for violence in a treatment setting. Assaultive behavior is also highly correlated with specific diagnoses. Substance abuse (alone or in combination with a mental illness) is the single most important risk factor for violence; the lifetime prevalence is 35% in individuals with substance abuse or dependence compared with 16% for those with schizophrenia or a major affective disorder and a notable 43.6% in those with a comorbid mental illness and substance abuse (Victoroff, 2017).

Novitsky and associates (2009) stated:

> The successful management of violence is predicated on an understanding of the dynamics of violence. A patient's threatening behavior is commonly an overreaction to feelings of impotence, helplessness, and perceived or actual humiliation. Aggression rarely occurs suddenly and unexpectedly. (p. 50)

Novitsky and associates (2009) described a **prodromal syndrome** characterized by anxiety and tension, verbal abuse and profanity, and increasing hyperactivity. These escalating behaviors usually do not occur in stages but most often overlap and sometimes occur simultaneously. Behaviors associated with this prodromal stage include rigid posture; clenched fists and jaws; grim, defiant affect; talking in a rapid, raised voice; arguing and demanding; using profanity and threatening verbalizations; agitation and pacing; and pounding and slamming.

Most assaultive behavior is preceded by a period of increasing hyperactivity. Behaviors associated with the prodromal syndrome should be considered emergent and demand immediate attention. Keen observation skills and background knowledge for accurate assessment are critical factors in predicting the potential for violent behavior. The Brøset Violence Checklist is presented in Box 15–1. It is a quick, simple, and reliable checklist that can be used to assess the risk for potential violence. Validity testing has shown a 63% accuracy for prediction of violence at a score of 2 and above (Almvik et al., 2000). De-escalation techniques are also included.

BOX 15–1 The Brøset Violence Checklist

Score 1 point for each behavior observed. At a score of ≥2, begin de-escalation techniques.

Behaviors	Score
Confusion	
Irritability	
Boisterousness	
Physical threats	
Verbal threats	
Attacks on objects	
TOTAL SCORE	

DE-ESCALATION TECHNIQUES

Calm voice	Helpful attitude
Walk outdoors or fresh air	Reduction in demands
Identify consequences	Decrease waiting times and request refusals
Group participation	
Open hands and non-threatening posture	Verbal redirection and limit setting
Relaxation techniques	Distract with a more positive activity (e.g., soft music or a quiet room)
Allow phone call	
Express concern	
Offer food or drink	Time-out/quiet time/open seclusion
Reduce stimulation and loud noise	Offer prn medication

If de-escalation techniques fail:

1. Suggest prn medications
2. Time-out or unlocked seclusion, which can progress to locked seclusion

Source: From Almvik, R., Woods, P., & Rasmussen, K. (2000). The Brøset violence checklist: Sensitivity, specificity, and interrater reliability. *Journal of Interpersonal Violence, 15*(12), 1284–1296, with permission. De-escalation techniques reprinted with permission from Barbara Barnes, Milwaukee County Behavioral Health Division.

Diagnosis and Outcome Identification

NANDA International does not include a separate nursing diagnosis for anger. The nursing diagnosis of maladaptive grieving may be used when anger is expressed inappropriately and the etiology is related to a loss.

The following nursing diagnoses may be considered for patients demonstrating inappropriate expression of anger or aggression:

■ Ineffective coping
■ Risk for self-directed or other-directed violence

Outcome Criteria

Outcome criteria include short- and long-term goals. Timelines are individually determined. The following criteria may be used for measurement of outcomes in the care of the patient needing assistance with management of anger and aggression.

The patient:

■ Recognizes when they are angry and seeks out staff/support person to talk about their feelings
■ Takes responsibility for own feelings of anger

■ Demonstrates the ability to exert internal control over feelings of anger
■ Demonstrates the ability to diffuse anger before losing control
■ Uses the tension generated by the anger in a constructive manner
■ Causes no harm to self or others
■ Uses steps of the problem-solving process rather than becoming violent as a means of seeking solutions

Planning and Implementation

In Table 15–2, a plan of care is presented for the patient who expresses anger inappropriately. Outcome criteria, appropriate nursing interventions, and rationales are included for each diagnosis. Cognitive behavior therapy (CBT) as a strategy for anger management and aggression reduction is an evidence-based treatment that, especially when incorporated in treatment for children and adolescents, has demonstrated effectiveness in reducing maladaptive aggression (Smeets et al., 2015; Sukhodolsky et al., 2016; Vacher et al., 2022). Although

Table 15–2 | CARE PLAN FOR THE INDIVIDUAL WHO EXPRESSES ANGER INAPPROPRIATELY

NURSING DIAGNOSIS: INEFFECTIVE COPING

RELATED TO: Negative role modeling and dysfunctional family system

EVIDENCED BY: Yelling, name calling, hitting others, and temper tantrums as expressions of anger

OUTCOME CRITERIA	NURSING INTERVENTIONS	RATIONALE
Patient is able to recognize anger in self and take responsibility before losing control.	1. Remain calm when dealing with an angry patient.	1. Anger expressed by the nurse will most likely incite increased anger in patients.
	2. Set verbal limits on behavior. Clearly delineate the consequences of inappropriate expression of anger and always follow through.	2. Consistency in enforcing the consequences is essential if positive outcomes are to be achieved. Inconsistency creates confusion and encourages testing of limits.
	3. Encourage the patient to keep a diary of angry thoughts and feelings, what triggered them, and how they were handled.	3. This activity provides a more objective measure of the problem. Introducing the patient to some basic principles of cognitive reflection not only encourages problem-solving in the short term but lays the groundwork for referral to longer-term CBT if this is identified as desirable.
	4. Avoid touching the patient when they become angry.	4. The patient may view touch as threatening and could become violent.

Continued

Table 15–2 | CARE PLAN FOR THE INDIVIDUAL WHO EXPRESSES ANGER INAPPROPRIATELY—cont'd

OUTCOME CRITERIA	NURSING INTERVENTIONS	RATIONALE
	5. Help the patient determine the real source of the anger.	5. Often, anger is displaced onto a safer object or person. If resolution is to occur, the first step is to identify the source of the anger.
	6. Help the patient find alternative ways of releasing tension, such as physical outlets, and more appropriate ways of expressing anger, such as seeking out staff when feelings emerge.	6. Patients will likely need assistance to problem solve more appropriate ways of behaving.
	7. Role model appropriate ways of expressing anger assertively, such as, "I dislike being called names. I get angry when I hear you saying those things about me."	7. Role modeling is one of the strongest methods of learning.

NURSING DIAGNOSIS: RISK FOR SELF-DIRECTED OR OTHER-DIRECTED VIOLENCE

RISK FACTORS: Having been nurtured in an atmosphere of violence; history of violence; substance intoxication

OUTCOME CRITERIA	NURSING INTERVENTIONS	RATIONALE
Patient will not harm self or others. Patient verbalizes anger rather than hit others.	1. Observe the patient for escalation of anger (called the *prodromal syndrome*): increased motor activity, pounding, slamming, tense posture, defiant affect, clenched teeth and fists, arguing, demanding, and challenging or threatening staff.	1. Violence may be prevented if risks are identified in time.
	2. When these behaviors are observed, first ensure that sufficient staff are available to help with a potentially violent situation. Attempt to defuse the anger beginning with the least restrictive means.	2. The initial consideration must be ensuring that adequate staff are present to assist in diffusing a potentially violent situation. Patient rights must be honored while preventing harm to patient and others.
	3. Techniques for dealing with aggression:	3. Aggression control techniques promote safety and reduce risk of harm to patient and others:
	a. Talking down. Say, "John, you seem very angry. Let's sit down and talk about it." (Be attentive to safe physical distance from the patient and the nurse's ability to exit [i.e., ensure that patient does not position self between a door and nurse].)	a. Promotes a trusting relationship and may prevent patient's anxiety from escalating while attending to the safety needs of the nurse as well.

Table 15–2	CARE PLAN FOR THE INDIVIDUAL WHO EXPRESSES ANGER INAPPROPRIATELY—cont'd		
OUTCOME CRITERIA	**NURSING INTERVENTIONS**	**RATIONALE**
	b. Physical outlets. Suggest exercise, walking, or engaging in another activity that provides an acceptable outlet for energy. Offer to stay with the patient during this activity.	b. Provides effective way for patient to release tension associated with high levels of anger. Staying with the patient offers an opportunity to provide support and to assess the patient's perception of the activity's effectiveness.
	c. Medication. If agitation continues to escalate, offer patient choice of taking medication voluntarily. If they refuse, reassess the situation to determine whether harm to self or others is imminent.	c. Tranquilizing medication may calm patient and prevent violence from escalating.
	d. Call for assistance. Remove self and other patients from the immediate area. Call violence code, push panic button, call for assault team, and follow other measures established by the institution. Sufficient staff to indicate a show of strength may be enough to de-escalate the situation, and the patient may agree to take the medication.	d. Patient and staff safety are of primary concern. Many states' accrediting bodies (such as The Joint Commission) and facilities require that staff members working with hospitalized psychiatric patients be trained or certified in psychiatric emergency interventions to ensure that the strategies used are in the best interest of staff and patient safety.
	e. Seclusion or restraints. If the patient is not calmed by talking down or by medication, use of mechanical restraints, seclusion, or both may be necessary. Be sure to have sufficient staff available to assist and appropriately deal with an out-of-control patient. Follow protocol for restraints or seclusion established by the institution. Restraints should be used as a last resort, after all other interventions have been unsuccessful and patient is clearly at risk of harm to self or others.	e. Patients who do not have internal control over their behavior may require external controls, such as seclusion, mechanical restraints, or both in order to prevent harm to self or others. However, these restrictive measures should be used only as a last resort after all other measures have been attempted and have failed.

Continued

Table 15–2 | CARE PLAN FOR THE INDIVIDUAL WHO EXPRESSES ANGER INAPPROPRIATELY—cont'd

OUTCOME CRITERIA	NURSING INTERVENTIONS	RATIONALE
	f. Observation and documentation. Hospital policy typically dictates the requirements for observation of the patient in restraints. Basic safety principles include that the patient in restraints should be observed throughout the period of restraint. Every 15 minutes, the patient should be monitored to ensure that circulation to extremities is not compromised (check temperature, color, pulses). Assist the patient with needs related to nutrition, hydration, and elimination. Position the patient so that comfort is facilitated, breathing is unobstructed, and aspiration prevented. (Patients should not be restrained in the prone position.) Document all observations.	f. Patient safety and well-being are nursing priorities.
	g. Ongoing assessment. As agitation decreases, assess the patient's readiness for restraint removal or reduction. With assistance from other staff members, remove one restraint at a time, while assessing the patient's response. This process minimizes the risk of injury to patient and staff.	g. Gradual removal of the restraints allows for testing of the patient's self-control. Patient and staff safety are of primary concern.
	h. Debriefing. It is important, when a patient loses control, for staff to follow up with a discussion about the situation. This discussion should occur among staff and with the patient (when the patient has regained control). The staff should discuss factors that necessitated the crisis intervention, factors that contributed to the failure of less restrictive interventions, and staff's thoughts about the safety and effectiveness of the intervention. When the patient has	h. Debriefing helps to diminish the emotional effect of the intervention. Mutual feedback is shared, and staff has an opportunity to process and learn from the event.

| **Table 15–2 | CARE PLAN FOR THE INDIVIDUAL WHO EXPRESSES ANGER INAPPROPRIATELY—cont'd** | | |
OUTCOME CRITERIA	NURSING INTERVENTIONS	RATIONALE
	regained control, a debriefing should occur in which the patient is encouraged to discuss thoughts about what contributed to the crisis situation and about staff interventions and to explore strategies to avert a crisis situation in the future. It is also important to discuss the situation with other patients who witnessed the episode so they understand and process what happened. Some patients may fear that they could be at risk for experiencing a crisis or that they might be in danger when someone else's behavior becomes aggressive.	

CBT is typically conducted by advanced practice nurses and other trained specialists, the generalist psychiatric nurse can incorporate principles of this modality in psychoeducation, which provides a foundation for referral to longer-term CBT.

Evaluation

Evaluation consists of reassessment to determine whether the nursing interventions have been successful in achieving the objectives of care. The following type of information may be gathered to determine the success of working with a patient exhibiting inappropriate expression of anger:

■ Is the patient able to recognize when they are angry now?
■ Can the patient take responsibility for these feelings and keep them in check without losing control?
■ Does the patient seek out staff or a support person to talk about feelings of anger when they occur?
■ Is the patient able to transfer tension generated by the anger into constructive activities?
■ Has harm to patient and others been avoided?
■ Is the patient able to solve problems adaptively without undue frustration and without becoming violent?

Summary and Key Points

■ Anger, a normal human emotion, is not necessarily a negative response.
■ When used appropriately, anger can provide positive assistance with problem-solving and decision making in everyday life situations.
■ Violence occurs when individuals lose control of their anger.
■ Anger is viewed as an emotional response to one's perception of a situation.
■ When denied or buried, anger can precipitate several psychophysiological disorders.
■ When anger is turned inward on the self, it can result in depression.
■ When expressed inappropriately, anger commonly interferes with interpersonal relationships.
■ When anger is suppressed, it often turns to resentment.
■ Anger generates a physiological arousal comparable to the stress response discussed in Chapter 1, "The Concept of Stress Adaptation."
■ Aggression is one way in which individuals express anger.
■ Aggression is a behavior intended to threaten or injure the victim's security or self-esteem.

■ Aggression can be physical or verbal, but it is virtually always designed to punish.

■ Aggression is a negative function or destructive use of anger.

■ Various predisposing factors to the way individuals express anger have been implicated. Some theorists suggest that the etiology is purely biological, whereas others believe it depends on psychological and environmental factors.

■ Some possible predisposing factors include role modeling, operant conditioning, neurophysiological disorders (e.g., brain tumors, trauma, or diseases), biochemical factors (e.g., increased levels of androgens or other alterations in hormone levels and neurotransmitter involvement), socioeconomic factors (e.g., living in poverty), and environmental factors (e.g., physical crowding,

uncomfortable temperature, use of alcohol or drugs).

■ Nurses must be aware of the symptoms associated with anger and aggression in order to make an accurate assessment.

■ Prevention is a key issue in the management of aggressive or violent behavior.

■ Elements identified as key risk factors in the potential for violence among acute psychiatric inpatients include (1) male gender, (2) substance use, (3) past history of violence, and (4) a diagnosis of schizophrenia.

■ Cognitive behavior therapy is an evidence-based treatment strategy for reducing maladaptive aggression, especially in the treatment of aggression in children and adolescents.

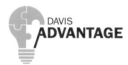 **DAVIS ADVANTAGE** | Go to **Davis Advantage** to complete your learning: strengthen understanding, apply your knowledge, and prepare for the Next Gen NCLEX®.

Review Questions

1. A client, age 27, was brought to the emergency department by two police officers. He smelled strongly of alcohol and was combative. His blood alcohol level was measured at 293 mg/dL. His girlfriend reported that he drinks excessively every day and is verbally and physically abusive. The nurse assigns the nursing diagnosis of "risk for other-directed violence." What would be appropriate outcome objectives for this diagnosis? (Select all that apply.)
   a. The client will not verbalize anger or hit anyone.
   b. The client will verbalize anger rather than hit others.
   c. The client will not harm self or others.
   d. The client will be restrained if he becomes verbally or physically abusive.

2. A client with a history of violence who has been hospitalized on the psychiatric unit becomes agitated and begins to threaten the staff and other clients. When all other interventions fail, the client is placed in restraints in the seclusion room. Which of the following are interventions for the client in restraints? (Select all that apply.)
   a. Check temperature and pulse of extremities.
   b. Document all observations.
   c. Explain to the client that restraint is punishment for violent behavior.
   d. Provide ongoing assessment and observation.
   e. Withhold food and fluids until the client is calm and can be released from restraints.

3. Which of these procedures is important immediately following an episode of violence on the unit? (Select all that apply.)
   a. Document all observations and occurrences.
   b. Conduct a debriefing with the staff.
   c. Explore with other clients their feelings associated with witnessing the incident.
   d. Warn the client that it could happen again if they become violent.

4. A client and his girlfriend had an argument during her visit to the psychiatric unit. Which behavior by the client would indicate he is learning to adaptively problem solve his frustrations?
    a. The client requests to be put in restraints to prevent hurting his girlfriend.
    b. When his girlfriend leaves, the client goes to the exercise room to try to release his anger with physical activity.
    c. The client says to the nurse, "I guess I'm going to have to dump that broad!"
    d. The client says to his girlfriend, "You'd better leave before I do something I'm sorry for."

5. Which of the following assessment data would the nurse consider as risk factors for possible violence in a client? (Select all that apply.)
    a. A diagnosis of somatization disorder
    b. A diagnosis of schizophrenia or bipolar disorder
    c. Substance intoxication
    d. Argumentative and demanding behavior
    e. Past history of violence

Clinical Judgment Questions

6. A client who was hospitalized with alcohol intoxication and violent behavior is sitting in the dayroom watching TV with the other clients when the nurse approaches with his 5 p.m. dose of haloperidol. The client says, "I feel in control now. I don't need any drugs." Which of these responses by the nurse demonstrates the best clinical judgment?
    a. Instruct the client that they must take the medication because of their history of violence.
    b. Instruct the client that if they will not take the medication orally, they will be restrained and given an intramuscular injection.
    c. Accept the client's refusal and document assessment of the client's mood and behavior.
    d. Secretly crush the medication into a beverage and offer it to the client.

7. A client with a history of violence is yelling in the dayroom and knocking over chairs. The nurse observes increased agitation, clenched fists, and loud, demanding voice. They are challenging and threatening staff and the other clients. The nurse's priority intervention would be to:
    a. Call for assistance.
    b. Draw up a syringe of prn haloperidol.
    c. Ask the client if they would like to talk about their anger.
    d. Tell the client if they do not calm down, they will have to be restrained.

8. When it has been assessed that a client is in control and no longer requires restraint, what should the nurse do next?
    a. Remove the restraints.
    b. Medicate the client before removing restraints.
    c. With assistance, remove one restraint and assess the client's level of self-control.
    d. Tell the client they will have to wait until the doctor comes in.

9. A client who has been in restraints is now calm. He apologizes to the nurse and says, "I hope I didn't hurt anyone." Which of these actions by the nurse demonstrates the best clinical judgment?
    a. Ignore the patient's comment to extinguish their aggressive behavior.
    b. Affirm to the patient that everyone loses control sometimes and tell him not to worry about it.
    c. Reinforce that it is fortunate that no one was hurt and assist the client to explore alternative behaviors when they become angry.
    d. Set firm limits with the client, instructing them that if they become angry again they will be secluded and restrained.

10. A client is noted to be pacing with clenched fists and saying, "I'm not putting up with this anymore. They've been trying to trick me all along." Which of these actions by the nurse is most appropriate at this point?
    a. Gently touch the client's shoulder and reassure them that no one is trying to trick them.
    b. Ask the client to describe what's upsetting them.
    c. Offer the client medication.
    d. Don't intervene but continue to watch the client from a distance.

References

Almvik, R., Woods, P., & Rasmussen, K. (2000). The Brøset Violence Checklist: Sensitivity, specificity, and interrater reliability. *Journal of Interpersonal Violence, 15*(12), 1284–1296. doi:10.1034/j.1600-0447.106.s412.22.x

American Psychological Association. (2013). *Violence in the media: Psychologists study TV and video game violence for potential harmful effects.* www.apa.org/action/resources/research-in-action/protect.aspx

American Psychological Association. (2022). *Controlling anger before it controls you.* www.apa.org/topics/anger/control.aspx

Archer, D. (2012). Environmental stressors and violence. *Psychology Today.* https://www.psychologytoday.com/blog/reading-between-the-headlines/201206/environmental-stressors-and-violence

Boland, R., & Verduin, M. L. (2022). *Kaplan & Sadock's synopsis of psychiatry.* (12th ed.). Wolters Kluwer.

Iozzino, L., Ferrari, C., Large, M., Nielssen, O., & Girolamo, G. (2015). Prevalence and risk factors of violence by psychiatric acute inpatients: A systematic review and meta-analysis. *PLoS ONE, 10*(6). doi:10.1371/journal.pone.0128536

Kassinove, H. (2023). *Anger: How to recognize and deal with a common emotion.* https://www.apa.org/news/press/releases/2012/05/anger

Merritt, P. (2017). *Neurophysiology of fear and aggression.* https://www.youtube.com/watch?v=L-hdPtzxOi8

Novitsky, M. A., Julius, R. J., & Dubin, W. R. (2009). Nonpharmacological management of violence in psychiatric emergencies. *Primary Psychiatry, 16*(9), 49–53.

Pavlov, K. A., Chistiakov, D. A., & Chekhonin, V. P. (2012). Genetic determinants of aggression and impulsivity in humans. *Journal of Applied Genetics, 53*(1), 61–82. doi:10.1007/s13353-011-0069-6.

Perry, B. (2016). *Aggression and violence: The neurobiology of experience.* https://bsahely.com/2016/05/11/aggression-and-violence-the-neurobiology-of-experience%e2%80%8f/

Smeets, K. C., Leeijen, A., Van Der Molen, M. J., Scheepers, F. E., Buitelaar, J. K., & Rommelse, N. (2015). Treatment moderators of cognitive behavior therapy to reduce aggressive behavior: A meta-analysis. *European Child Adolescent Psychiatry, 24:* 255–264. doi:10.1007/s00787-014-0592-1

Statistica. (2021). *Violent crime statistics in the U.S.* https://www.statista.com/topics/1750/violent-crime-in-the-us/#dossierKeyfigures

Sukhodolsky, D. G., Smith, S. D., McCauley, S. A., Ibrahim, K., & Piasecka, J. B. (2016). Behavioral interventions for anger, irritability, and aggression in children and adolescents. *Journal of Child and Adolescent Psychopharmacology, 26*(1), 58–64. https://doi.org/10.1089/cap.2015.0120

Vacher, C., Romo, L., Dereure, M., Soler, M., Picot, M. C., & Purper-Ouakil, D. (2022). Efficacy of cognitive behavioral therapy on aggressive behavior in children with attention deficit-hyperactivity disorder and emotion dysregulation: Study protocol of a randomized controlled trial. *Trials 23,* 124. https://doi.org/10.1186/s13063-022-05996-5

Vetulani, J. (2013). Neurochemistry of impulsiveness and aggression. *Psychiatria Polska, 47*(1), 103–115.

Victoroff, J. (2017). The neuropsychiatry of human aggression. In Sadock, B. A., Sadock, V. A., & Ruiz, P. (Eds.), *Comprehensive textbook of psychiatry* (10th ed.). Wolters Kluwer.

Zhang, Q., Cao, Y., & Tian, J. (2021). Effects of violent video games on aggressive cognition and aggressive behavior. *Cyberpsychology, Behavior, and Social Networking, 24*(1), 5–10. http://doi.org/10.10.89/cyber.2019.0676

Classical References

Warren, N. C. (1993). *Make anger your ally* (3rd ed.). Tyndale House Publishers.

Suicide Prevention 16

KEY TERMS

collaborative safety plan

suicide

suicide risk factors

suicide warning signs

CORE CONCEPTS

Caring: Therapeutic
relationship, patient-
centered care

Safety: Suicide risk
assessment, Suicide
prevention

Collaboration: Suicide
prevention

Evidence-Based
Practice: Suicide
prevention

Health Promotion:
Suicide risk
assessment

Professional Behavior:
Nursing process in
the care of patients
with suicidal thoughts
and behaviors

Clinical Judgment

OBJECTIVES

After reading this chapter, the student will be able to:

1. Discuss the epidemiology and risk factors related to suicide.
2. Describe the predisposing factors implicated in the development risk for suicidal behavior.
3. Differentiate between facts and myths regarding suicide.
4. Apply the nursing process in the care of patients exhibiting suicidal thoughts and behaviors.

Suicide is not a diagnosis or a disorder; it is a behavior. Specifically, **suicide** is the act of taking one's own life and is derived from the Latin words for "one's own killing." Many religions hold that suicide is a sin that is strictly forbidden. Cultural norms and attitudes also influence an individual's beliefs about suicide. Although some populations are considered at higher risk for suicide (such as American Indians and Alaska Natives; active and veteran military members; lesbian, gay, bisexual, or transgender individuals; people with disabilities; and people in prison or child welfare settings), suicide touches the lives of people of all ages, in all ethnic and racial groups, in all parts of the country. A complex interaction of factors such as mental illness, substance abuse, painful losses, exposure to violence, and social isolation are all influential in increasing these risks.

In the past decade, many state legislatures have debated the acceptability of physician-assisted suicide. Although it is legal in all of the United States for an individual or the individual's power of attorney to refuse life-preserving medical treatment, the majority of states have not legalized physician-assisted suicide. As of 2022, 10 states (California, Colorado, Hawaii, Maine, Montana, New Jersey, New Mexico, Oregon, Washington, and Vermont) plus the District of Columbia have legalized physician-assisted suicide (Compassion and Choices, 2022). Can suicide be a rational act? Many people in our society do not yet believe that it can.

In the field of psychiatry, suicide is considered an irrational act associated with mental illness and most commonly, but not exclusively, with depression or bipolar disorder. However, not everyone who takes their own life has a mental illness. Individuals in the community and in nonpsychiatric health-care settings may also be at risk. This chapter explores suicide from an epidemiological and etiological perspective. Care of the suicidal patient is presented in the context of the nursing process.

Historical Perspectives

In ancient Greece, individuals were said to have "committed" suicide because it was an offense against the state, and individuals who committed suicide were denied burial in community sites (Minois, 2001). In the culture of ancient Rome, individuals sometimes resorted to suicide to escape humiliation or abuse. In the Middle Ages, suicide was viewed as a selfish or criminal act (Minois, 2001). Individuals who "committed" suicide were often denied cemetery burial, and their property was confiscated and shared by the crown and the courts (MacDonald & Murphy, 1991). The issue of suicide changed during the Renaissance period. Although condemnation was still expected, the view became philosophical, allowing intellectuals to discuss the issue more freely.

Most philosophers of the 17th and 18th centuries condemned suicide, but some writers recognized a connection between suicide and melancholy or other severe mental disturbances (Minois, 2001). Suicide was illegal in England until 1961, and only in 1993 was it decriminalized in Ireland. With the decriminalization of suicide, many have advanced the idea that the term *committed suicide* should be removed from our vocabulary because it is inaccurate and potentially maintains a stigmatizing attitude toward this population.

Most religions consider suicide a sin against God. Judaism, Christianity, Islam, Hinduism, and Buddhism all condemn suicide. The Catholic church today still teaches that suicide is wrong, it is in opposition to proper love of self and love of God, and it wrongs others through the experience of loss and grief (Byron, 2016). But as Byron (2016) pointed out, some of the church's condemnation may have been rooted in a "denial of the responsibility to understand the pain that produces such an act," and he stresses the importance of encouraging those who "are hurting to open up," which, it is hoped, will remove some of the taboos of discussing suicide within the church. Likewise, replacing the term *committed* suicide (which has persisted in use long since its decriminalization) may also reduce the stigma and taboo that has historically been associated with discussing suicide.

Epidemiology

In 2020, the most recent year for which statistics have been recorded, 45,979 people died by suicide in the United States (Centers for Disease Control and Prevention[CDC], 2022b). This represents a decline in the trend of consistently increasing suicide rates from 2000 through 2018. Firearms is the most frequent means used (63%) followed by suffocation (27%), and in 2020 firearms became the primary means for females, which is a change from previous years (CDC, 2022c). Males have consistently had three to four times higher suicide rates than females. Although there has been an overall decline in rates among both groups, the incidence of suicide among females aged 10 to 24 increased. Male suicide rates have been consistently higher for those aged 75 and over (CDC, 2022c). In 2020, suicide was the 12th leading cause of death for all ages in the United States, changing from the 10th leading cause in 2019 due to the emergence of COVID-19 deaths and increases in deaths from chronic liver disease and cirrhosis (CDC, 2022c).

Many more people attempt suicide than die by suicide (about 12:1), and even more people seriously contemplate the act without carrying it out. Because statistics about numbers of suicide attempts reflect only those who have entered a treatment setting, the numbers could be much higher. With a steady increase in suicide rates from 2000 to 2018, suicide has been identified as a major health-care problem in the United States.

Historically, the suicide rate has been lower among military personnel than among the general population. However, in some time periods since the Iraq War began (including in 2010 and 2011) more soldiers died by suicide than died in combat (Nock et al., 2013). The suicide rate among active duty and military veterans increased by 16% (28.7/100,000) from 2019 to 2020, and this has been on the incline since 2015 when the rate was 20.3/100,000 (Myers, 2021). See Chapter 37, "Military Families," for further discussion.

Research continues with efforts to identify the best strategies for prevention and assessment of suicide risk, how to differentiate between those with suicidal ideation and those who attempt suicide, and evidence-based treatments and interventions. The federal government, through the Substance Abuse and Mental Health Services Administration, has endorsed the "Zero Suicide" movement, a partnership of several national organizations dedicated to identifying evidence-based strategies for suicide prevention. Within the next several years, our understanding of and approaches to treatment may dramatically change. We are certainly beginning to recognize that conventional interventions have not adequately addressed the complex needs of this population.

Many common assumptions about the individual expressing suicidal thoughts and behaviors are *not* supported by evidence. At the onset of discussing this topic it is important to separate evidence-based information from common myths. Some currently accepted facts and myths relating to suicide are presented in Table 16–1.

Risk Factors

Suicide risk factors are identified as factors that have statistically been correlated with a higher incidence of suicide. They should be differentiated from **suicide warning signs,** which are identified as factors

suggesting a more immediate concern. Both are included as part of a comprehensive assessment of overall risk for suicide.

Marital Status

Widows and widowers, in some studies, have been identified at higher risk for suicide, but a longitudinal study (Kposowa, 2000) found that being single or widowed had no effect on suicide rates. However, the evidence did support that divorced men are twice as likely as married men to die by suicide. In a more recent, large study Naess et al. (2021) found that

TABLE 16–1 **Facts and Myths About Suicide**	
MYTHS	**FACTS**
People who talk about suicide do not act on their ideas. Suicide happens without warning.	Eight of 10 people who kill themselves have given definite clues and warnings about their suicidal intentions. Very subtle clues may be ignored or disregarded by others.
You cannot stop a suicidal person. They are fully intent on dying.	Most suicidal people are very ambivalent about their feelings regarding living or dying. Most are "gambling with death" and see it as a cry for someone to save them.
Once a person is suicidal, they are suicidal forever.	Suicidal ideation and risk fluctuate over time and may be time limited. If provided adequate support and resources, a suicidal person can go on to lead a normal life. However, multiple suicide attempts may reflect greater chronicity of suicidal ideation. Reassessment over time is important to identify current risks.
Improvement after severe depression means that a person is no longer at risk of suicide.	Many suicides occur within about 3 months after the beginning of "improvement," when the individual has the energy to carry out suicidal intentions.
Suicide is inherited, or "runs in families."	Suicide is not inherited. However, suicide by a close family member increases an individual's risk factor for suicide.
All suicidal individuals are mentally ill, and suicide is the act of a psychotic person.	Although a majority of people who attempt suicide are extremely unhappy or clinically depressed, they are not necessarily psychotic. They are unable at that point in time to see an alternative solution to what they consider an unbearable problem.
Suicidal thoughts and attempts should be considered manipulative or attention-seeking behavior and should not be taken seriously.	All suicidal behavior must be approached with the gravity of the potential act in mind. Attention should be given to the possibility that the individual is issuing a cry for help.
People usually take their own lives by overdosing on drugs.	Gunshot wounds are the leading cause of death among suicide victims.
If an individual has attempted suicide, they will not do it again.	Between 50% and 80% of all people who ultimately kill themselves have at least one previous attempt.
Suicide always happens in an impulsive moment.	People often contemplate, imagine, plan strategies, write notes, post things on the Web. In-depth exploration and assessment may reveal these plans.
Young children (ages 5–12) cannot be suicidal.	Each year, 30 to 35 children younger than age 12 years take their own lives, and not all are clinically depressed.

Sources: Compiled from Fuller, K. (2020). *5 common myths about suicide debunked.* https://www.nami.org/Blogs/NAMI-Blog/September-2020/5-Common-Myths-About-Suicide-Debunked; National Alliance on Mental Illness. (2022). *Risk of suicide.* www.nami.org/Learn-More/Mental-Health-Conditions/Related-Conditions/Risk-of-Suicide; and The Samaritans. (2022). *Myths about suicide.* http://samaritansnyc.org/myths-about-suicide.

single status for any reason *was* associated with increased risk for suicide, but the highest risk for those never married were among those with low education and low income levels.

For those who are divorced and widowed, the stresses associated with major life changes and loss are influential. Evidence has demonstrated that a *change* in marital status increases the risk for suicidal behavior, particularly in the first year after the change and particularly among older people (Naess et al., 2021; Roškar et al., 2011; Yamauchi et al., 2013). Other research indicates that any transitional life events may increase the risk for suicidal thoughts and behaviors; however, men are less likely than women to engage social support connections and may wait until they experience suicidal thoughts and behaviors before engaging with their networks for support (Milton et al., 2020). Again, it should be noted that demographics such as marital status, age, and sex may inform about populations that are statistically at higher risk, but none of these factors are predictive of immediate risk. A thorough assessment of variables, including risk factors, warning signs, and a host of other data, is essential to identifying individuals at acute risk for attempting suicide.

Sex

More women than men attempt suicide, but men more often die by suicide. Although the risk for suicide is generally elevated both during inpatient psychiatric treatment and after discharge, one study found that the risk was significantly greater for women than men in that time period (Listabarth et al., 2020)

Age

Suicide risk and age are, in general, positively correlated, particularly with men. As noted previously, the suicide rate in females increased in 2020 for those aged 10 to 24 and the rate for men aged 75 and over remains consistently high, whereas the suicide rates for males between the ages of 45 and 74 decreased during the period from 2018 to 2020 (CDC, 2022c). Still, the greatest percentage (47.2%) of suicides occur within the age group of 35 to 64 years.

Although adolescents may statistically have a lower rate of suicide than some other age groups, it is still important to note that suicide has been the third-leading cause of death in this population over several years, and in 2013 became the second-leading cause of death, where it remained in 2020 (CDC, 2022b). Several factors put adolescents at risk for suicide, including impulsive and high-risk behaviors, untreated mood disorders (e.g., major depression

and bipolar disorder), access to lethal means (e.g., firearms), and substance abuse.

One study (Reyes et al., 2015) found a link between some modes of anger expression in adolescents and suicide risk; in particular, hopelessness and hostility modes of anger expression were associated with an increase in suicidal tendency. Among children younger than age 10, the statistics have historically demonstrated a low number of suicides, and some have argued that younger children are unable to intentionally consider and follow through with a suicide attempt. Anecdotal evidence has shown this is not always the case, with some therapists identifying 5- to 9-year-old children actively talking about suicide (Jobes, 2015). Research is beginning to emerge that supports real risk in young children (Duran & McGuinness, 2016). Bridge and associates (2015) studied a large sample of children ages 5 to 11 and found that, on average, 33 children per year die by suicide within this age group in the United States, predominately from suffocation and hanging. These researchers also noted that suicide was never coded as a cause of death for children younger than 5 years of age. However, when Whalen and associates (2015) studied children in the 3- to 7-year-old age group, they found about 11% with suicidal ideation. Increased risk was correlated with male sex, psychiatric illness in their mothers, and psychiatric illness in the child. In young girls ages 10 to 14 years, the incidence of self-inflicted injury has risen 18.8% every year between 2008 and 2015, and self-inflicted injury is one of the strongest risk factors for suicide (Mercado et al., 2017). Duran and McGuinness (2016) stressed that the implications for nursing are clear; direct inquiry about suicide ideas is a "necessary component in healthcare encounters with children," including those in primary care, in emergency departments, and with the school nurse.

It cannot be overstated, however, that although statistics reveal degrees of risk in certain age groups, screening for risk of suicide should be conducted for all individuals regardless of demographic characteristics.

Religion

Assessing religion's role in risk for suicide is complicated by variables such as degree of affiliation, participation, religious doctrine, and others. Further, although most studies have found religion to be protective, others have found it to be a risk factor (Lawrence et al., 2016). A systematic review of the research on religion and suicide risk (Lawrence et al., 2016) found that although religious affiliation is not protective against *suicide ideation*, it is protective against suicide attempts, and that religious service attendance is possibly protective against suicide. The authors of another study (Rasic et al., 2009) found that religious affiliation is associated with a decreased risk of suicide attempts in both the general population and in those with a mental illness independent of the availability of social support systems.

Socioeconomic Influences

Financial strain and unemployment have often been identified as risk factors for suicide. To what extent these factors act alone (as opposed to a complex interaction of several variables) requires further study. The CDC (2021) identified loss (including loss of employment) as one risk factor for suicide. Suicide rates are higher in rural areas and with a twofold greater use of firearms as the means (Ivey-Stephenson et al., 2017). Kim and associates (2016) studied the factors influencing a move from suicide ideation to suicide attempts and found that low education and unemployment significantly increased the prevalence of *attempts* among young adult men and women with suicide *ideation*. Because previous attempts are a leading risk factor for eventual suicide, assessing for suicide ideation in high-risk socioeconomic groups may be an important preventive measure.

Ethnicity

In 2020, the highest U.S. age-adjusted suicide rate was among Whites (15.05) and the second highest rate was among American Indians and Alaska Natives (14.53). Much lower rates were found among blacks or African Americans (7.40) and Asians and Pacific Islanders (6.79) (American Foundation for Suicide Prevention, 2022). Within the American Indian community, young adults are the highest-risk age group, and the rate of suicide is 2.5 times higher than the national average (National Indian Council on Aging, 2019).

One study examining suicide trends among school-age children younger than 12 (Bridge et al., 2015) found that suicide rates for black children 5 to 11 years of age nearly doubled over the period from 1993 to 2012, whereas the overall suicide rate in this age group remained relatively stable during the same time period. The use of hanging or suffocation as a means of taking one's own life also significantly increased in this population. A more recent study (Sheftall et al., 2021b) found that from 2003 to 2017 black youth experienced a significant upward trend in suicide with the largest annual percentage change in the 15- to 17-year age group and among girls. As of 2018, suicide became the second-leading cause of death in black children ages 10 to 14, and the third-leading cause of death in black adolescents ages 15 to 19 (Gordon, 2020). The contributing

factors to these recent trends are not well understood and will require further research, including a review of the effect of health-care disparities for select communities and populations.

Other Risk Factors

The majority of people who die by suicide have a diagnosable mental illness with numbers at least 10 times that of the general population (of those without a diagnosable mental illness, many suicides are related to crises associated with finances, relationships, discrimination, violence, terror, and war) (Bachman, 2018). The mental illnesses most commonly associated with suicide include depression, bipolar disorder, or substance use disorder.

In the latest edition of the *Diagnostic and Statistical Manual of Mental Disorders, Fifth Edition, Text Revision (DSM-5-TR)*, a new section, "Association With Suicidal Thoughts or Behavior" has been added for each diagnosis when there is evidence of associated risk (American Psychiatric Association, 2022). There are over 20 psychiatric disorders with this designation. The authors caution, however, that even among individuals with the same diagnosis, there is such a range of "relevant psychopathology" (p. 20) affecting the level of suicide risk, that clinicians should always conduct a thorough assessment of known risk factors and warning signs rather than rely solely on the presence (or absence) of a diagnosis known to have associated risks for suicide thoughts or behavior.

Studies support that individuals who have been hospitalized for a psychiatric illness have a higher risk of suicide than those with psychiatric illness in the general population and particularly in the first week and first month after hospitalization (Chung et al., 2019). This higher risk may be a reflection of the severity of their mental illness. Additional research supports that the increased risk of suicide in the period after discharge from psychiatric hospitalization is especially higher for those not connected to a system of care (Forte et al., 2019; Olfson et al., 2016).

Suicide risk may increase early in treatment with antidepressants. One possible reason is that as an individual's energy returns, they may have an increased ability to act out self-destructive wishes. Although suicide is often thought of as strictly related to depression, there is also a recognized risk of suicide among people with schizophrenia, bipolar disorders, personality disorders, eating disorders, anxiety disorders, and substance use disorders. A thorough suicide risk assessment should be conducted for anyone seeking mental health services.

Other major physical conditions have also been identified as contributing to increased risk for suicide (Ahmedani et al., 2017), with three conditions (traumatic brain injury, sleep disorders, and HIV/AIDS) conferring a twofold increase in risk. Severe insomnia is associated with increased suicide risk even in the absence of depression. Use of alcohol, and particularly a combination of alcohol and barbiturates, increases the risk of suicide. Withdrawal from stimulants increases suicide risk as the person begins to "crash." Psychosis, especially with command hallucinations (hearing voices telling one to harm or kill oneself), increases risk, as does having a chronic, painful, or disabling illness.

Several studies have indicated a higher risk factor for suicide among those in the LGBTQ+ community (Jadva et al., 2021; Janakiraman et al., 2020; Terrell et al., 2021; Williams et al., 2019; Yildiz, 2018). A report from the CDC (2016) identified that in a study of youth in grades 7 to 12, lesbian, gay, and bisexual youth were twice as likely as their heterosexual peers to attempt suicide (this study did not address the risk for transgender individuals). Another study, however, found that transgender individuals are also a high-risk population for suicide, with an alarming 41% lifetime prevalence (Stroumsa, 2014). A study of transgender and gender diverse individuals found that psychological distress had the strongest association with suicidal thoughts and behaviors; workplace discrimination, family rejection, health-care discrimination, and childhood bias-based victimization were lifetime risk factors (Cramer et al., 2022). See online Chapter 41, "Gender Dysphoria, Paraphilic Disorders, and Sexual Dysfunctions," for further discussion on this topic.

Higher risk is also associated with a family history of suicide, especially in a same-gender parent, and with individuals who have made previous suicide attempts. About one-half of individuals who kill themselves have previously attempted suicide. Because roughly equal numbers die by suicide on their first attempt, all individuals with suicide ideation should be assessed carefully for risk factors and warning signs. Significant losses, including relational, social, work, or financial, have also been identified as risk factors (CDC, 2021). In recent years, several suicides have been reported in the media among young people who are the victims of bullying. Pacer's National Bullying Prevention Center (2022) reported that 1 in 5 students report physical, emotional, or cyberbullying, and the most frequent reasons for being bullied include physical appearance, race/ethnicity, gender, disability, religion, or sexual orientation. Researchers have found a strong association between bullying and suicide-related behaviors, but the effects were mediated by other factors, including depression, substance abuse, and aggression (Reed et al., 2015).

Cyberbullying has also been associated with an increased risk of suicidal behavior among young people, and researchers found that both perpetrators and victims of cyberbullying had more suicidal ideation and were more likely to attempt suicide than those who had not experienced such forms of peer aggression (Bauman et al., 2013; John et al., 2018).

Predisposing Factors: Theories of Suicide

Psychological Theories

Psychological theories focus primarily on cognitive, emotional, and behavioral factors that are associated with risk for suicide. Although suicidal behavior is most commonly associated with depression, several other emotions and behaviors have been identified as influential. The following is a description of several of these psychological factors.

Anger Turned Inward

Freud (1957) believed that suicide was a response to intense self-hatred. The anger originates toward a love object but is ultimately turned inward against the self. In other words, Freud thought that suicide occurred as a result of an earlier repressed desire to kill someone else.

Hopelessness and Other Symptoms of Depression

Hopelessness has long been identified as a symptom of depression and an underlying factor in the predisposition to suicide. Although the many symptoms identified in suicide assessment tools attempt to assess for the seriousness of suicide ideation, current research is attempting to glean which symptoms might be more predictive of the move from ideation to attempts. In addition to hopelessness, the strength of the person's intention to die and the amount of suicide-specific rumination about suicide have also been identified as significant (Jobes, 2015; Rogers & Joiner, 2017). Further research has sought to identify the predictive value of state (temporary) hopelessness and trait (enduring) hopelessness (Burr et al., 2018). The researchers found that trait hopelessness was more positively associated with both suicide ideation and attempts.

History of Aggression and Violence

Outwardly directed aggression has been found to be associated with suicide attempts but not with suicide ideation, and among psychiatric patients, outwardly directed aggression was associated with planned rather than unplanned attempts (Swogger et al., 2014). Some evidence suggests that impulsive traits are higher in individuals with suicide ideation but not necessarily associated with more attempts

(Klonsky & May, 2015a). Ammerman and associates (2015) found that trait anger was associated with both suicidal and violent behavior and that emotional dysregulation was influential particularly for suicidal behavior.

Shame and Humiliation

Some individuals have viewed suicide as a "face-saving" mechanism—a way to prevent public humiliation after a social defeat such as a sudden loss of status or income. Both shame and humiliation may also interrupt one's sense of connectedness with others, and a sense of belonging and connectedness is considered protective against suicide. Evidence supports that the experience of shame is pronounced in trauma survivors (Taylor, 2015) and in females with borderline personality disorder (Wiklander et al., 2012). These findings may explain some of the influencing factors for increased risk of suicide in these populations.

Sociological Theories

Durkheim's Theory

Durkheim's classic work (1951) studied the individual's interaction with the society in which they lived. He believed that the more cohesive the society and the more that the individual felt an integrated part of society, the less likely they were to carry out suicide. Durkheim described three social categories of suicide:

1. **Egoistic suicide** is the response of the individual who feels separate from the mainstream of society. Integration is lacking, and the individual does not feel a part of any cohesive group (such as a family or a church).
2. **Altruistic suicide** is the opposite of egoistic suicide. The individual who is prone to altruistic suicide is excessively integrated into the group. The group is often governed by cultural, religious, or political ties, and allegiance is so strong that the individual will sacrifice their life for the group.
3. **Anomic suicide** occurs in response to changes in an individual's life (e.g., divorce, loss of job) that disrupt feelings of relatedness to the group. An interruption in the customary norms of behavior instills feelings of separateness and fears of being without support from the formerly cohesive group.

Connectedness continues to be identified as an important protective factor for suicide prevention and includes a sense of closeness with individuals, groups, families, schools, faith communities, community organizations, or cultural group (Suicide Prevention Resource Center, 2020).

Interpersonal Theory of Suicide

Thomas Joiner's (2005) interpersonal theory of suicide supports some of the same principles advanced by Durkheim that associates lack of a feeling of belonging with suicide risk. But Joiner's theory introduces the concept that suicide ideation and suicide attempts need to be understood as distinct processes. He proposed that low connectedness and a high sense of burden interact with each other to increase suicidal thoughts and desires, but those features in the presence of high capability for suicide are strongly associated with the move from ideation to lethal attempts. He advances the concept that people become less fearful (and therefore more capable) of self-destructive acts when they expose themselves repeatedly to painful or violent stimuli: a kind of "working up" to actually being capable of self-harm. The move from suicide ideation to attempts is not viewed as an impulsive act but rather a process of steps that, over time, create greater and greater risk.

The Three-Step Theory

Inspired by Joiner's theory, Klonsky and May (2015b) found that impulsivity is elevated both in people who have made suicide attempts and those who have suicidal thoughts and have never made an attempt. These researchers sought to identify the factors other than impulsivity that elevate suicide ideation to an active risk for attempts. Their research supported the following three-step trajectory:

1. Pain (usually psychological pain), when combined with hopelessness, significantly increases suicide ideation (for both men and women and across age groups).
2. Connectedness prevents suicide ideation from escalating in those at risk, but when pain and hopelessness exceed one's sense of connectedness to others, suicide ideation becomes active.
3. When strong, active suicide ideation is present, it leads to an attempt only if one has the capacity to make an attempt.

Biological Theories

Biological theories attempt to understand the biochemical and genetic influences in the risk for suicidal behavior. Current theories recognize that the complexity of suicide risk and behavior is likely a complex interaction of biological, psychological, interpersonal, and environmental factors.

Genetics

Twin studies have shown a much higher concordance rate for suicide risks in monozygotic twins than in dizygotic twins. Some studies with people who have attempted suicide have focused on the genotypic variations in the gene for tryptophan hydroxylase, with results indicating a significant association with suicidality (Zhang et al., 2010). Tryptophan hydroxylase is an enzyme associated with the synthesis of serotonin, and diminished serotonin has implications for both depression and suicidal behavior. Other research has identified a genetic variation in prefrontal cortex tissue that may be a biomarker for suicide risk when vulnerable individuals are exposed to a significant stressor (Sudak, 2017). More recently, researchers have identified DNA biomarkers with a strong connection to suicidality. These genome variants (not surprisingly) overlap with those of other psychiatric disorders (particularly depression and anxiety) but also with risk-taking behavior, smoking, and insomnia (Mullins et al., 2022; Strawbridge et al., 2019). Although these findings suggest the potential for a genetic predisposition toward suicidal behavior, more research is needed to clarify their role.

Neurochemical Factors

Studies have revealed altered levels of serotonin, glutamate, gamma-aminobutyric acid (GABA), and dopamine and increased levels of corticotropin-releasing hormone (CRH) (which triggers the release of cortisol) in individuals who died by suicide (Offord, 2020). These studies have supported the association of altered neurochemical levels with risk for suicide.

However, a meta-analysis examining biological factors found that they are, in general, weak predictors of a future *suicide attempt* or *death by suicide* (Chang et al., 2016). The only two biological factors that had statistical significance in this analysis were cytokines (anti-inflammatory response chemicals) and low levels of fish oil nutrients (including omega-3).

Application of the Nursing Process in the Care of Patients With Suicidal Ideation and Suicidal Behavior

Many research studies are being conducted that explore suicide from different vantage points to identify demographics, risk factors, predictors of risk for suicide attempts, and strategies for prevention. This research can help nurses become more aware of the phenomenon of suicide and understand the limitations of research in making a clinical judgment about a patient's actual risks versus statistical risks.

Influential organizations across the nation are also advancing the importance of improving the quality of care, documentation, and reporting of details around sentinel events related to acts of or deaths by suicide. Effective in July 2022, a new three-digit call number, **988**, simplifies contacting a national suicide crisis hotline (the existing National Suicide Prevention Lifeline). In addition to government-initiated national strategies for suicide prevention, The Joint Commission (2016) advanced standards that include requiring hospitals to conduct risk assessments "identifying specific patient characteristics and environmental features that may increase or decrease the risk of suicide." It is nurses practicing in general medical settings, including emergency departments and primary care practices, who are frontline practitioners in the fight to prevent suicide, so these assessment skills are critical wherever nurses are practicing. The American Psychiatric Nurses Association (APNA, 2022; Puntil et al., 2013) has taken a leadership role in identifying psychiatric-mental health nurse essential competencies for assessment and management of individuals at risk for suicide. The CDC (2011) advanced strategies for uniform definition and reporting about acts of self-directed violence to improve data collection and ultimately improve our understanding and prevention of suicide. At the heart of this wealth of information is the necessity for accurate, comprehensive suicide risk assessment that includes collaboration with the patient and other clinicians and is rooted in strategies to form a therapeutic relationship of trust and open communication.

Assessment

When nurses assess a patient's suicide ideation, it is important to identify and distinguish ideas (thoughts), plans (intentions), and attempts (behavior). Each of these assessment factors can provide information about a patient's level of risk. When the patient has attempted self-injury, it is important to distinguish between *suicidal self-injury* and *nonsuicidal self-injury*. The latter injury is often used as a method to release emotions, but it may also be a way of communicating the severity of distress that the patient is experiencing (Nock et al., 2013).

The following basic items should be considered when conducting a suicidal assessment: demographics; medical-psychiatric diagnoses; suicidal ideas or acts; interpersonal support system; analysis of the suicidal crisis; psychiatric, medical, and family history; and coping strategies.

Dr. David Satcher, as Surgeon General of the United States (1998–2002), spoke of risk factors and protective factors in his "Call to Action to Prevent Suicide" (U.S. Public Health Service, 1999). This report initiated a national movement toward research designed to better understand predictors of suicide risk and develop more effective evidence-based interventions. Current models have clarified risk factors as different from warning signs that are associated with a greater potential for suicide and suicidal behavior. Protective factors have been identified that are associated with reduced potential for suicide. Examples of protective factors are outlined in Box 16–1. Figure 16–1 presents a model for differentiating low, high, and imminent suicide risk. The goal of such models is not to predict a suicide attempt but to identify the level of intervention needed to prevent an attempt. Further, while risk assessment is part of a comprehensive psychosocial assessment and safety plan, there is good evidence that risk assessment scales, when used alone, have not had strong predictive value, and may provide a false sense of reassurance (Chan et al., 2016; Large et al., 2016). The importance of a comprehensive and collaborative approach cannot be overstated.

Demographics

The following demographics have been identified as associated with higher risk for suicide and therefore should be considered when assessing a patient for suicide risk. These include age, gender, race and ethnicity, sexual minorities, individuals with disabilities, veterans, selected occupations, and selected geographic areas, (CDC, 2022a). In addition, those experiencing transitional life events, financial strain, or have a family history of suicide may be at higher risk. Although demographics alone do not directly translate into an individual's risk, they provide

---

BOX 16–1 **Examples of Protective Factors**

Resilient temperament

Social competency

Skills in problem-solving, coping, and conflict resolution

Perception of social support from adults and peers

Positive expectations, optimism for the future; identification of future goals

Connectedness to family, school, community

Presence and involvement of caring adults (for adolescents)

Integration in social networks

Cultural and religious beliefs that discourage suicide and encourage preservation of life

Access to quality social services and clinical health care for mental, physical, and substance use disorders

Support through ongoing medical and mental health-care relationships

Restricted access to highly lethal means of suicide among people at risk

---

Crosby, A. E., Ortega, L., & Melanson, C. (2011). *Self-directed violence surveillance: Uniform definitions and recommended data elements, version 1.0.* Centers for Disease Control and Prevention, National Center for Injury Prevention and Control. www.cdc.gov/violenceprevention/pdf/Self-Directed-Violence-a.pdf

---

information as part of a comprehensive assessment of proximal or potentiating risk factors.

■ **Age:** Suicide was the second leading cause of death for people ages 10 to 14 and 25 to 34 in 2020, and men over the age of 75 had the highest rate (40.5/100,000) compared with other age groups (CDC, 2022a). Recent statistics identify that the highest percentage (47.2 %) of all suicides are among adults between the ages of 35 and 64. These statistics and evidence of suicide among children suggest that nurses should assess for suicide risk in all age groups.

■ **Gender:** Males are at higher risk for death by suicide than females, but females attempt suicide more frequently. As mentioned previously, males have consistently had three to four times higher suicide rates than females (CDC, 2022a).

■ **Ethnicity/race:** Age-adjusted suicide rates are highest among non-Hispanic American Indian/Alaska Native people (AI/AN) (23.9 per 100,000) and non-Hispanic white people (16.9 per 100,000) compared with other racial and ethnic groups, and in the period from 2019 to 2020 there were increased suicide rates for non-Hispanic black and non-Hispanic AI/AN people (CDC, 2022a)

■ **Sexual minorities:** Almost a quarter (23.4%) of high school students identifying as lesbian, gay, or bisexual reported attempting suicide in the prior 12 months. This rate is nearly four times higher than the rate reported among heterosexual students (6.4%) (CDC, 2022a)

■ **Individuals with disabilities**: Although there are limited data about risk factors among people with disabilities, a recent survey highlighted that in 2021, adults with disabilities were three times more likely to report suicidal ideation in the past month compared with people without disabilities (30.6% versus 8.3% in the general U.S. population) (CDC, 2022a).

■ **Veterans:** Veterans have an adjusted suicide rate that is 52.3% greater than the nonveteran U.S. adult population (CDC, 2022a). The most common method is firearms, which accounts for over 60% of all suicides among military members (Center for Deployment Psychology, n.d.).

■ **Occupation:** Health-care professionals (especially physicians), law enforcement officers, dentists, artists, mechanics, lawyers, and insurance agents have all been identified as occupational groups believed to incur greater risks for suicide. Potential contributing factors include occupations that involve high stress, isolation, lack of access to health-care resources, and repeated exposure to painful or violent stimuli. The most recent data on suicide rates by occupation (Peterson et al., 2020)

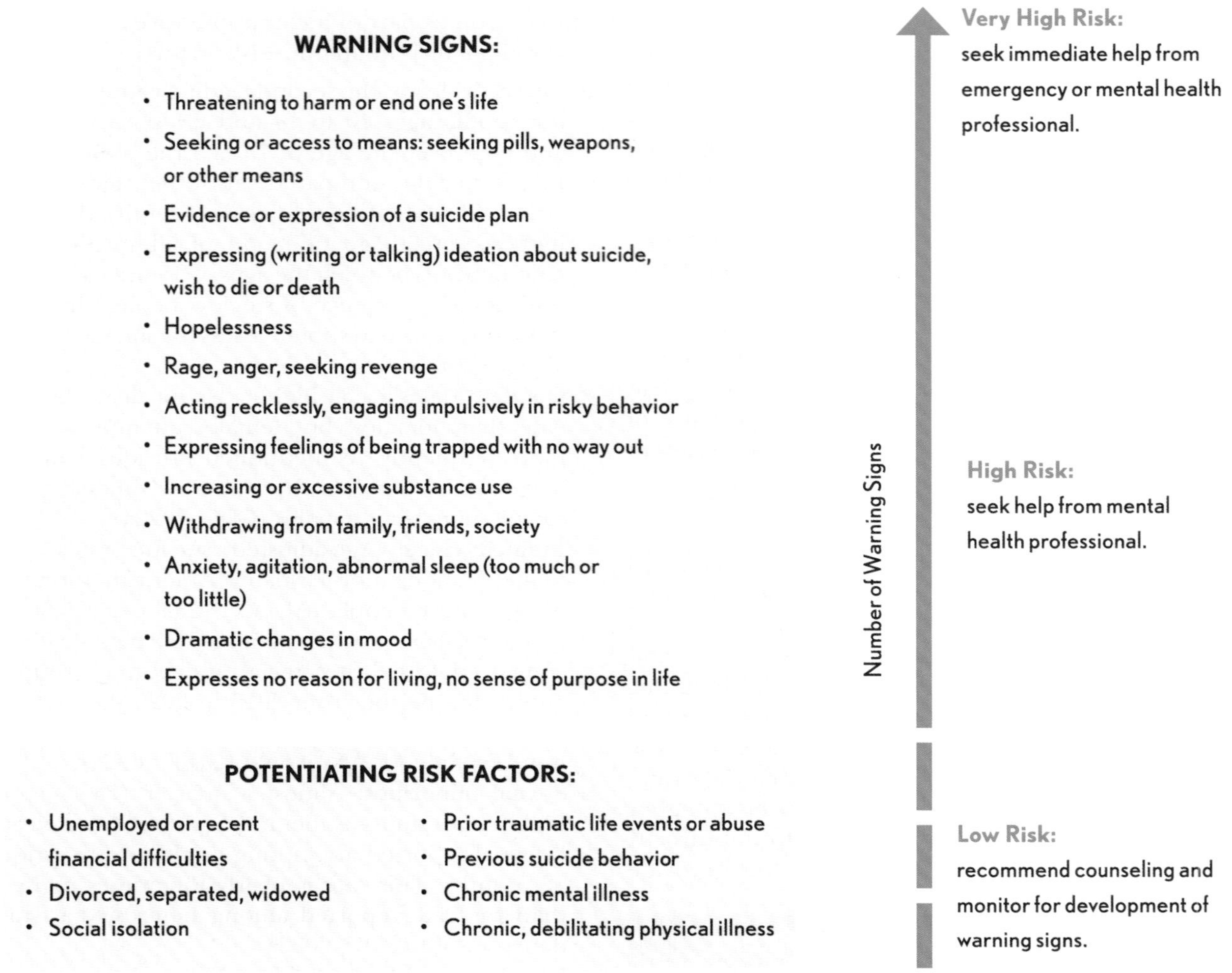

WARNING SIGNS:

- Threatening to harm or end one's life
- Seeking or access to means: seeking pills, weapons, or other means
- Evidence or expression of a suicide plan
- Expressing (writing or talking) ideation about suicide, wish to die or death
- Hopelessness
- Rage, anger, seeking revenge
- Acting recklessly, engaging impulsively in risky behavior
- Expressing feelings of being trapped with no way out
- Increasing or excessive substance use
- Withdrawing from family, friends, society
- Anxiety, agitation, abnormal sleep (too much or too little)
- Dramatic changes in mood
- Expresses no reason for living, no sense of purpose in life

Very High Risk: seek immediate help from emergency or mental health professional.

High Risk: seek help from mental health professional.

Number of Warning Signs

POTENTIATING RISK FACTORS:

- Unemployed or recent financial difficulties
- Divorced, separated, widowed
- Social isolation
- Prior traumatic life events or abuse
- Previous suicide behavior
- Chronic mental illness
- Chronic, debilitating physical illness

Low Risk: recommend counseling and monitor for development of warning signs.

FIGURE 16–1 Risk factors and warning signs for suicide. Reprinted with permission from the Ontario Hospital Association.

identified that highest rates were among construction workers, maintenance and repair workers, those in the arts and entertainment industry (including sports and the media), transportation workers, protective service workers, and healthcare support staff (particularly personal care aides and registered nurses).

■ **Geographic regions:** Suicide rates increase as population density decreases and an area becomes more rural (CDC, 2022a).

■ **Religion:** People with close religious affiliations may be at lower risk for attempting suicide if they believe, for example, that suicide is an unforgivable sin that is strictly forbidden within the religion. Conversely, people without close affiliations that impose restrictions about suicide may be at greater risk. It is important, therefore, to assess not just whether someone identifies with a particular religion but also their degree of affiliation.

■ **Family history:** A family history of suicide generally increases an individual's risk for suicidal ideation and behavior. In a recent novel study (Sheftall et al., 2021a) of risk factors among children aged 5 to 12, researchers found that children with suicidal ideation were more likely to have a parent with a history of a suicide attempt; however, more longitudinal research is needed to identify if this risk is predictive of suicide attempts later in life.

■ **Socioeconomic influences:** Financial strain and unemployment are identified as risk factors for suicide.

■ **Transitional life events:** Stressful transitional life events including divorce and widowhood may be associated with increased risk for suicide (Milton et al., 2020). It is important to collect data about transitional stressors, coping strategies, and availability of support networks.

Medical-Psychiatric Diagnosis

Assessment data must be gathered regarding any psychiatric or physical condition for which a patient is being treated. Mood disorders (major depression and bipolar disorders) are the disorders most commonly associated with suicide. Substance use disorders are also associated with an increased risk for suicide attempts. Other psychiatric disorders in which suicide risks have been identified include anxiety disorders, schizophrenia, anorexia nervosa, attention deficit-hyperactivity disorder, and borderline and antisocial personality disorders. Chronic and terminal physical illnesses have also been identified as potentiating risk factors.

Suicidal Ideas or Acts

An important part of the assessment of a patient's suicide risk is to determine the seriousness of the patient's intent to die. How serious is the patient's intent to die by suicide? How frequent are the patient's thoughts about suicide? Does the person have a plan? If so, do they have the means? How lethal are the means? Do they intend to carry out this plan? Has the individual ever attempted suicide before? These questions must be asked by the person conducting the assessment of the patient who is expressing suicidal ideation.

Individuals may provide both behavioral and verbal clues about their intention to act. Examples of behavioral clues that may indicate a decision to carry out suicidal intent include giving away prized possessions, getting financial affairs in order, writing suicide notes, and a sudden lift in mood.

Verbal clues may be both direct and indirect. Examples of direct statements include "I want to die" or "I'm going to kill myself." Examples of indirect statements include "This is the last time you'll see me," "I won't be around much longer for the doctor to worry about," or "I don't have anything worth living for anymore."

Rogers and Joiner's research (2017) provided evidence that suicide-specific rumination, that is, fixation on one's thoughts, intentions, and plans, may be an important predictor of suicidal behavior. Asking how frequently the patient is thinking about suicide ideas, intentions, and plans helps to discern this level of risk.

The lethality of the method identified by an individual with suicide ideation or by one who has already made an attempt provides meaningful information about the patient's intent to die. Use of firearms, hanging, and suffocation, for example, are considered highly lethal methods.

Other assessments include determining whether the individual has a plan, and if so, whether they have the means to carry out that plan. If the person states the suicide will be carried out with a gun, do they have access to a gun? Bullets? If pills are planned, what kind of pills? Are they accessible? Asking the patient, "How likely are you to carry out this plan?" may provide verbal confirmation of their level of intent.

Interpersonal Support System

Does the individual have support people on whom they can rely during a crisis situation? Lack of a meaningful network of satisfactory relationships may implicate an individual as a high risk for suicide during an emotional crisis.

Analysis of the Suicidal Crisis

Three aspects of assessment that enhance understanding of the patient's current suicidal crisis are evaluation of the patient's precipitating stressors, relevant history, and life-stage issues.

- **The precipitating stressor:** Adverse life events in combination with other risk factors, such as depression, may lead to suicide. Life stresses accompanied by an increase in emotional disturbance include the loss of a loved one either by death or by divorce, problems in major relationships, changes in social or occupational roles, or serious physical illness.
- **Relevant history:** Has the individual experienced numerous failures or rejections that would increase their vulnerability for a dysfunctional response to the current situation? Has the individual attempted suicide in the past? How recently? What was the method used in previous attempts?
- **Life-stage issues:** The ability to tolerate loss and disappointment is often compromised if those losses and disappointments occur during stages of life in which the individual struggles with developmental issues (e.g., adolescence, midlife).

Psychiatric, Medical, and Family History

The individual should be assessed for previous psychiatric treatment for depression, substance use disorder, or previous suicide attempts. A medical history should be obtained to determine the presence of chronic, debilitating, or terminal illness. Is there a history of depressive disorder in the family, and has a close relative died by suicide in the past?

Coping Strategies

How has the individual handled previous crisis situations? How does this situation differ from previous ones?

Presenting Symptoms

Several acronyms have been developed as mnemonic devices to summarize important factors that may increase a person's risk for suicidal behavior. One is the acronym IS PATH WARM? (American Association of Suicidology, 2019; Juhnke et al., 2007). The assessment items and patient descriptors for each letter are as follows:

Ideation: Has suicide ideas that are current and active, especially with an identified plan

Substance abuse: Has current or excessive use of alcohol or other mood-altering drugs

Purposelessness: Expresses thoughts that there is no reason to continue living

Anger: Expresses uncontrolled anger or feelings of rage

Trapped: Expresses the belief that there is no way out of the current situation

Hopelessness: Expresses a lack of hope and perceives little chance of positive change

Withdrawal: Expresses desire to withdraw from others or has begun withdrawing

Anxiety: Expresses anxiety, agitation, and/or changes in sleep patterns

Recklessness: Engages in reckless or risky activities with little thought of consequences

Mood: Expresses dramatic mood shifts

Mnemonic devices such as IS PATH WARM? can be helpful in remembering what types of presenting symptoms to assess for, but the overall assessment and management of suicidal behavior are far more complex and must consider available support systems, the individual's willingness to accept support, and their ability to establish a trusting therapeutic alliance with health-care professionals intervening on their behalf. Ultimately, a clinical judgment must be made about the patient's degree of risk so that appropriate measures can be taken to prevent an attempt. The Columbia Suicide Severity Rating Scale (Posner et al., 2011) is an evidence-based tool that assists in this process (Figure 16–2).

 The Collaborative Assessment and Management of Suicidality (CAMS) model is an evidence-based approach that focuses on the importance of patient-centered, problem-focused intervention to build an alliance with patients for collaboration in reducing risk for suicidal behavior (Jobes, 2012). This model focuses on assessment, which necessarily includes asking the patient to identify what is driving the desire to take their own life so that alternatives (identifying and capitalizing on motivations to live) can be explored. For all health-care professionals, this work begins with developing skills in asking basic and direct questions, such as "Are you having thoughts of hurting or killing yourself?"

Beyond the basic questions of whether or not a person has suicidal ideas, a plan, and access to means, there must be a recognition that patients are not always forthcoming or truthful in their answers to such questions. Several strategies for enhancing a collaborative, therapeutic relationship and communication about suicide assessment have been elaborated.

Columbia-Suicide Severity Rating Scale
Screen Version - Recent

	Past Month		Lifetime (Worst Point)	
Ask questions that are **bolded** and <u>underlined</u>.	Yes	No	Yes	No
Ask Questions 1 and 2				
1) *__Have you wished you were dead or wished you could go to sleep and not wake up?__*				
2) *__Have you actually had any thought of killing yourself?__*				
If YES to 2, ask questions 3, 4, 5, and 6. If NO to 2, go directly to question 6.				
3) *__Have you been thinking about how you might do this?__* E.g. "I thought about taking an overdose but I never made a specific plan as to when, where, or how I would actually do it...and I would never go through with it."				
4) *__Have you had these thoughts and had some intention of acting on them?__* As opposed to "I have the thought but I definitely will not do anything about them."				
5) *__Have you started to work out or worked out the details of how to kill yourself?__* *__Do you intend to carry out this plan?__*				

<u>**How long ago did the Worst Point Ideation occur?**</u> _____

	Yes	No
6) *__Have you ever done anything, started to do anything, or prepared to do anything to end your life?__*		
Examples: Collected pills, obtained a gun, gave away valuables, wrote a will or suicide note, took out pills but didn't swallow any, held a gun but changed your mind or it was grabbed from your hand, went to the roof but didn't jump; or actually took pills, tried to shoot yourself, cut yourself, tried to hang yourself, etc...		
If YES, ask: *__Was this within the past three months?__*		

☐ Low risk   ☐ Moderate risk   ▨ High risk

FIGURE 16-2 Columbia-Suicide Severity Rating Scale (C-SSRS). Reprinted with permission from The Columbia Lighthouse Project.

Because nurses are often at the front line of this assessment in medical-surgical departments, emergency departments, outpatient care, schools, and other health-care settings, they must be thoughtful, comprehensive, and conscientious in this pursuit regardless of the practice setting and whether or not the patient has been identified as having mental health issues. Shea (2009) stated that nurses need to assess not only what the patient is directly stating about their suicidal intent (stated intent), but also the amount of thinking, planning, and behaviors associated with suicide ideation (reflected intent) and the suicide intent that is withheld from the nurse (withheld intent). A summary of guiding principles in suicide risk assessment is included in Table 16–2.

One model for enhancing communication in suicide assessment is the Chronological Assessment of Suicide Events (CASE) approach. It is described as a flexible guide for interviewing that includes communication techniques designed to elicit and enhance detailed, valid feedback from patients about sensitive topics such as suicide. Several examples, as elaborated by Shea (2009), follow:

■ *Normalizing* communicates that the patient is not the only one who experiences suicidal ideation.

Example
"Sometimes when people are in a lot of emotional pain, they have thoughts of killing themselves. Have you had any thoughts like that?"

■ *Asking about behavioral events* rather than the patient's opinions may elicit more concrete information.

TABLE 16–2 Guiding Principles for Suicide Risk Assessment

PRINCIPLES	EXPLANATION
Screening for suicide risk should be conducted as an essential component of health assessment, and risk factors, warning signs, and threats should be taken seriously.	Screening includes identifying through detailed assessment the individual's unique situation to discern additional resources, consultations, and interventions needed to ensure client safety.
Establishment of a therapeutic relationship is foundational to effective suicide risk assessment.	Establishing trust through empathy and respect provides a safe environment for the client to tell their story.
Suicide risk assessment is complex and challenges the nurse to use many different communication strategies.	Assessment includes exploring the client's thoughts, feelings, and behaviors from a variety of perspectives.
Suicide risk assessment is an ongoing process, and the level of risk can increase or decrease over time.	Assessment should take place over time to look for fluctuations in risk factors and changes in stress level, intensity of ideation, intention to act on suicide ideation, and support systems.
Collaboration with the client and other sources of information facilitates confidence in clinical judgments.	Collaboration entails using information provided by other people who are familiar with the client from home, work, or school and other clinical team members. Collaboration also implies that all those involved in the client's care are working together.
Suicide risk assessment uses direct rather than indirect language.	Terminology such as "suicide" and "death" should be used rather than "not happy with living" or other indirect statements. Use of direct language also communicates to the client that these are acceptable topics to discuss.
Suicide risk assessment attempts to discern the underlying message.	It is important to discern when the client is communicating unbearable distress, feeling trapped, feeling hopeless, or feeling driven to avoid additional emotional or physical pain.
Suicide risk assessment considers cultural context.	Anyone, regardless of race, religion, or culture, may be at risk for suicide. Some cultural or religious prohibitions may influence someone's willingness to openly discuss personal feelings.
Suicide risk assessment is documented in detail.	Documentation includes risk factors, warning signs, underlying themes, level of risk, clinical judgments, and recommended interventions.

Source: Adapted from Perlman, C. M., Neufeld, E., Martin, L., Goy, M., & Hirdes, J. P. (2011). *Risk assessment inventory: A resource guide for Canadian healthcare organizations.* Hospital Association and Canadian Patient Safety Institute.

Example

"What did you do when you had those thoughts?" "How many pills did you take?" "What happened next?"

■ *Gentle assumptions* encourage further discussion by assuming there is more to tell.

Example

"What other times have you attempted suicide?"

■ *Denial of the specific* is helpful when a patient generally denies suicidal ideation. This strategy encourages more in-depth thought and response by asking questions that might trigger memories of specific events.

Example

After the patient denies suicidal ideation in response to a general question, the nurse asks more specifically, "Have you ever had thoughts of overdosing?" "Have you ever had thoughts about shooting yourself?"

■ *Chronologically exploring* the presenting suicide event, recent suicide events, past suicide events, and immediate suicide events can broaden the nurse's understanding of the patient's immediate suicidal intent in the context of their behavior over time.

Example

The nurse asks the patient about the event that precipitated this episode of care: "Tell me about the event that led you to be hospitalized," and then asks about any other recent events: "When was the last time you attempted suicide before this event? Tell me more about that event" (as well as their history of suicidal behavior over time). Finally, the nurse immediately explores current ideation and intent: "Tell me about your level of risk right now. Current ideas? Intensity? Intentions?"

Diagnosis and Outcome Identification

Nursing diagnoses for the suicidal patient may include the following:

■ Risk for suicidal behavior related to feelings of hopelessness and desperation
■ Hopelessness related to absence of support systems and perception of worthlessness
■ Ineffective coping related to extreme stress, crisis, feeling trapped, poorly developed coping skills, impulsivity

Outcome Criteria

Outcome criteria include short- and long-term goals. Timelines are individually determined. The criteria that follow may be used for measurement of outcomes in the care of the suicidal patient.

The patient:

1. Has experienced no physical harm to self
2. Develops a safety plan and sets realistic goals for self
3. Expresses optimism and hope for the future

Planning and Implementation

Table 16–3 provides a plan of care for the hospitalized patient who is suicidal. Nursing diagnoses are presented, along with outcome criteria, appropriate nursing interventions, and rationales for each.

Intervention With the Client Who Is Suicidal After Discharge or in an Outpatient Setting

In some instances, it may be determined that suicidal intent is low and that hospitalization is not required. Instead, the client with suicidal ideation may be treated in an outpatient setting. In addition, clients who have been hospitalized with acute risk for suicidal behavior continue to need follow-up and support postdischarge. Guidelines

---

Table 16–3 | CARE PLAN FOR THE SUICIDAL PATIENT

NURSING DIAGNOSIS: RISK FOR SUICIDAL BEHAVIOR
RELATED TO: Feelings of hopelessness and desperation

OUTCOME CRITERIA	NURSING INTERVENTIONS	RATIONALES
Patient will not harm self.	1. Ask the patient directly: "Have you thought about harming yourself in any way? If so, what do you plan to do? Do you have the means to carry out this plan? How strong are your intentions to die?" "How often do you think about suicide?"	1. The risk of suicide is greatly increased if the patient has developed a plan with lethal means and particularly if means are accessible for patient to execute the plan. Suicide-specific rumination is associated with suicide attempts.

Table 16–3 | CARE PLAN FOR THE SUICIDAL PATIENT—cont'd

OUTCOME CRITERIA	NURSING INTERVENTIONS	RATIONALES
	2. Create a safe environment for the patient. Remove all potentially harmful objects from patient's access (sharp objects, straps, belts, ties, glass items, alcohol). Supervise closely during meals and medication administration. Perform room searches as deemed necessary.	2. Patient safety is a nursing priority.
	3. Maintain close observation of the patient. Depending on level of suicide precaution, provide one-to-one supervision, constant visual observation, or every-15-minute checks at irregular intervals. Place the patient in a room close to nurse's station; do not assign to private room. Accompany to off-unit activities if attendance is indicated. May need to accompany to bathroom.	3. Close observation is necessary to ensure that the patient does not harm self in any way. Being alert for suicidal and escape attempts facilitates prevention or interruption of harmful behavior.
	4. Maintain special care in administration of medications.	4. Prevents saving up to overdose or discarding and not taking.
	5. Make rounds at frequent, *irregular* intervals (especially at night, toward early morning, at change of shift, or other predictably busy times for staff).	5. Prevents staff surveillance from becoming predictable. Being aware of the patient's location is important, especially when staff is busy and least available and observable.
	6. Encourage the patient to express honest feelings, including anger. Provide hostility release if needed.	6. Depression and suicidal behaviors may be viewed as anger turned inward on the self. If this anger can be verbalized in a nonthreatening environment, the patient may be able to eventually resolve these feelings.
Patient develops a safety plan for management of suicidal thoughts and urges.	1. Establish a trusting, therapeutic relationship to encourage open discussion of suicide.	1. Establishing trust and open communications encourages the patient to share thoughts and feelings.
	2. Collaborate with the patient to develop a safety plan that includes recognition of warning signs, coping strategies, supportive people and places, resources and contact information for crisis management, and plans to restrict access to lethal means.	2. Development of a comprehensive collaborative safety plan concretizes resources and management strategies. Actively engaging the patient in collaboration on the development of a safety plan promotes patient ownership and investment in the process.

Continued

Table 16–3 | CARE PLAN FOR THE SUICIDAL PATIENT—cont'd

OUTCOME CRITERIA	NURSING INTERVENTIONS	RATIONALES
	3. Assess verbal and nonverbal clues to identify the likelihood that the patient intends to follow through with the established safety plan and evaluate the patient's follow-through with safety plan measures while still hospitalized.	3. Assessment of patient safety includes analyzing congruence of verbal communication, nonverbal communication, and behavior.

NURSING DIAGNOSIS: HOPELESSNESS

RELATED TO: Absence of support systems and perception of worthlessness

EVIDENCED BY: Verbal cues (despondent content, "I can't"); flat affect; lack of initiative; suicidal ideas or attempts

OUTCOME CRITERIA	NURSING INTERVENTIONS	RATIONALES
Patient expresses hope and acceptance of life and situations over which they has no control.	1. Identify stressors in the patient's life that precipitated current crisis. Include assessing degree of emotional pain and hopelessness in relationship to feelings of connectedness or lack of connectedness with others.	1. It is important to identify contributing factors to assist the patient with stress management. Meaningful connections with others promotes hope and is identified as a protective factor against suicide.
	2. Determine coping behaviors previously used and the patient's perception of effectiveness then and now.	2. Identifying the patient's strengths encourages their use in the current crisis.
	3. Encourage the patient to explore and verbalize thoughts, feelings, and perceptions related to reasons for wanting to die as well as reasons for wanting to live.	3. Identification of feelings underlying behaviors helps the patient to begin the process of taking control of their own thoughts and feelings (to begin the process of reframing thoughts) and enables the nurse to help the patient focus on maximizing their reasons for wanting to live.
	4. 💬 Provide expressions of hope to the patient in a positive, low-key manner (e.g., "I know you feel you cannot go on, but I believe that things can get better for you. What you are feeling is temporary. It is okay if you don't see it just now.").	4. Although the patient feels hopeless, it is helpful to hear positive expressions from others. The patient's current state of mind may prevent them from identifying anything positive in life. It is important to accept the patient's feelings nonjudgmentally and to affirm their personal worth and value.
	5. Help the patient identify areas of life situation that are under their control.	5. The patient's emotional condition may interfere with the ability to problem solve. Assistance may be required to perceive benefits and consequences of available alternatives accurately.

Table 16–3 | CARE PLAN FOR THE SUICIDAL PATIENT—cont'd

OUTCOME CRITERIA	NURSING INTERVENTIONS	RATIONALES
	6. Identify sources that the patient may use after discharge when crises occur or feelings of hopelessness and possible suicidal ideation prevail. This includes local suicide hotlines and other available support services.	6. A collaboratively developed, concrete plan promotes hope in the face of a crisis.
	7. Assist the patient to explore and identify future-oriented goals.	7. Identifying goals encourages the patient to focus on hopefulness for the future.

NURSING DIAGNOSIS: INEFFECTIVE COPING

RELATED TO: Extreme stress, crisis, altered mental status, poorly developed coping skills, feeling trapped or hopeless, impulsivity

EVIDENCED BY: Verbal cues (despondent content, "I can't"); decreased affect; lack of initiative; suicidal ideas or attempts

OUTCOME CRITERIA	NURSING INTERVENTIONS	RATIONALES
Patient identifies coping strategies and expresses commitment to incorporate these as part of a plan to maintain personal safety.	1. Assist the patient to identify stressors and other warning signs that are associated with thoughts and plans for suicide.	1. Patient's awareness of triggers for increases in suicidal thinking, plans, and intentions promotes an understanding of situations requiring the implementation of the safety plan.
	2. Explore past coping skills that the patient identifies as effective.	2. Exploring the patient's perception of effective coping skills promotes active engagement in the process of identifying and carrying out a safety plan.
	3. Maintain a nonjudgmental attitude when discussing the patient's suicide ideas, plans, and intentions.	3. A nonjudgmental attitude promotes open communication and collaboration.
	4. Assist the patient to identify internal coping strategies for immediate response to a trigger event.	4. This promotes the patient's ability to develop a sense of personal control in response to suicide ideas.
	5. Assist the patient in identifying support systems, resources, and social activities that the patient can use to support ongoing personal safety.	5. External coping strategies, such as eliciting support from a family member or friend, community resources, and social activities that may help the patient minimize rumination about suicide, are all positive coping skills essential to a comprehensive safety plan.

for treatment of such clients on an outpatient basis include the following:

■ The person should have immediate access to support systems and be connected to a system of care, as the term after hospital discharge is a high-risk period. Arrangements must be made for the client to stay with family or friends. If this is not possible, hospitalization should be reconsidered.

■ A detailed **collaborative safety plan** should be developed that is an outgrowth of a comprehensive risk assessment and a collaborative, problem-solving discussion with the client. This intervention explores with the client what they will do to stay safe if there is a repeat of or increase in suicidal thoughts or urges. Box 16–2 provides more information on the essential components of a safety plan.

■ A safety plan should not be confused with a no-suicide contract. See Boxes 16–3 and 16–4 to learn about issues associated with developing an appropriate safety plan.

■ Enlist the help of family or friends to ensure that the home environment does not contain dangerous items, such as firearms or stockpiled drugs. Give support persons the telephone number of the counselor or an emergency contact person if the counselor is not available.

■ Appointments may need to be scheduled daily or every other day at first until the immediate suicidal crisis has subsided.

■ Establish rapport and promote a trusting relationship. It is important for the suicide counselor to

---

BOX 16–2 Essential Components of a Safety Plan

According to Stanley and Brown (2008, pp. 3–4), the essential components of a safety plan include nursing support and assistance for the following:

1. Recognizing warning signs that precede suicide crises
2. Identifying and employing internal coping strategies that the client can implement without needing to contact additional support people
3. Identifying supportive family members and friends with whom they can discuss suicide and who may help resolve a potential crisis
4. Identifying people and healthy social settings that they can use for general support and distraction from suicidal thoughts and urges
5. Identifying resources and contact information for mental health professionals and agencies when needed in an escalating crisis situation
6. Problem-solving with the client ways to reduce the potential for access to and use of lethal means

Once the safety plan is elaborated with the client, an evaluation of the appropriateness of the plan and a collaborative assessment of the likelihood that the client will implement this plan should be conducted.

Assessment for suicidal risk and responsive intervention must be ongoing, as suicidal ideas and intent may change over hours, days, or longer time periods. The need for revision of the safety plan may become evident. Critical times for reassessment of risk and reevaluation of the safety plan (Hoffman, 2013) include the following:

1. When there is a change in the client's clinical presentation or worsening of symptoms
2. When medications or treatments are changed
3. When significant others identify an increase in concern
4. When a client stops treatment

BOX 16–3 The Issue of No-Suicide Contracts

A critical issue that needs to be understood is that of no-suicide contracts, sometimes called *safety contracts,* which is a strategy used by some clinicians in the context of a long-term, therapeutic relationship in which the client "promises" to contact the clinician before acting on suicidal ideation. **No-suicide contracts are not the same as the development of a thorough safety plan. Contracting with a client is a controversial and often misused strategy** (Hoffman, 2013; Shea, 2009). **Evidence has not supported the efficacy of this method as a primary intervention** (Drew, 2001; Edwards & Sachman, 2010; Freedenthal, 2013; Rudd et al., 2006). In fact, it may even be counterproductive in clients with borderline or passive-aggressive pathology (Shea, 2009). Evidence does support the superiority of crisis response planning over the use of contracting for safety (Bryan et al., 2017). **Such contracts should *never* be used in short-term encounters with clients, such as in emergency departments or during brief hospital stays, or with clients who are unknown, agitated, psychotic, impulsive, or under the influence of drugs and alcohol** (Hoffman, 2013). **They should never be used with the presumption that they will deter a client from attempting suicide**. Shea adds that if clinicians use a safety contract with the belief that it will be a deterrent to suicide, they should understand that it **not only "guarantees nothing [but also] may yield a false sense of security" among clinicians** (2009, p. 21). The consequential danger is that clinicians may become less watchful or feel less need to reassess the client, thus missing critical signs of increasing suicide risk. Roberts (2020) cites American Psychiatric Association (APA) practice guidelines that advise against using no-suicide contracts independently or outside of a well-established patient-provider relationship. Nurses should avoid no-suicide contracting altogether. Even in the conduct of therapy, it should be used with great caution and for limited, specific assessment purposes.

In general, it is important to recognize that not all suicidal individuals are alike, so **interventions should be multifaceted, and suicide prevention plans should be comprehensive.** Many models and tools for suicide assessment have been developed. One such model, SAFE-T (Suicide Assessment Five-step Evaluation and Triage), summarizes the key elements in suicide assessment (Box 16–4).

BOX 16–4 SAFE-T: Suicide Assessment Five-Step Evaluation and Triage

1. Identify risk factors
   Note those that can be modified to reduce risk.
2. Identify protective factors
   Note those that can be enhanced.
3. Conduct suicide inquiry
   Evaluate suicidal thoughts, plans, behavior, and intent.
4. Determine risk level and intervention
   Choose appropriate intervention to address and reduce level of risk.
5. Document
   Record assessment of risk, rationale, intervention, and follow-up.

Source: Reprinted from U.S. Department of Health and Human Services, Substance Abuse and Mental Health Services Administration, www.samhsa.gov.

become a key person in the client's support system at this time.

■ Accept the client's feelings in a nonjudgmental manner.

CLINICAL PEARL Be direct. Talk openly and matter-of-factly about suicide. Listen actively and encourage expression of feelings, including anger.

■ Discuss the current crisis in the client's life using the problem-solving approach. Offer alternatives to suicide while at the same time empathizing with the client's pain that led to viewing suicide as an option (Jobes, 2012). An example of this kind of communication might be:

■ "I understand how this emotional pain you've been experiencing led you to consider suicide, but I'd like to explore with you some alternative ways to decrease your pain and to identify some reasons for continuing to live."

■ Help the client identify areas of life that are within their control and those that cannot be controlled. Discuss feelings associated with these control issues. It is important for the client to feel some control over their life situation in order to perceive a measure of self-worth.

■ The physician or nurse practitioner may prescribe antidepressants for an individual who is experiencing suicidal depression. It is wise to prescribe no more than a 3-day supply of the medication with no refills. The prescription can then be renewed at the client's next counseling session.

■ Psychological interventions that have demonstrated effectiveness in reducing suicidal behavior include dialectical behavior therapy, cognitive behavior

therapy, and CAMS (Jobes, 2015; Gotzsche & Gotzsche, 2017).

Single interventions, including hospitalization, medication alone, and no-suicide contracts, are not supported by evidence as effective in reducing suicides (Jobes, 2015). Clients need to be actively engaged as partners in each step of the assessment and intervention process. Evidence does support that early follow-up phone calls with patients who have been treated for a suicide attempt is an effective strategy for reducing suicide risk (Exbrayat et al., 2017; Stanley et al., 2018).

Information for Family and Friends of the Suicidal Client

The following suggestions are recommended for family and friends of an individual who is suicidal:

■ Take any hint of suicide seriously. Anyone expressing suicidal feelings needs immediate attention.

■ Do not keep secrets. If a suicidal person says, "Promise you won't tell anyone," do not make that promise. Suicidal individuals are ambivalent about dying, and suicidal behavior is a cry for help. It is that ambivalence that leads the person to confide to you the suicidal thoughts. Get help for the person and for yourself. To access the national suicide prevention hotline, simply dial **988**.

■ Be a good listener. If a person expresses suicidal thoughts or feels depressed, hopeless, or worthless, be supportive. Let the person know you are there for them and are willing to help the person seek professional help.

■ Many people find it awkward to put into words how another person's life is important for their own well-being, but it is important to stress that the person's life is important to you and to others. Emphasize in specific terms the ways in which the person's suicide would be devastating to you and others.

■ Express concern for an individual who expresses thoughts about suicide. The individual may make veiled comments or comments that sound as if they are joking, or the person may be withdrawn and reluctant to discuss their thoughts and feelings. In each case, ask questions, acknowledge the person's pain and feelings of hopelessness, and encourage the individual to talk to someone else if they do not feel comfortable talking with you.

■ Familiarize yourself with suicide intervention resources, such as mental health centers and suicide hotlines.

■ Ensure that access to firearms or other means of self-harm is restricted.

■ Communicate caring and commitment to providing support. Fleener (n.d.) offered the following specific suggestions for families and friends when *interacting* with someone who is suicidal:

- Acknowledge and accept the person's feelings and be an active listener.
- Try to give the person hope and remind the person that what they are feeling is temporary.
- Stay with the person. Do not leave the person alone. Go to where they are, if necessary.
- Show love and encouragement. Hold, hug, and touch the person. Allow the person to cry and express anger.
- Help the person seek professional help.
- Remove any items from the home with which the person may harm themselves.
- If there are children present, try to remove them from the home. Perhaps a friend or relative can assist by taking the children to their home. This type of situation can be extremely traumatic for children.
- Do *not* judge suicidal people, show anger toward them, provoke guilt in them, discount their feelings, or tell them to "snap out of it." This is a very real and serious situation to individuals experiencing suicidal ideation. They are in real pain. They feel the situation is hopeless and that there is no other way to resolve it aside from suicide.

Intervention With Families and Friends of Suicide Victims

Suicide of a family member can induce a whole gamut of feelings in the survivors. It has long been recognized that the bereavement process for families in which a member has taken their own life is complicated and requires an understanding by health-care providers of the unique burdens of this type of loss. Macnab (1993) identified the following symptoms that may be evident after the suicide of a loved one:

- A sense of guilt and responsibility
- Anger, resentment, and rage that can never find its "object"
- A heightened sense of emotionality, helplessness, failure, and despair
- A recurring self-searching: "If only I had done something," "If only I had not done something."
- A sense of confusion and search for an explanation: "Why did this happen?" "What does it mean?" "What could have stopped it?" "What will people think?"
- A sense of inner injury; the family feels wounded and does not know how they will ever get over it and get on with life
- A severe strain placed on relationships; a sense of impatience, irritability, and anger among family members
- A heightened feeling of vulnerability to illness and disease with this added burden of emotional stress

Read "Real People, Real Stories" for a better understanding of one person's lived experience of losing a child to suicide.

Strategies for assisting survivors of suicide victims include the following:

- Encourage the survivors to talk to each other about the suicide and respond to each other's viewpoints and reconstructing of events. Share memories.
- Be aware of any blaming or scapegoating of specific family members. Discuss how each person fits into the family situation, both before and after the suicide.
- Listen to feelings of guilt and self-persecution. Gently move the individuals toward the reality of the situation.
- Encourage the family members to discuss individual relationships with the lost loved one. Focus on both positive and negative aspects of the relationships. Gradually point out the irrationality of any idealized concepts of the deceased person. The family must be able to recognize both positive and negative aspects about the person before grief can be resolved.
- No two people grieve in the same way. It may appear that some family members are overcoming the grief faster than others. All family members must be made to understand that if this occurs, it is not because those family members care less—it is just that they grieve differently. Variables that enter into this phenomenon include individual past experiences, personal relationship with the deceased person, and individual temperament and coping abilities.
- Recognize how the suicide has caused disorganization in family coping. Reassess interpersonal relationships in the context of the event. Discuss coping strategies that have been successful in times of stress in the past, and work to reestablish these strategies within the family. Identify new adaptive coping strategies that can be incorporated.
- Identify resources that provide support: religious beliefs and spiritual counselors, close friends and relatives, support groups for survivors of suicide. One online connection that puts individuals in contact with survivors' groups specific to each state is the American Foundation for Suicide Prevention at www.afsp.org. A list of resources that provide information and help for issues regarding suicide is presented in Box 16–5.

Evaluation

Evaluation of the client who is suicidal is an ongoing process accomplished through continuous reassessment and determination of goal achievement. Once the immediate crisis has been resolved, extended

Real People, Real Stories: Surviving the Loss of a Loved One to Suicide

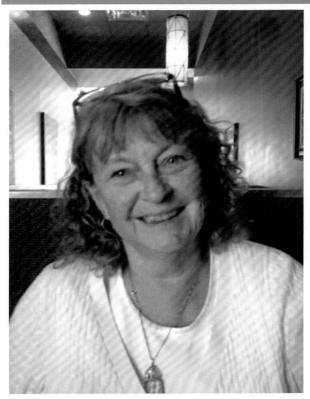

Losing a loved one to suicide results in a grief process often complicated by stigma, misinformation, lack of information, and sometimes a sense of alienation from others. Emmy's story describes her ongoing journey to grapple with the loss of her son to suicide.

Karyn: We've talked before but tell me more about your journey since Paul's death.

Emmy: My son Paul died in 1986 at age 17. The thing I remember most is that no one was talking about it. There were 10 students who died in his high school. Two others were known to be suicides.

Karyn: Do you mean no one was talking about it in the school system?

Emmy: Well, the students in Paul's class took up a collection that was for Paul, but the school couldn't decide how to use it, so it just sat there for the longest time. My other son heard they were going to use the money for supplies, so I went and talked to them to make sure that didn't happen. The school eventually built a memorial garden that became dedicated to all of the students who had died.

Paul died in June, and in August, when all the other students were returning to school, I got a call from a community suicide survivors counselor who told me she was holding a high school assembly to discuss suicide. I wanted her to talk to the ninth and tenth graders, but they wouldn't permit it. I thought the younger kids needed to talk about and learn about this too—they had been my younger son's classmates, and they were affected by it as well. When the suicide counselor

intervened, the teachers were told to watch Paul's friends for any evidence of "copycat" behavior, but that was all. I felt the school administration thought there was a stigma in talking about the cause of his death. I found out later that the seniors were talking about and memorializing Paul in their study halls. They were remembering him as a friend who was missed.

Karyn: How has your family coped with Paul's death?

Emmy: We didn't talk about Paul for the longest time; it was as if he didn't exist. We were very separate; we all went in our own directions. My husband started taking long bicycle trips, and he worked on a suicide hotline. I got very involved with offering a program for high school students called Listening POST (people offering students time), which allowed students to talk about anything they wanted to.

Karyn: I know you've told me that you're still close to several of Paul's peers.

Emmy: Oh yes, and their children too. But our family just became very separate. I don't even know how my other son got through his freshman year of high school. We went to a suicide survivors group as a family, and it was important to me as an outlet to talk, but we didn't talk as a family … and then we just stopped going, and the people who knew Paul didn't talk to us. I *so* wanted to talk to people who knew Paul.

After we stopped going to the survivors group, I started going to CoDA [Co-Dependents Anonymous] meetings, even though I don't think I'm codependent. It was more because I needed to talk … to understand how this happened. I felt like I wasn't there for him. … I was busy with my job and maybe I wasn't tuned in to his moods. I was always taught that boys don't like to talk about feelings.

Karyn: Yes, I guess I've been taught that, too.

Emmy: I just remember that night he told his dad and I that he loved us, he went to bed, and the next morning we found him. I just couldn't make sense of it. Years later, one of Paul's peers, who now has a teenage son, said he could finally tell me what he remembered. And there were signs. Apparently, he had said to some friends (while they were drinking alcohol), "Have you ever thought of killing yourself?" and they all laughed about it and nothing more was said. I also found out that he told an older peer, whom he had met at church camp, that he didn't want to live. The peer smacked him and told him if he ever had thoughts like that again that he [Paul] needed to come talk to him first. But they never told anyone else; they kept it among their peers. They thought they were all-knowing and never told an adult. He was hysterical when he found out what happened.

On that last weekend, he had been partying with his friends … there was alcohol involved … and the friend that was with him told me that someday he would tell me what went down that day. But it's 30 years later, and I still don't know. I know he was at the party with a girl, but I've never been able to find her or talk with her. She went to a different school.

Continued

Real People, Real Stories: Surviving the Loss of a Loved One to Suicide–cont'd

Karyn: And much of this information that you do know came 10 or more years after his death?

Emmy: Yes.

Karyn: What a long journey you've been on trying to put all the pieces together.

Emmy: (tearful) That's exactly it. Trying to put the pieces together, sort it out … but it never gets solved. … It's like being in a maze and you can't get out, and I had a lot of guilt.… Now I recognize that he just made some tragic bad choices.

Karyn: Appreciating that we don't "get over" such tremendous loss but rather amend our lives with some different understanding of love and loss, what has been most helpful in your healing?

Emmy: Yes, I think there was a point when I realized it was okay to feel some happiness. Being with people who don't know me makes it easier. My faith and fellowship group has been an important part of healing. CoDA was helpful because we talked about how different people process things, and I could understand better how people can get stuck. I used to say that my other son had lost his brother. I couldn't say that I had lost a son. When I had to fill out a health assessment at one point, and I had to respond to the question of how many pregnancies I'd had, that was the most difficult question … because I had to acknowledge … the

reality. And I involved myself with all the boys who were on the track team with Paul and the Listening POST and just talked about everything.

Karyn: What is the most important thing that nurses need to know?

Emmy: By the time we would have had any contact with nurses, it was too late. There were no ER, medical, or mental health visits before that. If they were to have an impact, it would have been in prevention in the schools. For example, I didn't know at that time to ask questions like, "Are you having thoughts of hurting yourself?" and "Do you have a plan in mind?" And Paul put on a different face for me. He wasn't solitary; he had lots of friends; he was active on the track team. …

Karyn: I think you're not alone with not having been taught about things like suicide assessment. Because, as you've said, historically people haven't talked about it. There is an organization called Red Flags National that promotes mental health education for students, parents, and teachers as a standard part of health education in schools.

Emmy: Yes. It needs to be talked about. It's been helpful for me to talk about it even now. I've never had to try to explain the story before.

To learn more about Red Flags National, go to www.redflags.org.

BOX 16–5 Resources Related to Suicide Prevention

National Suicide Hotline
1-800-SUICIDE (24/7)

National Suicide Prevention Lifeline
www.suicidepreventionlifeline.org
Dial **988**

American Association of Suicidology
www.suicidology.org

Depression and Bipolar Support Alliance (DBSA)
www.dbsalliance.org

American Foundation for Suicide Prevention
www.afsp.org

National Institute of Mental Health
www.nimh.nih.gov

National Alliance on Mental Illness
www.nami.org

American Psychiatric Association
www.psychiatry.org

Mental Health America
www.nmha.org

American Psychological Association
www.apa.org

Screening for Mental Health Stop a Suicide Today!
www.stopasuicide.org

Boys Town
www.boystown.org
1-800-448-3000 (24/7 national hotline)

Centre for Suicide Prevention (Canada)
www.suicideinfo.ca
1-833-456-4566 (24/7 helpline)

Samaritans (U.K. and Republic of Ireland)
www.samaritans.org
116-123 (24/7 helpline)

The Trevor Project
Confidential suicide hotline for LGBTQ youth
www.thetrevorproject.org
1-866-488-7386 (24/7 hotline)

Centers for Disease Control and Prevention
National Center for Injury Prevention and Control
Division of Violence Prevention
www.cdc.gov/injury/index.html

SAVE (Suicide Awareness Voices of Education)
www.save.org

Alliance of Hope: For Suicide Loss Survivors
www.allianceofhope.org

U.S. Department of Veterans Affairs
Veterans crisis line: 1(800)-273-8255 (press 1)

psychotherapy may be indicated. The long-term goals of individual or group psychotherapy for the client would be for them to:

- Develop and maintain a more positive self-concept and a sense of hopefulness.
- Learn more effective ways to express feelings to others.
- Achieve successful interpersonal relationships.
- Feel accepted by others and achieve a sense of belonging.

A person contemplating suicide feels worthless and hopeless. These goals serve to instill a sense of self-worth while offering a measure of hope and a meaning for living.

Summary and Key Points

- The majority of all people who attempt or die by suicide have a diagnosed mental disorder.
- Suicide is the second-leading cause of death among young Americans aged 10 to 14 and 25 to 34 years, and men aged 75 and older have the highest rate (40.5 per 100,000) compared with other age groups. Middle-aged adults (aged 35 to 64 years) account for 47.2% of all suicides in the United States, and suicide is the 9th leading cause of death for this age group.
- Evidence supports that transitional life changes such as recent change in relationship status (including breakups, divorce, and widowhood) are proximal risk factors.
- More women than men attempt suicide, but men succeed more often.
- Depressed men and women who consider themselves closely affiliated with a religion are less likely than their nonreligious counterparts to attempt suicide.
- Financial strain and unemployment are identified as risk factors for suicide.
- Age-adjusted suicide rates are highest among non-Hispanic AI/AN people (23.9 per 100,000) and non-Hispanic white people (16.9 per 100,000) compared with other racial and ethnic groups.
- Psychiatric disorders that predispose individuals to suicide include mood disorders (depression and bipolar disorders), substance use disorders, schizophrenia, anorexia nervosa, borderline and antisocial personality disorders, anxiety disorders, and attention deficit-hyperactivity disorders.
- Predisposing factors include internalized anger, hopelessness and other symptoms of severe depression, history of aggression and violence, shame and humiliation, developmental stressors, sociological influences, genetics, and neurochemical factors.
- Suicide risk assessment should be a patient-centered, collaborative process in the context of a therapeutic relationship and should chronologically explore presenting suicide events, recent events, past events, and immediate intentions.
- Assessment of the level of intervention needed includes identifying the number of proximal or potentiating risks as well as the number of warning signs.
- It is important for the nurse to determine the seriousness of the patient's suicidal intentions, the existence of a plan, and the availability and lethality of the method.
- Many tools exist to screen for risk factors and warning signs for suicide. The Columbia Suicide Severity Rating Scale is an evidence-based tool for assessing the degree of risk and making clinical judgments about what level of treatment is needed to help the patient remain free from self-injury or death by suicide. Risk assessment scales should not be used alone but in combination with a comprehensive psychosocial assessment.
- The suicidal person should not be left alone.
- A safety plan is developed with the patient following a comprehensive suicide risk assessment. A safety plan includes assisting the patient to recognize warning signs, identify and employ internal coping strategies, engage family members and friends as available support persons, identify people and social settings that can be used to distract from suicidal thoughts or urges, identify resources and contact information for crisis intervention, and problem solve ways to restrict access to lethal means.
- Once the crisis intervention is complete, the individual may require long-term psychotherapy, during which they work to:
  - Develop and maintain a more positive self-concept.
  - Learn more effective ways to express feelings.
  - Improve interpersonal relationships.
  - Achieve a sense of belonging and a measure of hope for living.
- Evidence-based psychological interventions include dialectical behavior therapy, cognitive behavior therapy, and the Collaborative Assessment and Management of Suicidality (CAMS) approach.

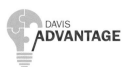
DAVIS
ADVANTAGE

Go to **Davis Advantage** to complete your learning: strengthen understanding, apply your knowledge, and prepare for the Next Gen NCLEX®.

Review Questions

1. Which of the following individuals demonstrates the highest number of risk factors for suicide?
   a. A client who reports they are in deep emotional pain, feels hopeless, and says "No one is there for me."
   b. A client who has been seeing a doctor for chronic, intractable pain and is taking pain medication.
   c. An American Indian client who just graduated from high school with honors.
   d. A physician who reports feeling "burnt out" and is considering retirement.

2. The nurse in the emergency department encounters a client who is expressing suicide ideation. Which of the following nursing considerations are important to good suicide risk assessment? (Select all that apply.)
   a. Collaborating with the client
   b. Asking the client specific questions about leisure activities
   c. Establishing trust and open communication with the client
   d. Asking the client specific questions about the strength of their intention to die
   e. Identifying whether the client has thought about a plan for trying to kill themselves

3. A client is hospitalized after a suicide attempt after breaking up with her boyfriend. Freudian psychoanalytic theory would explain the client's suicide attempt in which of the following ways?
   a. She feels hopeless about her future without her boyfriend.
   b. Without her boyfriend, she feels like an outsider with her peers.
   c. She is feeling intense guilt because her boyfriend broke up with her.
   d. She is angry at her boyfriend for breaking up with her and has turned the anger inward on herself.

4. Which of the following interventions are appropriate for a client on suicide precautions? (Select all that apply)
   a. Remove all sharp objects, belts, and other potentially dangerous articles from the client's environment.
   b. Accompany the client to off-unit activities.
   c. Reassess intensity of suicidal thoughts and urges on a regular basis.
   d. Put all of the client's possessions in storage and explain to her that she may have them back when she is off suicide precautions.

5. Success of long-term psychotherapy with a client (who attempted suicide after a breakup with his girlfriend) could be measured by which of the following behaviors?
   a. The client has a new girlfriend.
   b. The client has an increased sense of self-worth.
   c. The client does not take antidepressants anymore.
   d. The client told his old girlfriend how angry he was with her for breaking up with him.

Clinical Judgment Questions

6. A 27-year-old female client was admitted to the psychiatric unit from the medical intensive care unit where she was treated for taking a deliberate overdose of her antidepressant medication, trazodone (Desyrel). She says to the nurse, "My boyfriend broke up with me. We had been together for 6 years. I love him so much. I know I'll never get over him." Which is the best response by the nurse?
   a. "You'll get over him in time."
   b. "Forget him. There are other fish in the sea."
   c. "You must be feeling very sad about your loss."
   d. "Why do you think he broke up with you?"

7. The nurse identifies the primary nursing diagnosis for a client as "Risk for suicidal behavior related to feelings of hopelessness associated with loss of relationship." Which is the outcome criterion that would be most appropriate for this diagnosis?
   a. The client has experienced no self-harm.
   b. The client sets realistic goals.
   c. The client expresses some optimism and hope for the future.
   d. The client has reached a stage of acceptance in the loss of the relationship.

8. A client is hospitalized after a suicide attempt and says to the nurse, "When I get out of here, I'm going to try this again, and next time I'll choose a no-fail method." Which is the best response by the nurse?
   a. "You are safe here. We will make sure nothing happens to you."
   b. "You're just lucky your roommate came home when they did."
   c. "What exactly do you plan to do?"
   d. "I don't understand. You have so much to live for."

9. In determining the degree of suicidal risk with a client, the nurse assesses the following behavioral manifestations: severely depressed, withdrawn, statements of worthlessness, difficulty accomplishing activities of daily living, no close support systems. The nurse identifies the client's risk for suicide as which of the following?
   a. Low risk
   b. High risk
   c. Imminent risk
   d. Unable to be determined

10. A client who has been hospitalized after a suicide attempt is placed on suicide precautions on the psychiatric unit. The client admits that they are still feeling suicidal. Which of the following interventions are most appropriate in this instance? (Select all that apply.)
    a. Restrict access to any item that might be harmful by placing the client in a seclusion room.
    b. Check on the client every 15 minutes at irregular intervals, or assign a staff person to stay with them on a one-to-one basis.
    c. Obtain an order from the physician to give the client a sedative to calm them and reduce suicide ideas.
    d. Do not allow the client to participate in any unit activities while they are on suicide precautions.
    e. Ask the client specific questions about their thoughts, plans, and intentions related to suicide.

Communication Exercises

1. Mr. J. was brought to the emergency department by his brother, who is concerned about Mr. J.'s worsening depression. During the assessment, Mr. J. tells the nurse, "None of this matters. There's nothing that can make this any better." What would be an appropriate response by the nurse?

2. Mr. J. admits to the nurse that he has had suicidal ideas for the last couple of weeks. How would the nurse intervene with Mr. J. at this point?

3. Mr. J. tells the nurse that ever since his wife died 3 months ago, he does not want to go on living. What would be an example of empathic communication in response to this statement by Mr. J.?

🎬 MOVIE CONNECTIONS

Dead Poet's Society • It's Kind of a Funny Story • The Perks of Being a Wallflower • Girl, Interrupted • Cyberbully

References

Ahmedani, B. K., Peterson, E. L., Hu, Y., Rossom, R. C., Lynch, F., Lu, C. Y., Waitzfelder, B. E., Owen-Smith, A. A., Hubley, S., Prabhakar, D. L., Williams, L. K., Zeld, N., Mutter, E., Beck, A., Tolsma, D., & Simon, G. E. (2017). Major physical health conditions and risk of suicide. *American Journal of Preventive Medicine, 53*(3), 308–315. doi:10.1016/j.amepre.2017.04.001

American Association of Suicidology. (2019). *Warnings signs of acute suicide risk.* https://suicidology.org/wp-content/uploads/2019/07/Warning-Signs-Flyer.pdf

American Foundation for Suicide Prevention. (2022). *Suicide statistics.* https://afsp.org/suicide-statistics/

American Psychiatric Association. (2022). *Diagnostic and statistical manual of mental disorders, fifth edition, text revision (DSM-5-TR).* American Psychiatric Association.

American Psychiatric Nurses Association (APNA). (2022). *Psychiatric-mental health nursing essential competencies for the assessment and management of individuals at risk for suicide.* www.apna.org/i4a/pages/index.cfm?pageID=5684

Ammerman B. A., Klieman, E., Uyeji, L. L., & Knorr, A. C. (2015). Suicidal and violent behavior: The role of anger, emotion dysregulation, and impulsivity. *Personality and Individual Differences, 79.* DOI:10.1016/j.paid.2015.01.044

Bachmann S. (2018). Epidemiology of suicide and the psychiatric perspective. *International Journal of Environmental Research and Public Health, 15*(7), 1425. https://doi.org/10.3390/ijerph15071425

Bauman, S., Toomey, R. B., & Walker, J. L. (2013). Associations among bullying, cyberbullying, and suicide in high school students. *Journal of Adolescence, 36*(2), 341–350. doi:10.1016/j.adolescence.2012.12.001

Bridge, J. A., Asti, L., Horowitz, L. M., Greenhouse, J. B., Fontanella, C. A., Sheftall, A. H., & Campo, J. V. (2015). Suicide trends among elementary school–aged children in the United States from 1993 to 2012. *JAMA Pediatrics, 169*(7), 673–677. doi:10.1001/jamapediatrics.2015.0465

Bryan, C. J., Mintz, J., Clemans, T. A., Leeson, B., Burch, T. S., Williams, S. R., Maney, E., & Rudd, M. D. (2017). Effect of crisis response planning vs. contracts for safety on suicide risk in U.S. Army Soldiers: A randomized clinical trial. *Journal of Affective Disorders, 212,* 64–72, https://doi.org/10.1016/j.jad.2017.01.028.

Burr, E. M., Rahm-Knigge, R. L., & Conner, B. T. (2018). The differentiating role of state and trait hopelessness in suicidal ideation and suicide attempt. *Archives of Suicide Research, 22*(3), 510–517. doi: 10.1080/13811118.2017.1366960.

Byron, W. J. (2016). Do people who commit suicide go to hell? *Catholic Digest.* www.catholicdigest.com/articles/faith/knowledge/2007/04-01/do-people-who-commit-suicide-go-to-hell

Center for Deployment Psychology. (n.d.). *Suicide in the military.* https://deploymentpsych.org/disorders/suicide-main

Centers for Disease Control and Prevention (CDC). (2011). *Self-directed violence surveillance: Uniform definitions and recommended data elements.* https://stacks.cdc.gov/view/cdc/11997

Centers for Disease Control and Prevention (CDC). (2016). *Gay and bisexual men's health.* www.cdc.gov/msmhealth/suicide-violence-prevention.htm

Centers for Disease Control and Prevention. (2021). *Risk and protective factors.* https://www.cdc.gov/violenceprevention/suicide/riskprotectivefactors.html

Centers for Disease Control and Prevention (CDC). (2022a). *Facts about suicide.* https://www.cdc.gov/suicide/facts/index.html

Centers for Disease Control and Prevention (CDC). (2022b). *Suicide and self-harm injury.* https://www.cdc.gov/nchs/fastats/suicide.htm

Centers for Disease Control and Prevention (CDC). (2022c). *Suicide mortality in the United States: 2000–2020.* https://www.cdc.gov/nchs/products/databriefs/db433.htm

Chan, M., Bhatti, H., Meader, N., Stockton, S., Evans, J., O'Connor, R., Kapur, N., & Kendall, T. (2016). Predicting suicide following self-harm: Systematic review of risk factors and risk scales. *British Journal of Psychiatry, 209*(4), 277–283. https://doi.org/10.1192/bjp.bp.115.170050

Chang, B. P., Franklin, J. C., Ribeiro, J. D., Fox, K. R., Bentley, K. H., Kleiman, E. M., & Nock, M. K. (2016). Biological risk factors for suicidal behaviors: A meta-analysis. *Translational Psychiatry, 6*(9), e887. doi:10.1038/tp.2016.165

Chung, D., Hadzi-Pavlovic, D., Wang, M., Swaraj, S., Olfson, M., & Large, M. (2019). Meta-analysis of suicide rates in the first week and the first month after psychiatric hospitalization. *BMJ Open, 9*(3), e023883. https://doi.org/10.1136/bmjopen-2018-023883

Compassion and Choices. (2022). *States where medical aid in dying is authorized.* https://compassionandchoices.org/resources/states-or-territories-where-medical-aid-in-dying-is-authorized

Cramer, R. J., Kaniuka, A. R., Yada, F. N., Diaz-Garelli, F., Hill, R. M., Bowling, J., Macchia, J. M., & Tucker, R. P. (2022). An analysis of suicidal thoughts and behaviors among transgender and gender diverse adults. *Social Psychiatry and Psychiatric Epidemiology, 57*(1),195–205. doi: 10.1007/s00127-021-02115-8

Crosby, A. E., Ortega, L., & Melanson, C. (2011). *Self-directed violence surveillance: Uniform definitions and recommended data elements,* version 1.0. Centers for Disease Control and Prevention, National Center for Injury Prevention and Control. www.cdc.gov/violenceprevention/pdf/Self-Directed-Violence-a.pdf

Drew, B. (2001). Self-harm and no-suicide contract in psychiatric inpatient settings. *Archives of Psychiatric Nursing, 15*(3), 99–106. doi:10.1053/apnu.2001.23748

Duran, S., & McGuinness, T. M. (2016). Suicide in childhood. *Journal of Psychosocial Nursing, 54*(10), 27–30.

Edwards, S. J., & Sachman, M. D. (2010). No-suicide contracts, no-suicide agreements, and no-suicide assurances: A study of their nature, utilization, perceived effectiveness, and potential to cause harm. *Crisis, 31*(6), 290–302.

Exbrayat, S., Coudrot, C., Gourdon, X., Gay, A., Seos, J., Pellet, J., Trombert-Paviot, B., & Massoubre, C. (2017). Effect of telephone follow-up on repeated suicide attempt in patients discharged from an emergency psychiatry department: A controlled study. *BMC Psychiatry, 17,* 96. doi:10.1186/s12888-017-1258-6

Fleener, P. (n.d.). How to help a suicidal person. *Mental Health Today.* www.mental-health-today.com/suicide/sui2.htm

Forte, A., Buscajoni, A., Fiorillo, A., Pompili, M., & Baldessarini, R. J. (2019). Suicidal risk following hospital discharge: A review. *Harvard Review of Psychiatry, 27*(4), 209–216. https://doi.org/10.1097/HRP.0000000000000222

Freedenthal, S. (2013). *The use of no-suicide contracts.* www.speakingofsuicide.com/2013/05/15/no-suicide-contracts

Fuller, K. (2020). *5 common myths about suicide debunked.* https://www.nami.org/Blogs/NAMI-Blog/September-2020/5-Common-Myths-About-Suicide-Debunked

Gordon, J. A. (2020). *Addressing the crisis of black youth suicide.* Director's Messages. https://www.nimh.nih.gov/about/director/messages/2020/addressing-the-crisis-of-black-youth-suicide.shtml

Gotzsche, P. C., & Gotzsche, P. K. (2017). Cognitive behavioural therapy halves the risk of repeated suicide attempts: Systematic review. *Journal of the Royal Society of Medicine, 110*(10), 404–410. https://doi.org/10.1177/0141076817731904

Hoffman, R. (2013). Contracting for safety: A misused tool. *Pennsylvania Patient Safety Advisory, 10*(2), 82–84.

Ivey-Stephenson, A. Z., Crosby, A. E., Jack, S. P., Haileyesus, T., & Kresnow-Sedacca, M. (2017). Suicide trends among and within urbanization levels by sex, race/ethnicity, age group, and mechanism of death—United States, 2001–2015. *MMWR Surveillance Summary, 66*(SS-18), 1–16.

Jadva, V., Guasp, A., Bradlow, J. H., Bower-Brown, S., & Foley, S. (2021). Predictors of self-harm and suicide in LGBT youth: The role of gender, socioeconomic status, bullying and school experience, *Journal of Public Health,* 2021, 383. https://doi.org/10.1093/pubmed/fdab383

Janakiraman, R., Stanley, I. H., Duffy, M. E., Gai, A. R., Hanson, J. E., Gutierrez, P. M., & Joiner, T. E. (2020). Suicidal ideation severity in transgender and cisgender elevated-risk military service members at baseline and three-month follow-up. *Military Behavioral Health,* 1–9. DOI: 10.1080/21635781.2020.1742821

Jobes, D. A. (2015, September). Clinical suicidology: Innovations in assessment treatment of suicidal risk. Presentation at Psychiatric Grand Rounds, Summa Health Systems, Akron, OH.

Jobes, D. A. (2012). The collaborative assessment and management of suicidality (CAMS): An evolving evidence-based clinical approach to suicide risk. *Suicide and Life Threatening Behavior, 42*(6), 640–653. doi:10.1111/j.1943-278X.2012.00119.x

John, A., Glendenning, A. C., Marchant, A., Montgomery, P., Stewart, A., Wood, S., Lloyd, K., & Hawton, K. (2018). Self-harm, suicidal behaviours, and cyberbullying in children and young people: Systematic review. *Journal of Medical Internet Research, 20*(4), e129. https://doi.org/10.2196/jmir.9044

Joiner, T. E. (2005). *Why people die by suicide.* Harvard University Press.

Juhnke, G. A., Granello, P. F., & Lebrón-Striker, M. (2007). IS PATH WARM? A suicide assessment mnemonic for counselors. *ACA Professional Counseling Digest.* www.counseling.org/resources/library/ACA%20Digests/ACAPCD-03.pdf

Kim, J. L., Kim, J. M., Choi, Y., Lee, T., & Park, E. (2016). Effect of socioeconomic status on the linkage between suicidal ideation and suicide attempts. *Suicide and Life-Threatening Behavior, 46*(5), 588–597. doi:10.1111/sltb.12242

Klonsky, D. E., & May, A. M. (2015a). Impulsivity and suicide risk: Review and clinical implications. *Psychiatric Times, 32*(8).

http://www.psychiatrictimes.com/special-reports/impulsivity-and-suicide-risk-review-and-clinical-implications/page/0/2

Klonsky, D. E., & May, A. M. (2015b). The three-step theory (3ST): A new theory of suicide rooted in the "ideation-to-action" framework. *International Journal of Cognitive Therapy, 8*(2), 114–129. doi:10.1521/ijct.2015.8.2.114

Kposowa, A. (2000). Marital status and suicide in the National Longitudinal Mortality Study. *Journal of Epidemiology and Community Health, 54*(4), 254–261. doi:http://dx.doi.org/10.1136/jech.54.4.254

Large, M., Kaneson, M., Myles, N., Myles, H., Gunaratne, P., & Ryan, C. (2016). Meta-analysis of longitudinal cohort studies of suicide risk assessment among psychiatric patients: Heterogeneity in results and lack of improvement over time. *PLoS ONE, 11*(6), e0156322. https://doi.org/10.1371/journal.pone.0156322

Lawrence, R. E., Oquendo, M. A., & Stanley, B. (2016). Religion and suicide risk: A systematic review. *Archives of Suicide Research, 20*(1), 1–21. doi:10.1080/13811118.2015.1004494

Listabarth, S., Vyssoki, B., Glahn, A., Gmeiner, A., Pruckner, N., Vyssoki, S., Wippel, A., Waldhoer, T., & König, D. (2020). The effect of sex on suicide risk during and after psychiatric inpatient care in 12 countries—An ecological study. *European Psychiatry, 63*(1), E85. doi:10.1192/j.eurpsy.2020.83

Mercado, M. C., Holland, K., Leemis, R. W., Stone, D.M., & Wang, J. (2017). Trends in emergency department visits for nonfatal self-inflicted injuries among youth aged 10 to 24 years in the United States, 2001–2015. *Journal of the American Medical Association, 318*(19), 1931–1933. doi:10.1001/jama.2017.13317

Milton, A. C., Davenport T. A., Iorfino, F., Flego, A., Burns, J. M., & Hickie, I. B. (2020). Suicidal thoughts and behaviors and their associations with transitional life events in men and women: Findings from an international web-based sample. *JMIR Mental Health, 7*(9), e18383. doi: 10.2196/18383

Mullins, N., Kang, J. E., Camposo, A. I., Coleman, J. R. I., Edwards, A. C., Galfalvy, H., Levey, D. F., Lori, A., Shabalin, A., Starnawska, A., Su, M. H., Watson, H. J., Adams, M., Swapnil, A., Gandal, M., Hafferty, J. D., Hishimoto, A., Kim, M...Ruderferl, D. M. (2022). Dissecting the shared genetic architecture of suicide attempt, psychiatric disorders, and known risk factors. *Biological Psychiatry, 91*(3), 321–337. https://doi.org/10.1016/j.biopsych.2021.05.029

Myers, M. (2021). *Military suicides up 16 percent in 2020, but officials don't blame pandemic.* https://www.militarytimes.com/news/pentagon-congress/2021/09/30/military-suicides-up-15-percent-in-2020-but-officials-dont-blame-pandemic/

Naess, E. O., Mehlum, L., & Qin, P. (2021). Marital status and suicide risk: Temporal effect of marital breakdown and contextual difference by socioeconomic status. *SSM-Population Heath, 21.* https://doi.org/10.1016/j.ssmph.2021.100853

National Alliance on Mental Illness. (2022). *Risk of suicide.* www.nami.org/Learn-More/Mental-Health-Conditions/Related-Conditions/Risk-of-Suicide

National Indian Council on Aging. (2019). *American Indian suicide rate increases.* https://www.nicoa.org/national-american-indian-and-alaska-native-hope-for-life-day/

Nock, M. K., Deming, C. A., Fullerton, C. S., Gilman, S. E., Goldenberg, M., Kessler, R. C., McCarroll, J. E., & Ursan, R. J. (2013). Suicide among soldiers: A review of psychosocial risk and protective factors. *Psychiatry, 76*(2), 97–125. doi:10.1521/psyc.2013.76.2.97

Offord, C. (2020). What neurobiology can tell us about suicide. *The Scientist.* https://www.the-scientist.com/features/what-neurobiology-can-tell-us-about-suicide-66922

Olfson, M., Wall, M., Wang, S., Crystal, S., Liu, S.-M., Gerhard, T., & Blanco, C. (2016). Short-term suicide risk after psychiatric hospital discharge. *JAMA Psychiatry, 73*(11), 1119–1126. doi:10.1001/jamapsychiatry.2016.2035

Pacer's National Bullying Prevention Center. (2022). *Bullying statistics: By the numbers.* https://www.pacer.org/bullying/info/stats.asp

Perlman, C. M., Neufeld, E., Martin, L., Goy, M., & Hirdes, J. P. (2011). *Risk assessment inventory: A resource guide for Canadian healthcare organizations.* Hospital Association and Canadian Patient Safety Institute.

Peterson, C., Sussell, A., Li, J., Schumacher, P. K., Yeoman, K., & Stone, D. M. (2020). Suicide rates by industry and occupation—national violent death reporting system, 32 states, 2016. *MMWR Morbidity & Mortality Weekly Report, 69*, 57–62. https://doi.org/10.15585/mmwr.mm6903a1externalicon

Posner, K., Brown, G. K., Stanley, B., Brent, D. A., Yershova, K. V., Oquendo, M. A., Currier, G. W., Melvin, G. A., Greenhill, L., Shen, S., & Mann, J. J. (2011). The Columbia–Suicide Severity Rating Scale: Initial validity and internal consistency findings from three multisite studies with adolescents and adults. *American Journal of Psychiatry, 168*(12), 1266–1277. doi:10.1176/appi.ajp.2011.10111704

Puntil, C., York, J., Limandri, B., Greene, P., Arauz, E., & Hobbs, D. (2013). Competency-based training for PMH nurse generalists: Inpatient intervention and prevention of suicide. *Journal of the American Psychiatric Nurses Association, 19*(4), 205–210. doi:10.1177/1078390313496275

Rasic, D. T., Belik, S. L., Elias, B., Katz, L. Y., Enns, M., & Sareen, J. (2009). Spirituality, religion, and suicidal behavior in a nationally representative sample. *Journal of Affective Disorders, 114*(1), 32–40. doi:10.1016/j.jad.2008.08.007

Reed, K. P., Nugent, W., & Cooper, R. L. (2015). Testing a path model of relationships between gender, age, and bullying victimization and violent behavior, substance abuse, depression, suicidal ideation, and suicide attempts in adolescents. *Children and Youth Services Review, 55*, 128–137. https://doi.org/10.1016/j.childyouth.2015.05.016

Reyes, M. S., Cayubit, F. O., Angala, M. H., Bries, S. C., Capalungan, J. T., & McCutcheon, L. E. (2015). Exploring the link between adolescent anger expression and tendencies for suicide: A brief report. *North American Journal of Psychology, 17*(1), 113–118.

Roberts, C. (2020). *No-suicide contracts: Can they work?* https://www.mdedge.com/psychiatry/article/226013/depression/no-suicide-contracts-can-they-work?sso = true

Rogers, M. L., & Joiner, T. E. (2017). Suicide-specific rumination relates to lifetime suicide attempts above and beyond a variety of other suicide risk factors. *Journal of Psychiatric Research, 98.* doi:10.1016/j.jpsychires.2017.12.017

Roškar, S., Podlesek, A., Kuzmanić , M., Demšar, L.O., Zaletel, M., & Marušič , A. (2011). Suicide risk and its relationship to change in marital status. *Crisis, 32*(1), 24–30. doi:10.1027/0227-5910/a000054

Rudd, D. M., Mandrusiak, M., & Joiner, T. E. (2006). The case against no-suicide contract: The commitment to treatment statement as a practice alternative. *Journal of Clinical Psychology, 62*(2), 243–251. doi:10.1002/jclp.20227

Shea, S. C. (2009). Suicide assessment: Part 1: Uncovering suicidal intent: A sophisticated art. Part 2: Uncovering suicidal intent using the chronological assessment of suicide events. *Psychiatric Times, 26*(12), 1–26. www.psychiatrictimes.com/display/article/10168/1491291

Sheftall, A. H., Vakil, F., Armstrong, S. E., Rausch, J. R., Feng, X., Kerns, K. A., Brent, D. A., & Bridge, J. A. (2021a). Clinical risk factors, emotional reactivity/regulation and suicidal ideation in elementary school-aged children. *Journal of Psychiatric Research, 138*, 360–365. https://doi.org/10.1016/j.jpsychires.2021.04.021

Sheftall, A. H., Vakil, F., Ruch, D. A., Boyd, R. C., Lindsey, M. A., & Bridge, J. A. (2021b). Black youth suicide: Investigation of current trends and precipitating circumstances. *Journal of the American Academy of Child and Adolescent Psychiatry, 61*(5), 662–675. doi:https://doi.org/10.1016/j.jaac.2021.08.021

Stanley, B., & Brown, G. K. (2008). *The safety plan treatment manual to reduce suicide risk: Veteran version.* U.S. Department of Veterans Affairs.

Stanley, B., Brown, G. K., Brenner, L. A., Galfalvy, H. C., Currier, G. W., Knox, K. L., Chaudhury S. R., Bush A. L., & Green, K. L. (2018). Follow-up vs usual care of suicidal patients treated in the emergency department. *JAMA Psychiatry, 75*(9), 894–900. doi:10.1001/jamapsychiatry.2018.1776

Strawbridge, R., Ward, J., Ferguson, A, Graham, N., Shaw, R. J., Cullen, B., Pearsall, R., Lyall, R. M., Johnston, K. J. A., Niedzwiedz, C. L., Pell, J. P., Mackay, D., Martin, J. L., Lyall, D. M., Bailey, M. E. S., & Smith, D. J. (2019). Identification of novel genome-wide associations for suicidality in UK Biobank, genetic correlation with psychiatric disorders and polygenic association with completed suicide. *eBiomedicine, 41*, 517–525. doi:https://doi.org/10.1016/j.ebiom.2019.02.005

Stroumsa, D. (2014). The state of transgender health care: Policy, law, and medical frameworks. *American Journal of Public Health, 104*(3), 31–37. doi:10.2105/AJPH.2013.301789

Sudak, H. S. (2017). Suicide treatment. In Sadock, B. J., Sadock, V. A., & Ruiz, P. (Eds.), *Comprehensive textbook of psychiatry* (pp. 2618–2622). Wolters Kluwer.

Suicide Prevention Resource Center. (2020). *Promote social connectedness and support.* https://www.sprc.org/comprehensive-approach/social-connectedness

Swogger, M. T., Van Orden, K. A., & Conner, K. R. (2014). The relationship of outwardly directed aggression to suicidal ideation and suicide attempts across two high-risk samples. *Psychology of Violence, 4*(2), 184–195. https://doi.org/10.1037/a0033212

Taylor, T. F. (2015). The influence of shame on posttrauma disorders: Have we failed to see the obvious? *European Journal of Psychotraumatology, 6.* doi:10.3402/ejpt.v6.28847

Terrell, K. R., Zeglin, R. T., Palmer, R. E., Niemela, D. R. M., & Quinn, N. (2021). The tsunamic model of LGBTQ + deaths of despair: A systemic review to identify risk factors for deaths of despair among LGBTQ + people. *Journal of Homosexuality.* https://doi.org/10.1080/00918369.2021.1935620

The Joint Commission. (2016). *Sentinel Event Alert 56: Detecting and treating suicide ideation in all settings.* https://www.jointcommission.org/sea_issue_56

The Samaritans. (2022). *Myths about suicide.* http://samaritansnyc.org/myths-about-suicide

U.S. Department of Health and Human Services, substance Abuse and Mental Health Services Administration. (n.d.). *SAFE-T pocket card: Suicide assessment five-step evaluation and triage for clinicians.* https://store.samhsa.gov/product/SAFE-T-Pocket-Card-Suicide-Assessment-Five-Step-Evaluation-and-Triage-for-Clinicians/sma09-4432

Whalen, D., Dixon-Gordon, K., Belden, A., Barch, D., & Luby, J. (2015). Correlates and consequences of suicidal cognitions and behaviors in children ages 3 to 7 years. *Journal of the American Academy of Child & Adolescent Psychiatry, 54*(11), 926–937. doi:10.1016/j.jaac.2015.08.009

Wiklander, M., Samuelsson, M., Jokinen, J., Nilsonne, A., Wilczek, A., Rylander, G., & Åsberg, M. (2012). Shame-proneness in attempted suicide patients. *BMC Psychiatry, 12.* doi:10.1186/1471-244X-12-50

Williams, A. J., Arcelus, J., Townsend, E., & Michail, M. (2019). Examining risk factors for self-harm and suicide in LGBTQ + young people: A systematic review protocol. *BMJ Open, 9*(11), e031541. https://doi.org/10.1136/bmjopen-2019-031541

Yamauchi, T., Fujita, T., Tachimori, H., Takeshima, T., Inagaki, M., & Sudo, A. (2013). Age-adjusted relative suicide risk by marital and employment status over the past 25 years in Japan. *Journal of Public Health, 35*(1), 49–56. doi:10.1093/pubmed/fds054

Yıldız, E. (2018). Suicide in sexual minority populations: A systematic review of evidence-based studies, *Archives of Psychiatric Nursing, 32*(4), 650–659.

Zhang, Y., Zhang, C., Yuan, G., Yao, J., Cheng, Z., Liu, C., Liu, Q., Wan, G., Shi, G., Cheng, Y., Ling, Y., & Li, K. (2010). Effect of tryptophan hydroxylase-2 rs7305115 SNP on suicide attempts risk in major depression. *Behavioral and Brain Functions, 6*(49). https://doi.org/10.1186/1744-9081-6-49

Classical References

Durkheim, E. (1951). *Suicide: A study of sociology.* Free Press.

Freud, S. (1957). *Mourning and melancholia, Vol. 14* (standard ed.). Hogarth Press. (Original work published 1917.)

MacDonald, M., & Murphy, T. R. (1991). *Sleepless souls: Suicide in early modern England.* Oxford University Press.

Macnab, F. (1993). *Brief psychotherapy: An integrative approach in clinical practice.* Wiley.

Minois, G. (2001). *History of suicide: Voluntary death in Western culture.* Johns Hopkins University Press.

U.S. Public Health Service (USPHS). (1999). *The Surgeon General's call to action to prevent suicide.* USPHS.

Behavior Therapy 17

CORE CONCEPTS

Evidence-Based Practice:
  Behavior therapy

KEY TERMS

aversive stimulus

classical conditioning

conditioned response

conditioned stimulus

contingency contracting

covert sensitization

discriminative stimuli

extinction

flooding

modeling

negative reinforcement

operant conditioning

overt sensitization

positive reinforcement

Premack principle

reciprocal inhibition

shaping

stimulus generalization

systematic desensitization

time-out

token economy

unconditioned response

unconditioned stimulus

OBJECTIVES
After reading this chapter, the student will be able to:

1. Discuss the principles of classical and operant conditioning as foundations for behavior therapy.
2. Identify various techniques used in the modification of client behavior.

3. Implement the principles of behavior therapy using the steps of the nursing process.

A behavior is considered maladaptive when it is age-inappropriate, interferes with adaptive functioning, or is identified as culturally inappropriate. In the behavioral approach to therapy, behavior and personality develop through learning processes or, more precisely, through the interaction of the environment with an individual's genes. The basic assumption of this approach is that problematic behaviors occur when there has been inadequate learning and can therefore be corrected through the provision of appropriate learning experiences. The principles of behavior therapy as we know it today are based on the early studies of **classical conditioning** by Pavlov (1927) and **operant conditioning** by Skinner (1938). Although in this text the concepts are presented separately for reasons of clarification, behavioral change procedures are often combined with cognitive procedures (*cognitive behavior therapy*) and with issues related to emotional regulation (*dialectical behavior therapy*). Concepts of cognitive behavior therapy are presented in Chapter 18, "Cognitive Behavior Therapy."

Classical Conditioning

Classical conditioning is a process of learning introduced by the Russian physiologist Ivan Pavlov. In his experiments with dogs, during which he hoped to learn more about the digestive process, he inadvertently discovered that organisms can learn to respond in specific ways if they are conditioned to do so. Pavlov found that, as expected, the dogs salivated when they began to eat the food offered to them, a reflexive response that Pavlov called an **unconditioned response.** However, he also noticed that with time, the dogs began to salivate when the food came into their range of view, before it was even presented to them for consumption. Pavlov, concluding that this response was not reflexive but had been learned, called it a **conditioned response.** He carried the experiments even further by introducing an unrelated stimulus, one that had had no previous connection to the animal's food. He simultaneously presented the food with the sound of a bell. The animal responded with the expected reflexive salivation to the food. After several trials with the combined stimuli (food and bell), Pavlov found that the reflexive salivation occurred when the dog was presented with the sound of the bell in the absence of food.

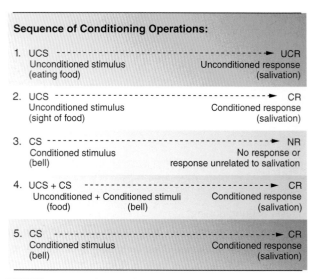

FIGURE 17–1 Pavlov's model of classic conditioning.

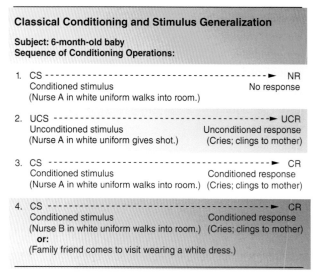

FIGURE 17–2 Example: Classical conditioning and stimulus generalization.

CORE CONCEPTS

Stimulus
A stimulus is an environmental event that interacts with and influences an individual's behavior.

Pavlov's discovery was important in terms of how learning can occur. Pavlov found that unconditioned responses (salivation) occur in response to unconditioned stimuli (eating food). He also found that, over time, an unrelated stimulus (sound of the bell) introduced with the **unconditioned stimulus** can elicit the same response alone, that is, the conditioned response. The unrelated stimulus is called the **conditioned stimulus.** The process by which the fear response is elicited from similar stimuli (all individuals in white uniforms) is called **stimulus generalization.** A graphic of Pavlov's classical conditioning model is presented in Figure 17–1. An example of the application of Pavlov's classical conditioning model to humans is shown in Figure 17–2.

Operant Conditioning

The focus of operant conditioning differs from that of classical conditioning. With classical conditioning, the focus is on behavioral responses elicited by specific objects or events. With operant conditioning, additional attention is given to the consequences of the behavioral response.

Operant conditioning was introduced by B. F. Skinner (1953), an American psychologist whose work was largely influenced by Edward Thorndike's (1911) law of effect; that is, that the connection between a stimulus and a response is strengthened or weakened by the consequences of the response. Several terms must be defined in order to understand the concept of operant conditioning.

As defined previously, stimuli are environmental events that interact with and influence an individual's behavior. Stimuli may precede or follow a behavior. A stimulus that follows a behavior (or response) is called a reinforcing stimulus, or *reinforcer.* The function is called *reinforcement.* When the reinforcing stimulus increases the probability that the behavior will recur, it is called a *positive reinforcer,* and the function is called **positive reinforcement. Negative reinforcement** increases the probability that a behavior will recur by removal of an undesirable reinforcing stimulus. A stimulus that follows a behavioral response and decreases the probability that the behavior will recur is called an **aversive stimulus,** or *punisher.* Examples of these reinforcing stimuli are presented in Table 17–1.

Stimuli that precede a behavioral response and predict that a particular reinforcement will occur are called **discriminative stimuli.** Discriminative stimuli are under an individual's control. The individual is able to *discriminate* between stimuli and *choose* according to the type of reinforcement they have come to associate with a specific stimulus. The following is an example of the concept of discrimination:

Example

Mrs. M. was admitted to the hospital from a nursing home 2 weeks ago. She has no family, and no one visits her. She is very lonely. Nurse A and Nurse B have taken care of Mrs. M. on a regular basis during her hospital stay. When she is feeling particularly lonely, Mrs. M. calls Nurse A to her room, for she has learned that Nurse A will stay and talk to her for a while, but Nurse B only takes care of her physical needs and leaves. She no longer seeks out Nurse B for emotional support and comfort. After several attempts, Mrs. M. is able to discriminate between stimuli. She can predict with assurance that calling Nurse A (and not Nurse B) will result in the reinforcement she desires.

CORE CONCEPTS

Behavior Therapy
A form of psychotherapy that aims to modify maladaptive behavior patterns by reinforcing more adaptive behaviors.

Techniques for Modifying Client Behavior

Shaping

In **shaping** the behavior of another, reinforcements are given for increasingly closer approximations to the desired response. For example, in eliciting speech from an autistic child, the teacher may first reward the child for (1) watching the teacher's lips, then (2) making any sound in imitation of the teacher, then (3) forming sounds similar to the word uttered by the teacher. Shaping has been shown to be an effective way of modifying behavior for tasks that a child has not mastered on command or are not in the child's repertoire. In a recent study (Martone et al., 2019), shaping was used effectively to increase food intake and acceptance of new foods in autistic children.

Modeling

Modeling refers to the learning of new behaviors by imitating the behavior in others. Role models are individuals who have qualities or skills that a person admires and wishes to imitate. Modeling occurs in various ways. Children imitate the behavior patterns of their parents, teachers, friends, and others. Adults and children alike model many of their behaviors after individuals observed on television and in movies. Unfortunately, modeling can result in maladaptive behaviors as well as adaptive ones.

In the practice setting, clients may imitate the behaviors of their care providers. This modeling can occur naturally in the therapeutic community environment. It can also occur in a therapy session in which the client watches a model demonstrate appropriate behaviors in a role-play of the client's problem. The client is then instructed to imitate the model's behaviors in a similar role-play and is positively reinforced for appropriate imitation.

Premack Principle

This technique, named for its originator, states that a frequently occurring response (R1) can serve as a positive reinforcement for a response (R2) that occurs less frequently (Premack, 1959). The **Premack principle** is applied by allowing R1 to occur only after R2 has been performed. That is, to encourage more of a particular behavior that an individual is not doing very often, a situation is created in which the person must perform that behavior *before* being permitted to do the "fun stuff" that they prefer to do. The person's preferred behavior becomes a reinforcement for accomplishing the desired behavior change. For

TABLE 17–1	**Examples of Reinforcing Stimuli**		
TYPES	**STIMULUS**	**BEHAVIORAL RESPONSE**	**REINFORCING STIMULUS**
Positive	Messy room	Child cleans their messy room.	Child gets allowance for cleaning room.
Negative	Messy room	Child cleans their messy room.	Child does not receive scolding from the mother.
Aversive	Messy room	Child does not clean their messy room.	Child receives scolding from the mother.

example, 13-year-old Jennie has been neglecting her homework for the past few weeks. She spends a lot of time on her cell phone talking to her friends. Applying the Premack principle, being allowed to talk on the cell phone to her friends could serve as a positive reinforcement for completing her homework.

In a recent review of the literature (Herrod et al., 2022), researchers affirmed the utility of incorporating the Premack principle in a variety of diverse situations and concluded that if implemented as first described, it should result in behavior change. They caution, though, that more rigorous research, particularly studies that establish the probability of responding as a prerequisite criterion, is needed. A schematic of the Premack principle for this situation is presented in Figure 17–3.

Extinction

Extinction is the gradual decrease in frequency or disappearance of a response when the positive reinforcement is withheld. A classic example of this technique is its use with children who have temper tantrums. The tantrum behaviors continue as long as the parent gives attention to them but decrease and often disappear when the parent simply walks away from the child and ignores the behavior.

Contingency Contracting

In **contingency contracting,** a contract is drawn up among all parties involved. The desired behavior change and specified reinforcers for performing this behavior are stated explicitly in writing. The negative consequences, or punishers, that will be rendered for not fulfilling the terms of the contract are also delineated. The contract is specific about how reinforcers and punishment will be presented; however, flexibility is important so that renegotiations can occur if necessary.

Token Economy

Token economy is a type of contingency contracting in which the reinforcers for desired behaviors are presented in the form of *tokens*. Essential to this technique is the prior determination of items and situations of significance to the client that can be employed as reinforcements. With this therapy, tokens are awarded when desired behaviors are performed and may be exchanged for designated privileges. For example, a client may be able to "buy" a snack for two tokens, a trip to the coffee shop or library for five tokens, or even a trip outside the hospital (if that is a realistic possibility) for another

designated number of tokens. The use of token economies was developed in the 1950s as a strategy for reinforcing desirable behaviors in long-term hospitalized patients with schizophrenia and, despite studies demonstrating their effectiveness in reinforcing adaptive behaviors, they have fallen out of favor over time (Dickerson et al., 2005). A more recent review of token economy (Doll et al., 2013) as a behavior modification strategy points out that most of the research predates the 1990s and that with more research on its use in contemporary settings and therapies, its current application may gain more favor with therapists. One study (Gholipour et al., 2012) found that token economies demonstrated some effectiveness in treating negative symptoms of schizophrenia. Currently, token economies are more often used to promote behavior change in children. A study of primary school students (Shakespeare et al., 2018) found that token economies were an effective tool in reducing disruptive behavior in classrooms, including violent behavior. A recent systematic review (Kim et al., 2021) concluded that token economies yielded large effect sizes as a tool in both general and special education classrooms. They have also been identified as an effective behavior modification strategy for children on the autism spectrum (Cihon et al., 2018).

Time-Out

Time-out is an aversive stimulus or punishment during which the client is removed from the environment where the unacceptable behavior is being exhibited. The client is usually isolated so that reinforcement from the attention of others is absent.

Reciprocal Inhibition

Also called *counterconditioning*, **reciprocal inhibition** decreases or eliminates a behavior by introducing a more adaptive behavior, but one that is incompatible with the unacceptable behavior (Wolpe, 1958). An example is the introduction of relaxation exercises to a phobic individual. Relaxation is practiced in the presence of anxiety so that in time, the individual is able to manage the anxiety in the presence of the phobic stimulus by engaging in relaxation exercises. Relaxation and anxiety are incompatible behaviors.

Overt Sensitization

Overt sensitization is a type of aversion therapy that produces unpleasant consequences for undesirable behavior. For example, disulfiram (Antabuse) is a

Discriminative stimulus - - - - - - - - - - -► R_2 - - - - - - - - - - - - - - -► R_1
(Homework assignment: (Completion of home-   (Talk to friends   **FIGURE 17–3** Example: Premack
To do or not to do)   work assignment)   on telephone)   principle.

drug given to individuals who wish to stop drinking alcohol. If an individual consumes alcohol while on Antabuse therapy, symptoms of severe nausea and vomiting, dyspnea, palpitations, and headache will occur. Instead of the euphoric feeling normally experienced from the alcohol (the positive reinforcement for drinking), the individual receives a severe punishment that is intended to extinguish the unacceptable behavior (drinking alcohol).

Covert Sensitization

Covert sensitization is a type of aversion therapy that relies on the individual's imagined unpleasant symptoms or negative consequences. The technique is under the client's control and can be used whenever and wherever it is required. The individual learns to visualize nauseating scenes and even to induce a mild feeling of nausea through mental imagery. This mental image is visualized when the individual is about to succumb to an attractive but undesirable behavior. It is most effective when paired with relaxation exercises that are performed instead of the undesirable behavior. The primary advantage of covert sensitization is that the individual does not actually perform the undesired behaviors but simply imagines them.

Systematic Desensitization

Systematic desensitization is a technique for assisting individuals to overcome their fear of a phobic stimulus. It was developed by Wolpe in the 1950s who later (1964) reported successfully treating a young male with a severe hand washing compulsion. McLeod (2021) described it as a process of counterconditioning. It is "systematic" in that there is a hierarchy of anxiety-producing events through which the individual progresses during therapy. An example of a hierarchy of events associated with a specific phobia of elevators may be as follows:

1. Discuss riding an elevator with the therapist.
2. Look at a picture of an elevator.
3. Walk into the lobby of a building and see the elevators.
4. Push the button for the elevator.
5. Walk into an elevator with a trusted person; disembark before the doors close.
6. Walk into an elevator with a trusted person. Allow doors to close, then open the doors and walk out.
7. Ride one floor with a trusted person, then walk back down the stairs.
8. Ride one floor with a trusted person and ride the elevator back down.
9. Ride the elevator alone.

As each of these steps is attempted, it is paired with relaxation exercises as an antagonistic behavior to anxiety. Generally, the desensitization procedures occur in the therapy setting, where the client is instructed to engage in relaxation exercises. When relaxation has been achieved, the client uses mental imagery to visualize the hierarchical step described by the therapist. If the client becomes anxious, the therapist again suggests relaxation exercises and presents a scene that is lower in the hierarchy. Therapy continues until the individual is able to progress through the entire hierarchy with manageable anxiety. The effects of relaxation in the presence of imagined anxiety-producing stimuli transfer to the real situation once the client has achieved relaxation capable of suppressing or inhibiting anxiety responses. A recent study demonstrated the effectiveness of future positive mental imagery as effective in reducing anticipatory anxiety associated with public speaking (Landkroon et al., 2022). However, some clients are not successful in extinguishing phobic reactions through imagery. For these clients, *real-life desensitization* may be required. In these instances, the therapist may arrange for the client to be exposed to the hierarchy of steps in the desensitization process, but in real-life situations. Relaxation exercises may or may not be a part of real-life desensitization.

Flooding

Flooding, sometimes called *implosive therapy,* is also used to desensitize individuals to phobic stimuli. It differs from systematic desensitization in that instead of working up a hierarchy of anxiety-producing stimuli, the individual is "flooded" with a continuous presentation (through mental imagery) of the phobic stimulus until it no longer elicits anxiety. Flooding is believed to produce faster results than systematic desensitization; however, some therapists report more lasting behavioral changes with systematic desensitization. Some questions have also been raised about the ethics of encouraging a patient to endure prolonged fear and psychological discomfort, and clients may avoid this type of therapy for that reason. Flooding is considered most effective in treating specific phobias; however, it is contraindicated with clients for whom intense anxiety would be hazardous, such as individuals with heart disease or fragile psychological adaptation (Boland & Verduin, 2022).

Role of the Nurse in Behavior Therapy

The nursing process is the vehicle for delivery of nursing care with the patient requiring assistance with behavior modification. The steps of the nursing process are illustrated in the following case study.

CASE STUDY

This example focuses on inpatient care, but these interventions can be modified and are applicable to various health-care settings, including partial hospitalization, community outpatient clinic, home health, and private practice.

ASSESSMENT

Zach, age 8, has been admitted to the child psychiatric unit of a university medical center after evaluation by a child psychiatrist. His parents, Tom and Deborah, are at an impasse, and their marriage is suffering because of constant conflict over their son's behavior at home and at school. Tom complains bitterly that Deborah is overly permissive with their son. Tom reports that Zach argues and has temper tantrums and insists on continuing games, books, and TV whenever Deborah puts him to bed so that an 8:30 p.m. bedtime regularly is delayed until 10:30 or later every night. Also, Deborah often cooks four or five different meals for her son's dinner if Zach stubbornly insists that he will not eat what has been prepared. At school, several teachers have complained that the child is stubborn and argumentative, is often disruptive in the classroom, and refuses to follow established rules.

When asked by the psychiatric nurse about other maladaptive behaviors, such as destruction of property, stealing, lying, or setting fires, the parents deny that these had been a problem. During the interview, Zach sits quietly without interrupting. He answers questions that are directed to him with brief responses and makes light of the problems described by his parents and reported by his teachers. The nurse conducts an assessment to rule out a history of trauma as an alternate explanation for his behavior and finds no evidence of trauma in Zach's history.

During his first 3 days on the unit, the following assessments are made:

1. Zach loses his temper when he cannot have his way. He screams, stomps his feet, and sometimes kicks the furniture.
2. Zach refuses to follow directions given by staff. He merely responds, "No, I won't."
3. Zach likes to engage in behaviors that annoy the staff and other children: belching loudly, scraping his fingernails across the blackboard, making loud noises when the other children are trying to watch television, opening his mouth when it is full of food.
4. Zach blames others when he makes a mistake. He spilled his milk at lunchtime while racing to get to a specific seat he knew Tony wanted. He blamed the accident on Tony, saying, "He made me do it! He tripped me!"

Upon completion of the initial assessments, the psychiatrist diagnoses Zach with oppositional defiant disorder.

DIAGNOSIS/OUTCOME IDENTIFICATION

Nursing diagnoses and outcome criteria for Zach include the following:

NURSING DIAGNOSES	OUTCOME CRITERIA
Noncompliance with therapy	Zach participates in and cooperates during therapeutic activities.
Defensive coping	Zach accepts responsibility for own behaviors and interacts with others without becoming defensive.
Impaired social interaction	Zach interacts with staff and peers using age-appropriate, acceptable behaviors.

PLANNING/IMPLEMENTATION

A contract for Zach's care is drawn up by the admitting nurse and others on the treatment team. Zach's contract is based on a system of token economies. He discusses with the nurse the kinds of privileges he would like to earn:

■ Having a can of pop for a snack (2 tokens)
■ Getting to watch 30 minutes of TV (5 tokens)
■ Getting to stay up later on Friday nights with the other clients (7 tokens)
■ Getting to play the video games (3 tokens)
■ Getting to walk with the nurse to the gift shop to spend some of his money (8 tokens)
■ Getting to go on the outside therapeutic recreation activities such as movies, the zoo, and picnics (10 tokens)

Tokens are awarded for appropriate behaviors:

■ Gets out of bed when the nurse calls him (1 token)
■ Gets dressed for breakfast (1 token)
■ Presents himself for *all* meals in an appropriate manner: no screaming, no belching, no opening his mouth when it is full of food, no throwing of food, staying in his chair during the meal, putting his tray away in the appropriate place when he is finished (2 tokens × 3 meals = 6 tokens)
■ Completes hygiene activities (1 token)
■ Accepts blame for own mistakes (1 token)
■ Does not fight; uses no obscene language; does not "sass" staff (1 token)
■ Remains quiet while others are watching TV (1 token)
■ Participates and is not disruptive in unit meetings and group therapy sessions (2 tokens)
■ Displays no temper tantrums (1 token)
■ Follows unit rules (1 token)
■ Goes to bed at designated hour without opposition (1 token)

Tokens are awarded at bedtime for absence of inappropriate behaviors during the day. For example, if Zach

CASE STUDY—cont'd

has no temper tantrums during the day, he is awarded 1 token. Likewise, if Zach has a temper tantrum (or exhibits other inappropriate behavior), he must pay back the token amount designated for that behavior. No other attention is given to inappropriate behaviors other than withholding and payback of tokens.

EXCEPTION: If Zach is receiving reinforcement from peers for inappropriate behaviors, staff has the option of imposing time-out or isolation until the behavior is extinguished.

The contract may be renegotiated at any time between Zach and staff. Additional privileges or responsibilities may be added as they develop and are deemed appropriate.

All staff members are consistent with the terms of the contract and do not allow Zach to manipulate. There are no exceptions without renegotiation of the contract.

NOTE: Parents meet regularly with the case manager from the treatment team. Effective parenting techniques are discussed, as are other problems identified within the marriage relationship. Parenting instruction coordinates with the pattern of behavior modification Zach is receiving on the psychiatric unit. The importance of follow-through is emphasized, along with strong encouragement that the parents maintain a united front in

disciplining Zach. Oppositional behaviors are nurtured by divided management.

EVALUATION

Reassessment is conducted to determine whether the nursing actions have been successful in achieving the objectives of Zach's care. Evaluation can be facilitated by gathering information using the following questions:

■ Does Zach participate in and cooperate during therapeutic activities?
■ Does he follow the rules of the unit (including mealtimes, hygiene, and bedtime) without opposition?
■ Does Zach accept responsibility for his own mistakes?
■ Is he able to complete a task without becoming defensive?
■ Does he refrain from interrupting when others are talking and from making noise in situations where quiet is in order?
■ Does he refrain from attempts to manipulate the staff?
■ Is he able to express anger appropriately without tantrum behaviors?
■ Does he demonstrate acceptable behavior in interactions with peers?

Summary and Key Points

- The basic assumption of behavior therapy is that problematic behaviors occur when there has been inadequate learning and can therefore be corrected through the provision of appropriate learning experiences.
- Today's principles of behavior therapy are based on research conducted by Pavlov and Skinner.
- Pavlov introduced a process that came to be known as *classical conditioning.*
- Pavlov demonstrated in his trials with laboratory animals that a neutral stimulus could acquire the ability to elicit a conditioned response through pairing with an unconditioned stimulus. He considered the conditioned response to be a new, learned response.
- Skinner, in his model of operant conditioning, gave additional attention to the consequences of the response as an approach to learning new behaviors.
- Skinner believed that the connection between a stimulus and a response is strengthened or weakened by the consequences of the response.
- Various techniques for modifying client behavior include the following:
  - Shaping: A technique in which reinforcements are given for increasingly closer approximations to the desired response

  - Modeling: The learning of new behaviors by imitating the behavior of others
  - Premack principle: The concept that a frequently occurring response can serve as a positive reinforcement for a response that occurs less frequently
  - Extinction: The gradual decrease in frequency or disappearance of a response when the positive reinforcement is withheld
  - Contingency contracting: A contract specifying a specific behavior change and the reinforcers to be given for performing the desired behaviors
  - Token economy: A type of contingency contracting in which the reinforcers for desired behaviors are presented in the form of tokens
  - Time-out: An aversive stimulus or punishment during which the client is removed from the environment where the unacceptable behavior is being exhibited
  - Reciprocal inhibition: A technique that decreases or eliminates a behavior by introducing a more adaptive behavior that is incompatible with the unacceptable behavior
  - Overt sensitization: A type of aversion therapy that produces unpleasant consequences for undesirable behavior

■ Covert sensitization: A type of aversion therapy that relies on an individual's imagined unpleasant symptoms or consequences for undesirable behaviors

■ Systematic desensitization: A technique for overcoming phobias in which there is a hierarchy of anxiety-producing events through which the individual progresses

■ Flooding (also called *implosion therapy*): A technique used to desensitize individuals to phobic stimuli by "flooding" them with a continuous presentation (through mental imagery) of the phobic stimulus until it no longer elicits anxiety

■ Nurses can implement behavior therapy techniques to help clients modify maladaptive behavior patterns.

■ The nursing process is a systematic method of directing care for clients who require this type of assistance.

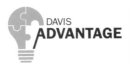 DAVIS ADVANTAGE | Go to **Davis Advantage** to complete your learning: strengthen understanding, apply your knowledge, and prepare for the Next Gen NCLEX®.

Review Questions

1. A positive reinforcer:
   a. Increases the probability that a behavior will recur.
   b. Decreases the probability that a behavior will recur.
   c. Has nothing to do with modifying behavior.
   d. Always results in positive behavior.

2. A negative reinforcer:
   a. Increases the probability that a behavior will recur.
   b. Decreases the probability that a behavior will recur.
   c. Has nothing to do with modifying behavior.
   d. Always results in unacceptable behavior.

3. An aversive stimulus or punisher:
   a. Increases the probability that a behavior will recur.
   b. Decreases the probability that a behavior will recur.
   c. Has nothing to do with modifying behavior.
   d. Always results in unacceptable behavior.

Situation: B.J. has been out with his friends. He is late getting home. He knows his wife will be angry and will yell at him for being late. He stops at the florist and buys a dozen red roses for her. Questions 4, 5, and 6 are related to this situation.

4. Which of the following behaviors represents positive reinforcement on the part of the wife?
   a. She meets him at the door, accepts the roses, and says nothing further about his being late.
   b. She meets him at the door, yelling that he is late, and makes him spend the night on the couch.
   c. She meets him at the door, expresses delight with the roses, and kisses him on the cheek.
   d. She meets him at the door and says, "How could you? You know I'm allergic to roses!"

5. Which of the following behaviors represents negative reinforcement on the part of the wife?
   a. She meets him at the door, accepts the roses, and says nothing further about his being late.
   b. She meets him at the door, yelling that he is late, and makes him spend the night on the couch.
   c. She meets him at the door, expresses delight with the roses, and kisses him on the cheek.
   d. She meets him at the door and says, "How could you? You know I'm allergic to roses!"

6. Which of the following behaviors represents an aversive stimulus on the part of the wife?
   a. She meets him at the door, accepts the roses, and says nothing further about his being late.
   b. She meets him at the door, yelling that he is late, and makes him spend the night on the couch.
   c. She meets him at the door, expresses delight with the roses, and kisses him on the cheek.
   d. She meets him at the door and says, "Didn't you remember I'm allergic to roses!"

Clinical Judgment Questions

7. The parents of a 14-year-old child ask the nurse for suggestions about how to promote homework completion and less time spent on social media. The nurse believes the Premack principle may be helpful. What should the nurse suggest to the parents?

   a. Tell the parents to reward their child each time homework is attempted, even if it is only for 5 minutes.

   b. Tell the parents to ignore this behavior, and eventually the child will start completing the homework without prompting.

   c. Tell the parents to draw up a contract stating what the consequences will be if homework is not completed.

   d. Tell the parents to explain to their child that TV is only permitted after the homework is completed.

8. A client has a fear of dogs. In helping them overcome this fear, the therapist is using systematic desensitization. List the following steps in the order in which the therapist would proceed.

   Have the client:

   a. Look at a real dog.

   b. Look at a stuffed toy dog.

   c. Pet a real dog.

   d. Pet the stuffed toy dog.

   e. Walk past a real dog.

   f. Look at a picture of a dog.

9. A client admitted to the psychiatric unit with anger management problems encountered another client stealing food from their plate. The client approaches the nurse and says, "I'm getting so angry I want to hit him, but I know I need to just walk away." Which response by the nurse would reinforce the client's response to this situation?

   a. Tell the client that walking away is not going to help them confront difficult situations.

   b. Tell the client that walking away is a healthy way to manage their anger.

   c. Tell the client that the staff will reprimand the other client who stole their food.

   d. Tell the client that their desire to lash out at someone behaving that way is normal.

References

Boland, R., & Verduin, M. L. (Eds). (2022). *Kaplan & Sadock's synopsis of psychiatry* (12th ed). Wolters Kluwer.

Cihon, J. H., Ferguson, J. L., Milne, C. M., Leaf, J. B., McEachin, J., & Leaf, R. (2018). A preliminary evaluation of a token system with a flexible earning requirement. *Behavior Analysis in Practice, 12*(3), 548–556. https://doi.org/10.1007/s40617-018-00316-3

Dickerson, F. B., Tenhula, W. N., & Green-Paden, L. D. (2005). The token economy for schizophrenia: Review of the literature and recommendations for future research. *Schizophrenia Research, 75*(2–3), 405–416. doi:10.1016/j.schres.2004.08.026

Doll, C., McLaughlin, T. F., & Barretto, A. (2013). The token economy: A recent review and evaluation. *International Journal of Basic and Applied Science, 2*(1), 131–149.

Gholipour, A., Abolghasemi, S. H., Gholinia, K., & Taheri, S. (2012). Token reinforcement therapeutic approach is more effective than exercise for controlling negative symptoms of schizophrenic patients: A randomized controlled trial. *International Journal of Preventive Medicine, 3*(7), 466–470.

Herrod, J. L., Snyder, S. K., Hart, J. B., Frantz, S. J., & Ayres, K. M. (2022). Applications of the Premack principle: A review of the literature. *Behavior Modification.* doi:10.1177/01454455221085249

Kim, J. Y., Fienup, D., Oh, A. E., & Wang, Y. (2021). Systematic review and meta-analysis of token economy practices in K-5 educational settings, 2000 to 2019. *Behavior Modification.* doi:10.1177/01454455211058077

Landkroon, E., van Dis, E. A. M., Meyerbröker, K., Salemink, E., Hagenaars, M. A., & Engelhard, I. M. (2022). Future-oriented positive mental imagery reduces anxiety for exposure to public speaking. *Behavior Therapy.* https://doi.org/10.1016/j.beth.2021.06.005

Martone, M. C. C., Martone, R. C., & Arantes, A. K. L. (2019). The use of shaping by relatives of autistic children to increase food intake. *European Journal of Behavior Analysis, 20*(2), 261–273. DOI: 10.1080/15021149.2019.1660953

McLeod, S. A. (2021). Systematic desensitization as a counter conditioning process. *Simply Psychology.* www.simplypsychology.org/Systematic-Desensitisation.html

Shakespeare, S., Peterkin, V. M. S., & Bourne, P. A. (2018). A token economy: An approach used for behavior modifications among disruptive primary school children. *MOJ Public Health, 7*(3), 89–99. DOI: 10.15406/mojph.2018.07.00212 DOI: 10.15406/mojph.2018.07.00212

Classical References

Pavlov, I. P. (1927). *Conditioned reflexes.* Oxford University Press.

Premack, D. (1959). Toward empirical behavior laws: I. Positive reinforcement. *Psychological Review, 66*(4), 219–233. doi:http://dx.doi.org/10.1037/h0040891

Skinner, B. F. (1938). *The behavior of organisms.* Appleton-Century-Crofts.

Skinner, B. F. (1953). *Science and human behavior.* Macmillan.

Thorndike, E. L. (1911). *Animal intelligence.* Macmillan.

Wolpe, J. (1958). *Psychotherapy by reciprocal inhibition.* Stanford University Press.

Wolpe, J. (1964). Behavior therapy in complex neurotic states. *The British Journal of Psychiatry, 110*(464): 28–34.

18

Cognitive Behavior Therapy

CORE CONCEPTS

Evidence-Based
  Practice: Cognitive
  behavior therapy

KEY TERMS

arbitrary inference

automatic thoughts

catastrophic thinking

decatastrophizing

dichotomous thinking

distraction

dysfunctional assumptions

magnification

minimization

overgeneralizations

personalization

schemas

selective abstraction

Socratic dialogue

OBJECTIVES
After reading this chapter, the student will be able to:

1. Discuss historical perspectives associated with cognitive behavior therapy.
2. Identify various indications for cognitive behavior therapy.
3. Describe goals, principles, and basic concepts of cognitive behavior therapy.
4. Discuss a variety of cognitive behavior therapy techniques.
5. Apply techniques of cognitive behavior therapy within the context of the nursing process.

Epictetus (55–135 AD), a Greek philosopher, is quoted as saying, "When something happens, the only thing in your power is your attitude toward it. It is not the things that disturb us, but our interpretation of their significance." One's attitude is a reflection of one's thoughts, and thoughts can have a significant effect on mood and behavior. This concept is the foundation on which the cognitive model and cognitive behavior therapy (CBT) is established. In CBT, the therapist uses various methods to create change in the client's thinking and belief system to bring about lasting emotional and behavioral change (Beck, 1995).

Cognitive therapy is based on the theory that distorted cognitions are at the foundation of many emotional, mental, and behavioral disorders. Clients with depression often seem to be consumed by negative thoughts about themselves and about how others see them; clients with anxiety disorders often have worried thoughts about past and future events; and clients with personality disorders often struggle with maladaptive thoughts about their relationships with others. Could helping clients change the way they think improve their mood and their behavior? There is much evidence to support that it can (Beck Institute for Cognitive Behavior Therapy, 2023; Brenes et al., 2015; Brent et al., 2015; David et al., 2018; Guille et al., 2015; Nakao et al., 2021; Rohan et al., 2015; Weck & Neng, 2015).

This chapter examines the historical development of the cognitive model, defines the goals of therapy, and describes various techniques of the cognitive approach. A discussion of the role of the nurse in the implementation of cognitive behavioral techniques with clients is presented.

Note: Aaron Beck, in the 1960s, originally developed a model for therapy called cognitive therapy. More recently, Beck's model has been broadened to include both cognitive and behavioral techniques and is called *cognitive behavior therapy (CBT)*. Both therapies are rooted in the cognitive model. In this chapter, these terms will be used interchangeably.

CORE CONCEPTS

Cognitive
Relating to the mental processes of thinking and reasoning.

Historical Background

Cognitive therapy has its roots in the early 1960s research on depression conducted by Aaron Beck (1963, 1964). Beck was trained in the Freudian psychoanalytic view of depression as "anger turned inward." In his clinical research, he began to observe a common theme of negative cognitive processing in the thoughts and dreams of his depressed clients (Beck & Weishaar, 2011).

Several theorists have taken from and expanded upon Beck's original concept. The common theme is the rejection of the passive listening used in psychoanalysis in favor of active, direct dialogues with clients (Beck & Weishaar, 2011). The work of contemporary behavioral therapists has also influenced the evolution of cognitive therapy. Behavioral techniques, such as expectancy of reinforcement and modeling, are based on cognitive processes. Lazarus and Folkman (1984), whose premises about *personal appraisal* and *coping* shape the conceptual framework of this book, have also substantially contributed to the cognitive approach to therapy. The model for cognitive therapy is based on an individual's cognition, or more specifically, an individual's personal cognitive appraisal of an event and the resulting emotions or behaviors. Personality—which undoubtedly influences our cognitive appraisal of an event—is shaped by the interaction between innate predisposition and the environment (Beck et al., 2015). Whereas some types of therapy may be directed toward improvement in coping strategies or adaptiveness of behavioral response, cognitive therapy is aimed at modifying distorted thinking about a situation. Because behavior and emotions are intimately linked to thoughts, this approach assumes that behavior and emotions will change as a result of changing one's thinking.

CORE CONCEPT

Cognitive Behavior Therapy
Cognitive behavior therapy (CBT) is based on the cognitive model, which advances the concept that a person's perceptions about a situation are more influential on their responses than the situation itself. Various techniques are incorporated to help clients learn how to change (reframe) their thinking and behavior in ways that will enhance mood, functioning, and sense of well-being (Beck Institute for Cognitive Behavior Therapy, 2023).

Indications for Cognitive Behavior Therapy

Cognitive therapy was originally developed for use with depression and is now used to treat a broad range of emotional disorders. CBT is one of the most researched psychosocial interventions. In a review of the literature (Nakao et al., 2021), researchers found evidence in several randomized controlled trials indicating that CBT was effective for a variety of mental problems including anxiety disorder, attention deficit-hypersensitivity disorder, bulimia nervosa, depression, and hypochondriasis; physical conditions including chronic fatigue syndrome, fibromyalgia, irritable bowel syndrome, and breast cancer; and behavioral problems including antisocial behaviors, drug abuse, gambling, overweight, and smoking. The proponents of CBT suggest that the emphasis of therapy must be varied and individualized for clients according to their specific diagnosis, symptoms, and level of functioning (Beck, 1995).

Goals and Principles of Cognitive Behavior Therapy

Beck and associates (1987) defined the goals of cognitive therapy as follows.

The client will:

1. Monitor their negative, automatic thoughts.
2. Recognize the connections between cognition, affect, and behavior.
3. Examine the evidence for and against distorted automatic thoughts.
4. Substitute more realistic interpretations for these biased cognitions.
5. Learn to identify and alter the dysfunctional beliefs that predispose them to distort experiences.

CBT is highly structured and short term, lasting from 12 to 16 weeks. A more recent approach to CBT treatment is intensive CBT (I-CBT), which involves longer sessions over a shorter period of time ranging from 1 day to 1 month. Evidence supports its effectiveness for obsessive-compulsive disorder (Jonsson et al., 2015), but more research is needed to evaluate its effectiveness for other disorders. I-CBT should not be confused with another recent approach, Internet CBT (i-CBT), which has also demonstrated effectiveness for the treatment of depression (Karyotaki et al., 2021) and anxiety (Aminoff et al., 2021; Axelsson et al., 2020). Although therapy must be tailored to the individual, the following principles underlie cognitive therapy for all patients (Beck Institute for Cognitive Therapy, 2023).

Principle 1. Cognitive behavior therapy is based on an ever-evolving formulation of the patient and their problems in cognitive terms. The therapist identifies the event that precipitated the distorted cognition. Current thinking patterns that serve to maintain the problematic behaviors are reviewed. The therapist then hypothesizes about certain developmental events and enduring patterns of cognitive appraisal that may have predisposed the patient to specific emotional and behavioral responses.

Principle 2. Cognitive behavior therapy requires a sound therapeutic alliance. A trusting relationship between therapist and patient must exist for cognitive therapy to succeed. The therapist must convey warmth, empathy, caring, and genuine positive regard. Development of a working relationship between therapist and patient is an individual process, and patients with various disorders will require varying degrees of effort to achieve this therapeutic alliance.

Principle 3. Cognitive behavior therapy emphasizes collaboration and active participation. Teamwork between therapist and patient is emphasized. They decide together what to work on during each session, how often they should meet, and what homework assignments should be completed between sessions.

Principle 4. Cognitive behavior therapy is goal-oriented and problem-focused. At the beginning of therapy, the patient is encouraged to identify what they perceive to be the problem or problems. With guidance from the therapist, goals are established as outcomes of therapy. Assistance in problem-solving is provided as required as the patient comes to recognize and correct distortions in thinking.

Principle 5. Cognitive behavior therapy initially emphasizes the present. Resolution of distressing situations that are based in the present usually leads to symptom reduction. It is therefore more beneficial to begin with current problems and delay shifting attention to the past until (1) the patient expresses a desire to do so, (2) the work on current problems produces little or no change, or (3) the therapist decides it is important to determine how dysfunctional ideas affecting the patient's current thinking originated.

Principle 6. Cognitive behavior therapy is educative, aims to teach the patient to be their own therapist, and emphasizes relapse prevention. From the beginning of therapy, the patient is taught about the nature and course of their disorder, about the cognitive model (i.e., how thoughts influence emotions and behavior), and about the process of cognitive therapy. The patient is taught how to set goals, plan behavioral change, and intervene on their own behalf.

Principle 7. Cognitive behavior therapy aims to be time limited. Patients often are seen weekly for a couple of months, followed by a number of biweekly sessions, then possibly a few monthly sessions. Some patients want periodic "booster" sessions every few months.

Principle 8. Cognitive behavior therapy sessions are structured. Each session has a set structure that includes (1) reviewing the patient's week, (2) collaboratively setting the agenda for this session, (3) reviewing the previous week's session, (4) reviewing the previous week's homework, (5) discussing this week's agenda items, (6) establishing homework for next week, and (7) summarizing this week's session. This format focuses attention on important items to maximize the use of therapy time.

Principle 9. Cognitive behavior therapy teaches patients to identify, evaluate, and respond to their dysfunctional thoughts and beliefs. Through gentle questioning and review of data, the therapist helps the patient identify their dysfunctional thinking, evaluate the validity of the thoughts, and devise a plan of action. These tasks are accomplished by helping the patient examine evidence that supports or contradicts the accuracy of the thoughts rather than directly challenging or confronting the belief.

Principle 10. Cognitive behavior therapy uses a variety of techniques to change thinking, mood, and behavior. Techniques from various therapies may be used within the cognitive framework. Emphasis in treatment is guided by the patient's particular disorder and directed toward modification of the dysfunctional cognitions that contribute to the maladaptive behavior associated with the disorder. Examples of disorders and the dysfunctional thinking for which cognitive therapy may be of benefit are discussed later in this chapter.

Basic Concepts

The most basic concept in CBT is that mood and behavior are primarily influenced by how we think about situations. Our thought processes are influenced by dysfunctional assumptions, automatic thoughts, and schemas (core beliefs).

Dysfunctional Assumptions

Dysfunctional assumptions are negative thoughts that are cognitive distortions and therefore cloud one's perception of reality. Because humans tend to hold on to negative thoughts easier than positive ones, these can become the foundation for irrational thought patterns (Vogel, 2022).

Automatic Thoughts

Automatic thoughts are those that occur rapidly in response to a situation and without rational analysis. These thoughts are often negative and based on erroneous logic. Beck and associates (1987) called these thoughts *cognitive errors.* Following are some examples of common cognitive errors:

Arbitrary Inference In a type of thinking error known as **arbitrary inference,** the individual automatically comes to a conclusion about an incident without the facts to support it or even despite contradictory evidence.

Example

Two months ago, Mrs. B. sent a wedding gift to the daughter of an old friend. She has not yet received acknowledgment of the gift. Mrs. B. thinks, "They obviously think I have poor taste" (instead of considering what other reasons there might be for a delay in the recipient's response).

Overgeneralization (Absolutistic Thinking) Sweeping conclusions are **overgeneralizations** made on the basis of one incident—an "all-or-nothing" kind of thinking.

Example

Frank submitted an article to a nursing journal, and it was rejected. Frank thinks, "No journal will ever be interested in anything I write."

Dichotomous Thinking An individual who is using **dichotomous thinking** views situations in terms of all-or-nothing, black-or-white, or good-or-bad.

Example

Frank submits an article to a nursing journal, and the editor returns it and asks Frank to rewrite parts of it. Frank thinks, "I'm a bad writer" (instead of recognizing that revision is a common part of the publication process).

Selective Abstraction A **selective abstraction** (sometimes referred to as a *mental filter*) is a conclusion based on only a selected portion of the evidence. The selected portion is usually the negative evidence or what the individual views as a failure, rather than any successes that have occurred.

Example

Jackie just graduated from high school with a 3.98/4.00 grade point average. She won a scholarship to the large state university near her home. She was active in sports and activities in high school and well liked by her peers. However, she is very depressed and dwells on the fact that she did not earn a scholarship to a prestigious Ivy League college to which she had applied (instead of considering her many other accomplishments).

Magnification Exaggerating the negative significance of an event is known as **magnification.**

Example

Nancy hears that her colleague at work is having a cocktail party over the weekend, and she is not invited. Nancy thinks, "She doesn't like me" (instead of considering that this may have been an event for a specific group of people).

Minimization Undervaluing the positive significance of an event is called **minimization.**

Example

Colin is feeling lonely. He telephones his son, Jon, who lives in a nearby town, and invites him to visit. Jon apologizes that he must go out of town on business and would not be able to visit at that time. While Jon is out of town, he calls his father twice, but Colin still feels unloved by his son (instead of acknowledging the positive efforts that his son made to keep in touch).

Catastrophic Thinking Always thinking that the worst will occur without considering the possibility of more likely positive outcomes is considered **catastrophic thinking.**

Example

On Janet's first day in her executive assistant job, her boss asked her to write a letter to another firm and put it on his desk for his signature. She did so and left for lunch. When she returned, the letter was on her desk with a minor typographical error circled in red and a note from her boss to correct the letter. Janet thinks, "This is it! I will surely be fired now!" (without considering that this may simply be her boss's way of orienting her to the expectations of the job).

Personalization With **personalization,** the person takes complete responsibility for situations without considering that other circumstances may have contributed to the outcome.

Example

Jack, who is a car salesman, has just given a 2-hour demonstration to Mrs. W. At the end of the demonstration, Mrs. W tells Jack that she appreciates his demonstration, but she won't be purchasing a car from him. Jack thinks, "I'm a lousy salesman" (instead of considering that Mrs. W may not have extra money to buy a new car at this time).

Schemas (Core Beliefs)

Beck and Weishaar (2011) defined cognitive **schemas** as:

> Structures that contain the individual's fundamental beliefs and assumptions. Schemas develop early in life from personal experience and identification with significant others. These concepts are reinforced by further learning experiences and, in turn, influence the formation of beliefs, values, and attitudes. (p. 284)

These schemas, or *core beliefs*, may be adaptive or maladaptive. They may be general or specific, and they may be latent, becoming evident only when triggered by a specific stressful stimulus. Schemas differ from automatic thoughts in that they are deeper cognitive structures that serve to screen information from the environment. For this reason, they are often more difficult to modify than automatic thoughts. However, the same techniques used for automatic thoughts can be used at the schema level. Schemas can be positive or negative and generally fall into two broad categories: those associated with *helplessness* and those associated with *unlovability* (Beck, 1995). Some examples of types of schemas are presented in Table 18–1.

Techniques of Cognitive Behavior Therapy

The three major components of CBT are didactic aspects, cognitive techniques, and behavioral interventions (Boland & Verduin, 2022).

Didactic (Educational) Aspects

A basic principle of CBT is to prepare the client to eventually become their own cognitive therapist. The therapist provides information to the client about what CBT is, how it works, and the structure of the cognitive process. Explanation about the expectations of both client and therapist is provided. Reading assignments are given to reinforce learning. Some therapists use audiotape or videotape sessions to teach clients about CBT. A full explanation about the relationship between depression (or anxiety, or whatever maladaptive response the client is experiencing) and distorted thinking patterns is an essential part of CBT.

Cognitive Techniques

Strategies used in CBT include recognizing and modifying automatic thoughts and recognizing and modifying schemas. Several techniques of CBT have been elaborated (Bettino, 2021; Freeman-Clevenger, 2014) and are described in the following sections.

Recognizing Automatic Thoughts and Schemas

Socratic Dialogue

In **Socratic dialogue** (also called *guided discovery*), the therapist questions the client to elaborate the "who, what, when, where, why, and how" of their situation. The client is asked to describe feelings associated with specific scenarios. Questions are primarily restatements of the client's own words in a way that may stimulate insight into possible dysfunctional thinking and produce dissonance about the validity of the thoughts.

Guided Relaxation and Behavioral Rehearsal

Guided relaxation is aimed at reducing autonomic response to anxiety. Techniques may include deep breathing, imagery, mindfulness meditation, and other exercises. These techniques also increase awareness of conscious control over breathing, anxiety symptoms, and thoughts.

Behavioral rehearsal, often accomplished through role-play, allows the client to practice a new way of responding to distressing situations and explore possible outcomes with the counselor before trying out the behavior in real-life situations. *Role-play* is a technique that should be used only when the relationship between client and therapist is strong and there is little likelihood of maladaptive transference. With role-play, the therapist assumes the role of an individual in a situation that produces a maladaptive response in the client. The situation is played out to elicit recognition of automatic thinking on the part of the client.

TABLE 18–1 **Examples of Types of Schemas**		
SCHEMA CATEGORY	**MALADAPTIVE/NEGATIVE**	**ADAPTIVE/POSITIVE**
Helplessness	No matter what I do, I will fail. I must be perfect. If I make one mistake, I will lose everything.	If I try and work very hard, I will succeed. I am not afraid of a challenge. If I make a mistake, I will try again.
Unlovability	I'm stupid. No one would love me. I'm nobody without a man.	I'm a lovable person. People respect me for myself.

Automatic Thought Records

This technique, one of the most frequently used methods of recognizing automatic thoughts, is taught to and discussed with the client in the therapy session. Thought recording is assigned as homework for the client outside of therapy. The client is asked to keep a written record of situations that occur and the automatic thoughts elicited by the situation. This process is called a *two-column thought recording*. Some therapists ask their clients to keep a three-column recording, which includes a description of the emotional response also associated with the situation, as illustrated in Table 18–2.

Modifying Automatic Thoughts and Schemas

Questioning the Evidence

With this technique, the client and therapist view the automatic thought as the hypothesis, and the client is assisted in questioning the facts associated with their cognitions.

Examining Options and Alternatives

To help the client see a broader range of possibilities than originally considered, the therapist guides the client in learning how to generate alternatives.

Decatastrophizing

With the technique of **decatastrophizing,** the therapist assists the client to examine the validity of an automatic negative thought. The client is assisted in examining "what is the worst thing that could happen?" and then to develop a plan of action. Even if some validity exists, the client is encouraged to review ways to cope adaptively and move beyond the current crisis.

Reattribution

Through Socratic questioning and testing of automatic thoughts, this technique aims to reverse negative attribution of clients from self-blame (common in depression) or placing blame solely on others (common in some personality disorders) to a more balanced attribution of responsibility.

Daily Record of Dysfunctional Thoughts (DRDT)

The DRDT is a tool commonly used in cognitive therapy to help clients identify and modify automatic thoughts. Two more columns are added to the three-column thought record presented earlier. Clients are then asked to rate the intensity of the thoughts and emotions on a 0% to 100% scale. The fourth column of the DRDT asks the client to describe a more rational cognition than the automatic thought identified in the second column and rate the intensity of the belief in the rational thought. In the fifth column, the client records any changes that have occurred as a result of modifying the automatic thought and the new rate of intensity associated with it. With this tool, the client is able to modify automatic thoughts by identifying them and formulating a more rational alternative. Table 18–3 presents an example of a DRDT as an extension to the three-column thought recording presented in Table 18–2.

Cognitive Rehearsal

This technique uses mental imagery to uncover potential automatic thoughts in advance of their occurrence in a stressful situation. A discussion identifies ways to modify these dysfunctional cognitions. The client is then given "homework" assignments to try these newly learned methods in real situations.

Behavioral Interventions

It is believed that in cognitive therapy, an interactive relationship exists between cognitions and behavior; that is, that cognitions affect behavior and behavior influences cognitions. With this concept in mind, several interventions are structured for the client to assist them to identify and modify maladaptive cognitions and behaviors.

The following procedures, which are behavior-oriented, are directed to help clients learn more adaptive behavioral strategies that will have a positive effect on cognitions (Bettino, 2021; Boland & Verduin, 2022; Freeman-Clevenger, 2014):

1. **Activity scheduling:** With this intervention, clients are asked to keep a daily log of their activities on an hourly basis and rate each activity, for mastery and pleasure, on a 0-to-10 scale. The schedule is then shared with the therapist and used to identify important areas needing concentration during therapy.

TABLE 18–2 **Three-Column Thought Recording**		
SITUATION	**AUTOMATIC THOUGHTS**	**EMOTIONAL RESPONSE**
My girlfriend broke up with me.	I'm a stupid person. No one would ever want to marry me.	Sadness; depression
I was turned down for a promotion.	Stupid boss! He doesn't know how to manage people. It's not fair!	Anger

TABLE 18–3 Sample Daily Record of Dysfunctional Thoughts (DRDT)

SITUATION	AUTOMATIC THOUGHT	EMOTIONAL RESPONSE	RATIONAL RESPONSE	OUTCOME: EMOTIONAL RESPONSE
My girlfriend broke up with me.	I'm a stupid person. No one would ever want to marry me. (95%)	Sadness; depression (90%)	I'm not stupid. Lots of people like me. Just because one person doesn't want to date me doesn't mean that no one would want to. (75%)	Sadness; depression (50%)
I was turned down for a promotion.	Stupid boss! He doesn't know how to manage people. It's not fair! (90%)	Anger (95%)	I guess I have to admit the other guy's education and experience fit the position better than mine. The boss was being fair because he filled the position based on qualifications. I'll try for the next promotion that fits my qualifications better. (70%)	Anger (20%) Disappointment (80%)

2. **Graded task assignments:** This intervention is used with clients who are facing a situation that they perceive as overwhelming. The task is broken down into subtasks that clients can complete one step at a time. Each subtask has a goal and a time interval attached to it. Successful completion of each subtask helps to increase self-esteem and decrease feelings of helplessness.

3. **Distraction:** When dysfunctional cognitions have been recognized, **distraction** can occur by engaging in activities that redirect the client's thinking and divert them from the intrusive thoughts or depressive ruminations that are contributing to the maladaptive responses.

4. **Miscellaneous techniques:** Relaxation exercises, assertiveness training, role modeling, social skills training, and contingency management contracts are all types of behavioral interventions used in cognitive therapy to help clients modify dysfunctional cognitions. Thought-stopping techniques (described in Chapter 13, "Assertiveness Training") may also be used to restructure dysfunctional thinking patterns.

Role of the Nurse in Cognitive Behavior Therapy

Many of the techniques used in CBT are well within the scope of nursing practice, from generalist through specialist levels. CBT requires an understanding of educational principles and the ability to use problem-solving skills to guide patients' thinking through a reframing process. The scope of contemporary psychiatric nursing practice is expanding, and although psychiatric nurses have been using some of these techniques to various degrees within their practices for years, it is important that knowledge and skills related to this type of therapy be promoted further. The value of CBT as a useful and cost-effective tool has been observed in many inpatient and community outpatient mental health settings.

Planning and Implementation

Table 18–4 presents a nursing care plan for a depressed, suicidal patient incorporating interventions associated with CBT that are within the scope of psychiatric nursing practice. These include providing psychoeducation, use of the therapeutic relationship, and counseling interventions (American Nurses Association, American Psychiatric Nurses Association, & International Society of Psychiatric-Mental Health Nurses, 2022). Rationales are presented for each intervention.

Evaluation

Reassessment is conducted to determine whether the nursing interventions have been successful in achieving the objectives of care. Evaluation can be facilitated by gathering information using the following questions:

1. Has self-harm been avoided?
2. Have suicidal ideations subsided?
3. Does the patient know where to seek help in a crisis?
4. Is the patient able to verbalize personal hope for the future?
5. Can the patient identify positive attributes about themselves?
6. Does the patient demonstrate motivation to move on with their life without fear of failure?

Table 18–4 | CARE PLAN FOR A PATIENT INCORPORATING COGNITIVE-FOCUSED INTERVENTIONS

NURSING DIAGNOSIS: RISK FOR SUICIDAL BEHAVIOR

RELATED TO: Depressed mood

OUTCOME CRITERIA	NURSING INTERVENTIONS	RATIONALE
Patient will not harm self.	1. Acknowledge the patient's feelings of despair and thoughts about suicide.	1. Acknowledging the patient's thoughts and feelings promotes self-awareness of thoughts associated with suicide.
	2. Convey warmth, accurate empathy, and genuineness.	2. Establishing a therapeutic alliance is foundational to a therapeutic, problem-solving relationship.
	3. Collaborate with the patient in conducting a thorough assessment of suicide risk. (See Chapter 16, "Suicide Prevention," for more information.)	3. Developing a collaborative assessment and plan for suicide prevention is foundational to working with any patient at risk for suicide.
	4. Encourage the patient to talk about reasons for wanting to die. Explore the patient's reasons for wanting to live.	4. This promotes the patient's awareness of thoughts and lays a foundation for helping the patient to reframe cognitive distortions.
	5. Encourage the patient to explore alternative ways of thinking and behaving.	5. Exploring alternatives initiates the process of cognitive reevaluation by looking at all possible alternatives.

NURSING DIAGNOSIS: CHRONIC LOW SELF-ESTEEM

RELATED TO: Lack of positive feedback and learned helplessness

EVIDENCED BY: A sense of worthlessness, lack of eye contact, social isolation, and negative/pessimistic outlook

OUTCOME CRITERIA	NURSING INTERVENTIONS	RATIONALE
Patient demonstrates increased self-esteem and perception of self as a worthwhile person.	1. Encourage the patient to discuss troubling or derogatory thoughts about self-worth.	1. This encourages patients to develop insight into their cognitive responses.
	2. Encourage the patient to analyze thoughts and explore alternative ways of thinking about self-worth.	2. This intervention encourages the patient to explore the validity of thoughts about self-worth and to begin correcting cognitive distortions.
	3. Educate the patient in mindfulness relaxation techniques.	3. Mindfulness relaxation promotes self-awareness of thoughts, feelings, and behaviors in the present (as opposed to ruminating about the past or worrying about the future).
	4. Reinforce patient's efforts to challenge negative thoughts and make observations about any noted improvement in mood and behavior.	4. Positive reinforcement promotes continued use of healthy coping strategies. Making observations about patient accomplishments and improvement in affect promotes positive self-esteem.

Summary and Key Points

- Cognitive behavior therapy (CBT) is founded on the premise that how people think significantly influences their feelings and behavior.
- The concept was initiated in the 1960s by Aaron Beck in his work with depressed clients. Since that time, it has been expanded for use with many emotional illnesses.
- CBT is short-term, highly structured, and goal-oriented therapy that consists of three major components: didactic, or educational, aspects; cognitive techniques; and behavioral interventions.
- Intensive CBT (I-CBT) involves longer sessions within a shorter time frame (a week or month) and evidence supports its benefit in the treatment of OCD.
- Internet-based CBT (i-CBT) is a recent treatment approach that has demonstrated effectiveness in the treatment of depression and anxiety.

- The therapist teaches the client about the relationship between their illness and the distorted thinking patterns. An explanation about CBT and how it works is provided.
- The therapist helps the client to recognize their negative automatic thoughts (sometimes called *cognitive errors*).
- Once these automatic thoughts have been identified, various cognitive and behavioral techniques are used to assist the client in modifying the dysfunctional thinking patterns.
- Independent homework assignments are an important part of the cognitive therapist's strategy.
- Many of the CBT techniques are within the scope of psychiatric-mental health nursing practice.
- As the role of the psychiatric nurse continues to expand, the knowledge and skills associated with a variety of therapies will need to be broadened. CBT is likely to be one in which nurses will become more involved.

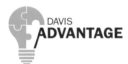

Go to **Davis Advantage** to complete your learning: strengthen understanding, apply your knowledge, and prepare for the Next Gen NCLEX®.

Review Questions

1. A nursing student failed the first test in nursing school and thinks, "Well, that's it! I'll never be a nurse." What automatic thought does this statement represent?
   a. Overgeneralization
   b. Magnification
   c. Catastrophic thinking
   d. Personalization

2. A college student is not accepted at the law school of their choice, and thinks, "I'm so stupid. No law school will ever accept me." What automatic thought does this statement represent?
   a. Overgeneralization
   b. Magnification
   c. Selective abstraction
   d. Minimization

3. Ashley's new in-laws came to dinner for the first time. When her mother-in-law left some food on her plate, Ashley thought, "I must be a lousy cook." What automatic thought does this statement represent?
   a. Dichotomous thinking
   b. Overgeneralization
   c. Minimization
   d. Personalization

4. Amal burned the toast and thinks, "I'm a totally incompetent person." What automatic thought does this statement represent?
   a. Selective abstraction
   b. Magnification
   c. Minimization
   d. Personalization

5. A client who is suffering from depression and suicidal ideation says, "I'm such a worthless person. I don't deserve to live." The therapist responds, "I would like for you to think about what problems suicide would solve." The therapist is using which of the following CBT techniques?
   a. Imagery
   b. Role-play
   c. Problem-solving
   d. Thought recording

6. The thought recording (two-column and three-column) cognitive therapy techniques help clients:
   a. Identify automatic thoughts.
   b. Modify automatic thoughts.
   c. Identify rational alternatives.
   d. All of the above.

7. A client tells the therapist, "I thought I would just die when my husband told me he was leaving me. If I had been a better wife, he wouldn't have fallen in love with another woman. It's all my fault." The therapist wants to use the technique of "examining the evidence." Which of the following statements reflects this technique?
   a. "How do you think you could have been a better wife?"
   b. "Okay, you say it's all your fault. Let's discuss why it might be your fault, and then we will look at why it may not be."
   c. "Let's talk about what would make you a happier person."
   d. "Would you have wanted him to stay if he didn't really want to?"

Clinical Judgment Questions

8. A client reports to the nurse, "My wife left me. No one else will ever love me. I'm going to be alone for the rest of my life." Which action by the nurse reflects an appropriate, cognitive-focused response?
   a. "What contributes to your thinking that you will be alone for the rest of your life?"
   b. "You're just overgeneralizing."
   c. "Why did your wife leave you?"
   d. "I'm sure there are other people that love you."

9. A client who was admitted to the psychiatric unit for depression tells the psychiatric nurse that they want to engage in CBT after discharge. Which action by the nurse is most appropriate at this point?
   a. Offer to begin CBT with the patient while they are hospitalized.
   b. Offer to explore referral to a therapist for this kind of treatment.
   c. Educate the client that CBT can only be completed while they are hospitalized.
   d. Educate the client that CBT is not effective for treating depression.

References

American Nurses Association (ANA), American Psychiatric Nurses Association, & International Society of Psychiatric-Mental Health Nurses. (2022). *Psychiatric-mental health nursing: Scope and standards of practice* (3rd ed.). ANA.

Aminoff, V., Sellén, M., Sörliden, E., Ludvigsson, M., Berg, M., & Andersson, G. (2021). Internet-based cognitive behavioral therapy for psychological distress associated with the Covid-19 pandemic: A pilot randomized controlled trial. *Frontiers in Psychology, 12,* 684540. doi:10.3389/fpsyg.2021.684540

Axelsson, E., Andersson, E., Ljótsson, B., Björkander, D., Hedman-Lagerlöf, M., & Hedman-Lagerlöf, E. (2020). Effect of Internet vs face-to-face cognitive behavior therapy for health anxiety: A randomized noninferiority clinical trial. *JAMA Psychiatry, 77*(9), 915–924. doi:10.1001/jamapsychiatry.2020.0940

Beck, A. T., Davis, D. D., & Freeman, A. (2015). *Cognitive therapy of personality disorders* (3rd ed.). Guilford Press.

Beck, A. T., & Weishaar, M. E. (2011). Cognitive therapy. In Corsini, R. J. & Wedding, D. (Eds.), *Current psychotherapies* (9th ed., pp. 276–309). Brooks/Cole.

Beck Institute for Cognitive Behavior Therapy. (2023). *Understanding CBT.* https://beckinstitute.org/about/understanding-cbt/

Bettino, K. (2021). *All about cognitive behavior therapy (CBT).* https://psychcentral.com/lib/in-depth-cognitive-behavioral-therapy

Boland, R., & Verduin, M. L. (Eds). (2022). *Kaplan & Sadock's synopsis of psychiatry* (12th ed). Wolters Kluwer.

Brenes, G. A., Danhauer, S. C., Lyles, M. F., Hogan, P. E., & Miller, M. E. (2015). Telephone-delivered cognitive behavioral therapy and telephone-delivered nondirective supportive therapy for rural older adults with generalized anxiety disorder: A randomized clinical trial. *JAMA Psychiatry, 72*(10), 1012–1020. doi:10.1001/jamapsychiatry.2015.1154

Brent, D. A., Brunwasser, S. M., Hollon, S. D., Weersing, V. R., Clarke, G. N., Dickerson, J. F.... Garber, J. (2015). Effect of a cognitive-behavioral prevention program on depression

6 years after implementation among at-risk adolescents: A randomized clinical trial. *JAMA Psychiatry, 72*(11), 1110–1118. doi:10.1001/jamapsychiatry.2015.1559

David, D., Cristea, I., & Hofmann, S. G. (2018). Why cognitive behavioral therapy is the current gold standard of psychotherapy. *Frontiers in Psychiatry, 9*(4). https://doi.org/10.3389/fpsyt.2018.00004

Freeman-Clevenger, S. M. (2014). Cognitive behavioral therapy. In Wheeler, K. (Ed.), *Psychotherapy for the advanced practice psychiatric nurse: A how-to guide for evidence-based practice* (2nd ed., pp. 313–345). New York: Springer.

Guille, C., Zhao, Z., Krystal, J., Nichols, B., Brady, K., & Sen, S. (2015). Web-based cognitive behavioral therapy intervention for the prevention of suicidal ideation in medical interns: A randomized controlled trial. *JAMA Psychiatry, 72*(12), 1192–1198. doi:10.1001/jamapsychiatry.2015.1880

Jonsson, H., Kristensen, M., & Arendt, M. (2015). Intensive cognitive behavioural therapy for obsessive-compulsive disorder: A systematic review and meta-analysis. *Journal of Obsessive, Compulsive, and Related Disorders, 6,* 83–96, 10.1016/j.jocrd.2015.04.004

Karyotaki E, Efthimiou O, Miguel C, Bermpohl, F. M., Furukawa, T. A., Cuijpers, J., & The Individual Patient Data Meta-Analyses for Depression (IPDMA-DE) Collaboration. (2021). Internet-based cognitive behavioral therapy for depression: A systematic review and individual patient data network meta-analysis. *JAMA Psychiatry, 78*(4), 361–371. doi:10.1001/jamapsychiatry.2020.4364

Nakao, M., Shirotsuki, K., & Sugaya, N. (2021). Cognitive–behavioral therapy for management of mental health and stress-related disorders: Recent advances in techniques and technologies. *BioPsychoSocial Medicine, 15*(16). https://doi.org/10.1186/s13030-021-00219-w

Rohan, K. J., Mahon, J. N., Evans, M., Ho, S. Y., Meyerhoff, J., Postolache, T. T., & Vacek, P. M. (2015). Randomized trial of cognitive-behavioral therapy versus light therapy for seasonal affective disorder: Acute outcomes. *American Journal of Psychiatry, 172*(9), 862–869. doi:10.1176/appi.ajp.2015.14101293

Vogel, K. (2022). *The basic principles of cognitive behavioral therapy.* https://psychcentral.com/pro/the-basic-principles-of-cognitive-behavior-therapy

Weck, F., & Neng, J. M. (2015). Response and remission after cognitive and exposure therapy for hypochondriasis. *Journal of Nervous and Mental Disorders, 203*(11), 883–885. doi:10.1097/NMD.0000000000000385

Classical References

Beck, A. T. (1963). Thinking and depression, I. Idiosyncratic content and cognitive distortions. *Archives of General Psychiatry, 9*(4), 324–333. doi:10.1001/archpsyc.1963.01720160014002

Beck, A. T. (1964). Thinking and depression, II. Theory and therapy. *Archives of General Psychiatry, 10*(6), 561–571. doi:10.1001/archpsyc.1964.01720240015003

Beck, A. T., Rush, A. H., Shaw, B. F., & Emery, G. (1987). *Cognitive therapy of depression.* Guilford Press.

Beck, J. S. (1995). *Cognitive therapy: Basics and beyond.* Guilford Press.

Lazarus, R. S., & Folkman, S. (1984). *Stress, appraisal, and coping.* Springer.

Electroconvulsive Therapy 19

CORE CONCEPTS

Professional Behavior: Nursing process in the care of patients receiving electroconvulsive therapy
Clinical Judgment

KEY TERMS

electroconvulsive therapy   grand mal seizure   informed consent

OBJECTIVES

After reading this chapter, the student will be able to:

1. Define *electroconvulsive therapy*.
2. Discuss historical perspectives related to electroconvulsive therapy.
3. Discuss indications, contraindications, mechanism of action, and side effects of electroconvulsive therapy.
4. Identify risks associated with electroconvulsive therapy.
5. Describe the role of the nurse in the administration of electroconvulsive therapy.

Electroconvulsive therapy (ECT) has long had a negative reputation. In the iconic depiction of this treatment in the movie *One Flew Over the Cuckoo's Nest,* it is a physically and emotionally brutal procedure imposed on unwilling patients in order to calm them. Today, ECT remains a controversial treatment for psychological disorders and the subject of impassioned debate among various factions within both the professional and lay communities.

In late 2018 the U.S. Food and Drug Administration (FDA) affirmed the safety of ECT in the treatment of depression and catatonia by downgrading the risk classification of ECT devices from class III (highest risk) to class II (lower risk) for those indications. The change in classification also stipulates several "special controls" that include requirements about the technical parameters for devices, labeling about adverse effects, practitioner training, and some aspects of clinical practice (Kellner, 2019). Kellner (2019) added

that the way the FDA identifies appropriate indications for use of ECT ("a severe major depressive episode associated with major depressive disorder or bipolar disorder in patients aged 13 years and older who have treatment resistance or who require a rapid response due to the severity of their psychiatric or medical condition") closely approximates the majority of its use in clinical practice in the United States.

Despite its controversial image, ECT has been used continuously for more than 50 years, longer than any other physical treatment for mental illness. Although typically reserved for individuals with treatment-resistant depression, the American Psychiatric Association (APA, 2019) reports that extensive research supports its effectiveness in the treatment of major depression with substantial improvements in approximately 80% of patients.

This chapter explores the historical perspectives, indications and contraindications, mechanism of action, side effects, and risks associated with ECT. The role of the nurse in the care of the patient receiving ECT is presented in the context of the nursing process.

Electroconvulsive Therapy, Defined

> ### CORE CONCEPTS
> **Electroconvulsive Therapy**
> **Electroconvulsive therapy** is the induction of a grand mal (generalized) seizure through the application of electrical current to the brain.

Seizures are characterized by a surge of electrical activity within the brain. With ECT, a **grand mal seizure,** more recently called a *tonic-clonic seizure* because of the characteristic muscle contractions that define this type of seizure, is induced in the patient by administering a dose of electrical current through electrodes placed either bilaterally (in the bifrontal or bifrontotemporal areas) or unilaterally on the right side of the frontotemporal area. Right unilateral ECT is associated with fewer cognitive side effects, and its efficacy can be ensured with adequate dosing strategies (Boland & Verduin, 2022). Although unilateral treatments were once conducted on the hemisphere of the nondominant hand, Boland and Verduin (2022) noted that the right hemisphere is involved in sustaining depressed mood regardless of handedness. The dose of electrical current is carefully controlled through the use of an ECT machine.

The amount of electrical stimulus applied is a point of controversy among clinicians. The dose of electrical stimulation must be strong enough to reach the patient's seizure threshold, but this threshold is highly variable among individuals. Further, a patient's seizure threshold may increase 25% to 200% during the course of ECT treatments. In this mechanism of action, ECT itself acts as an anticonvulsant because the seizure threshold increases as treatment progresses (Boland & Verduin, 2022).

Observing the patient is not always the best indicator of seizure activity. Movements are minimal because of the administration of a muscle relaxant before treatment. The tonic phase of the seizure usually lasts 10 to 20 seconds and may be identified by a rigid plantar extension of the feet. The clonic phase follows and is usually characterized by rhythmic movements of the muscles that decrease in frequency and finally disappear. Because of the muscle relaxant, movements may be observed merely as a rhythmic twitching of the toes. Monitoring electroencephalogram (EEG) activity during the treatment provides evidence of grand mal seizure activity.

Most clients require an average of 6 to 12 treatments, but some may require up to 20 treatments. Boland & Verduin (2022) indicated that treating manic episodes of bipolar disorder can take up to 20 treatments, schizophrenia can take more than 15 treatments, and the treatment of catatonia or delirium can take as little as 1 to 4 treatments. Treatments are usually administered every other day, three times per week. Treatments are performed on an inpatient basis for those who require close observation and care (e.g., clients who are suicidal, agitated, delusional, catatonic, or acutely manic). Those at less risk may receive therapy at an outpatient treatment facility.

Historical Perspectives

Inducing seizures to treat psychiatric illness was reported as early as the 16th century, although the mechanism of induction at that time was the administration of camphor. In the early 1900s, Hungarian neuropsychiatrist Ladislas Meduna observed that individuals with epilepsy had more than the average number of glial cells and that people with schizophrenia had fewer than average, sparking interest and further study into the clinical benefits of seizure induction. The first ECT treatment was performed in April 1938 by Italian psychiatrists Ugo Cerletti and Lucio Bini in Rome. Other somatic therapies were tried before that time, including insulin coma therapy and pharmacoconvulsive therapy.

Insulin coma therapy was introduced by the German psychiatrist Manfred Sakel in 1933. His therapy was used for clients with schizophrenia. The insulin injection treatments induced a hypoglycemic coma, which Sakel claimed was effective in alleviating schizophrenic symptoms. This therapy required vigorous medical and nursing intervention through the stages of induced coma. Some fatalities occurred when clients failed to respond to efforts directed at the termination of the coma. The efficacy of insulin coma therapy has been questioned, and its use has been discontinued in the treatment of mental illness.

Pharmacoconvulsive therapy was introduced in Budapest in 1934 by Ladislas Meduna (Fink, 2009). He induced seizures with intramuscular injections of camphor in oil in clients with schizophrenia. He based his treatment on clinical observation and theorized the existence of a biological antagonism between schizophrenia and epilepsy. By inducing seizures, schizophrenic symptoms could potentially be reduced. Because he discovered that camphor was unreliable for inducing seizures, he began using pentylenetetrazol (Metrazol). Some successes were reported in terms of reduction of psychotic symptoms, and until the advent of ECT in 1938, pentylenetetrazol was the most frequently used method for producing seizures in clients with psychosis. There was a brief resurgence of pharmacoconvulsive therapy in the late 1950s, when flurothyl (Indoklon), a potent inhalant convulsant, was introduced as an alternative for individuals who were unwilling to consent to ECT for the treatment of depression and schizophrenia. Pharmacoconvulsive therapy is no longer used in psychiatry.

Periodic recognition of the importance of ECT in the treatment of mental illness has been evident in the United States. After being initially accepted from 1940 to 1960, ECT was viewed as objectionable by both the psychiatric profession and the public for the next 20 years. A second wave of acceptance began around 1980 and has been increasing ever since. The period of unacceptability coincided with the introduction of tricyclic and monoamine oxidase inhibitor antidepressant drugs and ended when experts recognized that some individuals showed improvement with ECT after failing to respond to these other forms of therapy. ECT is now used as an alternative treatment for some individuals who do not respond to antidepressant therapy.

Currently, an estimated 100,000 people in the United States receive ECT treatments each year (Boland & Verduin, 2022). A large study of privately insured individuals (Wilkinson et al., 2018, Conclusions) concluded that ECT use in the United States is "exceptionally uncommon and is limited to patients with extensive multimorbidity and high levels of service use." The typical client is white, female, middle-aged, and from a middle- to upper-income background, receiving treatment in a private or university hospital for major depression, usually after drug therapy and other treatments have proved ineffective. Mainly because of the expense involved and the need for a team of highly skilled medical specialists, many public hospitals are unable to offer this treatment to their patients. Kellner (2019) estimated that only about 2% of psychiatrists in the United States actually practice ECT.

Indications

Major Depression

ECT has been shown to be effective in the treatment of severe depression, particularly among depressed clients who are also experiencing psychotic symptoms, catatonia, psychomotor retardation, and neurovegetative changes, such as disturbances in sleep, appetite, and energy. ECT typically is considered only after a trial of therapy with antidepressant medication has proved ineffective. It may be considered the treatment of choice when the need for treatment response is urgent, such as in patients who show extreme and pervasive suicidal intent or are refusing food and are nutritionally compromised (Mankad, 2019).

Mania

ECT is indicated in the treatment of acute manic episodes and is at least as effective as lithium (Boland & Verduin, 2022). At present, it is rarely used for this purpose because lithium and other pharmacotherapies are usually effective as a short- and long-term treatment. However, ECT has been shown to be effective in the treatment of manic clients who do not tolerate or fail to respond to lithium or other drug treatment or when life is threatened by dangerous behavior or exhaustion. A recent study concluded that bilateral ECT with high-energy dosing yielded a rapid remission of symptoms in delirious mania, which is a life-threatening condition (Reinfeld & Yacoub, 2022). ECT should not be used while a patient is receiving lithium because lithium lowers the seizure threshold and may cause prolonged seizures when combined with ECT (Boland & Verduin, 2022). ECT increases the seizure threshold progressively during treatment, and some evidence supports that increasing the seizure threshold is associated with improvement in manic symptoms (Elias et al., 2021)

Recent evidence has supported the use of ECT in the treatment of bipolar disorders with mixed states (concurrent depressive and manic features). This type of bipolar disorder is often more severe than other types, with lower interepisode remission and higher risk for suicide (Palma et al., 2016). Nonetheless, ECT is still used only when the patient has failed to respond to medication.

Schizophrenia

ECT can induce remission in some clients who present with acute schizophrenia, particularly those who have marked positive, catatonic, or affective (depression or mania) symptoms (Boland & Verduin, 2022). There is little evidence to support its efficacy in those with chronic symptoms of schizophrenia. Several researchers presented evidence showing that although ECT is safe and effective for clients with schizophrenia (Grover et al., 2018; Kellner, 2019; Sanghani et al., 2018), it is underused. Kellner advocated that globally, schizophrenia may be the leading indication for ECT but, again, in current practice, it is not commonly used.

Other Conditions

ECT has been reported as useful in episodic psychosis, atypical psychosis, obsessive-compulsive disorder, delirium, and medical conditions such as neuroleptic malignant syndrome, hypopituitarism, intractable seizure disorders, and Parkinson's disease, particularly when there is comorbid depression (Mankad, 2019; Boland & Verduin, 2022). For pregnant women and elderly individuals who are depressed, suicidal, and unable to take medication, ECT may be the treatment of choice. Oztav and associates (2015) reported that although the literature on safety of ECT in pregnancy is scarce, their research supported others' findings that it can be used safely. They also noted that 40% of pregnant patients treated with ECT in their study demonstrated full recovery. ECT is not effective in somatization disorders (unless there is comorbid depression), personality disorders, and anxiety disorders (Boland & Verduin, 2022).

Contraindications

There are no absolute contraindications for ECT. However, some patients may be considered at higher risk for adverse events that require attention and closer monitoring (Boland & Verduin, 2022; Prudic & Duan, 2017). High-risk conditions are chiefly cardiovascular and include myocardial infarction and cerebrovascular accident within the preceding 3 to 6 months, aortic or cerebral aneurysm, severe underlying hypertension, and congestive heart failure. Clients with cardiovascular problems are placed at risk because of the body's response to the seizure itself. The initial vagal response results in sinus bradycardia and a drop in blood pressure, followed immediately by tachycardia and a hypertensive response. These changes can be life-threatening to an individual with an already compromised cardiovascular system.

Patients with intracranial lesions may be at risk for edema or brain herniation after ECT, but these risks can be decreased by pretreatment with dexamethasone in cases in which the lesion is small (Boland & Verduin, 2022). Patients with increased intracranial pressure are at increased risk related to increased cerebral blood flow during seizures, but Boland & Verduin (2022) noted that risk can be lessened by controlling the patient's blood pressure during the treatment.

Other factors that place clients at risk during ECT include severe osteoporosis, acute and chronic pulmonary disorders, and high-risk or complicated pregnancy. Because oxytocin levels increase after ECT, there is an increased risk of intrauterine contractions and premature birth with an incidence of around 3% to 6% (Oztav et al., 2015).

Mechanism of Action

The exact mechanism by which ECT effects a therapeutic response is unknown. Many parts of the central nervous system are affected by ECT, including hormones, neuropeptides, neurotrophic factors, and nearly every neurotransmitter (Mankad, 2019). Affected neurotransmitters include serotonin, norepinephrine, and dopamine, which are the same biogenic amines that are affected by antidepressant drugs. Research on serotonin has yielded mixed results and the effect of ECT on serotonin levels remains controversial (Boland & Verduin, 2022). Other possible mechanisms of action, based on changes that occur during ECT, include an increase in gamma-aminobutyric acid (GABA) transmission and an increase of endogenous opioids, both of which may raise the seizure threshold (Mankad, 2019; Sharma et al., 2018). A longitudinal study of imaging research shows that the therapeutic response to ECT is associated with several effects on the brain, including decreased frontal perfusion, changes in metabolism, functional connectivity, volume, and neuronal chemical metabolites, all of which support anticonvulsant and neurotrophic effects of ECT (Abbott et al., 2014). Other studies have demonstrated increased GABA levels, increased sensitization of $5\text{-HT}_1\text{A}$ serotonin receptors, increased dopamine binding, and normalized dexamethasone suppression tests in patients who received ECT (Sharma et al., 2018). In another study, the researchers concluded that therapeutic response from ECT may be related to neuroplasticity in white matter microstructures, which are altered in major depression (Lyden et al., 2014).

Several studies have identified an increase in gray matter, particularly in the hippocampal and amygdala areas, after ECT (Depping et al., 2016; Pirnia et al., 2016; Sartorius et al., 2015). Because these areas of the brain show a decrease in volume in major depression, the study findings are being looked at with interest as an indication of neuroplasticity and the neurorestorative effects of ECT.

The results of studies relating to the mechanism underlying the effectiveness of ECT continue to be mixed and controversial. Its effectiveness may be a complex dynamic of several effects interacting with one another.

Side Effects

The most common side effects of ECT are temporary memory loss and confusion. Critics of the therapy argue that these changes represent irreversible brain damage. Proponents insist they are temporary and reversible. In one recent study that looked at long-term outcomes of ECT in clients with bipolar I disorder (Haghighi et al., 2016), the evidence supported that 2 years after ECT, cognitive skills and short-term memory were not impaired, whereas mood symptom recurrence had improved regardless of the level of mania.

Other cognitive deficits in the immediate post-ECT period include processing speed, attention, verbal and visual memory, spatial problem-solving, and executive functioning deficits, but Semovska and McLoughlin's meta-analysis demonstrated that most of those resolve within 3 days after treatment and some improve beyond baseline after 15 days (Sharma et al., 2018).

It has been argued that bilateral electrode placement may be more effective than right unilateral (RUL) placement but is associated with more cognitive side effects. However, evidence supports that a more aggressive stimulus in RUL placement improves its efficacy (Pulia et al., 2013).

Risks Associated With Electroconvulsive Therapy

Mortality

In 2011 the American Psychiatric Nurses Association (APNA) advanced a position statement in support of ECT for "severe depression that has been shown to be refractory to medication administration" (APNA, 2015). Studies indicated that the mortality rate from ECT is about 0.002% per treatment and 0.01% for each patient (Boland & Verduin, 2022). Although the occurrence is rare, the major cause of death with ECT is from cardiovascular complications (e.g., acute myocardial infarction or cerebrovascular accident), usually in individuals with previously compromised cardiac status. Assessment and management of cardiovascular disease *before* treatment is vital in the reduction of morbidity and mortality rates associated with ECT.

Memory Loss

Memory impairment almost always occurs to some degree during the course of ECT treatments, but follow-up studies indicate that most patients return to their cognitive baselines after 6 months (Boland & Verduin, 2022). Some clients do report persistent memory impairment and, in most cases, this impairment occurs among patients who showed little improvement with ECT (Boland & Verduin, 2022). Stimulation produced by sine wave (continuous) current resulted in greater short- and long-term deficits than that produced by short-pulse wave (intermittent) current. Sine waveforms are no longer recommended and have primarily been replaced by brief

and, more recently, ultrabrief pulse stimulations (Prudic & Duan, 2017). The risk of post-ECT cognitive deficits is also increased when there are baseline impairments in global cognitive functioning and concurrent use of lithium or medications with anticholinergic effects (Prudic & Duan, 2017). Although the overall risks of enduring memory loss are minimal, the physician should discuss this risk factor with all patients when obtaining informed consent.

Brain Damage

The question of brain damage secondary to ECT treatments has been advanced as a concern by critics of the procedure. The subject has been studied using a variety of brain imaging modalities, and virtually all conclude that there is no evidence of brain damage caused by ECT treatments (Boland & Verduin, 2022; McClintock & Husain, 2011). Previously cited studies on the neurorestorative effects of ECT have argued that this, too, is evidence in contradiction to ideas about brain-damaging effects of ECT.

The Role of the Nurse in Electroconvulsive Therapy

Nurses play an integral role in education, preparation for, and administration of ECT. They provide support before, during, and after the treatment to the patient and family and assist the medical professionals who are conducting the therapy. The nursing process provides a systematic approach to the provision of care for the patient receiving ECT.

Assessment

A complete physical examination must be conducted by the appropriate medical professional before the initiation of ECT. This evaluation should include a thorough assessment of cardiovascular and pulmonary status as well as laboratory blood and urine studies. A skeletal history and x-ray assessment should also be considered.

The nurse may be responsible for ensuring that **informed consent** has been obtained from the patient. Nurses do not actually obtain informed consent, which is the duty of the physician conducting the treatment. "No patient who has the capacity to give voluntary consent should be given ECT without his or her written consent," and clinicians should be aware of local, state, and federal laws governing the use of ECT (Mankad, 2019). If the depression is severe, the patient is clearly unable to consent to the procedure, and relevant laws allow it, permission may be obtained from family or another legally responsible individual. Consent is secured only after the patient or responsible individual acknowledges understanding of the procedure, including possible side effects and potential risks involved.

 The client and family must also understand that ECT is voluntary and that consent may be withdrawn at any time (APA, 2001; Fetterman & Ying, 2011). This kind of education supports patient-centered care.

Nurses may also be required to assess the following:

■ Evidence of suicidal ideation, plan, and means
■ Level of anxiety and fears associated with receiving ECT
■ Thought and communication patterns
■ Baseline memory for short- and long-term events
■ Patient and family knowledge of indications for, side effects of, and potential risks associated with ECT
■ Current and past use of medications
■ Baseline vital signs and history of allergies
■ The patient's ability to carry out activities of daily living

Diagnosis and Outcome Identification

Selection of appropriate nursing diagnoses for the patient undergoing ECT is based on the continual assessment before, during, and after treatment. Selected potential nursing diagnoses with outcome criteria for evaluation are presented in Table 19–1.

Planning and Implementation

ECT treatments are usually performed in the morning. The patient is given nothing by mouth (NPO) for 6 to 8 hours before the treatment. Some institutional policies require that the patient be placed on NPO status at midnight before the treatment day. The treatment team routinely consists of the psychiatrist, anesthesiologist, and two or more nurses.

Nursing interventions before the treatment include the following:

■ Ensuring that the physician and the anesthesiologist have obtained informed consent and that a signed permission form is included in the chart.
■ Ensuring that the most recent laboratory reports (complete blood count, urinalysis) and results of an electrocardiogram (ECG) and x-ray examination are available.
■ Taking and recording vital signs approximately 1 hour before treatment is scheduled. Have the patient void and remove dentures, eyeglasses or contact lenses, jewelry, and hairpins. Following institutional requirements, the patient should change into a hospital gown or, if permitted, into their own loose clothing or pajamas. At this point, it is best for the patient to remain in bed. Side rails may be raised unless prohibited by institutional policy or assessed as unsafe for the individual patient.
■ Administering the pretreatment medication as prescribed by the physician approximately 30 minutes before treatment. The usual order is for atropine sulfate or glycopyrrolate (Robinul) given intramuscularly. Either of these medications may be ordered to decrease secretions (to prevent

TABLE 19-1 Potential Nursing Diagnoses and Outcome Criteria for Patient Receiving ECT	
NURSING DIAGNOSES	**OUTCOME CRITERIA**
Anxiety (moderate to severe) related to impending therapy	Patient verbalizes a decrease in anxiety after explanation of procedure and expression of fears.
Deficient knowledge related to necessity for and side effects or risks of ECT	Patient verbalizes understanding of need for and side effects/risks of ECT after explanation.
Risk for injury related to risks associated with ECT	Patient undergoes treatment without sustaining injury.
Risk for aspiration related to altered level of consciousness immediately after treatment	Patient experiences no aspiration during ECT.
Decreased cardiac output related to vagal stimulation occurring during the ECT	Patient demonstrates adequate tissue perfusion during and after treatment (absence of cyanosis or severe change in mental status).
Impaired memory/acute confusion related to side effects of ECT	Patient maintains reality orientation after ECT treatment.
Self-care deficit related to incapacitation during postictal stage	Patient's self-care needs are fulfilled at all times.
Risk for activity intolerance related to post-ECT confusion and memory loss	Patient gradually increases participation in therapeutic activities to the highest level of personal capability.

aspiration) and counteract the effects of vagal stimulation (bradycardia) induced by ECT.

■ Staying with the patient to help allay fears and anxiety. Maintain a positive attitude about the procedure and encourage the patient to verbalize feelings.

In the treatment room, the patient is placed on the treatment table in a supine position, and the anesthesiologist intravenously administers a short-acting anesthetic. Methohexital (Brevital) is the most commonly used anesthetic, and it may be preferable due to its shorter duration; other alternatives include etomidate, ketamine, alfentanil, and propofol (Boland & Verduin, 2022). Boland and Verduin (2022) identified that the effective duration of seizures in the course of ECT is at least 25 seconds, and APA guidelines recommend a seizure duration of greater than 15 seconds (Luccarelli et al., 2021). Luccarelli and associates reported that, although a shorter-than-desired seizure duration might incline physicians to increase the treatment dose in subsequent treatments, their research found that it actually shortened the length of seizures. Porter and associates (2020) also noted, "for each treatment, the dose of electricity above threshold also has an impact on the degree of cognitive side-effects."

A muscle relaxant, usually succinylcholine chloride, is given intravenously to prevent severe muscle contractions during the seizure, thereby reducing the possibility of fractured or dislocated bones. Because succinylcholine paralyzes respiratory muscles as well, the patient is oxygenated with pure oxygen during and after the treatment, except for the brief interval of electrical stimulation, until spontaneous respirations return (Boland & Verduin, 2022). A blood pressure cuff may be placed on the lower leg and inflated above systolic pressure before the injection of the succinylcholine. Placement of a blood pressure cuff ensures that the seizure activity can be observed in one limb that is unaffected by the muscle relaxant.

An airway/bite block is placed in the patient's mouth, and the patient is positioned to facilitate airway patency. Electrodes are placed (either bilaterally or unilaterally) on the temples to deliver the electrical stimulation.

Nursing interventions during the treatment include the following:

■ Ensuring patency of airway and providing suctioning if needed.

■ Assisting the anesthesiologist with oxygenation as required.

■ Observing readouts on machines monitoring vital signs and cardiac functioning.

■ Providing support to the patient's arms and legs during the seizure.

■ Observing and recording the type and amount of movement induced by the seizure.

After the treatment, the anesthesiologist continues to oxygenate the patient with pure oxygen until spontaneous respirations return. Most patients awaken within 10 or 15 minutes of the treatment and are confused and disoriented; however, some patients will sleep for 1 to 2 hours after the treatment. All patients require close observation in this immediate posttreatment period.

Nursing interventions in the posttreatment period include the following:

■ Monitoring pulse, respirations, and blood pressure every 15 minutes for the first hour, during which time the patient should remain in bed.

■ Positioning the patient on their side to prevent aspiration.

■ Orienting the patient to time and place.

■ Describing what has occurred.

■ Providing reassurance that confusion will subside and memories should return after the course of ECT therapy.

■ Allowing the patient to verbalize fears and anxieties related to receiving ECT.

■ Staying with the patient until they are fully awake, oriented, and able to perform self-care activities without assistance.

■ Providing the patient with a highly structured schedule of routine activities to minimize confusion.

Evaluation

Evaluation of the effectiveness of nursing interventions is based on the achievement of the projected outcomes. Reassessment may be based on answers to the following questions:

■ Was the patient's anxiety maintained at a manageable level?

■ Was the patient/family teaching completed satisfactorily?

■ Did the patient/family verbalize understanding of the procedure, its side effects, and risks involved?

■ Did the patient undergo treatment without experiencing injury or aspiration?

■ Has the patient maintained adequate tissue perfusion during and after treatment? Have vital signs remained stable?

■ With consideration to the individual patient's condition and response to treatment, is the patient reoriented to time, place, and situation?

■ Have all of the patient's self-care needs been fulfilled?

■ Is the client participating in therapeutic activities to his or her maximum potential?

■ What is the patient's level of social interaction?

Careful documentation is an important part of the evaluation process. Some routine observations may be evaluated on flow sheets specifically identified for ECT. However, progress notes with detailed descriptions of patient behavioral changes are essential to evaluate improvement and help determine the number of treatments that will be administered. Continual reassessment, planning, and evaluation ensure that the patient receives adequate and appropriate nursing care throughout the course of therapy. Continuation treatment, defined as treatment for 6 months after remission from an acute episode of illness, is important because "at least half and upwards of 85% of ECT responders in some samples will relapse without continuation treatment, particularly in the first several weeks post-treatment" (Prudic & Duan, 2017, p. 3293). Continuation treatment may include psychotropic medication, medication and continuation ECT, or cognitive therapy. Some research has demonstrated that combining medications with continuation ECT or cognitive therapy is more effective than monotherapy (Prudic & Duan, 2017). Maintenance ECT, defined as ECT treatments after the 6-month continuation treatment period, may be administered either weekly, biweekly, or monthly for relapse prevention. Several controlled studies using maintenance ECT for up to 4 years have demonstrated positive outcomes for patients with depression (Prudic & Duan, 2017).

Other brain stimulation treatments, such as transcranial magnetic stimulation, cranial electrical stimulation, magnetic seizure therapy, and vagal nerve stimulation, provide alternatives that may also be beneficial in treatment-resistant cases, but more research is needed to identify effectiveness and best practices for their use.

 Studies, such as the one previously cited (Pulia et al., 2013), found that changes in the anesthetic agent (from propofol to methohexital) and increasing the dose of electric stimulus demonstrated improvements in the quality of their ECT procedures and efficacy. Pulia, the nurse involved in the research, highlights the active role that nurses can play when collaborating with other members of the health-care team to pursue quality improvement.

Summary and Key Points

- ECT is the induction of a grand mal seizure through the application of electrical current to the brain.
- ECT is a safe and effective treatment alternative for individuals with depression, mania, or schizoaffective disorder who do not respond to other forms of therapy.
- There are no absolute contraindications for ECT, but some conditions have associated increased risks and require close monitoring and attention. Individuals with cardiovascular problems are at higher risk for complications from ECT. Increased intracranial pressure and intracranial lesions impose higher risks for adverse events.
- Other factors that place patients at risk include severe osteoporosis, acute and chronic pulmonary disorders, and high-risk or complicated pregnancy.
- The exact mechanism of action of ECT is unknown, but there are multiple effects on central nervous system activity, including hormones, neuropeptides, neurotrophic factors, and nearly every neurotransmitter. Studies demonstrating an increase in gray matter, particularly in the hippocampal and amygdala areas, and increased connectivity in white matter microstructures suggest neuroplasticity and possibly neurorestorative effects of ECT.
- The most common side effects with ECT are temporary memory loss and confusion.
- Although it is rare, death must be considered a risk associated with ECT. When it does occur, the most common cause is cardiovascular complications.
- There is virtually no evidence supporting the idea that ECT causes permanent brain damage.
- The nurse assists with ECT using the steps of the nursing process before, during, and after treatment.
- Important nursing interventions include ensuring patient safety, managing patient anxiety, and providing adequate patient education.
- Nursing input into the ongoing evaluation of patient behavior is an important factor in determining the therapeutic effectiveness of ECT.

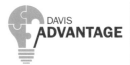 DAVIS **ADVANTAGE** | Go to **Davis Advantage** to complete your learning: strengthen understanding, apply your knowledge, and prepare for the Next Gen NCLEX®.

Review Questions

1. ECT is most commonly prescribed for which of the following?
   a. Bipolar disorder, manic
   b. Paranoid schizophrenia
   c. Major depression
   d. Obsessive-compulsive disorder

2. Which of the following best describes the average number of ECT treatments given and the timing of administration?
   a. One treatment per month for 6 to 12 months
   b. One treatment every other day, three times a week, for a total of 6 to 12 treatments
   c. One treatment three times per week for 6 to 12 months
   d. One treatment every day for a total of 10 to 20 treatments

3. Which of the following conditions increases the risk of adverse events associated with ECT? (Select all that apply.)
   a. Increased intracranial pressure
   b. Recent myocardial infarction
   c. Severe underlying hypertension
   d. Congestive heart failure
   e. Breast cancer

4. The most common side effects of ECT are:
   a. Permanent memory loss and brain damage.
   b. Fractured and dislocated bones.
   c. Myocardial infarction and cardiac arrest.
   d. Temporary memory loss and confusion.

5. Atropine sulfate is administered to a client receiving ECT for what purpose?
   a. To alleviate anxiety
   b. To decrease secretions
   c. To relax muscles
   d. As a short-acting anesthetic

6. Succinylcholine is administered to a client receiving ECT for what purpose?
   a. To alleviate anxiety
   b. To decrease secretions
   c. To relax muscles
   d. As a short-acting anesthetic

Clinical Judgment Questions

7. A client has been ordered ECT and asks the nurse, "Exactly how does ECT work?" Which of the following is the most accurate response by the nurse?
   a. "I'm not allowed to tell you that because that would be informed consent."
   b. "The exact mechanism is unknown, but there are several ways that ECT may have antidepressant effects."
   c. "The administration of a shock to the brain induces memory loss, which will make you forget you are depressed."
   d. "The neuroplasticity affected by seizure activity prevents further brain damage."

8. A client with major depression, who has not responded to antidepressant medication, has been referred for a course of ECT treatments. The client says to the nurse on admission, "I don't want to end up like McMurphy in *One Flew Over the Cuckoo's Nest*! I'm scared!" What is the client's priority nursing diagnosis at this time?
   a. Anxiety related to deficient knowledge about ECT
   b. Risk for injury related to risks associated with ECT
   c. Deficient knowledge related to negative media presentation of ECT
   d. Acute confusion related to side effects of ECT

9. A client, who has been hospitalized for ECT treatments, says to the nurse on admission, "I don't want to have ECT treatments because I heard they cause brain damage." Which of the following statements would be most appropriate by the nurse in response to the client's expression of concern?
    a. "I guarantee you won't have brain damage."
    b. "The doctor knows what he is doing. There's nothing to worry about."
    c. "There is no evidence that ECT causes brain damage but let's talk about what you can expect from the therapy."
    d. "I'm going to stay with you as long as you are scared."

10. What is the priority nursing intervention before starting ECT therapy?
    a. Take vital signs and record.
    b. Have the patient void.
    c. Administer succinylcholine.
    d. Ensure that the consent form has been signed.

References

Abbott, C. C., Gallegos, P., Rediske, N., Lemke, N. T., & Quinn, D. K. (2014). A review of longitudinal electroconvulsive therapy: Neuroimaging investigations. *Journal of Geriatric Psychiatry and Neurology, 27*(1), 33–46. doi:10.1177/0891988713516542

American Psychiatric Association. (2019). *What is electroconvulsive therapy?* https://www.psychiatry.org/patients-families/ect#:~:-text = Electroconvulsive%20therapy%20(ECT)%20is%20a, the%20patient%20is%20under%20anesthesia

American Psychiatric Association (APA). (2001). *The practice of electroconvulsive therapy: Recommendations for treatment, training, and privileging* (2nd ed.). APA.

American Psychiatric Nurses Association. (2015). *APNA position statement: Electroconvulsive therapy.* www.apna.org/i4a/pages/index.cfm?pageid=4448

Boland, R., & Verduin, M. L. (Eds.). (2022). *Kaplan & Sadock's synopsis of psychiatry* (12th ed.). Wolters Kluwer.

Depping, M. S., Nolte, H. M., Hirjak, D., & Thoman, P. A. (2016). Cerebellar volume change in response to electroconvulsive therapy in patients with major depression. *Progress in Neuro-Psychopharmacology and Biological Psychiatry.* doi:10.1016/j.pnpbp.2016.09.007

Elias, A., Thomas, N., & Sackeim, H. A. (2021). Electroconvulsive therapy in mania: A review of 80 years of clinical experience. *American Journal of Psychiatry, 178*(3), 229–39.

Fetterman, T .C., & Ying, P. (2011). Informed consent and electroconvulsive therapy. *Journal of the American Psychiatric Nurses Association, 17*(3), 219–222. doi:10.1177/1078390311408604

Fink, M. (2009). *Electroconvulsive therapy.* Oxford University Press.

Grover, S., Sahoo, S. Rabha, A., & Koirala, R. (2018). ECT in schizophrenia: A review of the evidence. *Acta Neuropsychiatrica, 31*(3), 1–13. doi:10.1017/neu.2018.32

Haghighi, M., Barikani, R., Jahangarda, L., Ahmeadpanaha, M., Bajoghli, H., Sadeghi Bahmani, D., Holsboer-Trachsler, E., & Brand, S. (2016). Levels of mania and cognitive performance two years after ECT in patients with bipolar I disorder—Results from a follow-up study. *Comprehensive Psychiatry, 69*(2016), 71–77. doi:http://dx.doi.org/10.1016/j.comppsych.2016.05.009

Kellner, C. H. (2019). The FDA on ECT: Supporting a vital treatment. *Psychiatric Times, 36*(6). https://www.psychiatrictimes.com/view/fda-ect-supporting-vital-treatment

Luccarelli, J., McCoy, T. H., Seiner, S. J., & Henry, M. E. (2021). Changes in seizure duration during acute course electroconvulsive therapy. *Brain Stimulation, 14*(4), 941–946. https://doi.org/10.1016/j.brs.2021.05.016.

Lyden, H., Espinoza, R.T., Pirnia, T., Clark, K., Joshi, S. H., Leaver, A. M., Woods, R. P., & Narr, K. L. (2014). Electroconvulsive therapy mediates neuroplasticity of white matter microstructure in major depression. *Translational Psychiatry, 4*(4), e380. doi:10.1038/tp.2014.21

Mankad, M. V. (2019). Electroconvulsive therapy. *Medscape.* http://emedicine.medscape.com/article/1525957-overview#a1

McClintock, S. M., & Husain, M. M. (2011). Electroconvulsive therapy does not damage the brain. *Journal of the American Psychiatric Nurses Association, 17*(3), 212–213. doi:10.1177/1078390311407667

Oztav, T., Arslan, M., Corekcioglu, S., Oflezer, C., Canbek, O., & Kurt, E. (2015). Safety of electroconvulsive therapy in pregnancy. *Journal of Mood Disorders, 5*(2), 47–52. doi:10.5455/jmood.20140811124733

Palma, M., Ferreira, B., Borja-Santos, N., Trancas, B., Monteiro, C., & Cardoso, G. (2016). Efficacy of electroconvulsive therapy in bipolar disorder with mixed features. *Depression Research and Treatment, 2016.* doi:http://dx.doi.org/10.1155/2016/8306071

Pirnia, T., Josh, S. H., Leaver, A., & Narr, K. (2016). Electroconvulsive therapy and structural neuroplasticity in neocortical, limbic and paralimbic cortex. *Translational Psychiatry, 6*(6). doi:10.1038/tp.2016.102

Porter, R. J., Baune, B. T., Morris, G., Hamilton, A., Bassett, D., Boyce, P., Hopwood, M. J., Mulder, R., Parker, G., Singh, A. B., Outhred, T., Das, P., & Malhi, G. S. (2020). Cognitive side-effects of electroconvulsive therapy: What are they, how to monitor them and what to tell patients. *British Journal of Psychiatry Open, 6*(3), e40. doi:10.1192/bjo.2020.17

Prudic, J., & Duan, Y. (2017). Electroconvulsive therapy. In Sadock, B. J., Sadock, V. A., & Ruiz, P. (Eds.), *Comprehensive textbook of psychiatry* (10th ed., pp. 3280–3298). Wolters Kluwer.

Pulia, K., Vaidya, P., Jayaram, G., Hayat, M. J., & Reti, I. M. (2013). ECT treatment outcomes following performance improvement changes. *Journal of Psychosocial Nursing and Mental Health Services, 51*(11), 20–25. doi:10.3928/02793695-20130628-02

Reinfeld, S., & Yacoub, A. (2022). An examination of electroconvulsive therapy and delivery of care in delirious mania. *The Journal of ECT.* doi:10.1097/YCT.0000000000000844

Sanghani, S. N., Petrides, G., & Kellner, C. H. (2018). Electroconvulsive therapy (ECT) in schizophrenia: A review of recent literature. *Current Opinion in Psychiatry, 31*, 213–222.

Sartorius, A., Boehringer, A., Demirakca, J., & Ende, G. (2015). Electroconvulsive therapy increases temporal gray matter volume and cortical thickness. *European Neuropsychopharmacology, 26*(3), 506–517. doi:10.1016/j.euroneuro.2015.12.036

Sharma, M. S., Ang-Rabeanes, M., Selek, S., Gajwani, P., & Soares, J. C. (2018). Neuromodulatory options for treatment-resistant depression. *Current Psychiatry, 17*(3), 26–37.

Wilkinson, S. T., Agbese, E., Leslie, D. L., & Rosenheck, R. A. (2018). Identifying recipients of electroconvulsive therapy: Data from privately insured Americans. *Psychiatric Services, 69*(5), 542–548. https://doi.org/10.1176/appi.ps.201700364

The Recovery Model

20

CORE CONCEPTS

Health Promotion:
  Recovery

Clinical Judgment

KEY TERMS

community

health

home

hope

purpose

Tidal Model

WRAP Model

Psychological Recovery
  Model

OBJECTIVES

After reading this chapter, the student will be able to:

1. Define *recovery*.
2. Discuss the 10 guiding principles of recovery as delineated by the Substance Abuse and Mental Health Services Administration.
3. Describe three models of recovery: Tidal Model, WRAP Model, and Psychological Recovery Model.
4. Identify nursing interventions to assist individuals with mental illness in the process of recovery.

For many years, it was believed that individuals with mental illnesses do not recover. Optimistically, the course of the illness was viewed in terms of maintenance, and pessimistically, with the expectation for deterioration. The medical model has primarily focused on the treatment of symptoms, largely with psychotropic medications. However, as Jacobs (2015) noted, despite these available treatments, people with severe mental illness "continue to have residual positive symptoms, negative symptoms and marked cognitive deficits" and as a result, have difficulty "getting their lives back on track." Research suggests that striving for and achieving recovery is, in fact, realistic for many individuals. Although critics of the recovery model argue that it contradicts the scientific medical model, other literature highlights the complementary and integrative potential of both models working collaboratively (Duckworth, 2015; Jacobs, 2015; Vera San Juan et al., 2021).

Vera San Juan and associates (2021), in their systematic review of the research on recovery practices, concluded that more research is needed to clarify a holistic model of recovery. Several aspects that have not been well defined in research include the roles and expectations of informal caregivers and cultural variability in definitions of recovery (most studies have defined recovery in terms of Western understandings of mental health). In addition, the authors found that, although a model that integrates the medical model with personal models of recovery can be complementary, users' testimonies reflect ongoing significant stigma and discrimination in psychiatric practice as barriers.

The concept of recovery is not new. It originally began in the addictions field and was used to describe the process of healing a substance-related disorder. The term has more recently been adopted by mental health professionals who suggest that recovery from mental illness is also possible.

CORE CONCEPT

Recovery
A process of moving toward improvement in health and quality of life.

What Is Recovery?

Several definitions of recovery as it applies to mental illness have been proposed. The Substance Abuse and Mental Health Services Administration (SAMHSA, 2017) suggested the following:

> Recovery from mental health disorders and substance use disorders is a process of change through which individuals improve their health and wellness, live a self-directed life, and strive to reach their full potential. Recovery is built on access to evidence-based clinical treatment and recovery support services for all populations.

Essential to understanding recovery definitions and models is the focus on recovery as an ongoing process rather than a set of interventions with a distinct endpoint.

SAMHSA (2017) suggested that a life in recovery is supported by four major dimensions:

1. **Health** is defined as overcoming or managing one's disease as well as living in a physically and emotionally healthy way.
2. **Home** is defined as a stable and safe place to live.
3. **Purpose** is defined as meaningful daily activities, such as a job, school, volunteerism, family caretaking, or creative endeavors, and the independence, income, and resources to participate in society.
4. **Community** is defined as relationships and social networks that provide support, friendship, love, and hope.

According to SAMHSA (2017), the process of recovery from mental illness and substance use disorders is highly personal and occurs via many pathways. It may include clinical treatment medications, faith-based approaches, peer support, family support, self-care, and other approaches. Recovery is characterized by continual growth and improvement in one's health and wellness that may involve setbacks. Because setbacks are a natural part of life, resilience becomes a key component of recovery. The President's New Freedom Commission on Mental Health

(2003) proposed a transformation within the mental health system to shift the paradigm of care of persons with serious mental illness from traditional medical psychiatric treatment toward the concept of recovery, and the American Psychiatric Association has endorsed a recovery model from a psychiatric services perspective (Sharfstein, 2005).

In a systematic review and synthesis of the various approaches to what has become known as the recovery model, Leamy and associates (2011) identified six recovery processes that form a common foundation for this model: connectedness, hope, optimism about the future, identity, meaning in life, and empowerment. The consumer is empowered to take primary control over decisions about their own care.

Guiding Principles of Recovery

As part of its Recovery Support Strategic Initiative, a year-long effort by SAMHSA and a wide range of partners in the behavioral health-care community and other fields, a working definition of recovery from mental health and substance use disorders (previously stated) was developed. In addition, guiding principles that support the recovery definition were delineated. These principles include the following (SAMHSA, 2012):

- **Recovery emerges from hope:** Hope entails the belief that recovery is a real possibility and that people can and do overcome the internal and external challenges, barriers, and obstacles that confront them. Hope is internalized and can be fostered by peers, families, providers, allies, and others. Hope is the catalyst of the recovery process.
- **Recovery is person-driven:** Self-determination and self-direction are the foundations for recovery as individuals define their own life goals and design their unique paths toward those goals. Individuals optimize their autonomy and independence to the greatest extent possible by leading, controlling, and exercising choice over the services and supports that assist their recovery and resilience. In so doing, they are empowered and provided the resources to make informed decisions, initiate recovery, build on their strengths, and gain or regain control over their lives.
- **Recovery occurs via many pathways:** Individuals are unique with distinct needs, strengths, preferences, goals, culture, and backgrounds (including trauma experiences) that affect and determine their pathways to recovery. Recovery is built on the multiple capacities, strengths, talents, coping abilities, resources, and inherent value of each

individual. Recovery pathways are highly personalized. They may include professional clinical treatment, use of medications, support from families and schools, faith-based approaches, peer support, and other approaches. Recovery is nonlinear and characterized by continual growth and improved functioning that may involve setbacks. Because setbacks are a natural, although not inevitable, part of the recovery process, it is essential to foster resilience for all individuals and families. Abstinence is the safest approach for those with substance use disorders. Use of tobacco and nonprescribed or illicit drugs is not safe for anyone. In some cases, recovery pathways can be enabled by creating a supportive environment. This is especially true for children, who may not have the legal or developmental capacity to set their own course.

■ **Recovery is holistic:** Recovery encompasses an individual's whole life, including mind, body, spirit, and community. This holistic view includes addressing self-care practices, family, housing, employment, education, clinical treatment for mental and substance use disorders, services and supports, primary health care, dental care, complementary and alternative services, faith, spirituality, creativity, social networks, transportation, and community participation. The array of services and supports available should be integrated and coordinated.

■ **Recovery is supported by peers and allies:** Mutual support and mutual aid groups, including the sharing of experiential knowledge and skills as well as social learning, play an invaluable role in recovery. Peers encourage and engage other peers and provide each other with a vital sense of belonging, supportive relationships, valued roles, and community. Through helping others and giving back to the community, individuals help themselves as well. Peer-operated support and services provide important resources to assist people along their journeys of recovery and wellness. In addictions recovery, peer support has long been recognized as foundational, especially in 12-step programs such as Alcoholics Anonymous. In mental health treatment, although formal peer support is a newer approach, the premises are similar. These individuals, sometimes called *peer support specialists,* may be trained or certified in supportive skills, but all share the experience of living with mental illness and can thus provide a unique perspective for support and trust in ongoing relationships. In a fully implemented recovery model, peer support specialists should be considered equal members of the treatment team (Getty, 2015). Professionals can also play an important role in the recovery process by providing clinical treatment and other services that support individuals in their chosen recovery paths. Although peers and allies play an important role for many in recovery, their role for children and youth may be slightly different. Peer supports for families are very important for children with behavioral health problems and can also play a supportive role for youth in recovery.

■ **Recovery is supported through relationships and social networks:** An important factor in the recovery process is the presence and involvement of people who believe in the person's ability to recover; who offer hope, support, and encouragement; and who suggest strategies and resources for change. Family members, peers, providers, faith groups, community members, and other allies form vital support networks. Through these relationships, people leave unhealthy or unfulfilling life roles behind and engage in new roles (e.g., partner, caregiver, friend, student, and employee) that lead to a greater sense of belonging, personhood, empowerment, autonomy, social inclusion, and community participation.

■ **Recovery is culturally based and influenced:** An individual's cultural background, with its many representations (including values, traditions, and beliefs), is key in determining a person's journey and unique pathway to recovery. Support services should be culturally grounded, attuned, sensitive, congruent, and competent, as well as personalized to meet each individual's unique needs. SAMHSA (2017) stressed that mental health and substance addiction services must not only respect and actively address the cultural and linguistic needs of diverse populations but should also reduce disparities in access to care.

■ **Recovery is supported by addressing trauma:** The experience of trauma (such as physical or sexual abuse, domestic violence, war, disaster, and other events) is often a precursor to or associated with alcohol and drug use, mental health problems, and related issues. Services and supports should be trauma-informed to foster safety (physical and emotional) and trust and should promote choice, empowerment, and collaboration.

■ **Recovery involves individual, family, and community strengths and responsibility:** Individuals, families, and communities have strengths and resources that serve as a foundation for recovery. In addition, individuals have personal responsibility for their own self-care and journeys of recovery and should be supported in speaking for themselves. Families and significant others have responsibilities to support their loved ones, especially children and youth in recovery. Communities have responsibilities to provide opportunities and resources to address discrimination and to foster social inclusion and recovery. Individuals in recovery also have a social responsibility and should have the ability to join with peers to speak collectively about their strengths, needs, wants, desires, and aspirations.

■ **Recovery is based on respect:** Community, systems, and societal acceptance and appreciation for people affected by mental health and substance use problems—including protecting their rights and eliminating discrimination—are crucial in achieving recovery. There is a need to acknowledge that taking steps toward recovery may require great courage. Self-acceptance, developing a positive and meaningful sense of identity, and regaining belief in one's self are particularly important.

The recovery model integrates services provided by professionals (e.g., medication, therapy, case management), services provided by consumers (e.g., advocacy, peer support programs, hotlines, mentoring), and services provided in collaboration (e.g., recovery education, crisis planning, community integration, consumer rights education) (Jacobson & Greenley, 2001). Jacobson and Greenley (2001) stated:

> Although many of these services may sound similar to services currently being offered in many mental health systems, it is important to recognize that no service is recovery-oriented unless it incorporates the attitude that recovery is possible and has the goal of promoting hope, healing, empowerment, and connection. (p. 485)

The concepts of consumer-driven care and empowerment are closely related to the concept of patient-centered care that has been advanced by the Institute of Medicine (2003) (now the National Academy of Medicine) as one of the key elements in improving the quality of health care in the future. As this cultural shift evolves, nurses will need to be thoughtful about language and attitudes that support patient-centered recovery models. For example, a traditional goal for a patient has been described as, "Patient will comply with prescribed medication regimen." In a patient-centered recovery model, a more appropriate goal might be stated as, "Patient will discuss preferences, advantages, and disadvantages of psychotropic medication in the management of their illness."

Models of Recovery

There are many evidence-based models of recovery. Three of these models, the Tidal Model, the Wellness Action Recovery Plan (WRAP), and the Psychological Recovery Model, are discussed in this chapter.

The Tidal Model

The Tidal Model was developed in the late 1990s by Phil Barker and Poppy Buchanan-Barker of Newcastle, United Kingdom. It is a mental health nursing recovery model that may be used as the basis for interdisciplinary mental health care (Barker & Buchanan-Barker, 2012). The authors use the power of metaphor to engage with the person in distress. The metaphor of *water* is used to describe how individuals in distress can become emotionally, physically, and spiritually *shipwrecked* (Barker & Buchanan-Barker, 2005) and the term "tidal" was chosen as a metaphor for the ebb and flow of the recovery process: like the rhythm of the waves in which change occurs slowly over time. The Tidal Model was the first recovery model to be developed by nurses in practice, drawing largely on nursing research, and in collaboration with users and consumers of mental health services (Barker & Buchanan-Barker, 2005; Brookes, 2006).

The **Tidal Model** uses a person-centered approach to help people manage problems of human living. Focus is on the individual's personal story, which is where their problems first appeared and where any growth, benefit, or recovery will be found (Barker & Buchanan-Barker, 2015).

Barker and Buchanan-Barker (2005) developed a set of essential values on which the model is based. These values, which they call the *10 Tidal Commitments*, provide practitioners with a philosophical focus for empowering people to make their own life changes rather than health-care professionals trying to manage or control "patient symptoms" (Buchanan-Barker & Barker, 2008). From these commitments, the authors developed the following Tidal Competencies, which reflect the ways the commitments are practiced in the clinical setting:

1. **Value the voice:** The person is encouraged to tell their story. "The person's story represents the beginning and endpoint of the helping encounter, embracing not only an account of the person's distress, but also the hope for its resolution" (Buchanan-Barker & Barker, 2008, p. 95). Practitioner competencies include a capacity to actively listen to the person's story and to help the person record the story in their own words.

2. **Respect the language:** Individuals are encouraged to speak their own words in their own unique way. "The language of the story—complete with its unusual grammar and personal metaphors—is the ideal medium for illuminating the way to recovery. We encourage people to speak their own words in their distinctive voice" (Buchanan-Barker & Barker, 2008, pp. 95–96). Practitioner competencies include helping individuals express

in their own language their understanding of personal experiences through the use of stories, anecdotes, and metaphors.

3. **Develop genuine curiosity:** Nurses and other caregivers "need to express genuine interest in the story so that they can better understand the storyteller and the story. Genuine curiosity reflects an interest in the person and the person's unique experience" (Buchanan-Barker & Barker, 2008, p. 96). Practitioner competencies include showing interest in the person's story, asking for clarification of certain points, and assisting the person in unfolding the story at their own pace.

4. **Become the apprentice:** The individual is the expert on their life story and must be the leader in deciding what needs to be done. "Professionals may learn something of the power of that story, but only if they apply themselves diligently and respectfully to the task by becoming apprentice-minded" (Buchanan-Barker & Barker, 2008, p. 96). Practitioner competencies include developing a plan of care for the individual based on their expressed needs or wishes and helping the individual identify specific problems and ways to address them.

5. **Use the available toolkit:** Attention is directed to the individual's strengths, which are the major tools in the recovery process. "The story contains examples of 'what has worked' for the person in the past or beliefs about 'what might work' for this person in the future. These represent the main tools that need to be used to unlock or build the story of recovery" (Buchanan-Barker & Barker, 2008, p. 96). Practitioner competencies include helping individuals identify what efforts may be successful in relation to solving identified problems and which people in the individual's life may be able to provide assistance.

6. **Craft the step beyond:** The individual and the practitioner decide together what needs to be done immediately. "Any 'first step' is a crucial step, revealing the power of change and potentially pointing toward the ultimate goal of recovery" (Buchanan-Barker & Barker, 2008, p. 96). Practitioner competencies include helping the individual determine what kind of change would represent a step toward recovery and what they need to do to take that first step in the progress toward that goal.

7. **Give the gift of time:** Change happens when the individual and practitioner spend quality time in a therapeutic relationship. "The challenge is using time for things that are important" (Young, 2010, p. 573). Practitioner competencies include acknowledging (and helping the individual understand) the importance of time dedicated to addressing the needs of the individual and the planning and implementing of care.

8. **Reveal personal wisdom:** People often do not realize their own personal wisdom, strengths, and abilities. "A key task for the professional is to help the person reveal and come to value that wisdom, so that it might be used to sustain the person throughout the voyage of recovery" (Buchanan-Barker & Barker, 2008, p. 97). Practitioner competencies include helping individuals identify personal strengths and weaknesses and develop self-confidence in their ability to help themselves.

9. **Know that change is constant:** Because change is a constant in everyone's life, important decisions and choices must be made along the path to recovery for growth to occur. Professional competencies include helping the individual develop awareness of the changes that are occurring and how they have influenced these changes. "The task of the professional helper is to develop awareness of how change is happening and to support the person in making decisions regarding the course of the recovery voyage" (Buchanan-Barker & Barker, 2008, p. 97).

10. **Be transparent:** Transparency is important in the team-building process between the individual and the professional helper. "Professionals are in a privileged position and should model confidence by being transparent at all times, helping the person understand exactly what is being done and why" (Buchanan-Barker & Barker, 2008, p. 97). Professional competencies include ensuring that the individual is aware of the significance of all interventions and that they receive copies of all documents related to the plan of care.

Young (2010) stated:

The Tidal Model is not a typical boxes-and-arrows diagram to use and follow. Instead, it is way of thinking, a paradigm for giving person-centered care that is strength-based, empowering, and relational. (p. 574)

The Wellness Recovery Action Plan (WRAP)

The **WRAP Model,** a system for monitoring, reducing, and eliminating uncomfortable or dangerous physical symptoms and emotional feelings, was developed in 1997 by a group of 30 individuals attending a mental health recovery skills seminar conducted by Mary Ellen Copeland in Vermont. This group (which included persons with psychiatric symptoms, family members, and care providers) determined the need for a system to incorporate the skills and strategies they were learning in the seminar into their everyday lives. Copeland (2001) stated:

> [WRAP] is a structured system for monitoring uncomfortable and distressing symptoms and, through planned responses, reducing, modifying or eliminating those symptoms. It also includes plans for responses from others when a person's symptoms have made it impossible to continue to make decisions, take care of him/herself and keep him/herself safe. (p. 129)

Copeland suggested that all a person needs to begin the program is a system for storing information (e.g., a notebook, computer, or tape recorder), and possibly a friend, health-care provider, or other support person to give assistance and feedback. The program is a stepwise process through which an individual is able to monitor and manage distressing symptoms that occur in daily life. Individuals may be assisted in the process by others (e.g., health-care professionals, significant others, friends), "but to be effective and empowering, the person experiencing the symptoms must develop the plan for himself/herself" (p. 129). Steps of the WRAP process are described in the following sections.

Step 1. Developing a Wellness Toolbox

In this first step, the individual creates a list of tools, strategies, and skills that they have used in the past (or has heard of in the past that they would like to try) to assist in relieving disturbing symptoms. Copeland (2001) offered several examples:

■ Talking to a friend or health-care professional
■ Peer counseling or exchange listening
■ Relaxation and stress reduction exercises
■ Guided imagery
■ Journaling
■ Physical exercise
■ Attending a support group
■ Doing something special for someone else
■ Listening to music

Step 2. Daily Maintenance List

The daily maintenance list is divided into three parts. In Part 1, the individual writes a description of how they feel (or would like to feel) when experiencing wellness (e.g., bright, cheerful, talkative, happy, optimistic, capable). This information is used as a reference point. In Part 2, using the wellness toolbox as a reference, the individual makes a list of things they need to do every day to maintain wellness. This activity is an important part of the plan and must be realistic so as not to set the individual up for failure or create additional frustration. Example items for Part 2 may include the following (Copeland, 2001):

■ Eat three healthy meals and three healthy snacks
■ Drink at least six 8-ounce glasses of water

■ Avoid caffeine, sugar, junk foods, and alcohol
■ Exercise for at least 30 minutes
■ Have 20 minutes of relaxation or meditation time
■ Write in my journal for at least 15 minutes
■ Take medications and vitamin supplements
■ Spend at least 30 minutes enjoying a fun, affirming, or creative activity

In Part 3 of this step, the individual keeps a list of things that need to be done. The individual reads this list daily as a reminder, and items may be considered for accomplishment on any given day at the individual's discretion. For Part 3, Copeland (2001) suggested items such as the following:

■ Spend time with counselor or case manager
■ Make an appointment with health-care professional
■ Spend time with friend or partner
■ Be in touch with my family
■ Spend time with children or pets
■ Buy groceries
■ Do the laundry
■ Write some letters
■ Remember someone's birthday or anniversary

Step 3. Triggers

This step is divided into two parts. In Part 1, the individual lists events or circumstances that, should they occur, would cause distress or discomfort. These triggers are situations to which the individual is susceptible or that have triggered or increased symptoms in the past. Copeland (2001) listed the following examples:

■ The anniversary dates of losses or trauma
■ Being exhausted
■ Work stress
■ Family friction
■ A relationship ending
■ Being judged, criticized, or teased
■ Financial problems
■ Physical illness
■ Sexual harassment or inappropriate sexual behavior
■ Substance abuse

In Part 2, the individual uses items from the wellness toolbox to develop a plan for what to do if triggers interfere with wellness.

Step 4. Early Warning Signs

This step is divided into two parts. Part 1 involves identification of subtle signs that indicate a possible worsening of the situation. Copeland (2001) stated, "Recognizing early warning signs and reviewing them regularly will help the person to become more aware of these early warning signs, allowing the person to take action before the signs worsen" (p. 136). Some types of early warning signs include anxiety, forgetfulness, lack of motivation, avoiding others or isolating, increased irritability, increase in smoking, using substances, or feeling worthless and inadequate. In Part 2, the individual develops a plan for responding to the early warning signs that result in relief or in preventing them from escalating. The plan may include items such as consulting a supporter or counselor, increasing focus on peer counseling, increasing time spent in relaxation exercises, or using other interventions from the wellness toolbox until warning signs diminish.

Step 5. Things Are Breaking Down or Getting Worse

This step is divided into two parts. In Part 1, the individual lists symptoms that indicate that the situation has worsened. In this stage, the symptoms are producing great discomfort, but the individual is still able to take some action on their own behalf. Immediate action is required to prevent a crisis from developing. Symptoms at this stage differ greatly from person to person, and Copeland (2001) stated, "What may mean 'things are breaking down' to one person may mean 'crisis' to another" (p. 137). She lists several examples of symptoms, which may include the following:

■ Irrational responses to events and the actions of others
■ Inability to sleep or sleeping all the time
■ Headaches
■ Not eating or overeating
■ Social isolation
■ Thoughts of self-harm
■ Substance abuse or chain smoking
■ Bizarre behaviors
■ Seeing things that are not there
■ Paranoia

In Part 2, the individual makes a plan that they think will help when the symptoms have worsened to this degree. The plan must be very specific and direct, with clear instructions. Some examples include the following (Copeland, 2001):

■ Call my health-care professional; ask for and follow directions.
■ Arrange for someone to stay with me around the clock until my symptoms subside.
■ Take action so that I cannot hurt myself if my symptoms get worse, such as giving my medication, checkbook, credit cards, and car keys to a previously designated friend for safekeeping.
■ Make sure I do everything on my daily checklist.
■ Have at least two peer counseling sessions daily.
■ Increase use of items from wellness toolbox (e.g., relaxation exercises, physical exercises, creative activities).

Step 6. Crisis Planning

This stage identifies symptoms indicating that individuals can no longer care for themselves, make independent decisions, or keep themselves safe. This stage is multifaceted and meant for use by caregivers on behalf of the individual who developed the plan. It is composed of the following parts (Copeland, 2001, p. 130):

■ Part 1: Gathers information that describes what the person is like when well.
■ Part 2: Identifies the symptoms that indicate when others need to take responsibility for the person's care.
■ Part 3: Provides names of supporters previously identified by the individual to speak on their behalf.
■ Part 4: Includes the name of health-care providers and phone numbers; medications currently using; allergies to medications; medications the individual would prefer to take, if additional medication is necessary; medications that the individual refuses to take.
■ Part 5: Includes the individual's preferred treatments and treatments that they wish to avoid.
■ Part 6: Identifies the individual's preferences in treatment facilities (e.g., home, community care, respite center).
■ Part 7: Identifies acceptable facilities if previous preferences cannot be executed. Facilities to avoid are also indicated.
■ Part 8: Includes an extensive description of what the individual expects from identified supporters who are acting on their behalf during a crisis.
■ Part 9: Consists of a list of indicators, developed by the individual, that communicates to supporters when their services are no longer required. The individual should update this plan periodically when they learn new information or changes their mind about certain situations. Assurance of the use of the crisis plan may be increased if it is notarized and signed in the presence of two witnesses. To further increase its potential for use, the person may appoint a durable power of attorney, although because of the variability of the legality of these documents from state to state, there is no guarantee that the plan will be followed.

Copeland stated:

WRAP is a systematic method for developing skills in self-management and empowerment. It provides a means for individuals with a mental illness to work more collaboratively with health-care providers. It is highly individualized and addresses the unique needs of the person and his/her situation. It is applicable to most any long-term illness/disability or problem situation. These benefits suggest that it can be used more widely and should be introduced as an option for individuals in need of a self-management system. (p. 149)

The Copeland Center for Wellness and Recovery (2020) offers resources for training in the WRAP Model and has established certification programs for peer support specialists and for programs that provide structured WRAP services.

The Psychological Recovery Model

Andresen et al. (2011) defined psychological recovery as "the establishment of a fulfilling, meaningful life and a positive sense of identity founded on hopefulness and self-determination. Psychological recovery is necessary whether mental illness is biologically based or the result of the exacerbation of emotional problems caused by stress" (p. 40). The **Psychological Recovery Model** does not emphasize the absence of symptoms; instead, it focuses on the person's self-determination in the course of their recovery process.

In examining a number of studies, Andresen and associates (2011) identified four components that were consistently evident in the recovery process:

■ **Hope:** Finding and maintaining hope that recovery can occur
■ **Responsibility:** Taking responsibility for one's life and well-being
■ **Self and identity:** Renewing the sense of self and building a positive identity
■ **Meaning and purpose:** Finding purpose and meaning in life

Andresen and associates (2011) conceptualized a five-stage model of recovery, which they defined by integrating into each stage the four components of the recovery process. An explanation of these stages is presented in the following paragraphs.

Stage 1. Moratorium

This stage is identified by dark despair and confusion. "It is called moratorium, because it seems 'life is on hold'" (p. 47).

■ **Hope:** In the moratorium stage, hopelessness prevails. Individuals may even perceive feelings of hopelessness from practitioners when treatment plans emphasize stabilization and maintenance, thereby conveying messages of no hope for recovery.
■ **Responsibility:** In the moratorium stage, the individual feels out of control and powerless to change.
■ **Self and identity:** In the moratorium stage, individuals feel "as though they no longer know who they are as a person" (p. 59). An individual's sense of identity as a valuable and functional member of society can be lost with a diagnosis of mental illness.

■ **Meaning and purpose:** The diagnosis of severe mental illness is a traumatic event that can challenge an individual's fundamental beliefs, creating a loss of meaning and purpose in life.

Stage 2. Awareness

In this stage, the individual realizes that a possibility for recovery exists. Andresen and associates (2011) state, "It involves an awareness of a possible self other than that of 'sick person': a self that is capable of recovery" (p. 47).

■ **Hope:** In the awareness stage, there is a dawn of hope that "life is not over." This feeling of hope may emanate from significant others, professionals, or family members. Individuals may also be inspired by others who have recovered. Hope may also be derived from strong inner determination and personal faith and spirituality.
■ **Responsibility:** In this stage, the individual develops an awareness of the need to take control of their life. Feelings of control and responsibility lead to a sense of personal empowerment that paves the way for recovery.
■ **Self and identity:** In the awareness stage, the individual comes to realize that they are a person independent of the illness. "The person realizes that there still exists an 'intact self' capable of taking action on one's own behalf" (p. 72).
■ **Meaning and purpose:** In the awareness stage, the individual strives for a personal comprehension of the illness, why it occurred, and what the implications of the illness are for their future. "Seeking a meaning of the illness can be explained by theories of cognitive control, in which one tries to understand unexplainable negative events by finding a reason for them" (p. 74).

Stage 3. Preparation

This stage begins with the individual's resolve to begin the work of recovery.

■ **Hope:** In the preparation stage, hope is manifested in the mobilization of personal and external resources to foster self-care and find pathways to goals. This stage includes identifying strengths and weaknesses, gathering knowledge and information, and seeking out available support systems.
■ **Responsibility:** Taking responsibility in the preparation stage involves learning about the effects of the illness and how to recognize, monitor, and manage symptoms. Taking charge of one's life also includes the ability to be independent and take care of basic needs.
■ **Self and identity:** Andresen and associates (2011) stated, "During the preparation stage, the person

takes stock of his or her skills and strengths in order to build on them to rediscover a positive sense of identity" (p. 81). The person is willing to take risks and try new activities to reestablish a sense of self. Lost aspects of self are rediscovered, new aspects are identified, and both are incorporated into a new self-identity.

■ **Meaning and purpose:** The basis for a meaningful life lies in solid core values. "Living according to one's valued directions gives meaning to the work of recovery, and for this reason, some people hold on tenaciously to their goals" (p. 83). Each individual must live by certain tenets that make life personally valuable and enriching. Individuals living with a severe mental illness may require a reordering of priorities and setting of new goals as part of their recovery.

Stage 4. Rebuilding

The hard work of recovery takes place in the rebuilding stage. The individual "takes the necessary steps to work toward his or her goals in rebuilding a meaningful life" (p. 87).

■ **Hope:** In the rebuilding stage, the individual has hope for and looks forward to a more fulfilling life. Realistic goals are set, and the individual is encouraged to pursue the recovery process at their own pace. With each success, hope is renewed.

■ **Responsibility:** "Through setting and working toward goals, the person begins to actively take control of his or her life; not only managing symptoms, but also enlisting social support, improving self-image, handling social pressures, and building social competence" (p. 90). Assuming control of treatment decisions and illness management is an essential part of the recovery process.

■ **Self and identity:** The individual elaborates and enhances their sense of identity, having succeeded in previous stages in developing a positive self-identity separate from the illness and a new sense of self-confidence by succeeding at new activities. In the rebuilding stage, the work of examining core values and working toward value-congruent goals reinforces a positive sense of identity and a commitment to recovery.

■ **Meaning and purpose:** Having realistic goals and a positive sense of identity provides a sense of purpose in life. Individuals need a reason to start each day. Andresen et al. (2011) stated, "Finding meaning [in life] is more than finding a valued occupation, but rather is more akin to finding a way to live. This may include, but is not limited to, vocational goals. It includes examining one's spirituality or philosophy of life. The journey is, in itself, a source of meaning for many" (p. 99).

Stage 5. Growth

The outcome of the psychological recovery process is growth. Although it is called the *final* stage of the Psychological Recovery Model, it is important to remember that this is a dynamic stage and personal growth is a continuous life process.

■ **Hope:** In the growth stage, the individual feels a sense of optimism and hope of a rewarding future. Skills that have been nurtured in the previous stages are applied with confidence, and the individual strives for higher levels of well-being.

■ **Responsibility:** Responsibility entails commitment to the recovery process even in the face of setbacks. In the growth phase, individuals exhibit confidence in managing their illnesses and are resilient when relapses occur. They are empowered by personal input and decision making regarding their treatment.

■ **Self and identity:** The individual in the growth stage has developed a strong, positive sense of self and identity. Andresen et al. (2011) stated, "Many consumers have reported feeling that they are a better person as a result of their struggle with the illness. [In one research study] participants reported developing personal qualities, including strength and courage; more confidence in the self; resourcefulness and responsibility; a new philosophy of life; compassion and empathy; a sense of self-worth; and being happier and more carefree" (pp. 108–109).

■ **Meaning and purpose:** Individuals who have reached the growth stage often report a more profound sense of meaning. Some describe having achieved a sense of serenity and peace; for others, it takes the form of a spiritual awakening. Some individuals find reward in educating others about the experience of mental illness and recovery.

Andresen and associates (2011) stated:

> Recovery from serious mental illness is more than staying out of the hospital or a return to some arbitrary level of functioning. It is more than merely coping with the illness. In [the growth] stage, the notion of wellbeing replaces that of wellness. While wellness implies the absence of illness, wellbeing refers to a more holistic psychological experience of fulfilling life. Although we may not expect everyone (including those who do not have a mental illness) to reach the highest levels of self-actualization, we can expect that all people have the opportunity to develop a positive sense of self and identity and to live a meaningful life filled with purpose and hope for the future. (p. 113)

Several recent qualitative studies have explored the perceived benefits and limitations of recovery-oriented approaches from users' perspectives (O'Keeffe et al., 2018; O'Keeffe et al., 2022; Wood & Alsawy, 2018). A common theme was discrepancy in perceptions about how well recovery approaches were implemented. Wood and Alsawy (2018) found common discrepancies in perceptions about timeliness, mutuality, strength of personal relationships, choice, and knowledge about what was happening. O'Keeffe and associates (2018) interviewed clients 20 years after their first psychotic episode who met criteria for "full functional recovery" and those that did not. They found that among those that did not experience recovery, a common theme was feeling abandoned to the recovery process. The authors concluded that flexibility in using evidence-based medical practices and recovery approaches is necessary and should be grounded in users' readiness and input. In their most recent study, O'Keeffe and associates (2022) found that users' perceptions about the meaning of recovery changed over time, highlighting the importance of ongoing discussion with clients about their perceptions on the meaning of recovery.

Nursing Interventions That Assist With Recovery

It is within the scope of nursing to assist individuals in many aspects of the mental health recovery process. Caldwell and associates (2010) stated:

> Professional nurses must play an active role in client recovery because they are employed in all aspects of service delivery systems, and most times professional nurses are responsible for the delivery and coordination of care. The professional nurse must be center stage in the development and implementation of any action plan involving client recovery. (p. 44)

Nurses have historically held the promotion of wellness within a collaborative nurse–patient relationship as a primary goal. Peplau (1991) described nursing as "a human relationship between an individual who is sick, or in need of health services, and a nurse especially educated to recognize and to respond to the need for help" (pp. 5–6). As previously noted, recovery models are inherently collaborative in that services are provided by professionals, by peers, and cooperatively by both. In addition to patient-centered collaboration, nurses play a key role in providing education about recovery approaches and in exploring potential consequences associated with the patient's decisions about their care, including the process to be implemented should they become a risk of harm to self or others. Examples of interventions and activities in which nurses and patient may collaborate in the patient's journey to recovery are outlined in Table 20–1.

Advocates for the recovery model stress its positive, hopeful, and empowering aspects that have been lacking in traditional medical models of treatment. Critics argue that an individual's subjective perception of recovery does not necessarily validate the quality of health-care interventions, particularly in cases where individuals (as in schizophrenia) may experience the symptom of anosognosia (in which they do not see themselves as having an illness despite apparent, significant symptoms). Duckworth (2015) promoted integrating recovery and medical models of treatment to ensure that scientific processes are used to validate outcomes associated with recovery models of intervention. He cited several examples of recovery-focused treatments that have been supported by research, such as the WRAP Model (previously discussed); dialectical behavioral therapy (DBT) for borderline personality disorders; cognitive enhancement therapy (CET) for improving cognition problems in patients with early stage psychosis; and the National Alliance on Mental Health's (NAMI) Family to Family Program, an education and peer support program for families experiencing mental illness.

TABLE 20–1	**Nurse–Patient Collaboration in the Mental Health Recovery Process**		
	TIDAL MODEL	**WRAP MODEL**	**PSYCHOLOGICAL RECOVERY MODEL**
Assessment	■ The patient tells their personal story ■ The nurse actively listens and expresses interest in the story ■ The nurse helps the patient record their story in patient's own language ■ The patient identifies specific problems they wish to address ■ The nurse and patient identify the patient's strengths and weaknesses	■ The patient develops a wellness toolbox by creating a list of tools, strategies, and skills that have been helpful in the past ■ The patient identifies strengths and weaknesses ■ The nurse provides assistance and feedback	■ The patient is feeling hopeless and powerless ■ The patient seeks the meaning of the illness ■ The nurse helps by offering hope ■ The patient begins to develop an awareness of the need to take control of and responsibility for their life

	TIDAL MODEL	WRAP MODEL	PSYCHOLOGICAL RECOVERY MODEL
TABLE 20-1	**Nurse–Patient Collaboration in the Mental Health Recovery Process—cont'd**		

Interventions	■ The nurse and patient determine what has worked in the past
	■ The patient suggests new tools they would like to try
	■ The patient decides what changes they would like to make and sets realistic goals
	■ The nurse and patient decide what must be done as the first step
	■ The nurse gives positive feedback for the patient's efforts to make life changes and for successes achieved
	■ The nurse encourages the patient to be as independent as possible but offers assistance when required
	■ The nurse gives the "gift of time"
		■ The patient creates a daily maintenance list:
		  ■ How they feel at their best
		  ■ What must be done daily to maintain wellness
		  ■ Reminder list of other things that need to be accomplished
		■ The patient identifies triggers that cause distress or discomfort and identifies what to do if triggers interfere with wellness
		■ The patient identifies signs of worsening symptoms and develops a plan to prevent escalation
		■ The patient identifies when symptoms have worsened and help is needed
		■ The patient identifies when they can no longer care for self and makes decisions (in writing) about treatment issues (what type, who will provide, who will represent patient's interests)
		■ The nurse offers support and provides feedback and assistance when needed
			■ The patient resolves to begin work of recovery
			■ The patient and nurse identify strengths and weaknesses
			■ The nurse assists patient to learn about the effects of the illness and how to recognize, monitor, and manage symptoms
			■ The patient identifies changes they wish to occur and sets realistic goals to rebuild a meaningful life
			■ The patient examines personal spirituality and philosophy of life in search of a meaning and purpose—one that gives them a "reason to start each day"

Outcomes	■ The patient acknowledges that change has occurred and is ongoing ■ The patient feels empowered to manage own self-care ■ The nurse is available for support	■ The patient develops skills in self-management ■ The patient develops self-confidence and hope for a brighter future	■ The patient develops a positive self-identity separate from the illness ■ The patient maintains a commitment to recovery in the face of setbacks ■ The patient feels a sense of optimism and hope of a rewarding future

Many nurse leaders see the changing health-care environment as an opportunity for nurses to expand their roles and assume key positions in education, prevention, assessment, and referral. Nurses are and will continue to be in key positions to assist individuals with mental illness to remain as independent as possible, to manage their illness within the community setting, and to strive to minimize the number of hospitalizations required. A vision of recovery from mental illness exists, and hope, trust, and self-determination should be incorporated into all treatment models.

Summary and Key Points

■ Recovery is characterized by continual growth and improvement in one's health and wellness that may involve setbacks.

■ SAMHSA identified four major dimensions that support a life in recovery: health, home, purpose, and community.

■ The President's New Freedom Commission on Mental Health (2003) proposed to transform the mental health system by shifting the paradigm of care of persons with serious mental illness from traditional medical psychiatric treatment toward the concept of recovery.

■ SAMHSA outlines 10 guiding principles that support recovery:
  ■ Recovery emerges from hope.
  ■ Recovery is person-driven.
  ■ Recovery occurs via many pathways.
  ■ Recovery is holistic.
  ■ Recovery is supported by peers and allies.
  ■ Recovery is supported through relationship and social networks.

- Recovery is culturally based and influenced.
- Recovery is supported by addressing trauma.
- Recovery involves individual, family, and community strengths and responsibility.
- Recovery is based on respect.
■ Many models of recovery exist. Three models discussed in this chapter are the Tidal Model, the Wellness Recovery Action Plan (WRAP) Model, and the Psychological Recovery Model.
■ Nurses work in key positions to assist individuals with mental illness in the recovery process. Interventions may be based on the three recovery models discussed in this chapter.

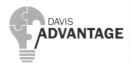

Go to **Davis Advantage** to complete your learning: strengthen understanding, apply your knowledge, and prepare for the Next Gen NCLEX®.

Review Questions

1. Which of the following is a true statement about mental health recovery? (Select all that apply.)
   a. Mental health recovery applies only to severe and persistent mental illnesses.
   b. Mental health recovery serves to provide empowerment to the consumer.
   c. Mental health recovery is based on the medical model.
   d. Mental health recovery is a collaborative process.

2. A nurse is assisting an individual with mental illness recovery using the Tidal Model. Which of the following is a component of this model?
   a. The wellness toolbox
   b. The daily maintenance list
   c. The individual's personal story
   d. Triggers

Clinical Judgment Questions

3. A nurse is assisting an individual with mental illness recovery using the Psychological Recovery Model. The client says to the nurse, "I have schizophrenia. Nothing can be done. I might as well die." In which stage of the Psychological Recovery Model should the nurse assess this individual to be?
   a. The awareness stage
   b. The preparation stage
   c. The rebuilding stage
   d. The moratorium stage

4. A nurse who is helping a client in the preparation stage of the Psychological Recovery Model might include which of the following interventions?
   a. Teach about the effects of the illness and how to recognize, monitor, and manage symptoms.
   b. Help the client identify triggers that cause distress or discomfort.
   c. Help the client establish a daily maintenance list.
   d. Listen actively while the client composes their personal story.

5. A client approaches the nurse and states, "I don't want to go to outpatient group therapy. I don't like groups." Which of these responses by the nurse supports a recovery model focus?
   a. "You need to attend weekly groups to support your ongoing recovery."
   b. "If you don't comply with treatment you will need to be hospitalized again."
   c. "Let's discuss some options for follow-up care and explore the advantages and disadvantages."
   d. "Your psychiatrist recommended this, but we can't force you to comply with treatment."

6. A client with bipolar disorder tells the nurse at the community mental health center that he stopped taking his medication and he is getting so much more done. His speech is rapid, and he admits that he hasn't gotten much sleep but states he is not tired. He doesn't want to be hospitalized because he is "about to save the world" with his new invention. Which of these interventions by the nurse is a priority?

a. Administer an intramuscular dose of his previously ordered medication.

b. Make arrangements for the client to be admitted to the psychiatric hospital.

c. Explore the advantages and disadvantages of medication adherence.

d. Assess the client for risk of harm to self and others.

7. A client is voluntarily admitted to the hospital with suicide ideation and tells the nurse, "I thought I was recovered from this depression, but this is my sixth episode. I guess I can't do anything right so I may as well just end it all." Which of these actions by the nurse is a priority?

a. Educate the client that depression is not an illness that one can recover from; they must instead learn how to manage it with a comprehensive treatment strategy.

b. Educate the client that recovery is a process that sometimes has setbacks and reinforce the individual's decision to seek hospitalization.

c. Assess the client's perception of what they've been doing that "is not right."

d. Assess why the client believes they are depressed.

Communication Exercises

1. Joshua comes to his appointment at the mental health clinic and states, "I can't sit still when I take those medications, so I don't want to take them anymore." Using principles of the recovery model, what are some options for responding to this client?

2. Kelly is a war veteran who was admitted to inpatient hospitalization with depression, alcohol addiction, and complaints of troubling nightmares. She states, at the admission assessment, "I don't trust any 'mental health gurus.' You can't possibly understand what I've been through." How will you respond, and what principles of the recovery model will guide your response?

References

Andresen, R., Oades, L. G., & Caputi, P. (2011). *Psychological recovery: Beyond mental illness.* Wiley.

Barker, P. J., & Buchanan-Barker, P. (2005). *The tidal model: A guide for mental health professionals.* Brunner-Routledge.

Barker, P. J., & Buchanan-Barker, P. (2012). Tidal model of mental health nursing. *Current Nursing.* https://currentnursing.com/nursing_theory/Tidal_Model.html

Barker, P. J., & Buchanan-Barker, P. (2015). *The tidal model: Reclaiming stories, recovering lives.* www.tidal-model.com

Brookes, N. (2006). Phil Barker: The tidal model of mental health recovery. In Tomey, A. M., & Alligood, M. R. (Eds.), *Nursing theorists and their work* (6th ed., pp. 696–725). Elsevier.

Buchanan-Barker, P., & Barker, P. J. (2008). The tidal commitments: Extending the value base of mental health recovery. *Journal of Psychiatric and Mental Health Nursing, 15*(2), 93–100. doi:10.1111/j.1365-2850.2007.01209.x

Caldwell, B. A., Sclafani, M., Swarbrick, M., & Piren, K. (2010). Psychiatric nursing practice and the recovery model of care. *Journal of Psychosocial Nursing, 48*(7), 42–48. doi:10.3928/02793695-20100504-03

Copeland Center for Wellness and Recovery. (2020). *Certified peer specialist training.* https://copelandcenter.com/our-services/certified-peer-specialist-training-cps

Copeland, M. E. (2001). Wellness recovery action plan: A system for monitoring, reducing and eliminating uncomfortable or dangerous physical symptoms and emotional feelings. In Brown, C. (Ed.), *Recovery and wellness: Models of hope and empowerment for people with mental illness* (pp. 127–150). Haworth Press.

Duckworth, K. (2015). *Science meets the human experience: Integrating the medical and recovery models.* https://www.nami.org/Blogs/NAMI-Blog/April-2015/Science-Meets-the-Human-Experience-Integrating-th#

Getty, S. M. (2015). Implementing a mental health program using the recovery model. *OT Practice 20*(3), 1–8.

Institute of Medicine. (2003). *Health professions education: A bridge to quality.* Institute of Medicine.

Jacobs, K. S. (2015). Recovery model of mental illness: A complementary approach to psychiatric care. *Indian Journal of Psychological Medicine, 37*(2), 117–119. doi:10.4103/0253-7176.155605

Jacobson, N., & Greenley, D. (2001). What is recovery? A conceptual model and explication. *Psychiatric Services, 52*(4), 482–485. doi:http://dx.doi.org/10.1176/appi.ps.52.4.482

Leamy, M., Bird, V., LeBoutillier, C., Williams, J., & Slade, M. (2011). Conceptual framework for personal recovery in mental health: Systematic review and narrative synthesis. *British Journal of Psychiatry, 199,* 445–452. doi:10.1192/bjp.bp.110.083733

O'Keeffe, D., Sheridan, A., Kelly, A., Doyle, R., Madigan, K., Lawlor, E., & Clarke, M. (2018). "Recovery" in the real world: Service user experiences of mental health service use and recommendations for change 20 years on from a first episode psychosis. *Administration and Policy in Mental Health, 45*(4), 635–648. https://doi.org/10.1007/s10488-018-0851-4

O'Keeffe, D., Sheridan, A., Kelly, A., Doyle, R., Madigan, K., Lawlor, E., & Clarke, M. (2022). A qualitative study exploring personal recovery meaning and the potential influence of clinical recovery status on this meaning 20 years after a first-episode psychosis. *Social Psychiatry & Psychiatric Epidemiology, 57*(3), 473–483. doi:10.1007/s00127-021-02121-w

President's New Freedom Commission on Mental Health. (2003). *Achieving the promise: Transforming mental health care in America.* govinfo.library.unt.edu/mentalhealthcommission/index.htm

Sharfstein, S. (2005). Recovery model will strengthen psychiatrist-patient relationship. *Psychiatric News, 40*(20), 3. doi:10.1176/pn.40.20.00400003

Substance Abuse and Mental Health Services Administration (SAMHSA). (2012). SAMHSA's working definition of recovery: 10 guiding principles of recovery. [Brochure]. SAMHSA.

Substance Abuse and Mental Health Services Administration (SAMHSA). (2017). *Recovery and recovery support.* https://www.samhsa.gov/recovery

Vera San Juan, N., Gronholm, P. C., Heslin, M., Lawrence, V., Bain, M., Okuma, A., & Evans-Lacko, S. (2021). Recovery from severe mental health problems: A systematic review of service user and informal caregiver perspectives. *Frontiers in Psychiatry, 12,* 712026. doi:10.3389/fpsyt.2021.712026

Wood L., & Alsawy S. (2018). Recovery in psychosis from a service user perspective: A systematic review and thematic synthesis of current qualitative evidence. *Community Mental Health Journal, 54*(6), 793–804. doi: 10.1007/s10597-017-0185-9

Young, B. B. (2010). Using the tidal model of mental health recovery to plan primary health care for women in residential substance abuse recovery. *Issues in Mental Health Nursing, 31*(9), 569–575. doi:10.3109/01612840.2010.487969

Classical References

Peplau, H. E. (1991). *Interpersonal relations in nursing: A conceptual frame of reference for psychodynamic nursing.* Springer.

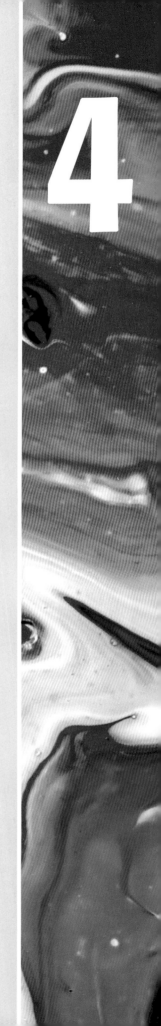

U N I T

4

Nursing Care of Patients With Alterations in Psychosocial Adaptation

21

Caring for Patients With Mental Illness and Substance Use Disorders in General Practice Settings

CORE CONCEPTS

Health Promotion:
Screening, referral

Professional Behavior:
Assessment,
Stigmatization

Caring: Patient-centered
care

KEY TERMS

diagnostic overshadowing
nonsuicidal self-injuring
behavior (NSSIB)
patient-centered care
retraumatization

screening
Screening, Brief Intervention,
and Referral to Treatment
(SBIRT)
social distancing

stigmatization
suicide prevention
trauma-informed care

OBJECTIVES
After reading this chapter, the student will be able to:

1. Recognize the effect of inadequate assessment, treatment, and referral for the patient with mental health and substance use disorders.
2. Discuss the evidence identifying the need for further mental health and substance use disorder education among health-care providers in primary care and other nonpsychiatric settings.
3. Describe essential elements in appropriate screening and referral of patients

with mental health and substance use disorders.
4. Analyze barriers that influence the screening, intervention, and referral process for patients with mental health and substance use concerns.
5. Describe essential aspects of the nurse's role in providing care for patients with psychiatric/mental health and substance use disorders in general practice.

The individual with mental illness has historically been misunderstood, misdiagnosed, and mistreated (see Chapter 2, "Mental Health and Mental Illness: Historical and Theoretical Concepts"). Current examples confirm that this problem is ongoing. In one case, a patient came into the emergency department with garbled speech that made their responses to questions difficult to comprehend. The patient was known to be a homeless person with chronic schizophrenia and was quickly transferred to a

psychiatric hospital. Once there, the patient's right-sided weakness, vital signs, and difficulty speaking were recognized as evidence of a cerebrovascular accident.

In another case, a hospitalized patient with schizophrenia reported to the nurse that there was a rock band playing music in his body and the drummer was playing in his chest; initially, these symptoms were identified as delusional thinking. However, after further assessment, it was determined that the patient was having a heart attack. Real examples of potentially fatal misdiagnoses like these are far too common.

Patients presenting with symptoms such as pain, lack of energy, and feelings of helplessness could be experiencing a variety of medical conditions, but these can also be signs of depression. If effective screening is not conducted, the patient may be at risk for worsening depression and suicide.

Nurses who choose to work in nonpsychiatric settings are *the* frontline responders in recognizing, intervening, and referring patients with neuropsychiatric illness for further treatment. Studies reveal, however, that attitudes, lack of education about the need for screening, and issues related to accessing services are all influential in lack of appropriate intervention to meet the needs of this population.

Clearly, there are genetic, neurological, neurochemical, and environmental influences in the etiology of mental illness that differentiate clinical illness from the range of emotions and behavior that are a part of general human experience. However, without specific education and appreciation for these symptoms as distressing signs of neurological illness, patients will continue to remain at risk for lack of treatment or mistreatment of both psychiatric and other medical disorders. Nurses must take the lead in educating other health-care professionals and the public, combating stigmatization of individuals with mental illness, recognizing neuropsychiatric symptoms, conducting appropriate screening, and collaborating effectively with other health-care providers to ensure appropriate referral when specialized mental health and addictions treatment are needed. This chapter explores the nurse's role and the evidence for education, screening, and referral needs in various nonpsychiatric settings.

The Need for Education of Health-Care Providers

Evidence supports that individuals with significant mental illness die anywhere from 10 to 25 years earlier than the general population, and most of those deaths are related to preventable or treatable causes (Gomes et al., 2015; Momen et al., 2022; Plana-Ripoll et al., 2019; Stefancic et al., 2021). The increased risk of mortality for individuals with mental illness may be related to **diagnostic overshadowing,** which describes a phenomenon in which a person's physical symptoms are attributed to their mental illness. For example, Gomes and associates reviewed studies showing that patients with both a mental illness and a cardiovascular condition received one-half as many follow-up interventions after a heart attack as those without a concurrent mental illness. This finding is

significant because many patients with mental illnesses are at greater risk for cardiovascular disease due to genetic, lifestyle, or environmental issues or to adverse effects from psychotropic medications.

Other studies have demonstrated that patients with mental illness who come to general health-care settings are at risk for lack of treatment or appropriate referral. This risk may be related to lack of knowledge about symptom detection (by patients and health-care providers), stigmatization, and lack of awareness about counseling and referral services (Bay et al., 2016; Betz et al., 2013; Hallyburton, 2022). These realities have led many people with mental illness to avoid seeking health care altogether. As we learn more about the progression and prognosis of illnesses such as schizophrenia, it has become apparent that early intervention is critical, because repeated psychotic episodes may have a cumulative damaging effect on the brain (see Chapter 24, "Schizophrenia Spectrum and Other Psychotic Disorders," for further discussion). The barriers to early intervention are compounded for individuals with schizophrenia because one of the neurological symptoms in this disorder is *anosognosia* (a lack of awareness or recognition of symptoms). During acute psychotic episodes, these individuals—who are suspicious of people and the surrounding environment and often unaware that they have a mental illness—may be brought to the emergency department against their will. It is not difficult to imagine how frightening this scenario might be for such an individual. Nurses in emergency settings play a key role in recognizing this patient as one who is experiencing significant neurological symptoms requiring immediate and ongoing care. Unfortunately, this patient may instead be stigmatized as one who is neither "really ill" nor requiring complex and compassionate intervention. The consequence of these attitudes for the patient is prolonged suffering and sometimes early death.

Nurses in any nonpsychiatric setting must also have a clear working knowledge of the effect of depressive disorders in treating other physical illnesses. Depression, a mental illness with multiple etiologies and symptoms, is estimated to affect 1 in 3 women and 1 in 5 men during their lifetime (Dattani, 2022) and is associated with many other chronic health conditions (National Institute of Mental Health [NIMH], 2021) (see Chapter 25, "Depressive Disorders," for further discussion). In addition, Boland and Verduin (2022) noted that bipolar disorder, which is characterized by bouts of depression and mania, most often starts with depression (75% of the time in women and 67% of the time in men) (see Chapter 26, "Bipolar and Related Disorders," for further discussion of these disorders). Knowledge of the distinction between depressive disorder and bipolar disorder has important implications for medication management and ongoing treatment. With such a high prevalence, the potentially disabling effects of untreated or mistreated illness, and the fact that suicide is a risk at all times in depressive illness, it seems apparent that all patients, in any encounter with health-care professionals, should be screened for evidence of depression and risk for suicide. But this has not been the case.

In addition, there are links between depression and many other diseases. Depression not only increases the risk for other illnesses but is associated with poorer outcomes. Evidence has demonstrated that depression is a risk factor for cardiovascular disease, metabolic syndrome, diabetes, dementia, asthma, arthritis, and hyperlipidemia (Bica et al., 2017). The risk of poorer outcomes has implications for both the medical condition and the depression and ultimately for the risk of suicide. Across the nation, the incidence of suicide has reached such epidemic proportions that it should be an assessment skill that every nurse is confident in performing (see Chapter 16, "Suicide Prevention," for further discussion of this topic). The importance of this knowledge base and appropriate screening may seem to be an obvious need in primary care and community settings, but it is equally important in medical settings within hospitals. Suicide in hospital settings is a sentinel event that is frequently reported to The Joint Commission, an organization that accredits hospitals and health-care systems. Williams and associates (2018) found that 25% of all inpatient suicides occur in nonbehavioral health settings and that lack of adequate risk assessment is influential. The authors excluded analysis of inpatient settings that were not hospitals (e.g., nursing homes, hospice facilities, and substance use rehabilitation centers), so the percentages of suicides in nonpsychiatric health-care settings may be higher than reported in this study.

Individuals affected by the national opioid epidemic and with other substance use disorders commonly seek care first in general medical and community practice settings before they are treated in psychiatric or addictions treatment settings. People often die of overdose before they ever reach an emergency department, which has prompted a nationwide effort to educate not only health-care professionals but the general public about how to recognize symptoms of overdose and administer treatment, such as naloxone and rescue breathing, to treat associated respiratory depression. (See Chapter 23, "Substance-Related and Addictive Disorders," for further discussion of this topic.)

Treatment for sleep disorders is often sought in primary care settings and sleep clinics, but it is essential to note that these disorders are contributing factors or sequelae associated with many psychiatric disorders. The *Diagnostic and Statistical Manual of Mental Disorders, Fifth Edition, Text Revision* (*DSM-5-TR;* American Psychiatric Association [APA], 2022) dedicates a chapter to the diagnosis of various sleep–wake disorders, noting that sleep disorders are often accompanied by depression, anxiety, and cognitive changes and are established risk factors for the development of mental illnesses, including substance use disorders. In addition, sleep disturbances may be an early symptom of a developing episode of mental illness that, with proper assessment and identification, allows for early intervention to prevent a full-blown episode. Perhaps most importantly, "multiple studies have found that the symptom of insomnia may increase the risk for suicidal thoughts, suicidal behavior, and death" (APA, 2022, p. 409).

Cognitive behavior therapy, specifically for the treatment of insomnia (CBT-I), is an evidence-based psychological treatment that has demonstrated effectiveness in treating primary insomnia and insomnia associated with comorbid depression, anxiety, post-traumatic stress disorder (PTSD), substance use disorders, and many other medical conditions (Alimoradi et al., 2022; Ham et al., 2020; Taylor & Pruiksma, 2014). It has been identified as the gold standard treatment for insomnia (without the side effects associated with sedative-hypnotic medication), but as Koffel and associates (2018) noted, systematic access barriers, lack of screening, and lack of knowledge about this evidence-based resource have limited referral for this treatment. It is clear that nurses play key educational, screening, and referral roles in community, primary, medical, and long-term care settings.

Psychiatric nursing is an essential component of basic undergraduate nursing curricula. *Every* nurse needs education about recognition of mental illnesses to perform competently in *any* nursing role. Studies have shown that when health-care professionals in nonpsychiatric settings are trained to feel confident in their ability to recognize the need for screening and use valid, reliable screening tools, rates of intervention and referral for mental health treatment improve. Although nurses typically enter general practice with general knowledge about mental illness recognition, communication strategies, and basic interventions, additional variables influence how these skills and knowledge are incorporated into practice. Three of these variables are the availability of screening tools, knowledge and accessibility of referral sources, and attitudes about the patient with mental illness or substance use disorders.

Screening

Many valid and reliable screening tools exist for identifying mental illnesses and substance use disorders. In psychiatry, the purpose of **screening** is to identify clinically significant symptoms that require further assessment and intervention. Tools that are completed by patient self-report are time efficient, but their use depends on the clinician's recognition of symptoms that support the need for screening and a belief that screening is essential for adequate identification and management of mental health and substance use issues.

Evidence supports that use of screening tools is better than clinical judgment alone in diagnosis of mental illness (Jackman et al., 2016; Mitchell et al., 2011; Préville et al., 2004; Singer et al., 2011) and may help reduce the risk that an individual's illness is missed completely or incorrectly identified (i.e., a false-negative result).

In one study, Horowitz and associates (2013) developed a two-item nursing screen for suicide risk in any medical setting. The need was identified after The Joint Commission issued a "Sentinel Event" alert highlighting the importance of suicide risk assessment in all medical settings. The screen asked the patient two questions: "In the past month, have you had thoughts about suicide?" and "Have you ever made a suicide attempt?" A "yes" response to either question prompted a third question, "Are you having thoughts of suicide right now?" Their study demonstrated improvement in identification of medical-surgical patients who may be at risk for suicide (4% were referred for additional evaluation) and highlighted the time efficiency of such screening tools (this tool took about 2 minutes to complete). Again, critical to the success of any strategy is the nurse's belief that this kind of screening is essential. Endorsement for the necessity of this screening by accrediting bodies such as The Joint Commission reinforces its essential role for nurses.

Fortunately, more research is being done to identify the need for better screening for mental illness and substance misuse in nonpsychiatric settings. The need for screening tools for depression and anxiety is particularly urgent. Roberge et al. (2016) conducted a qualitative study based on the recognition that depression and anxiety in patients seeking primary care for chronic diseases are linked to morbidity and mortality. Both patients and clinicians in this study identified a need for holistic care that includes screening and management of mental illness. Another study (Mollard et al., 2015) identified an increase in the incidence of postpartum depression among women in rural areas (a trend also seen internationally), and they concluded that nurses should be the lead change agents in improving policy around screening for depression in this population. A third study (Garcia de la Garza et al., 2021) noted that screening the general population for suicide risk is essential, because over a third of individuals making nonfatal suicide attempts do not seek mental health treatment. Research efforts have identified the need for improved neuropsychiatric screening in a variety of other settings as well, including home care, community care, long-term care, medical-surgical care, oncology care, geriatric care, and child-adolescent care (Bica et al., 2017; Grundberg, 2016; Koposov et al., 2017; Langdon et al., 2013; McGovern & Selwyn, 2014; Thompson et al., 2008).

Nurse managers are integral in promoting the importance of mental health and substance use screening by educating and equipping their staff nurses with screening tools that are valid, reliable, time efficient, and user friendly. Staff nurses must adopt an attitude that screening for mental illness is critical to their success in interventions for the physical illness that brought the patient to their nonpsychiatric setting and for referring patients to ongoing evaluation and treatment for the mental illness itself.

Many resources exist that identify valid and reliable screening tools for use in clinical practice settings. Moran and associates (2018), in a systematic review of the literature, identified 24 tools that are psychometrically tested and appropriate for use in primary care settings. The National Alliance on Mental Illness (NAMI) (2022) stresses the importance of screening youth and young adults:

> Approximately 50% of lifetime mental health conditions begin by age 14 and 75% begin by age 24. At the same time, the average delay between when symptoms first appear and intervention is approximately 11 years. Mental health screenings allow for early identification and intervention and help bridge the gap.

The American Academy of Pediatrics publishes materials and assessment tools for children, adolescents, and adults (American Academy of Pediatrics, 2022) that were chosen because of their evidence-based reliability and accessibility. Many screening tools are free to use and widely accessible, although some are copyrighted, proprietary, and associated with a fee for use.

Priority Issues for Screening in Any Health-Care Setting

The importance of screening for depression has already been discussed with regard to depression's prevalence, its link to the development of other diseases, and its association with poorer outcomes. Other issues that arise as part of a general health assessment may trigger the need for screening and further assessment, but some issues are considered so prevalent and so high risk that they are priorities to screen for in all patients. Three of these issues are trauma, suicide risk, and substance use disorders.

Trauma History

Screening for violence and trauma history is now well accepted as an essential psychosocial issue that should be conducted with patients when they first enter a health-care setting. Even in the early 1990s, violence and trauma were identified in nursing literature as growing areas of concern that are linked to a high risk for injury, unhealthy coping mechanisms, and other illnesses such as arthritis, irritable bowel syndrome, and chronic pain (Hoff & Rosenbaum, 1994), as well as having implications in surgical outcomes (Schofferman et al., 1992). Hoff and Rosenbaum (1994) also noted that although violence and trauma cross gender boundaries (as well as racial, ethnic, class, and national boundaries), most individuals affected by violence are women and children. Hoff and Ross (1993) estimated that up to 75% of female psychiatric patients have a current or past history of abuse. The classic study on adverse childhood experiences (ACEs) linked trauma in childhood to significant cognitive, social, psychological, and neurobiological changes that contribute to many physical and mental problems and early death (Felitti et al., 1998). These studies identified the critical importance of screening for trauma history. However, because many individuals with this history may be in denial, frightened about the consequences of sharing information, or experiencing guilt or shame, they may be reluctant to disclose information about their circumstances and history unless direct screening takes place. It is critical that nurses conduct screenings in private and communicate with a compassionate, nonjudgmental attitude. Pardee and associates (2017), in their review of ACE assessment tools, concluded that primary care nurse practitioners need more education and more efficient assessment tools to ensure that this type of screening is accomplished in primary care settings.

As research and nursing practice have focused more attention on the importance of screening for trauma and interpersonal violence history, we have also learned a great deal more about the significance of **trauma-informed care**—care that incorporates sensitivity to the effect of trauma history on current behavior and relationships. Patients are at risk for **retraumatization** if trauma screening is conducted without awareness or sensitivity to the effect of that trauma on the individual's current functioning (see Chapter 28, "Trauma- and Stressor-Related Disorders," and Chapter 34, "Survivors of Abuse or Neglect," for further discussion of these topics). Given the high prevalence of trauma, it is incumbent on nurses to practice trauma-informed care in every aspect of nursing intervention.

Risk for Suicide

National attention to the increasing suicide rates across the life span, among military personnel, and within specific ethnic groups and communities has raised awareness of the critical needs for screening and intervention among lay people and health-care providers alike. Military personnel with PTSD may present in medical settings with physical complaints, reports of nightmares, and substance use disorders, but unless health-care professionals specifically screen for suicide risk and warning signs, this potentially fatal risk may go undetected. The older adult with depression is another population that more often presents with physical complaints in primary care settings and may not even consider discussing depression, loneliness, or thoughts of suicide unless specifically asked.

Recent studies (Chen et al., 2020; Fuller-Thomson et al., 2020; Kõlves et al., 2021; Ramchand et al., 2021) have highlighted an increased risk for suicide among patients with Parkinson's disease; autism; women with attention deficit-hyperactivity disorder; and lesbian, gay, and bisexual adults, all of whom are more likely to be seen in primary care rather than in psychiatric settings. As with trauma victims, the facts that people at risk for suicide may not be forthcoming with this information; that suicide is a high-risk, potentially fatal problem; and that risk for suicide is a highly prevalent concern reinforce the need for universal screening.

One very important caution about screening for suicide risk that we are learning from ongoing research in **suicide prevention** is that although brief screening may open the door for discussion with a patient, it is not enough to prevent suicide in some individuals. In other words, just because a patient responds "no" to the question "Are you having thoughts of taking your own life?" does not mean that they are not at risk. Jobes (2015) suggested that in spite of the numerous brief screening tools that are available, they have been used more often as defensive medicine than actually contributing to suicide prevention. Defensive medicine refers to doing the minimum number of interventions needed to "meet the letter of the law." In this case, it would mean asking the patient the previously mentioned question, documenting that the patient denies suicidal ideation, and then assuming that we have "covered the necessary bases." As Jobes (2015) pointed out, research has demonstrated that brief screening may be inadequate because of the many variables that influence a person's decision to take their own life and the fact that ideation (as well as the intent to act on ideation) can change in intensity over time.

Patients in primary care settings with depression, substance misuse issues, or chronic pain should be recognized as having *identified risk factors* for suicide and should be screened carefully. In addition, given the current prevalence rates of suicide, nurses should develop the skill to carefully screen for suicide risk with every patient in every health-care setting. Establishing trust with the patient, developing a collaborative relationship, and displaying a willingness to discuss this issue from various vantage points (such as past history, recent history, immediate risk, and strength of the individual's intent to harm themselves) are all essential elements in identifying the need for referral and the level of care required for the patient's safety.

Nonsuicidal self-injuring behavior (NSSIB) is a related and complex phenomenon that is increasingly being seen in nonpsychiatric settings and challenges the nurse's skills to discern how to screen and when to refer for more intensive treatment. Kameg and associates (2013) reported that although NSSIB is typically a nonlethal, repetitive act used to reduce distress rather than end one's life, the individual who uses NSSIB is more likely to consider or attempt suicide than non–self-injurers. Therefore, individuals who exhibit NSSIB require screening for suicide risk. The authors also state that a patient who is identified as having comorbid psychiatric symptoms such as labile mood, dysphoria, anxiety, depersonalization, anhedonia, or borderline personality disorder should be referred to specialized mental health-care services. Those who exhibit NSSIB in response to command hallucinations should be considered in need of immediate medical attention. Several tools are available to screen for self-harm. Kameg and associates (2013) noted that the Self-Harm Inventory (Box 21–1) can be completed within 5 minutes and screens for borderline personality disorder symptoms as well as a variety of self-harm behaviors.

Substance Use Disorders

In the United States, rates of opioid misuse have reached epidemic levels, and rates of methamphetamine use have also increased significantly. Opioid addiction can lead to overdose, and methamphetamine withdrawal is associated with an increased risk for suicide. In addition, the numerous physical and psychological consequences of long-term alcohol use are well documented. All of these facts underscore the importance of screening for substance use disorders in nonpsychiatric settings. Although many tools exist to screen for substance misuse, the extent of their use in general practice settings varies. **Screening, Brief Intervention, and Referral to Treatment (SBIRT)** (SAMHSA, 2022) is an evidence-based approach that can be used in emergency departments, trauma centers, primary care, and other community settings. SAMHSA (2022) describes the SBIRT approach as follows:

■ Screening quickly assesses the severity of substance use and identifies the appropriate level of treatment.
■ Brief intervention focuses on increasing insight and awareness regarding substance use and motivation toward behavioral change.
■ Referral to treatment provides those identified as needing more extensive treatment with access to specialty care.

One study (Rahm et al., 2015) sought to identify why routine screening does not occur for an issue that has been so clearly identified as a public health concern. The authors, using SBIRT as the preferred model, asked primary care providers (including nurses, physicians, mental health specialists, and others) and patients to identify barriers to implementation of this approach. Although patients supported universal screening, they also noted that privacy concerns may be an issue. Privacy is an important consideration for nurses who are screening patients for substances of misuse. Many patients may deny using substances, particularly illegal substances, because they fear legal consequences. For example, many states consider substance use during pregnancy to be child abuse with legal consequences, and 25 states and the District of Columbia require health professionals to report suspected prenatal drug use (Guttmacher Institute, 2022), which may deter some women from seeking prenatal care. Establishment of trust, clear communication about why this information is being collected, and how it will be used are important first steps in the screening process.

The health-care providers in Rahm and associates' study (2015) noted that another barrier to implementation of screening processes for mental health issues and substance use disorders is competing workload

BOX 21–1 The Self-Harm Inventory

Instructions: Please answer the following questions by checking either "Yes" or "No." Check "Yes" only to those items where you have intentionally, or on purpose, tried to hurt yourself.

Yes   No   Have you ever intentionally, or on purpose, done any of the following:

_____   _____   1. Overdosed? (If yes, number of times _____)
_____   _____   2. Cut yourself on purpose? (If yes, number of times _____)
_____   _____   3. Burned yourself on purpose? (If yes, number of times _____)
_____   _____   4. Hit yourself? (If yes, number of times _____)
_____   _____   5. Banged your head on purpose? (If yes, number of times _____)
_____   _____   6. Abused alcohol?
_____   _____   7. Driven recklessly on purpose? (If yes, number of times _____)
_____   _____   8. Scratched yourself on purpose? (If yes, number of times _____)
_____   _____   9. Prevented wounds from healing?
_____   _____   10. Made medical situations worse on purpose (e.g., skipped medication)?
_____   _____   11. Been promiscuous (i.e., had many sexual partners)? (If yes, how many?_____)
_____   _____   12. Set yourself up in a relationship to be rejected?
_____   _____   13. Abused prescription medication?
_____   _____   14. Distanced yourself from God as punishment?
_____   _____   15. Engaged in emotionally abusive relationships? (If yes, number of _____relationships? _____)
_____   _____   16. Engaged in sexually abusive relationships? (If yes, number of relationships? _____)
_____   _____   17. Lost a job on purpose? (If yes, number of times _____)
_____   _____   18. Attempted suicide? (If yes, number of times _____)
_____   _____   19. Exercised an injury on purpose?
_____   _____   20. Tortured yourself with self-defeating thoughts?
_____   _____   21. Starved yourself to hurt yourself?
_____   _____   22. Abused laxatives to hurt yourself? (If yes, number of times _____)

Have you engaged in any other self-destructive behaviors not asked about in this inventory? If so, please describe below.

_____
_____
_____
_____

Used with permission from Sansone, R., & Sansone, L. (2010). Measuring self-harm behavior with the Self-Harm Inventory. Psychiatry, 7(4), 16–20.

demands. This finding suggests that the success of screening may be tied, at least in part, to workload issues or lack of clarity about how to prioritize tasks. Nurses face these concerns in most areas of practice. Recognizing the vital importance of screening and creating the structure to ensure that it occurs requires multidisciplinary collaboration, commitment, and support from health-care managers. Nurses are in a key position to educate others about the importance of screening for psychiatric and substance misuse issues in nonpsychiatric settings, and nurse leaders can help direct changes in screening requirements that address such critical public health-care needs.

CORE CONCEPT

Referral

Referral entails sending a patient to another health-care provider or specialty service for consultation or treatment.

Referral

Although structured screening of mental health issues has been identified as a critical first step in improving care for both mental illness and other medical illnesses, controversy exists over how much care should be provided in nonpsychiatric settings and when it is appropriate to refer to specialists for treatment. Grundberg (2016) concluded that if nonpsychiatric nurses are to be involved in early detection and interventions for mental health-related issues, these activities must be explicitly stated work objectives, and there must be effective collaboration between care providers. If nurses lack clarity about their roles and responsibilities in screening for and treatment of mental illnesses, referring the patient to needed services is unlikely to happen.

Several studies have found that providing training and education about evidence-based screening tools and referral pathways improved the referral process for mental health services (Allen et al., 2011; Brooker et al., 2007; Bruce et al., 2007; Hasche et al., 2013; Mulvaney-Day et al., 2018; Ruiz Escobar et al., 2021; Thompson et al., 2008). The process for referral to specialized mental health services is one in which the nurse must collaborate effectively with physicians, social workers, and other health-care providers within their practice setting and the setting to which they are referring a patient.

CORE CONCEPT

Patient-Centered Care
Patient-centered care is an approach to care provision that intends to "identify, respect, and care about patients' differences, values, preferences, and expressed needs; relieve pain and suffering; coordinate continuous care; listen to, clearly inform, communicate with, and educate patients; share decision making and management; and continuously advocate disease prevention, wellness, and promotion of healthy lifestyles, including a focus on population health" (Institute of Medicine, 2003).

The process of referral also involves collaboration with the patient. Patient collaboration is the essence of **patient-centered care.** The Institute of Medicine (2003) has stressed, in its landmark study of deaths associated with medical errors, that we must improve our understanding and application of this concept to improve the safety and quality of health care in the future. To apply the concepts of patient-centered care requires that nurses and other health-care professionals listen to patients, empower them in decision making around their care, and establish a collaborative partnership.

There are some circumstances in which providing care for a patient with psychiatric illness cannot be conducted collaboratively. Patients who are either strongly intent on hurting themselves or unaware that they have significant life-threatening symptoms of mental illness need to be referred to a more restrictive environment even when it is against their own will. Essential elements in this process include collaboration with other health-care professionals to increase confidence in making the difficult clinical judgment to involuntarily hospitalize the patient and thoughtful communication with the patient about the reasons for this referral.

Lauder and associates (2006), in their study of how nurses make clinical judgments about patients who are neglecting their self-care, cautioned that nurses need to be clear about the difference between severity of mental illness and capacity to make decisions.

Just because a patient has a severe mental illness does not necessarily mean that they are incapable of making decisions. Nurses should only be making referral (or any other) decisions *for* a patient when it is clear that the patient does not have the current capacity to make decisions in the interest of their personal safety and livelihood.

Two barriers to effective referral of patients with mental illness are lack of knowledge about available options for specialized treatment and difficulty accessing available resources. Some primary care settings and emergency departments have incorporated mental health specialists to either provide on-site intervention or to assist in the clinical judgment about referral to more intensive treatment. Nurses in nonpsychiatric settings must be familiar with mental health services and facilities within the community in which they practice to collaborate effectively and refer patients appropriately for ongoing care. SAMHSA (n.d.) provides an online locator map to identify mental health and addictions treatment services in localities throughout the United States. Box 21–2 lists some types of mental health and substance use disorder resources for referral.

CORE CONCEPT

Stigmatization
Stigmatization is the devaluing of a person because of a particular characteristic or illness. It is an attitude that is negative, discriminatory, and unethical. In the practice of health care, stigmatizing patients has the potential to inhibit the patient's ability to receive an accurate diagnosis and adequate treatment.

Stigma

Even with accessible, evidence-based screening tools and clear pathways for referral to mental health specialists, interventions can be derailed when the individual with mental illness is stigmatized. **Stigmatization,** an attitude of devaluing a person because of a particular characteristic or illness, has been identified as a barrier to effective mental illness treatment in primary care, emergency departments, medical-surgical settings, and even, at times, in psychiatric settings.

One of the negative outcomes of stigma is that individuals with mental illness or addiction may not seek treatment at all, which can have devastating consequences on the progression of the illness and may leave many other physical illnesses undetected

BOX 21–2 Types of Referral Resources for Mental Health and Addictions Treatment

SELF-HELP GROUPS

- 12-step programs such as Alcoholics Anonymous, Emotions Anonymous, and others provide ongoing peer support and education. Location and availability of AA meetings can be found online (www.aa.org). Some meetings are also conducted online.

MENTAL HEALTH-CARE PROFESSIONALS

- Psychiatrists (MDs) and Psychiatric-Mental Health Nurse Practitioners (PMH NPs) provide diagnostic, medication management, and counseling services and may conduct psychotherapy.
- Licensed Independent Social Workers (LISWs) provide counseling, case management, and advocacy.
- Psychologists (PhDs) provide counseling, individual and group psychotherapy, and psychological testing services.

COMMUNITY MENTAL HEALTH CENTERS

- Operated by community or county governments to provide public mental health services primarily to clients who cannot afford private services.
- Usually staffed with a broad range of mental health professionals and *peer support specialists* (individuals with mental illness who provide support in illness management and recovery), some of whom may have specialized training and certification.
- May provide a broad range of services for mental health and substance use disorders such as outpatient counseling, case management, intensive outpatient programs, and day programs.
- Often collaborate with and refer to area resources for support with employment, housing, and other care needs.

SUBSTANCE MISUSE AND ADDICTION TREATMENT CENTERS

- These treatment facilities usually have a broad range of mental health and addiction treatment health professionals, including certified chemical dependency counselors and physicians certified in addictions medicine.

- Services usually include detoxification (for safe withdrawal from addictive substances), intensive outpatient services (intensive group therapy, 3 to 5 days per week, and support with establishing relapse prevention plans), and/or residential treatment (inpatient rehabilitation; lengths of stay may range from several weeks to several months).

PHYSICIAN OR NURSE PRACTITIONER PRIMARY CARE

- Some primary care practices have incorporated mental illness management within their practice settings, particularly in areas where specialists are not readily accessible.

TELEMEDICINE

- Some mental health organizations provide counseling and medication management via teleconferencing interaction. Typically these services are provided by psychiatrists and nurse practitioners.

GENERAL HOSPITAL INPATIENT PSYCHIATRIC UNITS

- These units provide inpatient psychiatric care primarily for the purpose of assessment, monitoring and safety, medication management, and referral to outpatient mental health services for ongoing care.
- Typically staffed by a broad range of mental health professionals working as an interdisciplinary team that may include occupational or activities therapists, pastoral counselors, and mental health technicians, in addition to psychiatrists, nurses, and social workers.
- Lengths of stay typically average 3 to 5 days.

STATE PSYCHIATRIC HOSPITALS

- These are government-run inpatient treatment facilities with a broad range of mental health professionals as listed previously.
- Provide public mental health services for those unable to afford private services.
- Lengths of stay vary from several days to months or even years depending on patient needs.

---

and untreated. This problem occurs worldwide. In 2001 the World Health Organization (WHO) published a report recommending that mental health care be integrated into general health-care settings, including primary care settings, based on the premise that individuals with mental illness may avoid mental health services because of the associated stigma. Since then, research has informed us that several concerns still need to be addressed when the individual with mental illness seeks help in a nonpsychiatric setting; particularly knowledge gaps, clinical skills, and stigma (Beaulieu et al., 2017; Gwaikolo et al., 2017; Li et al., 2014a; Ng et al., 2017).

In one study, it was found that clients, on average, consulted more than three caregivers in a general hospital setting and that 75% did not get a diagnosis or treatment (Li et al., 2014b). Knowledge gaps in mental illnesses and attitudes toward the client manifesting symptoms of mental illness or substance addiction are primary influences.

Ng and associates (2017) specifically studied nurses' attitudes and found that previous psychiatric training, a desire to learn about neuropsychiatric illnesses, and positive contact with people who have mental illnesses were associated with less stigmatization. It is difficult to understand the lack of desire to be knowledgeable about a group of illnesses that have such a significant effect on all aspects of nursing care, but sometimes it is related to myths, fear, and stigma. Efforts to increase social contact and understand the *person* are important strategies to reduce stigma, but it first requires the nurse's willingness to engage meaningfully with people who have mental illnesses and addictions.

Social distancing is an aspect of stigma that refers to the tendency of health-care workers and others to avoid people with mental illness or addiction. This is different from the usage of the term that has become popularized as a strategy to reduce the spread of coronavirus disease (COVID-19). In the context of mental health, social distancing refers to a stigmatizing avoidance of patients when confronted with symptoms that are poorly understood or difficult to manage. Symptoms such as hallucinations, neglect of self-care, and agitation can be challenging for clinicians to manage when they feel frightened or ill equipped to intervene effectively. Reavely and Jorm (2015) found that individuals with mental illness reported similar avoidance behaviors from family and friends. These findings clarify the extent of the marginalization and disenfranchisement experienced by many individuals with mental illness and substance use disorders.

In a study of nurses in primary care settings (Ihalainen-en-Tamlander et al., 2016), researchers found that nurse's attitudes toward mental health patients were generally positive; however, less-experienced nurses or those without additional mental health training were more fearful and more likely to think mental health patients should be segregated. The authors highlight the importance of ongoing training, especially for less-experienced nurses, to increase confidence, reduce fear, and prevent the development of stigmatizing and distancing attitudes. Several studies validate that education programs, consultation with mental health professionals to increase comfort and skill level, and exposure to individuals with mental illness or substance use disorders are effective tools in reducing negative stereotyping, social distancing, and other stigmatizing attitudes and behaviors (Beaulieu et al., 2017; Flanagan et al., 2016; Li et al., 2014a; Ng et al., 2017). Student nurses who have been educated about mental illnesses, communication, and intervention strategies have developed an awareness of the problems associated with stigma. Often, they have had encounters with patients in treatment for mental illness or substance use disorders, and these nurses enter the workforce in a unique position to spearhead culture change. Many chapters within this text, particularly those with the "Real People, Real Stories" feature, provide important information to improve the nurse's knowledge and confidence in caring for patients with mental illness in any practice setting.

To effectively apply these skills and knowledge requires that nurses have a clear understanding of their role caring for such patients.

The Role of the Nurse in Caring for Patients With Psychiatric and Substance Use Disorders in Nonpsychiatric Settings

The nurse's role in caring for patients with psychiatric and substance use disorders in nonpsychiatric settings includes the following:

■ Examine one's personal beliefs and attitudes about individuals with mental illness and substance use disorders, focusing on contributing factors such as fear or lack of confidence in managing the patient's needs.

■ Develop awareness of how stigmatization negatively affects the provision of appropriate care and actively seek the knowledge and skills needed to increase confidence in patient care management.

■ Identify patients with potentially high-prevalence, high-risk mental health issues who require universal screening in any health-care setting.

■ Use evidence-based screening tools to identify patients needing further evaluation and referral to mental health or substance use disorder services.

■ Provide for patient safety, including continuous monitoring, while determinations are made about referral needs.

■ Establish a working knowledge of available mental health services for referral and collaborate with physicians, patients, and members of the health-care team to identify the most appropriate resources.

■ Engage patients throughout the assessment and referral process using a patient-centered approach that empowers patients in making decisions about care recommendations to the best of their ability.

All nurses will encounter patients with mental illnesses and substance use disorders, regardless of the practice setting. It is imperative that each nurse recognizes their role in reducing stigma personally and within the culture of the care team and provides the same attention to screening, intervention, and referral that is provided to patients with other chronic illnesses. This necessary foundation for nursing care addresses priority health-care needs, reduces poorer outcomes, improves individuals' quality of life, and minimizes the risks of premature death.

Summary and Key Points

■ In the United States and globally, individuals with psychiatric illness and substance use disorders are vulnerable to lack of or inadequate treatment, which is associated with poorer outcomes, undetected physical illnesses, and early death.

■ *Diagnostic overshadowing* is a process of wrongly assuming that a patient's medical symptoms are attributable to mental illness.

■ Three variables that influence nurses' responses to the patient with mental health and substance use disorders are lack of education and recognition of symptoms, lack of appropriate screening, and nurses' attitudes about patients with these illnesses.

■ Many evidence-based screening tools exist for the detection of mental illness or substance use disorders. Some are easily accessible, free to use, and time efficient.

■ Because of high prevalence and increased risk for morbidity and mortality, all patients should be screened for trauma history, substance use, and risk for suicide.

■ One of the identified barriers to adequate screening of patients for mental health issues in nonpsychiatric settings is competing workload demands. Nurses and nurse managers have a responsibility to prioritize mental illnesses and substance use disorders as critical public health issues.

■ Another identified barrier to appropriate screening and intervention is *social distancing*, which refers to the nurse's avoidance of patients with mental illnesses because of fear, lack of knowledge, lack of confidence in clinical skills, and stigma.

■ Nurses in nonpsychiatric settings must have a working knowledge of available resources for referral when mental health and substance misuse are identified. The Substance Abuse and Mental Health Services Administration provides online information about available mental health and addictions services for every locality in the United States.

■ *Referral* is a collaborative process with members of the health-care team, including the patient.

■ *Patient-centered care* requires that nurses listen to the patient, empower patients in decision making around their care, develop a collaborative partnership, and only make decisions *for* the patient (such as involuntary hospitalization) when the individual is clearly unable to and when it is necessary to protect their safety.

■ *Stigmatization* is the devaluing, marginalizing, and disenfranchising of certain patients because of symptoms or conditions. Stigmatizing patients with psychiatric and substance use disorders is an international concern contributing to patient neglect, inadequate treatment, avoidance of health-care professionals and treatment settings, and risk of early death.

■ The first step for every nurse in accomplishing safe, effective care for the patient with mental health and substance use disorders is reflection on one's own beliefs, attitudes, and behaviors, and actively making efforts to reduce stigma personally and within the culture of their practice setting.

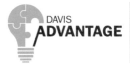

Go to **Davis Advantage** to complete your learning: strengthen understanding, apply your knowledge, and prepare for the Next Gen NCLEX®.

Review Questions

1. A client enters the emergency department and reports, "My bed is on fire, and my stomach, and we're all dead." The nurse's initial response is to call the psychiatric unit to secure an inpatient bed for this patient. The nurse's action is an example of:
   a. Prompt, appropriate referral.
   b. Patient-centered care.
   c. Stigmatization.
   d. Collaboration.

2. One of the outcomes of diagnostic overshadowing in clients with mental illness is:
   a. Better quality of life.
   b. Increased access to resources.
   c. More comprehensive care.
   d. Increased risk for death.

3. The nurse is reviewing discharge instructions with a client who is being discharged after a total knee replacement. Knowing that the client has a history of bipolar disorder, the nurse asks the client what needs they perceive they have for follow-up care related to this mental illness. This is an example of:
   a. Patient-centered care.
   b. Diagnostic overshadowing.
   c. Stigmatization.
   d. Discrimination.

4. Screening for substance use and suicide risk should be conducted in which of the following settings?
   a. Emergency departments
   b. Primary care settings
   c. Medical units
   d. All of the above

Clinical Judgment Questions

5. A client presents in the emergency department loudly proclaiming with rapid speech, "If I don't get more pain medication right now I'm going to call the attorney general and sue the entire health-care network." Which of the following should the nurse include in the initial screening and assessment? (Select all that apply.)
   a. Substance use
   b. Pain
   c. Mental illness
   d. Prior history of convictions
   e. Availability of an inpatient psychiatric bed

6. A client was admitted to the intensive care unit after a single-car accident in which they struck a cement wall. The individual is now responsive and wants to be discharged within the next couple of days. Which of the following are priorities for screening? (Select all that apply.)
   a. Traumatic brain injury
   b. Chronic pain
   c. Sexual dysfunction
   d. Depression and risk for suicide

7. The nurse manager recognizes a need to improve mental health and substance use screening and referral services for their clients in the public health clinic. Which of the following is a priority to begin an effective process for implementation?
   a. Provide a list of referral sources that are readily available to staff.
   b. Educate staff about the importance of prioritizing these public health concerns.
   c. Explore the literature for evidence-based screening tools.
   d. Inform the staff that they have been stigmatizing patients and this will not be tolerated.

8. A client on a medical unit is identified to be having suicidal ideation. Which of the following is a priority in managing their immediate care?
   a. Screen for depression
   b. Provide sedative medication
   c. Refer him to another setting
   d. Continuous monitoring and observation

References

Allen, J., Annells, M., Nunn, R., Petrie, E., Clark, E., Lang, L., & Robins, A. (2011). Evaluation of effectiveness and satisfaction outcomes of a mental health screening and referral clinical pathway for community nursing care. *Journal of Psychiatric and Mental Health Nursing, 18*(5), 375–385.

Alimoradi, Z., Jafari, E., Broström, A., Ohayon, M. M., Lin, C. Y., Griffiths, M. D., Blom, K., Jernelöv, S., Kaldo, V., & Pakpour, A. H. (2022). Effects of cognitive behavioral therapy for insomnia (CBT-I) on quality of life: A systematic review and meta-analysis, *Sleep Medicine Reviews, 64.* https://doi.org/10.1016/j.smrv.2022.101646

American Academy of Pediatrics. (2022). *Bright futures.* https://www.aap.org/en/practice-management/bright-futures

American Psychiatric Association (APA). (2022). *Diagnostic and statistical manual of mental disorders, fifth edition-text revision (DSM-5-TR).* American Psychiatric Association.

Bay, N., Bjørnestad, J., Johannessen, J. O., Larsen, T. K., & Joa, I. (2016). Obstacles to care in first-episode psychosis patients with a long duration of untreated psychosis. *Early Intervention in Psychiatry, 10*(1), 71–76. doi:10.1111/eip.12152

Beaulieu, T., Patten, S., Knaak, S., Weinerman, R., Campbell, H., & Lauria-Horner, B. (2017). Impact of skill-based approaches in reducing stigma in primary care physicians: Results from a double-blind, parallel-cluster, randomized controlled trial. *Canadian Journal of Psychiatry, 62*(5), 327–335.

Betz, M. E., Sullivan, A. F., Manton, A. P., Espinola, J. A., Miller, I., Camargo Jr, C. A., Boudreaux, E. D., & ED-SAFE Investigators. (2013). Knowledge, attitudes, and practices of emergency department providers in the care of suicidal patients. *Depression & Anxiety, 30*(10), 1005–1012.

Bica, T., Castelló, R., Toussaint, L. L., & Montesó-Curto, P. (2017). Depression as a risk factor of organic diseases: An international integrative review. *Journal of Nursing Scholarship, 49*(4), 389–399.

Boland, R., & Verduin, M. L. (Eds.). (2022). *Kaplan & Sadock's synopsis of psychiatry* (12th ed.). Wolters Kluwer.

Brooker, C., Ricketts, T., Bennett, S., & Lemme, F. (2007). Admission decisions following contact with an emergency mental health assessment and intervention service. *Journal of Clinical Nursing, 16*(7), 1313–1322.

Bruce, M. L., Brown, E. L., Raue, P. J., Mlodzianowski, A. E., Meyers, B. S., Leon, A. C., & Nassisi, P. (2007). A randomized trial of depression assessment intervention in home health care. *Journal of the American Geriatrics Society, 55*(11), 1793–1800.

Chen, Y., Yu, S., Hu, Y., Li, R. C., Artaud, F., Carcaillon-Bentata, L., Elbaz, A., & Lee, P. (2020). Risk of suicide among patients with Parkinson disease. *JAMA Psychiatry*. https://doi.org/10.1001/jamapsychiatry.2020.4001

Dattani, S. (2022). What is the lifetime prevalence of depression? *Our World Data*. https://ourworldindata.org/depression-lifetime-risk

Flanagan, E. H., Buck, T., Gamble, A., Hunter, C., Sewell, I., & Davidson, L. (2016). "Recovery speaks": A photovoice intervention to reduce stigma among primary care providers. *Psychiatric Services, 67*(5), 566–569. doi:10.1176/appi.ps.201500049

Fuller-Thomson, E., Rivière, R. N., Carrique, L., & Agbeyaka, S. (2020). The dark side of ADHD: Factors associated with suicide attempts among those with ADHD in a national representative Canadian sample. *Archives of Suicide Research*, 1–19. https://doi.org/10.1080/13811118.2020.1856258

Garcia de la Garza, A., Blanco, C., Olfson, M., & Wall, M. M. (2021). Identification of suicide attempt risk factors in a national US survey using machine learning. *JAMA Psychiatry, 78*(4), 398–406. https://doi.org/10.1001/jamapsychiatry.2020.4165

Gomes, J., Duraes, D., & Lima, G. (2015). Stigma kills. *European Psychiatry, 1*(30), 1863. doi:10.1016/S0924-9338(15)31427-9

Grundberg, Å. (2016). District nurses' perspectives on detecting mental health problems and promoting mental health among community-dwelling seniors with multimorbidity. *Journal of Clinical Nursing, 25*(17/18), 2590–2599.

Guttmacher Institute. (2022). *Substance use during pregnancy*. https://www.guttmacher.org/state-policy/explore/substance-use-during-pregnancy

Gwaikolo, W. S., Kohrt, B. A., & Cooper, J. L. (2017). Health system preparedness for integration of mental health services in rural Liberia. *BMC Health Services Research, 17*, 1–10.

Hallyburton, A. (2022). Diagnostic overshadowing: An evolutionary concept analysis on the misattribution of physical symptoms to preexisting psychological illnesses. *International Journal of Mental Health Nursing*. doi: 10.1111/inm.13034

Ham, O. K., Lee, B. G., Choi, E., & Choi, S. J. (2020). Efficacy of cognitive behavioral treatment for insomnia: A randomized

controlled trial. *Western Journal of Nursing Research, 42*(12), 1104–1112. doi:10.1177/0193945920914081

Hasche, L. K., Lee, M. J., Proctor, E. K., & Morrow-Howell, N. (2013). Does identification of depression affect community long-term care services ordered for older adults? *Social Work Research, 37*(3), 255–262.

Horowitz, L. M., Snyder, D., Ludi, E., Rosenstein, D. L., Kohn-Godbout, J., Lee, L., Cartledge, T., Farrrar, A., & Pao, M. (2013). Ask suicide-screening questions to everyone in medical settings: The asQ'em Quality Improvement Project. *Psychiatry, 54*(3), 239–247.

Ihalainen-Tamlander, N., Vähäniemi, A., Löyttyniemi, E., Suominen, T., & Välimäki, M. (2016). Stigmatizing attitudes in nurses towards people with mental illness: A cross-sectional study in primary settings in Finland. *Journal of Psychiatric and Mental Health Nursing, 23*(6–7), 427–437. doi:10.1111/jpm.12319

Institute of Medicine, Committee on the Health Professions Education Summit. (2003). *Health professions education: A bridge to quality*. National Academy of Sciences.

Jackman, K., Honig, J., & Bockting, W. (2016). Nonsuicidal self-injury among lesbian, gay, bisexual and transgender populations: An integrative review. *Journal of Clinical Nursing, 25*(23/24), 3438–3453.

Jobes, D. A. (2015, September). *Clinical suicidology: Innovations in assessment treatment of suicidal risk*. Presentation at Psychiatric Grand Rounds, Summa Health Systems, Akron, OH.

Kameg, K. M., Spencer Woods, A., Luther Szpak, J., & McCormick, M. (2013). Identifying and managing nonsuicidal self-injurious behavior in the primary care setting. *Journal of the American Association of Nurse Practitioners, 25*(4), 167–172.

Koffel, E., Bramoweth, A. D., & Ulmer, C. S. (2018). Increasing access to and utilization of cognitive behavioral therapy for insomnia (CBT-I): A narrative review. *Journal of General Internal Medicine, 33*, 955–962. https://doi.org/10.1007/s11606-018-4390-1

Kõlves, K., Fitzgerald, C., Nordentoft, M., Wood, S. J., & Erlangsen, A. (2021). Assessment of suicidal behaviors among individuals with autism spectrum disorder in Denmark. *JAMA Network Open, 4*(1), e2033565. https://doi.org/10.1001/jamanetworkopen.2020.33565

Koposov, R., Fossum, S., Frodl, T., NytrØ, O., Leventhal, B., Sourander, A., Quaglini, S., Molteni, M., Iglesia Vayá, M., Prokosch, H. U., Barbarini, N., Milham, M. P., Castellanos, F. X., & Skokauskas, N. (2017). Clinical decision support systems in child and adolescent psychiatry: A systematic review. *European Child & Adolescent Psychiatry, 26*(11), 1309–1317.

Langdon, R., Johnson, M., Carroll, V., & Antonio, G. (2013). Assessment of the elderly: It's worth covering the risks. *Journal of Nursing Management, 21*(1), 94–105.

Lauder, W., Ludwick, R., Zeller, R., & Winchell, J. (2006). Factors influencing nurses' judgments about self-neglect cases. *Journal of Psychiatric & Mental Health Nursing, 13*(3), 279–287.

Li, J., Li, J., Huang, Y., & Thornicroft, G. (2014a). Mental health training program for community mental health staff in Guangzhou, China: Effects on knowledge of mental illness and stigma. *International Journal of Mental Health Systems, 8*(1), 49.

Li, X., Zhang, W., Lin, Y., Zhang, X., Qu, Z., Wang, X., Zhang, Y., Xu, H., Zhao, S., Li, Y., & Tian, D. (2014b). Pathways to psychiatric care of patients from rural regions: A general-hospital-based study. *International Journal of Social Psychiatry, 60*(3), 280–289. doi:10.1177/0020764013485364

McGovern, A., & Selwyn, J. (2014). A quality improvement project: Improving recognition of low mood and depression in elderly inpatients. *Age & Ageing, 43*(suppl 2), ii7–ii7.

Mitchell, A. J., Hussain, N., Grainger, L., & Symonds, P. (2011). Identification of patient-reported distress by clinical nurse specialists in routine oncology practice: A multicentre UK study. *Psycho-Oncology, 20*(10), 1076–1083.

Mollard, E., Hudson, D. B., Ford, A., & Pullen, C. (2015). An integrative review of postpartum depression in rural U.S. communities. *Archives of Psychiatric Nursing, 30*(3), 418–424.

Momen, N. C., Plana-Ripoll, O., Agerbo, E., Christenson, M. K., Iburg, K. M., Laursen, T. M., Mortensen, P. B., Pedersen, C. B., Prior, A., Weye, N., & McGrath, J. J. (2022). Mortality associated with mental disorders and comorbid general medical conditions. *JAMA Psychiatry, 79*(5): 444–453. doi:10.1001/jamapsychiatry.2022.0347

Moran, G. E., Daniels, A. S., & Ghose, S. S. (2018). Screening for behavioral health conditions in primary care settings: A systematic review of the literature. *Journal of General Internal Medicine, 33*(3), 335–346. https://doi.org/10.1007/s11606-017-4181-0

Mulvaney-Day, N., Marshall, T., Downey Piscopo, K., Korsen, N., Lynch, S., Karnell, L. H., Moran, G. E., Daniels, A. S., & Ghose, S. S. (2018). Screening for behavioral health conditions in primary care settings: A systematic review of the literature. *Journal of General Internal Medicine, 33*(3), 335–346. https://doi.org/10.1007/s11606-017-4181-0

National Alliance on Mental Illness. (2022). *Mental health screening.* https://www.nami.org/Advocacy/Policy-Priorities/Intervene-Early/Mental-Health-Screening

National Institute of Mental Health (NIMH). (2021). *Chronic illness and mental health: Recognizing and treating depression.* https://www.nimh.nih.gov/health/publications/chronic-illness-mental-health

Ng, Y. P., Rashid, A., & O'Brien, F. (2017). Determining the effectiveness of a video-based contact intervention in improving attitudes of Penang primary care nurses toward people with mental illness. *PLoS ONE, 12*(11), 1–19.

Pardee, M. L., Kuzma, E., Dahlem, C. H., Boucher, N., & Darling-Fisher, C. (2017). Current state of screening high-ACE youth and emerging adults in primary care: Screening of high-ACE youth in primary care settings. *Journal of the American Association of Nurse Practitioners, 29.* doi:10.1002/2327-6924.12531

Plana-Ripoll, O., Pedersen, C. B., Agerbo, E., Holtz, Y., Erlangsen, A., Canudas-Romo, V., Andersen, P. K., Charlson, F. J., Christensen, M. K., Erskine, H. E., Ferrari, A. J., Iburg, K. M., Momen, N., Mortensen, P. B., Nordentoft, M., Santomauro, D. F., Scott, J. G., Whiteford, H. A., Weye, N., McGrath, J. J., & Laursen, T. M. (2019). A comprehensive analysis of mortality-related health metrics associated with mental disorders: A nationwide, register-based cohort study. *The Lancet.* doi:10.1016/S0140-6736(19)32316-5

Préville, M., Côté, G., Boyer, R., & Hébert, R. (2004). Detection of depression and anxiety disorders by home care nurses. *Aging & Mental Health, 8*(5), 400–409.

Rahm, A. K., Boggs, J. M., Martin, C., Price, D. W., Beck, A., Backer, T. E., & Dearing, J. W. (2015). Facilitators and barriers to implementing Screening, Brief Intervention, and Referral to Treatment (SBIRT) in primary care in integrated health care settings. *Substance Abuse, 36*(3), 281–288.

Ramchand, R., Schuler, M. S., Schoenbaum, M., Colpe, L., & Ayer, L. (2021). Suicidality among sexual minority adults: Gender, age, and race/ethnicity differences. *American Journal of Preventive Medicine.* https://doi.org/10.1080/13811118.2020.1856258

Reavely, N. J., & Jorm, A. F. (2015). Experiences of discrimination and positive treatment in people with mental health problems: Findings from an Australian national survey. *Australian and New Zealand Journal of Psychiatry, 49*(10), 906–913. doi:10.1177/0004867415602068

Roberge, P., Hudon, C., Pavilanis, A., Beaulieu, M., Benoit, A., Brouillet, H., Boulianne, I., De Pauw, A., Frigon, S., Gaboury, I., Gaudreault, M., Girard, A., Giroux, M., Grégoire, E., Langlois, L., Lemieux, M., Loignon, C., & Vanasse, A. (2016). A qualitative study of perceived needs and factors associated with the quality of care for common mental disorders in patients with chronic diseases: The perspective of primary care clinicians and patients. *BMC Family Practice, 17*, 1–14.

Ruiz Escobar, E., Pathak, S., & Blanchard, C. M. (2021). Screening and referral care delivery services and unmet health-related social needs: A systematic review. *Preventing Chronic Disease, 18*, E78. https://doi.org/10.5888/pcd18.200569

Sansone, R., & Sansone, L. (2010). Measuring self-harm behavior with the Self-Harm Inventory. *Psychiatry, 7*(4), 16–20.

Singer, S., Brown, A., Einenkel, J., Hauss, J., Hinz, A., Klein, A., Papsdorf, K., Stolzenburg, J. U., & Brähler, E. (2011). Identifying tumor patients' depression. *Supportive Care in Cancer, 19*(11), 1697–1703.

Stefancic, A., Bochichio, L., Svehaug, K., Alvi, T., & Cabassa, L. J. (2021). "We die 25 years sooner": Addressing physical health among persons with serious mental illness in supportive housing. *Community Mental Health Journal, 57*, 1195–1207 https://doi.org/10.1007/s10597-020-00752-y

Substance Abuse and Mental Health Services Administration (SAMHSA). (n.d.). *Findtreatment.gov.* https://findtreatment.gov/

Substance Abuse and Mental Health Services Administration (SAMHSA). (2022). *Screening, brief intervention, and referral to treatment (SBIRT).* https://www.samhsa.gov/sbirt/about

Taylor, D. J., & Pruiksma, K. E. (2014). Cognitive and behavioural therapy for insomnia (CBT-I) in psychiatric populations: A systematic review. *International Review of Psychiatry, 26*(2), 205–213. doi:10.3109/09540261.2014.902808

Thompson, P., Lang, L., & Annells, M. (2008). A systematic review of the effectiveness of in-home community nurse led interventions for the mental health of older persons. *Journal of Clinical Nursing, 17*(11), 1419–1427.

Williams, S. C., Schmaltz, S. P., Castro, G. M., & Baker, D. W. (2018). Incidence and method of suicide in hospitals in the United States. *The Joint Commission Journal on Quality and Patient Safety, 44*, 643–650.

Classical References

Felitti, V. J., Anda, R. F., Nordenberg, D., Williamson, D. F., Spitz, A. M., Edwards, V., Koss, M. P., & Marks, J. S. (1998). Relationship of childhood abuse and household dysfunction to many of the leading causes of death in adults—The Adverse Childhood Experiences (ACE) study. *American Journal of Preventive Medicine, 14*, 245–258.

Hoff, L. A., & Rosenbaum, L. (1994). A victimization assessment tool: Instrument development and clinical implications. *Journal of Advanced Nursing, 20,:* 627–634.

Hoff, L. A., & Ross, M. (1993). Curriculum guide for nursing: Violence against women and children. University of Ottawa, Faculty of Health Sciences, School of Nursing, Ottawa.

Schofferman, J., Anderson, D., Hines, R., Smith, G., & White, A. (1992). Childhood psychological trauma correlates with unsuccessful lumbar spine surgery. *Spine, 17*(Suppl.), 138–144.

World Health Organization (WHO). (2001). *The world health report 2001. Mental health: New understanding, new hope.* World Health Organization. https://apps.who.int/iris/bitstream/handle/10665/42390/WHR_2001.pdf?sequence=1&isAllowed=y

22 Neurocognitive Disorders

CORE CONCEPTS

Intracranial Regulation: Delirium, Dementia (major neurocognitive disorder)

Professional Behavior: Nursing process in the care of patients with neurocognitive disorders

Safety

Clinical Judgment

KEY TERMS

aphasia
apraxia
ataxia
confabulation

delirium
dementia
neurocognitive disorders (NCDs)

pseudodementia
sundowning

OBJECTIVES

After reading this chapter, the student will be able to:

1. Define and differentiate among various neurocognitive disorders (NCDs).
2. Discuss predisposing factors implicated in the etiology of NCDs.
3. Describe clinical symptoms and use the information to assess patients with NCDs.
4. Identify nursing diagnoses common to patients with NCDs and select appropriate nursing interventions for each.
5. Identify topics for patient and family teaching relevant to NCDs.
6. Discuss criteria for evaluating nursing care of patients with NCDs.
7. Describe various treatment modalities relevant to care of patients with NCDs.

Neurocognitive disorders (NCDs) include those in which a clinically significant deficit in cognition or memory exists, representing a notable change from a previous level of functioning. These disorders were previously identified in the *Diagnostic and Statistical Manual of Mental Disorders, Fourth Edition, Text Revision (DSM-IV-TR)* (American Psychiatric Association [APA], 2000) as "Dementia, Delirium, Amnestic, and Other Cognitive Disorders." In the *DSM-5-TR*, NCDs include delirium and the syndromes called major NCD or minor NCD, which are further specified according to the underlying cause (such as Alzheimer's disease [AD], Parkinson's disease [PD], or others) (APA, 2022).

This chapter presents predisposing factors, clinical symptoms, and nursing interventions for care of patients with NCDs. The objective is to provide quality care, respect patients' dignity, and promote quality of life while offering guidance and support to their families and primary caregivers.

CORE CONCEPT

Delirium

Delirium is a mental state characterized by an acute disturbance of cognition, manifested by short-term confusion, excitement, disorientation, and clouded consciousness. Hallucinations and illusions are common.

Delirium

Clinical Findings and Course

Delirium is characterized by a disturbance in attention and awareness and a change in cognition that develop rapidly over a short period (APA, 2022). Symptoms of delirium include difficulty sustaining and shifting attention. The person is very distractible and must be repeatedly reminded to focus attention. Disorganized thinking prevails and is reflected by speech that is rambling, irrelevant, pressured, and incoherent, and switches from subject to subject. Reasoning ability and goal-directed behavior are impaired. Disorientation to time and place is common, and impairment of recent memory is invariably evident. Misperceptions of the environment (illusions) and false perceptions (hallucinations) are prominent. Disturbances in the sleep–wake cycle also occur.

The individual's state of awareness may range from that of hypervigilance (heightened awareness to environmental stimuli) to stupor or semi-coma. Sleep may fluctuate between hypersomnolence (excessive sleepiness) and insomnia. Vivid dreams and nightmares are common.

Psychomotor activity may fluctuate between agitated, purposeless movements (e.g., restlessness, hyperactivity, striking out at nonexistent objects), and a vegetative state resembling catatonic stupor. Various forms of tremor are frequently present.

Emotional instability may be manifested by fear, anxiety, depression, irritability, anger, euphoria, or apathy. These emotions may be evidenced by crying, calls for help, cursing, muttering, moaning, acts of self-destruction, fearful attempts to flee, or attacks on others who are falsely viewed as threatening. Autonomic manifestations, such as tachycardia, sweating, flushed face, dilated pupils, and elevated blood pressure, are common.

The symptoms of delirium usually begin abruptly (e.g., after a head injury or seizure). At other times, they may be preceded by several hours or days of prodromal symptoms (e.g., restlessness, difficulty thinking clearly, insomnia or hypersomnolence, and nightmares). The slower onset is more common if the underlying cause is a systemic illness or metabolic imbalance.

The duration of delirium is usually brief (e.g., 1 week; rarely more than 1 month) and, after elimination of the underlying causes, symptoms usually diminish over a 3- to 7-day period. In some cases, however, resolution may take as long as 2 weeks (Boland & Verduin, 2022). The age of the person and duration of the delirium influence the rate of symptom resolution. Delirium is associated with a high mortality rate because of the seriousness of the precipitating medical conditions. At times, delirium may also shift into a more permanent cognitive disorder (e.g., major NCD).

Predisposing Factors

Delirium

Individuals most predisposed to delirium include those with serious medical, surgical, or neurological conditions. People older than age 65 are considered a high-risk group. Depression, falls, and elder abuse may also contribute to delirium. Other precipitating factors include the following (Boland & Verduin, 2022; Fabian & Solai, 2017):

■ Systemic infections
■ Febrile illness or hyperthermia
■ Metabolic disorders, such as electrolyte imbalances, hypercarbia, hypoglycemia, or hyponatremia
■ Hypoxia and chronic obstructive pulmonary disease (COPD)
■ Hepatic failure or renal failure
■ Head trauma
■ Seizures
■ Migraine headaches
■ Brain abscess or brain neoplasms
■ Stroke
■ Nutritional deficiency
■ Uncontrolled pain
■ Burns
■ Heat stroke
■ Orthopedic and cardiac surgeries
■ Social isolation, emotional stress, physical restraints, admission to an intensive care unit

Other Causes of Delirium

Substance Intoxication Delirium

In this subtype, the symptoms of delirium are caused by intoxication from certain substances, such as alcohol, amphetamines, cannabis, cocaine, hallucinogens, inhalants, opioids, phencyclidine, sedatives, hypnotics, anxiolytics, or other or unknown substances.

Substance Withdrawal Delirium

Withdrawal from certain substances can precipitate symptoms of delirium that are sufficiently severe to warrant clinical attention. These substances include alcohol; opioids; sedatives, hypnotics, or anxiolytics; and others.

Medication-Induced Delirium

Medications that have been known to precipitate delirium include anticholinergics, antihypertensives, corticosteroids, anticonvulsants, cardiac glycosides, analgesics, anesthetics, antineoplastic agents, antiparkinson drugs, H_2-receptor antagonists (e.g., cimetidine), and others (Boland & Verduin, 2022; Fabian & Solai, 2017). In addition, polypharmacy has been implicated in precipitating delirium.

Delirium Due to Another Medical Condition or to Multiple Etiologies

Evidence from the history, physical examination, or laboratory findings may indicate that symptoms of delirium are associated with another medical condition or attributable to more than one cause. For example, evidence supports a significant association between urinary tract infections and delirium, particularly among adults 65 years and older (Krinitski, 2021), and a recent study found that interleukin-6 levels (a mediator in inflammation) may be a contributing factor (Rashid et al., 2021). Current evidence supports that delirium is usually the result of many factors instead of just one (Fabian & Solai, 2017).

CORE CONCEPT

Neurocognitive
A term used to describe cognitive functions closely linked to particular areas of the brain that have to do with thinking, reasoning, memory, learning, and speaking.

Neurocognitive Disorder

NCD is classified in the *DSM-5-TR* (APA, 2022) as either mild or major, distinguished primarily by the severity of symptomatology. In some settings, mild NCD is called mild cognitive impairment (MCI) and is a focus of early intervention, which is critical to preventing or slowing the progression of the disorder. Major NCD constitutes what was previously described as dementia in the *DSM-IV-TR* (APA, 2000). In progressive neurodegenerative conditions, these two diagnoses may identify earlier and later stages of the same disorder. Either diagnosis may be appropriate (depending on the severity of symptoms) for certain other NCDs that are the result of reversible or temporary conditions. *DSM-5-TR* criteria for these disorders are presented in Box 22–1.

CORE CONCEPT

Dementia (major neurocognitive disorder)
Dementia is a general term for the impaired ability to remember, think, or make decisions that is severe enough to interfere with social, behavioral, occupational, and emotional functioning. Several different disease processes can culminate in dementia. Unlike delirium, the progression of cognitive decline occurs slowly, over time. In some cases, dementia may be reversible.

Clinical Findings, Epidemiology, and Course

An estimated 6.5 million people in the United States currently have AD, the most common form of NCD, and the prevalence (the number of people with the disease at any one time) increases dramatically with age, affecting about 5% of individuals between 65 and 74, 13.1% of individuals between 75 and 84, and 33.2% of individuals 85 and older (Alzheimer's Association, 2022). Although a small percentage of those with AD are under age 65, the majority (80%) are over age 75. Despite these age-related increases, AD is not a normal part of aging.

Almost two-thirds of Americans with AD are women, and there is a disproportionately higher prevalence in Black/African American and Hispanic/Latino people than among non-Hispanic White people. As the Alzheimer's Association notes, more research is needed to identify common risk factors in these higher-risk populations. By 2050 the number of people age 65 and older with Alzheimer's dementia is projected to reach 12.7 million (Alzheimer's Association, 2022).

The increase in AD incidence is not the result of an "epidemic." The greatest risk factor for AD is age, and the population of older adults in the United States continues to grow. Survival after diagnosis typically ranges from 4 to 8 years, with most of that time spent in the most severe stage of the disease. Some individuals live as long as 20 years, reflecting the uncertain course of AD. Despite these alarming statistics about AD, recent studies have indicated that dementia, in general, and newly developing cases of AD have been declining in the United States over the past few years (Alzheimer's Association, 2022; Langa et al., 2017). This trend may be related to improved treatment and education about risk factors associated with heart disease and stroke, which are responsible for some forms of dementia.

NCDs can be classified as either primary or secondary. Primary NCDs are those such as AD, in which the NCD itself is the major sign of an organic brain disease that is not directly related to any other organic illness. Secondary NCDs are caused by or related to another disease or condition, such as HIV disease or cerebral trauma.

In NCD, impairment is evident in abstract thinking, judgment, and impulse control. The conventional rules of social conduct are often disregarded. Behavior may be uninhibited and inappropriate. Personal appearance and hygiene are often neglected. Language may or may not be affected. Some individuals may have difficulty naming objects, or the language may seem vague and imprecise. In severe forms of NCD, the individual may not speak at all, which is called **aphasia.** The person may know their

BOX 22–1 **Comparison of Diagnostic Criteria for Neurocognitive Disorder**

Mild Neurocognitive Disorder

A. Evidence of modest cognitive decline from a previous level of performance in one or more cognitive domains (complex attention, executive function, learning and memory, language, perceptual-motor, or social cognition) based on:
1. Concern of the individual, a knowledgeable informant, or the clinician that there has been a mild decline in cognitive function; and
2. A modest impairment in cognitive performance, preferably documented by standardized neuropsychological testing, or, in its absence, another quantified clinical assessment.
B. The cognitive deficits do not interfere with capacity for independence in everyday activities (i.e., complex instrumental activities of daily living such as paying bills or managing medications are preserved, but greater effort, compensatory strategies, or accommodation may be required).
C. The cognitive deficits do not occur exclusively in the context of a delirium.
D. The cognitive deficits are not better explained by another mental disorder (e.g., major depressive disorder, schizophrenia).

Specify whether due to:
Note: Each subtype listed has specific diagnostic criteria and corresponding text, which follow the general discussion of major and mild neurocognitive disorders.

• Alzheimer's disease
• Frontotemporal degeneration
• Lewy body disease
• Vascular disease
• Traumatic brain injury
• Substance/medication use
• HIV infection
• Prion disease
• Parkinson's disease
• Huntington's disease
• Another medical condition
• Multiple etiologies
• Unknown etiology

Specify:

Without behavioral disturbance: If the cognitive disturbance is not accompanied by any clinically significant behavioral disturbance.

With behavioral disturbance *(specify disturbance):* If the cognitive disturbance is accompanied by a clinically significant behavioral disturbance (e.g., psychotic symptoms, mood disturbance, agitation, apathy, or other behavioral symptoms).

Major Neurocognitive Disorder

A. Evidence of significant cognitive decline from a previous level of performance in one or more cognitive domains (complex attention, executive function, learning and memory, language, perceptual-motor, or social cognition) based on:
1. Concern of the individual, a knowledgeable informant, or the clinician that there has been a significant decline in cognitive function; and
2. A substantial impairment in cognitive performance, preferably documented by standardized neuropsychological testing, or, in its absence, another quantified clinical assessment.
B. The cognitive deficits interfere with independence in everyday activities (i.e., at a minimum, requiring assistance with complex instrumental activities of daily living such as paying bills or managing medications).
C. The cognitive deficits do not occur exclusively in the context of a delirium.
D. The cognitive deficits are not better explained by another mental disorder (e.g., major depressive disorder, schizophrenia).

Specify whether due to:
Note: Each subtype listed has specific diagnostic criteria and corresponding text, which follow the general discussion of major and mild neurocognitive disorders.

• Alzheimer's disease
• Frontotemporal degeneration
• Lewy body disease
• Vascular disease
• Traumatic brain injury
• Substance/medication use
• HIV infection
• Prion disease
• Parkinson's disease
• Huntington's disease
• Another medical condition
• Multiple etiologies
• Unknown etiology

Specify current severity:

Mild: Difficulties with instrumental activities of daily living (e.g., housework, managing money)

Moderate: Difficulties with basic activities of daily living (e.g., feeding, dressing)

Severe: Fully dependent

Specify:

With agitation: If the cognitive disturbance is accompanied by clinically significant agitation.

With anxiety: If the cognitive disturbance is accompanied by clinically significant anxiety.

With mood symptoms: If the cognitive disturbance is accompanied by clinically significant mood symptoms (e.g., dysphoria, irritability, euphoria).

Continued

BOX 22–1 **Comparison of Diagnostic Criteria for Neurocognitive Disorder–cont'd**	
Mild Neurocognitive Disorder	**Major Neurocognitive Disorder**
	With psychotic disturbance: If the cognitive disturbance is accompanied by delusions or hallucinations.
	With other behavioral or psychological disturbance: If the cognitive disturbance is accompanied by other clinically significant behavioral or psychological disturbance (e.g., apathy, aggression, disinhibition, disruptive behaviors or vocalizations, sleep or appetite/eating disturbance).
	Without accompanying behavioral or psychological disturbance: If the cognitive disturbance is not accompanied by any clinically significant behavioral or psychological disturbance.

Source: Reprinted with permission from the Diagnostic and Statistical Manual of Mental Disorders, Fifth Edition, Text Revision, DSM-5-TR (Copyright 2022). American Psychiatric Association.

needs but may not know how to communicate those needs to a caregiver.

Personality change is common in NCD and may be manifested by either an alteration or accentuation of premorbid characteristics. For example, an individual who was previously very socially active may become apathetic and socially isolated. A previously neat person may become markedly untidy in their appearance. Conversely, an individual who had difficulty trusting others before the illness may exhibit extreme fear and paranoia as manifestations of the disorder.

The reversibility of NCD depends on the basic etiology of the disorder. Truly reversible NCD occurs in only a small percentage of cases and might be more appropriately termed *temporary*. Reversible causes of NCD (dementia or dementia-like symptoms) include some brain tumors, subdural hematomas, medication reactions, normal pressure hydrocephalus, vitamin/nutritional deficiencies (especially B_1, B_6, and B_{12}), poisoning, anoxia, central nervous system (CNS) infections, immune disorders, thyroid disorders, too much or too little sodium or calcium, and metabolic disorders (hypoglycemia) (Mayo Clinic, 2022b). In most people, NCD runs a progressive, irreversible course.

As the disease progresses, **apraxia,** the inability to carry out purposeful motor activities despite intact motor function and the inability to use objects properly, may develop. The individual may be irritable, moody, or exhibit sudden outbursts over trivial issues. The ability to work or care for personal needs independently will no longer be possible. These individuals can no longer be left alone because they do not comprehend their limitations and are at serious risk for accidents. Wandering away from the home or care setting often becomes a problem. In advanced

dementia, clinical features include profound memory deficits, minimal verbal communication, loss of ambulatory ability, inability to perform activities of daily living (ADLs), and incontinence. The most common clinical complications are eating problems and infections (Mitchell, 2015).

Several causes have been ascribed to NCD (see previous section "Predisposing Factors"), but AD accounts for 60% to 80% of all cases (Alzheimer's Association, 2022). The progression of symptoms associated with AD has been described in five stages (Alzheimer's Association, 2022):

Stage 1. Preclinical AD: In this stage of the illness, there are no apparent symptoms, such as decline in memory, despite changes that are beginning to occur in the brain. A positron emission tomography (PET) scan can be used to identify abnormal levels of beta-amyloid and decreased metabolism of glucose; cerebrospinal fluid (CSF) analysis can detect abnormal levels of beta-amyloid and changes in tau protein. However, these brain-related changes don't always culminate in progressive disease. Some individuals show evidence of beta-amyloid plaques at death but never had cognitive symptoms during their life.

Stage 2. MCI due to AD: In this stage, in addition to brain changes, subtle symptoms of memory loss, and language and thinking problems may be noticeable to the individual, family members, and friends, but not to others, and they may not interfere with the individual's ability to carry out everyday activities. These symptoms may indicate that the brain can no longer compensate for the damage and death of neurons caused by AD. However, some individuals with MCI revert to normal cognition without further decline. Others progress to dementia, which is characterized by noticeable memory, language, thinking, or behavioral symptoms that impair a person's ability to function in daily life, combined with biomarker evidence of Alzheimer's-related brain changes. As the disorder progresses there are typically multiple symptoms that change over time.

Stage 3. Mild dementia due to AD: In this stage, most people are able to function independently in many areas but are likely to require assistance with more challenging tasks and activities to maximize independence and remain safe. The individual may deny that a problem exists by covering up memory loss with **confabulation** (creating imaginary events to fill in memory gaps). Depression and social withdrawal are common.

Stage 4. Moderate dementia due to AD: In this stage, which is typically the longest stage, symptoms interfere with the completion of many ADLs. Symptoms include increasing confusion, difficulty completing multistep tasks (such as bathing and dressing), personality changes, behavioral changes (such as agitation and suspiciousness), difficulty recognizing loved ones, and sometimes incontinence. Symptoms often worsen in the late afternoon and evening—a phenomenon called **sundowning.**

Stage 5. Severe dementia due to AD: In this stage, symptoms interfere with most everyday activities. The individual loses interest in food, lacks awareness of mealtimes, or cannot remember if they have eaten and therefore will require assistance to maintain adequate nutrition. The person loses the ability to recognize family members and loved ones. They are likely to require 24-hour care. Symptoms may include greatly diminished ability to communicate, difficulty moving (sometimes to the point of being bed-bound), and difficulty swallowing. These symptoms increase risks for decubiti, contractures, blood clots, aspiration pneumonia, infections, and sepsis and may be contributing causes of death.

Predisposing Factors

NCDs are differentiated by their etiology, although they share common symptom presentation. Categories include NCDs due to:

- AD
- Frontotemporal degeneration
- Lewy body disease
- Vascular disease
- Traumatic brain injury
- Substance/medication use
- HIV infection
- Prion disease
- PD

- Huntington's disease
- Another medical condition
- Multiple etiologies
- Unspecified

Neurocognitive Disorder Due to Alzheimer's Disease

AD is characterized by the syndrome of symptoms identified as mild or major NCD and is categorized by the five stages described previously. The onset of symptoms is slow and insidious, and the course of the disorder is generally progressive and deteriorating. Memory impairment is a prominent feature.

Refinement of diagnostic criteria now enables clinicians to use specific clinical features to identify the disease with considerable accuracy. Examination by computed tomography (CT) scan or magnetic resonance imaging (MRI) reveals a degenerative pathology of the brain that includes atrophy, widened cortical sulci, and enlarged cerebral ventricles (Figs. 22–1 and 22–2). Microscopic examination reveals numerous neurofibrillary tangles and senile plaques in the brains of people with AD. These changes occur as a part of the normal aging process. However, in individuals with AD, they are found in dramatically increased numbers, and their profusion is concentrated in the hippocampus and certain parts of the cerebral cortex.

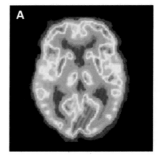
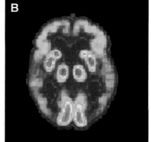
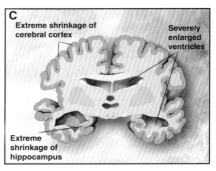

FIGURE 22–1 Changes in the Alzheimer's brain. A, Metabolic activity in a normal brain. B, Diminished metabolic activity in the Alzheimer's-diseased brain. C, Late-stage Alzheimer's disease with generalized atrophy and enlargement of the ventricles and sulci. (Source: Alzheimer's Disease Education & Referral Center, A Service of the National Institute on Aging.)

Brain Cross Sections

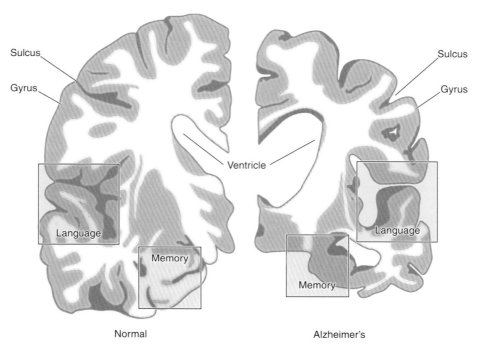

FIGURE 22–2 Neurobiology of Alzheimer's disease. (Source: American Health Assistance Foundation [2012]. https://www.brightfocus.org/alzheimers/infographic/brain-alzheimers-disease, with permission.)

NEUROTRANSMITTERS

A decrease in the neurotransmitter acetylcholine has been implicated in the etiology of Alzheimer's disease. Cholinergic sources arise from the brainstem and the basal forebrain to supply areas of the basal ganglia, thalamus, limbic structures, hippocampus, and cerebral cortex.

Cell bodies of origin for the serotonin pathways lie within the raphe nuclei located in the brainstem. Those for norepinephrine originate in the locus coeruleus. Projections for both neurotransmitters extend throughout the forebrain, prefrontal cortex, cerebellum, and limbic system. Dopamine pathways arise from areas in the midbrain and project to the frontal cortex, limbic system, basal ganglia, and thalamus. Dopamine neurons in the hypothalamus innervate the posterior pituitary.

Glutamate, an excitatory neurotransmitter, has largely descending pathways with highest concentrations in the cerebral cortex. It is also found in the hippocampus, thalamus, hypothalamus, cerebellum, and spinal cord.

AREAS OF THE BRAIN AFFECTED

Areas of the brain affected by Alzheimer's disease and associated symptoms include the following:
- Frontal lobe: Impaired reasoning ability; inability to solve problems and perform familiar tasks; poor judgment; inability to evaluate the appropriateness of behavior; aggressiveness.
- Parietal lobe: Impaired orientation ability; impaired visuospatial skills (unable to remain oriented within own environment).
- Occipital lobe: Impaired language interpretation; inability to recognize familiar objects.
- Temporal lobe: Inability to recall words; inability to use words correctly (language comprehension). In late stages, some people experience delusions and hallucinations.
- Hippocampus: Impaired memory. Short-term memory is affected initially. Later, the individual is unable to form new memories.
- Amygdala: Impaired emotions—depression, anxiety, fear, personality changes, apathy, paranoia.
- Neurotransmitters: Alterations in acetylcholine, dopamine, norepinephrine, serotonin, and others may play a role in behaviors such as restlessness, sleep impairment, mood, and agitation.

MEDICATIONS AND THEIR EFFECTS ON THE BRAIN

1. Cholinesterase inhibitors (e.g., donepezil, rivastigmine, and galantamine) act by inhibiting acetylcholinesterase, which slows the degradation of acetylcholine, thereby increasing concentrations of the neurotransmitter in the brain. Most common side effects include dizziness, gastrointestinal upset, fatigue, and headache.
2. *N*-methyl-d-aspartate (NMDA) receptor antagonists (e.g., memantine) act by blocking NMDA receptors from excessive glutamate, preventing continuous influx of calcium into the cells and ultimately slowing down neuronal degradation. Possible side effects include dizziness, headache, and constipation.
3. Human monoclonal antibody therapy (aducanumab) acts by preferentially binding to aggregated amyloid-β to reduce amyloid plaques and slow the progression of the disease. (Approved by the FDA in June 2021.)

Recent research points to a mutation in microtubule affinity regulating kinase (MARK 4) (an enzyme that is involved with many cell functions including cell division) as contributing to an accumulation and toxicity of tau proteins leading to neurodegeneration and pathogenesis in AD (Oba et al., 2020). Likely there are multiple contributing factors in the pathogenesis and progression of this disorder.

In 2018 the National Institute on Aging (NIA) and Alzheimer's Association redefined AD as the presence of three specific biomarkers (amyloid-beta [Aβ] plaques, tau neurofibrillary tangles, and neuronal damage) rather than by progression of cognitive symptoms (Sullivan, 2018). It is believed that this redefinition will, in the short term, clarify research and clinical drug trials, and in the long term may change the way AD is understood and treated. Other biomarkers, including lower levels of metabolites such as histamine, asparagine, aspartate, and citrulline (all involved in regulating inflammation), suggest that inflammation may be a key component in the pathology of this disease (Hampel et al., 2018). Recent research found that abnormal interleukin-6 levels (indicative of inflammation) and dysregulated interleukin-6 signaling is a key mechanism linking memory/cognitive impairment and metabolic dysregulation in AD (Lyra e Silva et al., 2021). Because biomarkers are present before cognitive symptoms appear, these findings promise the potential for preventive interventions and will, no doubt, be the focus of ongoing research.

A recent study found that individuals with AD and COVID-19 had roughly twice the mortality rate of those in the same age group without AD, and the findings were consistent whether the individuals were residing in a community or a nursing home (Gilstrap et al., 2022). Although the reasons for this association are not well understood, it is clear that individuals with AD have been a particularly vulnerable population in this pandemic.

Etiological Theories

The exact cause of AD is unknown, but experts believe that with the exception of rare cases in which genetic mutations cause AD, multiple factors rather than a single cause influence the development of this illness (Alzheimer's Association, 2022). Particularly in late-onset AD, the risk is influenced by multiple genes and environmental factors and their interaction with Aβ proteins in the transition to AD (Graziane & Sweet, 2017). As previously mentioned, recent research studies highlighted the effect of a mutation in MARK 4 as contributing to an accumulation and toxicity of tau proteins leading to neurodegeneration and pathogenesis in AD (Oba et al., 2020), and dysregulated interleukin-6 signaling is a key mechanism

linking memory/cognitive impairment and metabolic dysregulation in AD (Lyra e Silva et al., 2021). Several other research studies have led to hypotheses about contributing or causative factors:

- **Neurotransmitter alterations:** Research has indicated that in the brains of individuals with AD, the enzyme required to produce acetylcholine is dramatically reduced. The reduction seems to be greatest in the nucleus basalis of the inferior medial forebrain area (Boland & Verduin, 2022). The decrease in production of acetylcholine reduces the level of neurotransmitter that is released to cells in the cortex and hippocampus, resulting in cognitive process disturbances. Other neurotransmitters believed to be disrupted in AD include norepinephrine, serotonin, dopamine, and the amino acid glutamate. It has been proposed that in NCD, excess glutamate leads to overstimulation of the *N*-methyl-d-aspartate (NMDA) receptors, causing increased intracellular calcium and subsequent neuronal degeneration and cell death. Decreased levels of somatostatin and corticotropin have also been found in individuals with AD.

- **Plaques and tangles:** As mentioned previously, an overabundance of structures called *plaques* and *tangles* appear in the brains of individuals with AD. The plaques are made of a peptide called Aβ, derived from a larger protein called amyloid precursor protein (APP). Plaques are formed when Aβ peptides clump together and mix with molecules and other cellular matter. Tangles are formed from a special kind of cellular protein called *tau protein* that provides stability to the neuron. In AD, the tau protein is chemically altered. Strands of the protein become tangled, interfering with the neuronal transport system. It is unknown whether the plaques and tangles cause AD or are a consequence of the disease; it should be noted that both are seen in other disorders as well as in the normal brain with increasing age (Boland & Verduin, 2022). Plaques and tangles are thought to contribute to the destruction and death of neurons, leading to memory failure, personality changes, inability to carry out ADLs, and other features of the disease The plaques themselves can cause space-occupying lesions in the cortex, which contribute to inflammatory processes, synapse loss, and neuronal death (Graziane & Sweet, 2017). The number and density of these plaques (also called *amyloid plaques* or *senile plaques*) found in postmortem studies have been correlated with disease severity (Boland & Verduin, 2022).

- **Head trauma:** Individuals who have a history of head trauma are at risk for AD. Studies have shown that some individuals who experienced head trauma subsequently (after years) developed

AD (Graziane & Sweet, 2017). There is evidence that head trauma can increase inflammatory mediators and cause the deposition of Aβ plaques in the brain. The effects of traumatic brain injury on Aβ plaque development may also be mediated by genetic factors.

■ **Genetic factors:** A familial pattern is evident for some forms of AD, with as many as 40% of people with AD having a family history of the disease. Some families exhibit a pattern of inheritance that suggests autosomal dominant genetic transmission (Boland & Verduin, 2022). Some studies indicate that early-onset cases are more likely than late-onset cases to be familial, and that there is a link between AD and gene mutations found on chromosomes 21, 14, and 1 (Graziane & Sweet, 2017). Mutations on chromosome 21 cause the formation of abnormal APP. Mutations on chromosome 14 cause production of abnormal presenilin 1 (PS-1), and mutations on chromosome 1 lead to the formation of abnormal presenilin 2 (PS-2). Each of these mutations results in an increased amount of the Aβ protein that is a major component of the plaques associated with AD. Individuals with Down syndrome (who carry an extra copy of chromosome 21) have been found to be unusually susceptible to AD.

Late-onset AD is influenced by a gene known as apolipoprotein E (APOE), and particularly APOE epsilon 4, but in individuals with this genotype who do not have disease symptoms by age 65, only about 50% will develop AD (Graziane & Sweet, 2017). As research has continued, 20 additional influential genes have been identified, but their exact role in causing AD is still unclear. Although much of the research has focused on toxic amyloid and tau proteins in AD, some current research is exploring other molecular and cellular pathways that may be involved, including glial cell activation, inflammation, glucose transport systems, and abnormal neuronal circuit activity.

A study aimed at identifying biomarkers of AD before the onset of symptoms (Schindler et al., 2019) reported evidence that a blood test for amyloid levels, especially when considered along with age and presence of the APOE epsilon 4 gene variant, is 94% accurate in identifying people with early brain changes indicative of AD. Amyloid proteins begin to accumulate in the brain up to two decades before the onset of symptoms (Bhandari, 2019), and such a blood test, although not yet available for clinical use, could pave the way for identifying early prevention and treatment strategies. Other research found that individuals with the APOE4 gene variant showed hippocampal atrophy and cortical thinning in early AD, which suggests this may be a valuable biomarker

and a target for research into medication that slows the processes of deterioration in these structures (Abushakra et al., 2020).

Because previous research has demonstrated that ketone bodies have a protective effect on neurons, some research has focused on the effect of ketones in improving memory and learning. Several studies have reported the potential benefits of ketone-rich diets in slowing or improving cognitive decline in AD as blood sugar disorders have been associated with this disease (University Health News, 2019).

Vascular Neurocognitive Disorder

The cognitive symptoms in vascular NCD are caused by significant cerebrovascular disease. When blood flow in the brain is impaired, progressive intellectual deterioration occurs. Impairment may be located in large vessels or microvascular networks, and symptoms vary depending on the type, extent, and location of vascular lesion (APA, 2022). The disorder is more common in men than in women.

Vascular NCD typically has a more abrupt onset, and changes in thought processes occur in noticeable "steps" downward rather than as a gradual deterioration. At times, the symptoms seem to subside, and the individual exhibits fairly lucid thinking and better memory. The person may become optimistic that improvement is occurring, only to experience a further decline of functioning in a fluctuating pattern of progression. This irregular pattern of decline can be an intense source of anxiety for the individual with this disorder.

In vascular NCD, individuals experience small strokes that destroy many areas of the brain. The pattern of deficits varies depending on which regions of the brain have been affected. Certain focal neurological signs commonly seen with vascular NCD include weaknesses of the limbs, small-stepped gait, and difficulty with speech. Neuropsychiatric symptoms may include depression, anxiety, mania, apathy, catastrophic reactions, psychosis, or pathological laughing or crying (McCutcheon & Robinson, 2017).

Etiology

Vascular NCD is directly related to an interruption of blood flow to the brain. Symptoms result from death of nerve cells in regions nourished by diseased vessels. Various diseases and conditions that interfere with blood circulation have been implicated.

High blood pressure is thought to be one of the most significant factors in the etiology of multiple small strokes or cerebral infarcts. Hypertension leads to damage to the lining of blood vessels, which can result in rupture of the blood vessel with subsequent hemorrhage or an accumulation of fibrin in the vessel with intravascular clotting and inhibited blood flow. NCD also can result from infarcts related to occlusion of blood vessels by particulate matter that travels through the bloodstream to the brain. These emboli may be solid (e.g., clots, cellular debris, platelet aggregates), gaseous (e.g., air, nitrogen), or liquid (e.g., fat, after soft tissue trauma or fracture of long bones).

Cognitive impairment can occur with multiple small infarcts (sometimes called *silent strokes*) over time or with a single cerebrovascular event in a strategic area of the brain. An individual may have both vascular NCD and AD simultaneously. This condition is referred to as a *mixed* disorder, the prevalence of which is likely to increase as the population ages.

Frontotemporal Neurocognitive Disorder

Symptoms of frontotemporal NCD occur as a result of shrinking of the frontal and temporal anterior lobes of the brain. This type of NCD was identified as Pick's disease in the *DSM-IV-TR*. The cause of frontotemporal NCD is unknown, but a genetic factor appears to be involved. Symptoms tend to fall into two clinical patterns: (1) behavioral and personality changes and (2) speech and language problems. Common behavioral changes include "behavior that can be either impulsive (disinhibited) or bored and listless (apathetic) and includes inappropriate social behavior; lack of social tact; lack of empathy; distractibility; loss of insight into the behaviors of oneself and others; an increased interest in sex; changes in food preferences; agitation or, conversely, blunted emotions; neglect of personal hygiene; repetitive or compulsive behavior, and decreased energy and motivation" (National Institute of Neurological Disorders and Stroke [NINDS], 2019). Speech problems include impairment or loss of speech or increasing difficulty in using and understanding written and spoken language. Spatial skills and memory remain intact, but the disease progresses steadily and often rapidly, ranging from less than 2 years in some individuals to more than 10 years in others (NINDS, 2019).

Neurocognitive Disorder Due to Traumatic Brain Injury

According to *DSM-5-TR* criteria, this disorder is diagnosed based on evidence of:

> "an impact to the head or other mechanisms of rapid movement or displacement of the brain within the skull with one or more of the following: loss of consciousness, posttraumatic amnesia, disorientation and confusion, neurological signs (e.g., neuroimaging demonstrating injury; visual field cuts; anosmia; hemiparesis; hemisensory loss; cortical blindness; aphasia; apraxia; weakness; loss of balance; other sensory loss that cannot be accounted for by peripheral or other causes)" (APA, 2022, pp. 706–707).

Amnesia is the most common neurobehavioral symptom after head trauma. Other symptoms may include confusion and changes in speech, vision, and personality. Depending on the severity of the injury, these symptoms may eventually subside or may become permanent. Severe head injuries and multiple traumatic brain injuries increase one's risk for AD or other dementias, especially when there are other risk factors such as the presence of the APOE4 gene, which increases anyone's risk for AD (Mayo Clinic, 2023). Repeated head trauma, such as the type experienced by American football players and boxers, can result in chronic traumatic encephalopathy, a syndrome characterized by emotional lability, dysarthria, ataxia, and impulsivity.

Neurocognitive Disorder Due to Lewy Body Dementia

Dementia with Lewy bodies is now identified as the second most common cause of dementia in older adults after AD (Graziane & Sweet, 2017). Clinically, Lewy body NCD is fairly similar to AD; however, it tends to progress more rapidly, with earlier appearance of visual hallucinations and parkinsonian features.

Depression and delusions are also common symptoms in this population. Lewy body dementia gained public attention when an autopsy of famous comedian Robin Williams revealed that he had this disease. His widow reported that he had been seeking neurocognitive testing because he was aware of a decline in his mental capacities. He was also manifesting symptoms of depression and ultimately took his own life.

This disorder is distinguished by the presence of Lewy bodies—eosinophilic inclusion bodies—seen in the cerebral cortex and brainstem. Acetylcholinesterase (ACh) concentrations are reduced in the brains of people with Lewy body NCD, and consequently, cholinesterase inhibitors are likely to be more effective for this population than for those with Alzheimer's dementia (Crystal, 2018). These patients are highly sensitive to extrapyramidal effects of antipsychotic medications. The disease is progressive and irreversible and may account for as many as 25% of all NCD cases.

Neurocognitive Disorder Due to Parkinson's Disease

NCD is observed in as many as 80% of clients with PD (APA, 2022). This disease is characterized by a loss of nerve cells in the substantia nigra and diminished dopamine activity, resulting in involuntary muscle movements, slowness, and rigidity along with tremor in the upper extremities. In some instances, the cerebral changes that occur in NCD due to PD closely resemble those of AD.

Neurocognitive Disorder Due to HIV Infection

Infection with the HIV type 1 (HIV-1) can result in an NCD called *HIV-1-associated cognitive/motor complex.* A less severe form, known as *HIV-1-associated minor cognitive/motor disorder,* also occurs. The severity of symptoms is correlated with the extent of brain pathology. The immune dysfunction associated with HIV disease can lead to brain infections by other organisms, and HIV-1 also appears to cause NCD directly. In the early stages, neuropsychiatric symptoms may be manifested by barely perceptible changes in a person's normal psychological presentation. Severe cognitive changes, particularly confusion, changes in behavior, and sometimes psychoses, are not uncommon in the later stages.

With the advent of the highly active antiretroviral therapies (HAART), incidence rates of NCD due to HIV infection have declined. However, Moore and Marquine (2017) noted that several studies have detected elevated rates of NCDs in older adults who are HIV positive, suggesting that there may be additive negative effects for older HIV-positive individuals.

Substance/Medication-Induced Neurocognitive Disorder

NCD can occur as a result of substance reactions, overuse, or abuse. Symptoms are consistent with major or mild NCD and persist beyond the usual duration of intoxication and acute withdrawal (APA, 2022). Substances that have been associated with the development of NCDs include alcohol, sedatives, hypnotics, anxiolytics, and inhalants. Drugs that cause anticholinergic side effects and toxins, such as lead and mercury, have also been implicated.

Neurocognitive Disorder Due to Huntington's Disease

Huntington's disease (HD) is transmitted by a DNA error in a gene identified as huntingtin. The most vulnerable area of the brain is the striatum and damage to this area over time is responsible for the symptoms. The onset of symptoms (i.e., involuntary twitching of the limbs or facial muscles, mild cognitive changes, depression, and apathy) usually occurs between age 30 and 50 years. The individual usually declines into a profound state of cognitive impairment and **ataxia** (muscular incoordination). The average duration of the disease is 10 to 20 years depending on the severity of symptoms. As the disease progresses, the weakened individual usually dies secondary to pneumonia, heart failure, choking, or other complications (Huntington's Disease Society of America [HDSA], 2022). About 10% of the cases occur in children and adolescents, and the progression is typically more rapid than it is in adult-onset HD.

Neurocognitive Disorder Due to Prion Disease

Prion disease is a group of disorders caused by infectious agents called *prions* and characterized by its insidious onset and rapid progression. Manifestations include problems with coordination and other movement disturbances along with rapidly progressing dementia. Prion disease can only be definitely confirmed by brain biopsy or autopsy. Tests used for diagnostic purposes include CSF biomarkers of neuronal injury or CSF evidence of disease-causing prion proteins, MRI showing subcortical or cortical hyperintensity of gray matter, and electroencephalograms showing periodic sharp triphasic discharges (APA, 2022). From 5% to 15% of cases of prion disease have a genetic component. Symptoms may develop at any age in adults but typically occur between ages 40 and 60 years. The clinical course is extremely rapid, with the progression from diagnosis to death being less than 2 years. The most common form of prion disease in humans is Creutzfeldt-Jakob's disease (Johns Hopkins Medicine, n.d.).

Neurocognitive Disorder Due to Another Medical Condition

Many other medical conditions can cause NCD, including structural lesions, hypothyroidism, hyperparathyroidism, pituitary insufficiency, uremia, hepatic or renal failure encephalitis, brain tumor, pernicious anemia, thiamine deficiency, pellagra, uncontrolled epilepsy, cardiopulmonary insufficiency, fluid and electrolyte imbalances, CNS and systemic infections, systemic lupus erythematosus, and multiple sclerosis. The etiological factors associated with delirium and NCD are summarized in Box 22–2.

Application of the Nursing Process

Assessment

Nursing assessment of the patient with delirium or mild or major NCD is based on knowledge of the symptomatology associated with the disorders previously described in this chapter. Subjective and objective data are gathered by various members of the health-care team. Clinicians use a variety of methods for obtaining assessment information.

Patient History

Nurses play a significant role in acquiring the patient history, including the specific mental and physical changes that have occurred and the age at which the changes began. If the patient is unable to relate information adequately, the data should be obtained from family members or others who would be aware of the patient's physical and psychosocial history.

From the patient history, nurses should assess the following areas of concern: (1) type, frequency,

BOX 22–2 Etiological Factors Implicated in the Development of Delirium and/or Mild or Major Neurocognitive Disorder

Biological Factors

Hypoxia: Any condition leading to a deficiency of oxygen to the brain

Nutritional deficiencies: Vitamins (particularly B and C); protein; fluid and electrolyte imbalances

Metabolic disturbances: Porphyria; encephalopathies related to hepatic, renal, pancreatic, or pulmonary insufficiencies; hypoglycemia

Endocrine dysfunction: Thyroid, parathyroid, adrenal, pancreas, pituitary

Cardiovascular disease: Stroke, cardiac insufficiency, atherosclerosis

Primary brain disorders: Epilepsy, Alzheimer's disease, Pick's disease, Huntington's chorea, multiple sclerosis, Parkinson's disease

Infections: Encephalitis, meningitis, pneumonia, septicemia, neurosyphilis (dementia paralytica), HIV disease, acute rheumatic fever, Creutzfeldt-Jakob disease

Intracranial neoplasms

Congenital defects: Prenatal infections, such as first-trimester maternal rubella

Exogenous Factors

Birth trauma: Prolonged labor, damage from use of forceps, other obstetric complications

Cranial trauma: Concussion, contusions, hemorrhage, hematomas

Volatile inhalant compounds: Gasoline, glue, paint, paint thinners, spray paints, cleaning fluids, typewriter correction fluid, varnishes, and lacquers

Heavy metals: Lead, mercury, manganese

Other metallic elements: Aluminum

Organic phosphates: Various insecticides

Substance abuse/dependence: Alcohol, amphetamines, caffeine, cannabis, cocaine, hallucinogens, inhalants, nicotine, opioids, phencyclidine, sedatives, hypnotics, anxiolytics

Other medications: Anticholinergics, antihistamines, antidepressants, antipsychotics, antiparkinsonians, antihypertensives, steroids, digitalis

---

and severity of mood swings, personality and behavioral changes, and catastrophic emotional reactions; (2) cognitive changes, such as problems with attention span, thinking process, problem-solving, and memory (recent and remote); (3) language difficulties; (4) orientation to person, place, time, and situation; and (5) appropriateness of social behavior.

The nurse also should obtain information regarding current and past medication usage, history of other drug and alcohol use, and possible exposure to toxins. Knowledge regarding the history of related symptoms or specific illnesses (e.g., HD, AD, Pick's disease, or PD) in other family members may be useful.

Physical Assessment

Assessment of physical systems by both the nurse and the physician has two main emphases: signs of damage to the nervous system and evidence of diseases of other organs that could affect mental function. Diseases of various organ systems can induce confusion, loss of memory, and behavioral changes. These causes must be considered in diagnosing cognitive disorders. In the neurological examination, the patient is asked to perform maneuvers or answer questions that are designed to evaluate specific parts of the brain or peripheral nerves. Testing will assess mental status and alertness, muscle strength, reflexes, sensory perception, proprioception, language

skills, and coordination. Physical assessment should include looking for signs of abuse or neglect, screening for hearing or vision impairments, and conducting a mental status examination. An example of a mental status examination for a patient with NCD is presented in Box 22–3.

A battery of psychological tests may be ordered as part of the diagnostic examination. The results of these tests may be used to differentiate between NCD and **pseudodementia** (depression). Depression is one of the most common mental illnesses in the elderly, but it is often misdiagnosed and treated inadequately. Cognitive symptoms of depression may mimic NCD, and because of the prevalence of NCD in the elderly, providers are often too eager to make this diagnosis. A comparison of symptoms of NCD and pseudodementia is presented in Table 22–1. Nurses can assist in this assessment by carefully observing and documenting these sometimes subtle differences.

Diagnostic Laboratory Evaluations

The nurse also may be required to help the patient fulfill the physician's orders for special diagnostic laboratory evaluations. Many of these tests are conducted to rule out other factors associated with dementia and may include the following:

■ Evaluation of blood and urine samples to test for various infections

BOX 22–3 Mental Status Examination for Neurocognitive Disorder

Patient Name _____ Date _____

Age _____ Sex _____ Diagnosis _____

	MAXIMUM	CLIENT'S SCORE

1. **VERBAL FLUENCY**
   Ask patient to name as many animals as he/she can. (Time: 60 seconds) — 10 points — _____
   (Score 1 point/2 animals)

2. **COMPREHENSION**
   a. Point to the ceiling — 1 point — _____
   b. Point to your nose and the window — 1 point — _____
   c. Point to your foot, the door, and ceiling — 1 point — _____
   d. Point to the window, your leg, the door, and your thumb — 1 point — _____

3. **NAMING AND WORD FINDING**
   Ask the patient to name the following as you point to them:
   a. Watch stem (winder) — 1 point — _____
   b. Teeth — 1 point — _____
   c. Sole of shoe — 1 point — _____
   d. Buckle of belt — 1 point — _____
   e. Knuckles — 1 point — _____

4. **ORIENTATION**
   a. Date — 2 points — _____
   b. Day of week — 2 points — _____
   c. Month — 1 point — _____
   d. Year — 1 point — _____

5. **NEW LEARNING ABILITY**
   Tell the patient: "I'm going to tell you four words, which I want you to remember." Have the patient repeat the four words after they are initially presented, and then say that you will ask him/her to remember the words later. Continue with the examination, and at intervals of 5 and 10 minutes, ask the patient to recall the words. Three different sets of words are provided here.

		10 min	5 min.
a. Brown (Fun) (Grape)	2 points each:	_____	_____
b. Honesty (Loyalty) (Happiness)	2 points each:	_____	_____
c. Tulip (Carrot) (Stocking)	2 points each:	_____	_____
d. Eyedropper (Ankle) (Toothbrush)	2 points each:	_____	_____

6. **VERBAL STORY FOR IMMEDIATE RECALL**
   Tell the patient: "I'm going to read you a short story, which I want you to remember. Listen closely to what I read because I will ask you to tell me the story when I finish." Read the story slowly and carefully, but without pausing at the slash marks. After completing the paragraph, tell the patient to retell the story as accurately as possible. Record the number of correct memories (information within the slashes) and describe confabulation if it is present. (1 point = 1 remembered item [13 maximum points]) — 13 points — _____

   It was July/and the Rogers family, mom, dad, and four children/were packing up their station wagon/to go on vacation. They were taking their yearly trip/to the beach at Gulf Shores. This year they were making a special 1-day stop/at The Aquarium in New Orleans. After a long day's drive they arrived at the motel/only to discover that in their excitement/they had left the twins/and their suitcases/in the front yard.

BOX 22–3 Mental Status Examination for Neurocognitive Disorder—cont'd

7. VISUAL MEMORY (HIDDEN OBJECTS)

Tell the patient that you are going to hide some objects around the office (desk, bed) and that you want him/her to remember where they are. Hide four or five common objects (e.g., keys, pen, reflex hammer) in various places in the patient's sight. After a delay of several minutes, ask the patient to find the objects. (1 point per item found)

a. Coin	1 point	_____
b. Pen	1 point	_____
c. Comb	1 point	_____
d. Keys	1 point	_____
e. Fork	1 point	_____

8. PAIRED ASSOCIATE LEARNING

Tell the patient that you are going to read a list of words two at a time. The patient will be expected to remember the words that go together (e.g., big–little). When he/she is clear on the directions, read the first list of words at the rate of one pair per second. After reading the first list, test for recall by presenting the first recall list. Give the first word of a pair and ask for the word that was paired with it. Correct incorrect responses and proceed to the next pair. After the first recall has been completed, allow a 10-second delay and continue with the second presentation and recall lists.

Presentation Lists

1	2
a. High–Low	a. Good–Bad
b. House–Income	b. Book–Page
c. Good–Bad	c. High–Low
d. Book–Page	d. House–Income

Recall Lists

1	2		
a. House _____	a. High _____	2 points	_____
b. Book _____	b. Good _____	2 points	_____
c. High _____	c. House _____	2 points	_____
d. Good _____	d. Book _____	2 points	_____

9. CONSTRUCTIONAL ABILITY

Ask patient to reconstruct this drawing and to draw the other 2 items: 3 points   _____

Draw a daisy in a flowerpot	3 points	_____
Draw a clock with all the numbers and set the clock at 2:30.	3 points	_____

10. WRITTEN COMPLEX CALCULATIONS

a. Addition	108 $+\ 79$	1 point	_____
b. Subtraction	605 $-\ 86$	1 point	_____
c. Multiplication	108 $\times\ 36$	1 point	_____
d. Division	$559 \div 43$	1 point	_____

Continued

BOX 22–3 Mental Status Examination for Neurocognitive Disorder—cont'd

11. **PROVERB INTERPRETATION**

Tell the patient to explain the following sayings. Record the answers.

a. Don't cry over spilled milk.   2 points   _____

b. Rome wasn't built in a day.   2 points   _____

c. A drowning man will clutch at a straw.   2 points   _____

d. A golden hammer can break down an iron door.   2 points   _____

e. The hot coal burns, the cold one blackens.   2 points   _____

12. **SIMILARITIES**

Ask the patient to name the similarity or relationship between each of the two items.

a. Turnip..Cauliflower	2 points	_____
b. Car...Airplane	2 points	_____
c. Desk...Bookcase	2 points	_____
d. Poem...Novel	2 points	_____
e. Horse...Apple	2 points	_____

Maximum: 100 points   _____

Normal Individuals		Patients With Alzheimer's Disease	
Age-Group	**Mean Score (standard deviation)**	**Stage**	**Mean Score (standard deviation)**
40-49	80.9 (9.7)	I	57.2 (9.1)
50-59	82.3 (8.6)	II	37.0 (7.8)
60-69	75.5 (10.5)	III	13.4 (8.1)
70-79	66.9 (9.1)		
80-89	67.9 (11.0)		

Adapted from Strub, R. L., & Black, F. W. (2000). The mental status examination in neurology (4th ed.). F.A. Davis. With permission.

TABLE 22–1 A Comparison of Neurocognitive Disorder (NCD) and Pseudodementia (Depression)

SYMPTOM ELEMENT	NCD	PSEUDODEMENTIA (DEPRESSION)
Progression of symptoms	Slow	Rapid
Memory	Progressive deficits; recent memory loss greater than remote; may confabulate for memory "gaps"; no complaints of loss	More like forgetfulness; no evidence of progressive deficit; recent and remote loss equal; complaints of deficits; no confabulation (will more likely answer "I don't know")
Orientation	Disoriented to time and place; may wander in search of the familiar	Oriented to time and place; no wandering
Task performance	Consistently poor performance but struggles to perform	Performance is variable; little effort is put forth
Symptom severity	Worse as the day progresses	Better as the day progresses
Affective distress	Appears unconcerned	Communicates severe distress
Appetite	Unchanged	Diminished
Attention and concentration	Impaired	Intact

- Liver function studies to rule out hepatic disease
- Glucose tests to rule out diabetes or hypoglycemia
- Electrolytes to rule out imbalances
- Thyroid tests to rule out hypothyroidism
- Vitamin B$_{12}$ test to rule out nutritional deficiencies
- Drug and alcohol screening to rule out the presence of toxic substances

A rapid plasma reagin (RPR) test for syphilis and HIV testing should be included if the patient is at higher risk for these conditions. CT scanning produces an image of the size and shape of the brain, and MRI produces a computerized image of soft tissue in the brain. Both CT and MRI scans are useful in identifying areas of atrophy, such as those seen in AD, and may identify other pathological processes needed for differential diagnosis. A lumbar puncture may be performed to examine the CSF for evidence of CNS infection or hemorrhage if these conditions are suspected.

PET is used to reveal the metabolic activity of the brain, an evaluation some researchers believe is important for early diagnosis of AD. PET scan techniques can identify Aβ plaques and tau neurofibrillary tangles in the brain as well as decreases in glucose metabolism. Fluorodeoxyglucose (FDG) PET scans show areas of the brain where nutrients are poorly metabolized, indicating areas of degeneration.

Recently, a blood test for Aβ plaques has become available and received certification in the United States by the Centers for Medicare & Medicaid Services to allow distribution on the market. Even more recently, researchers (Reddy et al., 2022) found that incorporating plasma analysis of mRNA molecules could have predictive value for risk of AD and more specifically in high risk populations, such as African Americans.

Nursing Diagnosis and Outcome Identification

Using information collected during the assessment, the nurse completes the patient database, from which the selection of appropriate nursing diagnoses is determined. Table 22–2 presents a list of patient behaviors and the NANDA-I (Herdman et al., 2021) nursing diagnoses that correspond to those behaviors, which may be used in planning care for the patient with an NCD.

Outcome Criteria

The following criteria may be used for measurement of outcomes in the care of the patient with an NCD.

The patient:

- Has not experienced physical injury.
- Has not harmed self or others.
- Has maintained reality orientation to the best of their capability.
- Is able to communicate with their consistent caregiver.
- Fulfills ADLs with assistance (or for a patient who is unable to fulfill ADLs, has needs met as anticipated by the caregiver).
- Discusses positive aspects about self and life.

Planning and Implementation

Care for an individual with an NCD must focus on immediate needs and keeping the individual safe from harm.

TABLE 22–2 Assigning Nursing Diagnoses to Behaviors Commonly Associated with Neurocognitive Disorders	
BEHAVIORS	**NURSING DIAGNOSES**
Falls, wandering, poor coordination, confusion, misinterpretation of the environment (illusions, hallucinations), lack of understanding of environmental hazards, memory deficits	Risk for physical trauma
Disorientation, confusion, memory deficits, inaccurate interpretation of the environment, suspiciousness, paranoia	Disturbed thought processes Impaired memory
Having hallucinations (hears voices, sees visions, feels crawling sensation on skin)	Disturbed sensory perception*
Aggression (hitting, scratching, or kicking)	Risk for other-directed violence
Inability to name objects/people, loss of memory for words, difficulty finding the right word, confabulation, incoherent, screaming and demanding verbalizations	Impaired verbal communication
Inability to perform activities of daily living: feeding, dressing, hygiene, toileting	Self-care deficit (specify)
Expressions of shame and self-degradation, progressive social isolation, apathy, decreased activity, withdrawal, depressed mood	Situational low self-esteem Maladaptive grieving

*This nursing diagnosis has been resigned from the NANDA-I list of approved diagnoses but is used for purposes of this text.

Risk for Physical Trauma

Because the individual has impairments in cognitive and psychomotor functioning, it is important to ensure that the environment is as safe as possible to prevent injury. NANDA-I defines *Risk for physical trauma* as "susceptible to physical injury of a sudden onset and severity which require immediate attention" (Herdman et al., 2021, p. 492). Table 22–3 presents this nursing diagnosis in care plan format.

Patient Goals

Outcome criteria include short- and long-term goals. Timelines are individually determined.

Short-term goals

- Patient will call for assistance when ambulating or conducting other activities (if it is within their cognitive ability).
- Patient will maintain a calm demeanor, with minimal agitated behavior.
- Patient will remain free from physical injury.

Long-term goal

- Patient will not experience physical injury.

Interventions

Interventions for preventing injury in the cognitively impaired patient include the following:

- Arrange the furniture and other items in the room to accommodate the patient's disabilities. Ensure that frequently used items are stored within easy access.
- Keep the bed in its lowest position. If allowed by hospital regulation or accrediting body, limited use of bed rails may provide a measure of safety.
- A room near the nurse's station may be helpful to ensure that the patient can be closely observed. In some instances, one-to-one observation may be necessary, particularly for the delirious patient.
- Ensure that potentially dangerous items such as razors, glass items, or flammable materials are kept at the nurse's station and dispensed only when someone is available to stay with the patient while they are using these items.

Table 22–3 | CARE PLAN FOR THE PATIENT WITH A NEUROCOGNITIVE DISORDER

NURSING DIAGNOSIS: RISK FOR PHYSICAL TRAUMA

RELATED TO: Impairments in cognitive and psychomotor functioning

OUTCOME CRITERIA	NURSING INTERVENTIONS	RATIONALE
Short-Term Goals ■ Patient calls for assistance when ambulating or carrying out other activities (if it is within his or her cognitive ability). ■ Patient maintains a calm demeanor, with minimal agitated behavior. ■ Patient does not experience physical injury. **Long-Term Goal** ■ Patient does not experience physical injury.	The following measures may be instituted: a. Arrange furniture and other items in the room to accommodate patient's disabilities. b. Store frequently used items within easy access. c. Keep the bed in the lowest position from the floor when the patient is not being immediately attended to. Pad side rails and headboard if patient has history of seizures. Keep bed rails up when patient is in bed (if regulations permit). d. Assign room near nurses' station; observe frequently. e. Assist patient with ambulation. f. Keep a dim light on at night. g. Keep potentially dangerous objects, such as sharp objects or razors, in a secure location and supervise the patient in completing activities that may pose a risk for personal injury. h. Frequently orient the patient to place, time, and situation and incorporate validation therapy as appropriate. i. If the patient is prone to wander, provide an area within which wandering can be carried out safely. j. Soft restraints may be required if patient is very disoriented and hyperactive.	To ensure patient safety

■ Assist the patient with ambulation. Provide a cane or walker for balance and instruct the patient in its proper use. Transport the patient in a wheelchair when longer excursions are necessary.

■ Teach the patient to hold on to hand railing if one is available or to call for assistance when ambulating if they are cognitively able.

For the Agitated Patient

■ Maintain an environment of low stimulation for an individual with disruptions in cognitive processes. Irritability, hostility, aggression, and psychotic behaviors are troublesome symptoms that require management in individuals with cognitive disorders. These behaviors often make it difficult for family members to care for their loved ones and is a common cause for placement in an institution. Many families struggle with the idea of institutionalization but are not equipped to manage the overwhelming burden of caring for a person with an NCD. It is important to explore the advantages and disadvantages of institutional care with all families caring for agitated or aggressive loved ones.

■ Antipsychotics have historically been used to help manage behavioral symptoms in patients with NCD. Behavioral symptoms are common in patients with NCD at some point during the progression of the illness. However, treatment of nonpsychotic behavior with antipsychotics is an off-label use and could have legal implications. Conventional antipsychotics are also problematic because of their tendency to induce extrapyramidal side effects. Although antipsychotic medications are still used for this purpose by some physicians, the U.S. Food and Drug Administration (FDA) has issued *boxed warnings* for both typical and atypical antipsychotic medications in elderly patients with NCD-related psychosis due to their association with increased mortality in this patient population. Careful, ongoing physical and mental status assessment are important nursing interventions for the NCD patient being treated with antipsychotics.

■ Remain calm and undemanding and avoid pressing the individual to perform activities that they are refusing. Ijaopo (2017), in a review of nonpharmacological interventions, cited evidence that caregiver training in communication and patient-centered skills is not only effective in reducing patient agitation but the effects can be sustaining.

■ Nursing literature has highlighted novel, evidence-based interventions to reduce anxiety and agitation, including dance and other rhythmic movement therapy (Lapum & Bar, 2016). Other sources identify music therapy, aromatherapy, multisensory stimulation, animal-assisted therapy, physical activity, and therapeutic touch as possible nonpharmacologic interventions for mild to moderate agitation; however, the researchers noted that all interventions must be tailored to individual needs and duration. When an intervention is effective, it is typically short term (Ijaopo, 2017). Additionally, there is evidence that physical activity lowers Aβ-related cognitive decline and neurodegeneration, suggesting that this activity may be helpful in slowing progression of the disease (Rabin et al., 2019). In a systematic review and meta-analysis (Watt et al., 2019), the evidence supported that nonpharmacologic interventions were superior to pharmacological interventions for managing agitation and aggression in people with dementia.

For the Patient Who Wanders

Wandering behavior in NCD can cause great problems for caregivers. Several reasons have been proposed as to why individuals with NCD wander. Some clinicians associate wandering behavior with increased stress and anxiety or restless agitation. Others relate the behavior to stages of cognitive decline. When memory diminishes and fear sets in, individuals may wander in search of something that seems familiar to them. Increased walking at night corresponds with disruption of diurnal rhythm. Wandering is often a problem in midstage NCD and less so in later stages. Patients new to a nursing home may wander in an attempt to become oriented to new surroundings. Wandering behavior can also be attributed to physical causes, such as hunger, thirst, and urinary or fecal urgency. When the wandering behavior begins after a long period of stability, it may indicate that a new medical, psychiatric, or cognitive complication has occurred. Delirium may produce the abrupt onset of wandering behavior.

The goals of wandering therapy are to keep the individual safe, prevent intrusion into others' rooms, and determine contributing factors to the behavior. When caring for a patient who wanders, it is important to keep the following interventions in mind:

■ Keep the individual on a structured schedule of recreational activities and a strict feeding and toileting schedule.

■ Provide a safe, enclosed place for pacing and wandering.

■ Walk with the individual for a while and gently redirect them back to the care unit.

■ Ensure that outdoor exits are electronically controlled.

Disturbed Thought Processes/Impaired Memory and Disturbed Sensory Perception

In NCDs, disturbed thought processes, memory impairment, and disturbed sensory perceptions are evidenced by disorientation, confusion, and inaccurate interpretation of the environment, including illusions, delusions, and hallucinations. *Disturbed thought processes* are defined as disruptions in cognitive operations and activities. *Disturbed sensory perception* is defined as disrupted response to sensory stimuli accompanied by misinterpretation or false perceptions. *Impaired memory* is defined as the "persistent inability to remember or recall bits of information or skills" (Herdman et al., 2021, p. 333).

Patient Goals

Outcome criteria include short- and long-term goals. Timelines are individually determined.

Short-term goals

■ Patient uses measures provided (e.g., clocks, calendars, room identification) to maintain reality orientation.
■ Patient experiences fewer episodes of acute confusion.

Long-term goal

■ Patient maintains reality orientation to the best of their cognitive ability.

Interventions

For the Patient Who Is Disoriented

■ Try to keep the patient as oriented to reality as possible.
■ Use clocks and calendars with large numbers that are easy to read.
■ Place large, colorful signs on the doors to identify patients' rooms, bathrooms, activity rooms, dining rooms, and chapel.
■ Allow the patient to have as many of their personal items as possible. Even an old familiar chair in the room can provide a degree of comfort.
■ If possible, encourage family and close friends to be a part of the patient's care to promote feelings of security and orientation.
■ Provide the patient with radio, television, and music if they are diversions the patient enjoys; these may add a feeling of familiarity to the environment.
■ Ensure that noise level is controlled to prevent excess stimulation. Several studies have supported the benefits of using earplugs at night to reduce delirium (Hill, 2017; Litton et al., 2016; Van Rompaey et al., 2012).
■ Allow the patient to view old photograph albums and utilize reminiscence therapy. These are excellent ways to provide orientation to reality.
■ Maintain consistency of staff and caregivers to the best extent possible. Familiarity promotes comfort and feelings of security.
■ Continuously monitor for medication side effects. Physiological changes in the elderly can alter the body's response to certain medications. Toxic effects may intensify altered cognitive processes.

■ There has been criticism about reality orientation of individuals with NCD (particularly those with moderate to severe disease process), suggesting that constant relearning of material contributes to problems with mood and self-esteem (Spector et al., 2000). Alternatively, Scales and associates (2018) cited evidence that validation therapy has positive effects on agitation, apathy, irritability, and nighttime disturbance. They add that it has face validity as a patient-centered approach to care. See Box 22–4, Validation Therapy, for more information.

For the Patient With Delusions and Hallucinations

■ Minimize focus on delusional thinking. Do not disagree with made-up stories. Instead, gently correct the patient, offer reassurance that they are safe, and guide the conversation toward topics about real events and real people.
■ Never argue a point with the patient; to do so only serves to increase their anxiety and agitation.
■ Do not ignore reports of hallucinations when it is clear that the patient is experiencing them. It is important for the nurse to hear an explanation of the hallucination from the patient. These perceptions are very real and often very frightening to the patient. Unless they are appropriately managed, hallucinations can escalate into disturbing and even hostile behaviors. Visual and auditory hallucinations are the most common type in NCD. The physician may treat these manifestations with antipsychotic medication.
■ Assess for side effects of medications as a potential contributing factor to sensory perception disturbances.
■ Check to ensure that a patient's hearing aid is working properly and to ensure that faulty sounds are not being emitted.
■ Check eyeglasses to ensure that the individual is indeed wearing their own glasses.
■ Assess for other possible contributing factors to illusions or visual hallucination. Patients often see faces in patterns on fabrics or in pictures on the wall. A mirror can also be the cause of false perceptions. They may need to be moved or covered.
■ Provide reassurance that the patient is safe. It may be necessary to stay with the patient for a while until they are calm.
■ Never argue that the hallucination is not real. Try to let the patient know that, although you are not sharing the experience, you understand how distressing it is for them.
■ Distract the patient. Hallucinations are less likely to occur when the person is occupied or involved in what is going on around them. Focus on real situations and real people.

BOX 22–4 Validation Therapy

Validation therapy (VT), originated by Naomi Feil, a gerontological social worker, is a "method of communicating and being with disoriented very old people. It is a practical way of working that helps reduce stress, enhance dignity, and increase happiness. Validation is built on an empathetic attitude and a holistic view of individuals" (Validation Training Institute, 2022). The caregiver's approach involves listening nonjudgmentally with an openness to hearing what the patient is communicating and without correction, reorientation, or dismissal. Validation therapy validates the feelings and emotions of a person with NCD and may also integrate redirection techniques. Other important communication strategies include not lying, arguing, or contradicting what the patient says. Instead, listen with curiosity and ask questions to better understand what the patient is trying to communicate. For example, if the patient begins talking about their deceased spouse as if they were still alive, it is better not to communicate that the spouse is still alive (which would be a lie) but rather listen empathically and ask questions like "How did you meet your spouse?" or "What was your favorite thing to do together?"

EXAMPLE

 Mrs. W. (agitated): That old lady stole my watch! I know she did. She goes into people's rooms and takes our things. We call her "sticky fingers"!

Nurse: That watch is very important to you. Have you looked around the room for it? (***validating the patient's feelings***)

Mrs. W.: My husband gave it to me. He will be so upset that it is gone. I'm afraid to tell him.

Nurse: I'm sure you miss your husband very much. Tell me what it was like when you were together. What kinds of things did you do for fun? (***listening with curiosity and asking questions***)

Mrs. W.: We did a lot of traveling. To Italy, and England, and France. We ate wonderful food.

Nurse: Speaking of food, it is lunchtime, and I will walk with you to the dining room. (***redirection***)

Mrs. W.: Yes, I'm getting really hungry.

In this situation, the nurse validated Mrs. W.'s feelings about not being able to find her watch. She did not deny that it had been stolen, nor did she remind Mrs. W. that her husband was deceased. *(Remember: a concept of VT is that, on some level, Mrs. W. knows that her husband is dead.)* The nurse validated the emotions Mrs. W. was feeling about missing her husband. She brought up special times that Mrs. W. and her husband had spent together, which served to elevate Mrs. W.'s mood and self-esteem. Finally, she redirected Mrs. W. to the dining room to have her lunch. (The watch was eventually found in Mrs. W.'s medicine cabinet, where she had hidden it for safekeeping.) Through each of these communication strategies, the patient's perception of reality is validated and their self-esteem and dignity are preserved.

■ Assess whether or not the hallucinations are problematic for the patient. Not all hallucinations are upsetting.

Example

An elderly woman approaches the nurses' station and says, "I'm so perturbed. The woman in my room refuses to turn down my bed so that I can go to sleep." The nurse may respond, "I will walk to your room with you and see that your bed is turned down." The nurse chats with the patient about something that occurred during the day, and by the time they arrive at her room, there is no further mention of a woman in her room.

Impaired Verbal Communication

When individuals who are cognitively impaired begin to lose the ability to process verbal communication, the way that words are expressed becomes as important as what is said. NANDA-I defines *impaired verbal communication* as "decreased, delayed, or absent ability to receive, process, transmit, and/or use a system of symbols" (Herdman et al., 2021, p. 336).

Patient Goals

Outcome criteria include short- and long-term goals. Timelines are individually determined.

Short-term goals

■ Patient is able to make needs known to the primary caregiver.

■ Patient is able to understand basic communications in interactions with the primary caregiver.

Long-term goal

■ In later stages of the illness when the patient is unable to communicate, needs are anticipated and fulfilled by the primary caregiver.

Interventions

■ Use a calm and reassuring approach when interacting with the patient.

■ Use simple words, speak slowly and distinctly, and keep face-to-face contact with the patient.

■ Always identify yourself to the patient and call them by name at each meeting.

■ Use nonverbal gestures to help the patient understand what you want them to accomplish, if appropriate.

■ Ask only one question (or give only one direction) at a time and give the patient plenty of time to process the information and respond. The question may need to be rephrased if it is clear that the patient has not understood the meaning.

■ Always try to approach the patient from the front. An unexpected approach or touch from behind may startle and upset the patient and may even promote aggressive behavior.

■ Maintain consistency of staff and caregivers to the best extent possible. Consistency in staffing facilitates comfort and security and promotes an effective communication process with the patient.

■ If the patient becomes verbally aggressive, remain calm and provide validation for their feelings: "I know this is a hard time for you. You were always so busy and so active, and you took care of so many people. Maybe you could tell me about some of those people."

■ When it is appropriate, use touch and affection to communicate. Sometimes patients will respond to a hug or to a hand reaching for theirs when they will respond to nothing else.

Self-Care Deficit

It is important for patients to remain as independent as possible for as long as possible. They should be encouraged to accomplish ADLs to the best of their ability. NANDA-I defines *self-care deficit* as "inability to independently [bathe, put on or remove clothing, eat, perform tasks associated with bowel and bladder elimination]" (Herdman et al., 2021, pp. 316–319).

Patient Goals

Outcome criteria include short- and long-term goals. Timelines are individually determined.

Short-term goal

■ Patient participates in ADLs with assistance from the caregiver.

Long-term goals

■ Patient accomplishes ADLs to the best of their ability.
■ Unfulfilled needs are met by the caregiver.

Interventions

■ Provide a simple, structured environment for the patient, identify self-care deficits, and offer assistance as required.
■ Allow plenty of time for the patient to complete tasks.
■ Provide guidance and support for independent actions by talking the patient through the task one step at a time.

■ Provide a structured schedule of activities that does not change from day to day.
■ Ensure that ADLs follow the patient's usual routine as closely as possible.
■ Minimize confusion by providing for consistency in the assignment of daily caregivers.
■ Perform an ongoing assessment of the patient's ability to fulfill their nutritional needs, ensure personal safety, follow the medication regimen, and communicate the need for assistance with activities that they cannot accomplish independently. Anticipate needs that are not verbally communicated.
■ If the patient is to be discharged to family caregivers, assess those caregivers' ability to anticipate and fulfill the patient's unmet needs. Provide information to assist caregivers with this responsibility. Ensure that caregivers are aware of available community support systems from which they may seek assistance when required. Examples include adult day-care centers, housekeeping and homemaker services, respite care services, and the local chapter of a national support organization. Two helpful resources are the Alzheimer's Association and the Parkinson's Foundation.

Concept Care Mapping

The concept map care plan (see Chapter 8, "The Nursing Process in Psychiatric-Mental Health Nursing") is a diagrammatic teaching and learning strategy that allows visualization of interrelationships between medical diagnoses, nursing diagnoses, assessment data, and interventions. An example of a concept map care plan for a patient with an NCD is presented in Figure 22–3.

Patient and Family Education

The role of patient teacher is important in the psychiatric area, as it is in all areas of nursing. A list of topics for patient/family education relevant to NCDs is presented in Box 22–5.

Evaluation

In the final step of the nursing process, reassessment occurs to determine whether the nursing interventions have been effective in achieving the intended goals of care. Evaluation of the patient with an NCD is based on a series of short-term goals rather than on long-term goals. Resolution of identified problems may be unrealistic for this patient. For the patient with AD, for example, outcomes are measured in terms of slowing down the process rather than curing the problem. Evaluation questions may include the following:

■ Has the patient experienced injury?
■ Does the patient maintain orientation to time, person, place, and situation to the best of their cognitive ability?

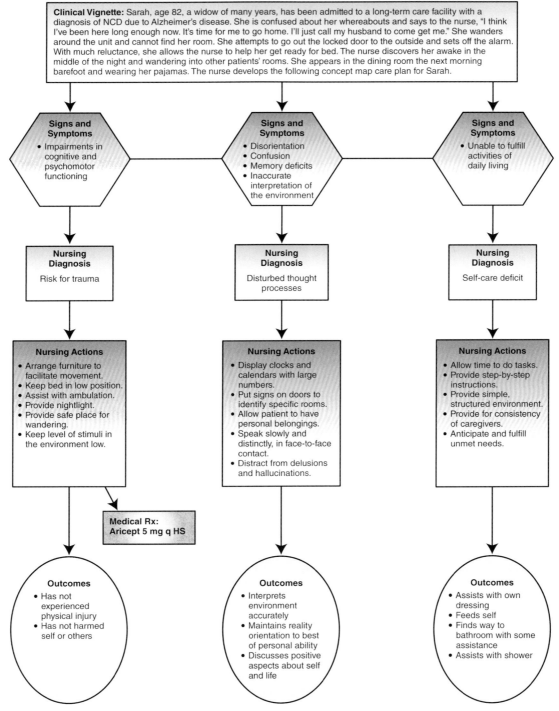

Clinical Vignette: Sarah, age 82, a widow of many years, has been admitted to a long-term care facility with a diagnosis of NCD due to Alzheimer's disease. She is confused about her whereabouts and says to the nurse, "I think I've been here long enough now. It's time for me to go home. I'll just call my husband to come get me." She wanders around the unit and cannot find her room. She attempts to go out the locked door to the outside and sets off the alarm. With much reluctance, she allows the nurse to help her get ready for bed. The nurse discovers her awake in the middle of the night and wandering into other patients' rooms. She appears in the dining room the next morning barefoot and wearing her pajamas. The nurse develops the following concept map care plan for Sarah.

Signs and Symptoms
• Impairments in cognitive and psychomotor functioning

Signs and Symptoms
• Disorientation
• Confusion
• Memory deficits
• Inaccurate interpretation of the environment

Signs and Symptoms
• Unable to fulfill activities of daily living

Nursing Diagnosis
Risk for trauma

Nursing Diagnosis
Disturbed thought processes

Nursing Diagnosis
Self-care deficit

Nursing Actions
• Arrange furniture to facilitate movement.
• Keep bed in low position.
• Assist with ambulation.
• Provide nightlight.
• Provide safe place for wandering.
• Keep level of stimuli in the environment low.

Nursing Actions
• Display clocks and calendars with large numbers.
• Put signs on doors to identify specific rooms.
• Allow patient to have personal belongings.
• Speak slowly and distinctly, in face-to-face contact.
• Distract from delusions and hallucinations.

Nursing Actions
• Allow time to do tasks.
• Provide step-by-step instructions.
• Provide simple, structured environment.
• Provide for consistency of caregivers.
• Anticipate and fulfill unmet needs.

Medical Rx:
Aricept 5 mg q HS

Outcomes
• Has not experienced physical injury
• Has not harmed self or others

Outcomes
• Interprets environment accurately
• Maintains reality orientation to best of personal ability
• Discusses positive aspects about self and life

Outcomes
• Assists with own dressing
• Feeds self
• Finds way to bathroom with some assistance
• Assists with shower

FIGURE 22–3 Concept map care plan for patient with major neurocognitive disorder.

■ Is the patient able to fulfill basic needs? Have those needs unmet by the patient been fulfilled by caregivers?

■ Is confusion minimized by familiar objects and structured, routine schedule of activities?

■ Do the prospective caregivers have information regarding the progression of the patient's illness?

■ Do caregivers have information regarding where to go for assistance and support in the care of their loved one?

■ Have the prospective caregivers received instruction in how to promote the patient's safety, minimize confusion and disorientation, and cope with difficult patient behaviors (e.g., hostility, anger, depression, agitation)?

BOX 22–5 Topics for Patient/Family Education Related to Neurocognitive Disorders

1. Nature of the illness
   a. Possible causes
   b. What to expect
   c. Symptoms
2. Management of the illness
   a. Ways to ensure patient safety
   b. How to maintain reality orientation
   c. Providing assistance with activities of daily living
   d. Nutritional information
   e. Difficult behaviors
   f. Medication administration
   g. Matters related to hygiene and toileting
3. Support services
   a. Financial assistance
   b. Legal assistance
   c. Caregiver support groups
   d. Respite care
   e. Home health care

■ Has the patient been able to maintain the best quality of life within the limitations posed by their illness?

Quality and Safety Education for Nurses (QSEN)

Several studies have demonstrated the positive outcomes associated with a particular patient-centered care approach for patients with dementia (Ballard et al., 2016, 2018, 2020; Whitaker et al., 2014). This program, called "Well-Being and Health for People with Dementia (WHELD)," is a nonpharmacological, psychosocial intervention that focuses on tailored person-centered activities, exercise, and social interaction for patients with dementia in long-term care settings. The evidence supported that training staff and incorporating these patient-centered interventions reduced patient agitation, reduced the need for antipsychotic medication, and improved quality of life in this population. Lack of medications to improve dementia and the dangers associated with antipsychotic use in elderly patients with dementia make these evidence-based interventions an important tool for quality nursing care in this population.

Medical Treatment Modalities

Delirium

The first step in the treatment of delirium should be the determination and correction of the underlying causes. Additional attention must be given to fluid and electrolyte status, hypoxia, anoxia, and diabetic problems. Staff members should remain with the patient at all times to monitor behavior and provide reorientation and assurance. The room should maintain a low level of stimuli.

Some physicians prefer not to prescribe medications for the patient with delirium, reasoning that additional agents may only compound the syndrome of brain dysfunction. However, psychosis with agitation and aggression demonstrated by the patient with delirium may require chemical or mechanical restraint for their personal safety. The choice of therapy is made with consideration for the patient's clinical condition and the underlying cause of the delirium. Low-dose antipsychotics are the most common medications used in delirium management. However, in a recent systematic review (Nikooie et al., 2019), researchers found no evidence of change in sedation status, duration of delirium, length of hospital stay, or mortality with either haloperidol or second generation antipsychotics versus placebo, and potentially harmful cardiac effects occurred more often.

Haloperidol (Haldol) is still used to treat psychotic features, but because it has been associated with prolongation of QT intervals, nurses must monitor the patient's cardiac status. Benzodiazepines are commonly used to treat delirium related to alcohol or benzodiazepine withdrawal. Melatonin, an over-the-counter (OTC) supplement, and ramelteon (Rozerem), a prescription medication for treatment of insomnia, have both been identified as potentially beneficial in prevention and treatment of delirium, because melatonin levels were found to be altered in patients with delirium (Alagiakrishnan, 2019).

Neurocognitive Disorder

Once a definitive diagnosis of NCD has been made, a primary consideration in the treatment of the disorder is the etiology. Focus must be directed to the identification and resolution of potentially reversible processes. Boland and Verduin (2022) noted that once dementia is apparent, it is essential to complete a clinical work-up to identify the syndrome and its causes because approximately 10% to 15% of people with dementia have potentially reversible conditions if treatment is initiated before irreversible damage takes place.

The need for general supportive care (with provisions for security, stimulation, nutrition, and treating the individual with patience and respect) has been recognized and accepted. Several pharmaceutical agents have been tried with varying degrees of success in the treatment of people with NCD. The six drugs that are currently FDA approved for the treatment of AD include donepezil, rivastigmine, galantamine, memantine, memantine combined with donepezil, and most recently, aducanumab. Selected drugs are described in the following sections according to the symptomatology for which they are indicated. A summary of medications for people with NCD is provided in Table 22–4.

TABLE 22–4 **Selected Medications Used in the Treatment of Clients With NCD**				
MEDICATION	**CLASSIFICATION**	**FOR TREATMENT OF**	**DAILY DOSAGE RANGE (mg)**	**SIDE EFFECTS**
Donepezil (Aricept)	Cholinesterase inhibitor	Cognitive impairment	5–10	Insomnia, dizziness, gastrointestinal (GI) upset, headache
Rivastigmine (Exelon)	Cholinesterase inhibitor	Cognitive impairment	6–12	Dizziness, headache, GI upset, fatigue
Galantamine (Razadyne)	Cholinesterase inhibitor	Cognitive impairment	8–24	Dizziness, headache, GI upset
Memantine (Namenda)	NMDA receptor antagonist	Cognitive impairment	5–20	Dizziness, headache, constipation
Memantine, extended-release + donepezil (Namzaric)	Anti-Alzheimer's agent	Moderate to severe Alzheimer's-type dementia	Memantine ER, 14–28 mg, and donepezil 10 mg, once daily	Headache, nausea, vomiting, dizziness, diarrhea, decreased appetite
Aducanumab (Aduhelm)	Amyloid-beta directed antibody	Alzheimer's disease	Titration is required for treatment initiation. The recommended maintenance dosage is 10 mg/kg administered as an intravenous infusion over approximately 1 hour every 4 weeks.	Amyloid-related imaging abnormalities (ARIA)-E: cerebral edema ARIA-H: microhemorrhage, ARIA-H superficial siderosis (indicative of iron overload)
Risperidone* (Risperdal)	Antipsychotic	Agitation, aggression, hallucinations, thought disturbances, wandering	1–4 (increase dosage cautiously)	Agitation, insomnia, headache, insomnia, extrapyramidal symptoms
Olanzapine* (Zyprexa)	Antipsychotic	Agitation, aggression, hallucinations, thought disturbances, wandering	5 (increase dosage cautiously)	Hypotension, dizziness, sedation, constipation, weight gain, dry mouth
Quetiapine* (Seroquel)	Antipsychotic	Agitation, aggression, hallucinations, thought disturbances, wandering	Initial dose 25 (titrate slowly)	Hypotension, tachycardia, dizziness, drowsiness, headache, constipation, dry mouth
Haloperidol* (Haldol)	Antipsychotic	Agitation, aggression, hallucinations, thought disturbances, wandering	1–4 (increase dosage cautiously)	Dry mouth, blurred vision, orthostatic hypotension, extrapyramidal symptoms, sedation
Pimavanserin (Nuplazid)	Antipsychotic	Hallucinations and delusions specifically associated with Parkinson's disease psychosis. *Note:* Pimavanserin is not approved for dementia-related psychosis unrelated to Parkinson's disease psychosis.	34 mg daily (17 mg, twice daily)	Peripheral edema, nausea, confusion, hallucinations, constipation, gait disturbance
Sertraline (Zoloft)	Antidepressant (SSRI)	Depression	50–100	Fatigue, insomnia, sedation, GI upset, headache, dizziness

Continued

TABLE 22–4 **Selected Medications Used in the Treatment of Clients With NCD—cont'd**				
MEDICATION	**CLASSIFICATION**	**FOR TREATMENT OF**	**DAILY DOSAGE RANGE (mg)**	**SIDE EFFECTS**
Paroxetine (Paxil)	Antidepressant (SSRI)	Depression	10–40	Dizziness, headache, insomnia, somnolence, GI upset
Nortriptyline (Pamelor)	Antidepressant (tricyclic)	Depression	30–50	Anticholinergic, orthostatic hypotension, sedation, arrhythmia
Lorazepam† (Ativan)	Antianxiety (benzodiazepine)	Anxiety	1–2	Drowsiness, dizziness, GI upset, hypotension, tolerance, dependence
Oxazepam† (Serax)	Antianxiety (benzodiazepine)	Anxiety	10–30	Drowsiness, dizziness, GI upset, hypotension, tolerance, dependence
Temazepam† (Restoril)	Sedative-hypnotic (benzodiazepine)	Insomnia	15	Drowsiness, dizziness, GI upset, hypotension, tolerance, dependence
Zolpidem (Ambien)‡	Sedative-hypnotic (nonbenzodiazepine)	Insomnia	5	Headache, drowsiness, dizziness, GI upset
Zaleplon (Sonata)‡	Sedative-hypnotic (nonbenzodiazepine)	Insomnia	5	Headache, drowsiness, dizziness, GI upset
Eszopiclone (Lunesta)‡	Sedative-hypnotic (nonbenzodiazepine)	Insomnia	1–2	Headache, drowsiness, dizziness, GI upset, unpleasant taste
Ramelteon (Rozerem)	Sedative-hypnotic (nonbenzodiazepine)	Insomnia	8	Dizziness, fatigue, drowsiness, GI upset
Trazodone	Antidepressant (heterocyclic)	Depression and insomnia	50	Dizziness, drowsiness, dry mouth, blurred vision, GI upset
Mirtazapine (Remeron)	Antidepressant (tetracyclic)	Depression and insomnia	7.5–15	Somnolence, dry mouth, constipation, increased appetite

*Although clinicians may still prescribe these medications in low-risk patients, no antipsychotics have been approved by the FDA for the treatment of patients with NCD-related psychosis. All antipsychotics include *boxed warnings* about the increased risk of death in elderly patients with NCD.
†Benzodiazepines should be used only for short-term treatment.
‡These sleep medications were found in one study to be associated with a 40% increase in fractures when used in patients with dementia (Priedt, 2018).

Cognitive Impairment

Cholinesterase inhibitors are often used for the treatment of mild to moderate cognitive impairment in AD and have demonstrated efficacy in treating patients with Lewy body dementia (Crystal, 2018). (Higher-dose donepezil has also been approved for moderate to severe AD.) Some of the clinical manifestations of AD are thought to result from a deficiency of the neurotransmitter acetylcholine. In the brain, acetylcholine is inactivated by the enzyme ACh. Donepezil (Aricept), rivastigmine (Exelon), and galantamine (Razadyne) act by inhibiting ACh, which slows the degradation of acetylcholine, thereby increasing concentrations of the neurotransmitter in the cerebral cortex. Because their action relies on functionally intact cholinergic neurons, the effects of these medications may lessen as the disease process advances, and there is no evidence that these medications alter the course of the underlying degenerative process.

Another medication, an NMDA receptor antagonist called memantine (Namenda), was approved by the FDA in 2003 for the treatment of moderate to severe AD. In a recent meta-analysis (Meng et al., 2019), memantine was also identified as beneficial in the treatment of cognitive impairment in PD and dementia with Lewy bodies.

High levels of glutamate in the brains of AD patients are thought to contribute to the symptomatology and decline in functionality. These high levels are caused by abnormal glutamate transmission. In normal neurotransmission, glutamate plays an essential role in learning and memory by triggering NMDA receptors to allow a controlled amount of calcium to flow into a nerve cell, creating the appropriate environment for information processing. In AD, there is a sustained release of glutamate, which results in a continuous influx of calcium into the nerve cells. This increased intracellular calcium concentration ultimately leads to disruption and death of the neurons.

Memantine may protect cells against excess glutamate by partially blocking NMDA receptors. In clinical trials, memantine has been shown to be effective in improving cognitive function and the ability to perform ADLs in individuals with moderate to severe AD. Although it does not stop or reverse the effects of the disease, it has been shown to slow progression of the decline in cognition and function. Because memantine's action differs from that of the cholinesterase inhibitors, consideration has been given to the coadministration of these medications. In 2014 the FDA approved one such drug, Namzaric, which is a combination of memantine and donepezil.

In June 2021, the FDA-approved aducanumab (Aduhelm), a human monoclonal antibody, as the first drug designed to treat an underlying cause of AD by targeting and reducing amyloid plaques, thereby slowing disease progression (Yang & Sun, 2021). Its approval has been the subject of controversy, and the FDA approval is conditional upon further research to determine the benefits of the drug and for which patients the drug will be most effective. "Unlike the other drugs approved to treat AD, aducanumab is associated with an increased risk of a serious condition called amyloid-related imaging abnormalities (ARIA), which can be an indicator of brain swelling" (Alzheimer's Association, 2022, p. 12).

A recent study (Coupland et al., 2019) found that anticholinergic drugs, including anticholinergic antidepressants, antipsychotics, antiepileptics, antiparkinson, and antimuscarinic drugs, *increased* the risk for dementia. The authors report that these findings highlight the importance of minimizing anticholinergic drug exposure in middle-aged and older adults. Anticholinergic side effects include confusion, blurred vision, constipation, dry mouth, dizziness, and difficulty urinating. Older people, and especially those with NCD, are particularly sensitive to these effects because of decreased cholinergic reserves. Many elderly individuals are also at increased risk for developing an anticholinergic toxicity syndrome because of the additive anticholinergic effects of multiple medications.

Current drug trials are under way to test for a vaccine against AD. Although some experts say they expect a vaccine will be available within the near future, other health experts suggest that it will be many years and possibly decades before a vaccine is available for humans (Ries, 2019). The rationales cited include that AD is a complex disease and the underlying pathology has not yet been clearly elucidated. More recently, Bakrania and associates (2021) developed a humanized antibody vaccine that attaches to certain Aβ protein variants. When administered in animal studies with mice, the researchers found it led to a striking reduction in amyloid-plaque formation, a rescue of brain glucose metabolism, a stabilization in neuron loss, and a rescue of memory deficiencies. Their hope is that evaluation of efficacy and safety in humans will soon lead to a vaccine for individuals with AD that will significantly alter the course of this illness.

Antipsychotics have been associated with increased mortality in patients with dementia and no antipsychotics have been approved by the FDA for the treatment of patients with NCD-related psychosis. All antipsychotics have a *boxed warning* about the increased risk of death in elderly patients with NCD. "The second generation antipsychotics risperidone, aripiprazole, and olanzapine have the best evidence for NCD-associated agitation and psychosis, but concerns about adverse effects (cardio- and cerebrovascular, metabolic, extrapyramidal) and modest efficacy limit their use" (Elie & Rej, 2018, p. 69). Although clinicians may still prescribe these medications, APA practice guidelines (2015) recommend prescribing antipsychotics only when the symptoms are severe and dangerous, the risks and benefits are discussed with patient and family, and the prescription is titrated up to the minimum effective dose.

Several herbs, vitamins, and other supplements have been studied for their potential benefits in the prevention and treatment of dementia. Of those studied, vitamin E has been advanced as potentially delaying the progression for those with mild to moderate disease, omega-3 fatty acids may lower the risk of developing dementia, and curcumin and gingko biloba have not demonstrated any benefits (Mayo Clinic, 2022a). Butler and associates (2018), in a systematic review of OTC supplements including vitamins C, D, E; omega-3 fatty acids; and gingko biloba, concluded that there is insufficient evidence to recommend any OTC supplement for cognitive protection in adults with normal cognition or MCI.

More recent research has focused on the chemical resveratrol, found in grape skins, cacao, and other foods. Several studies support its antioxidative, antiaging, and neuroprotective functions, and particularly its benefits for slowing cognitive decline associated with neurodegenerative diseases such as AD and PD (Griñán-Ferré et al., 2021; Kou & Chen,

2017; Loureiro et al., 2017; Turner et al., 2015). Zhang and associates (2021), in a detailed review of a multitude of research (citing over 200 studies) supporting the benefits of resveratrol, concluded that because many of the studies were conducted in animal models more research in humans is warranted and that "it is possible to recommend resveratrol as a promising agent for treating many human diseases" (p.16).

Nonpharmacologic treatments for cognitive impairment are also used for patients with NCD. These include cognitive rehabilitation (which includes education about cognitive strengths and weaknesses, cognitive stimulation, cognitive retraining, and compensatory strategies), music therapies, psychological therapies such as cognitive behavioral therapy (CBT), and mindfulness meditation (Alzheimer's Association, 2022). The goal of these treatments is primarily to reduce behavioral symptoms such as depression, anxiety, sleep disturbances, agitation, and aggression. Rabin and colleagues (2019) found that reducing vascular risk factors and increased physical activity reduced Aβ-related cognitive decline and gray matter volume loss, suggesting that these interventions may be beneficial in slowing the progression of AD.

Agitation, Aggression, Hallucinations, Thought Disturbances, and Wandering

Historically, physicians have prescribed antipsychotic medications to control agitation, aggression, hallucinations, thought disturbances, and wandering in people with NCD. The atypical antipsychotic medications, such as risperidone, olanzapine, quetiapine, and ziprasidone, were often favored because they were less likely to cause anticholinergic and extrapyramidal side effects. In 2005, however, after review of a number of studies, the FDA ordered *boxed warnings* on drug labels of all the atypical antipsychotics, citing an increased risk of death in elderly patients who display psychotic behaviors associated with NCD. Most of the deaths appeared to be cardiovascular related. In July 2008, based on the results of several studies, the FDA extended this warning to include all first generation antipsychotics as well, such as haloperidol and perphenazine. These findings pose a clinical dilemma for physicians who have found these medications to be helpful to their patients, and some have chosen to continue to use them in patients without significant cerebrovascular disease, in which previous behavioral programs have failed, and with consent from relatives or guardians who are clearly aware of the risks and benefits.

In 2016 a new drug, pimavanserin (Nuplazid), was approved by the FDA specifically for treatment of hallucinations and delusions in PD psychosis. The mechanism of action is unknown, but it is thought to provide benefit through its serotonin agonist and antagonist activities. It also carries a *boxed warning* for increased risk of death in elderly patients with dementia-related psychosis.

As previously mentioned, the WHELD Program of person-centered activities, social interaction, and exercise has demonstrated benefits for decreasing agitation, decreasing the use of antipsychotic medication, and improving quality of life for patients with dementia in long-term care settings (Ballard et al., 2018).

Depression

Depression is common among individuals with AD, particularly in the early stages. Recognizing the symptoms of depression in these individuals is often a challenge. Depression—which affects thinking, memory, sleep, and appetite and interferes with daily life—is sometimes difficult to distinguish from NCD. Clearly, the existence of depression in the person with NCD complicates and worsens the individual's functioning.

Antidepressant medication is sometimes used in the treatment of depression in those with NCD. Selective serotonin reuptake inhibitors (SSRIs) are considered the first-line drug treatment for depression in the elderly because of their favorable side-effect profile, although patients should be assessed for hyponatremia, because this is a risk associated with SSRI use in elderly patients. Tricyclic antidepressants are often avoided because of cardiac and anticholinergic side effects. Trazodone may be a good choice when used at bedtime for depression and insomnia. Dopaminergic agents (e.g., methylphenidate, amantadine, bromocriptine, and bupropion) may be helpful in the treatment of severe apathy.

Not only is depression common in AD, but evidence supports that individuals with depression—especially recurrent and chronic depression—are about two times more likely to develop AD than those who do not have depression (Herbert, 2016). Possible explanations for this increased risk have included common genetic links; disturbance in glucocorticoids that occurs in both AD and some forms of depression that inhibit hippocampal neurogenesis and plasticity; and cytokines, which are elevated in some forms of depression and are a known risk factor for AD (Herbert & Lucassen, 2016). Recent research (Harerimana et al., 2021) has, in fact, found genetic factors common to both AD and depression. The authors noted that although the shared genetic base is small, this connection may, at least in part, explain the increased risk for AD among individuals with recurrent depression and suggest that ineffectively treated depression may hasten the onset of AD symptoms.

Treating depression with medications in individuals with AD is complicated by the greater risks for adverse effects among older adults. In a systematic review of pharmacological versus nonpharmacological interventions for the treatment of depression in patients with AD, the authors concluded that "nondrug interventions were found to be more efficacious than drug interventions for reducing symptoms of depression in people with dementia without a major depressive disorder" (Watt et al., 2021, p. 1). They were unable to draw a conclusion about drug versus nondrug treatments in AD patients *with* a diagnosis of major depressive disorder because the studies they reviewed were dissimilar clinically and in methodology.

Anxiety

The progressive loss of mental functioning is a significant source of anxiety in the early stages of NCD. Encouraging patients to verbalize their feelings and fears associated with this loss may be useful in reducing the anxiety of individuals with NCD.

Some research suggests that anxiety may also be an early indicator of developing brain disease, and that older adults with MCI may progress more rapidly to AD when anxiety symptoms are also significant (Donovan et al., 2018).

Nonpharmacological treatments for anxiety include mindfulness meditation and other relaxation exercises. Antianxiety medications may be helpful but should not be used routinely or for prolonged periods. Benzodiazepines with shorter half-lives (e.g., lorazepam and oxazepam) are preferred to those longer-acting medications (e.g., diazepam), which promote a higher risk of oversedation and falls. Barbiturates are not appropriate as antianxiety agents because they frequently induce confusion and paradoxical excitement in elderly individuals.

Sleep Disturbances

Sleep problems are common in people with NCD and often intensify as the disease progresses. Wakefulness and nighttime wandering create distress and anguish in family members who are charged with protecting their loved one. Sleep disturbances are among the problems that most frequently initiate the need for client placement in a long-term care facility.

Some physicians treat sleep problems with sedative-hypnotic medications. Benzodiazepines may be useful for some individuals but are indicated for relatively brief periods only. Examples include flurazepam (Dalmane), temazepam (Restoril), and triazolam (Halcion). Daytime sedation, cognitive impairment, risk for falls, and paradoxical agitation in elderly clients are of particular concern with these medications. The nonbenzodiazepine sedative-hypnotics zolpidem (Ambien), zaleplon (Sonata), eszopiclone (Lunesta), and ramelteon (Rozerem) and the antidepressants trazodone (Desyrel) and mirtazapine (Remeron) may also be prescribed. Daytime sedation is a potential problem with these medications as well. As previously stated, barbiturates should not be used in elderly clients. Sleep problems are usually ongoing, and most clinicians prefer to use medications only to help an individual through a short-term stressful situation. Rising at the same time each morning; minimizing daytime sleep; participating in regular physical exercise no later than 4 hours before bedtime; getting proper nutrition; avoiding alcohol, caffeine, and nicotine; and retiring at the same time each night are behavioral approaches to sleep problems that may eliminate the need for sleep aids, particularly in the early stages of NCD. Because of the increased risk of adverse drug reactions in the elderly, many of whom are already taking multiple medications, pharmacological treatment of insomnia should be considered only after attempts at nonpharmacological strategies have failed.

CLINICAL JUDGMENT IN ACTION: CASE STUDY AND SAMPLE CARE PLAN

NURSING HISTORY AND ASSESSMENT

Recognizing cues: The nurse must demonstrate ability to recognize what information is most important to making an assessment (National Council of State Boards of Nursing [NCSBN], 2021). This information is italicized in the following:

Carmen is an 81-year-old widow who lives in the same small town in the same house that she shared with her husband until his death 16 years ago. She and her husband reared two daughters, Joan and Nancy, who live with their husbands in a large city about 2 hours away from Carmen. They have always visited Carmen every 1 or 2 months. She has four grown grandchildren who live in distant states and who see their grandmother on holidays.

About a year ago, Carmen's *daughters began to receive reports* from friends and other family members about incidents in which *Carmen was becoming forgetful (e.g., forgetting to go to a cousin's birthday party, taking a wrong turn and getting lost on the way to a niece's house [where she had driven many times], returning to church to search for something she thought she had forgotten [although she could not explain what it was], sending birthday gifts to people at the wrong times).* During visits, the

Continued

CLINICAL JUDGMENT IN ACTION: CASE STUDY AND SAMPLE CARE PLAN—cont'd

elder daughter, Joan, found **bills left unpaid, sometimes months overdue.** Housekeepers and yard workers reported to Joan that Carmen would forget she had paid them and try to pay them again, sometimes even a third time. She became very **confused when she would attempt to fill her weekly pillboxes, a task she had completed in the past without difficulty. Hundreds of dollars would disappear from her wallet, and she could not tell Joan what happened to the money.**

Joan and her husband subsequently moved to the small town where Carmen lived. They bought a home, and Joan visited her mother every day, took care of finances, and ensured that Carmen took her daily medications, although the daughter worked in a job that required occasional out-of-town travel. **As the months progressed, Carmen's cognitive abilities deteriorated. She burned food on the stove, left the house with the oven on, forgot to take her medication, got lost while driving in her car, missed appointments, and forgot the names of neighbors she had known for many years.** She began to **lose weight** because she was **forgetting to eat** her meals.

Carmen was evaluated by a neurologist, who **diagnosed her with neurocognitive disorder due to Alzheimer's disease.** Because they believed that Carmen needed 24-hour care, Joan and Nancy made the decision to place Carmen in a **long-term nursing facility.** In the nursing home, her condition has continued to deteriorate. Carmen **wanders** up and down the halls (day and night) and **has fallen twice,** once while attempting to get out of bed. She requires **assistance to shower and dress and has become incontinent of urine.** The nurses found her attempting to leave the building, saying, "I'm going across the street to visit my daughter." One morning at breakfast, she appeared in her pajamas in the communal dining room, not realizing that she had not dressed. She is **unable to form new memories and sometimes uses confabulation to fill in the blanks.** She **asks the same questions repeatedly,** sometimes **struggling for the right word.** She **can no longer provide the correct names of items in her environment. She has no concept of time.**

Joan visits Carmen daily and Nancy visits weekly, each offering support to the other in person and by phone. Carmen always seems pleased to see them but **can no longer call either of them by name. They are unsure if she knows who they are.**

Analyzing cues: The nurse must be able to interpret the information (NCSBN, 2021).

The nurse notes that Carmen's cognitive decline is progressive and she needs assistance with many ADLs. The nurse analyzes that Carmen's placement in a long-term care facility is an appropriate environment for 24-hour care, but even in this environment the patient remains at immediate risk for physical trauma, and Carmen's continued cognitive decline may be complicated by unfamiliar surroundings.

NURSING DIAGNOSES AND OUTCOME IDENTIFICATION

Generate solutions: The nurse must be able to connect their prioritized understanding of client needs to a course of action or plan of care (NCSBN, 2021).

From the assessment data, the nurse develops the following nursing diagnoses for Carmen:

1. Risk for physical trauma related to impairments in cognitive and psychomotor functioning; wandering; falls
   a. Outcome criteria: Carmen will remain free of injury during her nursing home stay.
   b. Short-term goals:
      ■ Carmen will not fall while wandering the halls.
      ■ Carmen will not fall out of bed.
2. Disturbed thought processes related to cerebral degeneration evidenced by disorientation, confusion, and memory deficits
   a. Outcome criteria: Carmen will maintain reality orientation to the best of her cognitive ability.
   b. Short-term goals:
      ■ Carmen will be able to find her room.
      ■ Carman will be able to communicate her needs to staff.
3. Self-care deficit related to cognitive impairments, disorientation, confusion, and memory deficits
   a. Outcome criteria: Carmen will accomplish ADLs to the best of her ability.
   b. Short-term goals:
      ■ Carmen will assist with dressing herself.
      ■ Carmen will cooperate with trips to the bathroom.
      ■ Carmen will wash herself in the shower with help from the nurse.

PLANNING AND IMPLEMENTATION

Take Action: The nurse must be able to identify what actions need to be taken and how they will be implemented (NCSBN, 2021).

RISK FOR PHYSICAL TRAUMA
The following nursing interventions may be implemented *to ensure patient safety:*

1. Arrange the furniture in Carmen's room so that it will accommodate free movement.
2. Store frequently used items within her easy reach.
3. Provide a "low bed" or possibly move her mattress from the bed to the floor to prevent falls from bed.
4. Attach a bed alarm to alert the nurse's station when Carmen has alighted from her bed.
5. Keep a dim light on in her room at night.
6. During the day and evening, provide a well-lighted area where Carmen can safely wander.
7. Ensure that all outside doors are electronically controlled.

CLINICAL JUDGMENT IN ACTION: CASE STUDY AND SAMPLE CARE PLAN—cont'd

8. Play soft music and maintain a low level of stimuli in the environment.

DISTURBED THOUGHT PROCESSES

The following nursing interventions may be implemented *to help maintain orientation and aid in memory and recognition:*

1. Use clocks and calendars with large numbers that are easy to read.
2. Put a sign on Carmen's door with her name on it and hang a personal item of hers on the door.
3. Ask Joan to bring some of Carmen's personal items for her room, even a favorite comfy chair if possible. Ask for some old photograph albums if they are available.
4. Keep the number of staff and caregivers to a minimum to promote familiarity.
5. Speak slowly and clearly while looking at Carmen's face.
6. Use reminiscence therapy with Carmen. Ask her to share happy times from her life with you. This technique helps decrease depression and boost self-esteem.
7. Mention the date and time in casual conversation. Refer to "spring rain," "summer flowers," "fall leaves." Emphasize holidays.
8. Correct misperceptions gently and matter-of-factly. Focus on real events and real people if false ideas should occur. Validate her feelings associated with current and past life situations.
9. Monitor for medication side effects, because toxic effects from certain medications can intensify altered thought processes.

SELF-CARE DEFICIT

The following nursing interventions may be implemented to ensure that all Carmen's needs are fulfilled.

1. Assess what Carmen can do independently and which tasks she needs assistance with.

2. Allow plenty of time for her to accomplish tasks that are within her ability. Clothing with easy removal or replacement, such as Velcro, facilitates independence.
3. Provide guidance and support for independent actions by talking her through tasks one step at a time.
4. Provide a structured schedule of activities that does not change from day to day.
5. Ensure that Carmen has snacks between meals.
6. Take Carmen to the bathroom regularly (according to her usual pattern, e.g., after meals, before bedtime, on arising).
7. To minimize nighttime wetness, offer fluid every 2 hours during the day and restrict fluid after 6 p.m.
8. To promote more restful nighttime sleep and less wandering at night, reduce naps during late afternoon and encourage sitting exercises, walking, and ball toss. Carbohydrate snacks at bedtime may also be helpful.

EVALUATION

Evaluate outcomes: The nurse must be able to evaluate actions taken and determine whether they have had a positive, neutral, or negative impact (NCSBN, 2021).

The outcome criteria identified for Carmen have been met. She has experienced no injury. She has not fallen out of bed. She continues to wander in a safe area. She can find her room by herself but occasionally requires some assistance when she is anxious and confused. She has some difficulty communicating her needs to the staff, but those who work with her on a consistent basis are able to anticipate her needs. All ADLs are being fulfilled, and Carmen assists with dressing and grooming, accomplishing about half on her own. Nighttime wandering has been minimized. Soft bedtime music helps to relax her.

Summary and Key Points

- Neurocognitive disorders constitute a large and growing public health concern.
- Delirium is a disturbance of awareness and change in cognition that develops rapidly over a short period. Level of consciousness is often affected, and psychomotor activity may fluctuate between agitated, purposeless movements and a vegetative state resembling catatonic stupor.
- The symptoms of delirium usually begin quite abruptly and often are reversible and brief.
- Delirium may be caused by a general medical condition, substance intoxication or withdrawal, ingestion of a medication, or exposure to a toxin. NCD is a syndrome of acquired, persistent

intellectual impairment ranging from mild to major, with compromised function in multiple spheres of mental activity, such as memory, language, visuospatial skills, emotion or personality, and cognition.

- Neurocognitive disorder is a syndrome of acquired, persistent intellectual impairment with compromised function in multiple spheres of mental activity, such as memory, language, visuospatial skills, emotion or personality, and cognition.
- Dementia (also described as major NCD in the *DSM-5-TR*) is a progressive decline of cognitive abilities in the presence of clear consciousness.
- Symptoms of NCD are insidious and develop slowly over time. In most clients, the disorder has a progressive, irreversible course.

- Causative factors for neurocognitive disorder include genetics, cardiovascular disease, infections, neurophysiological disorders, and other medical conditions.
- Nursing care of the patient with an NCD is presented around the six steps of the nursing process.
- Objectives of care for the patient experiencing an acute syndrome are aimed at eliminating the etiology, promoting patient safety, and facilitating a return to the highest possible level of functioning.
- Objectives of care for the patient experiencing a chronic, progressive disorder are aimed at preserving the dignity of the individual, promoting deceleration of the symptoms, maximizing functional capabilities, and maintaining the best quality of life within the limitations posed by illness.
- "Well-Being and Health for People with Dementia (WHELD)" is an evidence-based intervention for patients with dementia in long-term care settings that has demonstrated effectiveness in decreasing agitation, decreasing the need for antipsychotic medication, and improving the quality of life in this population.

- Nursing interventions are also directed toward helping the patient's family or primary caregivers learn about and cope with the chronic and progressive changes associated with NCD.
- Caregiver education about the disease process, expectations of patient behavioral changes, methods for facilitating care, and sources of assistance and support are important nursing intervention for families caring for a loved one with dementia. Caregiver burden can be significant as they struggle, both physically and emotionally, with the demands brought on by a disease process that is slowly taking their loved one away from them.
- Medical treatment of delirium focuses on identifying and correcting underlying causes.
- Medical treatment of NCD includes identifying and correcting reversible causes, pharmacotherapy, and general supportive care with attention to security, stimulation, nutrition, and treating the individual with patience and respect.
- The six drugs currently approved by the FDA for the treatment of cognitive decline in AD include donepezil, rivastigmine, galantamine, memantine, memantine ER with donepezil, and aducanumab.

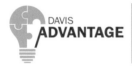

Go to **Davis Advantage** to complete your learning: strengthen understanding, apply your knowledge, and prepare for the Next Gen NCLEX®.

Review Questions

1. An example of a treatable (reversible) form of NCD is one that is caused by which of the following? (Select all that apply.)
   a. Multiple sclerosis
   b. Huntington's disease
   c. Electrolyte imbalance
   d. HIV disease
   e. Folate deficiency

2. A client has been diagnosed with NCD due to Alzheimer's disease. The cause of this disorder is which of the following?
   a. Multiple small brain infarcts
   b. Chronic alcohol abuse
   c. Cerebral abscess
   d. Unknown

3. Which of the following medications has been indicated for improvement in cognitive functioning in mild to moderate Alzheimer's disease? (Select all that apply.)
   a. Donepezil (Aricept)
   b. Rivastigmine (Exelon)
   c. Risperidone (Risperdal)
   d. Sertraline (Zoloft)
   e. Galantamine (Razadyne)

4. Which of the following factors is not associated with an increased incidence of neurocognitive disorder due to Alzheimer's disease?
   a. Multiple small strokes
   b. Family history of Alzheimer's disease
   c. Head trauma
   d. Advanced age

5. In addition to disturbances in cognition and orientation, individuals with Alzheimer's disease may also show changes in which of the following? (Select all that apply.)
   a. Personality
   b. Vision
   c. Speech
   d. Hearing
   e. Mobility

Clinical Judgment Questions

6. A client, who has neurocognitive disorder due to Alzheimer's disease, says to the nurse, "I have a date tonight. I always have a date on Christmas." Which of the following is the most appropriate response?
   a. "Don't be silly. It's not Christmas."
   b. "Today is Tuesday, October 21. We will have supper soon, and then your daughter will come to visit."
   c. "Who is your date with?"
   d. "I think you need some more medication. I'll bring it to you now."

7. A client who has NCD due to Alzheimer's disease has trouble sleeping and wanders around at night. Which of the following nursing actions would be *best* to promote sleep in this client?
   a. Ask the doctor to prescribe flurazepam (Dalmane).
   b. Ensure that the client gets an afternoon nap so they will not be overtired at bedtime.
   c. Make the client a cup of tea with honey before bedtime.
   d. Ensure that the client gets regular physical exercise during the day.

8. The night nurse finds a client with Alzheimer's disease wandering the hallway at 4 a.m. and trying to open the door to the side yard. Which of the following is the best initial response by the nurse?
   a. "That door leads out to the patio. It's nighttime. You don't want to go outside now."
   b. "You look confused. What is bothering you?"
   c. "This is the patio door. Are you looking for the bathroom?"
   d. "Are you lonely? Perhaps you'd like to go back to your room and talk for a while."

9. A client with neurocognitive disease due to Alzheimer's disease is admitted to the hospital. Which of the following actions by the nurse is a priority?
   a. Ensuring that she receives food she likes to prevent hunger
   b. Ensuring that the environment is safe to prevent injury
   c. Ensuring that she meets the other patients to prevent social isolation
   d. Ensuring that she takes care of her own ADLs to prevent dependence

10. Which of the following interventions is most appropriate in helping a client with Alzheimer's disease with ADLs? (Select all that apply.)
    a. Perform ADLs for her while she is in the hospital.
    b. Provide her with a written list of activities she is expected to perform.
    c. Provide step-by-step instructions and plenty of time to perform independently as many ADLs as possible.
    d. Tell her that if her morning care is not completed by 9 a.m., it will be performed for her by the nurse's aide so that she can attend group therapy.

TEST YOUR CLINICAL REASONING AND CLINICAL JUDGMENT SKILLS

Joe, a 62-year-old accountant, began having difficulty remembering details necessary to perform his job. He was also having trouble at home, failing to keep his finances straight, and forgetting to pay bills. It became increasingly difficult for him to function properly at work, and eventually he was forced to retire. His cognitive deterioration continued, and behavioral problems soon began. He became stubborn, verbally and physically abusive, and suspicious of almost everyone in his environment. His wife and son convinced him to see a physician, who recommended hospitalization for testing.

At Joe's initial evaluation, he was fully alert and cooperative but obviously anxious and fidgety. He thought he was at his accounting office, and he could not state what year it was. He could not say the names of his parents or siblings, nor did he know who was currently the president of the United States. He could not perform simple arithmetic calculations, write a proper sentence, or copy a drawing. He interpreted proverbs concretely and had difficulty stating similarities between related objects.

Laboratory serum studies revealed no abnormalities, but a CT scan showed marked cortical atrophy. The physician's diagnosis was neurocognitive disorder due to Alzheimer's disease.

Answer the following questions related to Joe:

1. Identify the pertinent assessment data from which nursing care will be devised.
2. What is the primary nursing diagnosis for Joe?
3. How would outcomes be identified?

Communication Exercises

1. Mrs. B. is a patient on the Alzheimer's unit. The nurse hears her yelling, "Waitress! Waitress! Why can't I get some service around here?"

   How should the nurse respond appropriately to this statement by Mrs. B.?

2. Mrs. B., who had breakfast an hour ago, says to the nurse, "I've been waiting and waiting for my breakfast. On the farm, we always had breakfast by 6 o'clock. Those were the good old days."

   How should the nurse respond appropriately to this statement by Mrs. B.?

 MOVIE CONNECTIONS

The Notebook (Alzheimer's disease) • *Away From Her* (Alzheimer's disease) • *Iris* (Alzheimer's disease) • *Still Alice* (early onset Alzheimer's disease)

References

Abushakra, S., Porsteinsson, A. P., Sabbagh, M., Bracoud, L., Schaerer, J., Power, A., Hey, J. A., Scott, D., Suhy, J., & Tola, M. (2020). APOE ε4/ε4 homozygotes with early Alzheimer's disease show accelerated hippocampal atrophy and cortical thinning that correlates with cognitive decline. *Alzheimer's & Dementia: Translational Research & Clinical Interventions, 6*(1), e12117.

Alagiakrishnan, K. (2019). *Delirium medications.* http://emedicine.medscape.com/article/288890-medication

Alzheimer's Association. (2022). *2022 Alzheimer's disease facts and figures.* https://www.alz.org/media/Documents/alzheimers-facts-and-figures.pdf

American Psychiatric Association (APA). (2000). *Diagnostic and statistical manual of mental disorders* (4th ed.). *Text revision.* APA.

American Psychiatric Association (APA). (2015). *The American Psychiatric Association practice guideline on the use of antipsychotics to treat agitation or psychosis in patients with dementia.* http://psychiatryonline.org/doi/book/10.1176/appi.books.9780890426807

American Psychiatric Association (APA). (2022). *Diagnostic and statistical manual of mental disorders, fifth edition, text revision (DSM-5-TR).* APA.

Bakrania, P., Hall, G., Bouter, Y., Bouter, C., Beindorff, N., Cowan, R., Davies, S., Price, J., Mpamhanga, C., Love, E., Matthews, D., Carr, M. D., & Bayer, T. A. (2021). Discovery of a novel pseudo β-hairpin structure of N-truncated amyloid-β for use as a vaccine against Alzheimer's disease. *Molecular Psychiatry.* https://doi.org/10.1038/s41380-021-01385-7

Ballard, C., Corbett, A., Orrell, M., Williams, G., Moniz-Cook, E., Romeo, R., Woods, B., Garrod, L., Testad, I., Woodward-Carlson, B., Wenborn, J., Knapp, M., & Fossey J. (2018). Impact of person-centered care training and person-centered activities on quality of life, agitation, and antipsychotic use in people with dementia living in nursing homes: A cluster randomized controlled trial. *PLoS Med, 15*(2), e1002500. https://doi.org/10.1371/journal.pmed.1002500

Ballard, C., Orrell, M., Moniz-Cook, E., Woods, R., Whitaker, R., Corbett, A., Aarsland, D., Murray, J., Lawrence, V., Testad, I., Knapp, M., Romeo, R., Zala, D., Stafford, J., Hoare, Z., Garrod, L., Sun, Y., McLaughlin, E., Woodward-Carlton, B., Williams, G., & Fossey, J. (2020). Improving mental health and reducing antipsychotic use in people with dementia in care homes: The WHELD research programme including two RCTs. *Programme Grants for Applied Research, 8*(6). https://doi.org/10.3310/pgfar08060

Ballard, C., Orrell, M., Yong Zhong, S., Moniz-Cook, E., Stafford, J., Whittaker, R., Woods, B., Corbett, A., Garrod, L., Khan, Z., Woodward-Carlton, B., Wenborn, J., & Fossey, J. (2016). Impact of antipsychotic review and nonpharmacological intervention on antipsychotic use, neuropsychiatric symptoms, and mortality in people with dementia living in nursing homes: A factorial cluster-randomized controlled trial by the Well-Being and Health for People With Dementia (WHELD) Program. *American Journal of Psychiatry, 173*(3), 252–262. https://doi.org/10.1176/appi.ajp.2015.15010130

Bhandari, T. (2019). Blood test is highly accurate at identifying Alzheimer's before symptoms arise [press release]. Washington University School of Medicine in St. Louis; August 1, 2019.

Boland, R., & Verduin, M. L. (2022). *Kaplan & Sadock's synopsis of psychiatry* (P. Ruiz, Ed.). (12th ed.). Wolters Kluwer.

Butler, M., Nelson, V. A., Davila, H., Ratner, E., Fink, H. A., Hemmy, L. S., McCarten, J. R., Barclay, T. R., Brasure, M., & Kane, R. L. (2018). Over-the-counter supplement interventions to prevent cognitive decline, mild cognitive impairment, and clinical Alzheimer-type dementia: A systematic review. *Annals of Internal Medicine, 168*(1), 52–62. doi:10.7326/M17-1530

Coupland, C. A., Hill, T., Dening, T., Morriss, R., Moore, M., & Hippisley-Cox, J. (2019). Anticholinergic drug exposure and the risk of dementia: A nested case-control study. *JAMA Internal Medicine, 179*(8), 1084–1093. doi:10.1001/jamainternmed.2019.0677

Crystal, H. A. (2018). Dementia with Lewy bodies: Treatment and management. *Medscape.* emedicine.medscape.com/article/1135041-treatment

Donovan, N. J., Locascio, J. J., Marshall, G. A., Gatchel, J., Hanseeuw, B. J., Rentz, D. M., Johnson, K. A., & Sperling, R. A. (2018). Harvard aging brain study. Longitudinal association of amyloid beta and anxious-depressive symptoms in cognitively normal older adults. *American Journal of Psychiatry, 175*(6), 530–537. doi:10.1176/appi.ajp.2017.17040442

Elie, D., & Rej, S. (2018). Pharmacological management of neuropsychiatric symptoms in patients with major neurocognitive disorders. *Journal of Psychiatry & Neuroscience, 43*(1), 69–70. https://doi.org/10.1503/jpn.170117

Fabian, T. J., & Solai, L. K. (2017). Neurocognitive disorders. In Sadock, B. J., Sadock, V. A., & Ruiz, P. (Eds.), *Comprehensive textbook of psychiatry* (pp. 1178–1191). Wolters Kluwer.

Gilstrap, L., Zhou, W., Alsan, M., Nanda, A., & Skinner, J. S. (2022). Trends in mortality rates among medicare enrollees with Alzheimer disease and related dementias before and during the early phase of the COVID-19 pandemic. *JAMA Neurology, 79*(4), 342–348. doi:10.1001/jamaneurol.2022.0010

Graziane, J. A., & Sweet, R. A. (2017). Dementia. In Sadock, B. J., Sadock, V. A., & Ruiz, P. (Eds.), *Comprehensive textbook of psychiatry* (pp. 1191–1221). Wolters Kluwer.

Griñán-Ferré, C., Bellver-Sanchis, A., Izquierdo, V., Corpas, R., Roig-Soriano, J., Chillón, M., Andres-Lacueva, C., Somogyvári, M., Sőti, C., Sanfeliu, C., & Pallàsa, M. (2021). The pleiotropic neuroprotective effects of resveratrol in cognitive decline and Alzheimer's disease pathology: From antioxidant to epigenetic therapy. *Ageing Research Reviews, 67.* https://doi.org/10.1016/j.arr.2021.101271

Hampel, H., O'Bryant, S. E., Molinuevo, J. L., Zetterberg, H., Masters, C. L., Lista, S., Kiddle, S. J., Batrla, R., & Blennow, K. (2018). Blood-based biomarkers for Alzheimer disease: Mapping the road to the clinic. *Nature Reviews. Neurology, 14*(11), 639–652. doi:10.1038/s41582-018-0079-7

Harerimana, N. V., Liu, Y., Gerasimov, E. S., Duong, D., Beach, T. G., Reiman, E. M., Schneider, J. A., Boyle, P., Lori, A., Bennett, D. A., Lah, J. J., Levey, A. I., Seyfried, N. T., Wingo, T. S., & Wingo, A. P. (2021). Genetic evidence supporting a causal role of depression in Alzheimer's disease. *Biological Psychiatry.* doi:10.1016/j.biopsych.2021.11.025

Herbert, J. (2016). Depression is a risk for Alzheimer's: We need to know why. *Psychology Today.* https://www.psychologytoday.com/us/blog/hormones-and-the-brain/201604/depression-is-risk-alzheimer-s-we-need-know-why

Herbert, J., & Lucassen, P. J. (2016). Depression as a risk factor for Alzheimer's disease: Genes, steroids, cytokines and neurogenesis—What do we need to know? *Frontiers in Neuroendocrinology, 41,* 153–171. doi:10.1016/j.yfrne.2015.12.001

Herdman, T. H., Kamitsuru, S., & Lopes, C. T. (Eds.). (2021). *NANDA International, Inc. nursing diagnoses: Definitions and classification 2021–2023* (12th ed.). Thieme.

Hill, L. (2017). Earplugs could be an effective sleep hygiene strategy to reduce delirium in the ICU. *Evidence-Based Nursing, 20,* 20.

Huntington's Disease Society of America (HDSA). (2022). *What is Huntington's disease? Overview of Huntington's disease.* https://hdsa.org/what-is-hd/overview-of-huntingtons-disease/

Ijaopo, E. O. (2017). Dementia-related agitation: A review of nonpharmacological interventions and analysis of risks and benefits of pharmacotherapy. *Translational Psychiatry, 7*(10), e1250. https://doi.org/10.1038/tp.2017.199

Johns Hopkins Medicine. (n.d.). Prion diseases. *Health Library.* www.hopkinsmedicine.org/healthlibrary/conditions/nervous_system_disorders/prion_diseases_134,56

Krinitski, D., Kasina, R., Klöppel, S., & Lenouvel, E. (2021) Associations of delirium with urinary tract infections and asymptomatic bacteriuria in adults aged 65 and older: A systematic review and meta_analysis. *Journal of the American Geriatrics Society, 69*(11), 3312–3313. https://doi.org/10.1111/jgs.17418

Kou, X., & Chen, N. (2017). Resveratrol as a natural autophagy regulator for prevention and treatment of Alzheimer's disease. *Nutrients, 9*(9), 927. doi:10.3390/nu9090927

Langa, K. M., Larson, E. B., Crimmins, E. M., Faul, J. D., Levine, D. A., Kabeto, M. U., & Weir, D. R. (2017). A comparison of the prevalence of dementia in the United States in 2000 and 2012. *JAMA Internal Medicine, 177*(1), 51–58. doi:10.1001/jamainternmed. 2016.6807

Lapum, J. L., & Bar, R. J. (2016). Dance for individuals with dementia. *Journal of Psychosocial Nursing, 54*(3), 31–34. doi:10.3928/02793695-20160219-05

Litton, E., Carnegie, V., Elliott, R., & Webb, S. A. (2016). The efficacy of earplugs as a sleep hygiene strategy for reducing delirium in the ICU: A systematic review and meta-analysis. *Critical Care Medicine.* doi: 10.3310/signal-000209

Loureiro, J. A., Andrade, S., Duarte, A., Neves, A. R., Queiroz, J. F., Nunes, C., Sevin, E., Fenart, L., Gosselet, F., Coelho, M. A. N., & Pereira, M. C. (2017). Resveratrol and grape extract-loaded solid lipid nanoparticles for the treatment of Alzheimer's disease. *Molecules, 22,* 277. https://doi.org/10.3390/molecules22020277

Lyra e Silva, N. M., Gonçalves, R. A., Pascoal, T. A., Lima-Filho, R. A. S., Resende, E., Vieira, E. L. M., Teixeira, A. L., de Souza, L. C., Peny, J. A., Fortuna, J. T. S., Furigo, I. C., Hashiguchi, D., Miya-Coreixas, V. S., Clarke, J. R., Abisambra, J. F., Longo, B. M., Donato Jr., J., Fraser, P. E., Rosa-Neto, P., Caramelli, P..... De Felice, F. G. (2021). Proinflammatory interleukin-6 signaling links cognitive impairments and peripheral metabolic alterations in Alzheimer's disease. *Translational Psychiatry 11,* 251. https://doi.org/10.1038/s41398-021-01349-z

Mayo Clinic. (2022a). *Alzheimer's disease: Diagnosis and treatment.* https://www.mayoclinic.org/diseases-conditions/alzheimers-disease/diagnosis-treatment/drc-20350453%99s-disease-vaccine-be-reality

Mayo Clinic. (2022b). *Dementia: Symptoms and causes.* https://www.mayoclinic.org/diseases-conditions/dementia/symptoms-causes/syc-20352013

Mayo Clinic. (2023). *Alzheimer's disease: Symptoms and causes.* https://www.mayoclinic.org/diseases-conditions/alzheimers-disease/symptoms-causes/syc-20350447

McCutcheon, S. T., & Robinson, R. G. (2017). Neuropsychiatric aspects of cerebrovascular disease. In Sadock, B. J., Sadock, V. A., & Ruiz, P. (Eds.), *Comprehensive textbook of psychiatry* (pp. 474–489). Wolters Kluwer.

Meng, Y. H., Wang, P. P., Song, Y. X., & Wang, J. H. (2019). Cholinesterase inhibitors and memantine for Parkinson's disease dementia and Lewy body dementia: A meta-analysis. *Experimental and Therapeutic Medicine, 17*(3), 1611–1624. https://doi.org/10.3892/etm.2018.7129

Mitchell, S. (2015). Advanced dementia. *New England Journal of Medicine, 372*(26), 2533–2540. doi:10.1056/NEJMcp1412652

Moore, R. C., & Marquine, M. J. (2017). HIV and aging. In Sadock, B. J., Sadock, V. A., & Ruiz, P. (Eds.), *Comprehensive textbook of psychiatry* (pp. 4268–4274). Wolters Kluwer.

National Council of State Boards of Nursing (NCSBN). (2021). *Next generation NCLEX®: comparison between case studies and stand-alone items.* https://www.ncsbn.org/public-files/NGN_Fall21_English_Final.pdf

National Institute of Neurological Disorders and Stroke. (2019). NINDS frontotemporal dementia information page. National Institutes of Health. https://www.ninds.nih.gov/Disorders/All-Disorders/Frontotemporal-Dementia-Information-Page

Nikooie, R., Neufeld, K. J., Oh, E. S., Wilson, L. M., Zhang, A., Robinson, K. A., & Needham, D. M. (2019). Antipsychotics for treating delirium in hospitalized adults: A systematic review. *Annals of Internal Medicine.* doi:10.7326/M19-1860.

Oba, T., Saito, T., Asada, A., Shimizu, S., Iijima, K. M., & Ando, K. (2020). Microtubule affinity–regulating kinase 4 with an Alzheimer's disease-related mutation promotes tau accumulation and exacerbates neurodegeneration. *Molecular Bases of Disease Neurobiology, 295*(50), P17138–17147. https://doi.org/10.1074/jbc.RA120.014420

Priedt, R. (2018). *Sleeping pills may be risky for dementia patients.* https://www.webmd.com/alzheimers/news/20180725/sleeping-pills-may-be-risky-for-dementia-patients

Rabin, J. S., Klein, H., Kirn, D. R., Schultz, A. P., Yang, H. S., Hampton, O., Jiang, S., Buckley, R. F., Viswanathan, A., Hedden, T., Pruzin, J., Yau, W. W., Guzmán-Vélez, E., Quiroz, Y. T., Properzi, M., Marshall, G. A., Rentz, D. M., Johnson, K. A., Sperling, R. A., & Chhatwal, J. P. (2019). Associations of physical activity and β-amyloid with longitudinal cognition and neurodegeneration in clinically normal older adults. *JAMA Neurology.* doi:10.1001/jamaneurol.2019.1879

Rashid, M. H., Sparrow, N. A., Anwar, F., Guidry, G., Covarrubias, A. E., Pang, H., Bogguri, C., Karumanchi, S. A., & Lahiri. S. (2021). Interleukin-6 mediates delirium-like phenotypes in a murine model of urinary tract infection. *Journal of Neuroinflammation, 18*(1). doi:10.1186/s12974-021-02304-x

Reddy, J. S., Jin, J., Lincoln, S. J., Ho, C. C. G., Crook, J. E., Wang, X., Malphrus, K. G., Nguyen, T., Tamvaka, N., Grieg-Custo, M. T., Lucas, J. A., Graff-Radford, N. R., Ertekin-Taner, N., & Carrasquillo, M. M. (2022). Transcript levels in plasma contribute substantial predictive value as potential Alzheimer's disease biomarkers in African Americans. *eBioMedicine.* doi:https://doi.org/10.1016/j.ebiom.2022.103929

Ries, J. (2019). *An Alzheimer's vaccine won't be approved anytime soon, here's why.* https://www.healthline.com/health-news/dont-bet-on-an-alzheimers-vaccine-anytime-soon#Alzheimer%E2%80%99s-is-a-complex-disease-and-difficult-to-treat

Scales, K., Zimmerman, S., & Miller, S. J. (2018). Evidence-based nonpharmacological practices to address behavioral and psychological symptoms of dementia. *The Gerontologist, 58*(supp 1), S88–S102. https://doi.org/10.1093/geront/gnx167

Schindler, S. E., Bollinger, J. G., Ovod, V., Mawuenyega, K. G., Li, Y., Gordon, B. A., Holtzman, D. M., Morris, J. C., Benzinger, T. L. S., Xiong, C., Fagan, A. M., & Bateman, R. J. (2019). High-precision plasma β-amyloid 42/40 predicts current and future brain amyloidosis. *Neurology,* August 1, 2019 [Epub ahead of print]. doi:10.1212/WNL.0000000000008081

Spector, A., Davies, S., Woods, B., & Orrell, M. (2000). Reality orientation for dementia: A systematic review of the evidence of effectiveness from randomized controlled trials. *The Gerontologist, 40*(2), 206–212. doi:https://doi.org/10.1093/geront/40.2.206

Strub, R. L., & Black, F. W. (2000). *The mental status examination in neurology* (4th ed.). F.A. Davis.

Sullivan, M. (2018). Alzheimer's: Biomarkers, not cognition, will now define disorder. *Clinical Psychiatry News.* https://www.mdedge.com/clinicalneurologynews/article/163073/alzheimers-cognition/alzheimers-biomarkers-not-cognition-will

Turner, R. S., Thomas, R. G., Craft, S., van Dyck, C. H., Mintzer, J., Reynolds, B. A., Brewer, J. B., Rissman, R. A., Raman, R., Aisen, P. S., & Alzheimer's Disease Cooperative Study. (2015). A randomized, double-blind, placebo-controlled trial of resveratrol for Alzheimer disease. *Neurology, 85*(16), 1383–1391. doi:10.1212/WNL.0000000000002035

University Health News. (2019). *Ketogenic diet shows promising results for all dementia stages.* https://universityhealthnews.com/daily/memory/ketogenic-diet-shows-promising-results-for-all-dementia-stages/

Validation Training Institute. (2022). *What is validation?* https://vfvalidation.org/get-started/what-is-validation/

Van Rompaey, B., Elseviers, M. M., Van Drom, W., Fromont, V., & Jorens, P. G. (2012). The effect of earplugs during the night on the onset of delirium and sleep perception: A randomized controlled trial in intensive care patients. *Critical Care, 16*(3), R73. doi:10.1186/cc11330

Watt, J., Goodarzi, Z., Veroniki, A. A., Nincic, V., Kahn, P.A., Ghassemi, M., Lai, Y., Treister, V. A., Thompson, Y., Schneider, R., Tricco, A. C., & Strauss, S. E. (2021). Comparative efficacy of interventions for reducing symptoms of depression in people with dementia: systematic review and network meta-analysis. *BMJ, 372.* doi:https://doi.org/10.1136/bmj.n532

Watt, J. A., Goodarzi, Z., Veroniki, A. A., Nincic, V., Khan, P. A., Ghassemi, M., Thompson, Y, Tricco, A. C. & Straus, S. E. (2019). Comparative efficacy of interventions for aggressive and agitated behaviors in dementia. *Annals of Internal Medicine, 171*(9), 633–42. doi:10.7326/M19-0993

Whitaker, R., Fossey, J., Ballard, C., Orrell, M., Moniz-Cook, E., Woods, R. T., Murray, J., Stafford, J., Knapp, M., Romeo, R., Carlton, B. W., Testad, I., & Khan, Z. (2014). Improving well-being and health for people with dementia (WHELD): Study protocol for a randomised controlled trial. *BioMed Central, 15*(284). doi:10.1186/1745-6215-15-284

Yang, P., & Sun, F. (2021). Aducanumab: The first targeted Alzheimer's therapy. *Drug Discoveries and Therapeutics, 15*(3), 166–168. doi:10.5582/ddt.2021.01061. PMID: 34234067

Zhang, L. X., Li, C. X., Kakar, M. U., Khan, M. S., Wu, P. F., Amir, R. M., Dai, D. F., Naveed, M., Li, Q. Y., Saeed, M., Shen, J. Q., Rajput, S. A., & Li, J. H. (2021). Resveratrol (RV): A pharmacological review and call for further research. *Biomedicine & Pharmacotherapy, 143,* 1–20. https://doi.org/10.1016/j.biopha.2021.112164

Substance-Related and Addictive Disorders

23

CORE CONCEPTS

Addiction

Communication

Collaboration

Professional Behavior: Nursing process in the care of patients with substance use disorders

Stress and Coping

Safety: Intoxication and Withdrawal

Clinical Judgment

KEY TERMS

addiction

Alcoholics Anonymous (AA)

amphetamines

ascites

blacking out

cannabis

codependency

detoxification

disulfiram

dual diagnosis

esophageal varices

Gamblers Anonymous (GA)

hepatic encephalopathy

intoxication

Korsakoff's psychosis

medication-assisted treatment

misuse

opioids

peer assistance programs

phencyclidine (PCP)

tolerance

Wernicke's encephalopathy

withdrawal

OBJECTIVES

After reading this chapter, the student will be able to:

1. Define *addiction, intoxication,* and *withdrawal.*
2. Discuss predisposing factors implicated in the etiology of substance-related and addictive disorders.
3. Identify symptomatology and use the information in assessment of patients with various substance-related and addictive disorders.
4. Identify nursing diagnoses common to patients with substance-related and addictive disorders and select appropriate nursing interventions for each.
5. Identify topics for patient and family teaching relevant to substance-related and addictive disorders.
6. Describe relevant outcome criteria for evaluating nursing care of patients with substance-related and addictive disorders.
7. Discuss the issue of substance-related and addictive disorders within the nursing profession.
8. Define *codependency,* and identify behavioral characteristics associated with the disorder.
9. Discuss treatment of codependency.
10. Describe various modalities relevant to treatment of individuals with substance-related and addictive disorders.

Substance-related disorders comprise two groups: substance-use disorders (addiction) and substance-induced disorders (intoxication, withdrawal, delirium, neurocognitive disorder, psychosis, bipolar disorder, depressive disorder, obsessive-compulsive disorder, anxiety disorder, sexual dysfunction, and sleep disorders). This chapter discusses addiction, intoxication, and withdrawal. The remainder of the substance-induced disorders are discussed in the chapters with which they share symptomatology (e.g., substance-induced depressive disorder is discussed in Chapter 25, "Depressive Disorders," and substance-induced anxiety disorder is discussed in Chapter 27, "Anxiety, Obsessive-Compulsive, and Related Disorders"). Also included in this chapter is a discussion of gambling disorder, a nonsubstance addiction disorder.

Drugs are a pervasive part of our society. Certain mood-altering substances, such as alcohol, caffeine, and nicotine, are socially acceptable and used moderately by many adult Americans. Society has even developed a relative indifference to an occasional misuse of these substances despite documentation of their negative effects on health.

A wide variety of substances are produced for medicinal purposes. These include central nervous system (CNS) stimulants (e.g., amphetamines) and CNS depressants (e.g., sedatives, tranquilizers), as well as numerous over-the-counter (OTC) preparations designed to relieve nearly every kind of human ailment, real or imagined.

Some historically illegal substances have achieved a degree of social acceptance by certain subcultures. Marijuana, for example, although by no means harmless, has been legalized in many states for medicinal use, recreational purposes, or both. The long-term effects of its use are still being studied, whereas the potentially dangerous effects of other illegal substances (e.g., lysergic acid diethylamide [LSD], phencyclidine [PCP], cocaine, and heroin) have been well documented. Dramatic increases in both prescription and illegally purchased **opioids** (a group of drugs that includes natural opioids, semi-synthetics, and synthetics with morphine-like action, [American Psychiatric Association (APA), 2022]) have prompted national attention and initiatives in response to an alarming number of associated deaths.

This chapter discusses the physical and behavioral manifestations and personal and social consequences related to the **misuse** (overuse with potentially harmful consequences) or **addiction** (physical, mental, and behavioral reliance) to alcohol, other CNS depressants, CNS stimulants, opioids, hallucinogens, and cannabis and those related to the nonsubstance addiction to gambling. The term *misuse* is equivalent to the term *abuse* but is replacing the latter term in many contexts to reduce the shaming and stigmatization associated with individuals being described as *abusers*. Variations in attitudes regarding substance consumption and patterns of use are explored. For example, drinking alcohol is considered by many to be a part of the culture of college life, while substance misuse is especially prevalent among individuals between the ages of 18 and 24. Substance-related disorders are diagnosed more commonly in men than in women, but the gender ratios vary with the class of the substance.

Codependency is described in this chapter, along with substance use disorder treatment. The issue of substance impairment within the nursing profession is also explored. Nursing care for individuals with substance use and addictive disorders is presented in the context of the six steps of the nursing process. Various medical and other treatment modalities are also discussed.

Substance Use Disorder, Defined

> **CORE CONCEPT**
> **Addiction**
> A compulsive or chronic requirement. The need is so strong as to generate distress (either physical or psychological) if left unfulfilled.

Substance Addiction

The *Diagnostic and Statistical Manual of Mental Disorders, Fifth Edition, Text Revision (DSM-5-TR)* (APA, 2022) lists diagnostic criteria for addiction to specific substances, including alcohol, caffeine, cannabis, hallucinogens, inhalants, opioids, sedative-hypnotics or anxiolytics, stimulants, and tobacco (nicotine). Individuals are considered to have a substance use disorder when use interferes with the ability to fulfill role obligations at work, school, or home. Often, the individual would like to control the use of the substance but attempts to do so fail and use continues to increase. Intense cravings lead to excessive time spent trying to procure more of the substance or recover from the effects of its use. Use of the substance causes problems with interpersonal relationships, and the individual may become socially isolated. Individuals with substance use disorders often participate in hazardous activities when they are impaired by the substance, and they continue to use the substance despite knowing that its use is contributing to a physical or psychological problem. The term "drug dependence" or "physical dependence" is used to describe aspects of substance use that may lead to addiction: **tolerance** (the amount needed to achieve the desired effect continually increases), increased use, and the physical and mental symptoms of withdrawal when drug use is abruptly stopped. Addiction is evident when there is evidence of physical dependence *and* the priority focus of one's thinking and behavior is obtaining the substance to the point (and in spite) of disruptions in social, occupational, and other aspects of functioning.

Substance-Induced Disorder, Defined

CORE CONCEPT
Intoxication
A state of disturbance in cognition, perception, behavior, level of consciousness, judgment, and other functions that is directly attributable to the effects of a psychoactive drug. It may be marked by a physical and mental state of exhilaration and emotional frenzy or lethargy and stupor.

Substance Intoxication

Intoxication is defined as the development of a reversible syndrome of symptoms after excessive use of a substance. The symptoms are drug specific and occur during or shortly after ingestion of the substance. The CNS is directly affected, and disruption in physical and psychological functioning occurs. Judgment is disturbed, resulting in inappropriate and maladaptive behavior, and social and occupational functioning are impaired.

CORE CONCEPT
Withdrawal
The physiological and mental readjustment that accompanies the discontinuation of an addictive substance.

Substance Withdrawal

Withdrawal occurs upon abrupt reduction or discontinuation of a substance that has been used regularly over a prolonged period of time. The substance-specific syndrome includes clinically significant physical signs and symptoms as well as psychological changes such as disturbances in thinking, feeling, and behavior.

Classes of Psychoactive Substances

The following classes of psychoactive substances are associated with substance use and substance-induced disorders:

1. Alcohol
2. Caffeine
3. Cannabis
4. Hallucinogens
5. Inhalants
6. Opioids
7. Sedative hypnotic, or anxiolytics
8. Stimulants
9. Tobacco (nicotine)

Predisposing Factors to Substance-Related Disorders

Many factors have been implicated in the predisposition to improperly use and become addicted to substances. At present, no single theory can adequately explain the etiology of this problem. Undoubtedly, a complex interaction among various factors influences a person's susceptibility.

Biological Factors
Genetics

Hereditary factors appear to be involved in the development of some substance use disorders, especially alcoholism. Children of alcoholics are four times more likely than other children to become alcoholics (American Academy of Child and Adolescent Psychiatry, 2022). Twin studies have demonstrated that monozygotic (one egg, genetically identical) twins have a higher rate for concordance of alcoholism than dizygotic (two eggs, genetically nonidentical) twins (Schuckit, 2017). Furthermore, biological offspring of alcoholic parents have a significantly greater incidence of alcoholism than offspring of nonalcoholic parents, whether the child was reared by the biological parents or by nonalcoholic adoptive parents (Schuckit, 2017). Research continues to discover genetic influences in addiction, but currently scientists estimate that genetics account for 40% to 60% of a person's vulnerability (National Institute on Drug Abuse [NIDA], 2020b). Some of this vulnerability may be related to heritable personality traits, such as high novelty seeking and low harm avoidance, both of which have been linked to substance use disorders (Iannucci & Weiss, 2017). Other variables include lifestyle influences such as diet, exercise, and types of social activities (e.g., frequency of engaging in social activities that include regular substance use).

Neurobiology

There is good evidence that changes in brain structure and brain neurochemistry occur in the process of developing an addiction, but whether these changes wholly explain etiology remains controversial. Alcohol has demonstrated effects on almost all neurotransmitters, but those most strongly linked to substance use disorders include opioid, catecholamine (especially dopamine), glutamate (especially those binding to *N*-methyl-D-aspartate [NMDA]), and gamma-aminobutyric acid (GABA) systems (Volkow & Boyle, 2018; Wang et al., 2019). Structures within the brain that are most associated with the drive toward compulsive substance use include the basal ganglia (which plays a role in pleasure and habit formation), the extended amygdala (which responds to stressors such as anxiety or perceived threats), and the prefrontal cortex (which is involved in thinking, problem-solving, judgment, and impulse control) (NIDA, 2020a). Once activated, the neuronal pathways that sense pleasure and reward are believed responsible for pleasurable sensations associated with the substance, as well as creating a "memory" that triggers a desire for repeated use of the substance. These pathways are referred to as the *brain-reward circuitry*. Over time, the brain tries to compensate for this excessive activation by lowering levels of these neurotransmitters, and the result is that an individual begins to feel sick when they stop or attempt to curtail use of the substance. At this point, the substance user needs to continue use of the substance simply to feel less sick.

Skeptics of neurobiological theories of addiction (and some of them are from within the scientific community) argue that biological findings may be overinterpreted and, because drug-dependent individuals are able to change their behavior, addiction is more likely a complex interaction of several factors than a single neurobiological process. Heilig and associates (2021) argued that identifying addiction as a disease of the brain is a valid construct and that a neurobiological basis for this disease is "fundamentally sound" although also influenced by a variety of other factors. They conclude that the debate reveals the need for multidisciplinary research that integrates neuroscientific, behavioral, clinical, and sociocultural perspectives for a disorder that is multifaceted within a population that has variable predisposing factors.

Psychological Factors
Developmental Influences

Psychodynamic theory suggests that individuals with punitive superegos turn to drugs to diminish unconscious anxiety and increase feelings of power and self-worth. Boland and Verduin (2022) stated, "As a form of self-medication, alcohol may be used to control panic, opioids to diminish anger, and amphetamines to alleviate depression. Some addicts have great difficulty recognizing their inner emotional states, a condition called *alexithymia*" (p. 275).

The landmark study on adverse childhood experiences (ACEs) (Felitti et al., 1998) found that the breadth of exposure to childhood trauma (which includes many forms of psychological, physical, or sexual abuse) shows a strong graded relationship to multiple risk factors for many leading causes of death in adulthood, including substance use disorders. They theorize that chronic trauma during childhood disrupts cognitive functioning, impairing a child's ability to cope with negative emotions, and the more adverse experiences, the greater the likelihood of a variety of health consequences in adulthood. Since the original study, several other studies have found links between childhood adverse experiences and increased lifetime prevalence for illicit drug use, dependency, and addiction (Dube et al., 2003; LeTendre & Reed, 2017); earlier onset of alcohol use (Rothman et al., 2008); increased prescription drug use (Forster et al., 2017); higher risk of mental and substance use disorders in adults over 50 years of age (Choi et al., 2017); and increased prevalence ratios for tobacco use among adolescents and adults (Fernandes et al., 2021; Ford et al., 2011; Maia-Silva et al., 2021).

Personality Factors

Certain personality traits have been associated with an increased tendency toward addictive behavior. Some clinicians believe low self-esteem, frequent depression, passivity, antisocial personality traits, the inability to relax or to defer gratification, and the inability to communicate effectively are common in individuals who misuse substances. These personality characteristics are not necessarily *predictive* of addictive behavior, yet for reasons not completely understood, they often accompany addiction. In some cases, the substance user may be self-medicating to treat symptoms of depression or anxiety.

Cognitive Factors

Irrational thinking patterns have long been identified as a central problem in addiction. Whether these thought patterns contribute to the development of or simply perpetuate an existing addiction is unclear, but the influence they hold is widely accepted. Twerski (1997) described these thought patterns as "addictive thinking" and suggests that when unchallenged, they may culminate in additional addictions even when a person stops using the drug to which they first became addicted. Some examples of irrational thinking patterns often associated with addiction include denial ("I'm not really addicted"), projection ("It's my wife's fault that I take drugs"), and rationalization ("I have to take drugs because I am in pain"). Exploring these thought patterns and their influence on problematic behavior, which is the basis of cognitive behavior therapy (CBT), has been identified as beneficial in addiction treatment (NIDA, 2018).

Sociocultural Factors

Social Learning

The effects of modeling, imitation, and identification on behavior can be observed from early childhood onward. The family appears to be an important influence in relation to substance use. Studies have shown that children and adolescents are more likely to use substances if their parents provide a model for substance use and misuse. Peers often exert substantial influence on the child or adolescent who is being encouraged to use substances for the first time. Modeling may continue to be a factor in substance use once the individual enters the workforce, particularly if the setting provides plenty of leisure time with coworkers, and drinking is valued as a way to express group cohesiveness.

Conditioning

Conditioning is a term describing a learned response that occurs after repeated exposure to a stimulus. Substance misuse can become a learned response from the substance itself and from the environment where use occurs. Many substances create a pleasurable experience that encourages the user to repeat it; thus, it is the intrinsically reinforcing properties of addictive drugs that "condition" the individual to repeatedly seek out their use.

The environment in which the substance is taken also contributes to the reinforcement. If the environment is pleasurable, substance use is usually increased. In addition, as the substance induces a state of pleasure, the user often associates that environment with these feelings and thus with drug use. Aversive stimuli within an environment are thought to be associated with a decrease in substance use within that environment.

Cultural and Ethnic Influences

Factors within an individual's culture help establish patterns of substance use by molding attitudes, influencing patterns of consumption based on cultural acceptance, and determining the availability of the substance. However, it is important to remember that a person's risk for addiction is multifaceted and cannot be tied solely to ethnic or cultural factors. For centuries, the French and Italians have considered wine an essential part of the family meal, even for children. The incidence of alcohol addiction is low, and acute intoxication from alcohol is not common. Conversely, alcohol problems in Ireland, where alcohol is a part of the social culture and pubs are considered hubs for social activity, are among the highest internationally; Alcohol Action Ireland (2022) reported that 40% of drinkers engage in heavy episode drinking at least monthly and 25% engage in heavy episode drinking weekly; the prevalence of alcohol use disorder is one in seven adults.

Decreased function of alcohol-metabolizing enzymes (alcohol dehydrogenase and aldehyde dehydrogenase) in some people of Asian heritage can lead to more rapid intoxication and toxic symptoms (Boland & Verduin, 2022). These changes cause alcohol to be converted quickly to acetaldehyde and decrease the rate at which acetaldehyde is oxidized. As a result of these changes, acetaldehyde rapidly accumulates in the body, producing unpleasant symptoms such as flushing, headaches, nausea, and palpitations when alcohol is consumed. However, whether these genetic variations influence higher or lower prevalence of substance use disorders has been a subject of debate.

The Dynamics of Substance-Related Disorders

Alcohol Use Disorder

Profile of the Substance

Alcohol is a natural substance formed by the reaction of fermenting sugar with yeast spores. Although there are many types of alcohol, the kind in alcoholic beverages is known scientifically as ethyl alcohol and chemically as C_2H_5OH. Its abbreviation, ETOH, is sometimes seen in medical records and other documents and publications.

By strict definition, alcohol is classified as a food because it contains calories; however, it has no nutritional value. Different alcoholic beverages are produced by using different sources of sugar for the fermentation process. For example, beer is made from malted barley, wine from grapes or berries, whiskey from malted grains, and rum from molasses. Distilled beverages (e.g., whiskey, scotch, gin, vodka, and other "hard" liquors) derive their names from the further concentration of the alcohol through a process called *distillation.*

The alcohol content varies by type of beverage. For example, most American beers contain 3% to 6% alcohol, wines average 10% to 20%, and distilled beverages range from 40% to 50% alcohol. For consistency, the average-sized drink, regardless of beverage, is considered to have 0.5 ounce of alcohol. This amount is present in 12 ounces of beer, 3 to 5 ounces of wine, and a cocktail with 1 ounce of whiskey. If consumed at the same rate, all would have an equal effect on one's body.

Alcohol exerts a depressant effect on the CNS, resulting in behavioral and mood changes proportional to the alcoholic concentration in the blood. Most states consider legal intoxication as a blood alcohol level of 0.08%.

The body burns alcohol at the rate of about 0.5 ounce per hour, so behavioral changes would not be expected to occur in an individual who slowly consumed only one average-sized drink per hour. Other factors influence these effects, however, such as an individual's physical size and whether or not the stomach contains food at the time of alcohol consumption. Alcohol is also thought to have a more profound effect when an individual is emotionally stressed or fatigued.

Most alcohol is metabolized in the liver, and the outcome of this process is the production of acetaldehyde. Acetaldehyde is then broken down by aldehyde dehydrogenase. Increased exposure to acetaldehyde leads to CNS depression, and prolonged exposure is associated with many detrimental health effects. At high levels, acetaldehyde causes the release of histamines and catecholamines, which can affect blood pressure and produce flushing, nausea, and vomiting. Although acetaldehyde oxidation generally occurs rapidly, in individuals who have genetic variations that affect alcohol dehydrogenase and aldehyde dehydrogenase, the process occurs more slowly, which may result in negative physical reactions to alcohol. These genetic variations are more common in Asian (Japanese, Chinese, and Korean) individuals (Schuckit, 2017).

Historical Aspects

The use of alcohol can be traced back to the Neolithic age, with known consumption of beer and wine around 6400 BC. With the introduction of distillation by the Arabs in the Middle Ages, alchemists believed that alcohol was the answer to all of their ailments. The word *whiskey,* meaning "water of life," became widely known.

In America, American Indian and Alaska Native (AI/AN) people had been drinking beer and wine before the arrival of the first immigrants from European countries. Refinement of the distillation process made beverages with high alcohol content readily available. By the early 1800s, one renowned physician of the time, Benjamin Rush, identified excessive, chronic alcohol consumption as a disease and an addiction. The strong religious mores on which the United States was founded soon led to the Temperance movement, which sought to prohibit the sale of alcoholic beverages. By the middle of the 19th century, 13 states had passed prohibition laws. The most notable prohibition of alcohol in the United States was from 1920 to 1933. The mandatory restrictions on national social habits resulted in the creation of profitable underground markets that led to flourishing criminal enterprises. Conversely, millions of dollars in federal, state, and local revenues from taxes and import duties on alcohol were lost. Although today alcohol is legal in the United States and the majority of people do not become physically addicted, there is a high prevalence of physical illness, injury, and loss of life secondary to alcohol misuse.

Patterns of Use

According to the 2020 National Survey of Drug Use and Health (Substance Abuse and Mental Health Services Administration [SAMHSA], 2021a) the prevalence of alcohol use is 8.2% among those ages 12 to 17 years and 54.2% for adults 18 years and older. There has been a significant decline in alcohol use among young adults (ages 18 to 26 years) since 2016. Overall, about 11% of Americans meet criteria for an alcohol use disorder. Why do people drink? In the United States, people use alcoholic beverages to enhance the flavor of food with meals; at social gatherings to encourage relaxation and conviviality among guests; and to promote a feeling of celebration on special occasions such as weddings, birthdays, and anniversaries. An alcoholic beverage (wine) is also used as part of the sacred ritual in some religious ceremonies. Therapeutically, alcohol is the major ingredient in many OTC and prescription medicines that are prepared in concentrated form. Therefore, alcohol can be harmless and enjoyable—sometimes even beneficial—if it is used responsibly and in moderation.

Like any other mind-altering drug, however, alcohol has the potential for misuse. Indeed, it currently accounts for the largest percentage of substance use disorders (74%) in the United States (SAMHSA, 2021a). It is estimated that, annually, 95,000 deaths are related to excessive alcohol use, and it is the third-leading lifestyle-related cause of death in the United States (the first is tobacco and the second is poor diet and physical inactivity) (National Institute on Alcohol Abuse and Alcoholism [NIAAA], 2022). In addition, alcohol use is a factor in more than one-half of all homicides, suicides, and traffic accidents. Incidents of domestic violence are commonly alcohol related. Heavy drinking contributes to illness in each of the top three causes of death: heart disease, cancer, and stroke.

An emerging trend is a phenomenon called high-intensity drinking, which is defined as consuming alcohol at levels that are two or more times the gender-specific binge drinking thresholds. Compared with people who did not binge drink, people who drank alcohol at twice the gender-specific binge drinking thresholds were 70 times more likely to have an alcohol-related emergency department visit, and those who consumed alcohol at three times the gender-specific binge thresholds were 93 times more likely to have an alcohol-related ED visit (NIAAA, 2022). It is estimated that up to 40% of hospital beds in the United States are being used to treat health conditions related to alcohol consumption. Fetal alcohol syndrome (FAS), caused by prenatal exposure to alcohol, is the most common, known preventable or environmental cause of intellectual disability (Lee et al., 2022). Jellinek's classic work (1952) outlined four phases through which the alcoholic's pattern of drinking progresses. Although some variability among individuals is to be expected within this model, the main point is to describe alcoholism as a progressive illness and a "vicious circle" associated with obsessive drinking (Hazelden Betty Ford Foundation, 2021).

Phase I. The Prealcoholic Phase

This phase is characterized by drinking to relieve anxiety, forget about stressors, or, in general, to feel better about oneself. Tolerance develops and the amount required to achieve the desired effect steadily increases.

Phase II. The Early Alcoholic Phase

Blacking out—brief periods of amnesia that occur during or immediately after a period of drinking—is a sign of this phase. Now the alcohol is no longer a source of pleasure or relief for the individual but rather a drug that is *required* by the individual. Common thinking and behaviors include sneaking drinks or secret drinking, obsessive thinking about alcohol, preoccupation with protecting and maintaining the supply of alcohol, rapid gulping of drinks, further blackouts, lying, and use of defense mechanisms such as denial and rationalization.

Phase III. The Crucial Phase

In this phase, the individual has lost control of their use of alcohol, and physiological addiction is clearly evident. This loss of control has been described as the inability to choose whether or not to drink. Binge drinking, lasting from a few hours to several weeks, is common. The NIAAA defines binge drinking as "a pattern of drinking that brings blood alcohol concentration (BAC) levels to 0.08 g/dL. This typically occurs after 4 drinks for women and 5 drinks for men—in about 2 hours" (NIAAA, 2022). These episodes are characterized by sickness, loss of consciousness, squalor, and degradation. In this phase, the individual is extremely ill. Anger and aggression are common manifestations. Drinking is the total focus, and individuals are willing to risk losing everything that was once important to maintain the addiction. By this phase of the illness, it is not uncommon for the individual to have experienced the loss of job, marriage, family, friends, and most especially, self-respect.

Phase IV. The Chronic Phase

This phase is characterized by emotional and physical disintegration. The individual is usually intoxicated more often than they are sober. Emotional disintegration is evidenced by profound helplessness and self-pity. Impairment in reality testing may result in psychosis. Life-threatening physical manifestations may be evident in virtually every system of the body. Unmanaged withdrawal from alcohol results in a syndrome of symptoms that includes hallucinations, tremors, convulsions, severe agitation, and panic. Depression and suicidal ideation are not uncommon. For long-term heavy drinkers, abrupt withdrawal of alcohol can be fatal.

Effects on the Body

Alcohol can induce a general, nonselective, reversible depression of the CNS. About 20% of the alcohol content in a single drink is absorbed directly and immediately into the bloodstream through the stomach wall. Unlike other "foods," alcohol does not have to be digested. The blood carries the alcohol directly to the brain, where it acts on the brain's central control areas, depressing brain activity. The other 80% of the drink's alcohol content is processed slightly more slowly through the upper intestinal tract and into the bloodstream. Only moments after alcohol is consumed, it can be found in all tissues, organs, and secretions of the body. The rapidity of absorption is influenced by various factors. For example, absorption is delayed when the drink is sipped rather than gulped, when the stomach contains food, and when the drink is wine or beer rather than a distilled beverage.

At low doses, alcohol produces relaxation, loss of inhibition, lack of concentration, drowsiness, slurred speech, and sleep. Chronic misuse results in multisystem physiological impairments. These complications include (but are not limited to) those outlined in the following sections.

Peripheral Neuropathy

Peripheral neuropathy, characterized by nerve damage, results in pain, burning, tingling, or prickly sensations of the extremities. Researchers believe it is the direct result of deficiency in the B vitamins, particularly thiamine. Nutritional deficiencies are common in chronic alcoholics due to insufficient intake of nutrients and because the toxic effect of alcohol results in malabsorption of nutrients. The process is often reversible with abstinence from alcohol and restoration of nutritional deficiencies, but for some individuals, pain and numbness may be permanent

(Schuckit, 2017). With chronic alcohol use permanent muscle wasting and paralysis can occur.

Alcoholic Myopathy

Alcoholic myopathy may occur as an acute or chronic condition. In the acute condition, also called *acute alcoholic necrotizing myopathy* or *alcoholic rhabdomyolysis,* the individual experiences a sudden onset of muscle pain, swelling, and weakness along with myoglobinuria, evidenced by a red tinge in the urine. Creatine kinase may be elevated before the appearance of symptoms. Experimental studies have suggested that alcohol use and malnourishment are necessary to produce this syndrome (Lanska, 2022). Muscle symptoms are usually generalized, but pain and swelling may selectively involve the calves or other muscle groups. Laboratory studies show elevations of the enzymes creatine phosphokinase (CPK), lactate dehydrogenase (LDH), aldolase, and aspartate aminotransferase (AST). The symptoms of chronic alcoholic myopathy include a gradual wasting and weakness in skeletal muscles. Neither the pain and tenderness nor the elevated muscle enzymes seen in acute myopathy are evident in the chronic condition.

Alcoholic myopathy is thought to be a result of the same B vitamin deficiency that contributes to peripheral neuropathy. Improvement occurs with abstinence from alcohol and the return to a nutritious diet with vitamin supplements.

Wernicke's Encephalopathy

Wernicke's encephalopathy represents the most serious form of thiamine deficiency in alcoholics. Symptoms include paralysis of the ocular muscles, diplopia, ataxia, somnolence, and stupor. If thiamine replacement therapy is not given quickly, death will ensue.

Korsakoff's Psychosis

Korsakoff's psychosis is identified by a syndrome of confusion, loss of recent memory, and confabulation in alcoholics. It is frequently encountered in individuals recovering from Wernicke's encephalopathy. In the United States, the two disorders are usually considered together and are called *Wernicke-Korsakoff syndrome.* Treatment is parenteral or oral thiamine replacement.

Alcoholic Cardiomyopathy

The effect of alcohol on the heart is an accumulation of lipids in the myocardial cells, resulting in enlargement and a weakened condition. The clinical findings of alcoholic cardiomyopathy are generally caused by congestive heart failure or arrhythmia. Symptoms include decreased exercise tolerance, tachycardia, dyspnea, edema, palpitations, and nonproductive cough. Laboratory studies may show elevation of the enzymes CPK, AST, alanine aminotransferase (ALT), and LDH. Changes may be observed by electrocardiogram, and congestive heart failure may be evident on chest x-ray films.

The treatment is total permanent abstinence from alcohol. Treatment of congestive heart failure may include rest, oxygen, digitalization, sodium restriction, and diuretics. Prognosis is encouraging if treated in the early stages. The death rate is high for individuals with advanced symptomatology.

Esophagitis

Esophagitis—inflammation and pain in the esophagus—occurs because of the toxic effects of alcohol on the esophageal mucosa and because of frequent vomiting associated with alcohol misuse.

Gastritis

The effects of alcohol on the stomach include inflammation of the stomach lining characterized by epigastric distress, nausea, vomiting, and distention. Alcohol breaks down the stomach's protective mucosal barrier, allowing hydrochloric acid to erode the stomach wall. Damage to blood vessels may result in hemorrhage.

Pancreatitis

Pancreatitis may be categorized as *acute* or *chronic.* Acute pancreatitis usually occurs a day or two after a binge of excessive alcohol consumption. Symptoms include constant, severe epigastric pain, nausea and vomiting, and abdominal distention. The chronic condition leads to pancreatic insufficiency resulting in steatorrhea, malnutrition, weight loss, and diabetes mellitus.

Alcoholic Hepatitis

Alcoholic hepatitis is inflammation of the liver caused by long-term heavy alcohol use. Clinical manifestations include an enlarged and tender liver, nausea and vomiting, lethargy, anorexia, elevated white blood cell count, fever, and jaundice. **Ascites** (fluid accumulation in the abdomen) and weight loss may be evident in more severe cases. With treatment—which includes strict abstinence from alcohol, proper nutrition, and rest—the individual can experience complete recovery. Severe cases can lead to cirrhosis or **hepatic encephalopathy** (abnormalities in brain function brought on by severe liver disease).

Cirrhosis of the Liver

Cirrhosis of the liver may be caused by anything that results in chronic injury to the liver. It is the end stage of alcoholic liver disease and results from long-term chronic alcohol misuse. There is widespread destruction of liver cells, which are replaced by fibrous (scar) tissue. Clinical manifestations include nausea and vomiting, anorexia, weight loss, abdominal pain, jaundice, edema, anemia, and blood coagulation abnormalities. Treatment includes abstention from alcohol, correction of malnutrition, and supportive care to prevent complications of the disease. Complications of cirrhosis include the following:

- **Portal hypertension:** Elevation of blood pressure through the portal circulation results from defective blood flow through the cirrhotic liver.
- **Ascites:** This condition, in which an excessive amount of serous fluid accumulates in the abdominal cavity, occurs in response to portal hypertension. The increased pressure results in the seepage of fluid from the surface of the liver into the abdominal cavity.
- **Esophageal varices:** Veins in the esophagus that become distended because of excessive pressure due to defective blood flow through the cirrhotic liver are termed **esophageal varices**. As this pressure increases, these varicosities can rupture, resulting in hemorrhage and sometimes death.
- **Hepatic encephalopathy:** This serious complication occurs in response to the inability of the diseased liver to convert ammonia to urea for excretion. The continued rise in serum ammonia results in progressively impaired mental functioning, apathy, euphoria or depression, sleep disturbance, increasing confusion, and progression to coma and eventual death. Treatment includes complete abstention from alcohol, reduction of protein in the diet; avoidance of medications broken down by the liver or medications with ammonium (including certain antacids); and reduction of intestinal ammonia using neomycin, rifaximin, or lactulose (National Library of Medicine [NLM], 2022).

Leukopenia

The production, function, and movement of the white blood cells are impaired in chronic alcoholism. This condition, called *leukopenia,* places the individual at high risk for contracting infectious diseases and for complicated recovery.

Thrombocytopenia

Platelet production and survival are impaired as a result of the toxic effects of alcohol, which increases the risk of hemorrhage. Abstinence from alcohol rapidly reverses this deficiency.

Sexual Dysfunction

Alcohol interferes with the normal production and maintenance of female and male hormones, and long-term alcohol use can interfere with the liver's ability to metabolize estrogenic compounds (Boland & Verduin, 2022). For women, this can mean changes in the menstrual cycle and a decrease in or loss of fertility. For men, the altered hormone levels result in diminished libido, decreased sexual performance, and impaired fertility. Gynecomastia may develop secondary to testicular atrophy.

Use During Pregnancy

Fetal Alcohol Spectrum disorders

Prenatal exposure to alcohol can result in a broad range of disorders to the fetus, known as *fetal alcohol spectrum disorders (FASDs),* the most involved of which is *FAS*. People with FAS have CNS problems, as well as minor facial feature and growth problems. They often have a hard time in school and trouble getting along with others (Centers for Disease Control and Prevention [CDC], 2022a). There may be problems with learning, memory, attention span, communication, vision, hearing, or a combination of these. Other FASDs include alcohol-related neurodevelopmental disorder (ARND) and alcohol-related birth defects (ARBDs) that might include problems with the heart, kidneys, bones, or hearing (CDC, 2022a).

There is no safe amount and no safe time to drink alcohol during pregnancy because alcohol can damage a fetus at any stage of development (CDC, 2022a). Therefore, alcohol consumption should be avoided by women who are pregnant or trying to become pregnant. Few estimates of the prevalence for FASDs are available, but experts estimate that the numbers may be as high as 1% to 5% of the population (CDC, 2022a). The common feature in the development of FASD is women who drink alcohol during pregnancy: heavy drinking and binge drinking increases the risk (CDC, 2022a).

Boland & Verduin (2022) reported that women with alcohol-related disorders have a 35% risk of having a child with defects. Children with FASDs may have the following characteristics or exhibit the following behaviors (CDC, 2022a):

- Abnormal facial features
- Small head size
- Shorter-than-average height
- Low body weight
- Poor coordination
- Hyperactive behavior
- Difficulty paying attention
- Poor memory
- Difficulty in school
- Learning disabilities
- Speech and language delays
- Intellectual disability or low IQ
- Poor reasoning and judgment skills
- Sleep and sucking problems as a baby
- Vision or hearing problems
- Problems with the heart, kidneys, or bones

Neuroimaging of children with FASDs shows abnormalities in multiple regions of the brain, particularly structural anomalies in white matter tracts within different parts of the corpus callosum (Zhang et al., 2019). Children with FASDs are often at risk for psychiatric disorders, most commonly attention deficit-hyperactivity disorder, mood disorders, and oppositional defiant disorder (Denny et al., 2017). A diagnosis of specifically FAS requires the following criteria be met (NIAAA, 2021):

■ Evidence of prenatal alcohol exposure (PAE)
■ Evidence of CNS abnormalities (structural or functional)
■ A specific pattern of three facial abnormalities: narrow eye openings, a smooth area between the lip and the nose (vs. the normal ridge), and a thin upper lip (see Figure 23–1)
■ Growth deficits either prenatally, after birth, or both

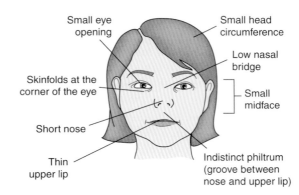

FIGURE 23–1 Facial features that may be present in fetal alcohol syndrome. (From the National Institute of Alcohol Abuse and Alcoholism of the National Institutes of Health, Washington, DC.)

Real Nurses, Real Advice

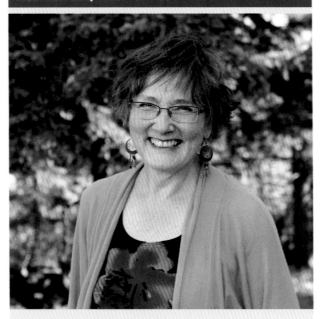

Based on analysis of recent Behavioral Risk Factor Surveillance Survey (BRFSS) data, 1 in 7 American women drink alcohol during their pregnancy (Gosdin et al., 2022). PAE is the leading cause of preventable birth defects and intellectual disability. Most of those who experience an FASD do not have visible defects. They are brain-based disabilities that manifest over time as attention, learning, behavioral, and social symptoms. Nurses can play a key role in FASD prevention by reminding their patients that there is no safe amount, no safe type, and no safe time to consume alcohol during pregnancy.

Marilyn Pierce-Bulger, APRN (MN, FNP-BC, CNM)
President, Board of Directors, Alaska Center for FASD

Children with FASDs require lifelong care and treatment. There is no cure, but it can be prevented. The Collaborative for Alcohol-Free Pregnancy, a joint effort of the CDC along with FASD Practice and Implementation Centers and National Partners (CDC, 2022a), stresses the importance of using evidence-based tools such as alcohol screening and brief intervention (SBI) to prevent alcohol-exposed pregnancy and risky alcohol use. Nurses who work with women of childbearing age or who are pregnant can play a vital role in ensuring that this type of screening is conducted. Online training and resources for nurses and other health-care professionals are available through the CDC (2023).

Alcohol Intoxication

Behavioral and cognitive symptoms of alcohol intoxication include disinhibition of sexual or aggressive impulses, mood lability, impaired judgment, impaired social or occupational functioning, slurred speech, incoordination, unsteady gait, nystagmus, and flushed face. Several physical symptoms associated with alcohol intoxication include CNS depression, hypoglycemia, hypothermia, hyper- or hypotension, and vomiting, among others. Intoxication usually is evident at blood alcohol levels between 100 and 200 mg/dL. Death has been reported at levels ranging from 400 to 700 mg/dL.

Alcohol Withdrawal

Within 4 to 12 hours of cessation of or reduction in heavy and prolonged alcohol use (several days or longer), the following withdrawal symptoms may appear: coarse tremor of hands, tongue, or eyelids; nausea or vomiting; malaise or weakness; tachycardia; sweating; elevated blood pressure; anxiety; depressed mood or irritability; transient hallucinations or illusions; headache; and insomnia. About 5% of hospital patients with alcohol-related disorders develop *alcohol withdrawal delirium*, also known as DTs (delirium tremens), a medical emergency that, if left untreated, confers a 20% mortality rate (Boland & Verduin, 2022). Concomitant medical problems may increase this risk. The onset of delirium is usually on the second or third day after decrease or discontinuation of alcohol use. Symptoms include those described under the syndrome of delirium (see Chapter 22, "Neurocognitive Disorders").

Sedative, Hypnotic, or Anxiolytic Use Disorder

Profile of the Substance

The sedative, hypnotic, and anxiolytic compounds are drugs of diverse chemical structures that are capable of inducing varying degrees of CNS depression, from tranquilizing relief of anxiety to anesthesia, coma, and even death. They are generally categorized as (1) barbiturates, (2) nonbarbiturate hypnotics, and (3) antianxiety agents. Effects produced by these substances depend on size of dose and potency of drug administered. Table 23–1 presents a selected list of drugs included in these categories. Generic names are followed in parentheses by the trade names. Common street names for each category are also included.

Several principles have been identified that are fairly typical among all CNS depressants:

1. **The effects of CNS depressants are additive with one another and with the behavioral state of the user.** For example, when these drugs are used in combination with each other or with alcohol, the depressive effects are compounded. These intense depressive effects are often unpredictable and can even be fatal. Similarly, a person who is mentally depressed or physically fatigued may have an exaggerated response to a dose of the drug that would only slightly affect a person in a normal or excited state. The U.S. Food and Drug Administration (FDA, 2016) began requiring boxed warnings (commonly referred to as *black box warnings*), its strongest warning label, for benzodiazepines, opioid analgesics, and opioid cough products, based on evidence that the combination of opioids and benzodiazepines carries a particularly high risk for excessive sleepiness, respiratory depression, coma, and death.

2. **CNS depressants are capable of producing physiological dependence.** If large doses of CNS depressants are repeatedly administered over a

TABLE 23–1	Sedative, Hypnotic, and Anxiolytic Drugs	
CATEGORIES	**GENERIC (TRADE) NAMES**	**COMMON STREET NAMES**
Barbiturates	Amobarbital (Amytal) Pentobarbital (Nembutal) Secobarbital (Seconal) Butabarbital (Butisol) Phenobarbital	Blue birds, blue angels, yellow jackets, yellow birds, GB, lillys, pinks, reds Pheno, sleepers
Nonbarbiturate hypnotics	Chloral hydrate Estazolam Flurazepam Temazepam (Restoril) Triazolam (Halcion) Quazepam (Doral) Eszopiclone (Lunesta) Ramelteon (Rozerem) Zaleplon (Sonata) Zolpidem (Ambien) Suvorexant (Belsomra) Tasimelteon (Hetlioz)	Peter, Mickey, sleepers Green devils, tummies Halcyon daze A-minus, nappien, no-go, tic tacs
Antianxiety agents	Alprazolam (Xanax) Chlordiazepoxide (Librium) Clonazepam (Klonopin) Clorazepate (Tranxene) Diazepam (Valium) Lorazepam (Ativan) Oxazepam (Serax) Meprobamate (Miltown)	Bars, footballs, zannies Green and whites, roaches K-pin Vs (Valium; color designates strength), blues, mothers little helpers Zzz dolls, dollies (meprobamate)
Club drugs	Flunitrazepam (Rohypnol) Gamma hydroxybutyric acid (gamma hydroxybutyrate; GHB)	Date rape drug, roofies, R-2, rope, forget me pill; G, liquid X, grievous bodily harm, easy lay

prolonged duration, a period of CNS hyperexcitability occurs upon withdrawal of the drug. The response can be quite severe, even leading to convulsions and death.

3. **CNS depressants are capable of producing psychological dependence.** CNS depressants have the potential to generate a psychic drive for periodic or continuous administration of the drug to achieve maximum functioning or feeling of well-being.

4. **Cross-tolerance and cross-dependence may exist between various CNS depressants.** Cross-tolerance refers to a condition in which an individual becomes resistant to the effects of one drug because they have developed tolerance to another drug with similar pharmacological activity. Cross-dependence is a condition in which an individual can become dependent on more than one substance because of their similar activity and effects.

Historical Aspects

Anxiety and insomnia, two of the most common human afflictions, were treated during the 19th century with opiates, bromide salts, chloral hydrate, paraldehyde, and alcohol (Julien, 2014). Because opiates were known to produce physical addiction, the bromides carried the risk of chronic bromide poisoning, and chloral hydrate and paraldehyde had an objectionable taste and smell, alcohol became the prescribed depressant drug of choice. However, some people refused to use alcohol either because they did not like the taste or for moral reasons, and others tended to take more than prescribed. Therefore, a search for a better sedative drug continued.

Although barbituric acid was first synthesized in 1864, it was not until 1912 that phenobarbital was introduced into medicine as a sedative drug, the first of the structurally classified group of drugs called barbiturates (Julien, 2014). Since that time, more than 2,500 barbiturate derivatives have been synthesized, but fewer than a dozen remain in medical use. Illicit use of these drugs for recreational purposes grew throughout the 1930s and 1940s.

Efforts to create depressant medications that were not barbiturate derivatives accelerated. By the mid-1950s, the market for depressants had been expanded by the appearance of the nonbarbiturates glutethimide, ethchlorvynol, methyprylon, and meprobamate. Benzodiazepines were introduced around 1960 with the marketing of chlordiazepoxide (Librium), followed shortly by its derivative diazepam (Valium). The use of these drugs and others within their group grew rapidly, and they are prescribed widely in medical

practice. Their margin of safety is greater than that of barbiturates and the other nonbarbiturates. However, prolonged use of even moderate doses is likely to result in physical and psychological addiction, with a characteristic syndrome of withdrawal that can be severe.

Patterns of Use

Boland & Verduin (2022) reported that about 15% of all persons in the United States have had a benzodiazepine prescribed by a physician. Of all the drugs used in clinical practice, the sedative, hypnotic, and anxiolytic drugs are among the most widely prescribed.

Two patterns that lead to addiction are described. The first pattern begins with an individual whose physician originally prescribed the CNS depressant to treat anxiety or insomnia. Independently, the individual increases the dosage or frequency from that which was prescribed. Use of the medication is justified based on treating symptoms, but as tolerance grows, more of the drug is required to produce the desired effect. Substance-seeking behavior is evident as the individual seeks prescriptions from several physicians to maintain sufficient supplies.

The second pattern involves people in their teens or early 20s who use illegally obtained substances in the company of their peers. The initial objective is to achieve a feeling of euphoria. The drug is usually used intermittently during recreational gatherings. This pattern of intermittent use leads to regular use and extreme levels of tolerance. Combining use with other substances is not uncommon. Physical and psychological addiction leads to intense substance-seeking behaviors, most often through illegal channels.

Effects on the Body

The sedative, hypnotic, and anxiolytic compounds induce a general depressant effect; that is, they depress the activity of the brain, nerves, muscles, and heart tissue. The primary action of sedatives, hypnotics, and anxiolytics is on nervous tissue. However, large doses may affect other organ systems. They reduce the rate of metabolism in a variety of tissues throughout the body and depress any system that uses energy. Large doses are required to produce these effects. In lower doses, these drugs appear more selective in their depressant actions by exerting their action on the centers within the brain that are concerned with arousal (e.g., the ascending reticular activating system, in the reticular formation, and the diffuse thalamic projection system).

These drugs are capable of producing all levels of CNS depression—from mild sedation to death. The level is determined by dosage and potency of the drug used. In Figure 23–2, a continuum

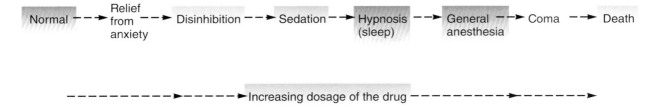

FIGURE 23–2   Continuum of CNS depression with increasing doses of sedative, hypnotic, or anxiolytic drugs.

demonstrates how increasing doses of these drugs affect the level of CNS depression.

The following is a discussion of the physiological effects of these medications.

Effects on Sleep and Dreaming

Barbiturate use decreases the amount of sleep time spent dreaming. During drug withdrawal, dreaming becomes vivid and excessive. Rebound insomnia and increased dreaming (termed *rapid-eye-movement [REM] rebound*) are not uncommon with abrupt withdrawal from long-term use of these drugs as sleeping aids.

Respiratory Depression

Barbiturates are capable of inhibiting the reticular activating system, resulting in respiratory depression that may lead to lethal overdose. In addition, additive effects can occur with the concurrent use of other CNS depressants, also effecting a life-threatening situation.

Cardiovascular Effects

Hypotension may be a problem with large doses. Only a slight decrease in blood pressure is noted with normal oral dosage. High dosages of barbiturates also compromise cardiac contractility and vascular tone, which may result in cardiovascular collapse. Individuals with congestive heart failure are more susceptible to these effects (Lafferty, 2017).

Renal Function

In doses high enough to produce anesthesia and an overdose, barbiturates may reduce urine output (oliguria). At the usual sedative-hypnotic dosage, however, there is no evidence of direct action on the kidneys.

Hepatic Effects

Barbiturates stimulate the production of liver enzymes. Increases in cytochrome P450 isoenzymes inhibit the metabolism of many medications, including antipsychotics, antidepressants, anticonvulsants, and steroid hormones, and accelerate metabolism of the barbiturates themselves (Dubovsky, 2017). Preexisting liver disease may predispose an individual to additional liver damage with excessive barbiturate use.

Body Temperature

High doses of barbiturates can greatly decrease body temperature. It is not significantly altered with normal dosage levels.

Sexual Function

CNS depressants tend to produce a biphasic response. There is an initial increase in libido, presumably from the primary disinhibitory effects of the drug, followed by impaired sexual pleasure. In men, this initial response is followed by a decreased ability to maintain an erection.

Sedative, Hypnotic, or Anxiolytic Intoxication

The *DSM-5-TR* (APA, 2022) describes sedative, hypnotic, or anxiolytic intoxication as the presence of clinically significant maladaptive behavioral or psychological changes that develop during, or shortly after, use of one of these substances. These maladaptive changes may include inappropriate sexual or aggressive behavior, mood lability, impaired judgment, or impaired social or occupational functioning. Other symptoms that may develop with excessive use of CNS depressants include slurred speech, incoordination, unsteady gait, nystagmus, impairment in attention or memory, and stupor or coma.

"Club drugs" in this category include gamma hydroxybutyric acid (GHB) and flunitrazepam (Rohypnol). Like all depressants, they can produce a state of disinhibition, excitement, drunkenness, and amnesia. They have been widely implicated as "date rape" drugs, because their presence is easily disguised in drinks. They produce anterograde amnesia, the inability to remember events experienced.

Sedative, Hypnotic, or Anxiolytic Withdrawal

Withdrawal from sedatives, hypnotics, or anxiolytics produces a characteristic syndrome of symptoms that develops after a marked decrease in or cessation of intake after several weeks or more of regular use (APA, 2022). The onset of symptoms depends on the drug from which the individual is withdrawing. With short-acting sedative-hypnotics (e.g., alprazolam, lorazepam), symptoms may begin between 12 and 24 hours after the last dose, reach peak intensity between 24 and 72 hours, and subside in 5 to 10 days. Withdrawal symptoms from substances with longer half-lives (e.g., diazepam, phenobarbital, chlordiazepoxide) may begin within 2 to 7 days, peak on the fifth to eighth day, and subside in 10 to 16 days.

Severe withdrawal is most likely to occur when a substance has been used at high dosages for prolonged periods. However, withdrawal symptoms also have been reported with moderate dosages taken over a relatively short duration. Withdrawal symptoms include autonomic hyperactivity (e.g., sweating or pulse rate greater than 100), increased hand tremor, insomnia, nausea or vomiting, hallucinations, illusions, psychomotor agitation, anxiety, or grand mal seizures, and delirium.

Stimulant Use Disorder
Profile of the Substance

CNS stimulants are identified by the behavioral stimulation and psychomotor agitation they induce. They differ widely in molecular structure and mechanism of action. The amount of CNS stimulation caused by a certain drug depends on both the area in the brain or spinal cord that is affected by the drug and the cellular mechanism fundamental to the increased excitability. The *DSM-5-TR* (APA, 2022) categorizes caffeine-related disorders and tobacco-related disorders as separate and distinct diagnoses. For purposes of this text, these substances are discussed with the stimulant-related disorders.

Groups within this category are classified according to similarities in their mechanism of action. The *psychomotor stimulants* induce stimulation by augmentation or potentiation of the neurotransmitters norepinephrine, epinephrine, or dopamine. The *general cellular stimulants* (caffeine and nicotine) exert their action directly on cellular activity. Caffeine inhibits the enzyme phosphodiesterase, allowing increased levels of adenosine 3´, 5´-cyclic phosphate (cAMP), a chemical substance that promotes increased rates of cellular metabolism. Nicotine stimulates ganglionic synapses. This results in increased acetylcholine, which stimulates nerve impulse transmission to the entire autonomic nervous system. A selected list of drugs included in these categories is presented in Table 23–2.

The two most prevalent and widely used stimulants are caffeine and nicotine. Caffeine is readily

TABLE 23–2 **CNS Stimulants**		
CATEGORIES	**GENERIC (TRADE) NAMES**	**COMMON STREET NAMES**
Amphetamines	Dextroamphetamine (Dexedrine) Methamphetamine (Desoxyn) 3,4-methylenedioxyamphetamine (MDMA)* Amphetamine + dextroamphetamine (Adderall)	Dexies, uppers, truck drivers Meth, speed, crystal, ice, crank, chalk, fire, glass Adam, ecstasy, Eve, XTC, Molly Beans, pep pills, speed, uppers, study buddies, smart pills
Synthetic stimulants	3,4-methylenedioxypyrovalerone (MDPV)* 4-methylmethcathinone (mephedrone, 4-MMC)* Methylone* Ethylone Dibutylone Alpha-PVP	Bath salts (also called blue silk, cloud 9, ivory wave, vanilla sky, white lightning, and others), flakka, gravel
Nonamphetamine stimulants	Phendimetrazine (Bontril) Benzphetamine (Didrex) Diethylpropion (Tenuate) Phentermine (Adipex-P; Ionamin) Sibutramine (Meridia)† Methylphenidate (Ritalin) Dexmethylphenidate (Focalin) Modafinil (Provigil)	Diet pills Vitamin R, kibbles and bits, study buddies
Cocaine	Cocaine hydrochloride	Coke, blow, toot, snow, lady, flake, crack
Caffeine	Coffee, tea, colas, chocolate	Java, mud, brew, cocoa
Nicotine	Cigarettes, cigars, pipe tobacco, snuff	Weeds, fags, butts, chaw, cancer sticks

*Cross-listed with the hallucinogens.
†No longer marketed in the United States.

available in every supermarket and grocery store as a common ingredient in coffee, tea, colas, chocolate, and energy drinks. Nicotine is the primary psychoactive substance found in tobacco products. When used in moderation, these stimulants tend to relieve fatigue and increase alertness. They are a generally accepted part of our culture; however, with increased social awareness regarding the health risks associated with tobacco products, their use has become stigmatized in some circles.

The more potent stimulants, because of their potential for physiological dependence, are under regulation by the Controlled Substances Act. These controlled stimulants are available for therapeutic purposes by prescription only; however, they are also clandestinely manufactured and widely distributed on the illicit market. More recently, the synthetic stimulants mephedrone, 3,4-methylenedioxypyrovalerone (MDPV), methylone, and others have become available, and because their chemical structures had been altered, they were not initially identifiable as a controlled substance or regulated by the federal government. Known as "bath salts," street names include *blue silk, cloud 9, ivory wave, vanilla sky, white knight, white lightning, stardust,* and *purple wave.* In October 2011 the U.S. Drug Enforcement Administration (DEA) issued emergency scheduling of these substances to make their possession and sales illegal (except as authorized by law). They are currently designated as schedule I substances, the most restrictive category under the Controlled Substances Act. This action was taken in response to reports of episodes of violent behavior associated with use of the substance.

Another synthetic cathinone, alpha-PVP (commonly known as *flakka, gravel, $5 insanity,* or *the zombie drug*), whose chemical structure is similar but not identical to bath salts, has appeared in the United States. This drug can be snorted, injected, eaten, and vaporized for inhalation in e-cigarettes. Vaporization is a particularly dangerous route because of its immediate absorption, and deaths have been reported secondary to overdose, suicide, and heart attack.

Flakka was considered a significant health hazard in 2014 and 2015, but no deaths were reported in 2016, after China (the sole provider of this drug) banned the production and exportation of alpha-PVP (Storrs, 2016). Although flakka use has declined, flakka-related erratic behavior and sometimes criminal activity continue to surface in some areas of the United States. Palomar and associate's research (2019) estimated the prevalence of use among high school seniors was "rare" (0.8 %) but note that use may be under-reported because flakka is often added to the party drug known as XTC or Molly and the user may not be aware of its presence.

Complicating the arena of illicit stimulant use is the fact that when one synthetic stimulant is banned, it is often replaced by another (Storrs, 2016). For example, when China banned methylone (a drug similar to flakka) in 2014, it was replaced by ethylone; after ethylone was banned, a similar drug called dibutylone surfaced. This pattern creates an ongoing challenge for the FDA and DEA to identify and take action on each new synthetic variant as it comes to public attention (usually through significant health consequences or deaths). New synthetic drugs may also be difficult to identify because standard drug screens do not recognize these chemicals.

Historical Aspects

Cocaine is the most potent stimulant derived from nature. It is extracted from the leaves of the coca plant, which has been cultivated in the Andean highlands of South America since prehistoric times. Natives of the region chew the leaves of the plant for refreshment and relief from fatigue.

Coca leaves must be mixed with lime to release the cocaine alkaloid. The chemical formula for the pure form of the drug was developed in 1960. Physicians began using the drug as an anesthetic in eye, nose, and throat surgeries, and it was used in the United States in a morphine-cocaine elixir designed to relieve the suffering associated with terminal illness. These therapeutic uses are now obsolete.

Cocaine has achieved a degree of acceptability within some social circles. It is illicitly distributed as a white crystalline powder, often mixed with other ingredients to increase its volume and create more profit. The drug is most commonly "snorted," and chronic users may manifest symptoms that resemble the congested nose of a common cold. The intensely pleasurable effects of the drug create the potential for extraordinary psychological addiction.

Another form of cocaine commonly used in the United States is made by processing powdered cocaine with ammonia or sodium bicarbonate and water and heating it to remove the hydrochloride. The term *crack,* the street name for this form of the drug, refers to the crackling sound heard when the mixture is smoked. Because this type of cocaine can be easily vaporized and inhaled, its effects have an extremely rapid onset. See "Real People, Real Stories" for Alan's experience with crack cocaine and alcohol addiction.

Amphetamine was first prepared in 1887. Various derivatives of the drug soon followed, and clinical use of the drug began in 1927. **Amphetamines** were used extensively for medical purposes through the 1960s, but recognition of their potential for misuse and addiction has sharply decreased clinical use.

Real People, Real Stories: Alan Brunner on Substance Use Disorder

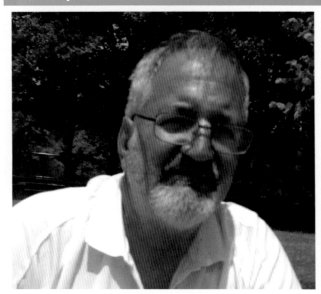

Substance use disorders often follow a progressive pattern that develops over a long period of time. Alan's story is an example of that process. See also Chapter 7, "Therapeutic Communication," for an interaction with Alan that incorporates motivational interviewing. Reflect on important issues for primary prevention education. Consider examples of interventions that are ineffective or unhealthy for the user and the care provider. Incorporate an understanding of codependency in this reflection.

Karyn: Tell me about when you first used drugs or alcohol.

Alan: I was 15 years old when I first started smoking pot and 16 when I had my first drink. The pot use went from occasional use to several times a week by the time I was a senior in high school. I knew that was a problem, but the drinking progressed much more gradually. For years, I only drank on weekends. For a while, my buddy and I would share a quart on the weekend. Eventually, we each had our own quart, then two quarts each. I only drank beer. Once when I was teenager, I drank a fifth of vodka, and I got extremely sick. My mom didn't try to rescue me or help me feel better or cover for me. I just had to live through the consequences, and that was probably a good thing; I never drank vodka again. But the beer drinking became more often and at higher amounts. Even so, it took another 35 years to recognize that it was a problem!

Karyn: Was there any history of alcoholism in your family?

Alan: Oh yeah... several relatives. My dad had a drinking problem, and that led to my parents divorcing when I was 14 years old. When I was 19, I moved in with my dad, and then I started drinking during the week, too—because he did. My dad always worked and had a strong work ethic, even though he was a heavy drinker, so I thought, "As long as I'm able to drink and it's not interfering with work, then it's not a problem." I also

remember thinking, "It's just beer, and I would never use the 'strong' or 'bad' drugs, like cocaine—I would NEVER do that."

Karyn: So your beer drinking increased while you were living with your father?

Alan: Initially, yes, but then I was surrounding myself with people and friends who liked to drink. I moved in with a friend, and we usually drank a case of beer each night. Then I started an auto repair business with a friend who was a heavy drinker, and we had beer at the shop. Pretty soon we weren't leaving the shop until all the beer was gone. Then I got involved with auto racing, and that was an environment with lots of alcohol and cocaine.

Karyn: I remember you said you were using cocaine. Is that when the use started?

Alan: No, actually I had become friends with a deacon at my church, probably because we both liked to drink. He was the one that introduced me to cocaine.

Karyn: So you started using cocaine along with drinking?

Alan: Yeah, even though I had said I would never do that. But I discovered that if I did cocaine, I had a lot more energy and I could stay awake longer, so I could be a much "better" drinker. (chuckles)

Karyn: Tell me about when you recognized that your use was a problem.

Alan: Well, eventually, I was drinking at home because it was a waste of "good drinking time" to get together with other people. So largely, I was sitting at home in the dark drinking by myself, and the beer never even made it into the fridge. The cocaine was putting me in the company of some very bad people. I knew I had to somehow get away from that... and when I started using cocaine, I said, "One thing I'll never do is crack," but then I started doing that, and that's when things completely fell apart.

Karyn: Fell apart?

Alan: I was racking up a lot of legal problems. I had some DUIs and reckless operation charges before that, but now I'm getting drug possession charges, paraphernalia charges, driving with a suspended license, driving with expired license plates, more DUIs, disorderly conduct charges. And the crack—that drug rips out your soul! You're always chasing the high that you got the first time you used it, and you never find that, so you keep using more. That's why one of my friends called crack "gotta" because you gotta have it. ... And you don't care about ANYTHING else—you don't care if you die.

Karyn: You told me you've been clean and sober for 7 years. How did you turn the corner?

Alan: I had such a huge legal mess that my lawyer was recommending I just accept the jail time (3 to 10 days) and be done with it, but the judge offered treatment in lieu of jail, and I told him that's what I wanted because I knew I needed it. I was told, though, that if I violated the treatment program, I would spend a year in jail, so

Real People, Real Stories: Alan Brunner on Substance Use Disorder—cont'd

I knew I was taking a big risk by going into treatment. But I knew it was the only way out—and I knew I needed it.

Karyn: So what is your relapse prevention plan?

Alan: I have an AA sponsor, and I go to meetings sometimes, but not as often as I used to. I never allow myself to become too proud about my sobriety because I know all it would take is one drink. As long as I remember that, I'm vulnerable. … I don't get too cocky. I've also had a lot of support from family, especially my mom. She supported me every step of the way in treatment. Having supportive people around you is essential. The relationship I had been in for many years broke up largely because she was telling my counselors that she wanted me to cut down but she wasn't in favor of abstinence—she was quite a partier, too. Staying in that relationship, I believed (and my counselors believed), was putting my sobriety at risk.

Karyn: What do you think is important for health-care providers to know or to do to help someone who has a substance use problem?

Alan: First of all, a person has to want help. You can't fix another person, and you can't help someone who doesn't want help.

Karyn: I agree, that is so important. I think health-care providers (and family caregivers) are vulnerable sometimes to thinking they can fix any health problem, which can culminate in interventions that are ineffective and unhealthy for the user and for the care provider.

Alan: Yes, and I would also say that health-care providers need to know how to recognize symptoms of problematic substance use.

Karyn: Like?

Alan: Like someone having "the shakes," someone not looking at you when they are answering questions, blaming other people for their circumstances and consequences, talking in circles. Don't ever ask someone, "Are you an alcoholic or a drug addict?" because we'll always say no unless we're in recovery—the denial is so strong. I also think not being too judgmental is important so you can find ways to open the door to discuss the issues. If someone is too "hard-nosed" and judgmental, I think it reinforces the denial. Asking a question like "Have you ever been drinking and couldn't remember events around that time?" is good because having blackouts is a good indication of an alcohol problem. You may not be able to "fix" someone, but you can "plant seeds" and hope that the information and education will have an impact at some point. I think that's why people who are recovering themselves can be so effective as health-care providers because they can share their own story of addiction and, since most people think they are completely unique, hearing someone else's story about having been in the same place you are now may turn on a light switch and help people recognize their own need for treatment.

Today, they are prescribed only to treat narcolepsy (a rare disorder resulting in an uncontrollable desire for sleep), hyperactivity disorders in children, and certain cases of obesity. Clandestine production of amphetamines for distribution on the illicit market has become a thriving business. Methamphetamine can be smoked, snorted, injected, or taken orally. The effects include an intense rush from smoking or intravenous injection and a slower onset of euphoria as a result of snorting or oral ingestion. Another form of the drug, crystal methamphetamine, is produced by slowly recrystallizing powder methamphetamine from a solvent such as methanol, ethanol, isopropanol, or acetone. This colorless, odorless, large-crystal form of D-methamphetamine is commonly called *glass* or *ice* because of its appearance. Crystal meth is usually smoked in a glass pipe like crack cocaine.

Although methamphetamine use is widespread, particularly on college campuses, its use has perhaps been overshadowed by the nationwide opioid epidemic with its associated deaths. An alarming recent trend has been the increasing use of methamphetamines in combination with opioids. Ellis and associates, as cited by Dotinga (2018), reported that the use of crystal meth increased by 82% in the last decade and combined use of opioids and methamphetamine almost doubled during the same time period. Ellis and associates note that individuals with opioid-use disorder sometimes use amphetamines to create a state of arousal to counteract the sedative effects of opioids. The use of combinations of drugs increases the risk of adverse effects and overdose. It also underscores the importance of assessing for multisubstance use in any individual presenting with substance use issues.

The earliest history of caffeine is unknown and is shrouded by legend and myth. Caffeine was first discovered in coffee in 1820 and in tea 7 years later. Both beverages have been widely accepted and enjoyed as a "pick-me-up" by many cultures.

Tobacco use has a long history; Mayan carved drawings dated between 600 and 1,000 AD are the earliest evidence that appears to depict smoking tobacco. Introduced in Europe in the mid-16th century, its use grew rapidly and by the end of the 16th century, it was being used all over Europe. In the early 17th century, tobacco was being grown in India, China, Japan, Southeast Asia, the Middle

East, and West Africa. Tobacco came to America with the settlement of the earliest colonies. Today, it is grown in many countries of the world, and although smoking is decreasing in most industrialized nations, it continues to be a serious problem in developing areas. Nicotine use, the active chemical in tobacco, is increasing among youth through e-cigarettes (vaping).

Patterns of Use

Because of their pleasurable effects, CNS stimulants have a high potential for misuse. In 2020, the National Survey on Drug Use and Health (NSDUH) identified that 1.9% of respondents reported having used cocaine in the past year (a small decline from the previous year), 0.2% reported using crack, and 0.9 % reported taking methamphetamines (SAMHSA, 2021a). Over 1.5 million Americans had a methamphetamine use disorder. Additionally, recent research (Roehler et al., 2021) reports that nonfatal stimulant overdoses have increased in all age-groups under 25 years of age including those under 10 years of age. Overdose deaths have increased for both cocaine and methamphetamines; methamphetamine overdose deaths quadrupled from 2011 to 2017, and in 2020 during the COVID-19 pandemic, overdose deaths from psychostimulants (like methamphetamine) increased by almost 35% (CDC, 2020).

Many individuals who misuse or are addicted to CNS stimulants began using the substance for the appetite-suppressant effect in an attempt at weight control. Increasingly higher doses are consumed in an effort to maintain the pleasurable effects. With continued use, these effects diminish as dysphoric effects increase. A persistent craving for the substance remains even in the face of unpleasant adverse effects from continued use.

CNS stimulant use is usually characterized by either episodic or chronic daily or near-daily use. Individuals who use the substances on an episodic basis often "binge" on the drug with consumption of very high dosages followed by a day or two of recuperation. This recuperation period is characterized by extremely intense and unpleasant symptoms and is thus often called a "crash."

The daily user may take large or small doses and may use the drug several times a day or only at a specific time during the day. The amount consumed usually increases over time as tolerance develops. Chronic users tend to rely on CNS stimulants to feel more powerful, more confident, and more decisive. They often fall into a pattern of taking "uppers" in the morning and "downers," such as alcohol or sleeping pills, at night.

The average American consumes two cups of coffee (about 200 mg of caffeine) per day. Caffeine is consumed in various amounts by about 90% of the population. At a level of 500 to 600 mg of daily caffeine consumption, symptoms of anxiety, insomnia, and depression are not uncommon, and caffeine dependence and withdrawal can occur. Caffeine consumption is prevalent among children as well as adults. Energy drinks have some of the highest caffeine contents of all beverages, and a study by Attipoe and associates (2016) found that several energy drinks had different levels of caffeine (±15%) than what was reported on the label. In addition, many beverages have multiple servings in one bottle and some beverages do not list the caffeine content on the label. Individuals may be at risk for consuming far more caffeine than they expected. Table 23–3 lists some common sources of caffeine.

Although tobacco use has been declining, the NSDUH reports 23.3% of Americans aged 12 and older used tobacco products in the prior year and 6.5% engaged in nicotine vaping (SAMHSA, 2021a). Since 1964, when the results of the first public health report on smoking were issued, the percentage of total smokers has been on the decline but the percentage of women and teenage smokers has declined more slowly than that of adult men. Even though tobacco use is on the decline, people with severe mental illness and those in addiction treatment continue to have higher rates of use than the general population (SAMHSA, 2021b).

The dangers of secondhand smoke continue to be identified as a significant health hazard. The CDC (2021c) reported that, annually, secondhand smoke claims the lives of almost 50,000 nonsmokers from heart disease, stroke, and lung cancer. Additionally, smoking increases the risk of infant mortality from sudden infant death syndrome.

Vaping, the use of a device to heat and release chemicals that can then be inhaled, is a current trend. One such device is the e-cigarette, which typically contains nicotine. In addition to its addiction potential, nicotine is known to be harmful to developing brains and, therefore, particularly dangerous to teens and pregnant women. Its use has become common among youth (in 2021, about 1 of every 35 middle school students [2.8%] reported that they had used electronic cigarettes in the past 30 days), significantly surpassing conventional cigarette smoking (CDC, 2022b). Vaping of *marijuana* among teenagers has also been on the rise. Reports of serious respiratory illness secondary to vaping have raised additional safety concerns. The CDC (2022b) reported:

> The FDA has alerted the public to thousands of reports of serious lung illnesses associated with vaping, including dozens of deaths... Many of the suspect products tested by the states or federal health officials

TABLE 23–3 **Common Sources of Caffeine**	
SOURCE	**CAFFEINE CONTENT (mg)**
FOOD AND BEVERAGES	
8 oz brewed coffee	90–165
8 oz instant coffee	63–110
8 oz decaffeinated coffee	2–5
1 oz espresso	47–64
8 oz brewed tea	25–48
8 oz instant tea	30
8 oz green tea	25–29
8–12 oz cola drinks	22–54
8–24 oz energy drinks	142–375
2 oz high-energy drinks	215–240
1.93 oz 10-hour energy shot	422
5–6 oz cocoa	20
8 oz chocolate milk	2–7
1 oz chocolate bar	22
PRESCRIPTION MEDICATIONS	
APCs (aspirin, phenacetin, caffeine)	32
Cafergot	100
Fiorinal	40
Migralam	100
OVER-THE-COUNTER ANALGESICS	
Anacin, Empirin, Midol, Vanquish	32
Excedrin Migraine (aspirin, acetaminophen, caffeine)	65
OVER-THE-COUNTER STIMULANTS	
NoDoz tablets	100
Vivarin	200
Caffedrine	250

Sources: Juliano, L. M., & Griffiths, R. R. (2017). Caffeine-related disorders. In Sadock, B. A., Sadock, V. A., & Ruiz, P. (Eds.), *Comprehensive textbook of psychiatry* (10th ed., pp. 1291–1303). Wolters Kluwer; Mayo Clinic. (2022). *Caffeine content for coffee, tea, soda, and more.* https://www.mayoclinic.org/healthy-lifestyle/nutrition-and-healthy-eating/in-depth/caffeine/art-20049372

have been identified as vaping products containing THC, the main psychotropic ingredient in marijuana. Some of the patients reported a mixture of THC and nicotine; and some reported vaping nicotine alone. While the CDC and FDA continue to investigate possible other contributing substances, CDC has identified a thickening agent—Vitamin E acetate—as a chemical of concern among people with e-cigarette or vaping associated lung injuries. They recommend that people should not use any product containing Vitamin E acetate, or any vaping products containing THC.

Effects on the Body

CNS stimulants are a group of pharmacological agents that are capable of exciting the entire nervous system. This is accomplished by increasing the activity or augmenting the capability of the neurotransmitter agents directly involved in bodily activation and behavioral stimulation. Physiological responses vary according to the potency and dosage of the drug.

Central Nervous System Effects

Stimulation of the CNS results in tremor, restlessness, anorexia, insomnia, agitation, and increased motor activity. Amphetamines, nonamphetamine stimulants, and cocaine produce increased alertness, decreased fatigue, elation and euphoria, and subjective feelings of greater mental agility and muscular power. Chronic use of these drugs may result in compulsive behavior, paranoia, hallucinations, and aggressive behavior.

Cardiovascular/Pulmonary Effects

Amphetamines can induce increased systolic and diastolic blood pressure, increased heart rate, and cardiac arrhythmias. These drugs also relax bronchial smooth muscle.

Cocaine intoxication typically produces an increase in myocardial demand for oxygen and an increase in heart rate. Severe vasoconstriction may occur and can result in myocardial infarction, ventricular fibrillation, and sudden death. Inhaled cocaine can cause pulmonary hemorrhage, chronic bronchiolitis, and pneumonia. Nasal rhinitis is a result of chronic cocaine snorting.

Caffeine ingestion can result in increased heart rate, palpitations, extrasystoles, and cardiac arrhythmias. Caffeine induces dilation of pulmonary and general systemic blood vessels and constriction of cerebral blood vessels.

Nicotine stimulates the sympathetic nervous system, increasing heart rate, blood pressure, and cardiac contractility, thereby increasing myocardial oxygen consumption and demand for blood flow. Contractions of gastric smooth muscle associated with hunger are inhibited, thereby producing a mild anorectic effect.

Gastrointestinal and Renal Effects

Gastrointestinal (GI) effects of amphetamines are somewhat unpredictable; however, a decrease in GI tract motility commonly results in constipation.

Contraction of the bladder sphincter makes urination difficult. Caffeine exerts a diuretic effect on the kidneys. Nicotine stimulates the hypothalamus to release antidiuretic hormone, reducing the excretion of urine. Because nicotine increases the tone and activity of the bowel, it may occasionally cause diarrhea.

Most CNS stimulants induce a small rise in metabolic rate and various degrees of anorexia. Amphetamines and cocaine can cause a rise in body temperature.

Sexual Function

CNS stimulants appear to increase sexual urges in both men and women. Women, more frequently than men, report that stimulants increase sexual desire and orgasms. Some men may experience sexual dysfunction with the use of stimulants. For the majority of individuals, however, these drugs exert a powerful aphrodisiac effect.

Stimulant Intoxication

Stimulant intoxication produces maladaptive behavioral and psychological changes that develop during or shortly after use of these drugs. Amphetamine and cocaine intoxication typically produces euphoria or affective blunting; changes in sociability; hypervigilance; interpersonal sensitivity; anxiety, tension, or anger; stereotyped behaviors; or impaired judgment. In severe amphetamine intoxication, symptoms may include memory loss, psychosis, and violent aggression. Physical effects include tachycardia or bradycardia, pupillary dilation, elevated or lowered blood pressure, perspiration or chills, nausea or vomiting, weight loss, psychomotor agitation or retardation, muscular weakness, respiratory depression, chest pain, cardiac arrhythmias, confusion, seizures, dyskinesias, dystonias, or coma (APA, 2022).

Intoxication from caffeine usually occurs after consumption well in excess of 250 mg but may occur with low doses in children, the elderly, or those not previously exposed to caffeine. Symptoms include restlessness, nervousness, excitement, insomnia, flushed face, diuresis, GI disturbance, muscle twitching, rambling flow of thought and speech, tachycardia or cardiac arrhythmia, periods of inexhaustibility, and psychomotor agitation (APA, 2022).

Stimulant Withdrawal

Stimulant withdrawal is the presence of a characteristic withdrawal syndrome that develops within a few hours to a few days after cessation of or marked reduction in prolonged (generally high dose) stimulant use (APA, 2022). This syndrome is often referred to as "crashing," an apt description because the symptoms include fatigue, cramps, depression, headaches, and nightmares. The dysphoria can be intense enough to result in increased risk for suicide. Peak withdrawal symptoms usually occur within 2 to 4 days of abstinence.

Caffeine withdrawal syndrome can occur after abrupt cessation of (or substantial reduction in) caffeine intake after prolonged daily use (APA, 2022). The symptoms begin within 24 hours after the last consumption and may include headache, fatigue, drowsiness, dysphoric mood, irritability, difficulty concentrating, flu-like symptoms, nausea, vomiting, and muscle pain and stiffness.

Withdrawal from nicotine results in dysphoric or depressed mood; insomnia; irritability, frustration, or anger; anxiety; difficulty concentrating; restlessness; decreased heart rate; and increased appetite or weight gain (APA, 2022). A mild syndrome of nicotine withdrawal can appear when a smoker switches from regular cigarettes to low-nicotine cigarettes (Boland & Verduin, 2022).

Inhalant Use Disorder
Profile of the Substance

Inhalant disorders are induced by inhaling the aliphatic and aromatic hydrocarbons found in substances such as fuels, solvents, adhesives, aerosol propellants, and paint thinners. Specific examples of these substances include gasoline, varnish remover, lighter fluid, airplane glue, rubber cement, cleaning fluid, spray paint, shoe conditioner, and typewriter correction fluid. Toluene (methylbenzene, toluol, phenylmethane) is a common ingredient in many inhaled substances, including paints, glues, and gasoline, and is responsible for the mind-altering effects that occur after inhalation.

Historical Aspects

Use of inhalants for altered consciousness or religious rituals dates back to ancient times. In the early 19th century, ether, chloroform, and nitrous oxide were inhaled for recreational purposes. By the 1960s, the inhaling of substances for recreational effects had spread to a wide range of products, including shoe polish, paints and paint thinners, lighter fluid, and gasoline.

Patterns of Use

Inhalant substances are readily available, legal, and inexpensive—three factors that make them attractive to children, teens, and young adults. Younger teens more commonly inhale glue, gasoline, and spray paints. In older teens, nitrous oxide (also known as "whippets") use is more common, and in adults, nitrites, such as amyl nitrites (also called "poppers") are common inhalants used for mind-altering effects.

The Monitoring the Future Study (Johnston et al., 2022), which monitors trends in adolescent drug use, found that inhalant use has declined over the last decade with some fluctuations among different age groups. In 2021, a gradual decline was seen in all age groups 12 years old or older. A worrisome finding in this survey was a significant decline (since 2015) in the number of adolescents who believe that experimental use of inhalants is harmful. Past education and advertising campaigns about the risks associated with inhalant use have contributed to the decline in use over the last decade (Johnston et al., 2022), and this education may need to be reintroduced and reinforced with today's adolescents. Nurses who work with children and adolescents can play a significant role in providing that education.

Methods of use include "huffing"—a procedure in which a rag soaked with the substance is applied to the mouth and nose and the vapors inhaled. Another common method is called "bagging," in which the substance is placed in a paper or plastic bag from which it is inhaled by the user. The substance may also be inhaled directly from the container or sprayed in the mouth or nose. Boland and Verduin (2022) reported that "inhalant use among adolescents is associated with an increased likelihood of conduct disorder or antisocial personality disorder" (p. 327). Tolerance to inhalants has been reported with heavy use. A mild withdrawal syndrome has been documented but does not appear to be clinically significant. Among children with inhalant use disorder, the products may be used several times a week, often on weekends and after school. Adults with inhalant use disorder may use the substance at varying times each day or binge on the substance over a period of several days.

Effects on the Body

Inhalants are absorbed through the lungs and reach the CNS very rapidly. The behavioral actions of inhalants are variable depending on the inhalant being used, but many have effects similar to CNS depressants (Howard et al., 2017). Inhalants initially create rapid excitation followed by drowsiness, incoordination, and disinhibition. The effects are relatively brief, lasting from several minutes to a few hours, depending on the specific substance and amount consumed.

Central Nervous System Effects

Inhalants can cause both central and peripheral nervous system damage. Symptoms of neurological damage such as ataxia, peripheral and sensorimotor neuropathy, speech problems, and tremor can occur. Other CNS effects that have been reported with heavy inhalant use include ototoxicity, encephalopathy, parkinsonism, and damage to the protective sheath around certain nerve fibers in the brain and peripheral nervous system. These effects are particularly damaging to youth because their nervous systems are still developing. Chronic use has been associated with the development of several mental illnesses, including anxiety and psychotic disorders. Inhalant use in pregnant women has been linked to fetal development disorders, malformations, and death. Infants are at risk for *fetal solvent syndrome* (similar to FAS), a syndrome of behavioral, language, and developmental impairments that may include hyperactivity and aggression (Howard et al., 2017).

Respiratory Effects

Respiratory effects of inhalant use range from coughing and wheezing to dyspnea, emphysema, and pneumonia. There is increased airway resistance due to inflammation of the passages. Death can occur from asphyxiation, from suffocation when plastic bags are put over one's head to inhale substances, and from *sudden sniffing death,* which causes a sudden fatal cardiac arrest secondary to rapid and irregular heart rhythms.

Gastrointestinal Effects

Abdominal pain, nausea, and vomiting may occur. A rash may be present around the individual's nose and mouth. Unusual breath odors are common. Chronic inhalant use has been associated with liver failure (and renal failure) as well as liver tumors.

Renal System Effects

Acute and chronic renal failure and hepatorenal syndrome may occur. Renal toxicity from toluene exposure has been reported, manifesting in renal tubular acidosis, hypokalemia, hypophosphatemia, hyperchloremia, azotemia, sterile pyuria, hematuria, and proteinuria (McKeown, 2022).

Inhalant Intoxication

The *DSM-5-TR* defines inhalant intoxication as "clinically significant problematic behavioral or psychological changes that developed during or shortly after intended or unintended inhalation of a volatile hydrocarbon substance" (APA, 2022). Symptoms are similar to alcohol intoxication and may include the following (APA, 2022; Howard et al., 2017):

- Dizziness; ataxia
- Euphoria; excitation; disinhibition
- Nystagmus; blurred vision; double vision
- Slurred speech
- Hypoactive reflexes
- Psychomotor retardation; lethargy
- Generalized muscle weakness
- Stupor or coma (at higher doses)

Inhalant Withdrawal

Mild withdrawal symptoms may occur after chronic, long-term use. Reported symptoms include restlessness, nausea and vomiting, runny nose and watery eyes, poor attention and concentration, and mood changes. The *DSM-5-TR*, however, does not include inhalant withdrawal as a diagnosis because they believe the symptoms are considered either too mild or too inconsistent to be included (Patterson, 2022).

Opioid Use Disorder

Profile of the Substance

The term *opioid* refers to a group of compounds that includes (APA, 2022):

- Natural opioids (such as morphine and codeine)
- Semisynthetics (heroin, oxycodone, hydrocodone, hydromorphone, oxymorphone)
- Synthetics with morphine-like action (methadone, meperidine, tramadol, fentanyl, carfentanyl)

Opioids exert both sedative and analgesic effects, and their major medical uses are for the relief of pain, treatment of diarrhea, and relief of coughing. Under close supervision, opioids are indispensable in the practice of medicine. They are the most effective agents known for the relief of intense pain. They also induce a pleasurable effect that promotes misuse. And because opioids are capable of inducing tolerance, their use may lead to significant physiological and psychological dependence. The physiological and psychological dependence that occurs with opioids, as well as the development of profound tolerance, contribute to the development of addiction characterized by the individual's ongoing quest for more of the substance, regardless of the means. The United States is currently facing an unprecedented death toll associated with opioid overdose.

Opioids are popular drugs of misuse because they desensitize an individual to both psychological and physiological pain and induce a sense of euphoria. Lethargy and indifference to the environment are common manifestations.

Individuals who are addicted to opioids usually spend much of their time acquiring the substance to sustain their addiction. Individuals who are addicted to opioids are seldom able to hold a steady job that will support their need and often must secure funds from friends, relatives, or whomever they have not yet alienated with their addiction-related behavior. It is not uncommon for individuals addicted to opioids to resort to illegal means of obtaining funds, such as burglary, robbery, prostitution, or selling drugs.

Methods of administration of opioid drugs include oral ingestion, snorting, smoking, and subcutaneous, intramuscular, and intravenous injection. A selected list of opioid substances is presented in Table 23–4.

Historical Aspects

In its crude form, opium is a brownish-black gummy substance obtained from the ripened pods of the opium poppy. References to the use of opiates have been found in the Egyptian, Greek, and Arabian cultures as early as 3,000 BC. The drug became widely used both medicinally and recreationally throughout

TABLE 23–4 **Opioids and Related Substances**		
CATEGORIES	**GENERIC (TRADE) NAMES**	**COMMON STREET NAMES**
Opioids of natural origin	Opium (ingredient in various antidiarrheal agents) Morphinan (Astramorph) Codeine (ingredient in various analgesics and cough suppressants) Kratom (opioid-like)	Black stuff, poppy, tar, big O M, white stuff, Miss Emma Terp, schoolboy, syrup, cody Herbal speedball, Thang, Kakuam, Thom, Ketum, Biak
Opioid derivatives	Heroin Hydromorphone (Dilaudid) Oxycodone (Percodan; OxyContin) Hydrocodone (Vicodin)	H, horse, junk, brown sugar, smack, skag, TNT, Harry DLs, 4s, lords, little D Perks, perkies, Oxy, O.C. Vike
Synthetic opiate-like drugs	Meperidine (Demerol) Methadone (Dolophine) Pentazocine (Talwin) Fentanyl (Fentora) Carfentanil Desomorphine U-47700 Sufentanil Tramadol	Doctors Dollies, done Ts Apache, China girl, China town, dance fever, goodfella, jackpot Krokodil Pink, pinky, U4 Trammies, chill pills, ultras

Europe during the 16th and 17th centuries. Most of the opium supply came from China, where the drug was introduced by Arab traders in the late 17th century. Morphine, the primary active ingredient of opium, was isolated in 1803 by the European chemist Friedrich Sertürner. Since that time, morphine rather than crude opium has been used throughout the world for the medical treatment of pain and diarrhea. This process was facilitated in 1853 by the development of the hypodermic syringe, which made it possible to deliver undiluted morphine quickly into the body for rapid relief from pain.

This development also created a new variety of opioid user in the United States: one who was able to self-administer the drug by injection. In addition, the large influx of Chinese immigrants into the United States during this era introduced opium smoking to this country. By the early part of the 20th century, opium addiction was widespread.

In response to the concerns over the prevalence of opium addiction, in 1914 the U.S. government passed the Harrison Narcotic Act, which created strict controls on the accessibility of opioids. Until that time, these substances were freely available to the public without a prescription. The Harrison Act banned the use of opioids for nonmedicinal purposes and drove the use of heroin underground. To this day, the beneficial uses of these substances are widely acclaimed within the medical profession, but the illicit trafficking of the drugs for recreational purposes continues to resist most efforts at control.

Historically, the term "opiate" referred to naturally occurring (or slightly modified) components of opium, and the term "opioid" described synthetic opiates. However, more recently, the term "opioid" has been used to describe the entire class of drugs. In this discussion, these terms are used interchangeably.

Patterns of Use

The development of opioid addiction may follow one of two typical behavior patterns. The first occurs in the individual who has obtained the drug by prescription from a physician for the relief of a medical problem. Misuse and addiction occur when the individual increases the amount and frequency of use, justifying the behavior as symptom treatment. They become obsessed with obtaining more and more of the substance, seeking out several physicians to replenish and maintain supplies and eventually turning to illegal sources (including heroin) if unable to acquire additional prescriptions.

The second pattern of behavior occurs among individuals who use the drugs for recreational purposes and obtain them from illegal sources. Opioids may be used alone to induce the euphoric effects or in combination with stimulants or other drugs to enhance the euphoria or counteract the substance's depressant effects. Tolerance develops and addiction occurs, leading the individual to procure the substance by whatever means is required to support the habit.

The CDC reports that, on average, 136 Americans die per day from an opioid overdose (CDC, 2021b). Drug overdose deaths have been climbing steadily since 1999 and in 2020 (even though the NSDUH [SAMHSA, 2021a] noted a slight decline in those reporting opioid use over the past year) opioid overdose deaths rose 30% (CDC, 2021a). Although several factors are influential in this ongoing rise in the death toll, the COVID-19 pandemic certainly confounded the problem with individuals reporting some difficulties accessing care or delays in obtaining prescriptions during 2020 (SAMHSA, 2021a). Opioids account for 70.6% of all drug overdose deaths and most of those involve synthetic opioids (CDC, 2021b).

Efforts have been made in some states to exert stricter controls on opiate prescription practices, and 2012 marked the first year of a trend toward a decline in prescription rates nationally. However, beginning in 2010, an increase in heroin use, and in 2013, an increase in the use of synthetic opioids (e.g., illicitly manufactured fentanyl and carfentanil), are evidence that the opioid epidemic and associated deaths are ongoing problems. The chemical structure of illegally manufactured fentanyl continues to change and is sometimes found mixed with heroin, counterfeit pills, and cocaine (CDC, 2021b).

The mixture of fentanyl with heroin is particularly lethal. When heroin is mixed with fentanyl, it may cause accidental overdose because fentanyl is 30 to 50 times more potent than pure heroin. Carfentanil (carfentanyl), a potent drug used mainly in the capture of wild animals (100 times more potent than fentanyl and 10,000 times more potent than morphine), has been responsible for rapid accidental overdose and often death when ingested along with heroin (National Institutes of Health [NIH], 2022).

Late in 2018, the FDA approved a sublingual tablet form of sufentanil (5 to 10 times more potent than fentanyl) and although intended for the treatment of severe acute pain in certified, medically supervised health-care settings, critics argue that it adds one more very potent opioid to the arsenal of those that may be diverted, easily administered, and potentially fatal (Brooks, 2018). Much like the trend with synthetic amphetamines discussed earlier in this chapter, a new synthetic opiate, U-47700 (although discovered in the 1970s), surfaced in 2015 and was responsible for 46 fatalities in 2016.

The substance underwent emergency classification as a schedule I drug to allow the DEA more time to collect data on the substance (Duffy, 2016). U-47700 is 10 times more potent than morphine. It is found in counterfeit oxycodone tablets and is the key ingredient in a street drug called "gray death" (Kyei-Baffour & Lindsley, 2020).

Kratom, a plant from Southeast Asia that triggers opiate-like effects, surfaced in the United States and was subsequently banned; however, this decision was reversed when researchers argued that it might help them develop tools to overcome opioid and alcohol addiction, as well as chronic pain (MPR, 2016). Two of the over 40 alkaloids that have been isolated from kratom leaves (mitragynine and 7-hydroxymitragynine) have opioid-like properties, and potency at the mu opioid receptors for these has been found to exceed that of morphine (Stanciu et al., 2020). The FDA has not yet approved or regulated kratom, and a recent CDC report (2019) identified 91 deaths (during 2016–2017) associated with its use. Currently, the DEA lists kratom as a chemical of concern. It is being evaluated for placement into controlled substance scheduling, although some states have already banned its use and identified it as a schedule I substance (Drugs.com, 2022).

At present, opioid misuse and death by overdose remain a national epidemic, but several national initiatives to address this public health crisis have been identified. A National Practice Guideline for use of medications to treat opioid use disorder has been established (American Society of Addiction Medicine [ASAM], 2020). For the first time in U.S. history, in 2016 the Surgeon General declared illicit drug use and misuse of prescription drugs a national health-care priority and committed to the need for additional research and treatment options. In 2018 the Surgeon General advanced a public health advisory urging more Americans to carry naloxone (a narcotic antagonist) kits to assist (along with rescue breathing) in preventing opiate overdose and death. Some state programs, such as Project Dawn in Ohio, are providing naloxone education and distribution of rescue kits free of charge to individuals who are willing to carry them for responding to opioid overdose victims. In 2018 the NIH launched the Helping End Addiction Long-term (HEAL) initiative, identifying 15 areas of critical focus for research and development to address the opiate epidemic. These areas include research on longer-acting naloxone-type drugs, better responses to chronic pain management, better management of neonatal opiate withdrawal (NIDA, [2019a] reports that the equivalent of every 15 minutes a baby is born in opiate withdrawal), and better access to and efficacy of treatment options (Twachtman, 2018). All of these efforts underscore the gravity of this ongoing national public health issue.

Effects on the Body

Opiates may be classified as *narcotic analgesics*. They exert their major effects primarily on the CNS, eyes, and GI tract. Chronic morphine use or acute morphine toxicity is manifested by a syndrome of sedation, chronic constipation, decreased respiratory rate, and pinpoint pupils. The intensity of symptoms is largely dose dependent. The following physiological effects are common with opioid use.

Central Nervous System Effects

All opioids, opioid derivatives, and synthetic opioid-like drugs affect the CNS. Common manifestations include euphoria, mood changes, and mental clouding. Other common CNS effects include drowsiness and pain reduction. Pupillary constriction occurs in response to the stimulation of the oculomotor nerve. CNS depression of the respiratory centers within the medulla results in respiratory depression. The antitussive response is caused by suppression of the cough center within the medulla. Nausea and vomiting commonly associated with opiate ingestion are related to the stimulation of the centers within the medulla that trigger this response.

Gastrointestinal Effects

These drugs exert a profound effect on the GI tract. Both stomach and intestinal tone increase, whereas peristaltic activity of the intestines is diminished. These effects lead to a marked decrease in the movement of food through the GI tract. This notable therapeutic effect is used in the treatment of severe diarrhea; no drugs have yet been developed that are more effective than opioids for this purpose. However, constipation and even fecal impaction may be a serious problem for the chronic opioid user. Loperamide (Imodium), an antidiarrheal drug with small amounts of opioids, has surfaced as a drug of misuse, with users taking anywhere from 50 to over 100 pills to achieve a high. Not only does this increase the risk for significant constipation and other GI effects, but it has been associated with deaths secondary to overdose.

Cardiovascular Effects

In therapeutic doses, opioids have minimal effect on the action of the heart. Morphine is used extensively to relieve pulmonary edema and the pain of myocardial infarction in cardiac patients. At high doses, opioids induce hypotension, which may be caused by direct action on the heart or by opioid-induced histamine release. Although most opioids do not affect cardiac conductivity, "methadone and buprenorphine can prolong QTc, especially when used in patients at risk for QTc prolongation" (Chen & Ashburn, 2015, p. S27). Misuse of loperamide has been linked to cardiac dysrhythmias and death because at very high doses (needed to achieve other than antidiarrheal effects), this medication is highly cardiotoxic (Davenport, 2016).

Sexual Function

Opioid use causes decreased sexual function and diminished libido, and long-term use has been associated with erectile dysfunction. Delayed ejaculation, impotence, and orgasm failure (in both men and women) may occur.

Opioid Intoxication

Opioid intoxication constitutes clinically significant problematic behavioral or psychological changes that develop during, or shortly after, opioid use (APA, 2022). Symptoms include initial euphoria followed by apathy, dysphoria, psychomotor agitation or retardation, and impaired judgment. Physical symptoms include pupillary constriction (or dilation due to anoxia from severe overdose), drowsiness, slurred speech, and impairment in attention or memory. Symptoms are consistent with the half-life of most opioid drugs and usually last for several hours. Severe opioid intoxication can lead to *respiratory depression,* coma, and death.

Opioid Withdrawal

Opioid withdrawal produces a syndrome of symptoms that develops after cessation of or reduction in heavy and prolonged use of an opiate or related substance. Symptoms include dysphoric mood, nausea or vomiting, muscle aches, lacrimation or rhinorrhea, pupillary dilation, piloerection, sweating, diarrhea, yawning, fever, and insomnia. With short-acting drugs such as heroin, withdrawal symptoms occur within 6 to 8 hours after the last dose, peak within 1 to 3 days, and gradually subside over a period of 5 to 10 days. With longer-acting drugs such as methadone, withdrawal symptoms begin within 1 to 3 days after the last dose, peak between days 4 and 6, and are complete in 14 to 21 days. Withdrawal from the ultrashort-acting meperidine begins quickly, reaches a peak in 8 to 12 hours, and is complete in 4 to 5 days.

Hallucinogen Use Disorder
Profile of the Substance

Hallucinogenic substances can distort an individual's perception of reality, alter sensory perception, and induce hallucinations. For this reason, they have sometimes been referred to as "mind-expanding drugs." Some of the effects of these substances have been likened to those of a psychotic break. The hallucinations experienced by an individual with schizophrenia, however, are most often auditory, whereas substance-induced hallucinations are usually visual. Drugs that are considered hallucinogens include several diverse groups:

■ Ergolines (such as LSD)
■ Phenylalkylamines (such as mescaline)
■ Indolamines (such as psilocybin)
■ Methylenedioxymethamphetamine (MDMA)
■ Dimethyltryptamine (DMT)

Perceptual distortions have been reported by some users as spiritual, as giving a sense of depersonalization (observing oneself having the experience), or as feeling at peace with self and the universe. Others, who describe their experiences as "bad trips," report feelings of panic and a fear of dying or going insane. A common danger reported with hallucinogenic drugs is that of flashbacks, or a spontaneous recurrence of the hallucinogenic state without ingestion of the drug. These can occur months after the drug was last taken.

Recurrent use can produce tolerance, encouraging users to resort to increasingly higher dosages. No evidence of physical addiction is detectable when the drug is withdrawn; however, recurrent use appears to induce a psychological addiction to the insight-inducing experiences that a user may associate with episodes of hallucinogen use (Boland & Verduin, 2022). This psychological addiction varies according to the drug, the dose, and the individual user. Hallucinogens are highly unpredictable in the effects they may induce each time they are used.

Many hallucinogenic substances have structural similarities. Some are produced synthetically; others are natural products of plants and fungi. A selected list of hallucinogens is presented in Table 23–5.

Historical Aspects

Hallucinogens have been used throughout history in many cultures for religious and mystical experiences, including in Aztec, Mexican Indian, and Hindu ceremonies (Parish, 2015). Use of the peyote cactus as part of religious ceremonies in the southwestern part of the United States still occurs today, although this ritual use has greatly diminished.

LSD was first synthesized in 1943 by Dr. Albert Hoffman as a clinical research tool to investigate the biochemical etiology of schizophrenia. It soon reached the illicit market, and its misuse began to overshadow the research effort.

The misuse of hallucinogens reached a peak in the late 1960s, waned during the 1970s, and returned to

TABLE 23-5	Hallucinogens	
CATEGORIES	**GENERIC (TRADE) NAMES**	**COMMON STREET NAMES**
Naturally occurring hallucinogens	Mescaline (the primary active ingredient of the peyote cactus)	Cactus, mesc, mescal, half moon, big chief, bad seed, peyote
	Psilocybin and psilocin (active ingredients of *Psilocybe* mushrooms)	Magic mushroom, God's flesh, shrooms
	Ololiuqui (morning glory seeds)	Heavenly blue, glories, pearly gates, flying saucers
	Salvia divinorum	Salvia, Sally D, magic mint
Synthetic compounds	Lysergic acid diethylamide (LSD)—synthetically produced from a fungal substance found on rye or a chemical substance found in morning glory seeds	Acid, cube, big D, California sunshine, microdots, blue dots, sugar, orange wedges, peace tablets, purple haze, cupcakes
	Dimethyltryptamine (DMT) and diethyltryptamine (DET)—chemical analogues of tryptamine	Businessman's trip
	2,5-Dimethoxy-4-methylamphetamine (DOM)	STP (serenity, tranquility, peace)
	Phencyclidine (PCP)	Angel dust, hog, peace pill, rocket fuel
	Ketamine (Ketalar)	Special K, vitamin K, kit kat
	3,4-Methylene-dioxyamphetamine (MDMA)*	XTC, ecstasy, Adam, Eve
	Methoxy-amphetamine (MDA)	Love drug, Molly
	3,4-methylenedioxypyrovalerone (MDPV)*	Sally, sass, sassafras
	4-methylmethcathinone (mephedrone, 4-MMC)*	Bath salts (also called blue silk, cloud 9, ivory wave, vanilla sky, white knight, and others)
	Methylone*	MCAT, bubbles, white magic, meph, drone, M-smack

*Cross-listed with the CNS stimulants.

favor in the 1980s with the so-called designer drugs (e.g., MDMA, also known as "Molly" or "ecstasy," and methoxyamphetamine [MDA]). Another hallucinogen, **PCP**, originally was developed in the 1950s as an anesthetic, but this use was discontinued because of serious adverse effects. It continues to be used illegally and is often combined with cannabis. A number of deaths have been directly attributed to the use of PCP, and numerous accidental deaths have occurred as a result of overdose and the behavioral changes the drug precipitates. A derivative of PCP, ketamine, is also used as a preoperative anesthetic and misused for its psychedelic properties. It produces effects similar to but somewhat less intense than those of PCP. Ketamine has been advanced as having potential benefits in the treatment of depression and post-traumatic stress disorder (PTSD). In 2019, the FDA approved a nasal spray formulation of esketamine (Spravato) for use in treatment-resistant depression. Its use is restricted to certified medical clinics and requires a risk evaluation and mitigation strategy (REMS).

Several therapeutic uses of LSD have been proposed, including the treatment of chronic alcoholism and the reduction of intractable pain, such as occurs in malignant disease. In one systematic review of research on the therapeutic benefits of LSD for depression and anxiety, the authors concluded that evidence supports immediate antidepressant and antianxiety effects that endured for several months when taken in a controlled setting (Muttoni et al., 2019). They caution, though, that the number and size of the studies thus far have been small. In another systematic review, the authors concluded that the evidence is strongest for the use of LSD in alcohol treatment (Fuentes et al., 2020). Clearly there is current interest in the potential benefits of LSD in psychiatry, but more research is needed.

Patterns of Use

Use of hallucinogens is usually episodic. Because cognitive and perceptual abilities are so markedly affected by these substances, the user must set aside time from normal daily activities for indulgence. According to a national study in 2020, 2.6% of Americans 12 years and older reported using hallucinogens in the last year (SAMHSA, 2021a).

LSD, like other hallucinogens, does not lead to the development of physical addiction or withdrawal symptoms. However, tolerance for LSD and other hallucinogens develops quickly and to a high degree. In fact, tolerance is complete after 3 to 4 consecutive days of use. Recovery from tolerance also occurs very rapidly (in 4 to 7 days), so the individual is able to achieve the desired effect from the drug repeatedly and often.

PCP is usually taken episodically, in binges that can last for several days. However, some chronic users take the substance daily. Physical addiction does not occur with PCP; however, psychological addiction characterized by craving for the drug has been reported in chronic users, as has the development of tolerance. Tolerance apparently develops quickly with frequent use.

Psilocybin is an ingredient of the *Psilocybe* mushroom indigenous to the United States and Mexico. Ingestion of these mushrooms produces an effect similar to that of LSD but of a shorter duration. This hallucinogenic chemical can now be produced synthetically.

Mescaline is the only hallucinogenic compound used legally for religious purposes today by members of the Native American Church of the United States. It is the primary active ingredient of the peyote cactus. Neither physical nor psychological addiction occurs with the use of mescaline, although as with other hallucinogens, tolerance can develop quickly with frequent use.

Salvia is an herb from the mint family that has hallucinogenic effects when dried leaves are chewed, extracted juices are consumed, or smoke from the leaves is inhaled. This particular hallucinogen is advertised and sold over the Internet because it is not currently regulated by the Controlled Substances Act, but some states have limited or banned its use, possession, or sale. The DEA lists it as a drug of concern.

Among the most potent hallucinogens of the current drug culture are those categorized as amphetamine derivatives. These include 2,5-dimethoxy-4-m ethylamphetamine (DOM, STP), MDMA, and MDA. At lower doses, these drugs produce the "high" associated with CNS stimulants. At higher doses, hallucinogenic effects occur. These drugs have existed for many years but were rediscovered in the mid-1980s. Because of the rapid increase in recreational use, the DEA imposed an emergency classification of MDMA as a schedule I drug in 1985. MDMA, or ecstasy, is a synthetic drug with both stimulant and hallucinogenic qualities. It has a chemical structure similar to methamphetamine and mescaline and has become widely available throughout the world. Because of its growing popularity, the demand for this drug has led to tablets and capsules being sold as ecstasy that are not pure MDMA. Many contain drugs such as methamphetamine, PCP, amphetamine, ketamine, and *p*-methoxyamphetamine (PMA; a stimulant with hallucinogenic properties; more toxic than MDMA). This practice has increased the dangers associated with MDMA use. Overdose deaths rose from 2019 to 2020, and although most of these were related to synthetic opioids, methamphetamine overdose deaths have been on the rise as well.

Effects on the Body

The effects produced by the various hallucinogenics are highly unpredictable. The variety of effects may be related to dosage, the mental state of the individual, and the environment in which the substance is used. Some common effects have been reported (APA, 2022; Boland & Verduin, 2022; Julien, 2014).

Physiological Effects

■ Nausea and vomiting
■ Chills
■ Pupil dilation
■ Increased pulse, blood pressure, and temperature
■ Mild dizziness
■ Trembling
■ Loss of appetite
■ Insomnia
■ Sweating
■ A slowing of respirations
■ Elevation in blood sugar

Psychological Effects

■ Heightened response to color, texture, and sounds
■ Heightened body awareness
■ Distortion of vision
■ Sense of slowed time
■ All feelings magnified: love, lust, hate, joy, anger, pain, terror, despair
■ Fear of losing control
■ Paranoia, panic
■ Euphoria, bliss
■ Projection of self into dreamlike images
■ Serenity, peace
■ Depersonalization
■ Derealization
■ Increased libido

The effects of hallucinogens are not always pleasurable for the user. Two types of toxic reactions are known to occur. The first is the *panic reaction* or "bad trip." Symptoms include intense anxiety, fear, and stimulation. The individual hallucinates and fears going insane. Paranoia and acute psychosis may be evident.

The second type of toxic reaction to hallucinogens is the *flashback*. This phenomenon refers to the transient, spontaneous repetition of a previous LSD-induced experience that occurs without taking the substance. The *DSM-5-TR* (APA, 2022) refers to this as *hallucinogen persisting perception disorder*. Various studies have reported a range from 15% to 80% of hallucinogen users reporting having experienced flashbacks (Boland & Verduin, 2022). These episodes typically last for a few minutes or less.

Hallucinogen Intoxication

Symptoms of hallucinogen intoxication develop during or shortly after hallucinogen use. Maladaptive behavioral or psychological changes include marked anxiety or depression, ideas of reference (a type of delusional thinking that all activity within one's environment is "referred to" [about] one's self), fear of losing one's mind, paranoid ideation, and impaired judgment (APA, 2022). Perceptual changes occur while the individual is fully awake and alert and include intensification of perceptions, depersonalization, derealization, illusions, hallucinations, and synesthesias (APA, 2022). Because hallucinogens are sympathomimetics, they can cause tachycardia, hypertension, sweating, blurred vision, papillary dilation, and tremors.

Symptoms of PCP intoxication are unpredictable. Specific symptoms are dose related and may be manifested by impulsiveness, impaired judgment, assaultiveness, and belligerence, or the individual may appear calm, stuporous, or comatose. Physical symptoms include vertical or horizontal nystagmus, hypertension, tachycardia, ataxia, diminished pain sensation, muscle rigidity, and seizures. Symptoms of ketamine intoxication appear similar to those of PCP.

General effects of MDMA (ecstasy) include increased heart rate, blood pressure, and body temperature; dehydration; confusion; insomnia; and paranoia. Overdose can result in panic attacks, hallucinations, severe hyperthermia, dehydration, and seizures. Death can occur from kidney or cardiovascular failure.

Hallucinogen Withdrawal

A clinically significant pattern of withdrawal from hallucinations has not been consistently documented in humans (APA, 2022) and therefore is not included in the *DSM-5-TR* as a relevant aspect of hallucinogen use disorder. However, some drugs with hallucinogenic properties such as MDMA or other methamphetamines are associated with a withdrawal syndrome that may include mood disturbances, malaise, poor concentration, irritability, sleep disturbances, and other symptoms.

Cannabis Use Disorder
Profile of the Substance

Cannabis has been legalized in several states for recreational and medicinal use, although on a federal level, the DEA identifies it as a schedule I controlled substance. The major psychoactive ingredient of this class of substances is delta-9-tetrahydrocannabinol (THC). It occurs naturally in the plant *Cannabis sativa*, which grows readily in warm climates. Technically, the term cannabis refers to all products from the *C. sativa* plant, which contains roughly 540 chemical substances, but the term cannabis is often used interchangeably with marijuana (NIH, 2019a). Marijuana, the most

prevalent type of cannabis preparation, is composed of the dried leaves, stems, and flowers of the plant. Hashish is a more potent concentrate of the resin derived from the flowering tops of the plant. Hash oil is a very concentrated form of THC made by boiling hashish in a solvent and filtering out the solid matter. NIDA (2019b) reported that smoking THC-rich resins is on the rise. The practice, called "dabbing," can deliver very large amounts of THC to the body and has been associated with contributing to various medical emergencies. Cannabis products are usually smoked in the form of loosely rolled cigarettes or may be inhaled through the use of vaporizers to reduce the irritants and toxins associated with smoking. Cannabis can also be taken orally when it is prepared in food, but about two to three times the amount of cannabis must be ingested orally to equal the potency obtained by the inhalation of its smoke (Boland & Verduin, 2022). Vaping THC has become more prevalent among teenagers with the rising popularity of vaping devices (NIH, 2019b), and one study found that the majority of lung injuries associated with vaping, some of which were fatal, were among those vaping marijuana or cannabis oils (Butt et al., 2019).

At moderate dosages, cannabis produces effects resembling alcohol and other CNS depressants. By depressing higher brain centers, they release lower centers from inhibitory influences. There has been some controversy in the past over the classification of these substances. They are not narcotics, although they are legally classified as controlled substances. They are not hallucinogens, although in very high dosages they can induce hallucinations. They are not sedative-hypnotics, although they most closely resemble these substances. Like sedative-hypnotics, their action occurs in the ascending reticular activating system.

Psychological addiction has been shown to occur with cannabis, and tolerance can occur. Controversy has existed about whether physiological addiction occurs with cannabis. In the past, symptoms of cannabis withdrawal were not considered clinically significant enough for inclusion in the *DSM*. However, the *DSM-5* Substance-Related Disorders Work Group determined that subsequent research has provided significant data to support cannabis withdrawal as a valid and reliable syndrome that can negatively affect abstinence attempts of heavy cannabis users. The diagnosis of Cannabis Withdrawal has been included in the *DSM-5-TR* (APA, 2022).

Synthetic cannabinoids, on the other hand, have been clearly identified as potentially addictive (NIDA, 2020b). Although some of these chemicals are illegal to buy, sell, or possess, manufacturers often sidestep the laws by altering their chemical formulas. Standard drug tests cannot easily detect many of these chemicals. Common cannabis preparations are presented in Table 23–6.

Historical Aspects

Products of *C. sativa* have been used therapeutically for nearly 5,000 years (Julien, 2014). Cannabis was first employed in China and India as an antiseptic and an analgesic. Its use later spread to the Middle East, Africa, and Eastern Europe.

In the United States, medical interest in the use of cannabis arose during the early part of the 19th century. Many articles were published espousing its use for varied reasons. The drug was almost as commonly used for medicinal purposes as aspirin is today and could be purchased without a prescription in any drug store. It was purported to have antibacterial and anticonvulsant capabilities, decrease intraocular pressure, decrease pain, help in the treatment of asthma, increase appetite, and generally raise one's morale.

The drug fell out of favor primarily because of the significant variation in potency within batches of medication caused by the variations in the THC content of different plants. Other medications were favored for their greater degree of solubility and faster onset of action than cannabis products. A federal law put an end to its legal use in 1937, after an association between marijuana and criminal activity became evident. In the 1960s, marijuana became the symbol of the "antiestablishment" generation and reached its peak as an illicit recreational drug.

Research continues into the possible therapeutic uses of cannabis. It has been shown to be effective for relieving nausea and vomiting associated with cancer chemotherapy when other antinausea medications fail. It has also been used in the treatment of chronic pain, glaucoma, multiple sclerosis, acquired immune deficiency syndrome, and epilepsy. Cannabidiol (CBD), a chemical in cannabis that has very small amounts of THC and which may block the psychoactive properties of THC, is being studied for its potential use in many medical disorders, including schizophrenia, dystonias, and Parkinson's disease. One small study (Leweke et al., 2021) reported improvements in cognition with CBD use among participants with schizophrenia, but in a systematic review (Ahmed et al., 2021) the researchers found evidence that THC worsened symptoms and there was insufficient evidence of effect for THC or CBD to recommend medical cannabis in the treatment of schizophrenia.

Advocates who praise the therapeutic usefulness and support the legalization of cannabis persist within the United States today. Such groups as the Alliance for Cannabis Therapeutics (ACT) and the National Organization for the Reform of Marijuana Laws (NORML) have lobbied extensively to allow individuals with medical conditions easier access to the drug. The medical use of marijuana is legal in several states, as is recreational use. However, the DEA still considers marijuana a schedule I controlled substance. Even the Farm Bill of 2018, which legalizes the sale of hemp and hemp products in the United States, does not legalize all hemp-derived CBD products; for example, it is not legal to include CBD in food or dietary supplements even though some CBD products are labeled as such (Evans, 2020).

Two medications that have components of the marijuana plant or related synthetic compounds are currently FDA approved. Dronabinol, a synthetic compound in the medication Marinol, is approved for nausea and vomiting associated with cancer treatment and for severe weight loss associated with AIDS. Nabilone, a chemical similar to THC and found in the medication Cesamet, is a similar FDA-approved drug. A third medication, Sativex, is an oromucosal spray containing THC and CBD. It can be prescribed in the United States only with a special exemption from the FDA for use in select patients and it is currently in Phase III drug trials to explore its potential benefits in cancer treatment. In 2018 the first cannabis-based drug (Epidiolex) became FDA approved for the treatment of epilepsy.

Patterns of Use

Among people aged 12 or older in 2020, 17.9% (or about 49.6 million people) reported using cannabis in the past 12 months and 5.1% reported having a cannabis use disorder in the past year (NIDA, 2021). Many people incorrectly regard cannabis as a

TABLE 23–6	**Cannabinoids**	
CATEGORY	**COMMON PREPARATIONS**	**STREET NAMES**
Cannabis	Marijuana Hashish	Joint, weed, pot, grass, Mary Jane, Texas tea, locoweed, MJ, hay, stick Hash, bhang, ganja, charas
Synthetic cannabinoids	New psychoactive substances (NPS) powders or liquids To be inhaled (smoked or vaped)	K2, Spice, Black Mamba, Joker, Kush, Kronic

substance of low potential for adverse effects. This lack of knowledge has promoted use of the substance by individuals who believe it is harmless. Tolerance, although it tends to decline rapidly, does occur with chronic use. As tolerance develops, physical addiction also occurs, resulting in a withdrawal syndrome upon cessation of drug use.

One controversy that exists regarding marijuana (particularly because of several statewide trends toward legalization) is whether its use is a "gateway" to the use of other illicit drugs. NIDA (2021) reported that although some research shows that marijuana use is likely to precede use of other drugs and the development of addiction to other substances (including nicotine), "the majority of people who use marijuana do not go on to use other, 'harder' substances." More research is needed to clarify these associations as well as the effect of social environments on increasing one's tendency to try other drugs.

Effects on the Body

The following is a summary of some of the effects that have been attributed to marijuana usage. Undoubtedly, as research continues, evidence of additional physiological and psychological effects will be made available.

Cardiovascular Effects

Cannabis ingestion induces tachycardia and orthostatic hypotension (NIDA, 2021). With the decrease in blood pressure, myocardial oxygen supply is decreased. Tachycardia in turn increases oxygen demand. Marijuana raises the heart rate for up to 3 hours after smoking.

Respiratory Effects

Marijuana produces a greater amount of "tar" than its equivalent weight in tobacco. Because of the method by which marijuana is smoked—that is, the smoke is held in the lungs for as long as possible to achieve the desired effect—larger amounts of tar are deposited in the lungs, promoting deleterious effects.

Although the initial reaction to marijuana is bronchodilation, thereby facilitating respiratory function, chronic use results in obstructive airway disorders. Frequent marijuana users often have laryngitis, bronchitis, cough, and hoarseness.

Reproductive Effects

Some studies have shown that, with heavy marijuana use, men may have a decrease in sperm count, motility, and structure (Payne et al., 2019). In women, heavy marijuana use may result in a suppression of ovulation, disruption in menstrual cycles, and alteration of hormone levels. Children exposed to marijuana during fetal development have a higher incidence of attention, problem-solving, and memory problems than unexposed children (NIDA, 2021).

Central Nervous System Effects

Acute CNS effects of marijuana are dose related. Many people report a feeling of being high—the equivalent of being "drunk" on alcohol. Symptoms include feelings of euphoria, relaxed inhibitions, disorientation, depersonalization, and relaxation. At higher doses, sensory alterations may occur, including impairment in judgment of time and distance, recent memory, and learning ability. Physiological symptoms may include tremors, muscle rigidity, and conjunctival redness. Toxic effects are generally characterized by panic reactions. Very heavy usage has been shown to precipitate an acute psychosis that is self-limited and short-lived once the drug is removed from the body (Julien, 2014).

Heavy, long-term cannabis use is also associated with a condition called *amotivational syndrome*. Amotivational syndrome is defined as lack of motivation to persist in or complete a task that requires ongoing attention. Persons are described as "apathetic, anergic, usually gaining weight, and appearing slothful" (Boland & Verduin, 2022, p. 289). Evidence supports that long-term use also impairs cognitive functions of memory, attention, and organization; these impairments may also contribute to some of the symptoms apparent in amotivational syndrome.

Sexual Function

Marijuana is reported to enhance the sexual experience in both men and women. The intensified sensory awareness and the slowness of time perception are thought to increase sexual satisfaction. Marijuana also enhances sexual function by releasing inhibitions for certain activities that would normally be restrained.

Cannabis Intoxication

Cannabis intoxication is evidenced by the presence of clinically significant behavioral or psychological changes that develop during or shortly after cannabis use. Symptoms include impaired motor coordination, euphoria, anxiety, a sensation of slowed time, impaired judgment and memory, and social withdrawal. Physical symptoms include conjunctival injection (red eyes), increased appetite, dry mouth, and tachycardia. The impairment of motor skills lasts for 8 to 12 hours and interferes with the operation of motor vehicles. These effects are additive to those of alcohol, which is commonly used in combination with cannabis. Cannabis intoxication delirium is marked by significant cognitive impairment and difficulty performing tasks. Higher doses also impair level of consciousness.

Marijuana when taken alone is not associated with death from overdose, but large amounts of THC (and THC content has been increasing over the last decade) can result in symptoms such as anxiety, paranoia, and (in rare cases) extreme psychotic reactions (NIDA, 2019b). Synthetic cannabinoids, on the other hand, are associated with toxic reactions, elevated blood pressure, reduced blood supply to the heart, kidney damage, and seizures, all of which may be life-threatening; the risk of fatality is increased when combined with synthetic opioids (NIDA, 2020b). Because the strengths are variable (up to 100 times more potent than THC), the risks of using these substances are unpredictable. Symptoms include agitation, high blood pressure, shaking and seizures, nausea and vomiting, hallucinations and paranoia, and violent behavior.

Cannabis Withdrawal

The *DSM-5-TR* (APA, 2022) describes a syndrome of symptoms that occurs upon cessation of heavy, prolonged cannabis use. Symptoms occur within 1 week after cessation of use and may include any of the following:

■ Irritability, anger, or aggression
■ Nervousness, restlessness, or anxiety
■ Sleep difficulty (e.g., insomnia, disturbing dreams)
■ Decreased appetite or weight loss
■ Depressed mood
■ Physical symptoms, such as abdominal pain, tremors, sweating, fever, chills, or headache

Tables 23–7 and 23–8 include summaries of the psychoactive substances, including symptoms of intoxication, withdrawal, use, overdose, possible therapeutic uses, and trade and common names by which they may be referred. The dynamics of substance use disorders using the transactional model of stress and adaptation are presented in Figure 23–3.

Application of the Nursing Process

Assessment

In the preintroductory phase of relationship development, the nurse must examine their feelings about working with a patient who misuses substances. If the nurse views these behaviors as morally wrong, and they have internalized these attitudes from very early in life, it may be difficult to suppress judgmental feelings. The role that alcohol or other substances has played (or plays) in the life of the nurse most certainly will affect the way in which they interact with a patient who has a substance use disorder.

How are attitudes examined? Some individuals may have sufficient ability for introspection to recognize whether they have unresolved issues related to substance misuse. For others, it may be more helpful to discuss these issues in a group situation, where insight may be gained from feedback regarding the perceptions of others.

Whether alone or in a group, the nurse may gain a greater understanding about attitudes and feelings related to substance misuse by responding to the following types of questions. As written here, the questions are specific to alcohol, but they could be adapted for any substance.

■ What are my drinking patterns?
■ If I drink, why do I drink? When, where, and how much?
■ If I don't drink, why do I abstain?
■ Am I comfortable with my drinking patterns?
■ If I decided not to drink any more, would that be a problem for me?
■ What did I learn from my parents about drinking?
■ Have my attitudes changed as an adult?
■ What are my feelings about people who become intoxicated?
■ Does it seem more acceptable for some individuals than for others?
■ Do I ever use terms such as "sot," "drunk," or "boozer" to describe some individuals who overindulge, yet I overlook it in others?
■ Do I ever overindulge myself?
■ Has the use of alcohol (by me or others) affected my life in any way?
■ Do I see alcohol/drug misuse as a sign of weakness? A moral problem? An illness?

Unless nurses fully understand and accept their own attitudes and feelings, they cannot be empathetic toward patients' problems. Patients in recovery need to know they are accepted for themselves, regardless of past behaviors. Nurses must be able to separate the person from the behavior and to accept that individual with unconditional positive regard.

Motivational Interviewing

Motivational interviewing is an approach that can be used in the assessment and intervention process for people with any disorder, although it first gained popularity in treatment of patients with substance use disorders. It uses skills such as empathy, validation, open-ended questions, and reflection to explore the individual's motivation, strengths, and readiness for change. Some of the preceding questions could easily be reframed to explore the patient's attitudes

TABLE 23–7 Psychoactive Substances: A Profile Summary

CLASS OF DRUGS	SYMPTOMS OF USE	THERAPEUTIC USES	SYMPTOMS OF OVERDOSE	TRADE NAMES OR CHEMICAL NAMES	COMMON NAMES
CNS DEPRESSANTS					
Alcohol	Relaxation, loss of inhibitions, lack of concentration, drowsiness, slurred speech, sleep	Antidote for methanol consumption; ingredient in many pharmacological concentrates	Nausea, vomiting; shallow respirations; cold, clammy skin; weak, rapid pulse; coma; possible death	Ethyl alcohol, beer, gin, rum, vodka, bourbon, whiskey, liqueurs, wine, brandy, sherry, champagne	Booze, alcohol, liquor, drinks, cocktails, highballs, nightcaps, moonshine, white lightning, firewater
Other (barbiturates and nonbarbiturates)	Same as alcohol	Relief from anxiety and insomnia; as anticonvulsants and anesthetics	Anxiety, fever, agitation, hallucinations, disorientation, tremors, delirium, convulsions, possible death	Seconal, Amytal, Nembutal Valium Librium Noctec Miltown	Red birds, yellow birds, blue birds Blues/yellows Green and whites Mickies Downers
CNS STIMULANTS					
Amphetamines and related drugs	Hyperactivity, agitation, euphoria, insomnia, loss of appetite	Management of narcolepsy, hyperkinesia, and weight control	Cardiac arrhythmias, headache, convulsions, hypertension, rapid heart rate, coma, possible death	Dexedrine, Didrex, Tenuate, Bontril, Ritalin, Focalin, Meridia, Provigil	Uppers, pep pills, wake-ups, bennies, eye-openers, speed, black beauties, sweet As
Cocaine	Euphoria, hyperactivity, restlessness, talkativeness, increased pulse, dilated pupils, rhinitis		Hallucinations, convulsions, pulmonary edema, respiratory failure, coma, cardiac arrest, possible death	Cocaine hydrochloride	Coke, flake, snow, dust, happy dust, gold dust, girl, Cecil, C, toot, blow, crack
Synthetic stimulants	Agitation, insomnia, irritability, dizziness, decreased ability to think clearly, increased heart rate, chest pains	treatment resistant PTSD (MDMA)	Paranoia, nausea, vomiting, seizures, heart attack, stroke, increased heart rate, increased blood pressure, nosebleeds, hallucinations, aggressive behavior	MDMA (3,4-methylenedioxy-methamphetamine) Mephedrone, MDPV (3-4 methylenedioxypyrovalerone) Methylone Ethylone, Dibutylone Alpha-PVP	Bath salts, bliss, vanilla sky, ivory wave, purple wave, molly

TABLE 23–7 Psychoactive Substances: A Profile Summary—cont'd

CLASS OF DRUGS	SYMPTOMS OF USE	THERAPEUTIC USES	SYMPTOMS OF OVERDOSE	TRADE NAMES OR CHEMICAL NAMES	COMMON NAMES
OPIOIDS	Euphoria, lethargy, drowsiness, lack of motivation, constricted pupils	As analgesics; antidiarrheals, and antitussives; methadone in substitution therapy; heroin has no therapeutic use	Shallow breathing, slowed pulse, clammy skin, pulmonary edema, respiratory arrest, convulsions, coma, possible death	Heroin Morphine Codeine Dilaudid Demerol Dolophine Percodan Talwin Opium Carfentanil Sufentanil	Snow, stuff, H, harry, horse M, morph, Miss Emma Schoolboy Lords Doctors Dollies Perkies Ts Big O, black stuff
HALLUCINOGENS	Visual hallucinations, disorientation, confusion, paranoid delusions, euphoria, anxiety, panic, increased pulse	LSD has been proposed in the treatment of chronic alcoholism, and in the reduction of intractable pain	Agitation, extreme hyperactivity, violence, hallucinations, psychosis, convulsions, possible death	LSD PCP Mescaline DMT STP, DOM MDMA Ketamine MDPV	Acid, cube, big D Angel dust, hog, peace pill Mesc Businessman's trip Serenity and peace Ecstasy, XTC Special K, vitamin K, kit kat Bath salts
CANNABINOIDS	Relaxation, talkativeness, lowered inhibitions, euphoria, mood swings	Marijuana has been used for relief of nausea and vomiting associated with antineoplastic chemotherapy and to reduce eye pressure in glaucoma	Fatigue, paranoia, delusions, hallucinations, possible psychosis	Cannabis Hashish	Marijuana, pot, grass, joint, Mary Jane, MJ Hash, rope, Sweet Lucy
SYNTHETIC CANNABINOIDS	Highly variable: from elevated mood and relaxation to extreme anxiety, confusion, paranoia, hallucinations	Pain management in multiple sclerosis, diabetic neuropathy, nausea and vomiting	Rapid heart rate, vomiting, violent behavior, suicidal thoughts	Many chemical names	Fake weed, K2, Spice, Black Mamba, Kush, Joker Kronic (over 500 street names for various chemical formulas)

TABLE 23–8   Summary of Symptoms Associated With the Syndromes of Intoxication and Withdrawal

CLASS OF DRUGS	INTOXICATION	WITHDRAWAL	COMMENTS
Alcohol	Aggressiveness, impaired judgment, impaired attention, irritability, euphoria, depression, emotional lability, slurred speech, incoordination, unsteady gait, nystagmus, flushed face	Tremors, nausea/vomiting, malaise, weakness, tachycardia, sweating, elevated blood pressure, anxiety, depressed mood, irritability, hallucinations, headache, insomnia, seizures	Alcohol withdrawal may begin within 4–6 hours after last drink. May progress to delirium tremens on second or third day. Use of Librium or Serax is common for substitution therapy.
Amphetamines and related substances	Fighting, grandiosity, hypervigilance, psychomotor agitation, impaired judgment, tachycardia, pupillary dilation, elevated blood pressure, perspiration or chills, nausea and vomiting	Anxiety, depressed mood, irritability, craving for the substance, fatigue, insomnia or hypersomnia, psychomotor agitation, paranoid and suicidal ideation	Withdrawal symptoms usually peak within 2–4 days, although depression and irritability may persist for months. Antidepressants may be used.
Caffeine	Restlessness, nervousness, excitement, insomnia, flushed face, diuresis, gastrointestinal complaints, muscle twitching, rambling flow of thought and speech, cardiac arrhythmia, periods of inexhaustibility, psychomotor agitation	Headache	Caffeine is contained in coffee, tea, colas, cocoa, chocolate, some over-the-counter analgesics, "cold" preparations, and stimulants.
Cannabis	Euphoria, anxiety, suspiciousness, sensation of slowed time, impaired judgment, social withdrawal, tachycardia, conjunctival redness, increased appetite, hallucinations	Restlessness, irritability, insomnia, loss of appetite, depressed mood, tremors, fever, chills, headache, stomach pain	Intoxication occurs immediately and lasts about 3 hours. Oral ingestion is more slowly absorbed and has longer-lasting effects.
Cocaine	Euphoria, fighting, grandiosity, hypervigilance, psychomotor agitation, impaired judgment, tachycardia, elevated blood pressure, pupillary dilation, perspiration or chills, nausea/vomiting, hallucinations, delirium	Depression, anxiety, irritability, fatigue, insomnia or hypersomnia, psychomotor agitation, paranoid or suicidal ideation, apathy, social withdrawal	Large doses of the drug can result in convulsions or death from cardiac arrhythmias or respiratory paralysis.
Inhalants	Belligerence, assaultiveness, apathy, impaired judgment, dizziness, nystagmus, slurred speech, unsteady gait, lethargy, depressed reflexes, tremor, blurred vision, stupor or coma, euphoria, irritation around eyes, throat, and nose	Body aches, cravings, depression, headaches, insomnia, nervousness, tremors, panic attacks, seizures	Intoxication occurs within 5 minutes of inhalation. Symptoms last 60–90 minutes. Large doses can result in death from CNS depression or cardiac arrhythmia.
Nicotine	Nausea, vomiting, headache, rapid heart rate and respirations, increased blood pressure, dizziness, confusion	Craving for the drug, irritability, anger, frustration, anxiety, difficulty concentrating, restlessness, decreased heart rate, increased appetite, weight gain, tremor, headaches, insomnia	Symptoms of withdrawal begin within 24 hours of last drug use and decrease in intensity over days, weeks, or sometimes longer.
Opioids	Euphoria, lethargy, somnolence, apathy, dysphoria, impaired judgment, pupillary constriction, drowsiness, slurred speech, constipation, nausea, decreased respiratory rate and blood pressure	Craving for the drug, nausea/vomiting, muscle aches, lacrimation or rhinorrhea, pupillary dilation, piloerection or sweating, diarrhea, yawning, fever, insomnia	Withdrawal symptoms appear within 6–8 hours after last dose, reach a peak in the second or third day, and subside in 5–10 days. Times are shorter with meperidine and longer with methadone.

TABLE 23-8	Summary of Symptoms Associated With the Syndromes of Intoxication and Withdrawal—cont'd		
CLASS OF DRUGS	**INTOXICATION**	**WITHDRAWAL**	**COMMENTS**
Phencyclidine and related substances	Belligerence, assaultiveness, impulsiveness, psychomotor agitation, impaired judgment, nystagmus, increased heart rate and blood pressure, diminished pain response, ataxia, dysarthria, muscle rigidity, seizures, hyperacusis, delirium		Delirium can occur within 24 hours after use of phencyclidine or may occur up to a week after recovery from an overdose of the drug.
Sedatives, hypnotics, and anxiolytics	Disinhibition of sexual or aggressive impulses, mood lability, impaired judgment, slurred speech, incoordination, unsteady gait, impairment in attention or memory disorientation, confusion	Nausea/vomiting, malaise, weakness, tachycardia, sweating, anxiety, irritability, orthostatic hypotension, tremor, insomnia, seizures	Withdrawal may progress to delirium, usually within 1 week of last use. Long-acting barbiturates or benzodiazepines may be used in withdrawal substitution therapy.

and feelings. Through this process, the individual is empowered to become an active partner in treatment goals while exploring reasons for resistance to behavior change. For example, rather than telling a person that they must abstain from alcohol and attend 12-step meetings, the health-care professional helps the individual articulate what they want to achieve and then facilitates the process of exploring the advantages and disadvantages of desired behavior change. See Chapter 6, "Relationship Development" and Chapter 7, "Therapeutic Communication" for more discussion of this approach and a sample interview using motivational interviewing.

 Motivational interviewing is a patient-centered approach that encourages empowerment and active engagement, and as such, it articulates well with two current trends in psychiatric-mental health nursing care: recognizing the importance of patient-centered care as an essential nursing competency (Institute of Medicine, 2003) and the recovery model (see Chapter 20, "The Recovery Model," for further discussion of this model).

Assessment Tools

Nurses often perform the admission interview. A variety of assessment tools are appropriate for use in chemical dependency units. A nursing history and assessment tool was presented in Chapter 8, "The Nursing Process in Psychiatric-Mental Health Nursing." With some adaptation, it is an appropriate instrument for creating a database on patients who misuse substances. Box 23–1 presents a drug history and assessment that could be used in conjunction with the general biopsychosocial assessment.

The Clinical Institute Withdrawal Assessment of Alcohol Scale, Revised (CIWA-Ar) is a tool used by many hospitals to assess risk and severity of withdrawal from alcohol. It may be used for initial assessment as well as ongoing monitoring of alcohol withdrawal symptoms. A copy of the CIWA-Ar is presented in Box 23–2.

Many screening tools exist for determining whether an individual has a problem with substances. SAMHSA recommends an integrated public health approach known as SBIRT to accomplish early intervention and identifying people at risk for substance use disorders. SBIRT is an acronym for **S**creening, **B**rief **I**ntervention, **R**eferral, and **T**reatment. Many screening tools and other resources to accomplish this approach are available on SAMHSA's Web site (SAMHSA, 2022). Some psychiatric units administer these surveys to all admitted patients to help determine whether there is a secondary alcohol problem in addition to the psychiatric problem for which the individual is being admitted (sometimes called **dual diagnosis**). These tools can be adapted for use in diagnosing problems with other drugs as well.

Dual Diagnosis

The NIH (2018) reported that 7.7 million adults with a substance use disorder also have a co-occurring mental illness, which represents 37.9% of all adults with a substance use disorder. If the patient is diagnosed with both mental illness and a coexisting substance disorder, they may be assigned to a special program that targets both problems. Traditional counseling approaches use more confrontation than is considered appropriate for individuals with dual diagnoses. Most dual diagnosis programs take a supportive, less confrontational approach.

Peer support groups are an important part of the treatment program. Group members offer

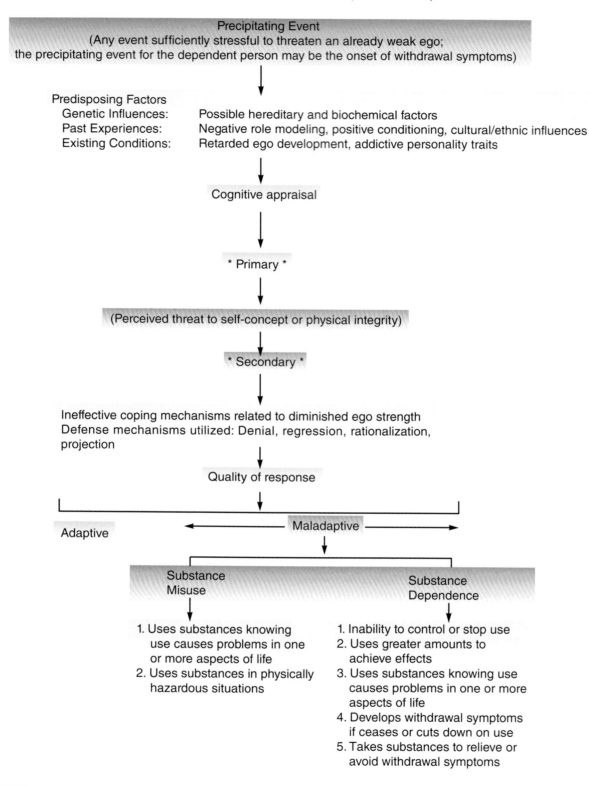

FIGURE 23–3   The dynamics of substance use disorders using the transactional model of stress and adaptation.

BOX 23–1 **Drug History and Assessment***

1. When you were growing up, did anyone in your family drink alcohol or take other kinds of drugs?
2. If so, how did the substance use affect the family situation?
3. When did you have your first drink/drugs?
4. How long have you been drinking/taking drugs on a regular basis?
5. What is your pattern of substance use?
   a. When do you use substances?
   b. What do you use?
   c. How much do you use?
   d. Where are you and with whom when you use substances?
6. When did you have your last drink/drug? What was it and how much did you consume?
7. Does using the substance(s) cause problems for you? Describe. Include family, friends, job, school, other.
8. Have you ever experienced injury as a result of substance use?
9. Have you ever been arrested or incarcerated for drinking/using drugs?
10. Have you ever tried to stop drinking/using drugs? If so, what was the result? Did you experience any physical symptoms, such as tremors, headache, insomnia, sweating, or seizures?
11. Have you ever experienced loss of memory for times when you have been drinking/using drugs?
12. Describe a typical day in your life.
13. Are there any changes you would like to make in your life? If so, what are they?
14. What plans or ideas do you have for seeing that these changes occur?

To be used in conjunction with general biopsychosocial nursing history and assessment tool (see Chapter 8, "The Nursing Process in Psychiatric-Mental Health Nursing").

BOX 23–2 **Clinical Institute Withdrawal Assessment of Alcohol Scale, Revised**

Patient: Date: Time:

PULSE OR HEART RATE, TAKEN FOR 1 MINUTE:

NAUSEA AND VOMITING—Ask "Do you feel sick to your stomach? Have you vomited?" Observation.

0 no nausea and no vomiting
1 mild nausea with no vomiting
2
3
4 intermittent nausea with dry heaves
5
6
7 constant nausea, frequent dry heaves and vomiting

TREMOR—Arms extended and fingers spread apart. Observation.

0 no tremor
1 not visible, but can be felt fingertip to fingertip
2
3
4 moderate, with patient's arms extended
5
6
7 severe, even with arms not extended

BLOOD PRESSURE:

TACTILE DISTURBANCES—Ask "Have you any itching, pins and needles sensations, any burning, any numbness, or do you feel bugs crawling on or under your skin?" Observation.
0 none
1 very mild itching, pins and needles, burning or numbness
2 mild itching, pins and needles, burning or numbness
3 moderate itching, pins and needles, burning or numbness
4 moderately severe hallucinations
5 severe hallucinations
6 extremely severe hallucinations
7 continuous hallucinations

AUDITORY DISTURBANCES—Ask "Are you more aware of sounds around you? Are they harsh? Do they frighten you? Are you hearing anything that is disturbing to you? Are you hearing things you know are not there?" Observation.
0 not present
1 very mild harshness or ability to frighten
2 mild harshness or ability to frighten
3 moderate harshness or ability to frighten
4 moderately severe hallucinations
5 severe hallucinations
6 extremely severe hallucinations
7 continuous hallucinations

Continued

BOX 23–2 Clinical Institute Withdrawal Assessment of Alcohol Scale, Revised–cont'd

PAROXYSMAL SWEATS—Observation.

0 no sweat visible
1 barely perceptible sweating, palms moist
2
3
4 beads of sweat obvious on forehead
5
6
7 drenching sweats

ANXIETY—Ask "Do you feel nervous?" Observation.

0 no anxiety, at ease
1 mild anxious
2
3
4 moderately anxious, or guarded, so anxiety is inferred
5
6
7 equivalent to acute panic states as seen in severe delirium or acute schizophrenic reactions

AGITATION—Observation

0 normal activity
1 somewhat more than normal activity
2
3
4 moderately fidgety and restless
5
6
7 paces back and forth during most of the interview, or constantly thrashes about

_____
_____
_____
_____
_____
_____

VISUAL DISTURBANCES—Ask "Does the light appear to be too bright? Is its color different? Does it hurt your eyes? Are you seeing anything that is disturbing to you? Are you seeing things you know are not there?" Observation.

0 not present
1 very mild sensitivity
2 mild sensitivity
3 moderate sensitivity
4 moderately severe hallucinations
5 severe hallucinations
6 extremely severe hallucinations
7 continuous hallucinations

HEADACHE, FULLNESS IN HEAD—Ask "Does your head feel different? Does it feel like there is a band around your head?" Do not rate for dizziness or lightheadedness. Otherwise, rate severity.

0 not present
1 very mild
2 mild
3 moderate
4 moderately severe
5 severe
6 very severe
7 extremely severe

ORIENTATION AND CLOUDING OF SENSORIUM—Ask "What day is this? Where are you? Who am I?"

0 oriented and can do serial additions
1 cannot do serial additions or is uncertain about date
2 disoriented for date by no more than 2 calendar days
3 disoriented for date by more than 2 calendar days
4 disoriented for place/or person

Total CIWA-Ar Score _____
Rater's Initials _____
Maximum Possible Score 67*

___

*The CIWA-Ar is not copyrighted and may be reproduced freely. This assessment for monitoring withdrawal symptoms requires approximately 5 minutes to administer. The maximum score is 67 (see instrument). Patients scoring less than 10 do not usually need additional medication for withdrawal.
From Sullivan, J. T., Sykora, K., Schneiderman, J., Naranjo, C. A., & Sellers, E. M. (1989). Assessment of alcohol withdrawal: The revised Clinical Institute Withdrawal Assessment for Alcohol scale (CIWA-Ar). *British Journal of Addiction, 84*(11), 1353–1357.

encouragement and practical advice to each other. Psychodynamic therapy can be useful for some individuals with dual diagnoses by exploring the personal history of how psychiatric disorders and substance misuse have reinforced one another and how the cycle can be broken. Cognitive and behavioral therapies are helpful in training people to monitor moods and thought patterns that lead to substance

misuse. Teaching patients about coping skills and stress management also promotes skills in maintaining abstinence and dealing with substance cravings. (See Chapter 30, "Eating Disorders," for Vic's discussion of his dual diagnosis, alcohol use disorder, and anorexia nervosa, in "Real People, Real Stories.")

Individuals with dual diagnoses should be educated about 12-step recovery programs (e.g.,

Alcoholics Anonymous [AA] or Narcotics Anonymous). Some people are resistant to attending 12-step programs, and they often do better in support groups specifically designed for people with psychiatric disorders and substance use disorders.

Generally, 12-step and substance misuse education groups are integrated into regular programming for the psychiatric patient with a dual diagnosis. An individual in a psychiatric facility or day treatment program will attend a substance use-related group periodically in lieu of another scheduled activity therapy. Topics are directed toward areas that are unique to people with mental illness, such as mixing medications with other substances, as well as topics that are common to those with a primary substance use disorder. Individuals are encouraged to discuss their personal problems.

Continued attendance at 12-step group meetings is encouraged upon discharge from treatment. Family involvement is enlisted, and preventive strategies are outlined. Individual case management is common, and success is often promoted by this close supervision.

Diagnosis and Outcome Identification

The next step in the nursing process is to identify appropriate nursing diagnoses by analyzing the data collected during the assessment phase. The individual who misuses or is dependent on substances undoubtedly has many unmet physical and emotional needs. Table 23–9 presents a list of patient behaviors and the NANDA-I nursing diagnoses (Herdman et al., 2021) that correspond to those behaviors, which may be used in planning care for the patient with a substance use disorder.

Outcome Criteria

The following criteria may be used for measurement of outcomes in the care of the patient with substance-related disorders.

The patient:

- Has not experienced physical injury
- Has not caused harm to self or others
- Accepts responsibility for own behavior
- Acknowledges association between personal problems and use of substance(s)
- Demonstrates more adaptive coping mechanisms that can be used in stressful situations (instead of taking substances)
- Shows no signs or symptoms of infection or malnutrition
- Exhibits evidence of increased self-worth by attempting new projects without fear of failure and by demonstrating less defensive behavior toward others
- Verbalizes importance of abstaining from use of substances in order to maintain optimal wellness

TABLE 23–9	Assigning Nursing Diagnoses to Behaviors Commonly Associated With Substance Use Disorders
BEHAVIORS	**NURSING DIAGNOSES**
Makes statements such as, "I don't have a problem with (substance). I can quit any time I want to." Delays seeking assistance; does not perceive problems related to use of substances; minimizes use of substances; unable to admit effect of disease on life pattern	Denial
Misuse of substances; destructive behavior toward others and self; inability to meet basic needs; inability to meet role expectations; risk taking	Ineffective coping
Loss of weight, pale conjunctiva and mucous membranes, decreased skin turgor, electrolyte imbalance, anemia, drinks alcohol instead of eating	Imbalanced nutrition: Less than body requirements/Deficient fluid volume
Risk factors: Malnutrition, altered immune condition, failing to avoid exposure to pathogens	Risk for infection
Criticizes self and others, self-destructive behavior (misuse of substances as a coping mechanism), dysfunctional family background	Chronic low self-esteem
Denies that substance is harmful; continues to use substance despite obvious consequences	Deficient knowledge
FOR THE PATIENT WITHDRAWING FROM CNS DEPRESSANTS:	
Risk factors: CNS agitation (tremors, elevated blood pressure, nausea and vomiting, hallucinations, illusions, tachycardia, anxiety, seizures)	Risk for injury/Acute substance withdrawal syndrome (or risk for)
FOR THE PATIENT WITHDRAWING FROM CNS STIMULANTS:	
Risk factors: Intense feelings of lassitude and depression; "crashing," suicidal ideation	Risk for suicidal behavior/Acute substance withdrawal syndrome (or risk for)

Planning and Implementation

Implementation of nursing care with patients who misuse substances is a long-term process, often beginning with **detoxification** (weaning off a substance to prevent acute withdrawal symptoms) and progressing to total abstinence. The following sections present a group of selected nursing diagnoses, with short- and long-term goals and nursing interventions for each.

Risk for Injury

Risk for injury is defined as "susceptible to physical damage due to environmental conditions interacting with the individual's adaptive and defensive resources, which may compromise health" (Herdman et al., 2021, p. 480).

Patient Goals

Outcome criteria include short- and long-term goals. Timelines are individually determined.

Short-term goal

■ Patient's condition will stabilize within 72 hours.

Long-term goal

■ Patient will not experience physical injury.

Interventions
For the patient in substance withdrawal

■ Assess the patient's level of disorientation to determine specific requirements for safety.
■ Obtain a drug history, if possible. It is important to determine the type of substance(s) used, the time and amount of last use, the length and frequency of use, and the amount used on a daily basis.
■ Because subjective history is often not accurate, obtain a urine sample for laboratory analysis of substance content.
■ It is important to keep the patient in as quiet an environment as possible. Excessive stimuli may increase agitation. A private room is ideal.
■ Observe patient behaviors frequently. If the seriousness of the condition warrants, it may be necessary to assign a staff person on a one-to-one basis.
■ Accompany and assist the patient when ambulating and use a wheelchair for transporting the patient long distances.
■ Pad the headboard and side rails of the bed with thick towels to protect the patient in case of a seizure.
■ Suicide precautions may need to be instituted for the patient withdrawing from CNS stimulants.
■ Ensure that smoking materials and other potentially harmful objects are stored away from the patient's access.
■ Frequently orient the patient to reality and the surroundings.

■ Monitor the patient's vital signs every 15 minutes initially and less frequently as acute symptoms subside.
■ Follow the medication regimen as ordered by the physician. Common psychopharmacological intervention for substance intoxication and withdrawal is presented later in this chapter in the section "Treatment Modalities for Substance-Related Disorders."

Denial

Denial is defined as a "conscious or unconscious attempt to disavow the knowledge or meaning of an event to reduce anxiety and/or fear, leading to the detriment of health" (Herdman et al., 2021, p. 418). Table 23–10 presents this nursing diagnosis in care plan format.

Patient Goals

Outcome criteria include short- and long-term goals. Timelines are individually determined.

Short-term goal

■ Patient will focus on behavioral outcomes associated with substance use.

Long-term goal

■ Patient will verbalize acceptance of responsibility for their own behavior and acknowledge association between substance use and personal problems.

Interventions

■ Begin by working to develop a trusting nurse–patient relationship. Be honest and keep all promises.
■ Convey an attitude of acceptance to the patient. Ensure that they understand, "It is not *you* but your *behavior* that is unacceptable." An attitude of acceptance helps to promote the patient's feelings of dignity and self-worth.
■ Provide information to correct misconceptions about substance misuse. The patient may rationalize their behavior with statements such as, "I'm not an alcoholic. I can stop drinking any time I want. Besides, I only drink beer" or "I only smoke pot to relax before class. So what? I know lots of people who do. Besides, you can't get hooked on pot." Many myths abound regarding use of specific substances. Factual information presented in a matter-of-fact, nonjudgmental way explaining what behaviors constitute a substance use disorder may help the patient focus on their own behaviors as an illness that requires help.
■ Identify recent maladaptive behaviors or situations that have occurred in the patient's life and discuss how use of substances may have been a

Table 23–10 | CARE PLAN FOR A PATIENT WITH A SUBSTANCE USE DISORDER

NURSING DIAGNOSIS: DENIAL

RELATED TO: Lack of coping skills to manage anxiety

EVIDENCED BY: Statements indicating no problem with substance use

OUTCOME CRITERIA	NURSING INTERVENTIONS	RATIONALE
Short-Term Goal ■ Patient diverts attention away from external issues and focuses on behavioral outcomes associated with substance use. **Long-Term Goal** ■ Patient verbalizes acceptance of responsibility for own behavior and acknowledges association between substance use and personal problems.	1. Begin by working to develop a trusting nurse-patient relationship. Be honest. Keep all promises. 2. Convey an attitude of acceptance to the patient. Ensure that they understand "It is not *you* but your *behavior* that is unacceptable." 3. Provide information to correct misconceptions about substance misuse. The patient may rationalize their behavior with statements such as "I'm not an alcoholic. I can stop drinking any time I want. Besides, I only drink beer," or "I only smoke pot to relax before class. So what? I know lots of people who do. Besides, you can't get hooked on pot." 4. Identify recent maladaptive behaviors or situations that have occurred in the patient's life and discuss how use of substances may have been a contributing factor. 5. Use confrontation with caring. Do not allow the patient to fantasize about their lifestyle (e.g., "It is my understanding that the last time you drank alcohol, you…" or "The laboratory report shows that you were under the influence of alcohol when you had the accident that injured three people"). 6. Do not accept rationalization or projection as the patient attempts to make excuses or blame other people or situations for their behavior. 7. Encourage participation in group activities.	1. Trust is the basis of a therapeutic relationship. 2. An attitude of acceptance promotes feelings of dignity and self-worth. 3. Many myths abound regarding use of specific substances. Factual information presented in a matter-of-fact, nonjudgmental way explaining what behaviors constitute substance-related disorders may help the patient focus on their own behaviors as an illness that requires help. 4. The first step in decreasing use of denial is for patient to see the relationship between substance use and personal problems. 5. Confrontation interferes with the patient's ability to use denial; a caring attitude preserves self-esteem and reduces the need for the patient to use defense mechanisms to reduce anxiety. 6. Rationalization and projection prolong denial that problems exist in the patient's life because of substance use. 7. Peer feedback is often more accepted than feedback from authority figures. Peer pressure can be a strong factor, as can association with individuals who are experiencing or who have experienced similar problems.

Continued

Table 23–10	CARE PLAN FOR A PATIENT WITH A SUBSTANCE USE DISORDER–cont'd	
OUTCOME CRITERIA	NURSING INTERVENTIONS	RATIONALE
	8. Offer immediate positive recognition of the patient's expressions of insight gained regarding illness and acceptance of responsibility for own behavior.	8. Positive reinforcement enhances self-esteem and encourages repetition of desirable behaviors.
	9. Employ motivational interviewing techniques to begin an exploration of the patient's motivations and readiness for change.	9. Using a patient-centered approach that includes techniques such as reflection, open-ended questions, clarification, and validation encourages the patient to actively engage in problem-solving.

contributing factor. The first step in decreasing denial is for the patient to see the relationship between substance use and personal problems.

■ Use confrontation with caring. Do not allow the patient to fantasize about their lifestyle. Confrontation interferes with the patient's ability to use denial; a caring attitude preserves self-esteem and reduces the need for the patient to rely on defense mechanisms to reduce anxiety.

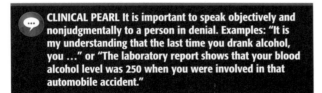

> **CLINICAL PEARL** It is important to speak objectively and nonjudgmentally to a person in denial. Examples: "It is my understanding that the last time you drank alcohol, you ..." or "The laboratory report shows that your blood alcohol level was 250 when you were involved in that automobile accident."

■ Acknowledge the use of rationalization or projection as the patient attempts to make excuses for or blame their behavior on other people or situations. Rationalization and projection prolong the patient's denial that problems exist secondary to substance use.

■ Encourage participation in group activities. Peer feedback is often more accepted than feedback from authority figures. Peer pressure from individuals who are experiencing or who have experienced similar problems can be powerfully influential in confronting denial as well.

■ Offer immediate positive recognition of the patient's expressions of insight regarding illness and acceptance of responsibility for their own behavior. Positive reinforcement enhances self-esteem and encourages the repetition of desirable behaviors.

Ineffective Coping

Ineffective coping is defined as "a pattern of invalid appraisal of stressors, with cognitive and/or behavioral efforts, that fails to manage demands related to well-being" (Herdman et al., 2021, p. 408).

Patient Goals

Outcome criteria include short- and long-term goals. Timelines are individually determined.

Short-term goal

■ Patient will express true feelings about using substances as a method of coping with stress.

Long-term goal

■ Patient will be able to verbalize use of adaptive coping mechanisms, instead of substance misuse, in response to stress.

Interventions

■ Spend time with the patient and establish a trusting relationship.

■ Set limits on manipulative behavior. Be sure that the patient knows what is acceptable, what is not, and the consequences for violating the limits set. Ensure that all staff maintain consistency with this intervention. Encourage the patient to verbalize feelings, fears, and anxieties. Answer any questions they may have regarding the disorder. Verbalization of feelings in a nonthreatening environment may help the patient come to terms with long-unresolved issues.

■ Explain the effects of substance misuse on the body. Emphasize that the prognosis is closely related to abstinence. Many patients lack knowledge about the deleterious effects of substance misuse on the body.

■ Explore with the patient the options available to assist with stressful situations rather than resorting to substance use (e.g., contacting various members of AA or Narcotics Anonymous, physical exercise, relaxation techniques, meditation). The patient may have persistently resorted to chemical use and thus possess little or no knowledge of adaptive responses to stress.

■ Provide positive reinforcement for evidence of gratification delayed appropriately. Encourage the patient to be as independent as possible in performing their self-care. Provide positive feedback for independent decision making and effective use of problem-solving skills.

Dysfunctional Family Processes

Dysfunctional family processes is defined as "family functioning which fails to support the well-being of its members" (Herdman et al., 2021, p. 373).

Patient Goals

Outcome criteria include short- and long-term goals. Timelines are individually determined.

Short-term goals

■ Family members will participate in individual family programs and support groups.

■ Family members will identify ineffective coping behaviors and consequences.

■ Family will initiate and plan for necessary lifestyle changes.

Long-term goal

■ Family members will take action to change self-destructive behaviors and alter behaviors that contribute to the individual's addiction.

Interventions

■ Review family history; explore roles of family members, current level of functioning, circumstances involving alcohol use, strengths, and areas of growth. Explore how family members have coped with the person's addiction (e.g., denial, repression, rationalization, hurt, loneliness, projection). Family members who enable may have the same feelings as the patient and use ineffective methods for dealing with the situation, necessitating help in learning new and effective coping skills.

■ Determine the extent of enabling behaviors evidenced by family members; explore these behaviors with each individual and the patient. Enabling behaviors are those that inhibit rather than promote change. Family and friends may enable continued substance use because the user has convinced them that this is the most helpful way to show their love. The substance user often relies on others to cover up for their inability to cope with daily responsibilities, but this scenario is less likely to promote the need for change.

■ Provide information about enabling behavior and addictive disease characteristics for both the user and nonuser. Achieving awareness and knowledge of behaviors (e.g., avoiding and shielding, taking over responsibilities, rationalizing, and subserving) provides an opportunity for individuals to begin the process of change.

■ Identify and discuss the possibility of sabotage behaviors by family members. Even though family members may verbalize a desire for the individual to become substance free, the reality of interactive dynamics is that they may unconsciously not want the individual to recover, as this would affect the family members' role in the relationship. Additionally, they may receive sympathy or attention from others (secondary gain).

■ Assist the patient's partner to understand that the patient's abstinence and drug use are not the partner's responsibility, and that the patient's use of substances may or may not change despite involvement in treatment. Partners must come to realize and accept that the only behavior they can control is their own.

■ Involve the family in plans for discharge from treatment. Substance misuse and addiction is a family illness. Because the family has been so involved in dealing with the substance use behavior, family members need help adjusting to the new behavior of sobriety/abstinence. Encourage involvement with self-help associations, such as AA, Al-Anon, Alateen, Codependents Anonymous (CoDA), and professional family therapy. These organizations put the patient and family in direct contact with support systems necessary for continued sobriety and assist with problem resolution.

Concept Care Mapping

The concept map care plan (see Chapter 8, "The Nursing Process in Psychiatric-Mental Health Nursing") is a diagrammatic teaching and learning strategy that allows visualization of interrelationships between medical diagnoses, nursing diagnoses, assessment data, and treatments. An example of a concept map care plan for a patient with a substance use disorder is presented in Figure 23–4.

Patient and Family Education

The role of patient teacher is important in the psychiatric area, as it is in all areas of nursing. A list of topics for patient and family education relevant to substance-related disorders is presented in Box 23–3. Sample patient teaching guides are available online.

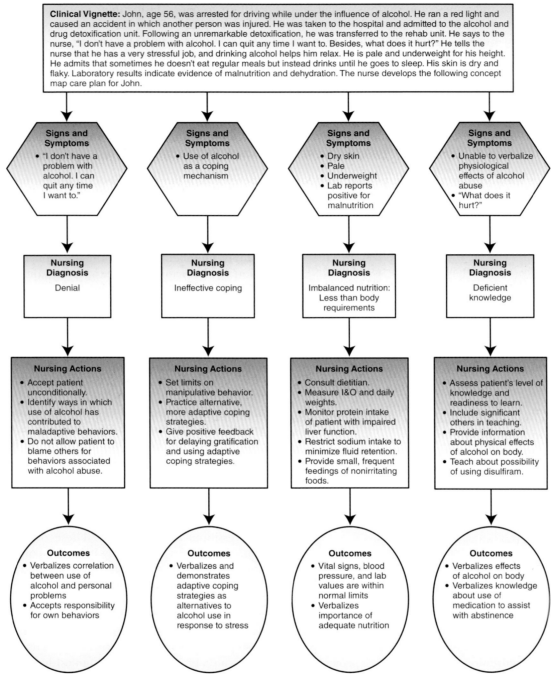

Clinical Vignette: John, age 56, was arrested for driving while under the influence of alcohol. He ran a red light and caused an accident in which another person was injured. He was taken to the hospital and admitted to the alcohol and drug detoxification unit. Following an unremarkable detoxification, he was transferred to the rehab unit. He says to the nurse, "I don't have a problem with alcohol. I can quit any time I want to. Besides, what does it hurt?" He tells the nurse that he has a very stressful job, and drinking alcohol helps him relax. He is pale and underweight for his height. He admits that sometimes he doesn't eat regular meals but instead drinks until he goes to sleep. His skin is dry and flaky. Laboratory results indicate evidence of malnutrition and dehydration. The nurse develops the following concept map care plan for John.

Signs and Symptoms
- "I don't have a problem with alcohol. I can quit any time I want to."

Signs and Symptoms
- Use of alcohol as a coping mechanism

Signs and Symptoms
- Dry skin
- Pale
- Underweight
- Lab reports positive for malnutrition

Signs and Symptoms
- Unable to verbalize physiological effects of alcohol abuse
- "What does it hurt?"

Nursing Diagnosis
Denial

Nursing Diagnosis
Ineffective coping

Nursing Diagnosis
Imbalanced nutrition: Less than body requirements

Nursing Diagnosis
Deficient knowledge

Nursing Actions
- Accept patient unconditionally.
- Identify ways in which use of alcohol has contributed to maladaptive behaviors.
- Do not allow patient to blame others for behaviors associated with alcohol abuse.

Nursing Actions
- Set limits on manipulative behavior.
- Practice alternative, more adaptive coping strategies.
- Give positive feedback for delaying gratification and using adaptive coping strategies.

Nursing Actions
- Consult dietitian.
- Measure I&O and daily weights.
- Monitor protein intake of patient with impaired liver function.
- Restrict sodium intake to minimize fluid retention.
- Provide small, frequent feedings of nonirritating foods.

Nursing Actions
- Assess patient's level of knowledge and readiness to learn.
- Include significant others in teaching.
- Provide information about physical effects of alcohol on body.
- Teach about possibility of using disulfiram.

Outcomes
- Verbalizes correlation between use of alcohol and personal problems
- Accepts responsibility for own behaviors

Outcomes
- Verbalizes and demonstrates adaptive coping strategies as alternatives to alcohol use in response to stress

Outcomes
- Vital signs, blood pressure, and lab values are within normal limits
- Verbalizes importance of adequate nutrition

Outcomes
- Verbalizes effects of alcohol on body
- Verbalizes knowledge about use of medication to assist with abstinence

FIGURE 23–4 Concept map care plan for patient with alcoholism.

Evaluation

The final step of the nursing process involves reassessment to determine whether the nursing interventions have been effective in achieving the intended goals of care. Evaluation of the patient with a substance-related disorder may be accomplished by using information gathered from the following reassessment questions:

■ Has detoxification occurred without complications?
■ Is the patient still in denial?

■ Does the patient accept responsibility for their own behavior? Have they acknowledged a personal problem with substances?
■ Has a correlation been made between personal problems and the use of substances?
■ Does the patient still make excuses or blame others for use of substances?
■ Has the patient remained substance free during treatment?
■ Does the patient cooperate with treatment?

BOX 23–3 Topics for Patient and Family Education Related to Substance Use Disorders

NATURE OF THE ILLNESS
1. Effects of (substance) on the body
   a. Alcohol
   b. Other CNS depressants
   c. CNS stimulants
   d. Hallucinogens
   e. Inhalants
   f. Opioids
   g. Cannabinoids
2. Ways in which use of (substance) affects life.

MANAGEMENT OF THE ILLNESS
1. Activities to substitute for (substance) in times of stress
2. Relaxation techniques
   a. Progressive relaxation
   b. Tense and relax
   c. Deep breathing
   d. Autogenics
3. Problem-solving skills
4. The essentials of good nutrition

SUPPORT SERVICES
1. Financial assistance
2. Legal assistance
3. Alcoholics Anonymous (or other support group specific to another substance)
4. One-to-one support person

■ Does the patient refrain from manipulative behavior and violation of limits?

■ Is the patient able to verbalize motivation toward alternative adaptive coping strategies to substitute for substance use? Has the use of these strategies been demonstrated? Does positive reinforcement encourage the repetition of these adaptive behaviors?

■ Has nutritional status been restored? Does the patient consume a diet adequate for their size and level of activity? Is the patient able to discuss the importance of adequate nutrition?

■ Has the patient remained free of infection during hospitalization?

■ Is the patient able to verbalize the effects of substance misuse on the body?

The Chemically Impaired Nurse

Substance misuse and addiction have the potential for impairment in an individual's social, occupational, psychological, and physical functioning. This impairment becomes an especially serious problem when the person is responsible for the lives of others each day. A recent study found that 18% of nurses screened positive for substance use problems and 6.6% met criteria for a substance use disorder (Trinkoff et al., 2022). Alcohol is the most widely misused drug, followed closely by narcotics. Nurses who misuse substances have an added vulnerability because they are often handling controlled substances when providing patient care.

For years, the impaired nurse was protected, promoted, transferred, ignored, or fired. These types of responses promoted the growth of the problem. The most effective are programs that involve early reporting and treatment of chemical addiction as a disease, with a focus on public safety and rehabilitation of the nurse.

How does one identify the impaired nurse? It is easy to overlook what *might* be a problem. Denial, on the part of the impaired nurse as well as nurse colleagues, is still the strongest defense for not confronting substance misuse. Some states have mandatory reporting laws that require observers to report substance-impaired nurses to the state board of nursing. These laws are difficult to enforce, and hospitals are not always compliant with mandatory reporting. Some hospitals may choose not to report to the state board of nursing if the impaired nurse is actively seeking treatment and is not placing patients in danger.

Several signs of substance impairment in nurses have been identified. They are not easy to detect and will vary according to the substance used. There may be high absenteeism if the person's source is outside the work area, or the individual may rarely miss work if the substance source is at work. There may be an increase in "wasting" of drugs, higher incidences of incorrect narcotic counts, and a higher record of signing out drugs than for other nurses.

Poor concentration, difficulty meeting deadlines, inappropriate responses, and poor memory or recall usually occur late in the disease process. The person may also have problems with relationships. Other possible signs include irritability, mood swings, tendency to isolate, elaborate excuses for behavior, unkempt appearance, impaired motor coordination, slurred speech, flushed face, inconsistent job performance, and frequent use of the restroom. They may frequently medicate other nurses' patients, and there may be patient complaints of inadequate pain control. Discrepancies in documentation may occur. Ideally, suspicious behavior is recognized by peers and intervention sought before the impaired nurse reaches late stages of the disease process. As uncomfortable as it may be to tell a supervisor about suspected impairment in a colleague, it is in the interest of the nurse's health and critically important to ensuring patient safety.

If suspicious behavior occurs, it is important to keep careful, objective records. Confrontation with the impaired nurse will undoubtedly result in hostility and denial. Confrontation should not occur solely between peers but rather should involve a supervisor or other nurse manager and should include the offer of assistance in seeking treatment. When a report is made to the state board of nursing, it should be a factual documentation of specific events and actions, not a diagnostic statement of impairment.

State boards generally decide each case on an individual basis. A state board may deny, suspend, or revoke a license based on a report of chemical impairment by a nurse. Several state boards of nursing have passed diversionary laws that allow impaired nurses to avoid disciplinary action by agreeing to seek treatment. Some administer the treatment programs themselves, and others refer the nurse to community resources or state nurses' association assistance programs. Treatment may entail successful completion of inpatient, outpatient, group, or individual counseling treatment program(s); evidence of regular attendance at nurse support groups or a 12-step program; random negative drug screens; and employment or volunteer activities during the suspension period. When a nurse is deemed safe to return to practice, they may be closely monitored for several years and required to undergo random drug screenings. The nurse also may be required to practice under specifically circumscribed conditions for a designated period of time.

In 1982 the American Nurses Association (ANA) House of Delegates adopted a national resolution to assist impaired nurses. Since that time, the majority of state nurses' associations have developed (or are developing) programs for nurses who are impaired by substances or psychiatric illness. The individuals who administer these efforts are nurse members of the state associations, as well as nurses who are in recovery themselves. For this reason, they are called **peer assistance programs.**

Peer assistance programs strive to intervene early, reduce hazards to clients, and increase prospects for the nurse's recovery. Most states provide either a hotline number that the impaired nurse or intervening colleague may call or phone numbers of peer assistance committee members. Typically, a contract is drawn up detailing the method of treatment, which may be obtained from various sources, such as employee assistance programs, AA, Narcotics Anonymous, private counseling, or outpatient clinics. Guidelines for monitoring the course of treatment are established. Peer support is provided through regular contact with the impaired nurse, usually for 2 years. Peer assistance programs serve to assist impaired nurses to recognize their impairment, obtain necessary treatment, and regain accountability within their profession. Most states either provide or

have provisions to accept other designated peer assistance programs as alternatives to discipline from the state board as long as the impaired nurse is adhering to the requirements of the program.

Codependency

The concept of **codependency** arose from a need to define the dysfunctional behaviors that are evident among members of the family of a chemically addicted person. The term has been expanded to include all individuals from families that harbor secrets of physical or emotional abuse or pathological conditions. Living under these conditions results in unmet needs for autonomy and self-esteem and a profound sense of powerlessness. The codependent person is able to achieve a sense of control only through fulfilling the needs of others. Personal identity is relinquished and boundaries with the other person become blurred. The codependent person disowns their own needs and wants to respond to external demands and the demands of others. Codependence has been called "a dysfunctional relationship with oneself."

The traits associated with a codependent personality are varied. In a relationship, the codependent person derives self-worth from that of the partner, whose feelings and behaviors determine how the codependent should feel and behave. In order for the codependent to feel good, their partner must be happy and behave in appropriate ways. If the partner is not happy, the codependent feels responsible for *making* the partner happy. The codependent's home life is fraught with stress. Ego boundaries are weak, and behaviors are often enmeshed with those of the pathological partner. Denial that problems exist is common. Feelings are kept in control, and anxiety may be released in the form of stress-related illnesses or compulsive behaviors such as eating, spending, working, or use of substances.

Selected characteristics of the codependent individual (Beatty, 2011) include the following:

■ Taking care of others at the expense of one's own needs

■ Feeling responsible for fixing other people's problems

■ Having low self-esteem; expecting to perform perfectly but never feeling "good enough"

■ Desperately seeking approval from others; often identified as "people pleasers"

■ Generally unhappy and seeking things outside oneself to attempt to fulfill unmet needs

■ Tending to have come from dysfunctional families where there was abuse or neglect

■ Having weak boundaries that lead to feelings of resentment, lack of trust, and anger toward others

The Codependent Nurse

Certain characteristics of codependence have been associated with the profession of nursing. A shortage of nurses combined with the increasing ranks of seriously ill patients may result in nurses providing care to and fulfilling everyone's needs but their own. Many health-care workers who were reared in homes with a chemically addicted person or otherwise dysfunctional family are at risk for having unresolved codependent tendencies reactivated. Nurses who assumed the "fixer" role in their dysfunctional families of origin during childhood may attempt to resume that role in their caregiving professions. They are attracted to a profession in which they are needed but nurture feelings of resentment for receiving so little in return. Their emotional needs go unmet, but they continue to deny that these needs exist. Instead, these unmet emotional needs may be manifested through use of compulsive behaviors, such as work or spending excessively, or addictions, such as to food or substances.

Codependent nurses have a need to be in control. They often strive for an unrealistic level of achievement. Their self-worth comes from the feeling of being needed by others and maintaining control over the environment. They nurture the dependence of others and accept the responsibility for the happiness and contentment of others. They rarely express their true feelings, and they do what is necessary to preserve harmony and maintain control. They are at high risk for physical and emotional burnout.

Treating Codependency

Cermak (1986) identified four stages in the recovery process for individuals with codependent personality:

Stage I: The Survival Stage In this first stage, codependent individuals must begin to let go of the denial that problems exist or that their personal capabilities are unlimited. This initiation of abstinence from blanket denial may be a very emotional and painful period.

Stage II: The Reidentification Stage Reidentification occurs when individuals are able to glimpse their true selves through a break in the denial system. They accept the label of codependent and take responsibility for their own dysfunctional behavior. Codependents tend to enter reidentification only after being convinced that it is more painful not to do so. They accept their limitations and are ready to face the issues of codependence.

Stage III: The Core Issues Stage In this stage, the recovering codependent must face the fact that relationships cannot be managed by force of will. Each

partner must be independent and autonomous. The goal of this stage is to detach from the struggles of life that exist because of prideful and willful efforts to control things that are beyond the individual's power to control.

Stage IV: The Reintegration Stage This is a stage of self-acceptance and willingness to change when codependents relinquish the power *over others* that was not rightfully theirs but reclaim the *personal* power that they do possess. Integrity is achieved out of awareness, honesty, and connection with one's spiritual consciousness. Control is achieved through self-discipline and self-confidence.

Self-help groups have been found helpful in the treatment of codependency. Groups developed for families of chemically addicted people, such as Al-Anon, may be of assistance. Groups specific to codependency also exist. One of these groups, which bases its philosophy on the Twelve Steps of Alcoholics Anonymous (see the section that follows), is Co-Dependents Anonymous (CoDA, n.d.).

Treatment Modalities for Substance-Related Disorders

Alcoholics Anonymous

AA is a major self-help organization for the treatment of alcoholism. It was founded in 1935 by two alcoholics—a stockbroker, Bill Wilson, and a physician, Bob Smith—who discovered that they could remain sober through mutual support. They accomplished this not as professionals, but as peers who were able to share their common experiences. Soon they were working with other alcoholics, who in turn worked with others. The movement grew, and remarkably, individuals who had been treated unsuccessfully by professionals were able to maintain sobriety through helping one another.

Today, AA chapters exist in virtually every community in the United States. The self-help groups are based on the concept of peer support—acceptance and understanding from others who have experienced the same problems. The only requirement for membership is a desire on the part of the alcoholic person to stop drinking. Each new member is assigned a support person from whom they may seek assistance when the temptation to drink occurs.

The sole purpose of AA is to help members stay sober. When sobriety has been achieved, they are expected to help other alcoholic people. The Twelve Steps that embody the philosophy of AA provide specific guidelines on how to attain and maintain sobriety (Box 23–4).

BOX 23–4 **Alcoholics Anonymous**

THE TWELVE STEPS

1. We admitted we were powerless over alcohol—that our lives have become unmanageable.
2. Came to believe that a Power greater than ourselves could restore us to sanity.
3. Made a decision to turn our will and our lives over to the care of God as we understood Him.
4. Made a searching and fearless moral inventory of ourselves.
5. Admitted to God, to ourselves, and to another human being the exact nature of our wrongs.
6. Were entirely ready to have God remove all these defects of character.
7. Humbly asked Him to remove our shortcomings.
8. Made a list of all persons we had harmed and became willing to make amends to them all.
9. Made direct amends to such people wherever possible except when to do so would injure them or others.
10. Continued to take personal inventory and when we were wrong promptly admitted it.
11. Sought through prayer and meditation to improve our conscious contact with God as we understood Him, praying only for knowledge of His will for us and the power to carry that out.
12. Having had a spiritual awakening as the result of these steps, we tried to carry this message to alcoholics and to practice these principles in all our affairs.

THE TWELVE TRADITIONS

1. Our common welfare should come first; personal recovery depends on AA unity.
2. For our group purpose there is but one ultimate authority—a loving God as He may express Himself in our group conscience. Our leaders are but trusted servants; they do not govern.
3. The one requirement for AA membership is a desire to stop drinking.
4. Each group should be autonomous except in matters affecting other groups or AA as a whole.
5. Each group has but one primary purpose—to carry its message to the alcoholic who still suffers.
6. An AA group ought never endorse, finance, or lend the AA name to any related facility or outside enterprise, lest problems of money, property, and prestige divert us from our primary purpose.
7. Every AA group ought to be fully self-supporting, declining outside contributions.
8. Alcoholics Anonymous should remain forever nonprofessional, but our service centers may employ special workers.
9. Alcoholics Anonymous, as such, ought never be organized; but we may create service boards of committees directly responsible to those they serve.
10. Alcoholics Anonymous has no opinion on outside issues; hence, the Alcoholics Anonymous name ought never be drawn into public controversy.
11. Our public relations policy is based on attraction rather than promotion; we need always maintain personal anonymity at the level of press, radio, and films.
12. Anonymity is the spiritual foundation of all our traditions, ever reminding us to place principles before personalities.

The Twelve Steps and Twelve Traditions are reprinted with permission of Alcoholics Anonymous World Services, Inc. (AAWS). Permission to reprint the Twelve Steps and Twelve Traditions does not mean that AAWS has reviewed or approved the contents of this publication, or that AA necessarily agrees with the views expressed herein. AA is a program of recovery from alcoholism only. Use of the Twelve Steps and Twelve Traditions in connection with programs and activities which are patterned after AA, but which address other problems, or in any other non-AA context, does not imply otherwise.

AA accepts alcoholism as an illness and promotes total abstinence as the only cure, emphasizing that the alcoholic person can never safely return to social drinking. They encourage the members to seek sobriety, taking 1 day at a time. The Twelve Traditions are the statements of principles that govern the organization.

AA has been the model for various self-help groups associated with addiction problems. Although AA is, perhaps, the most well-known self-help recovery support service, there are others such as Women for Sobriety and SMART (Self-Management and Recovery Training). Some of the groups and the memberships for which they are organized are listed in Table 23–11. Nurses need to be accurately informed about available self-help groups and their importance as a treatment resource on the health-care continuum so that they can be used as a referral source for patients with substance use disorders.

Pharmacotherapy

Disulfiram (Antabuse): Alcohol Deterrent Therapy

Disulfiram (Antabuse) is a drug that can be administered as a deterrent to drinking to individuals who misuse alcohol. Ingestion of alcohol while taking disulfiram results in a syndrome of symptoms that produce substantial discomfort for the individual and even result in death if the blood alcohol level is high. The reaction varies according to the sensitivity of the individual and how much alcohol was ingested.

Disulfiram works by inhibiting the enzyme aldehyde dehydrogenase, thereby blocking the oxidation

TABLE 23–11 **Addiction Self-Help Groups**	
GROUP	**MEMBERSHIP**
Adult Children of Alcoholics (ACOA)	Adults who grew up with an alcoholic in the home
Al-Anon	Families of alcoholics
Alateen	Adolescent children of alcoholics
Children Are People	School-age children with an alcoholic family member
Cocaine Anonymous	Cocaine addicts
Codependents Anonymous (CoDA)	Families of those with alcohol or other substance use disorders
Families Anonymous	Parents of children who misuse substances
Fresh Start	Nicotine addicts
Gamblers Anonymous	Gambling addicts
Narcotics Anonymous	Narcotics addicts
Nar-Anon	Families of narcotics addicts
Overeaters Anonymous	Food addicts
Pills Anonymous	Polysubstance addicts
Pot Smokers Anonymous	Marijuana smokers
Smokers Anonymous	Nicotine addicts
Women for Sobriety	Female alcoholics
SMART (Self-Management and Recovery Training) and CRAFT (Community Reinforcement and Family Training) group meetings	Individuals, family, and friends with many types of addictions, e.g., Alcohol, Eating Disorders, Marijuana, Gambling, Prescription Drugs, Heroin, Sex Addiction, Smoking

of alcohol at the stage when acetaldehyde is converted to acetate. The resulting acetaldehyde accumulation in the blood is thought to produce the symptoms associated with the disulfiram-alcohol reaction. These symptoms persist as long as alcohol is being metabolized. The rate of alcohol elimination does not appear to be affected.

Symptoms of disulfiram-alcohol reaction can occur within 5 to 10 minutes of ingestion of alcohol. Mild reactions can occur at blood alcohol levels as low as 5 to 10 mg/dL. Symptoms are fully developed at approximately 50 mg/dL and may include flushed skin, throbbing in the head and neck, respiratory difficulty, dizziness, nausea and vomiting, sweating, hyperventilation, tachycardia, hypotension, weakness, blurred vision, and confusion. With a blood alcohol level of approximately 125 to 150 mg/dL, severe reactions can occur, including respiratory depression, cardiovascular collapse, arrhythmias, myocardial infarction, acute congestive heart failure, unconsciousness, convulsions, and death.

Disulfiram should not be administered until it has been determined that the client has abstained from alcohol for at least 12 hours. If disulfiram is discontinued, it is important for the client to understand that the sensitivity to alcohol may last for as long as 2 weeks. Consuming alcohol or alcohol-containing substances during this time could result in the disulfiram-alcohol reaction.

The client receiving disulfiram therapy should be aware of and avoid alcohol-containing substances. These products, such as liquid cough and cold preparations, vanilla extract, aftershave lotions, colognes, mouthwash, nail polish removers, and isopropyl alcohol, are capable of producing the symptoms described if ingested or even rubbed on the skin. The individual must read labels carefully and inform any doctor, dentist, or other health-care professional from whom assistance is sought that they are taking disulfiram. In addition, the client must carry a card explaining participation in disulfiram therapy, possible consequences of the therapy, and symptoms that may indicate an emergency.

The client must be assessed carefully before beginning disulfiram therapy. A thorough medical screening is performed before therapy commences, and written informed consent is usually required. The drug is contraindicated in clients at high risk for alcohol ingestion. It is also contraindicated for psychotic clients and clients with severe cardiac, renal, or hepatic disease.

Disulfiram therapy is not a cure for alcoholism. It provides a measure of control for the individual who desires to avoid impulse drinking. Clients receiving disulfiram therapy are encouraged to seek other assistance with their problem, such as AA or another support group, to aid in the recovery process.

Vitamin Replacement in Alcohol Use Disorder

Multivitamin therapy in combination with daily injections or oral administration of thiamine is common protocol. Thiamine is commonly deficient in chronic alcoholics. Replacement therapy is required to prevent neuropathy, confusion, and encephalopathy.

Medication-Assisted Treatment

Medication-assisted treatment refers to the use of a medication to decrease the intensity of symptoms in an individual who is withdrawing from or who is experiencing the effects of excessive use of alcohol and other drugs and to decrease cravings by administering a controlled dose of another medication. A discussion of the types of medication-assisted treatment for specific withdrawal syndromes follows.

Alcohol Withdrawal

Benzodiazepines are widely used drugs for medication-assisted treatment in alcohol withdrawal. Benzodiazepines act similarly to alcohol in their effects but can be administered in controlled doses to prevent adverse effects of alcohol withdrawal. Chlordiazepoxide (Librium), oxazepam (Serax), lorazepam (Ativan), and diazepam (Valium) are the most commonly used agents. The approach to treatment with benzodiazepines for alcohol withdrawal is to start with relatively high doses and reduce the dosage by 20% to 25% each day until withdrawal is complete. Additional doses may be given for breakthrough signs or symptoms. In people with liver disease, accumulation of the longer-acting agents (chlordiazepoxide and diazepam) may be problematic, and use of the shorter-acting benzodiazepines (lorazepam or oxazepam) is more appropriate.

Anticonvulsant medications are also used in treating alcohol withdrawal (e.g., carbamazepine, valproic acid, phenobarbital, or gabapentin) to prevent withdrawal seizures. These drugs are particularly useful in individuals who have had repeated episodes of alcohol withdrawal. Repeated episodes of withdrawal appear to "kindle" even more serious withdrawal episodes, including the production of withdrawal seizures that can result in brain damage (Julien, 2014).

These anticonvulsants have been used successfully in both acute withdrawal and to reduce longer-term craving. Rosenson and associates (2013) found that a single IV dose of phenobarbital along with symptom-guided lorazepam for management of acute withdrawal reduced intensive care unit (ICU) admissions and did not have any adverse effects.

Alcohol Abstinence

The narcotic antagonist naltrexone (ReVia [oral], Vivitrol [injection]) was approved by the FDA in 1994 for the treatment of alcohol addiction. Naltrexone, which was approved in 1984 for the treatment of heroin addiction, works on the same receptors in the brain that produce the feelings of pleasure when heroin or other opiates bind to them but does not produce the same "narcotic high" and is not habit forming. Although alcohol does not bind to these same brain receptors, a meta-analysis of research studies (Del Re et al., 2013) concluded that naltrexone affords a small but significant effect in percent days of abstinence and relapse to drinking. In comparison to placebo-treated individuals, participants on naltrexone therapy showed significantly lower overall relapse rates and fewer drinks per drinking day among those who did resume drinking. In 2004 the FDA approved acamprosate (Campral), which is indicated for the maintenance of abstinence from alcohol in patients with alcohol addiction who are abstinent at treatment initiation. The mechanism of action of acamprosate in maintenance of alcohol abstinence is not completely understood. It is hypothesized to restore the normal balance between neuronal excitation and inhibition by interacting with glutamate and GABA neurotransmitter systems. Acamprosate is ineffective in those who have not undergone detoxification and not achieved alcohol abstinence before beginning treatment. It is recommended for concomitant use with psychosocial therapy.

An OTC antioxidant, *N*-acetylcysteine, has demonstrated in animal studies to be beneficial in reducing alcohol-seeking and withdrawal symptoms and preventing alcohol toxicity. However, only one study in humans has shown that it may decrease use in adolescents who are using alcohol and marijuana concurrently (Tomko et al., 2018). More research is needed, and *N*-acetylcysteine is currently not approved by the FDA for treatment of substance use disorders.

Opiate Intoxication

Examples of drugs in the opioid classification include opium, morphine, codeine, heroin, hydromorphone, oxycodone, and hydrocodone. Synthetic opiate-like narcotic analgesics include meperidine, methadone, pentazocine, tramadol, fentanyl, carfentanil, sufentanil, and U-47700.

Opiate intoxication is treated with narcotic antagonists such as naloxone (Narcan) or naltrexone (ReVia, Vivitrol) to prevent relapse. In 2015 the FDA approved an intranasal form of naloxone hydrochloride under a fast-track approval process in response to the continued increase in deaths associated with drug overdose, particularly from respiratory depression and arrest. It is reported to work within 2 minutes but must be given quickly to prevent death (Brown, 2015). *Naloxone* nasal spray can cause severe withdrawal in patients who are opioid dependent. A current concern identified by the recent NIH initiative, HEAL, is a need for stronger, more effective naloxone options because overdoses secondary to fentanyl and carfentanil do not always respond to existing medications. *Naltrexone* is used after opioid intoxication to prevent relapse, but because it is potent blocker of opioids, the individual must be free of opioids for at least 7 to 14 days to avoid sudden withdrawal symptoms. The physician may order a naloxone challenge test before use of naltrexone to ensure a negative challenge test.

Opiate Withdrawal

Opiate withdrawal symptoms, as discussed previously, last for varying amounts of time, depending on the type of opiate. Withdrawal therapy includes rest, adequate nutritional support, and medication-assisted treatment with drugs such as methadone or buprenorphine. Although not all patient treatment plans will include medication-assisted treatment, there is evidence that it is beneficial in reducing withdrawal symptoms, and recent studies have supported that addition of this treatment reduces overall mortality risks (Jancin, 2018). Methadone, if ordered, is given on the first day in a dose sufficient to suppress withdrawal symptoms. The dose is then gradually tapered over a specified time. As the dose of methadone diminishes, renewed abstinence symptoms may be ameliorated by the addition of clonidine. Some patients are maintained on medication-assisted treatment indefinitely, although this was not the original intent for these drugs. Grossman, as cited by Jancin (2018), reported that studies repeatedly demonstrate that when treatment stops, the risk of relapse increases. Methadone can only be administered in methadone clinics that are overseen at state and federal levels.

In 2002 the FDA approved two forms of the drug buprenorphine for treating opiate addiction. Buprenorphine is an opioid partial agonist (whereas methadone is an opioid agonist, similar to morphine). It is considered to be somewhat safer and causes fewer side effects, making it especially attractive for people who are mildly or moderately addicted. Individuals are able to access treatment with buprenorphine in office-based settings, providing an alternative to methadone clinics. Physicians who prescribe buprenorphine must be certified to do so by the Society of Addiction Medicine, the American Academy of Addiction Psychiatry, the APA, or other associations deemed appropriate. The number of patients to whom individual physicians may provide outpatient buprenorphine treatment was previously limited to 100, but in response to the growing opioid epidemic, a new federal rule became effective in August 2016 increasing the allowable number to 275 patients, with stipulations about necessary credentialing in addictions medicine or addictions psychiatry and allowable practice settings. Currently, buprenorphine/naloxone combinations (in sublingual tablets or film, buccal film, extended-release, and long-acting injectable forms) and injectable naltrexone are all options for medication-assisted treatment of opioid addiction.

Clonidine (Catapres) also has been used to suppress opiate withdrawal symptoms. As monotherapy, it is not as effective as substitution with methadone, but it is nonaddicting and serves as a bridge to enable the individual to stay opiate free long enough to facilitate termination of methadone maintenance.

In 2018 the FDA approved lofexidine (Lucemyra), the first nonopioid medication specifically for the management of opioid withdrawal symptoms. It is used to facilitate abrupt discontinuation of opioids in adults. Lofexidine is a selective alpha-2-adrenergic receptor agonist that reduces the release of norepinephrine and is believed to be beneficial in easing withdrawal symptoms. It was originally being evaluated as an antihypertensive, but research was halted when it was found to be less effective than clonidine. It may be more desirable than clonidine in the management of opiate withdrawal because it has fewer side effects (DrugBank, 2021). The FDA approved this medication on fast-track status and is requiring additional postmarket studies. Future studies will be conducted to evaluate its benefits in neonatal opiate withdrawal. Currently, it is only approved for 14 days of treatment in adults.

Barbiturate Withdrawal

Medication-assisted treatment for CNS depressant withdrawal (particularly barbiturates) is most commonly used with the long-acting barbiturate phenobarbital (Luminal). The dosage required to suppress withdrawal symptoms is administered. When stabilization has been achieved, the dose is gradually decreased by 30 mg/day until withdrawal is complete. Long-acting benzodiazepines are commonly used for medication-assisted treatment when the misused substance is a nonbarbiturate CNS depressant.

Stimulant Intoxication

Treatment of stimulant intoxication usually begins with minor tranquilizers such as chlordiazepoxide and progresses to major tranquilizers such as haloperidol (Haldol). Antipsychotics should be administered with caution because of their propensity to lower the seizure threshold. Repeated seizures are treated with IV diazepam.

Stimulant Withdrawal

Withdrawal from CNS stimulants does not constitute a medical emergency such as that observed with CNS depressants like alcohol or benzodiazepines. Treatment is usually aimed at reducing drug craving and managing severe depression. The individual is placed in a quiet atmosphere and allowed to sleep and eat as much as is needed or desired. Suicide precautions may need to be instituted. Antidepressant therapy may be helpful in treating symptoms of depression.

Hallucinogens and Cannabinoids

Medication-assisted treatment is not required with these drugs, and there are no FDA-approved medications for the treatment of these substance use disorders. When adverse reactions such as anxiety or panic occur, benzodiazepines (e.g., diazepam or chlordiazepoxide) may be prescribed to prevent harm to the patient or others. Psychotic reactions may be treated with antipsychotic medications.

Counseling

Counseling on a one-to-one basis is often used to help the client who misuses substances. The relationship is goal directed, and the length of the counseling may vary from weeks to years. The focus is on current reality, development of a working treatment relationship, and strengthening ego assets. The counselor must be warm, kind, and nonjudgmental yet able to set limits firmly. Research consistently demonstrates that personal characteristics of counselors are highly predictive of client outcomes. In addition to technical counseling skills, many important therapeutic qualities affect the outcome of counseling, including insight, respect, genuineness, concreteness, and empathy (SAMHSA, 2014). Often counselors in substance use disorders treatment are themselves engaged in an ongoing recovery program from alcohol or drug addiction or both. Having the shared experience of addiction is considered an opportunity to develop connection and compassion with the client, and there is typically more self-disclosure about the counselors' own journey than is typical in psychiatric settings.

Counseling of the client who misuses substances involves various phases, each of which is of indeterminate length. In the first phase, an assessment is conducted. Factual data are collected to determine whether the client does indeed have a problem with substances; that is, that substances are regularly impairing effective functioning in one or more significant life areas.

After the assessment, in the working phase of the relationship, the counselor assists the individual to accept that the use of substances causes problems in significant life areas and that they are not able to prevent these problems. The client states a desire to make changes. The strength of the denial system is determined by the duration and extent of substance-related adverse effects in the person's life. Thus, those individuals with minor substance-related problems of recent origin have less difficulty with this stage than those with long-term extensive impairment. The individual also works to gain self-control and abstain from substances.

Once the problem has been identified and sobriety achieved, the client must have a concrete and workable plan for getting through the early weeks of abstinence. Anticipatory guidance through role-playing helps the individual practice how they will respond when substances are readily obtainable and the impulse to partake is strong.

Counseling often includes the family or specific family members. In family counseling, the therapist tries to help each member see how they have affected and been affected by the substance misuse behavior. Family strengths are mobilized, and family members are encouraged to move in a positive direction. Referrals are often made to self-help groups such as Al-Anon, Nar-Anon, Alateen, Families Anonymous, and Adult Children of Alcoholics.

Group Therapy

Group therapy has long been regarded as a powerful agent of change with those who misuse substances. In groups, individuals are able to share their experiences with others going through similar problems. They are able to "see themselves in others" and thus confront their defenses about giving up the substance. They may recognize similar attitudes and defenses in others. Groups also give individuals the capacity to communicate needs and feelings directly.

In task-oriented education groups, the leader is charged with presenting material associated with substance misuse and its effects on the person's life. Other educational groups that may be effective include assertiveness techniques and relaxation training. Teaching groups differ from psychotherapy groups, whose focus is on helping individuals understand and manage difficult feelings and situations, particularly as they relate to substance use.

Therapy groups and self-help groups such as AA complement each other. Whereas the self-help group focus is on achieving and maintaining sobriety, in the therapy group the individual may learn more adaptive ways of coping, how to deal with problems that may have arisen from or were exacerbated by the former substance use, and ways to improve quality of life and function more effectively without substances.

Nonsubstance Addictions

Gambling Disorder

Gambling disorder is defined by the *DSM-5-TR* as persistent and recurrent problematic gambling behavior leading to clinically significant impairment or distress (APA, 2022). The preoccupation with and impulse to gamble often intensifies when the individual is under stress. Many impulsive gamblers describe a physical sensation of restlessness and anticipation that can be relieved only by placing a bet. Winning stimulates reward centers in the brain, increasing feelings of power and decreasing anxiety. The problem gambler increasingly uses gambling to try to cope with stress and regain a sense of control.

As the need to gamble increases, the individual is forced to obtain money by any means available, such as borrowing money from illegal sources or pawning personal items (or items that belong to others). As gambling debts accrue, or out of a need to continue gambling, the individual may desperately resort to forgery, theft, or even embezzlement. Family relationships are disrupted, and impairment in occupational functioning may occur because of absences from work in order to gamble.

Gambling behavior usually begins in adolescence; however, compulsive behaviors rarely occur before young adulthood. The disorder generally runs a chronic course, with periods of waxing and waning that are largely dependent on psychosocial stress. Although comprehensive statistics are lacking, available information estimates that 1% to 2% of the general population are problem gamblers (Boland & Verduin, 2022). It is more common among men than women.

Various personality disorder traits have been associated with pathological gambling. In a systematic review and meta-analysis (Dowling et al., 2015), the most prevalent included narcissistic, antisocial, avoidant, obsessive-compulsive, and borderline traits. The researchers conclude that in any treatment setting for gambling disorders, screening, and treatment for these common comorbid conditions must be addressed. Common comorbidities include depression, suicide ideation, substance use disorders, and PTSD. Gambling problems may be episodic and increase during periods of stress or depression, or the behavior may be persistent (APA, 2022).

Predisposing Factors to Gambling Disorder

Biological Influences

Genetic Familial and twin studies show an increased prevalence of pathological gambling in family members of individuals diagnosed with the disorder. Black and associates (2014) found that first-degree relatives of pathological gamblers were eight times more likely to develop the same condition, which suggests an underlying genetic predisposition.

Physiological Studies of dopamine receptor systems have implicated this neurotransmitter in the development of addictive personality traits, including pathological gambling (Weiss & Pontone, 2014). Support for this association comes from studies that demonstrated a correlation between the development of pathological gambling behaviors after individuals were treated with dopamine receptor agonist drugs (Lanteri et al., 2018; Scavone et al., 2019).

Biochemical theories suggest that, ironically, both winning and losing (perhaps related to the excitement of taking a risk) may stimulate the reward and pleasure centers of the brain. This response could contribute to persistent and repeated desire to gamble even when one is not winning.

Psychosocial Influences

Boland and Verduin (2022) reported that the following may be predisposing factors to the development of pathological gambling: "loss of a parent by death, separation, divorce, or desertion before the child is 15 years of age; inappropriate parental discipline (absence, inconsistency, or harshness); exposure to and availability of gambling activities for the adolescent; a family emphasis on material and financial symbols; and a lack of family emphasis on saving, planning, and budgeting." (p. 332)

Treatment Modalities for Gambling Disorder

Because most pathological gamblers deny that they have a problem, treatment is difficult. Most gamblers only seek treatment due to legal difficulties, family pressures, or other psychiatric complaints. Behavior therapy, CBT, motivational interviewing, 12-step programs (Gamblers Anonymous), and self-help strategies such as bibliotherapy (the use of stories or other texts to support recovery) have all been used with pathological gambling with various degrees of success. About one-third of individuals with gambling disorders recover without need for treatment (Rash et al., 2016). Some medications have been used with effective results in the treatment of pathological gambling. Selective serotonin reuptake inhibitors (SSRIs) and clomipramine have been used to treat obsessive-compulsive disorders and may have benefits for those with gambling disorder who have comorbid obsessive-compulsive traits.

Lithium, carbamazepine, and naltrexone have also been shown effective.

Possibly the most effective treatment of pathological gambling is participation by the individual in **Gamblers Anonymous (GA)**. This self-help group is modeled on AA.

CLINICAL JUDGMENT IN ACTION: CASE STUDY AND SAMPLE CARE PLAN

NURSING HISTORY AND ASSESSMENT

Recognizing cues: The nurse must demonstrate ability to recognize what information is most important to making an assessment (National Council of State Boards of Nursing [NCSBN], 2021). This information is italicized in the following collection of data.

The police bring Dan to the emergency department of the local hospital around 9 p.m. His wife, Cassandra, called 911 when *Dan became violent,* and she began to fear for her safety. Dan was *fired from his job* as a foreman in a manufacturing plant for refusing to follow his supervisor's directions on a project. When cleaning up after his move, *several partially used liquor bottles were found in his work area.*

Cassandra reports that Dan *has been drinking since he came home shortly after noon today.* He bloodied her nose and punched her in the stomach when she poured the contents of a bottle he was drinking down the kitchen sink. The police responded to her call and brought Dan to the hospital in handcuffs. By the time they arrive at the hospital, Dan has calmed down and appears drugged and drowsy. *His blood alcohol level measures 247 mg/dL.* He *acknowledges that his drinking has "gotten out of control" and he expresses remorse for his violent behavior.* He admits that he *drinks daily because if he doesn't he feels sick.* He is admitted to the detoxification unit of the hospital with a diagnosis of alcohol intoxication.

Cassandra tells the admitting nurse that she and Dan have been married for 12 years. He was a social drinker before they were married, but his *drinking has increased over the years.* He has been under a lot of stress at work; hates his job, his boss, and his coworkers; and is *depressed a lot of the time.* He *never had a loving relationship with his parents, who are now deceased.* For the *past few years, his pattern has been to come home, start drinking immediately, and drink until he passes out for the night.* She states that she has tried to get him to go for help with his drinking, but he refuses and says that he doesn't have a problem. Cassandra begins to cry and says to the nurse, "We can't go on like this. I don't know what to do!"

Analyzing cues: The nurse must be able to interpret the information (NCSBN, 2021).

The nurse interprets that this episode of drinking is not an isolated incident and the patient's report that he feels sick when he doesn't drink suggests the presence of withdrawal symptoms. The nurse interprets that Cassandra's report of Dan being depressed a lot of the time warrants further assessment.

Prioritize hypotheses: The nurse must be able to identify the client's most important needs (NCSBN, 2021).

The nurse conducts further assessment and determines that although Dan admits to feeling depressed, he denies suicide ideation or previous attempts. They collaborate to develop a plan for safe detoxification from alcohol and relapse prevention.

NURSING DIAGNOSES AND OUTCOME IDENTIFICATION

Generate solutions: The nurse must be able to connect their prioritized understanding of client needs to a course of action or plan of care (NCSBN, 2021).

From the assessment data, the nurse develops the following nursing diagnoses for Dan:

1. Risk for injury related to alcohol withdrawal.
   a. Short-term goal: Dan's condition will stabilize within 72 hours.
   b. Long-term goal: Dan will not experience physical injury.
2. Ineffective coping related to low self-esteem, weak ego development, and underlying fears and anxieties.
   a. Short-term goal: Dan will focus immediate attention on behavioral changes required to achieve sobriety.
   b. Long-term goal: Dan will accept responsibility for his drinking behaviors and acknowledge the association between his drinking and personal problems.

PLANNING AND IMPLEMENTATION

Take Action: The nurse must be able to identify what actions need to be taken and how they will be implemented (NCSBN, 2021).

RISK FOR INJURY

The following nursing interventions may be implemented *to ensure patient safety:*

1. Assess Dan's level of disorientation; frequently orient him to reality and his surroundings.
2. Obtain a drug history.
3. Obtain a urine sample for analysis.
4. Place Dan in a quiet room (private, if possible).

5. Ensure that smoking materials and other potentially harmful objects are stored away.
6. Observe Dan frequently. Take vital signs every 15 to 30 minutes.
7. Monitor for signs of withdrawal within a few hours after admission. Watch for signs of
   ■ Increased heart rate
   ■ Tremors
   ■ Headache
   ■ Diaphoresis
   ■ Agitation; restlessness
   ■ Nausea
   ■ Fever
   ■ Convulsions
8. Follow medication regimen, as ordered by physician (commonly a benzodiazepine, thiamine, multivitamin).

INEFFECTIVE COPING

The following nursing interventions may be implemented *to help Dan accept responsibility for the behavioral consequences associated with his drinking and to develop more effective coping skills:*

1. Develop Dan's trust by spending time with him, being honest, and keeping all promises.
2. Ensure that Dan understands that it is not *him* but his *behavior* that is unacceptable.
3. Provide Dan with accurate information about the effects of alcohol. Do this in a matter-of-fact, nonjudgmental way.
4. Point out recent negative events that have occurred in Dan's life and associate the use of alcohol with these events. Help him to see the association.
5. Use confrontation with caring: "Yes, your wife called the police. You were physically abusive. She was afraid. And your blood alcohol level was 247 when you were brought in. You were obviously not in control of your behavior at the time."
6. Don't accept excuses for his drinking. Point out rationalization and projection behaviors. These behaviors prolong denial that he has a problem. He must directly accept responsibility for his drinking (not make excuses and blame it on the behavior of others). He must come to understand that only *he* has control of his behavior.
7. Encourage Dan to attend group therapy during treatment and AA after treatment. Peer feedback is a strong factor in helping individuals recognize their problems and ultimately remain sober.
8. Encourage Cassandra to attend Al-Anon meetings. She can benefit from the experiences of others who have experienced and are experiencing the same types of problems as she is.
9. Help Dan to identify ways that he can cope besides using alcohol, such as exercise, sports, and relaxation. He should choose what is most appropriate for him and be given positive feedback for efforts made toward change.

EVALUATION

Evaluate outcomes: The nurse must be able to evaluate actions taken and determine whether they have had a positive, neutral, or negative effect (NCSBN, 2021).

The outcome criteria identified for Dan have been met. He experienced an uncomplicated withdrawal from verbalizes understanding of the relationship between his personal problems and his drinking and accepts responsibility for his own behavior. He verbalizes understanding that alcohol addiction is an illness that requires ongoing support and treatment, and he regularly attends AA meetings. Cassandra regularly attends Al-Anon meetings.

Summary and Key Points

■ An individual is considered to be addicted to a substance when they are unable to control its use, even knowing that it interferes with normal functioning; when increasing amounts of the substance are required to produce the desired effects; and when characteristic withdrawal symptoms develop upon cessation or drastic decrease in use of the substance.

■ *Substance intoxication* is defined as the development of a reversible syndrome of maladaptive behavioral or psychological changes due to the direct physiological effects of a substance on the CNS and develop during or shortly after ingestion of (or exposure to) a substance.

■ *Substance withdrawal* is the development of a substance-specific maladaptive behavioral change, with physiological and cognitive concomitants, due to the cessation of or reduction in heavy and prolonged substance use.

■ The etiology of substance use disorders is unknown. Various contributing factors have been implicated, such as genetics, biochemical changes, developmental influences, personality factors, social learning, conditioning, and cultural and ethnic influences.

■ Although multiple factors influence the development of a substance use disorder, it is clearly a disease of the brain.

■ Seven classes of substances are presented in this chapter in terms of a profile of the substance,

■ historical aspects, patterns of use and misuse, and effects on the body. They include alcohol, other CNS depressants, CNS stimulants, opioids, hallucinogens, inhalants, and cannabinoids.

■ The nurse uses the nursing process as the vehicle for delivery of care of the patient with a substance-related disorder.

■ The nurse must first examine their own feelings regarding personal substance use and substance use by others. Only the nurse who can be accepting and nonjudgmental of substance-use behaviors will be effective in working with these patients.

■ Specialized care is given to patients with dual diagnoses of mental illness and substance use disorders.

■ Addiction to substances is a problem for many members of the nursing profession. Most state boards of nursing and state nurses' associations have established avenues for peer assistance to provide help to impaired members of the profession.

■ Individuals who are reared in families with chemically addicted people learn patterns of dysfunctional behavior that carry over into adult life. One of these dysfunctional behavior patterns is *codependence*. Codependent individuals sacrifice their own needs for the fulfillment of the needs of others in order to achieve a sense of control. Many nurses also have codependent traits.

■ Treatment modalities for substance-related disorders include self-help groups, deterrent therapy, individual counseling, and group therapy. Medication-assisted treatment is frequently implemented for individuals experiencing substance intoxication or substance withdrawal or to prevent relapse. Treatment modalities are implemented on an inpatient basis or in outpatient settings, depending on the severity of the impairment.

■ Gambling disorder is defined by the *DSM-5-TR* as persistent and recurrent problematic gambling behavior leading to clinically significant impairment or distress. Gambling disorder may have a genetic component; other etiologies include abnormalities in serotonergic, noradrenergic, and dopaminergic neurotransmitter systems. A number of psychosocial influences have also been implicated in the predisposition to gambling disorder, including dysfunctional family patterns.

■ Behavior therapy, cognitive therapy, motivational interviewing, 12-step programs (Gamblers Anonymous), and self-help strategies such as bibliotherapy have been used with gambling disorder with various degrees of success. Medications such as SSRIs, clomipramine, lithium, carbamazepine, and naltrexone have also been tried.

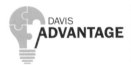 DAVIS **ADVANTAGE** | Go to **Davis Advantage** to complete your learning: strengthen understanding, apply your knowledge, and prepare for the Next Gen NCLEX®.

Review Questions

1. A client is admitted to the hospital after an extended period of binge alcohol drinking. His wife reports that he has been a heavy drinker for several years. Laboratory reports reveal he has a blood alcohol level of 250 mg/dL. He is placed on the chemical addiction unit for detoxification. When would the first signs of alcohol withdrawal symptoms be expected to occur?
   a. Several hours after the last drink
   b. 2 to 3 days after the last drink
   c. 4 to 5 days after the last drink
   d. 6 to 7 days after the last drink

2. Symptoms of alcohol withdrawal include:
   a. Euphoria, hyperactivity, and insomnia.
   b. Depression, suicidal ideation, and hypersomnia.
   c. Diaphoresis, nausea and vomiting, and tremors.
   d. Unsteady gait, nystagmus, and profound disorientation.

3. Which of the following medications is the physician most likely to order for a client experiencing alcohol withdrawal syndrome?
   a. Haloperidol (Haldol)
   b. Chlordiazepoxide (Librium)
   c. Methadone (Dolophine)
   d. Cannabidiol (Epidiolex)

4. A client who has been admitted to the chemical dependence treatment unit after being disciplined for drinking on the job states to the nurse, "I don't have a problem with alcohol. I can handle my booze better than anyone I know." Which defense mechanism is the client using?
   a. Denial
   b. Projection
   c. Displacement
   d. Rationalization

5. A client who has been admitted to the alcohol rehabilitation unit after being fired for drinking on the job states to the nurse, "I don't have a problem with alcohol. My boss is a jerk! I haven't missed any more days than my coworkers." What is the nurse's best response?
   a. "Maybe your boss is mistaken."
   b. "You are here because your drinking was interfering with your work."
   c. "Get real! You're an alcoholic and you know it!"
   d. "Why do you think your boss is a jerk?"

Clinical Judgment Questions

6. A client who has been admitted to intensive outpatient treatment for substance use disorder arrives for group therapy and appears groggy with constricted pupils. The client denies using substances. Which of the following would be the best intervention at this time?
   a. Ask the client to empty their pockets.
   b. Smell the client's breath for evidence of alcohol.
   c. Conduct a drug screen to assess for presence of opioids.
   d. Discharge the client for failure to comply with treatment expectations.

7. A client admitted to the inpatient detoxification program for alcohol withdrawal approaches the nurse complaining of nausea and feeling shaky. The nurse notices that the client has hand tremors and appears diaphoretic. Which of these nursing interventions is a priority?
   a. Check the client's temperature.
   b. Send a urine sample to the laboratory for a random drug screen.
   c. Ask the client if there is anything that they are particularly stressed about.
   d. Administer prn benzodiazepine that was ordered for management of withdrawal symptoms.

8. A client comes into the emergency department stating that they are "crashing" and feel like they would "be better off dead." Which of these nursing interventions is a priority?
   a. Instruct the client not to worry; these are temporary signs of withdrawal and should go away in a few days.
   b. Request an order for amphetamines to ease the client's withdrawal symptoms.
   c. Assess the client's risk for suicide.
   d. Instruct the physician that the client may need naloxone.

9. A client is brought to the emergency department unconscious by a friend who says the individual was injecting heroin. The client is assessed to have a weak pulse. Which of these interventions are priorities?
   a. Administer naloxone and rescue breathing.
   b. IV benzodiazepines and continuous monitoring of vital signs.
   c. Ask the friend how much heroin the person took and confirm with a laboratory drug screen.
   d. Initiate cardiopulmonary resuscitation and prepare to use an external defibrillator.

10. A client admitted to the emergency department smells strongly of alcohol, and his wife reports he has been a heavy drinker for the last 25 years. After the nurse completes an assessment, the physician asks if there are any physical signs of long-term chronic alcohol misuse. Which of these findings should the nurse include in reporting to the physician? (Select all that apply.)
   a. The client reports weak leg muscles, and his gait is unsteady.
   b. The client's abdomen is distended.
   c. The client reports he was coughing up some blood.
   d. The client reports he has double vision.
   e. Blood tests reveal a low white blood cell count.

IMPLICATIONS OF RESEARCH FOR EVIDENCE-BASED PRACTICE

Daviet, R., Aydogan, G., Jagannathan, K., Spilka, N., Koellinger, P. D., Kranzler, H. R., Nave, G., & Wetherill, R. R. (2022). Associations between alcohol consumption and gray and white matter volumes in the UK Biobank. *Nature Communications, 13,* 1175. https://doi.org/10.1038/s41467-022-28735-5

DESCRIPTION OF THE STUDY: Previous research has demonstrated an association between heavy alcohol consumption and brain atrophy, neuronal loss, and loss of white matter. Researchers in this study examined the associations between alcohol intake and brain structure in generally healthy middle-aged and older adults (N = 36,678) to determine whether there were negative associations between alcohol intake and brain structures at lower levels of alcohol intake.

RESULTS OF THE STUDY: This study found that there were, indeed, negative associations between drinking as little as one to two drinks per day and changes in brain macrostructure and microstructure that were already apparent at this consumption level and became stronger as alcohol intake increased.

IMPLICATIONS FOR NURSING PRACTICE: Nurses play an active role in educating patients about health-related behaviors. Studies such as this guide the nurse in making evidence-based recommendations.

TEST YOUR CLINICAL REASONING AND CLINICAL JUDGMENT SKILLS

Kelly, age 23 years, is a first-year law student engaged to a surgical resident at the local university hospital. She has been struggling to do well in law school because she wants to make her parents, two prominent local attorneys, proud of her. She had never aspired to do anything but go into law, and that is also what her parents expected her to do.

Kelly's midterm grades were not as high as she had hoped, so she increased the number of hours of study time, staying awake all night several nights a week to study. She started drinking large amounts of coffee to stay awake but still found herself falling asleep as she tried to study at the library and in her apartment. As final examinations approached, she began to panic that she would not be able to continue the pace of studying she felt she needed to make the grades she hoped for.

One of Kelly's classmates told her that she needed some "speed" to give her that extra energy to study. Her classmate said, "All the kids do it. Hardly anyone I know gets through law school without it." She gave Kelly the name of a source.

Kelly contacted the source, who supplied her with enough amphetamines to see her through final examinations. Kelly was excited, because she had so much energy, did not require sleep, and was able to study the additional hours she thought she needed for the examinations. However, when the results were posted, Kelly had failed two courses and would have to repeat them in summer school if she was to continue with her class in the fall. She continued to replenish her supply of amphetamines from her contact until he told her he could not get her anymore. She became frantic and stole a prescription blank from her fiancé and forged his name for more pills.

She started taking increasing amounts of the medication to achieve the high she wanted to feel. Her behavior became erratic. Yesterday, her fiancé received a call from a pharmacy to clarify an order for amphetamines that Kelly had written. He insisted that she admit herself to the chemical addiction unit for detoxification.

On the unit, she appears tired and depressed, moves very slowly, and wants to sleep all the time. She keeps saying to the nurse, "I'm a real failure. I'll never be an attorney like my parents. I'm too dumb. I just wish I could die."

Answer the following questions related to Kelly:

1. What is the primary nursing diagnosis for Kelly?
2. Describe important nursing interventions to be implemented with Kelly.
3. In addition to physical safety, what would be the primary short-term goal the nurses would strive to achieve with Kelly?

Communication Exercises

1. Tom is a patient on the alcohol treatment unit. He says to the nurse, "My boss and my wife ganged up on me. They think I have a drinking problem. I don't have a drinking problem! I can quit any time I want to!"

    How would the nurse respond appropriately to this statement by Tom?

2. Tom says to the nurse, "My head hurts. I didn't sleep very well last night. I'm getting shaky and it's hot in here! I could sure use a cup of coffee and a cigarette."

    How would the nurse respond appropriately to this statement by Tom?

3. Tom says, "Sure, I missed a couple days of work. Everyone gets sick now and then. I don't think my wife cares about what happens to me. She and my boss got together and decided I needed to be here, or I lose my job!"

    How would the nurse respond appropriately to this statement by Tom?

MOVIE CONNECTIONS

Affliction (alcoholism) • *Days of Wine and Roses* (alcoholism) • *I'll Cry Tomorrow* (alcoholism) • *When a Man Loves a Woman* (alcoholism) • *Clean and Sober* (addiction–cocaine) • *28 Days* (alcoholism) • *Lady Sings the Blues* (addiction–heroin) • *I'm Dancing as Fast as I Can* (addiction–sedatives) • *The Rose* (polysubstance addiction) • *Ben Is Back* (polysubstance addiction) • *Beautiful Boy* (amphetamine addiction) • *Six Balloons* (heroin addiction) • *A Star Is Born* (alcoholism)

References

Ahmed, S., Roth, R. M., Stanciu, C. N., & Brunette, M. F. (2021). The impact of THC and CBD in schizophrenia: A systematic review. *Frontiers in Psychiatry, 12,* 694394. https://doi.org/10.3389/fpsyt.2021.694394

Alcohol Action Ireland. (2022). *Alcohol facts: Overview of alcohol-related harm.* https://alcoholireland.ie/facts/alcohol-related-harm-facts-and-statistics/

American Academy of Child and Adolescent Psychiatry. (2022). *Facts for families: Children of alcoholics.* https://www.aacap.org/AACAP/Families_and_Youth/Facts_for_Families/FFF-Guide/Children-Of-Alcoholics-017.aspx

American Psychiatric Association (APA). (2022). *Diagnostic and statistical manual of mental disorders fifth edition, text revision (DSM-5-TR).* APA.

American Society of Addiction Medicine. (2020). *The ASAM national practice guideline for the treatment of opioid use disorder: Focused update.* http://eguideline.guidelinecentral.com/i/1224390-national-practice-guideline-for-the-treatment-of-opioid-use-disorder-2020-update/0?

Attipoe, S., Leggit, J., & Deuster, P. A. (2016). Caffeine content in popular energy drinks and energy shots. *Military Medicine, 181* (9), 1016–1020. https://doi.org/10.7205/MILMED-D-15-00459

Beatty, M. (2011). *Codependent no more.* Hazelden.

Black, D., Coryell, W., Crowe, R., McCormick, B., Shaw, M., & Allen, J. A. (2014). Direct, controlled, blind family study of DSM-IV pathological gambling. *Journal of Clinical Psychiatry, 75*(3), 215–221. doi:10.4088/JCP.13m08566

Boland, R., & Verduin, M. L. (2022). *Kaplan & Sadock's synopsis of psychiatry* (P. Ruiz, Ed.). (12th ed.). Wolters Kluwer.

Brooks, M. (2018). *FDA goes ahead with approval of sufentanil despite controversy.* www.medscape.com/viewarticle/904330

Brown, T. (2015). *FDA approves Narcan nasal spray to treat opioid overdose.* www.medscape.com/viewarticle/854716

Butt, Y. M., Smith, M. L., Tazelaar, H. D., Vaszer, L. T., Swanson, K. L., & Mayo Clinic. (2019). Pathology of vaping-associated lung injury. *New England Journal of Medicine, 381,* 1780–1781. https://doi.org/10.1056/NEJMc1913069

Centers for Disease Control and Prevention (CDC). (2019). *Notes from the field: Unintentional Drug overdose deaths with kratom detected — 27 states, July 2016–December 2017.* https://www.cdc.gov/mmwr/volumes/68/wr/mm6814a2.htm

Centers for Disease Control and Prevention (CDC). (2020). *Overdose deaths accelerating during covid-19.* https://www.cdc.gov/media/releases/2020/p1218-overdose-deaths-covid-19.html

Centers for Disease Control and Prevention (CDC). (2021a). *Drug Overdose Deaths in the U.S. Up 30% in 2020.* https://www.cdc.gov/nchs/pressroom/nchs_press_releases/2021/20210714.htm

Centers for Disease Control and Prevention (CDC). (2021b). *Opiate overdose: Understanding the epidemic.* https://www.cdc.gov/drugoverdose/epidemic/index.html

Centers for Disease Control and Prevention (CDC). (2021c). *General information about secondhand smoke.* https://www.cdc.gov/tobacco/data_statistics/fact_sheets/secondhand_smoke/general_facts/index.htm

Centers for Disease Control and Prevention (CDC). (2022a). *Fetal alcohol spectrum disorders (FASDs).* www.cdc.gov/ncbddd/fasd/index.html

Centers for Disease Control and Prevention (CDC). (2022b). *Youth and tobacco use.* https://www.cdc.gov/tobacco/data_statistics/fact_sheets/youth_data/tobacco_use/index.htm

Centers for Disease Control and Prevention (CDC). (2023). *Online training and resources: Collaborative for alcohol-free pregnancy.* https://ww https://www.cdc.gov/ncbddd/fasd/searchable-training?Topics=Collaborative%20for%20Alcohol-Free%20Pregnancy%20Courses

Chen, A., & Ashburn, M. A. (2015). Cardiac effects of opioid therapy. *Pain Medicine, 16,* S27–S31. doi:10.1111/pme.12915

Choi, N. G., DiNitto, D. M., Marti, C. N., & Choi, B. Y. (2017). Association of adverse childhood experiences with lifetime mental and substance use disorders among men and women aged 50 + years. *International Psychogeriatrics, 29*(3), 359–372. doi:10.1017/S1041610216001800

Co-Dependents Anonymous (CoDA) (n.d.). https://coda.org/

Davenport, L. (2016). Abuse of OTC antidiarrheal meds linked to cardiac deaths. *Medscape.* https://www.medscape.com/viewarticle/863232

Daviet, R., Aydogan, G., Jagannathan, K., Spilka, N., Koellinger, P. D., Kranzler, H. R., Nave, G., & Wetherill, R. R. (2022). Associations between alcohol consumption and gray and white matter volumes in the UK Biobank. *Nature Communications, 13,* 1175. https://doi.org/10.1038/s41467-022-28735-5

Del Re, A. C., Maisel, N., Blodgett, J., & Finney, J. (2013). The declining efficacy of naltrexone pharmacotherapy for alcohol use disorders over time: A multivariate meta-analysis. *Alcoholism: Clinical and Experimental Research, 37*(6), 1064–1068.

Denny, L., Coles, S., & Blitz, R. (2017). Fetal alcohol syndrome and fetal alcohol spectrum disorders. *American Family Physician, 96*(8), 515–522A.

Dotinga, R. (2018). Methamphetamine use climbing among opioid users. *Clinical Psychiatry News.* https://www.mdedge.com/psychiatry/article/169254/addiction-medicine/methamphetamine-use-climbing-among-opioid-users?utm_source=News_CPN_eNL_070418_F&utm_medium=e-mail&utm_content=Opioid%20users%20turn%20to%20meth

Dowling, N. A., Cowlishaw, S., Jackson, A. C., Merkouris, S. S., Francis, K. L., & Christensen, D. R. (2015). The prevalence of comorbid personality disorders in treatment-seeking problem gamblers: A systematic review and meta-analysis. *Journal of Personality Disorders, 29*(6), 735–754. doi:10.1521/pedi_2014_28_168

DrugBank. (2021). *Lofexidine.* https://www.drugbank.ca/drugs/DB04948

Drugs.com. (2022). *Kratom.* https://www.drugs.com/illicit/kratom.html

Dube, S. R., Felitti, V. J., Dong, M., Chapman, D. P., Giles, W. H., Anda, R. F. (2003). Childhood abuse, neglect, and household dysfunction and the risk of illicit drug use: The adverse childhood experiences study. *Pediatrics, 111*(3), 564–572.

Dubovsky, S. L. (2017). Barbiturates and similar acting substances. In Sadock, B. A., Sadock, V. A., & Ruiz, P. (Eds.), *Comprehensive textbook of psychiatry* (10th ed., pp. 2984–2991). Wolters Kluwer.

Duffy, S. (2016). *DEA classifies deadly synthetic opioid as Schedule I.* www.empr.com/news/dea-classifies-deadly synthetic-opioid-as-schedule-i/article/572194

Evans, D. G. (2020). Medical fraud, mislabeling, contamination: all common in CBD products. *Missouri Medicine, 117*(5), 394–399.

Fernandes, G. S., Spiers, A., Vaidya, N., Zhang, Y., Sharma, E., Holla, B., Heron, J., Hickman, M., Murthy, P., Chakrabarti, A., Basu, D., Subodh, B. N., Singh, L., Singh, R., Kalyanram, K., Kartik, K., Kumaran, K., Krishnaveni, G., Kuriyan, R., Kurpad, S.,….& Benegal, V. (2021). Adverse childhood experiences and substance misuse in young people in India: Results from the multisite cVEDA cohort. *BMC Public Health 21,* 1920. https://doi.org/10.1186/s12889021-11892-5

Ford, E. S., Anda, R. F., Edwards, V. J., Perry, G. S., Zhao, G., Li, C., & Croft, J. B. (2011). Adverse childhood experiences and smoking status in five states. *Preventive Medicine 53*(3), 188–193. doi:10.1016/j.ypmed.2011.06.015

Forster, M., Gower, A. L., Borowsky, I. W., & McMorris, B. J. (2017). Associations between adverse childhood experiences, student-teacher relationships, and nonmedical use of prescription medications among adolescents. *Addictive Behaviors: 68,* 30–34. doi:10.1016/j.addbeh.2017.01.004

Fuentes, J. J., Fonseca, F., Elices, M., Farré, M., & Torrens, M. (2020). Therapeutic use of LSD in psychiatry: A systematic review of randomized-controlled clinical trials. *Frontiers in Psychiatry, 10*(943). https://doi.org/10.3389/fpsyt.2019.00943

Gosdin, L. K., Deputy, N. P., Kim, S. Y., Dang, E. P., & Denny, C. H. (2022). Alcohol consumption and binge drinking during pregnancy among adults aged 18–49 years—United States, 2018–2020. *MMWR 71*(1), 10–13. DOI: http://dx.doi.org/10.15585/mmwr.mm7101a2

Hazelden Betty Ford Foundation. (2021). *Stages of Alcoholism.* https://www.hazeldenbettyford.org/articles/stages-of-alcoholism

Herdman, T. H., Kamitsuru, S., & Lopes, C. T. (Eds.). (2021). *NANDA International, Inc. nursing diagnoses: Definitions and classification 2021–2023.* (12th ed.). Thieme.

Heilig, M., MacKillop, J., Martinez, D., Rehm, J., Leggio, L., & Vanderhuren, L. (2021). Addiction as a brain disease revised: why it still matters, and the need for consilience. *Neuropsychopharmacology, 46,* 1715–1723 (2021). https://doi.org/10.1038/s41386-020-00950-y

Howard, M. O., Bowen, S. E. & Garland, E. L. (2017). Inhalant-related disorders. In Sadock, B. A., Sadock, V. A., & Ruiz P. (Eds.), *Comprehensive textbook of psychiatry* (10th ed., pp. 1328–1342). Wolters Kluwer.

Iannucci, R. A., & Weiss, R. D. (2017). Stimulant-related disorders. In Sadock, B. A., Sadock, V. A., & Ruiz P. (Eds.), *Comprehensive textbook of psychiatry* (10th ed., pp. 1280–1290). Wolters Kluwer.

Institute of Medicine. (2003). *Health professions education: A bridge to quality.* Institute of Medicine.

Jancin, B. (2018). How to prescribe effectively for opioid use disorder. https://www.mdedge.com/internalmedicine/article/171003/addiction-medicine/how-prescribe-effectively-opioid-use-disorder *Family Practice News.* https://www.mdedge.com/familypracticenews/article/171003/addiction-medicine/how-prescribe-effectively opioid-use-disorder

Johnston, L. D., Miech, R. A., O'Malley, P. M., Bachman, J. G., Schulenberg, J. E., & Patrick, M. E. (2022*). Monitoring the Future national survey results on drug use 1975–2021: Overview, key findings on adolescent drug use.* Institute for Social Research, University of Michigan.

Juliano, L. M., & Griffiths, R. R. (2017). Caffeine-related disorders. In Sadock, B. A., Sadock, V. A., & Ruiz P. (Eds.), *Comprehensive textbook of psychiatry* (10th ed., pp. 1291–1303). Wolters Kluwer.

Julien, R. M. (2014). *A primer of drug action: A comprehensive guide to actions, uses and side effects of psychoactive drugs* (13th ed.). Worth Publishers.

Kyei-Baffour, K., & Lindsley, C. W. (2020). DARK classics in chemical neuroscience: U-47700. *ACS Chemical Neuroscience, 11*(23), 3928–3936. https://doi.org/10.1021/acschemneuro.0c00330

Lafferty, K. A. (2017). *Barbiturate toxicity.* https://emedicine.medscape.com/article/813155-overview#a5

Lanska, D. (2022). Alcoholic myopathy. *Medlink Neurology.* www.medlink.com/article/alcoholic_myopathy

Lanteri, P. F., Leguia, A., Doladé, N. G., García, G. C., & Figueras, A. (2018). Drug-induced
gambling disorder: A not so rare but underreported condition. *Psychiatry Research, 269,* 593–595. https://doi.org/10.1016/j.psychres.2018.09.008

Lee, K., Cascella, M., & Marwaha, R. (2022). *Intellectual Disability.* https://www.ncbi.nlm.nih.gov/books/NBK547654/

LeTendre, M. L., & Reed, M. B. (2017). The effect of adverse childhood experience on clinical diagnosis of a substance use disorder: Results of a nationally representative study. *Substance Use & Misuse, 52*(6), 689–697. https://doi.org/10.1080/10826084.2016.1253746

Leweke, F. M., Rohleder, C., Gerth, C. W., Hellmich, M., Pukrop, R., & Koethe, D. (2021). Cannabidiol and amisulpride improve cognition in acute schizophrenia in an explorative, double-blind, active-controlled, randomized clinical trial. *Frontiers in Pharmacology, 12,* 614811. doi: 10.3389/fphar.2021.614811

Maia-Silva, K. M., Zamel, N., Selby, P., Fontes, C. J. F., & Santos, U. P. (2021). Tobacco smoking associated with adverse childhood experiences in a Brazilian community university sample: A case-control study. *Children and Youth Services Review, 120*, 105438. https://doi.org/10.1016/j.childyouth.2020. 105438

Mayo Clinic. (2022). *Caffeine content for coffee, tea, soda, and more.* https://www.mayoclinic.org/healthy-lifestyle/nutrition-and-healthy-eating/in-depth/caffeine/art-20049372

McKeown, N. J. (2022). Toluene toxicity. *Medscape Reference: Drugs, diseases, and procedures.* http://emedicine.medscape.com/article/818939-overview

MPR. (2016). *DEA reverses decision to ban kratom.* www.empr.com/news/dea-reverses-decision-to-ban-kratom/article/559547

Muttoni, S., Ardissino, M., & John, C. (2019). Classical psychedelics for the treatment of depression and anxiety: A systematic review. *Journal of Affective Disorders, 258*, 11–24. https://doi.org/10.1016/j.jad.2019.07.076

National Council of State Boards of Nursing (NCSBN). (2021, Fall). *Next generation NCLEX® News: Comparison between case studies and stand-alone items.* https://www.ncsbn.org/public-files/NGN_Fall21_English_Final.pdf https://www.ncsbn.org/NGN_Fall21_English_Final.pdf

National Institute on Alcohol Abuse and Alcoholism (NIAAA). (2021). *Drug misuse and addiction.* https://www.drugabuse.gov/publications/drugs-brains-behavior-science-addiction/drug-misuse-addiction

National Institute on Alcohol Abuse and Alcoholism (NIAAA). (2022). *Alcohol facts and statistics.* https://www.niaaa.nih.gov/publications/brochures-and-fact-sheets/alcohol-facts-and-statistics

National Institute on Drug Abuse (NIDA). (2018). *National institute on drug abuse (NIDA) principles of drug addiction treatment: A research-based guide (Third Edition)* https://nida.nih.gov/sites/default/files/675-principles-of-drug-addiction-treatment-a-research-based-guide-third-edition.pdfhttps://www.drugabuse.gov/publications/principles-drug-addiction-treatment-research-based-guide-third-edition/evidence-based-approaches-to-drug-addiction-treatment/behavioral-therapies/cognitive-behavioral-therapy

National Institute on Drug Abuse (NIDA). (2019a). *Dramatic increases in maternal opioid use and neonatal abstinence syndrome.* https://www.drugabuse.gov/related-topics/trends-statistics/infographics/dramatic-increases-in-maternal-opioid-use-neonatal-abstinence-syndrome

National Institute on Drug Abuse (NIDA). (2019b). *Marijuana: Drug facts.* https://www.drugabuse.gov/publications/drugfacts/marijuana

National Institute on Drug Abuse (NIDA). (2020a). *Drug Misuse and Addiction.* https://nida.nih.gov/publications/drugs-brains-behavior-science-addiction/drug-misuse-addiction

National Institute on Drug Abuse (NIDA). (2020b). *Synthetic cannabinoids.* https://www.drug abuse.gov/publications/drugfacts/synthetic-cannabinoids-k2spice

National Institute on Drug Abuse (NIDA). (2021). *Marijuana research report.* https://www.drugabuse.gov/publications/research-reports/marijuana/what-marijuana

National Institutes of Health (NIH). (2018). *Comorbidity: Substance use and other mental disorders.* https://www.drugabuse.gov/drug-topics/trends-statistics/infographics/comorbidity-substance-use-other-mental-disorders

National Institutes of Health (NIH). (2019a). *Cannabis (marijuana) and cannabinoids: What you need to know.* https://www.nccih.nih.gov/health/cannabis-marijuana-and-cannabinoids-what-you-need-to-know

National Institutes of Health (NIH). (2019b). *Tobacco, nicotine and vaping.* https://nida.nih.gov/research-topics/tobacconicotine-vaping

National Institutes of Health (NIH). (2022). *Carfentanil.* https://pubchem.ncbi.nlm.nih.gov/compound/Carfentanil

National Library of Medicine (NLM). (2022). *Loss of brain function—Liver disease.* www.nlm.nih.gov/medlineplus/ency/article/000302.htm

Palomar, J. J., Rutherford, C., & Keyes, K. M. (2019). "Flakka" use among high school seniors in the United States. *Drug and Alcohol Dependence, 196*, 86–90. https://doi.org/10.1016/j.drugalcdep.2018.12.014.

Parish, B. S. (2015). *Hallucinogen use.* http://emedicine.medscape.com/article/293752-overview

Patterson. E. (2022). *What is inhalant withdrawal and detoxification like?* https://www.withdrawal.net/inhalant/

Payne, K. S., Mazur, D. J., Hotaling, J. M., & Pastusza, A. W. (2019). Cannabis and male fertility: A systematic review. *Journal of Urology, 202*(4), 674–681.

Rash, C. J., Weinstock, J., & Van Patten, R. (2016). A review of gambling disorder and substance use disorders. *Dovepress, 7*, 3–13. doi:https://doi.org/10.2147/SAR.S83460

Roehler, D. R., Olsen, E. O., Mustaquim, D., & Vivolo-Kantor, A. M. (2021). Suspected nonfatal drug-related overdoses among youth in the US: 2016–2019. *Pediatrics 147*(1), e2020003491. https://doi.org/10.1542/peds.2020-003491

Rosenson, J., Clements, C., Simon, B., Vieaux, J., Graffman, S., Vahidnia, F., Cisse, B., Lam, J., & Alter, H. (2013). Phenobarbital for acute alcohol withdrawal: A prospective randomized double-blind placebo-controlled study. *The Journal of Emergency Medicine, 44*(3), 592–598.

Rothman, E. F., Edwards, E. M., Heeren, T., & Hingson, R. W. (2008). Adverse childhood experiences predict earlier age of drinking onset: Results from a representative US sample of current or former drinkers. *Pediatrics 122*(2), e298–e304.

Scavone, C., Stelitano, B., Rafaniello, C., Rossi, F., Sportiello, L., & Capuano, A. (2019). Drugs-induced pathological gambling: An analysis of Italian spontaneous reporting system. *Journal of Gambling Studies 36*, 85–96. https://doi.org/10.1007/s10899-019-09828-1

Schuckit, M. A. (2017). Alcohol-related disorders. In Sadock, B. A., Sadock, V. A., & Ruiz, P. (Eds.), *Comprehensive textbook of psychiatry* (10th ed., pp. 1264–1279). Wolters Kluwer.

Stanciu, C. N., Hybki, B. G., & Penders, T. M. (2020). Kratom: What we know and what to tell your patients. *Current Psychiatry, 19*(3), 37–42.

Storrs, C. (2016). Is street drug flakka gone for good? www.cnn.com/2016/04/18/health/flakka-drug-disappearance/index.html

Substance Abuse and Mental Health Services Administration (SAMHSA). (2014). *Clinical supervision and professional development of the substance abuse counselor.* Treatment Improvement Protocol (TIP) Series 52, DHHS Publication No. SMA 09-4435. SAMHSA.

Substance Abuse and Mental Health Services Administration (SAMHSA). (2021a). *2020 national survey of drug use and health.* https://www.samhsa.gov/data/release/2020-national-survey-drug-use-and-health-nsduh-releases

Substance Abuse and Mental Health Services Administration (SAMHSA). (2021b). *Alcohol, tobacco, and other drugs.* https://www.samhsa.gov/find-help/atod

Substance Abuse and Mental Health Services Administration (SAMHSA). (2022). *Resources for screening, brief intervention, and referral to treatment (SBIRT).* https://www.samhsa.gov/sbirt/resources

Tomko, R. L., Jones, J. L., Gilmore, A. K., Brady, K. T., Back, S. E., & Gray, K. M. (2018). *N*-acetylcysteine: A potential treatment for substance use disorders. *Current Psychiatry, 17*(6), 31–41.

Trinkoff, A. M., Selby, V. L., Han, K., Baek, H., Steele, J., Edwin, H. S., Yoon, J. M., & Storr, C. L. (2022). The prevalence of substance use and substance use problems in registered nurses: Estimates from the nurse worklife and wellness study. *Journal of Nursing Regulation, 12*(4), 35–46. doi:https://doi.org/10.1016/S2155-8256(22)00014-X

Twachtman, G. (2018). *NIH launches HEAL initiative to combat opioid crisis.* https://www.mdedge.com/psychiatry/article/167889/addiction-medicine/nih-launches-heal-initiative-combat-opioid-crisis

U.S. Food and Drug Administration (FDA). (2016). *FDA requires strong warnings for opioid analgesics, prescription opioid cough products, and benzodiazepine labeling related to serious risks and death from combined use.* https://www.fda.gov/NewsEvents/Newsroom/PressAnnouncements/ucm518697.htm

Volkow, N. D., & Boyle, M. (2018). Neuroscience of addiction: Relevance to prevention and treatment. *American Journal of Psychiatry, 175*(8), 729–740. https://doi.org/10.1176/appi.ajp.2018.17101174

Wang, W., Zeng, F., Hu, Y., & Li, X. (2019). A mini-review of the role of glutamate transporter in drug addiction. *Frontiers in Neurology.* https://doi.org/10.3389/fneur.2019.01123

Weiss, H. D., & Pontone, G. M. (2014). Dopamine receptor agonist drugs and impulse control disorders. *JAMA Internal Medicine, 174*(12), 1935–1937. doi:10.1001/jamainternmed.2014.4097

Zhang, C., Paolozza, A., Tseng, P. H., Reynolds, J. N., Munoz, D. P., & Itti, L. (2019). Detection of children/youth with fetal alcohol spectrum disorder through eye movement, psychometric, and neuroimaging data. *Frontiers in Neurology, 10*(80). https://doi.org/10.3389/fneur.2019.00080

Classical References

Cermak, T. L. (1986). *Diagnosing and treating codependence.* Hazelden Publishing.

Felitti, V. J., Anda, R. F., Nordenberg, D., Williamson, D. F., Spitz, A. M., Edwards, V., Koss, M. P., & Marks, J. S. (1998). Relationship of childhood abuse and household dysfunction to many of the leading causes of death in adults: The adverse childhood experiences (ACE) study. *American Journal of Preventive Medicine, 14*(4), 245–258.

Jellinek, E. M. (1952). Phases of alcohol addiction. *Quarterly Journal of Studies on Alcohol, 13*(4), 673–684. doi:http://dx.doi.org/10.15288/QJSA.1952.13.673

Sullivan, J. T., Sykora, K., Schneiderman, J., Naranjo, C. A., & Sellers, E. M. (1989). Assessment of alcohol withdrawal: The revised Clinical Institute Withdrawal Assessment for Alcohol scale (CIWA-Ar). *British Journal of Addiction, 84*(11), 1353–1357. doi:10.1111/j.1360-0443.1989.tb00737.x

Twerski, A. (1997). *Addictive thinking: Understanding self-deception* (2nd ed.) Hazelden.

Schizophrenia Spectrum and Other Psychotic Disorders

24

KEY TERMS

anhedonia

anosognosia

catatonia

circumstantiality

clang associations

delusions

echolalia

echopraxia

hallucinations

illusions

loose association

magical thinking

negative symptoms

neologisms

neuroleptic malignant syndrome (NMS)

paranoid delusions

perseveration

positive symptoms

psychosis

schizophrenia

serious mental illness (SMI)

social skills training

tangentiality

waxy flexibility

word salad

OBJECTIVES
After reading this chapter, the student will be able to:

1. Discuss the concepts of schizophrenia and other psychotic disorders.
2. Identify predisposing factors in the development of these disorders.
3. Describe various types of schizophrenia and other psychotic disorders.
4. Identify symptomatology associated with these disorders and use this information in patient assessment.
5. Formulate nursing diagnoses and outcomes of care for patients with schizophrenia and other psychotic disorders.

6. Identify topics for patient and family teaching relevant to schizophrenia and other psychotic disorders.
7. Describe appropriate nursing interventions for behaviors associated with these disorders.
8. Describe relevant criteria for evaluating nursing care of patients with schizophrenia and other psychotic disorders.
9. Discuss modalities relevant to treatment of schizophrenia and other psychotic disorders.

The term *schizophrenia* was coined in 1908 by the Swiss psychiatrist Eugen Bleuler, derived from the Greek *skhizo* ("split') and *phren* ("mind"). Over the years, much debate has surrounded the concept of schizophrenia. Various definitions of the disorder have evolved, and numerous treatment strategies been proposed, but none has proven to be uniformly effective or sufficient. The *Diagnostic and Statistical Manual of Mental Disorders, Fifth Edition, Text Revision (DSM-5-TR)* (American Psychiatric Association [APA], 2022) supports this concept by describing schizophrenia as one of the schizophrenia spectrum disorders. Although current consensus points to schizophrenia as a neurodevelopmental disorder (Álvarez et al., 2015), schizophrenia spectrum disorders may have several etiological influences including genetic predisposition, biochemical dysfunction, physiological factors, and psychosocial stress. Tripathi and colleagues (2018) believe that the neurodevelopmental hypothesis falls short in explaining the magnitude of brain changes that occur in schizophrenia. They suggest that these changes can better be explained as "the cumulative effect of neurodevelopmental abnormality, change in neuroplasticity, and alteration in neuronal maturation" (p. 8). Although research is ongoing, there may never be a single treatment that cures the disorder. Effective treatment requires a comprehensive, multidisciplinary effort, including pharmacotherapy and various forms of psychosocial care, such as housing, living skills, **social skills training** (training in verbal and nonverbal skills needed for effective interpersonal relationships), rehabilitation and recovery, and family therapy. Emerging evidence indicates that a comprehensive, patient-centered approach offers hope for a recovery process and improved quality of life in this population.

Of all the mental illnesses, schizophrenia is likely responsible for longer hospitalizations, greater chaos in family life, more exorbitant costs to individuals and governments, and more fear than any other. **Serious mental illness (SMI)** is defined as a mental, behavioral, or emotional disorder resulting in serious functional impairment, which substantially interferes with or limits one or more major life activities, and studies have shown that people with an SMI like schizophrenia have, on average, a 25-year shorter life span than the general population (Chesney, et al., 2014; Druss et al., 2011; Roberts et al., 2017). Because schizophrenia is such an enormous threat to life and happiness and because its causes are an unsolved puzzle, it has also probably been studied more than any other mental disorder.

Risk for suicide is a major concern among patients with schizophrenia. About 20% of people with schizophrenia attempt suicide, and current evidence suggests that about 5% to 6% die by suicide, with many more having significant suicidal ideation (APA, 2022). This chapter explores various theories of predisposing factors implicated in the development of schizophrenia. Symptomatology associated with different diagnostic categories of the disorder is discussed. Nursing care is presented in the context of the six steps of the nursing process. Various dimensions of medical treatment are explored.

Nature of the Disorder

CORE CONCEPT

Psychosis

A severe mental condition in which there is disorganization of the personality, deterioration in social functioning, and loss of contact with, or distortion of, reality is termed **psychosis**. There may be evidence of hallucinations (false sensory perceptions not associated with real external stimuli) and delusions (fixed, false beliefs). Psychosis can occur with or without the presence of organic impairment.

Schizophrenia is a disabling psychological disorder. Characteristically, disturbances in thought processes, perception, and affect invariably result in a severe deterioration of social and occupational functioning.

The estimated lifetime prevalence of schizophrenia is about 0.3% to 0.7% in the general population (APA, 2022). Symptoms generally appear in late adolescence or early adulthood, although they may occur in middle or late adult life. Early-onset schizophrenia refers to symptoms that begin in childhood and adolescence before age 18 years. This condition, although rare, is recognized as a progressive neurodevelopmental disorder with a chronic and severely symptomatic course. Some studies have indicated that schizophrenia occurs more often and earlier in men than in women (B. Miller, 2020).

Phases of Schizophrenia

The pattern of development of schizophrenia may be viewed in four phases: premorbid, prodromal, active psychotic (acute schizophrenic episode), and residual.

Phase I: Premorbid Phase

Premorbid signs are those that occur before there is clear evidence of illness and may include distinctive personality traits or behaviors. Premorbid personality and behavioral indications may include being very shy and withdrawn, having poor peer relationships, doing poorly in school, and demonstrating asocial behavior. Boland and Verduin (2022) stated:

> In the typical, but not invariable, premorbid history of schizophrenia, patients had schizoid or schizotypal personalities characterized as quiet, passive and introverted; as children, they had few friends. Preschizophrenic adolescents may have no close friends and no dates and may avoid team sports. They may enjoy [solitary activities] to the exclusion of social activities. (p. 349)

Current research is focused on the premorbid phase in hopes that identification of potential biomarkers and at-risk individuals may prevent transition to illness or provide early intervention (García-Gutiérrez et al., 2020).

Phase II: Prodromal Phase

Prodromal signs are differentiated from premorbid signs in that prodromal symptoms more clearly manifest as signs of developing schizophrenia than do premorbid signs. The prodromal phase of schizophrenia begins with a change from premorbid functioning and extends until the onset of frank psychotic symptoms. This phase can be as brief as a few weeks or months, but most studies indicate that the average length of the prodromal phase is between 2 and 5 years. During this phase, the individual begins to show signs of significant deterioration in function. Fifty percent of this population complain of depressive symptoms (APA, 2022). Social withdrawal is not uncommon, and signs of cognitive impairment may begin to emerge. Some adolescent patients develop sudden onset of obsessive-compulsive behavior during the prodromal phase (Boland & Verduin, 2022).

Recognition of the behaviors associated with the prodromal phase provides an opportunity for early intervention with a possibility for improvement in long-term outcomes. Current treatment guidelines suggest therapeutic interventions that offer support with identified problems, cognitive therapies to minimize functional impairment, family interventions to improve coping, and involvement with a patient's school to reduce the possibility of failure. Some controversy exists about the benefit of pharmaceutical therapy during the prodromal phase; however, evidence supports that comprehensive treatment started at the time of the first psychotic episode is associated with better outcomes (Kane et al., 2015).

Phase III: Active Psychotic Phase (Acute Schizophrenic Episode)

Schizophrenia is a chronic illness but is characterized by acute episodes in which symptoms are more pronounced. In the active phase of the disorder, psychotic symptoms are typically prominent. Box 24–1 describes the *DSM-5-TR* (APA, 2022) diagnostic criteria for schizophrenia.

Phase IV: Residual Phase

Schizophrenia is characterized by periods of remission and exacerbation and consequently is described as episodic despite being a chronic illness. A residual phase usually follows the active phase of the illness, during which symptoms of the active phase (symptoms described in phase III) are either absent or no longer prominent. Positive symptoms (e.g., delusions and hallucinations) may be improved, but negative symptoms (e.g., deficits in normal functions) may remain (Box 24–2), and flat affect and impairment in role functioning are common during this phase. It has long been thought that these negative symptoms are pervasive and stable, but current research has challenged that belief with evidence that negative symptoms can improve over time (Savill et al., 2015), although admittedly they are difficult to treat. Residual impairment often increases with additional episodes of active psychosis.

Prognosis

Outcomes in schizophrenia are difficult to predict and are highly variable, but long-term follow-up studies indicate that significant clinical improvement occurs in about 44% of patients with schizophrenia (Os & Reininghaus, 2017). Associated factors include good premorbid functioning, later age at onset, female sex, abrupt onset of symptoms with an obvious precipitating factor (as opposed to gradual, insidious onset of symptoms), lower depression scores, low baseline levels of aggression, rapid resolution of active-phase symptoms, minimal residual symptoms, absence of structural brain abnormalities, ability to live independently at baseline, no family history of schizophrenia, and good family support (Boland & Verduin, 2022; Frankenburg, 2020; Shrivastava et al., 2010).

Predisposing Factors

The cause of schizophrenia is still uncertain. Most likely, no single factor can be implicated in the etiology; rather, the disease probably results from a combination of influences including biological, psychological, and environmental factors.

Biological Factors

Refer to Chapter 3, "Concepts of Psychobiology," for a more thorough review of the biological implications of psychiatric illness.

BOX 24–1 DSM-5-TR Criteria for the Diagnosis of Schizophrenia

A. Two (or more) of the following, each present for a significant portion of time during a 1-month period (or less if successfully treated). At least one of these must be (1), (2), or (3):
   1. Delusions
   2. Hallucinations
   3. Disorganized speech (e.g., frequent derailment or incoherence)
   4. Grossly disorganized or catatonic behavior
   5. Negative symptoms (i.e., diminished emotional expression or avolition)[A5]

B. For a significant portion of the time since the onset of the disturbance, level of functioning in one or more major areas, such as work, interpersonal relations, or self-care, is markedly below the level achieved before the onset (or when the onset is in childhood or adolescence, there is failure to achieve expected level of interpersonal, academic, or occupational functioning).

C. Continuous signs of the disturbance persist for at least 6 months. This 6-month period must include at least 1 month of symptoms (or less if successfully treated) that meet Criterion A (i.e., active-phase symptoms) and may include periods of prodromal or residual symptoms. During these prodromal or residual periods, the signs of the disturbance may be manifested by only negative symptoms or by two or more symptoms listed in Criterion A present in an attenuated form (e.g., odd beliefs, unusual perceptual experiences).

D. Schizoaffective disorder and depressive or bipolar disorder with psychotic features have been ruled out because either (1) no major depressive or manic episodes have occurred concurrently with the active-phase symptoms; or (2) if mood episodes have occurred during active-phase symptoms, they have been present for a minority of the total duration of the active and residual periods of the illness.

E. The disturbance is not attributable to the physiological effects of a substance (e.g., a drug of abuse, a medication) or another medical condition.

F. If there is a history of autism spectrum disorder or a communication disorder of childhood onset, the additional diagnosis of schizophrenia is made only if prominent delusions or hallucinations, in addition to the other required symptoms of schizophrenia, are also present for at least 1 month (or less if successfully treated).

Specify if: The following course specifiers are only to be used after a 1-year duration of the disorder and if they are not in contradiction to the diagnostic course criteria.

First episode, currently in acute episode: First manifestation of the disorder meeting the defining diagnostic symptom and time criteria. An acute episode is a time period in which the symptom criteria are fulfilled.

First episode, currently in partial remission: Partial remission is a period of time during which an improvement after a previous episode is maintained and in which the defining criteria of the disorder are only partially fulfilled.

First episode, currently in full remission: Full remission is a period of time after a previous episode during which no disorder-specific symptoms are present.

Multiple episodes, currently in acute episode: Multiple episodes may be determined after a minimum of two episodes (i.e., after a first episode, a remission and a minimum of one relapse).

Multiple episodes, currently in partial remission

Multiple episodes, currently in full remission

Continuous: Symptoms fulfilling the diagnostic symptom criteria of the disorder are remaining for the majority of the illness course, with subthreshold symptom periods being very brief relative to the overall course.

Unspecified

Specify if: with catatonia.

Specify current severity.

Reprinted with permission from the *Diagnostic and Statistical Manual of Mental Disorders, Fifth Edition, Text Revision (DSM-5-TR)* (Copyright © 2022). American Psychiatric Association. All Rights Reserved.

Genetics

The body of evidence supporting a genetic vulnerability to schizophrenia is growing. Studies show that relatives of individuals with schizophrenia have a much higher probability of developing the disease than does the general population. Whereas the lifetime risk for developing schizophrenia is about 0.3% to 0.7%, studies have shown that first-degree relatives of an identified patient have up to a 9% greater risk of developing schizophrenia than relatives of controls (Os & Reininghaus, 2017).

The most compelling evidence for a genetic component in schizophrenia comes from twin studies. In monozygotic (identical) twins there is a 50% concordance rate for schizophrenia, which is four to five times the concordance rate in dizygotic twins or other first-degree relatives (Boland & Verduin, 2022). Identical twins reared apart have the same

BOX 24–2 **Positive and Negative Symptoms of Schizophrenia***

POSITIVE SYMPTOMS

Delusions (Fixed, False Beliefs)

Persecutory—belief that one is going to be harmed by other(s)

Referential—belief that cues in the environment are specifically referring to them

Grandiose—belief that they have exceptional greatness

Somatic—beliefs that center on one's body functioning

Erotomanic—belief that someone of higher status or celebrity is in love with them

Hallucinations (Sensory Perceptions Without External Stimuli)

Auditory (most common in schizophrenia)

Visual

Tactile

Olfactory

Gustatory

(Note: Hallucinations may be a normal part of religious experience in some cultural contexts.)

Disorganized Thinking (Manifested in Speech)

Loose association

Tangentiality

Circumstantiality

Incoherence (includes word salad)

Neologisms

Clang associations

Echolalia

Grossly Disorganized or Abnormal Motor Behavior (Including Catatonia)

Hyperactivity

Hypervigilance

Hostility

Agitation

Childlike silliness

Catatonia (ranging from rigid or bizarre posture and decreased responsivity to complete lack of verbal or behavioral response to the environment)

Catatonic excitement (excessive and purposeless motor activity)

Stereotyped, repetitive movements

Unusual mannerisms or postures

NEGATIVE SYMPTOMS

Deficits in several areas of cognitive function, including dysfunction in working memory, attention, processing speed, reasoning, planning, abstract thinking, and problem-solving, may manifest as the following negative symptoms.

Lack of Emotional Expression

Blunted affect

Lack of movement in head and hands that add expression in communication

Lack of intonation in speech

Decreased or Lack of Motivation to Complete Purposeful Activities (Avolition)

Neglect of activities of daily living

Decreased Verbal Communication (Alogia)

Decreased Interest in Social Interaction and Relationship (Asociality)

Withdrawal

Poor rapport

Diminished Ability for Abstract Thinking (Concrete Thinking)

Concrete interpretation of events and communication from others

---

*Positive symptoms refer to symptoms that are present ("added") in people with schizophrenia and not typically present in people without the disease. Negative symptoms are referred to as deficits or impairments (things "taken away" by the illness) in individuals with schizophrenia.

Sources: American Psychiatric Association (APA). (2022). *Diagnostic and statistical manual of mental disorders, fifth edition, text revision (DSM-5-TR)*. APA; Kay, S. R., Fiszbein, A., & Opler, L. A. (1987). The positive and negative syndrome scale (PANSS) for schizophrenia. *Schizophrenia Bulletin, 13*(2), 261–276.

rate of development of the illness as do those reared together. Because in about one-half of the cases only one of a pair of identical twins develops schizophrenia, genetic makeup cannot be solely responsible for causing this disease. Os and Reininghaus (2017) suggested that additive and interacting combinations of genes, environmental factors, and the moderation of gene expression through interaction with environmental factors are probably all influential.

How schizophrenia is inherited is uncertain. Current research is focused on determining which gene or genes are important in the predisposition to schizophrenia and what other biomarkers may predict risk for this illness. Okazaki and associates (2016) studied gene expression in peripheral blood samples of patients admitted with acute psychosis and found that a specific combination of genes (*CDK4, MCM7,* and *POLD4*) differentiated these patients from controls. This finding suggests that the combination could be a genetic biomarker for schizophrenia and may also clarify aspects of pathophysiology in schizophrenia. The authors conclude that the messenger ribonucleic acid (mRNA) expression changes that occur in *CDK4* are potential biomarkers for both trait (stable features) and state (temporary change) symptoms in schizophrenia. The strongest genetic associations to date have been variations in the major histocompatibility complex (MHC), particularly C4 alleles that are involved in synaptic pruning that occurs during adolescence and young adulthood (Boland & Verduin, 2022).

Research is ongoing to identify genetic influences in schizophrenia that will hone our understanding of the multivariate influences in the development of this disease and perhaps identify treatment implications.

Biochemical Factors

The oldest and most thoroughly explored biological theory to explain schizophrenia attributes a pathogenic role to abnormal brain biochemistry. Notions of a "chemical disturbance" as an explanation for mental illness were suggested by some theorists as early as the mid-19th century.

The Dopamine Hypothesis

This theory suggests that schizophrenia or schizophrenia-like symptoms may be caused by an excess of dopamine-dependent neuronal activity in the brain (Fig. 24–1). This excess activity may be related to increased production or release of the substance at nerve terminals, increased receptor sensitivity, too many dopamine receptors, or a combination of these mechanisms.

Pharmacological support for this hypothesis came from the observation that amphetamines, which increase levels of dopamine, induced symptoms that mimic those of psychosis. First generation antipsychotics (e.g., chlorpromazine or haloperidol) lower brain levels of dopamine by blocking dopamine receptors (particularly at D2 receptors), thus reducing psychotic symptoms, including those induced by amphetamines. Postmortem brain studies of individuals with schizophrenia reveal alterations in the presynaptic and postsynaptic dopaminergic system, and more recent in vivo studies using positron emission tomography (PET) and single-photon emission computed tomography (SPECT) imaging have revealed increased dopamine synthesis capacity in patients with schizophrenia (Howes et al., 2015). People with **positive symptoms** such as delusions and hallucinations (referred to as *positive* symptoms because they are "added" to the clinical picture) respond with greater efficacy to dopamine-reducing drugs than do people with **negative symptoms** (deficits in normal functions such as apathy, poverty of ideas, and loss of drive). More information about positive and negative symptoms is listed in Box 24–2.

Over time we have learned that there are several different types of dopamine receptors (D1, D2, D3, D4, and D5), and research continues to identify the specific role of each in the course of schizophrenia as well the implications for treatment. Clozapine, for example, an atypical antipsychotic with a unique clinical profile, has more affinity for D4 receptors. D3 receptors, found in several areas of the brain, have been identified as relevant in the expression of negative symptoms. Although dopamine receptors have been a large focus of research, at least in part because of their relevance in drug pharmacological treatment, there are several other neurotransmitter dysregulations apparent in individuals with schizophrenia. These are discussed in the following section.

Other Biochemical Hypotheses

Abnormalities in the neurotransmitters norepinephrine, serotonin, acetylcholine, and gamma-aminobutyric acid and in the neuroregulators, such as prostaglandins and endorphins, have all been implicated in the predisposition to schizophrenia. Excess of serotonin has been hypothesized to be responsible for both positive and negative symptoms of schizophrenia, and the effectiveness of medications such as clozapine (a strong serotonin antagonist) lends support to this hypothesis. Recent research has implicated the neurotransmitter glutamate in the etiology of schizophrenia. The *N*-methyl-D-aspartate (NMDA) receptor is activated by the neurotransmitters glutamate and glycine. Psychopharmacological studies have shown that glutamate antagonists (e.g., phencyclidine [PCP], ketamine) can produce schizophrenia-like symptoms in individuals who do not have the disorder (Beck et al., 2020). In one study, participants experiencing ketamine-induced schizophrenia-like psychotic symptoms were treated with a drug trial of a glycine transporter-1 inhibitor (D'Souza et al., 2012). This medication was shown to reduce psychotic symptoms induced by the NMDA receptor antagonism of ketamine, so it is hoped that it may also benefit schizophrenia treatment. Despite evidence of a glutamate link to schizophrenia (Hu et al., 2014), more research is needed on the implications for treatment. Previous studies have focused on reducing glutamate levels in patients who have advanced illness, but current research has identified that glutamate levels may be more important in the *transition* to psychosis. This theory is supported by the fact that first episodes of psychosis are often precipitated by stress, and glutamate increases under stress (Bossong et al., 2019). When glutamate levels are very high, the hippocampus becomes hypermetabolic and then begins to atrophy. Hippocampal atrophy has been identified as a significant finding in many individuals with schizophrenia. Future research may find that interventions targeting glutamate are beneficial in high-risk individuals or those in early stages of illness to prevent onset or slow the progression of the disease (Bossong et al., 2019).

Current conventional antipsychotic medications mainly target the dopamine receptors in the brain.

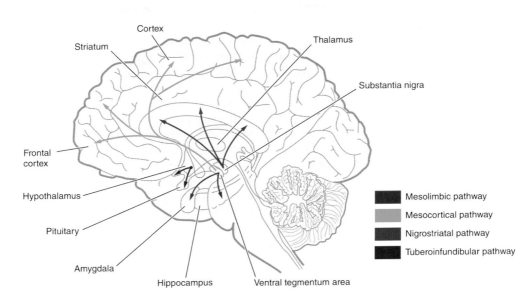

FIGURE 24–1   Neurobiology of schizophrenia.

NEUROTRANSMITTERS

A number of neurotransmitters have been implicated in the etiology of schizophrenia: dopamine, norepinephrine, serotonin, glutamate, and gamma-aminobutyric acid (GABA). The dopaminergic system has been most widely studied and closely linked to the symptoms associated with the disease.

AREAS OF THE BRAIN AFFECTED

Four major dopaminergic pathways (the pathways that transmit dopamine to different areas of the brain) have been identified:

• *Mesolimbic pathway:* Originates in the ventral tegmentum area (VTA) and projects to areas of the limbic system, including the nucleus accumbens, amygdala, and hippocampus. The mesolimbic pathway is associated with functions of memory, emotion, arousal, and pleasure. Excess activity in the mesolimbic tract has been implicated in the positive symptoms of schizophrenia (e.g., hallucinations, delusions). Dopamine blockade in this pathway is the target of antipsychotic medication to reduce hallucinations and delusions.

• *Mesocortical pathway:* Originates in the VTA and projects into the cortex. The mesocortical pathway is concerned with cognition, social behavior, planning, problem-solving, motivation, and reinforcement in learning. Negative symptoms of schizophrenia (e.g., flat affect, apathy, lack of motivation, and anhedonia) have been associated with diminished activity in the mesocortical tract.

• *Nigrostriatal pathway:* Originates in the substantia nigra and terminates in the striatum of the basal ganglia. This pathway is associated with the function of motor control. Degeneration in this pathway is associated with Parkinson's disease, and because typical antipsychotics may also block dopamine here, drug-induced Parkinson-like extrapyramidal side effects (EPS) and tardive dyskinesia occur.

• *Tuberoinfundibular pathway:* Originates in the hypothalamus and projects to the pituitary gland. It is associated with endocrine function, digestion, metabolism, hunger, thirst, temperature control, and sexual arousal. Dopamine blockade in this pathway is associated with an increase in prolactin levels (hyperprolactinemia), which can result in galactorrhea (milk discharge from the nipples) in both men and women, erectile disorder, and anorgasmia.

ANTIPSYCHOTIC MEDICATIONS

Type	Receptor Affinity	Associated Side Effects
First generation (typical) antipsychotics such as 　Phenothiazines 　Haloperidol Provide relief of psychosis, improvement in positive symptoms, worsening of negative symptoms.	Strong D2 (dopamine) Varying degrees of affinity for: 　ACh (acetylcholine) 　α_1 (norepinephrine) H$_1$ (histamine) Weak 5-HT (serotonin)	EPS, hyperprolactinemia, neuroleptic malignant syndrome Anticholinergic effects Tachycardia, tremors, insomnia, postural hypotension Weight gain, sedation
Second generation (atypical) antipsychotics such as: 　Clozapine, olanzapine, quetiapine, aripiprazole, risperidone, iloperidone, ziprasidone, paliperidone, asenapine, lurasidone Provide relief of psychosis, improvement in positive symptoms, improvement in negative symptoms.	Strong 5-HT Low to moderate D2 Varying degrees of affinity for: 　ACh 　α-adrenergic 　H$_1$	Low potential for ejaculatory difficulty Sexual dysfunction, gastrointestinal disturbance, headache Low potential for EPS Anticholinergic effects Tachycardia, tremors, insomnia, postural hypotension Weight gain, sedation

Newer second generation antipsychotics have a strong affinity for serotonergic receptors. The glutamate model of schizophrenia suggests possibilities for new biomarkers signaling early illness and for new approaches to prevention and early treatment.

Physiological Factors

A number of potential physiological factors have been identified in the medical literature. However, their specific mechanisms and implications in the etiology of schizophrenia are unclear. Current theories suggest that it "is likely that these genetic risks, environmental risks and vulnerability factors are cumulative and interactive with each other and with critical periods of neurodevelopmental vulnerability" (Davis et al., 2016, p. 185).

Viral Infection

Boland and Verduin (2022) reported that epidemiological data indicate a high incidence of schizophrenia after prenatal exposure to influenza. They stated:

> Other data supporting a viral hypothesis are an increased number of physical anomalies at birth, an increased rate of pregnancy and birth complications, seasonality of birth consistent with viral infection, geographical clusters of adult cases, and seasonality of hospitalizations. (p. 360)

The effect of autoimmune antibodies in the brain is being studied within the field of psychoneuroimmunology, and evidence suggests that these antibodies may be responsible for the development of at least some cases of schizophrenia after infection from a neurotoxic virus (particularly prenatal exposure to *Toxoplasma gondii*) (Torrey, 2022). Torrey notes that *T. gondii* is known to cause delusions, hallucinations, and other psychotic symptoms and is transmitted to humans commonly through undercooked meats and exposure to cat feces. Cytokines (chemicals that manage the immune system) are found to be dysregulated in many patients with schizophrenia and research supports growing evidence that this dysregulation is influential in the pathogenesis of schizophrenia, perhaps through the effect of multiple avenues including genetics, childhood trauma, and disturbances in the gut microbiome (Dawidowski et al., 2021).

Anatomical Abnormalities

With the use of neuroimaging technologies, structural brain abnormalities have been observed in individuals with schizophrenia. Ventricular enlargement is the most consistent finding; however, some reduction in gray matter is also reported. As previously discussed, reduction in the volume of the hippocampus observed in neuroimaging studies may signal risk for transition to a first psychotic episode (Harrisberger et al., 2016).

Studies that focus on risk for a first psychotic episode are important, as early treatment is associated with better outcomes. Ultimately, it is hoped that these studies will also point to preventive strategies.

Magnetic resonance imaging has revealed reduced symmetry in lobes of the brain and reductions in size of structures within the limbic system in individuals with schizophrenia. Considerable evidence from post-mortem studies has shown abnormalities in the prefrontal cortex, and people who have had prefrontal lobotomies are reported to manifest with many symptoms common to schizophrenia, including flat affect and cognitive deterioration (Boland & Verduin, 2022).

Diffusion tensor imaging studies have identified widespread white matter abnormalities in schizophrenia (Viher et al., 2016). These abnormalities in white matter microstructure appear to be primarily associated with negative symptoms and psychomotor behavior abnormalities.

Long-term studies of patients with schizophrenia have noted brain volume reduction, particularly in the temporal and preventricular areas (Veijola et al., 2014). It has been postulated that long-term antipsychotic medication use may contribute to this reduction, but the implications are unclear. Veijola and associates (2014) found that symptom severity, level of functional ability, and decline in cognitive abilities were not correlated with this reduction in brain volume.

Electrophysiology

Several studies have evaluated 40-Hz auditory steady-state response, a measure of electrical activity in the brain, and identified neural circuit dysfunctions in people with schizophrenia. A recent meta-analysis (Thunè et al., 2016) of these studies demonstrates robust evidence of such dysfunction in schizophrenia. The meaning of these circuit dysfunctions is not well understood, but they may indicate another biomarker for identifying risk or illness.

Physical Conditions

Several medical conditions are known to cause acute psychotic episodes, including Huntington's disease, hypothyroidism or hyperthyroidism, hypoglycemia, calcium imbalances, temporal lobe epilepsy, Wilson's disease, central nervous system (CNS) neoplasms, encephalitis, meningitis, neurosyphilis, and stroke. See Box 24–3 for a list of many medical conditions associated with psychosis.

Psychological Factors

Early conceptualizations of schizophrenia focused on family relationship factors as major influences in the development of the illness, probably in light of the conspicuous absence of information related to a biological connection. These early theories

BOX 24–3 General Medical Conditions That May Cause Psychosis

Acute intermittent porphyria
Brain abscesses
Cerebrovascular disease
CNS infections
CNS trauma
Cushing's syndrome
Deafness
Encephalitis
Fluid or electrolyte imbalances
Hepatic disease
Herpes encephalitis
Huntington's disease
Hypoadrenocorticism
Hypoparathyroidism or hyperparathyroidism
Hypothyroidism or hyperthyroidism
Meningitis
Metabolic conditions (e.g., hypoxia; hypercarbia; hypoglycemia)
Migraine headache
Neoplasms
Neurosyphilis
Normal pressure hydrocephalus
Renal disease
Systemic lupus erythematosus
Temporal lobe epilepsy
Vitamin deficiency (e.g., B$_{12}$)
Wilson's disease

Compiled from American Psychiatric Association (APA). (2022). *Diagnostic and statistical manual of mental disorders, fifth edition, text revision (DSM-5-TR)*. APA; Boland, R., & Verduin, M. L. (2022). *Kaplan & Sadock's synopsis of psychiatry (P. Ruiz, Ed.)*. (12th ed.). Wolters Kluwer.

implicated poor parent-child communication, particularly condemning the mother as "schizophrenogenic" (inducing schizophrenia in her child) related to a troublesome communication style known as *double-bind communication*. This theory is no longer accepted. Researchers now focus their studies on schizophrenia as a brain disorder. Although family relationships are not involved in the etiology of the illness, the symptoms in schizophrenia can contribute to significant disruption in communication and relationships among family members, so psychosocial factors should always be part of a comprehensive assessment. Further, evidence suggests that childhood trauma, and particularly multiple traumatizations, are associated (in combination with many other influences) with the development of schizophrenia in vulnerable populations (Álvarez et al., 2015; Davis

et al., 2016; Popovic et al., 2019). Trauma-informed care should also be part of a comprehensive psychosocial assessment and intervention for this patient.

Environmental Influences

Sociocultural Factors

Many studies have attempted to link schizophrenia to social class. Epidemiological statistics have shown that more individuals from lower socioeconomic classes experience symptoms associated with schizophrenia than do those from higher socioeconomic groups (Os & Reininghaus, 2017). These studies consistently find that lack of material resources (including housing and access to health care) and fragmented social relationships increase the risk for schizophrenia, whereas social cohesion and ethnic density (the concentration of a given ethnic group in a particular area) are protective.

An alternative view is that of the *downward drift hypothesis*, which suggests that because of the characteristic symptoms of the disorder, individuals with schizophrenia have difficulty maintaining gainful employment and "drift down" to a lower socioeconomic level (or fail to rise out of a lower socioeconomic group). Proponents of this view consider poor social conditions to be a consequence rather than a cause of schizophrenia.

Stressful Life Events

No scientific evidence indicates that stress causes schizophrenia. It is probable, however, that stress may contribute to the severity and course of the illness. It is known that extreme stress can precipitate psychotic episodes, so it may also precipitate symptoms in an individual who possesses a genetic vulnerability to schizophrenia. Stressful life events also may be associated with exacerbation of schizophrenic symptoms and increased rates of relapse.

Cannabis and Genetic Vulnerability

Studies of genetic vulnerability for schizophrenia have linked certain genes (*COMT* and *ATK1*) to increased risk for psychosis, particularly for adolescents with this genetic vulnerability who use cannabinoids (Radhakrishnan et al., 2014). Both cannabis and synthetic cannabinoids can induce schizophrenia-like symptoms. In people with a preexisting psychosis, cannabinoids can exacerbate symptoms. Individuals with schizophrenia who continue to use cannabis experience shorter periods of remission and more frequent relapses (J. Miller, 2020). More importantly, the increased risk for psychotic disorders such as schizophrenia with cannabis use suggests the influence of lifestyle factors in the expression of genes and supports the theory that multiple factors play a role in the causality of this illness.

Theoretical Integration and the Transactional Model

Although no single theory or hypothesis has been postulated that substantiates a clear-cut explanation for the disease, accumulating evidence supports the concept of multiple causation in the development of schizophrenia. Evidence gathered from a systematic review of the literature on schizophrenia (Matheson et al., 2014) summarized these influences:

> Patients have relatively poor cognitive functioning, and subtle, but diverse, structural brain alterations, altered electrophysiological functioning and sleep patterns, minor physical anomalies, neurological soft signs, and sensory alterations. There are markers of infection, inflammation or altered immunological parameters; and there is increased mortality from a range of causes. Risk for schizophrenia is increased with cannabis use, pregnancy and birth complications, prenatal exposure to *Toxoplasma gondii*, childhood CNS viral infections, childhood adversities, urbanicity, and immigration (first and second generation), particularly in certain ethnic groups. Developmental motor delays and lower intelligence quotient in childhood and adolescence are apparent. (p. 3387)

Despite the wealth of research and knowledge that we have about schizophrenia, much more is needed before we will fully understand this illness.

One way to conceptualize the pathway to acute illness is through exploring influencing factors and the individual's response to these stressors. The dynamics of schizophrenia using the transactional model of stress and adaptation are presented in Figure 24–2.

Other Schizophrenia Spectrum and Psychotic Disorders

The *DSM-5-TR* (APA, 2022) identifies a spectrum of psychotic disorders organized to reflect a gradient of psychopathology from least to most severe. The degree of severity is determined by the level, number, and duration of psychotic signs and symptoms.

Several disorders may carry the additional specification of *With Catatonic Features*. **Catatonia** refers to a significant motor disturbance that may range from stupor (no motor activity) to excessive motor activity and agitation. The disorders in which catatonia may appear include brief psychotic disorder, schizophreniform disorder, schizophrenia, schizoaffective disorder, and substance-induced psychotic disorder. It may also be applied to neurodevelopmental disorder, major depressive disorder, and bipolar disorders I and II (APA, 2022).

The *DSM-5-TR* initiates the spectrum of disorders with Schizotypal Personality Disorder. For purposes of this textbook, this disorder is presented in Chapter 31, "Personality Disorders."

Delusional Disorder

Delusional disorder is characterized by the presence of delusions experienced for at least 1 month (APA, 2022). Hallucinations are not prominent (or may not be present), and behavior is not bizarre. The *DSM-5-TR* states that a specifier may be added to denote whether the delusions include bizarre content (i.e., if the thought is "clearly implausible, not understandable, and not derived from ordinary life experiences" [p. 105]). Subtypes of delusional disorders include erotomanic, grandiose, jealous, persecutory, somatic, and mixed. These are discussed further in the section "Application of the Nursing Process."

Brief Psychotic Disorder

This disorder is identified by the sudden onset of psychotic symptoms that may or may not be preceded by a severe psychosocial stressor. These symptoms last at least a day but less than a month, and there is an eventual full return to the premorbid level of functioning (APA, 2022). The individual experiences emotional turmoil or overwhelming perplexity or confusion. Evidence of impaired reality may include incoherent speech, delusions, hallucinations, bizarre behavior, and disorientation. Catatonic features may also be associated with this disorder.

Substance/Medication-Induced Psychotic Disorder

The prominent hallucinations and delusions associated with this disorder are directly attributable to substance intoxication or withdrawal or exposure to a medication or toxin. This diagnosis is made when delusions and/or hallucinations predominate during or soon after intoxication, withdrawal, or exposure to a substance or medication and they are severe enough to warrant clinical attention (APA, 2022). The medical history, physical examination, or laboratory findings provide evidence that the appearance of the symptoms occurred in association with substance intoxication or withdrawal or exposure to a medication or toxin. Substances believed to induce psychotic disorders are presented in Box 24–4. Catatonic features may also be associated with this disorder.

Psychotic Disorder Due to Another Medical Condition

The essential features of this disorder are prominent hallucinations and delusions that can be directly attributed to another medical condition (APA, 2022). The diagnosis is not made if the symptoms occur during the course of delirium. A number of medical conditions that can cause psychotic symptoms are presented in Box 24–3.

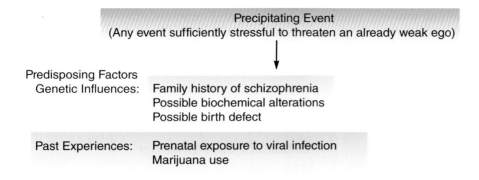

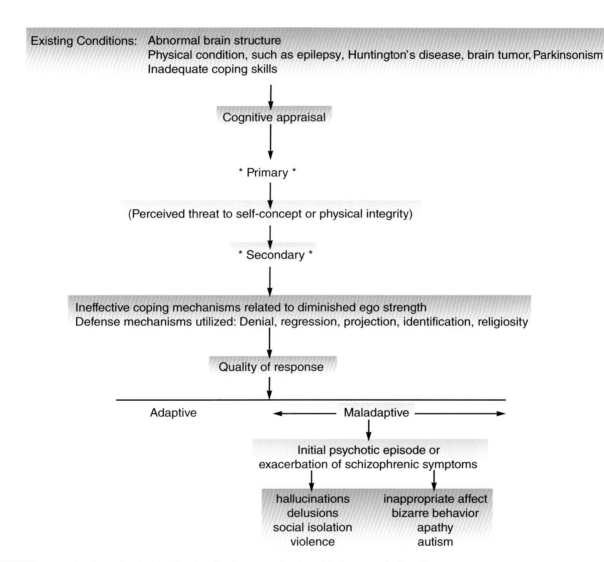

FIGURE 24–2 The dynamics of schizophrenia using the transactional model of stress and adaptation.

Catatonic Disorder Due to Another Medical Condition

This diagnosis is made when symptomatology evidenced from medical history, physical examination, or laboratory findings is directly attributable to the physiological consequences of another medical condition (APA, 2022). Types of medical conditions associated with catatonia include metabolic disorders (e.g., hepatic encephalopathy, diabetic ketoacidosis, hypothyroidism and hyperthyroidism, hypoadrenalism and hyperadrenalism, hypercalcemia, and

Drugs of abuse	Alcohol
	Amphetamines and related substances
	Cannabis
	Cocaine
	Hallucinogens
	Inhalants
	Opioids
	Phencyclidine and related substances
	Sedatives, hypnotics, and anxiolytics
Medications	Anesthetics and analgesics
	Anticholinergic agents
	Anticonvulsants
	Antidepressant medication
	Antihistamines
	Antihypertensive agents
	Antimicrobial medications
	Antineoplastic medications
	Antiparkinsonian agents
	Cardiovascular medications
	Corticosteroids
	Disulfiram
	Gastrointestinal medications
	Muscle relaxants
	Nonsteroidal anti-inflammatory agents
Toxins	Anticholinesterase
	Organophosphate insecticides
	Nerve gases
	Carbon dioxide
	Carbon monoxide
	Volatile substances (e.g., fuel, paint, gasoline, toluene)

Compiled from American Psychiatric Association (APA). (2022). *Diagnostic and statistical manual of mental disorders, fifth edition, text revision (DSM-5-TR)*. APA; Freudenreich, O. (2010). Differential diagnosis of psychotic symptoms: Medical "mimics." *Psychiatric Times, 27*(12), 52–61.

vitamin B_{12} deficiency) and neurological conditions (e.g., epilepsy, tumors, cerebrovascular disease, head trauma, and encephalitis) (APA, 2022).

Schizophreniform Disorder

The essential symptoms of this disorder are identical to those of schizophrenia but the duration, including prodromal, active, and residual phases, is at least 1 month but less than 6 months (APA, 2022). If the diagnosis is made while the individual is still symptomatic but has been so for less than 6 months, it is qualified as "provisional." The diagnosis is changed to schizophrenia if the clinical picture persists beyond 6 months. Schizophreniform disorder is

thought to have a good prognosis if at least two of the following features are present: the individual's affect is not blunted or flat, there is a rapid onset of psychotic symptoms (within 4 weeks) from the time the unusual behavior is noticed, there is confusion or perplexity, and there is good premorbid social and occupational functioning (APA, 2022). Catatonic features may also be associated with this disorder.

Schizoaffective Disorder

This disorder is manifested by signs and symptoms of schizophrenia along with a strong element of symptomatology associated with the mood disorders (depression or mania). The individual may appear depressed, with psychomotor retardation and suicidal ideation, or symptoms may include euphoria, grandiosity, and hyperactivity. A defining factor in the diagnosis of schizoaffective disorder is the presence of hallucinations and/or delusions that occur for at least 2 weeks in the absence of a major mood episode (APA, 2022). However, prominent mood disorder symptoms must be evident for most of the time. The prognosis for schizoaffective disorder is generally better than that for other schizophrenic disorders but worse than that for mood disorders alone. Catatonic features may also be associated with this disorder.

Application of the Nursing Process

Schizophrenia—Background Assessment Data

The diagnostic criteria for schizophrenia were presented earlier in this chapter. As previously stated, symptoms may present in phases, with schizophrenia representing the active phase of the disorder. Symptoms associated with the active phase are discussed in this section.

In the first step of the nursing process, the nurse gathers a database from which nursing diagnoses are derived, and a plan of care is formulated. This step of the nursing process is important because problem identification, objectives of care, and outcome criteria cannot be accurately determined without an accurate assessment.

Assessment of the patient with schizophrenia is a complex process and is based on information gathered from multiple sources. Patients in an acute episode of their illness may not be able to make significant contributions to their history. Data may be obtained from family members, if possible; from old medical records, if available; or from other individuals who are able to report on the progression of the patient's behavior.

The nurse must be familiar with behaviors common to the disorder to obtain an adequate assessment of the patient with schizophrenia. This includes positive and negative symptoms. Most but not all individuals exhibit a mixture of both types of symptoms.

The seven domains of cognitive dysfunction that are common in schizophrenia are working memory; attention; speed of processing thoughts; verbal learning; and substantial deficit in reasoning, abstract thinking, and problem-solving. Tripathi and associates (2018) estimated that 98% of patients with schizophrenia have these cognitive deficits, which can aggravate other symptoms and dramatically interfere with one's quality of life. To date, pharmacological treatments generally have been ineffective in treating these symptoms.

It is important to note that not all patients with schizophrenia experience all of these symptoms. Bora (2015) noted that in individuals who develop cognitive deficits, the age of onset is variable, and MacCabe and associates (2013) identified that a subgroup of individuals with schizophrenia have no cognitive impairment even in adulthood. Many factors contribute to functional impairment and decline beyond the symptoms themselves, including comorbid metabolic conditions, chronic substance use, stress, frequency and intensity of episodes, residual symptoms, and social defeat (Bora, 2015). A summary of positive and negative symptoms is presented in Box 24–2.

Positive Symptoms

Positive symptoms are abnormal symptoms that are common manifestations of schizophrenia and referred to as positive because they are "added to" rather than deficits in the clinical picture.

Disturbances in Thought Content

Delusions **Delusions** are fixed, false beliefs that are irrational and that the individual maintains are true despite evidence to the contrary. These beliefs are not explainable as part of the person's usual religious or cultural precepts. Delusions are subdivided according to their content. Some of the more common ones are listed here:

■ **Persecutory delusions:** These are the most common type of delusion in which individuals believe they are being persecuted or malevolently treated in some way. Frequent themes include being plotted against, cheated or defrauded, followed and spied on, poisoned, or drugged. The individual may obsess about and exaggerate a slight rebuff (either real or imagined) until it becomes the focus of a delusional system. Repeated complaints may be directed at legal authorities. The individual feels threatened and believes that others intend harm or persecution toward them in some way (e.g., "The FBI has bugged my room and intends to kill me"; "The government put a chip in my brain to erase my memories"). These may also be referred to as **paranoid delusions**, which describe the extreme suspiciousness of others and of their actions or perceived intentions (e.g., "I won't eat this food. I know it has been poisoned"). Aggression or violence may occur because the individual believes that they must defend themselves against someone or something perceived to be a threat.

■ **Grandiose delusions:** The individual has an exaggerated feeling of importance, power, knowledge, or identity. They may believe that they have a special relationship with a famous person or even assume the identity of a famous person (believing that the actual person is an imposter). Grandiose delusions of a religious nature may lead to assumption of the identity of a deity or religious leader (e.g., "I am Jesus Christ").

■ **Delusions of reference:** Events within the environment are referred by the psychotic person to themselves (e.g., "Someone is trying to get a message to me through the articles in this magazine [or newspaper or TV program]; I must break the code so that I can receive the message") and these beliefs become fixed (as with other delusions) despite evidence to the contrary. *Ideas of reference* are less rigid than delusions of reference. For example, an individual with ideas of reference may think that other people in the room who are giggling must be laughing about them, but with additional information can acknowledge that there could be other explanations for their laughter.

■ **Delusions of control or influence:** The individual believes certain objects or people have control over their behavior (e.g., "The dentist put a filling in my tooth; I now receive transmissions through the filling that control what I think and do") or the person believes that their thoughts or behaviors have control over specific situations or people (e.g., the mother who believes that if she scolds her son in any way, he will die). This type of delusion is similar to **magical thinking**, which is common in children (e.g., "The sky is raining because I'm sad").

■ **Somatic delusions:** The individual has a false idea about the functioning of their body. They may believe that they have some type of general medical condition or that there has been an alteration in a body organ or its function (e.g., "The doctor says I'm not pregnant, but I know I am"; "There is an alien force that is eating my brain").

■ **Nihilistic delusions:** The individual has a false idea that the self, a part of the self, others, or the world is nonexistent or has been destroyed (e.g., "The world no longer exists"; "I have no heart").

■ **Erotomanic delusions:** Individuals with erotomanic delusions falsely believe that someone, usually of a higher status, is in love with them. Famous people are often the subjects of erotomanic delusions.

Sometimes the delusion is kept secret, but some individuals may follow, contact, or otherwise try to pursue the object of their delusion.

■ **Jealous delusions:** The content of jealous delusions centers on the idea that the person's sexual partner is unfaithful. The idea is irrational and without cause, but the individual with the delusion searches for evidence to justify the belief. The sexual partner is confronted (and sometimes physically attacked) regarding the imagined infidelity. The imagined "lover" of the sexual partner also may be the object of the attack. Attempts to restrict the autonomy of the sexual partner in an effort to stop the imagined infidelity are common.

Disturbances in Thought Processes Manifested in Speech

Loose Associations Thinking is characterized by speech in which ideas shift from one unrelated subject to another. Typically, the individual with **loose associations** is unaware that the topics are unconnected. When the condition is severe, speech may be incoherent (e.g., "We wanted to take the bus, but the airport took all the traffic. Driving is the ticket when you want to get somewhere. We have it all in our pockets").

Neologisms **Neologisms** are newly invented words that are meaningless to others but have symbolic meaning to the individual (e.g., "She wanted to give me a ride in her new *uniphorum*").

Clang Associations The choice of words is governed by sounds, often taking the form of rhyming, which forms **clang associations.** For instance, "It is very cold. I am cold and bold. The gold has been sold."

Word Salad **word salad** is a group of words that appear to be put together randomly, without any logical connection (e.g., "Most forward action grows life double plays circle uniform").

Circumstantiality With **circumstantiality,** the individual delays in reaching the point of a communication because of unnecessary and tedious details. The point or goal is usually met but only with numerous interruptions by the interviewer to keep the person on track.

Tangentiality **Tangentiality** refers to a veering away from the topic of discussion and demonstrates difficulty in maintaining focus and attention.

Perseveration The individual who exhibits **perseveration** persistently repeats the same word or idea in response to different questions. It is the manifestation of a thought-processing disturbance in which the person gets stuck on a particular thought.

Echolalia **Echolalia** refers to repeating words or phrases spoken by another. In toddlers, this repetition is a normal phase in development, but in children with autism, echolalia may persist beyond the toddler years. In adulthood, echolalia is a significant neurological symptom of thought disturbance that occurs in schizophrenia, strokes, and other neurological disorders.

Disturbances in Perception

Hallucinations **Hallucinations,** or false sensory perceptions not associated with real external stimuli, may involve any of the five senses. Types of hallucinations include the following:

■ **Auditory:** Auditory hallucinations are false perceptions of sound. Most commonly, these are voices, but the individual may report clicks, rushing noises, music, and other noises. Command hallucinations are "voices" that issue commands to the individual. They are potentially dangerous when the commands are for violence to self or others. Auditory hallucinations are the most common type in schizophrenia.

■ **Visual:** These are false visual perceptions that may consist of formed images, such as those of people, or of unformed images, such as flashes of light. Visual hallucinations occur 27% of the time in individuals with schizophrenia (and 15% in affective psychosis). They typically co-occur with auditory hallucinations and are associated with poorer outcomes (Waters et al., 2014).

■ **Tactile:** Tactile hallucinations are false perceptions of the sense of touch, often of something on or under the skin. One specific tactile hallucination is *formication,* the sensation that something is crawling on or under the skin.

■ **Gustatory:** This is a false perception of taste. Most commonly, gustatory hallucinations are described as unpleasant tastes.

■ **Olfactory:** Olfactory hallucinations are false perceptions of the sense of smell.

Illusions **Illusions** are misperceptions or misinterpretations of real external stimuli. These may occur in the prodromal, active, and residual phases of schizophrenia and may co-occur with delusions.

Echopraxia The individual who exhibits **echopraxia** imitates movements made by others. The mechanisms underlying echopraxia in schizophrenia are not well understood, but current evidence suggests that it may involve a disturbance in mirror neuron activity in the presence of social cognition impairments and self-monitoring deficits, culminating in imitative psychomotor behavior (Urvakhsh et al., 2014). Imitative behavior is a natural human response, but when it occurs frequently and involuntarily it could be echopraxia (Drake, 2021). Echopraxia may also occur in several other conditions including Tourette's syndrome, brain injuries, epilepsy, autoimmune conditions, major neurocognitive disorder, and in those on the autism spectrum.

Negative Symptoms

Disturbances in Affect

Affect describes the visual manifestations associated with an individual's feeling state or emotional tone.

Inappropriate Affect Affect is inappropriate when the individual's emotional tone is incongruent with the circumstances (e.g., a young woman who laughs when told of the death of her mother).

Bland or Flat Affect Affect is described as bland when the emotional tone is very weak. The individual with flat affect appears to be void of emotional tone (or overt expression of feelings).

Apathy

The person with schizophrenia often demonstrates an indifference to or disinterest in the environment. The bland or flat affect is a manifestation of the emotional apathy.

Avolition

Impaired volition has to do with the inability to initiate goal-directed activity. In the individual with schizophrenia, this may take the form of inadequate interest, lack of motivation, neglect of activities of daily living including personal hygiene and appearance, or inability to choose a logical course of action in a given situation.

Lack of Interest or Skills in Interpersonal Interaction

Some patients with acute schizophrenia cling to others and intrude on the personal space of others, exhibiting behaviors that are not socially and culturally acceptable. Others may exhibit ambivalence in social relationships or may withdraw from relationships altogether (asociality).

Lack of Insight

Anosognosia is defined as an individual's lack of awareness of having an illness or disorder even when symptoms appear obvious to others. The *DSM-5-TR* identifies this symptom as the "most common predictor of nonadherence to treatment, and it predicts higher relapse rates, increased number of involuntary treatments, poorer psychosocial functioning, aggression, and poorer course of illness" (APA, 2022, p. 116).

Anergia

Anergia is a deficiency of energy. The individual with schizophrenia may lack sufficient energy to carry out activities of daily living or to interact with others.

Inability to Experience Pleasure

This distressing symptom, called **anhedonia,** is also common in major depression and may increase one's risk for suicide.

Lack of Abstract Thinking Ability

Lack of abstract thinking ability, called concrete thinking, is manifested in literal interpretations of the environment and represents a regression to an earlier level of cognitive development. Abstract thinking may be impaired in some individuals with schizophrenia (as well as autism spectrum disorders, brain injuries, major neurocognitive disorders, and intellectual disability disorders). For example, a person with this deficit would have great difficulty describing the abstract meaning of sayings such as "I'm climbing the walls" or "It's raining cats and dogs."

Associated Features

Waxy Flexibility

Waxy flexibility describes a condition in which the individual with schizophrenia allows body parts to be placed in bizarre or uncomfortable positions. This symptom is associated with catatonia. Once placed in position, the arm, leg, or head remains in that position for long periods, regardless of how uncomfortable it is for the person. For example, the nurse may position the patient's arm in an outward position to take a blood pressure measurement. When the cuff is removed, the patient maintains the arm in the position in which it was placed to take the reading. Waxy flexibility may also occur in other disorders including autism, Parkinson's disease, Wilson's disease, encephalitis, systemic lupus erythematosus, liver or kidney transplants, medication withdrawal, or drug-induced psychosis (Wiginton, 2022).

Posturing

Posturing is manifested by the voluntary assumption of inappropriate or bizarre postures.

Pacing and Rocking

Pacing back and forth and body rocking (a slow, rhythmic, backward-and-forward swaying of the trunk from the hips, usually while sitting) are common psychomotor behaviors of the patient with schizophrenia.

Regression

Regression is the retreat to an earlier level of development. Regression, a primary defense mechanism of schizophrenia, may be maladaptive coping to reduce insecurity, fear, or anxiety. It provides the basis for many of the behaviors associated with schizophrenia.

Regression has also been noted to occur in many mental disorders including borderline personality disorder, major depressive disorders, dissociative disorders, and dementia.

Eye Movement Abnormalities

Eye movement abnormalities may manifest in several ways including difficulty maintaining focus on a stationary object and difficulty with smooth pursuit of a moving object. Research (Benson et al., 2012) has found that simple eye movement tests can distinguish the abnormalities common in schizophrenia with exceptional accuracy.

Diagnosis and Outcome Identification

Using information collected during the assessment, the nurse completes the patient database, from which the selection of appropriate nursing diagnoses is determined. Table 24–1 presents a list of patient behaviors and the nursing diagnoses that correspond to those behaviors, which may be used in planning care for patients with psychotic disorders.

Outcome Criteria

The following criteria may be used for measurement of outcomes in the care of the patient with schizophrenia.

The patient:

■ Demonstrates an ability to relate satisfactorily to others
■ Recognizes distortions of reality
■ Has not harmed self or others
■ Perceives self realistically
■ Demonstrates the ability to perceive the environment correctly
■ Maintains anxiety at a manageable level

TABLE 24–1	Assigning Nursing Diagnoses to Behaviors Commonly Associated With Psychotic Disorders
BEHAVIORS	**NURSING DIAGNOSES**
Impaired communication (inappropriate responses), disordered thought sequencing, rapid mood swings, poor concentration, disorientation, stops talking in midsentence, tilts head to side as if listening	Disturbed sensory perception*
Delusional thinking; inability to concentrate; impaired volition; inability to problem-solve, abstract, or conceptualize; extreme suspiciousness of others; inaccurate interpretation of the environment	Disturbed thought processes
Withdrawal; sad, dull affect; need-fear dilemma; preoccupation with own thoughts; expression of feelings of rejection or of aloneness imposed by others; uncommunicative; seeks to be alone	Social isolation
Risk factors: Aggressive body language (e.g., clenching fists and jaw, pacing, threatening stance); verbal aggression; catatonic excitement; command hallucinations; rage reactions; history of violence; overt and aggressive acts; goal-directed destruction of objects in the environment; self-destructive behavior; active, aggressive suicidal acts	Risk for violence: Self-directed or other-directed
Loose association of ideas, neologisms, word salad, clang associations, echolalia, verbalizations that reflect concrete thinking, poor eye contact, difficulty expressing thoughts verbally, inappropriate verbalization	Impaired verbal communication
Difficulty carrying out tasks associated with hygiene, dressing, grooming, eating, and toileting	Self-care deficit
Neglectful care of the ill family member regarding basic human needs or illness treatment, extreme denial or prolonged overconcern regarding family member's illness, depression, hostility and aggression	Interrupted family processes
Inability to take responsibility for meeting basic health practices, history of lack of health-seeking behavior, lack of expressed interest in improving health behaviors, demonstrated lack of knowledge regarding basic health practices, anosognosia (lack of insight about illness)	Ineffective health maintenance
Unsafe, unclean, disorderly home environment; household members express difficulty in maintaining their home in a safe and comfortable condition	Impaired home maintenance

*This diagnosis has been resigned from the NANDA-I list of approved diagnoses. It is used in this instance because it is most compatible with the identified behaviors.
Source: Adapted from Herdman, T. H., Kamitsuru, S., & Lopes, C. T. (Eds.). (2021). *NANDA International, Inc. nursing diagnoses: Definitions and classification, 2021–2023* (12th ed.). Thieme.

- Relinquishes the need for delusions and hallucinations
- Demonstrates the ability to trust others
- Uses appropriate verbal communication in interactions with others
- Performs self-care activities independently

Planning and Implementation

The following section presents a group of selected nursing diagnoses, with short- and long-term goals and nursing interventions for each. In general, nursing interventions should be directed toward establishing trust, because suspiciousness is a common symptom in this disorder.

 Use of a passive rather than a directive communication approach, which offers the patient with paranoia the opportunity to make their own decisions about activities, treatment goals, and other aspects of care, helps establish trust while incorporating a patient-centered approach. For example, saying, "Would you like to attend group now?" is a less directive approach than saying "You need to go to group now."

Nurses must be aware of their own attitudes to avoid perpetuating stigmatization of this patient, which is frequently cited by individuals as a reason they have avoided seeking treatment. One way to reduce stigma is to become familiar with real people who suffer from this disorder rather than relying on fictitious representations (and sometimes misrepresentations) of this population in popular media.

Real Nurses, Real Advice

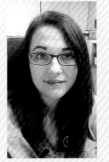

"The delusions, paranoia, and voices are very real to the patient with schizophrenia, so making sure not to devalue their experience is very important. It can also be a frightening experience so approaching slowly, staying at least an arm's length away, and speaking in a calming voice lets them know that you are there to help. Many times they just want someone to listen and treat them like a person first instead of always seeing their illness first."

–Sarah Taylor, Psychiatric Nursing Supervisor

(See the "Real People, Real Stories" introduction to Dr. Fred Frese.)

Some institutions use a case management model to coordinate care (see Chapter 8, "The Nursing Process in Psychiatric-Mental Health Nursing," for a more detailed explanation). In case management models, the plan of care may take the form of a critical pathway. In general, team approaches to the care of this patient have been identified as essential to positive outcomes and recovery.

 One of the QSEN competencies identifies the importance of teamwork and collaboration.
Nurses must collaborate effectively with other team members (including social workers, case managers, psychiatrists, chaplains, and counselors) to identify and respond to the complex care needs of this patient.

Disturbed Sensory Perception: Auditory/Visual

Disturbed sensory perception has been resigned as a nursing diagnosis by NANDA International (NANDA-I), but it is retained in this text because of its appropriateness in describing specific behaviors. The diagnosis is defined as sensory perceptions that are inconsistent with external stimuli and may include auditory, visual, tactile, olfactory, or gustatory perceptions. The following nursing interventions speak specifically to auditory hallucinations, the most common type occurring in schizophrenia. Table 24–2 presents this nursing diagnosis in care plan format.

Patient Goals

Outcome criteria include short- and long-term goals. Timelines are individually determined.

Short-term goal

- Patient will discuss content of hallucinations with nurse or therapist within 1 week.

Long-term goal

- Patient will be able to define and test reality, reducing or eliminating the occurrence of hallucinations.

This goal may not be realistic for the individual with severe and persistent illness who has experienced auditory hallucinations for many years. A more realistic goal may be:

- Patient will verbalize understanding that the voices are a result of their illness and demonstrate ways to interrupt the hallucination.

Interventions

- Observe the patient for signs of hallucinations (listening pose, laughing or talking to self, stopping in midsentence). Ask, "Are you hearing other voices?" "Are you able to distinguish those voices

Real People, Real Stories: Dr. Fred Frese

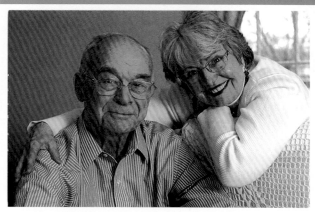

People with schizophrenia continue to be disenfranchised, misunderstood, and stigmatized. Even within health care, evidence has shown that some settings have been hostile to people with serious mental illnesses. One way to begin combating stigmatization of people with mental illness is to get to know them personally. Dr. Fred Frese, who died in 2018, was a licensed psychologist and an internationally renowned speaker, writer, and advocate in the field of mental illness.

Karyn: Could you share a little bit about your history with schizophrenia?

Dr. Frese: I was 25 when I had my first episode. I was in the Marines and—I know I had seen the movie *The Manchurian Candidate* previously—and I began to think that the Vietnamese were using the same strategies from the movie to control us. When I let my commanding officer know my theories, I was hospitalized involuntarily, and for the next 10 years I was in and out of hospitals—mostly involuntarily—taking various medications, living many different places, and not employed.

Karyn: Were you getting any treatments or intervention that you thought were helpful to your recovery?

Dr. Frese: Well, at that time it was thought that schizophrenia was not an illness from which one could recover. Even recently, I've heard some folks who have a family member with schizophrenia say, "There's no way that anyone with this illness can get better." But that's starting to change, and now that the government, through SAMHSA (Substance Abuse and Mental Health Services Administration) is backing the recovery model approach, I think health care will improve. I remember being told that my brain was going to progressively deteriorate and that I would never be able to function on my own. All in all, I probably spent about a year of my life in hospitalizations. Once the laws changed and I knew you had to be of imminent harm to yourself or others in order to be hospitalized involuntarily, I talked some of the health professionals out of admitting me. During the last attempt to hospitalize me, I actually escaped and ran away, even though I was in pretty bad shape.

Karyn: So since you were knowledgeable about the laws, you could essentially be your own self-advocate and argue your case, so to speak?

Dr. Frese: Yes, and by that time, I was in grad school and had secured a job at what is now the Department of Mental Health and Addiction Services. I remember I was living in the hallway of some university housing, and one of the students, who saw me day after day just hanging around and not really doing anything, suggested that I might be eligible for a government job because of my military background. When I applied, the receptionist saw my history of mental health commitments and said I would never get the job, but I did. The last time I went to the hospital, I went voluntarily because I knew I needed more medication, but they thought I needed to be hospitalized and I didn't; so I ran away.

Karyn: Sounds like you were managing a lot of stuff—grad school, working—and, at the same time, episodically struggling with symptoms of illness. You were working in the field of mental health, too. Was the work environment supportive?

Dr. Frese: Not always. It seemed like even among my coworkers, when something strange happened, they thought it was something wrong with me.

Karyn: What do you mean by "something strange"?

Dr. Frese: Like one time when they perceived I was spending too much time interacting with patients, they assumed I was "going off again," and next thing I knew, they called a "blue alert" and wanted to hospitalize me. But that time, the medical director just told me to take some time off. I never did find out why they called that blue alert.

Karyn: So you haven't been hospitalized for a very long time, and you are internationally renowned for all of your work and advocacy in the field of mental health. What do you think has contributed most to your recovery?

Dr. Frese: No, I haven't been hospitalized since I got married. I think that has been central in my recovery: having a person who you trust to give you feedback and let me know when I need more medication.

Karyn: What role do medications play in recovery?

Dr. Frese: It's very individual. We need more research to identify who, among people with schizophrenia, will benefit most by continuous medication versus episodic, reduced doses, or no medication. Genetic research is hopeful, but we're not there yet. It's hard to advise any individual what to do without knowing their individual circumstances, and even knowing, it can be very hard.

Karyn: What do you think is most important for future nurses to know about what they should do or say when they encounter someone with schizophrenia in a health-care setting, such as ER, for example?

Real People, Real Stories: Dr. Fred Frese—cont'd

Dr. Frese: Even though Freud's theories about psychoanalysis and insight-oriented therapy have been shown in research to be not only not helpful in the treatment of people with schizophrenia but potentially harmful, these ideas continue to influence the thinking of health-care professionals. I would tell nurses to wean themselves away from psychoanalytic concepts in treating people with schizophrenia. There continue to be assumptions that something bad must have happened in this patient's childhood, and the family is probably to blame. It's not a good way to forge relationships and may prejudge or isolate the people that can provide invaluable support.

So I would say to future nurses, don't make assumptions about me because you see a diagnosis or the kind of medication I'm on, and don't try to blame anyone for my symptoms. Treat me with civility and respect, don't respond to me with shock and disbelief, bullying, or laughing at me. Listening to the patient is the best way to establish and maintain a relationship. Even if the patient is saying something that doesn't make any sense to you, the best response is, "That's very interesting; tell me more."

Table 24–2 | CARE PLAN FOR THE PATIENT WITH SCHIZOPHRENIA

NURSING DIAGNOSIS: DISTURBED SENSORY PERCEPTION: AUDITORY/VISUAL

RELATED TO: Panic anxiety, extreme loneliness, and withdrawal into the self

EVIDENCED BY: Inappropriate responses, disordered thought sequencing, rapid mood swings, poor concentration, disorientation

OUTCOME CRITERIA	NURSING INTERVENTIONS	RATIONALE
Short-Term Goal ■ Patient discusses content of hallucinations with nurse or therapist within 1 week. **Long-Term Goals** ■ Patient is able to define and test reality, reducing or eliminating the occurrence of hallucinations. *Note:* This goal may not be realistic for the individual with severe and persistent illness who has experienced auditory hallucinations for many years. A more realistic goal may be: ■ Patient verbalizes understanding that the voices are a result of their illness and demonstrates ways to interrupt the hallucination.	1. Observe for signs of hallucinations (listening pose, laughing or talking to self, stopping in midsentence). Ask, "Are you hearing something else?" Or "Are you hearing other voices?" 2. Avoid touching the patient without warning them that you are about to do so. 3. An attitude of acceptance will encourage the patient to share the content of the hallucination with you. Ask, "What do you hear the voices saying to you?" 4. Do not reinforce the hallucination. Use "the voices" instead of words such as "they" that imply validation. Let client know that you do not share the perception. Say, "Even though I realize the voices are real to you, I do not hear any voices speaking."	1. Early intervention may prevent aggressive response to command hallucinations. Because the patient may not recognize these voices as hallucinations, it is better to ask the patient about what they are hearing rather than use the word "hallucinations." 2. The patient may perceive touch as threatening and may respond in an aggressive manner. 3. This question is important to prevent possible injury to the patient or others from command hallucinations. 4. It is important for the nurse to be honest, and the patient must accept the perception as unreal before hallucinations can be eliminated.

Continued

Table 24–2 | CARE PLAN FOR THE PATIENT WITH SCHIZOPHRENIA–cont'd

OUTCOME CRITERIA	NURSING INTERVENTIONS	RATIONALE
	5. Help the patient understand the connection between increased anxiety and the presence of hallucinations.	5. If the patient can learn to interrupt escalating anxiety, hallucinations may be prevented.
	6. Try to distract the patient from the hallucination.	6. Involvement in interpersonal activities and explanation of the actual situation facilitates reality orientation.
	7. For some patients, auditory hallucinations persist after the acute psychotic episode has subsided. Listening to the radio or watching television helps distract some patients from attention to the voices. Others have benefited from an intervention called *voice dismissal.* With this technique, the patient is taught to say loudly, "Go away!" or "Leave me alone!" in a conscious effort to dismiss the auditory perception.	7. These activities assist the patient in exerting some conscious control over the hallucination.

NURSING DIAGNOSIS: IMPAIRED VERBAL COMMUNICATION

RELATED TO: Panic anxiety, regression, withdrawal, disordered, unrealistic thinking

EVIDENCED BY: Loose association of ideas, neologisms, word salad, clang association, echolalia, verbalizations that reflect concrete thinking, poor eye contact

OUTCOME CRITERIA	NURSING INTERVENTIONS	RATIONALE
Short-Term Goal ■ Patient demonstrates the ability to remain on one topic, using appropriate, intermittent eye contact for 5 minutes with the nurse or therapist. Long-Term Goal ■ By time of discharge from treatment, patient demonstrates ability to carry on a verbal communication in a socially acceptable manner with health-care providers and peers.	1. Attempt to decode incomprehensible communication patterns. Seek validation and clarification by stating, "Is it that you mean...?" or "I don't understand what you mean by that. Would you please explain it to me?"	1. These techniques reveal how the patient is being perceived by others and conveys the nurse's desire to establish meaningful communication
	2. Maintain staff assignments as consistently as possible.	2. Consistency facilitates trust and understanding between patient and nurse.
	3. The technique of verbalizing the implied is used with the patient who is mute (unable or unwilling to speak). Example: "That must have been a very difficult time for you when your mother left. You must have felt very alone."	3. This approach conveys empathy and may encourage the patient to disclose painful issues.

Table 24–2 | CARE PLAN FOR THE PATIENT WITH SCHIZOPHRENIA—cont'd

OUTCOME CRITERIA	NURSING INTERVENTIONS	RATIONALE
	4. Anticipate and fulfill the patient's needs until functional communication pattern returns.	4. Patient safety and comfort are nursing priorities.
	5. Orient the patient to reality as required. Call patient by name. Validate those aspects of communication that help differentiate between what is real and not real.	5. These techniques may facilitate restoration of functional communication patterns in the patient.
	6. Explanations must be provided at the patient's level of comprehension. Example: "Pick up the spoon, scoop some mashed potatoes into it, and put it in your mouth."	6. Because concrete thinking prevails, abstract phrases and clichés must be avoided, as they are likely to be misinterpreted.

NURSING DIAGNOSIS: SELF-CARE DEFICIT

RELATED TO: Withdrawal, regression, panic anxiety, perceptual or cognitive impairment, inability to trust

EVIDENCED BY: Difficulty carrying out tasks associated with hygiene, dressing, grooming, eating, toileting

OUTCOME CRITERIA	NURSING INTERVENTIONS	RATIONALE
Short-Term Goal ■ Patient verbalizes a desire to perform activities of daily living (ADLs) by end of 1 week. **Long-Term Goal** ■ Patient is able to perform ADLs in an independent manner and demonstrates a willingness to do so by time of discharge from treatment.	1. Provide assistance with self-care needs as required. Some patients who are severely withdrawn may require total care.	1. Patient safety and comfort are nursing priorities.
	2. Encourage the patient to perform as many activities as possible independently. Provide positive reinforcement for independent accomplishments.	2. Independent accomplishment and positive reinforcement enhance self-esteem and promote repetition of desirable behaviors.
	3. Use concrete communication to show the patient what is expected. Provide step-by-step instructions for assistance in performing ADLs. Example: "Take your pajamas off and put them in the drawer. Take your shirt and pants from the closet and put them on. Comb your hair and brush your teeth."	3. Because concrete thinking prevails, explanations must be provided at the patient's concrete level of comprehension.
	4. Creative approaches may need to be taken with a patient who is not eating, such as allowing the patient to open their own canned or packaged foods; family style serving may also be an option.	4. These techniques may be helpful with the patient who is paranoid and may be suspicious that they are being poisoned with food or medication.
	5. If toileting needs are not being met, establish a structured schedule for the patient.	5. A structured schedule helps the patient establish a pattern so they can develop a habit of toileting independently.

from my voice?" Early intervention may prevent aggressive responses to command hallucinations (such as voices telling the patient to hurt or kill themselves).

■ Avoid touching the patient or ask for permission before doing so. The patient may perceive touch as threatening and respond in an aggressive or defensive manner.

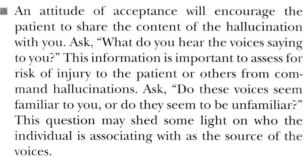 ■ An attitude of acceptance will encourage the patient to share the content of the hallucination with you. Ask, "What do you hear the voices saying to you?" This information is important to assess for risk of injury to the patient or others from command hallucinations. Ask, "Do these voices seem familiar to you, or do they seem to be unfamiliar?" This question may shed some light on who the individual is associating with as the source of the voices.

> **CLINICAL PEARL** Do not reinforce the hallucination. Use "the voices" instead of words such as "they" that imply validation. Let the patient know that you do not share the perception. For example, saying, "Even though I realize that the voices are real to you, I do not hear any voices speaking" conveys honesty and respect for the patient's experience as real, and it provides a foundation for exploration of management and coping strategies.

■ Assess the patient's level of anxiety and help them understand that increased anxiety may trigger hallucinations. If the patient can learn to interrupt escalating anxiety, these episodes may be minimized or prevented.

■ Try to distract the patient from the hallucination. Involvement in interpersonal activities and explanation of the actual situation will help the patient focus on reality.

■ For some patients, auditory hallucinations persist after the acute psychotic episode has subsided. Listening to the radio or watching television helps provide distraction from the voices. Others have benefited from an intervention called *voice dismissal*. With this technique, the patient is taught to say loudly, "Go away!" or "Leave me alone!" thereby exerting some conscious control over the behavior.

■ Assess for suicide risk. Some individuals have taken their own lives to escape from pervasive, troubling, or frightening hallucinations.

Disturbed Thought Processes

Disturbed thought processes are evidenced by behaviors that indicate the presence of delusional thinking, suspiciousness, and inaccurate interpretation of the environment. The diagnosis is defined as a disruption in cognitive operations and activities.

Patient Goals

Outcome criteria include short- and long-term goals. Timelines are individually determined.

Short-term goal

■ By the end of 2 weeks, patient will recognize and verbalize that symptoms escalate at times of increased anxiety.

Long-term goal

Depending on chronicity of the disease process, choose the most realistic long-term goal for the patient:

■ By time of discharge from treatment, patient's verbalizations will reflect reality-based thinking with no evidence of delusional ideation.

■ By time of discharge from treatment, patient will be able to differentiate between delusional thinking and reality.

Interventions

■ Convey acceptance of the patient's need for the false belief but indicate that you do not share the belief. The patient must understand that you do not view the idea as real.

■ Do not argue or deny the belief. Arguing with the patient or denying the belief serves no useful purpose, because delusional ideas are not eliminated by this approach, and the development of a trusting relationship may be impeded.

> **CLINICAL PEARL** Use reasonable doubt as a therapeutic technique. For example, when a patient says, "The FBI is wiretapping directly into my brain," the nurse may respond, "I understand that you believe this is true, but I personally find it hard to accept."

■ Reinforce and focus on reality. Although initially encouraging the patient to describe their delusional thoughts may be helpful to understand the patient's experience and to establish trust, discourage long ruminations about irrational thinking. Talk about real events and real people. See Box 24–5 for a list of interventions that may be helpful when working with a highly suspicious patient.

Risk for Violence: Self-Directed or Other-Directed

Risk for self- or other-directed violence is defined by NANDA-I as "susceptible to behaviors in which an individual demonstrates that he or she can be physically, emotionally, and/or sexually harmful either to self or to others" (Herdman et al., 2021, pp. 522–523).

BOX 24–5 Interventions for Patients With Suspicious Ideation

Patients who are prone to suspicious ideation are vulnerable to misinterpreting information and social cues in their environment, which can be a barrier to communication and relationship building. The following are some interventions to promote positive communication and establishment of trusting relationships.

- To promote the development of trust, use the same staff as much as possible; be honest and keep all promises.
- Avoid physical contact. Ask the patient's permission before using touch to perform a procedure, such as taking blood pressure. Patients with suspicious ideation often perceive touch as threatening and may respond in an aggressive or defensive manner.
- Avoid laughing, whispering, or talking quietly where the patient can see you but cannot hear what is being said.
- Extremely suspicious patients may believe they are being poisoned and refuse to eat food from an individually prepared tray. It may be necessary to provide canned food with a can opener or serve food family style.
- They may believe they are being poisoned with their medication and attempt to discard the tablets or capsules. Mouth checks may be necessary after medication administration to verify whether the patient is actually swallowing the pills.
- Competitive activities may be threatening to suspicious patients. Activities that encourage a one-to-one relationship with the nurse or therapist are best.
- Maintain an assertive, matter-of-fact, yet genuine approach. Approaches that are overly directive or cheerful may increase the patient's suspiciousness.

Patient Goals

Outcome criteria include short- and long-term goals. Timelines are individually determined.

Short-term goals

- Within [a specified time], patient will be able to recognize signs of increasing anxiety and agitation and report to staff (or other care provider) for assistance with intervention.
- Patient will not harm self or others.

Long-term goal

- Patient will not harm self or others.

Interventions

- Maintain a low level of environmental stimuli (low lighting, few people, simple decor, low noise level). Anxiety levels often increase in a stimulating environment. A suspicious, agitated patient may perceive individuals and noise as threatening.

- Observe the patient's behavior frequently while carrying out routine activities to avoid creating suspicion. Close observation is necessary so that intervention can occur if required to ensure the patient's (and others') safety.
- Assess for presence of suicidal ideation or command hallucinations that may be instructing the patient to harm self or others and remove all dangerous objects from the patient's environment so that they may not use them to harm self or others.

CLINICAL PEARL Intervene at the first sign of increased anxiety, agitation, or verbal or behavioral aggression. Offer empathetic response to the patient's feelings: "You seem anxious [or frustrated, or angry] about this situation. How can I help?" Validation of the patient's feelings conveys a caring attitude, and offering assistance reinforces trust.

- Maintain a calm attitude. As the patient's anxiety increases, offer some alternatives: participating in physical activity (e.g., exercise), talking about the situation, taking antianxiety medication. Offering alternatives gives the patient some control over the situation.
- Have sufficient staff available to indicate a show of strength to patient if it becomes necessary. The presence of adequate numbers of staff demonstrates control over the situation and also provides physical security for individual staff members.
- If the patient is not calmed by "talking down" or by medication and is posing an imminent threat to the safety of self or others, use of restraint may be necessary. The least restrictive method must be selected when planning interventions for an aggressive or violent patient. Restraints should be used only as a last resort, after all other interventions have been unsuccessful, and only if the patient is clearly at risk of harm to self or others.
- If restraint is deemed necessary, ensure that sufficient staff is available to assist. Follow protocol established by the institution. As the patient's agitation decreases, assess their readiness for restraint removal or reduction. Remove one restraint at a time while assessing the patient's response. This procedure minimizes the risk of injury to the patient and staff.

Impaired Verbal Communication

Impaired verbal communication is defined by NANDA-I as "decreased, delayed, or absent ability to receive, process, transmit, and/or use a system of symbols" (Herdman et al., 2021, p. 336). This care plan is also presented in Table 24–2.

Patient Goals

Outcome criteria include short- and long-term goals. Timelines are individually determined.

Short-term goal

■ Patient will demonstrate ability to remain on one topic, using appropriate, intermittent eye contact, for 5 minutes with the nurse or therapist.

Long-term goal

■ By time of discharge from treatment, patient will demonstrate ability to carry on a verbal communication in a socially acceptable manner with health-care providers and peers.

Interventions

■ Facilitate trust and understanding by maintaining staff assignments as consistently as possible. In a nonthreatening manner, explain to the patient how their behavior and verbalizations are viewed by and may alienate others.

CLINICAL PEARL Attempt to decode incomprehensible communication patterns. Seek validation and clarification by stating, "Is it that you mean... ?" or "I don't understand what you mean by that. Would you please explain it to me?" These techniques reveal to the patient how they are being perceived by others and demonstrate active listening and interest in understanding what the patient is trying to communicate.

■ Anticipate and fulfill the patient's needs until functional communication has been established.
■ Orient the patient to reality as required. Call the patient by name. Validate those aspects of communication that help differentiate between what is real and not real. These techniques may facilitate restoration of functional communication patterns.

CLINICAL PEARL If the patient is unable or unwilling to speak (mutism), using the technique of verbalizing the implied is therapeutic. For example, say "That must have been very difficult for you when your mother left. You must have felt very alone." This approach conveys empathy, facilitates trust, and eventually may encourage the patient to discuss painful issues.

■ Because concrete thinking may be a symptom, abstract phrases, clichés, and joking must be avoided, as they are likely to be misinterpreted. Explanations must be provided at the patient's level of comprehension.

CLINICAL PEARL Speak plainly and use clear language to minimize misinterpretation by the patient. For example, "Pick up the spoon, scoop some mashed potatoes into it, and put it in your mouth."

Concept Care Mapping

The concept map care plan (see Chapter 8, "The Nursing Process in Psychiatric-Mental Health Nursing") is a diagrammatic teaching and learning strategy that allows visualization of interrelationships between medical diagnoses, nursing diagnoses, assessment data, and treatments. An example of a concept map care plan for a patient with schizophrenia is presented in Figure 24–3.

Patient/Family Education

The role of patient teacher is important in the psychiatric area, as it is in all areas of nursing. A list of topics for patient and family education relevant to schizophrenia is presented in Box 24–6.

Evaluation

In the final step of the nursing process, a reassessment is conducted to determine whether the nursing actions have been successful in achieving the objectives of care. Evaluation of the nursing actions for the patient with exacerbation of schizophrenic psychosis may be facilitated by gathering information using the following types of questions:

■ Has the patient established trust with at least one staff member?
■ Is the anxiety level maintained at a manageable level?
■ Is delusional thinking still prevalent?
■ Is hallucinogenic activity evident? Does the patient share content of hallucinations, particularly if commands are heard?
■ Is the patient able to interrupt escalating anxiety with adaptive coping mechanisms?
■ Is the patient easily agitated?
■ Is the patient able to interact with others appropriately?
■ Does the patient voluntarily attend therapy activities?
■ Is verbal communication comprehensible?
■ Is the patient adhering to prescribed medications? Does the patient verbalize the importance of taking medication regularly and on a long-term basis? Does the patient verbalize understanding of possible side effects and when to seek assistance from the physician?
■ Does the patient spend time with others rather than isolating themselves?
■ Is the patient able to carry out all activities of daily living independently?
■ Is the patient able to verbalize resources from which they may seek assistance outside the hospital?
■ Does the family have information regarding support groups in which they may participate and from which they may seek assistance in dealing with their family member who is ill?

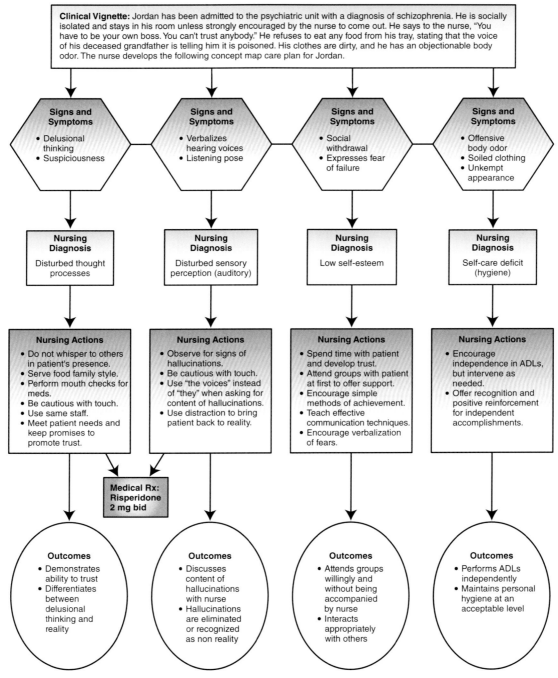

Clinical Vignette: Jordan has been admitted to the psychiatric unit with a diagnosis of schizophrenia. He is socially isolated and stays in his room unless strongly encouraged by the nurse to come out. He says to the nurse, "You have to be your own boss. You can't trust anybody." He refuses to eat any food from his tray, stating that the voice of his deceased grandfather is telling him it is poisoned. His clothes are dirty, and he has an objectionable body odor. The nurse develops the following concept map care plan for Jordan.

Signs and Symptoms
- Delusional thinking
- Suspiciousness

Signs and Symptoms
- Verbalizes hearing voices
- Listening pose

Signs and Symptoms
- Social withdrawal
- Expresses fear of failure

Signs and Symptoms
- Offensive body odor
- Soiled clothing
- Unkempt appearance

Nursing Diagnosis
Disturbed thought processes

Nursing Diagnosis
Disturbed sensory perception (auditory)

Nursing Diagnosis
Low self-esteem

Nursing Diagnosis
Self-care deficit (hygiene)

Nursing Actions
- Do not whisper to others in patient's presence.
- Serve food family style.
- Perform mouth checks for meds.
- Be cautious with touch.
- Use same staff.
- Meet patient needs and keep promises to promote trust.

Nursing Actions
- Observe for signs of hallucinations.
- Be cautious with touch.
- Use "the voices" instead of "they" when asking for content of hallucinations.
- Use distraction to bring patient back to reality.

Nursing Actions
- Spend time with patient and develop trust.
- Attend groups with patient at first to offer support.
- Encourage simple methods of achievement.
- Teach effective communication techniques.
- Encourage verbalization of fears.

Nursing Actions
- Encourage independence in ADLs, but intervene as needed.
- Offer recognition and positive reinforcement for independent accomplishments.

Medical Rx: Risperidone 2 mg bid

Outcomes
- Demonstrates ability to trust
- Differentiates between delusional thinking and reality

Outcomes
- Discusses content of hallucinations with nurse
- Hallucinations are eliminated or recognized as non reality

Outcomes
- Attends groups willingly and without being accompanied by nurse
- Interacts appropriately with others

Outcomes
- Performs ADLs independently
- Maintains personal hygiene at an acceptable level

FIGURE 24–3 Concept map care plan for patient with schizophrenia.

■ If the patient lives alone, do they have a source for assistance with home maintenance and health management?

Quality and Safety Education for Nurses (QSEN)

The Institute of Medicine (now the National Academy of Medicine), in its report *Health Professions Education: A Bridge to Quality* (Institute of Medicine [IOM], 2003), challenged faculties of medicine, nursing, and other health professions to ensure that their graduates have achieved a core set of competencies to meet the needs of the 21st-century health-care system. These competencies include *providing patient-centered care, working in interdisciplinary teams, employing evidence-based practice, applying quality improvement, maintaining safety,* and *utilizing informatics.* Patient-centered care is foundational to the recovery model (see Chapter 20, "The

BOX 24–6 Topics for Patient/Family Education Related to Schizophrenia

NATURE OF THE ILLNESS
1. What to expect as the illness progresses
2. Symptoms associated with the illness
3. Ways for family to respond to behaviors associated with the illness

MANAGEMENT OF THE ILLNESS
1. Connection of exacerbation of symptoms to times of stress
2. Appropriate medication management
3. Side effects of medications
4. Importance of not stopping medications
5. When to contact health-care provider
6. Relaxation techniques
7. Social skills training
8. Daily living skills training

SUPPORT SERVICES
1. Financial assistance
2. Legal assistance
3. Caregiver support groups
4. Respite care
5. Home health care
6. Residential treatment options

Recovery Model"), which has been advanced as an important framework for empowering patients with SMIs such as schizophrenia. This model promotes active patient engagement in treatment with a focus on achieving the patient's full recovery potential. However, to maintain *patient safety* and because some patients lack insight about their need for treatment, decisions may need to be made for them in their best interest. Supporting the patient's recovery necessitates the use of several resources and disciplines, which may include housing and financial assistance, medication management, peer support, spiritual counsel, and case management services. It is essential that nurses working with this population have a good understanding of the available support services for patients with schizophrenia and that they effectively work within interdisciplinary teams to meet this patient's complex needs.

Treatment Modalities for Schizophrenia and Other Psychotic Disorders

The prognosis for schizophrenia has often been reported in a paradigm of thirds. About one-third of people with schizophrenia achieve significant and lasting improvement. They may never experience another episode of psychosis after the initial occurrence. One-third may achieve some improvement with intermittent relapses and residual disability. Their occupational level may have decreased because of their illness, or they may be socially isolated. Finally, one-third experience severe and permanent incapacity. They often do not respond to medication and remain severely ill for much of their lives. Men typically have poorer outcomes than women; women respond better to treatment with antipsychotic medications. Although the paradigm of thirds provides a general guideline for understanding the variable course and prognosis in schizophrenia, Jablensky (2017) noted that with each successive decade there has been a trend toward a less deteriorating course in schizophrenia, which may be attributed to both treatment advances, early intervention, and changes in attitudes about this illness.

Psychological Treatments

Individual Psychotherapy

Individual, recovery-oriented psychotherapy and cognitive therapies are evidence-based interventions in the treatment of the person with schizophrenia, but they should be adjuncts to a multifaceted team approach. The primary focus in all cases must reflect efforts to decrease anxiety and increase trust.

Establishing a relationship is often particularly difficult because although the individual with schizophrenia often experiences loneliness and isolation, they struggle with closeness and trust. The individual is likely to respond to attempts at closeness with suspicion, anxiety, aggression, or regression. Successful intervention may be achieved with honesty, simple directness, and a manner that respects the person's privacy and human dignity. Exaggerated warmth and professions of friendship are likely to be met with confusion and suspicion.

Once a therapeutic interpersonal relationship has been established, reality orientation is maintained through exploration of the person's behavior within relationships. Education is provided to help the individual identify sources of real or perceived danger and ways of reacting appropriately. Methods for improving interpersonal communication, emotional expression, and frustration tolerance are attempted.

Group Therapy

Group therapy for individuals with schizophrenia has been shown to be effective, particularly with outpatients and when combined with drug treatment. Boland and Verduin (2022) stated:

Group therapy for persons with schizophrenia generally focuses on real-life plans, problems, and relationships. Some investigators doubt that dynamic interpretation and insight therapy are valuable for typical patients with schizophrenia. But group therapy is effective in reducing social isolation, increasing the sense of cohesiveness, and improving reality testing for patients with schizophrenia. (p. 355)

Group therapy in inpatient settings is less productive. Inpatient treatment usually occurs when symptomatology and social disorganization are at their most intense. At this time, the lowest level of stimulation is most beneficial for the patient. Because group therapy can be intensive and highly stimulating, it may be counterproductive early in treatment.

Group therapy for schizophrenia has been most useful over the long-term course of the illness. The social interaction, sense of cohesiveness, identification, and reality testing achieved within the group setting have proven to be highly therapeutic processes for individuals with this illness. Groups that offer a supportive environment appear to be more helpful than those that follow a more confrontational approach.

Behavior Therapy

Behavior modification has a history of qualified success in reducing the frequency of bizarre, disturbing, and socially unacceptable behaviors and increasing appropriate behaviors (Liberman, 1972; Marzillier & Birchwood, 1981). Features associated with positive outcomes include the following:

- Clearly defining goals and how they will be measured
- Attaching positive and negative reinforcements to adaptive and maladaptive behavior (token economies are an example)
- Using simple, concrete instructions and prompts to elicit the desired behavior

Behavior therapy can be a powerful treatment tool for helping patients change undesirable behaviors. In the treatment setting, the health-care provider can use praise and other positive reinforcements to help the patient with schizophrenia reduce the frequency of maladaptive or deviant behaviors. A limitation of this type of therapy is the inability of some individuals with schizophrenia to apply what they have learned from the treatment setting to the community setting.

More recently, evidence supports the use of cognitive behavior therapy (CBT) as an adjunctive treatment for symptoms of schizophrenia (Kart et al., 2021), but the researchers note that CBT is more effective in individuals with more flexible beliefs, good insight, and a shorter duration of illness. They also note that more research is needed to evaluate its effectiveness in treating negative symptoms.

Social Treatments
Social Skills Training

Social skills training is used to help individuals manage struggles with interpersonal relationships and communication, which are often complicated by an inability to perceive responses in others accurately. Mueser et al. (2001) described this training as follows:

The basic premise of social skills training is that complex interpersonal skills involve the smooth integration of a combination of simpler behaviors, including *nonverbal behaviors* (e.g., facial expression, eye contact); *paralinguistic features* (e.g., voice loudness and affect); *verbal content* (i.e., the appropriateness of what is said); and *interactive balance* (e.g., response latency, amount of time talking). These specific skills can be systematically taught, and, through the process of *shaping* (i.e., rewarding successive approximations toward the target behavior), complex behavioral repertoires can be acquired. (p. 6)

Social dysfunction is a hallmark of schizophrenia. Impairment in interpersonal relations is included as part of the defining diagnostic criteria for the condition in the *DSM-5-TR* (APA, 2022). Considerable attention is now being given to enhancement of social skills for this population.

The educational procedure in social skills training focuses on role-playing. A series of brief scenarios are selected. These should be typical of situations patients experience in their daily lives and graduated in terms of level of difficulty. The health-care provider may serve as a role model for some behaviors. For example, "See how I sort of nod my head up and down and look at your face while you talk." This demonstration is followed by the patient's role-playing. Immediate feedback is provided regarding the patient's presentation. With repetition, the patient's response gradually becomes smooth and effortless.

Progress is directed toward the individual's needs and limitations. The focus is on small units of behavior, and the training proceeds very gradually. Highly threatening issues are avoided, and emphasis is placed on functional skills that are relevant to activities of daily living. *Milieu therapy*, which focuses on the individual's interaction within a social environment, may provide opportunities for social skills training.

Cognitive Remediation Therapy

As mentioned previously, many of the cognitive deficits common in schizophrenia have not been particularly responsive to existing pharmacological treatments. However, some evidence suggests that cognitive remediation therapies, which include social cognition training, can be an effective treatment. Cognitive remediation is based on behavioral training aimed at helping the patient to mend areas of cognitive dysfunction, including attention, memory, social cognition, and executive functions. The intervention entails repetitive drills and practice. The evidence supports that this training results in significant improvements in memory, attention, problem-solving, cognition, social cognition, independent living skills, and social adjustment (Tripathi et al., 2018).

Family Therapy

Schizophrenia is an illness that can puzzle, disrupt, and sometimes tear apart families. Even when families appear to cope well, there is a notable effect on the mental and physical health of the family when a family member has this illness.

The importance of the expanded role of family in the aftercare of those with schizophrenia has been recognized, thereby stimulating interest in family intervention programs designed to support the family system, prevent or delay relapse, and help to maintain the patient in the community. These psychoeducational programs treat the family as a resource rather than a stressor, with the focus on practical problem-solving and specific behaviors for coping with stress. These programs recognize the biological basis for schizophrenia and the effect that stress has on the individual's ability to function. By providing the family with information about the illness and suggestions for effective coping, psychoeducational programs reduce the likelihood of the patient's relapse and the possible emergence of mental illness in previously nonaffected relatives.

Mueser and associates (2001) stated that although models of family intervention with schizophrenia differ in their characteristics and methods, effective treatment programs share several features:

■ All programs are long term (usually 9 months to 2 years or more).
■ They all provide the patient and family with information about the illness and its management.
■ They focus on improving adherence to prescribed medications.
■ They strive to decrease stress in the family and improve family functioning.

Asen (2002) suggested the following interventions with families of individuals with schizophrenia:

■ Forming a close alliance with the caregivers
■ Lowering the emotional climate within the family by reducing stress and burden on family members
■ Increasing the ability of family members to anticipate and solve problems
■ Reducing the expressions of anger and guilt by family members

■ Maintaining reasonable expectations for how the ill family member should perform
■ Encouraging family members to set appropriate limits while retaining some degree of separateness
■ Promoting desirable changes in the family members' behaviors and belief systems

Family therapy typically consists of a brief program of family education about schizophrenia and a more extended program of family contact designed to reduce overt manifestations of conflict and improve patterns of family communication and problem-solving. The response to this type of therapy has been dramatic. Studies confirm that more positive outcomes in the treatment of the person with schizophrenia can be achieved by including the family system in the program of care (Caqueo-Urízar et al., 2015).

Assertive Community Treatment

Assertive community treatment (ACT) is an evidence-based program of case management that takes a team approach in providing comprehensive, community-based psychiatric treatment, rehabilitation, and support to persons with serious and persistent mental illness such as schizophrenia. Other terms for this type of treatment include mobile treatment teams and community support programs. Assertive programs of treatment are individually tailored for each client, intended to be proactive, and include teaching basic living skills, helping clients work with community agencies, and assisting clients in developing a social support network. Vocational expectations are emphasized, and supported work settings (i.e., sheltered workshops) are an important part of the treatment program. Other services include treatment for substance misuse and addictions, psychoeducational programs, family support and education, mobile crisis intervention, and attention to health-care needs.

Responsibilities are shared by multiple team members, including psychiatrists, nurses, social workers, vocational rehabilitation therapists, and addictions counselors. Services are provided in the person's home; within the neighborhood; in local restaurants, parks, or stores; or wherever assistance by the client is required. These services are available to the client 24 hours a day, 365 days a year, and ACT is considered a long-term intervention strategy. One study looked at the impact of a *Housing First* intervention (an intervention that prioritizes rapid rehousing for homeless individuals with schizophrenia) and found that when this type of intervention was combined with ACT, medication adherence improved from less than 50% to 78%. Additionally, these combined interventions improved clients' integration in the community, increased residential stability, and decreased criminal convictions (Rezansoff et al., 2016).

ACT has been shown to reduce the number of hospitalizations and decrease costs of care for these clients. Although it has been called "paternalistic" and "coercive" by its critics, ACT has provided much-needed services and increased quality of life for many clients who are unable to manage in a less-structured environment. One limitation is that treatment programs of this kind are time and labor intensive.

Recovery Model

Research provides support for recovery as an objective within reach for individuals with schizophrenia (Lysaker et al., 2010). Lysaker and associates (2010) stated:

> Recovery from schizophrenia, in the sense of a state in which persons experience no difficulties associated with the illness, can occur but the modal outcome seems to be one in which difficulties linked to symptoms, social function, and work appear periodically but can be successfully confronted. (p. 40)

Conceptual models of recovery from mental illness are presented in Chapter 20, "The Recovery Model." The recovery model has been used primarily in caring for individuals with SMI, such as schizophrenia and bipolar disorder. However, concepts of the model are amenable to use with all individuals experiencing emotional conditions that require assistance and desiring to take control and manage their lives more independently.

Weiden (2010) identified two types of recovery with schizophrenia: functional and process. Functional recovery focuses on the individual's level of functioning in such areas as relationships, work, independent living, and other activities. They may or may not be experiencing active symptoms of schizophrenia. With process recovery, there is no defined endpoint. Recovery continues throughout the individual's life and involves collaboration between client and clinician. The individual identifies goals based on personal values or what they define as giving meaning and purpose to life. The clinician and client work together to develop a treatment plan in alignment with the goals set forth by the client. In the process recovery model, the individual may still be experiencing symptoms. Weiden (2010) stated:

> Patients do not have to be in remission, nor does remission automatically have to be a desired (or likely) goal when embarking on a recovery-oriented treatment plan. As long as the patient (and family) understands that a process recovery treatment plan is not to be confused with a promise of "cure" or even "remission," then one does not overpromise.

The concept of recovery in schizophrenia remains controversial among clinicians, and many challenges lie ahead for continued study. Recovery models have similarities with ACT in that they both necessarily engage the support of multiple resources, but recovery models also highlight the dimension of active engagement and empowerment of the client in decision making. Some argue that this approach is difficult to implement with clients who lack insight about their illness or the need for treatment. Further, there is a lack of consistency in what constitutes "recovery," and many concepts exist.

 One of the identified QSEN competencies is patient-centered care and, despite the controversies about the recovery model approach, the hope is that as these models become better studied and more clearly defined, they will provide a treatment approach that is comprehensive, protective, and supportive of patient-centered care.

RAISE (Recovery After an Initial Schizophrenic Episode)

The RAISE approach to treatment for schizophrenia is based on a large National Institute of Mental Health (NIMH) initiative that began in 2008. Research findings published in 2015 have demonstrated several benefits of this approach. Kane and associates (2015) described the RAISE approach as follows:

> The premise of the NIMH RAISE-ETP (Early Treatment Program) is to combine state-of-the-art pharmacological and psychosocial treatments delivered by a well-trained, multidisciplinary team, in order to significantly improve the functional outcome and quality of life for first episode psychosis patients. The RAISE approach incorporates many elements from other treatment approaches, including community treatment, recovery model approaches, family approaches, and comprehensive care models. It adds the dimension of early intervention at the first episode of psychosis. The research findings after 5 years of studying this approach are promising for improving care to this population when intervention begins at the earliest onset of psychotic symptoms. Positive outcomes have included greater adherence to treatment programs; greater improvement in symptoms, interpersonal relationships, and quality of life; more involvement in employment or educational pursuits; and less frequent hospitalizations than are seen for clients involved in more traditional treatment approaches (Kane et al., 2015).

The hope for this approach to treatment is that through early and comprehensive intervention, the long-term debilitating consequences of schizophrenia can be averted or minimized.

Psychopharmacological Treatment

Chlorpromazine (Thorazine) was first introduced in the United States in 1952. At that time, it was used in conjunction with barbiturates in surgical anesthesia. With increased use, the drug's psychic properties were recognized, and by 1954 it was marketed as an antipsychotic medication in the United States. The manufacture and sale of other antipsychotic drugs followed in rapid succession.

Antipsychotic medications are also called *neuroleptics,* and historically were referred to as major tranquilizers. They are effective in the treatment of acute and chronic manifestations of schizophrenia and in maintenance therapy to prevent exacerbation of schizophrenic symptoms. A meta-analysis of studies (Takeuchi et al., 2017) evaluating the benefits of maintenance antipsychotic medication found significant worsening of symptoms over the course of a year in patients who did not continue taking medication.

As mentioned earlier, the efficacy of antipsychotic medications is enhanced by adjunct psychosocial therapy. Because the psychotic manifestations of the illness subside with use of the drugs, individuals on medication are generally more cooperative with the psychosocial therapies. However, it takes several weeks for the antipsychotics to effectively treat positive symptoms, which often leads to discontinuation of the medication. Patients and families need to be educated about the importance of waiting, often for several weeks, to determine whether medications will be effective.

These medications are classified as either *typical* (first generation, with more dopaminergic activity) or *atypical* (second generation, with some serotonergic activity,). Examples of commonly used antipsychotic agents are presented in Table 24–3. A description of these medications follows. More detailed information is available in Chapter 4, "Psychopharmacology."

Indications

Antipsychotic medications are used in the treatment of schizophrenia and other psychotic disorders. Selected agents are used in the treatment of bipolar mania (olanzapine, aripiprazole, chlorpromazine, quetiapine, risperidone, asenapine, ziprasidone, cariprazine).

Action

Typical antipsychotics work by blocking postsynaptic dopamine receptors in the basal ganglia, hypothalamus, limbic system, brainstem, and medulla. They demonstrate varying affinity for cholinergic, alpha$_1$-adrenergic, and histaminic receptors. Antipsychotic effects may also be related to inhibition of dopamine-mediated transmission of neural impulses at the synapses.

Atypical antipsychotics are weaker dopamine receptor antagonists than conventional antipsychotics but more potent antagonists of the serotonin (5-hydroxytryptamine) type 2A (5HT$_2$A) receptors. They also exhibit antagonism for cholinergic, histaminic, and adrenergic receptors. Positive symptoms respond relatively well to treatment with both typical (first generation) and atypical (second generation) antipsychotic medication. Boland and Verduin (2022) identified that positive symptoms tend to become less severe over time, whereas the negative or "deficit" symptoms are socially debilitating and may increase in severity. Atypical antipsychotics have been advanced as being more effective than first generation antipsychotics in treating negative symptoms (particularly cariprazine), but researchers continue to search for medications that will specifically treat the cognitive deficits that are most problematic for patients with schizophrenia. These deficits include those of memory, attention, language, and executive functions, which can dramatically affect an individual's overall functional ability. A detailed discussion of contraindications, precautions, side effects, and drug interactions associated with antipsychotic medications is available in Chapter 4, "Psychopharmacology."

Side Effects

The effects of these medications are related to blockage of receptors for which they exhibit various degrees of affinity. Blockage of the dopamine receptors is thought to be responsible for controlling positive symptoms of schizophrenia. Dopamine blockage also results in extrapyramidal symptoms (EPS) and prolactin elevation (galactorrhea; gynecomastia). (A list of medications commonly used to treat EPS is included in Table 24–4.) Cholinergic blockade causes anticholinergic side effects (dry mouth, blurred vision, constipation, urinary retention, tachycardia). Blockage of the alpha$_1$-adrenergic receptors produces dizziness, orthostatic hypotension, tremors, and reflex tachycardia. Histamine blockade is associated with weight gain and sedation.

The plan of care should include monitoring for the side effects of antipsychotic medications and educating the patient and family about safety precautions when taking antipsychotic medication. (A list of side effects and relevant nursing interventions is included in Chapter 4, "Psychopharmacology.")

There have been two recent and novel developments in psychopharmacological treatments for patients with schizophrenia. The first is a formulation of aripiprazole (Abilify MyCite) with a tracking sensor that allows the patient (and others) to monitor medication adherence. Approved in late

TABLE 24–3 **Antipsychotic Agents**

CATEGORIES	GENERIC (TRADE NAME)	DAILY DOSAGE RANGE (mg)
Typical antipsychotic agents (first generation; conventional)	Chlorpromazine	40–400
	Fluphenazine	2.5–10
	Haloperidol (Haldol)	1–30 (PO)
	Loxapine	20–250
	Loxapine (inhaled)	10 mg single use inhaler
	Perphenazine	12–64
	Pimozide (Orap) (For motor tics in Tourette's)	1–10
	Prochlorperazine	15–150
	Thiothixene (Navane)	6–30
	Trifluoperazine	4–40
Atypical antipsychotic agents (second generation; novel)	Aripiprazole (Abilify)	10–30
	(Abilify MyCite; with tracking sensor)	2–30
	Aripiprazole lauroxil (Aristada)	441–662 monthly, 882 every 6 weeks, 1064 every 2 months (IM injection)
	Asenapine (Saphris)	10–20
	Asenapine transdermal (Secuado)	3.8–7.6 patch
	Brexpiprazole (Rexulti)	2–4
	Cariprazine (Vraylar)	1.5–6
	Clozapine (Clozaril)	300–900
	Iloperidone (Fanapt)	12–24
	Lurasidone (Latuda)	40–80
	Olanzapine (Zyprexa)	5–20
	Olanzapine/samidorphan (Lybalvi)	5/10–20/10
	Paliperidone (Invega)	6–12
	(Invega Sustenna—once a month)	39–234 (IM)
	(Invega Trinza—once every 3 months)	273–819 (IM)
	Quetiapine (Seroquel)	300–400
	Risperidone (Risperdal)	4–8
	Risperidone, long-acting (Perseris)	90 or 120 subcutaneously (once a month)
	Ziprasidone (Geodon)	40–160

2017, this formulation has spurred controversy and debate about the benefits versus the potential intrusiveness of such a monitoring device. The second novel treatment is valbenazine (Ingrezza), a drug for the treatment of tardive dyskinesia. Tardive dyskinesia, a movement disturbance that is more prevalent with first generation antipsychotics, is particularly troubling because it has been a permanent, incurable side effect. Valbenazine works by reducing dopamine release at the synaptic cleft and has demonstrated effectiveness in reducing abnormal involuntary movements such as tardive dyskinesia. Future research will determine its long-term effectiveness. Currently, the cost for this treatment may limit its accessibility for many with chronic, SMI and those without insurance coverage.

Patient and Family Education Related to Antipsychotics

The patient receiving antipsychotic medication should:

■ Use caution when driving or operating dangerous machinery. Drowsiness and dizziness can occur.
■ Not stop taking the drug abruptly after long-term use. To do so might produce withdrawal symptoms, such as nausea, vomiting, dizziness, gastritis, headache, tachycardia, insomnia, and tremulousness.

TABLE 24-4 Antiparkinsonian Agents Used to Treat Extrapyramidal Side Effects of Antipsychotic Drugs

Indication	Used to treat parkinsonism of various causes and drug-induced extrapyramidal reactions.
Action	Restores the natural balance of acetylcholine and dopamine in the CNS. The imbalance is a deficiency in dopamine that results in excessive cholinergic activity.
Contraindications/ precautions	Antiparkinsonian agents are contraindicated in individuals with hypersensitivity. Anticholinergics should be avoided by individuals with angle-closure glaucoma; pyloric, duodenal, or bladder neck obstructions; prostatic hypertrophy; or myasthenia gravis. Caution should be used in administering these drugs to clients with hepatic, renal, or cardiac insufficiency; elderly and debilitated clients; those with a tendency toward urinary retention; or those exposed to high environmental temperatures.
Common side effects	Anticholinergic effects (dry mouth, blurred vision, constipation, paralytic ileus, urinary retention, tachycardia, elevated temperature, decreased sweating), nausea/GI upset, sedation, dizziness, orthostatic hypotension, exacerbation of psychoses.

CHEMICAL CLASS	GENERIC (TRADE NAME)	DAILY DOSAGE RANGE (mg)
Anticholinergics	Benztropine (Cogentin)	1–8
	Biperiden (Akineton)	2–6
	Trihexyphenidyl	1–15
Antihistamines	Diphenhydramine (Benadryl)	25–200
Dopaminergic agonists	Amantadine	200–300
VMAT2 inhibitor (for tardive dyskinesia)	Valbenazine	40–80
	Deutetrabenazine	6–48

CNS: central nervous system; GI: gastrointestinal; VMAT2: vesicular monoamine transporter type 2.

■ Use sunblock lotion and wear protective clothing when spending time outdoors. Skin is more susceptible to sunburn, which can occur in as little as 30 minutes.

■ Report weekly (if receiving clozapine therapy) to have blood levels drawn and to obtain a weekly supply of the drug.

■ Report immediately to the physician the occurrence of any of the following symptoms: sore throat, fever, malaise, unusual bleeding, easy bruising, persistent nausea and vomiting, severe headache, rapid heart rate, difficulty urinating, muscle twitching, tremors, dark-colored urine, excessive urination, excessive thirst, excessive hunger, weakness, pale stools, yellow skin or eyes, muscular incoordination, or skin rash.

■ Rise slowly from a sitting or lying position to prevent a sudden drop in blood pressure.

■ Take frequent sips of water, chew sugarless gum, or suck on hard candy if dry mouth is a problem. Good oral care (frequent brushing and flossing) is important.

■ Consult the physician regarding smoking while on antipsychotic therapy. Smoking increases the metabolism of antipsychotics, requiring an adjustment in dosage to achieve a therapeutic effect.

■ Dress warmly in cold weather and avoid extended exposure to very high or low temperatures. Body temperature is harder to maintain with this medication.

■ Avoid drinking alcohol while on antipsychotic therapy. These drugs potentiate each other's effects.

■ Avoid taking other medications (including over-the-counter products) without the physician's approval. Many medications contain substances that interact with antipsychotics in a way that may be harmful.

■ Be aware of possible risks of taking antipsychotics during pregnancy. Antipsychotics are thought to cross the placental barrier; if so, a fetus could experience adverse effects of the drug. Neonates are at increased risk for EPS and withdrawal after delivery when exposed to antipsychotics during the third trimester. Inform the physician immediately if pregnancy occurs, is suspected, or is planned.

■ Be aware of side effects of antipsychotic drugs. Refer to written materials furnished by health-care providers for safe self-administration.

■ Continue to take the medication, even if feeling well and as though it is not needed. Symptoms may return if medication is discontinued.

■ Carry a card or other identification at all times describing medications being taken.

Smoking Cessation

Smoking cigarettes has long been identified as a particular health risk for people with schizophrenia because the prevalence is three times that of the general population. It is estimated that as many as 88% of those with schizophrenia and 70% of those with bipolar disorder are smokers (Kranjac, 2016). Some people report increased ability to concentrate when smoking tobacco, which has led to clinical trials of drugs that increase nicotine levels. However, to date, these drugs have not been proven to be effective. In addition to the obvious health risks of chronic lung diseases and cancers, smoking decreases the effectiveness of some psychotropic medications. Varenicline (Chantix), a nicotine agonist used as a smoking deterrent, was once thought to increase symptoms and even suicide risk in those with SMI. However, a recent meta-analysis (Wu et al., 2016) concluded that varenicline is effective for assisting with smoking cessation in this population and that "there was no clear evidence of neuropsychiatric or other adverse events compared with placebo" (p. 1554). In any scenario, assessing the patient's motivation to stop smoking and exploring viable treatment options, including psychological interventions, is an important component of treatment.

CLINICAL JUDGMENT IN ACTION: CASE STUDY AND SAMPLE CARE PLAN

NURSING HISTORY AND ASSESSMENT

Recognizing cues: The nurse must demonstrate the ability to recognize what information is most important to making an assessment (National Council of State Boards of Nursing [NCSBN], 2021). This information is italicized in the following.

Frank is 22 years old. He joined the Marines just out of high school at age 18 for a 3-year enlistment. His final year was spent in Afghanistan. When his enlistment was up, he returned to his hometown and married a young woman with whom he had been a high school classmate. Frank has *always been quiet, somewhat withdrawn, and had very few friends.* He was the only child of a single mom who never married, and he does not know his father. His mother was killed in an automobile accident the spring before he enlisted in the Marines.

During the past year, he has become increasingly isolated and withdrawn. He is without regular employment but finds work as a day laborer when he can. His wife, Suzanne, works as a secretary and is the primary wage earner. Lately, *Frank has become very suspicious of Suzanne and sometimes follows her to work. He also drops in on her at work and accuses her of having affairs with some of the men in the office.*

Last evening when Suzanne got home from work, Frank was *hiding in the closet.* She didn't know he was home. When she started to undress, he jumped out of the closet *holding a large kitchen knife and threatened to kill her "for being unfaithful."* Suzanne managed to flee their home and ran to the neighbor's house and called the police.

Frank told the police that he *received a message over the radio from his Marine commanding officer telling him that he couldn't allow his wife to continue to commit adultery, and the only way he could stop it was to kill her.* The police took Frank to the emergency department of the VA Hospital, where he was *admitted to the psychiatric unit.* Suzanne is helping with the admission history.

Suzanne tells the nurse that she has never been unfaithful to Frank and she doesn't know why he believes that she has. Frank tells the nurse that he has been *"taking orders from my commanding officer through my car radio ever since I got back from Afghanistan."* He survived a helicopter crash in Afghanistan in which all were killed except Frank and one other man. Frank says, "I have to follow my CO's orders. *God saved me to annihilate the impure."*

After an evaluation, the psychiatrist diagnoses Frank with schizophrenia. He orders olanzapine 10 mg PO to be given daily and olanzapine 10 mg IM q6h prn for agitation.

Analyzing cues: The nurse must be able to interpret the information (NCSBN, 2021).

The nurse interprets that Frank's suspicious ideation and his behavior toward his wife raise the risk for violence toward others. The statements by Frank about receiving messages through the radio is evidence of auditory hallucinations and his statement about God saving him to annihilate the impure is interpreted as both a delusion (fixed false belief) and a command hallucination.

Prioritize hypotheses: The nurse must be able to identify the client's most important needs (NCSBN, 2021).

Continued

CLINICAL JUDGMENT IN ACTION: CASE STUDY AND SAMPLE CARE PLAN—cont'd

The nurse identifies that the patient, while admitted to the hospital, remains at risk for violence related to suspicious ideation, command hallucinations, and delusions. In addition to safety concerns, the nurse recognizes that establishing trust will be a priority intervention. Although there may be unresolved grief and service-related post-trauma issues that require further assessment, the nurse prioritizes safety and patient stabilization as priorities at present.

NURSING DIAGNOSES AND OUTCOME IDENTIFICATION

Generate solutions: The nurse must be able to connect their prioritized understanding of client needs to a course of action or plan of care (NCSBN, 2021).

From the assessment data, the nurse develops the following nursing diagnoses for Frank:

1. Risk for other-directed violence related to command hallucinations; and history of violence.
   a. Short-term goals:
      - Frank will seek out staff when anxiety and agitation start to increase.
      - Frank will not harm self or others.
   b. Long-term goal: Frank will not harm self or others.
2. Disturbed sensory perception: Auditory hallucinations related to increased anxiety and agitation and withdrawal into self
   a. Short-term goals:
      - Frank will discuss the content of the hallucinations with the nurse.
      - Frank will maintain anxiety at a manageable level.
   b. Long-term goal: Frank will be able to define and test reality, reducing or eliminating the occurrence of hallucinations.

PLANNING AND IMPLEMENTATION

Take Action: The nurse must be able to identify what actions need to be taken and how they will be implemented (NCSBN, 2021).

RISK FOR OTHER-DIRECTED VIOLENCE

1. Establish trust through open, honest, communication and encourage Frank to discuss concerns within his comfort level.
2. Monitor Frank's behavior frequently, but in a manner of carrying out routine activities so as not to create suspiciousness on his part.
3. Watch for the following signs (considered the prodrome to aggressive behavior): increased motor activity, pounding, slamming, tense posture, defiant affect, clenched teeth and fists, arguing, demanding, and challenging or threatening staff.
4. If Frank becomes aggressive, maintain a calm attitude. Try talking. Offer medication. Provide physical activities.
5. If these interventions fail, engage other staff members to provide physical crisis intervention as needed.

6. Utilize restraints only as a last resort and if Frank is clearly at risk of harm to himself or others.
7. Assess for presence of suicide risk and collaborate with the patient to develop a personal safety plan as needed.

DISTURBED SENSORY PERCEPTION: AUDITORY

1. Monitor Frank's behavior for signs that he is hearing voices: listening pose, talking and laughing to self, stopping in midsentence.
2. If these behaviors are observed, ask Frank, "Are you hearing the voices again?"
3. Encourage Frank to share the content of the hallucinations. This information is important for early intervention in case the content contains commands to harm himself or others.
4. Say to Frank, "I understand that the voice is real to you, but I do not hear any voices speaking." It is important for him to learn the difference between what is real and what is not real.
5. Try to help Frank recognize that the voices often appear at times when he becomes anxious about something and his agitation increases.
6. Help him to recognize this increasing anxiety and teach him methods to keep it from escalating.
7. Use distracting activities to bring him back to reality. Involvement with real people and real situations will help to distract him from the hallucination.
8. Teach him to use *voice dismissal.* When he hears the CO's (or others') voice, he should shout, "Go away!" or "Leave me alone!" These commands may help to diminish the sounds and give him a feeling of control over the situation.

EVALUATION

Evaluate outcomes: The nurse must be able to evaluate actions taken and determine whether they have had a positive, neutral, or negative effect (NCSBN, 2021).

The outcome criteria identified for Frank have been met. When feeling especially anxious or becoming agitated, he seeks out staff for comfort and for assistance in maintaining his anxiety at a manageable level. He currently denies suicide ideation. He is experiencing fewer auditory hallucinations and has learned to use voice dismissal to interrupt the behavior. He has begun to discuss traumas associated with military combat, ongoing grief issues over the loss of his mother, and is beginning to recognize his position in the grief process. He has been referred to a psychologist for outpatient counseling, outpatient psychiatrist visits for medication management, and a vocational rehabilitation specialist to explore employment opportunities. Suzanne has begun attending family support meetings through the local chapter of The National Alliance on Mental Illness.

Summary and Key Points

- Schizophrenia is a disorder that includes thought disturbances along with emotional and behavioral symptoms that result in a significant amount of personal, emotional, and social cost if untreated. Early diagnosis and intervention are associated with better outcomes.

- For many years, there was little agreement about the definition of schizophrenia. The *DSM-5-TR* (APA, 2022) identifies specific criteria for diagnosis of the disorder that include at least delusions, hallucinations, or disorganized speech and may also include grossly disorganized or catatonic behavior and negative symptoms.

- The initial symptoms of schizophrenia most often occur in early adulthood. Development of the disorder can be viewed in four phases: (1) premorbid, (2) prodromal, (3) active psychotic (schizophrenia), and (4) residual.

- The cause of schizophrenia remains unclear. Most likely no single factor can be implicated; rather, the disease probably results from a complex interaction of genetic, biochemical, psychological, and environmental factors.

- A spectrum of schizophrenic and other psychotic disorders has been identified. These include (on a gradient of psychopathology from least to most severe): schizotypal personality disorder, delusional disorder, brief psychotic disorder, substance-induced psychotic disorder, psychotic disorder associated with another medical condition, catatonic disorder associated with another medical condition, schizophreniform disorder, schizoaffective disorder, and schizophrenia.

- Nursing care of the patient with schizophrenia is accomplished using the six steps of the nursing process.

- Nursing assessment is based on knowledge of symptomatology related to thought content and form, perception, affect, sense of self, volition, interpersonal functioning and relationship to the external world, and psychomotor behavior.

- Symptoms of schizophrenia are categorized as *positive* (an excess or distortion of normal functions) or *negative* (a diminution or loss of normal functions).

- Antipsychotic medications remain the mainstay of treatment for psychotic disorders. Atypical antipsychotics have become the first line of pharmacological treatment. They have a more favorable side-effect profile than the conventional (typical) antipsychotics.

- Individuals with schizophrenia require long-term integrated treatment with pharmacological and other interventions. Some of these include individual psychotherapy, group therapy, behavior therapy, social skills training, milieu therapy, family therapy, and assertive community treatment. For the majority of people, the most effective treatment appears to be a combination of psychotropic medication and psychosocial therapy.

- Some clinicians are choosing a course of therapy based on a model of recovery, similar to that which has been used for many years with addiction. The basic premise of a recovery model is empowerment of the client. The recovery model is designed to allow clients primary control over decisions about their own care and to enable persons with mental health problems to live a meaningful life in a community of their choice while striving to achieve their full potential.

- Families generally require support and education about psychotic illnesses. The focus is on coping with the diagnosis, understanding the illness and its course, teaching about medication, and learning ways to manage symptoms.

- The most current, evidence-based approach to treatment, RAISE, demonstrates that early intervention at the first episode of psychosis can significantly improve outcomes.

- There is a risk for suicide among patients with schizophrenia, so suicide risk assessment should always be considered an essential evaluation component.

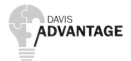

Go to **Davis Advantage** to complete your learning: strengthen understanding, apply your knowledge, and prepare for the Next Gen NCLEX®.)

Review Questions

1. Recent research on the RAISE approach to the treatment of schizophrenia incorporates which of the following elements as important to improving outcomes? (Select all that apply.)
   a. Early intervention at the first episode of psychosis
   b. Support for employment or educational pursuits
   c. Rapid high-dose loading with antipsychotic medication
   d. Court-ordered sanctions for treatment
   e. Recovery-focused psychotherapy

2. Which of the following is the primary goal in working with an actively psychotic, suspicious client?
   a. Promote interaction with others.
   b. Decrease the client's anxiety and increase trust.
   c. Improve the client's relationship with their parents.
   d. Encourage participation in therapy activities.

3. A client with schizophrenia has physician's orders for haloperidol (Haldol) 5 mg IM STAT and then 3 mg PO tid; 2 mg benztropine PO bid prn. Why is benztropine ordered?
   a. To treat extrapyramidal symptoms
   b. To prevent neuroleptic malignant syndrome
   c. To decrease psychotic symptoms
   d. To induce sleep

4. A client on the psychiatric unit tells the nurse that the CIA is looking for him and will kill him if they find him. The client's false belief is an example of a:
   a. Delusion of persecution.
   b. Delusion of reference.
   c. Delusion of control or influence.
   d. Delusion of grandeur.

5. The primary focus of family therapy for clients with schizophrenia and their families is:
   a. To discuss problem-solving and adaptive behaviors for coping with stress.
   b. To introduce the family to others with the same problem.
   c. To keep the client and family in touch with the health-care system.
   d. To promote family interaction and increase understanding of the illness.

6. A client recently admitted to the hospital reports to the nurse, "I don't understand why I was brought here. I was simply hanging out in my apartment and the police said I had to come with them." This is an example of what symptom of schizophrenia?
   a. Delusions of reference
   b. Loose association
   c. Anosognosia
   d. Auditory hallucinations

Clinical Judgment Questions

7. Which of the following assessments by the nurse would convey a need for prn benztropine?
   a. Increased level of agitation
   b. Complaints of a sore throat
   c. A yellowish cast to the skin
   d. Muscle spasms

8. A client on the psychiatric unit tells the nurse that the CIA has planted a tracking device in their brain to kill them. The most appropriate response by the nurse is:
   a. "That's ridiculous. No one is going to hurt you."
   b. "The CIA isn't interested in people like you."
   c. "Why do you think the CIA wants to kill you?"
   d. "I know you believe that, but it's really hard for me to believe."

9. The nurse is interviewing a client on the psychiatric unit. The client tilts their head to the side, stops talking in midsentence, and listens intently. Which is the most appropriate follow-up assessment based on this information?

 a. Ask the client if they are experiencing loose associations.

 b. Ask the client if they need more medication.

 c. Ask the client if they are hearing something or someone other than the nurse's voice.

 d. Ask the client if their neck is stiff.

10. A client reports to the nurse that their foot is on fire and they think the demons are trying to burn off their flesh. The priority nursing intervention for this symptom is to:

 a. Administer prn haloperidol as ordered.

 b. Evaluate the client's foot to rule out physical causes for his complaint.

 c. Administer prn benztropine as ordered.

 d. Ask the client if they would like to speak with a chaplain.

11. When a client suddenly becomes aggressive and violent on the unit, which of the following approaches would be best for the nurse to use *first*?

 a. Provide large motor activities to relieve the client's pent-up tension.

 b. Administer a dose of prn haloperidol to keep the client calm.

 c. Call for sufficient help to manage the situation safely.

 d. Convey to the client that their behavior is unacceptable and will not be permitted.

12. A client who is diagnosed with schizophrenia has been socially isolated and hearing voices telling them to kill their parents. The client has been admitted to the psychiatric unit from the emergency department. Which is the most important initial intervention for this client?

 a. Give an injection of haloperidol.

 b. Assess the client to evaluate their safety toward themselves and others.

 c. Place the client in restraints.

 d. Order the client a nutritious diet.

IMPLICATIONS OF RESEARCH FOR EVIDENCE-BASED PRACTICE

Stroup, T. S., Olfson, M., Huang, C., Wall, M. M., Goldberg, T., Devanand, D. P., & Gerhard, T. P. (2021). Age-specific prevalence and incidence of dementia diagnoses among older U.S. adults with schizophrenia. *JAMA Psychiatry*, 78(6), 632–641. https://doi.org/10.1001/jamapsychiatry.2021.0042

DESCRIPTION OF THE STUDY: This study sought to estimate the age-specific prevalence and incidence of dementia in older adults with schizophrenia by comparing them to older adults without schizophrenia. This was a retrospective cohort study of 8,011,773 Medicare recipients 66 years and older. It is known that the risk of dementia among those with schizophrenia is high, and this study sought to clarify the magnitude and timing of this increased risk.

RESULTS OF THE STUDY: At 66 years of age, the prevalence of diagnosed dementia was 27.9% among individuals with schizophrenia compared with 1.3% in the group without serious mental illness (SMI). By 80 years of age, the prevalence of dementia diagnoses rose to 70.2% in the group with schizophrenia and 11.3% in the group without SMI. The annual incidence of dementia diagnoses per 1,000 person-years at 66 years of age was 52.5 among individuals with schizophrenia and 4.5 among individuals without SMI and increased to 216.2 and 32.3, respectively, by 80 years of age.

IMPLICATIONS FOR NURSING PRACTICE: Several symptoms of schizophrenia overlap with those of dementia, so differential diagnosis can be a challenge. One of the most prominent symptoms in dementia, however, is recent memory loss, and when nurses assess this to be prominent in the older adult with schizophrenia, the nurse can play an active role in collaborating with team members to recommend further testing. Nurses also play an active role in educating patients and families regarding lifestyle factors that may decrease risks for dementia such as weight management, diabetes management, and strategies to reduce risk for cardiovascular disease. Careful assessment and collaboration with team members has treatment implications as well, because antipsychotic medication use in the patient with dementia has been associated with many risks, including sudden death.

TEST YOUR CLINICAL REASONING AND CLINICAL JUDGMENT SKILLS

Sara, a 23-year-old single woman, has just been admitted to the psychiatric unit by her parents. They explain that over the past few months she has become increasingly withdrawn. She stays in her room alone but lately has been heard talking and laughing to herself.

Sara left home for the first time at age 18 to attend college. She performed well during her first semester, but when she returned after Christmas, she began to accuse her roommate of stealing her possessions. She started writing to her parents that her roommate wanted to kill her and that her roommate was turning everyone against her. She said she feared for her life. She started missing classes and stayed in her bed most of the time. Sometimes she locked herself in her closet. Her parents took her home, and she was hospitalized and diagnosed with schizophrenia. She has since been maintained on antipsychotic medication while taking a few classes at the local community college.

Sara tells the admitting nurse that she quit taking her medication 4 weeks ago because the pharmacist who fills the prescriptions is plotting to have her killed. She believes he is trying to poison her. She says she got this information from a television message. As Sara speaks, the nurse notices that she sometimes stops in midsentence and listens; sometimes she cocks her head to the side and moves her lips as though she is talking.

Answer the following questions related to Sara:

1. From the assessment data, what would be the most immediate nursing concern in working with Sara?
2. What is the nursing diagnosis related to this concern?
3. What interventions must be accomplished before the nurse can be successful in working with Sara?

Communication Exercises

1. Hal, a patient on the psychiatric unit, has a diagnosis of schizophrenia. He lives in a halfway house, where last evening he began yelling, "Aliens are on the way to take over our bodies! The message is coming through loud and clear!" The residence supervisor became frightened and called 911. As Hal is being admitted to the psychiatric unit he tells the nurse, "I'm special! I get messages from a higher being! We are in for big trouble!"

   How would the nurse respond appropriately to this statement by Hal?

2. The nurse notices that Hal is sitting off by himself in a corner of the dayroom. He appears to be talking to himself and tilts his head to the side as if listening to something.

   How would the nurse intervene with Hal in this situation?

3. Hal says to the nurse, "We must choose to take a ride and slip and slide."

   How would the nurse respond appropriately to this statement by Hal?

MOVIE CONNECTIONS

I Never Promised You a Rose Garden (schizophrenia) • *A Beautiful Mind* (schizophrenia) • *The Fisher King* (schizophrenia) • *Bennie & Joon* (schizophrenia) • *Out of Darkness* (schizophrenia) • *Conspiracy Theory* (paranoia) • *The Fan* (delusional disorder) • *The Soloist* (schizophrenia) • *Of Two Minds* (schizophrenia)

References

Álvarez, M. J., Masramon, H., Peña, C., Pont, M., Gourdier, C., Roura-Poch, P., & Arrufat, F. (2015). Cumulative effects of childhood traumas: Polytraumatization, dissociation, and schizophrenia. *Community Mental Health Journal, 51*(1), 54–62. doi:10.1007/s10597-014-9755-2

American Psychiatric Association (APA). (2022). *Diagnostic and statistical manual of mental disorders, fifth edition, text revision (DSM-5-TR).* APA.

Asen, E. (2002). Outcome research in family therapy: Family intervention for psychosis. *Advances in Psychiatric Treatment, 8,* 230–238. doi:10.1192/apt.8.3.230

Beck, K., Hindley, G., Borgan, F., Ginestet, C., McCutcheon, R., Brugger, S., Driesen, N., Ranganathan, M., D'Souza, D. C., Taylor, M., Krystal, J. H., & Howes, O. D. (2020). Association of ketamine with psychiatric symptoms and implications for its therapeutic use and for understanding schizophrenia: A systematic review and meta-analysis. *JAMA Network Open, 3*(5), e204693. doi:10.1001/jamanetworkopen.2020.4693

Benson, P. J., Beedie, S. A., Shephard, E., Giegling, I., Rujescu, G., St. Clair, D. (2012). Simple viewing tests can detect eye movement abnormalities that distinguish schizophrenia cases from controls with exceptional accuracy. *Biological Psychiatry, 72*(9), 716–724.

Boland, R., & Verduin, M. L. (2022). *Kaplan & Sadock's synopsis of psychiatry* (P. Ruiz, Ed.). (12th ed.). Wolters Kluwer.

Bora, E. (2015). Neurodevelopmental origin of cognitive impairment in schizophrenia. *Psychological Medicine, 45*(1), 1–9. doi:10.1017/S0033291714001263

Bossong, M. G., Antoniades, M., Azis, M., Samson, C., Quinn, B., Bonoldi, I., Modinos, G., Perez, J., Howes, O. D., Stone, J. M., Allen, P., & McGuire, P. (2019). Association of hippocampal glutamate levels with adverse outcomes in individuals at clinical high risk for psychosis. *JAMA Psychiatry, 76*(2):199-207. doi: 10.1001/jamapsychiatry.2018.3252

Caqueo-Urízar, A., Rus-Calafell, M., Urzúa, A., Escudero, J., & Gutiérrez-Maldonado, J. (2015). The role of family therapy in the management of schizophrenia: Challenges and solutions. *Neuropsychiatric Disease and Treatment, 11,* 145–151. doi:10.2147/NDT.S51331

Chesney, E., Goodwin, G. M., & Fazel, S. (2014). Risks of all-cause and suicide mortality in mental disorders: A metareview. *World Psychiatry.* https://doi.org/10.1002/wps.20128

Davis, J., Eyre, H., Jacka, F. N., Dodd, S., Dean, O., McEwen, S., Debnath, M., McGrath, J., Maes, M., Amminger, P., McGorry, P. D., Pantelis, C., & Berk, M. (2016). A review of vulnerability and risks for schizophrenia: Beyond the two hit hypothesis. *Neuroscience and Biobehavioral Reviews, 65,* 185–194. https://doi.org/10.1016/j.neubiorev.2016.03.017

Dawidowski, B., Górniak, A., Podwalski, P., Lebiecka, Z., Misiak, B., & Samochowiec, J. (2021). The Role of cytokines in the pathogenesis of schizophrenia. *Journal of Clinical Medicine, 10*(17), 3849. https://doi.org/10.3390/jcm10173849

D'Souza, D. C., Singh, N., Elander, J., Carbuto, M., Pittman, B., Udo de Haes, J., Sjogren, M., Peeters, P., Ranganathan, M., & Schipper, J. (2012). Glycine transporter inhibitor attenuates the psychotomimetic effects of ketamine in healthy males: Preliminary evidence. *Neuropsychopharmacology, 37,* 1036–1046.

Drake, K. (2021). *Echopraxia in schizophrenia, autism, and Tourette syndrome.* https://psychcentral.com/health/echopraxia#what-is-echopraxia

Druss, B. G., Zhao, L., Von Esenwein, S., Morrato, E. H., & Marcus, S. C. (2011). Understanding excess mortality in persons with mental illness: 17-year follow up of a nationally representative US survey. *Medical Care, 49*(6), 599–604.

Frankenburg, F. R. (2020). What factors affect the prognosis of schizophrenia? *Medscape.* https://www.medscape.com/answers/288259-13995/what-factors-affect-the-prognosis-of-schizophrenia

Freudenreich, O. (2010). Differential diagnosis of psychotic symptoms: Medical "mimics." *Psychiatric Times, 27*(12), 52–61.

García-Gutiérrez, M. S., Navarrete, F., Sala, F., Gasparyan, A., Austrich-Olivares, A., & Manzanares, J. (2020). Biomarkers in psychiatry: Concept, definition, types and relevance to the clinical reality. *Frontiers in Psychiatry, 11,* 432. doi: 10.3389/fpsyt.2020.00432

Harrisberger, F., Smieskova1, R., Vogler, C., Egli, T., Schmidt, A., Lenz, C., Simon, A. E., Riecher-Rössler, A., Papassotiropoulos, A., & Borgwardt, S. (2016). Impact of polygenic schizophrenia-related risk and hippocampal volumes on the onset of psychosis. *Translational Psychiatry, 6,* e868. doi:10.1038/tp.2016.143

Herdman, T. H., Kamitsuru, S., & Lopes, C. T. (Eds.). (2021). *NANDA International, Inc. nursing diagnoses: Definitions and classification, 2021–2023* (12th ed.). Thieme.

Howes, O., McCutcheon, R., & Stone, J. (2015). Glutamate and dopamine in schizophrenia: An update for the 21st century. *Journal of Psychopharmacology (Oxford, England), 29*(2), 97–115. https://doi.org/10.1177/0269881114563634

Hu, W., MacDonald, M. L., Elswick, D. E., & Sweet, R. A. (2014). The glutamate hypothesis of schizophrenia: Evidence from human brain tissue studies. *Annals of the New York Academy of Sciences, 1338*(1), 38–57 [Abstract]. doi:10.1111/nyas.12547

Institute of Medicine. (2003). *Health professions education: A bridge to quality.* National Academies Press.

Jablensky, A. (2017). Worldwide burden of schizophrenia. In Sadock, B. J., Sadock, V. A., & Ruiz, P. (Eds.), *Comprehensive textbook of psychiatry* (pp. 1425–1437). Wolters Kluwer.

Kane, J. M., Schooler, N. R., Marcy, P., Correll, C. U., Brunette, M. F., Mueser, K. T., Rosenheck, R. A., Addington, J., Estroff, S. E., Robinson, J., Penn, D. L., & Robinson, D. G. (2015). The RAISE early treatment program for first-episode psychosis: Background, rationale, and study design. *The Journal of Clinical Psychiatry, 76*(3), 240–246. https://doi.org/10.4088/JCP.14m09289

Kart, A., Özdel, K., & Türkçapar, M. H. (2021). *Noro Psikiyatri Arsivi, 58*(Suppl 1), S61–S65. https://doi.org/10.29399/npa.27418

Kranjac, D. (2016). *Pharmacotherapy for smoking cessation in adults with neuropsychiatric illness.* www.psychiatryadvisor.com/addiction/smoking-cessation-in-adults-with-neuropsychiatric-illness/article/518385

Lysaker, P. H., Roe, D., & Buck, K. D. (2010). Recovery and wellness amid schizophrenia: Definitions, evidence, and the implications for clinical practice. *Journal of the American Psychiatric Nurses Association, 16*(1), 36–42. doi:10.1177/1078390309353943

MacCabe, J. H., Wicks, S., Löfving, S., David, A. S., Berndtsson, Å., Gustafsson, J-E, Allebeck, P., & Dalman, C. (2013). Decline in cognitive performance between ages 13 and 18 years and the risk for psychosis in adulthood: A Swedish longitudinal cohort study in males. *JAMA Psychiatry, 70*(3), 261–270. doi:10.1001/2013.jamapsychiatry.43

Matheson, S. L., Shepherd, A. M., & Carr, V. J. (2014). How much do we know about schizophrenia and how well do we know it? Evidence from the Schizophrenia Library. *Psychological Medicine—London, 44*(6), 3387–3405. doi:10.1017/S0033291714000166

Miller, B. (2020). Schizophrenia: Clinical considerations in men versus women. *Psychiatric Times.* https://www.psychiatrictimes.com/view/schizophrenia-clinical-considerations-men-versus-women

Miller, J. (2020). Schizophrenia: A broad Rx. *Psychiatric Times.* https://www.psychiatrictimes.com/view/schizophrenia-a-broad-rx

Mueser, K. T., Bond, G. R., & Drake, R. E. (2001). Community-based treatment of schizophrenia and other severe mental disorders: Treatment outcomes. *Medscape Psychiatry & Mental Health eJournal.* www.medscape.com/viewarticle/430529

National Council of State Boards of Nursing (NCSBN). (2021). *Next generation NCLEX®: Comparison between case studies and stand-alone items.* https://www.ncsbn.org/public-files/NGN_Fall21_English_Final.pdf

Okazaki, S., Boku, S., Otsuka, I., Mouri, K., Aoyama, S., Shiroiwa, K., Sora, I., Fujita, A., Shirai, Y., Shirakawa, O., Kokai, M., & Hishimoto, A. (2016). The cell cycle-related genes as biomarkers for schizophrenia. *Progress Neuropsychopharmacology and Biological Psychiatry, 70*(suppl. 9), 85–91. doi:10.1016/j.pnpbp.2016.05.005

Os, J. V., & Reininghaus, U. (2017). The clinical epidemiology of schizophrenia. In Sadock, B. J., Sadock, V. A., & Ruiz, P. (Eds.), *Comprehensive textbook of psychiatry* (10th ed., pp. 1445–1457). Wolters Kluwer.

Popovic, D., Schmitt, A., Kaurani, L., Senner, F., Papiol, S., Malchow, B., Fischer, A., Schulze, T. G., Koutsouleris, N., & Falkai, P. (2019). Childhood trauma in schizophrenia: Current findings and research perspectives. *Frontiers in Neuroscience. 13,* 274. doi: 10.3389/fnins.2019.00274

Radhakrishnan, R., Wilkinson, S. T., & D'Souza, D. C. (2014). Gone to pot—A review of the association between cannabis and psychosis. *Frontiers in Psychiatry, 5*(54). doi:10.3389/fpsyt.2014.00054

Rezansoff, S., Moniruzzaman, A., Fazel, S., McCandless, L., Procyshyn, R., & Somers, J. M. (2016). Housing First improves adherence to antipsychotic medication among formerly homeless adults with schizophrenia: Results of a randomized controlled trial. *Schizophrenia Bulletin.* doi:10.1093/schbul/sbw136

Roberts, L. W., Louie, A. K., Guerrero, A., Balon, R., Beresin, E. V., Brenner, A., & Coverdale, J. (2017). Premature mortality among people with mental illness: Advocacy in academic psychiatry. *Academic Psychiatry, 41*(4), 441–446.

Savill, M., Banks, C., Khanom, H., & Priebe, S. (2015). Do negative symptoms of schizophrenia change overtime? A meta-analysis of longitudinal data. *Psychological Medicine, 45,* 1613–1627. doi:10.1017/S0033291714002712

Shrivastava, A., Shah, N., Johnston, M., Stitt, L., & Thakar, M. (2010). Predictors of long-term outcome of first-episode schizophrenia: A ten-year follow-up study. *Indian Journal of Psychiatry, 52*(4), 320–326. https://doi.org/10.4103/0019-5545.74306

Stroup, T. S., Olfson, M., Huang, C., Wall, M. M., Goldberg, T., Devanand, D. P., & Gerhard, T. P. (2021). Age-specific prevalence and incidence of dementia diagnoses among older us adults with schizophrenia. *JAMA Psychiatry, 78*(6), 632–641. https://doi.org/10.1001/jamapsychiatry.2021.0042

Takeuchi, H., Kantor, N., Sanches, M., Fervaha, G., Agid, O., & Remington, G. (2017). One-year symptom trajectories in patients with stable schizophrenia maintained on antipsychotics versus placebo: Meta-analysis. *British Journal of Psychiatry, 211*(3). doi:10.1192/bjp.bp.116.186007

Thunè, H., Recasens, M., & Uhlhaas, P. J. (2016). The 40-Hz auditory steady-state response in patients with schizophrenia: A meta-analysis. *JAMA Psychiatry.* http://jamanetwork.com/journals/jamapsychiatry/article-abstract/2566207

Tripathi, A., Kar, S. K., & Shukla, R. (2018). Cognitive deficits in schizophrenia: Understanding the biological correlates and remediation strategies. *Clinical Psychopharmacology and Neuroscience, 16*(1), 7–17. https://doi.org/10.9758/cpn.2018.16.1.7

Torrey, E. F. (2022). Cats, toxoplasmosis, and psychosis: Understanding the risks. *Current Psychiatry, 21*(5), 15–19.

Urvakhsh, M. M., Thirthalli, J., Aneelraj, D., Jadhav, P., Gangadhar, B. N., & Keshavan, M. S. (2014). Mirror neuron dysfunction in schizophrenia and its functional implications: A systematic review. *Schizophrenia Research, 160*(1–3), 9–19. doi:http://dx.doi.org/10.1016/j.schres.2014.10.040

Veijola, J., Guo, J. Y., Moilanen, J. S., Jaaskelainen, E., Miettunen, J., Kyllonen, M., Haapea, M., Huhtaniska, S., Alaräisänen, A., Mäki, P., Kiviniemi, V., Nikkinen, J., Starck, T., Remes, J. J., Tanskanen, P., Tervonen, O., Wink, A. M., Kehagia, A., Suckling, J., … Murray, G. (2014). Longitudinal changes in total brain volume in schizophrenia: Relation to symptom severity, cognition and antipsychotic medication. *PLoS ONE, 9*(7), e101689. doi:10.1371/journal.pone.0101689

Viher, P.V., Stegmayer, K., Giezendanner, S., Federspiel, A., Bohlhalter, S., Vanbellingen, T., Weist, R., Strik, W., & Walthera, S. (2016). Cerebral white matter structure is associated with DSM-5 schizophrenia symptom dimensions. *Neuroimage: Clinical, 12*(suppl. 7), 93–99. doi:http://dx.doi.org/10.1016/j.nicl.2016.06.013

Waters, F., Collerton, D., Ffytche, D. H., Jardri, R., Pins, D., Dudley, R., Blom, J. D., Mosimann, U. P., Eperjesi, F., Ford, S., & Laroi, F. (2014). Visual hallucinations in the psychosis spectrum and comparative information from neurodegenerative disorders and eye disease. *Schizophrenia Bulletin, 40*(suppl. 4), 233–245. doi:10.1093/schbul/sbu036

Weiden, P. J. (2010). Is recovery attainable in schizophrenia? *Medscape Psychiatry & Mental Health.* www.medscape.com/viewarticle/729750

Wiginton, K. (2022). *What is waxy flexibility?* https://www.webmd.com/schizophrenia/waxy-flexibility-schizophrenia

Wu, Q., Gilbody, S., Peckham, E., Brabyn, S., & Parrott, S. (2016). Varenicline for smoking cessation and reduction in people with severe mental illnesses: Systematic review and meta-analysis. *Addiction, 111*(9), 1554–1567. Epub 2016 Jun 9. doi:10.1111/add.13415.

Classical Reference

Kay, S. R., Fiszbein, A., & Opler, L. A. (1987). The positive and negative syndrome scale (PANSS) for schizophrenia. *Schizophrenia Bulletin, 13*(2), 261–276.

Liberman, R. P. (1972). Behavioral modification of schizophrenia: A review. *Schizophrenia Bulletin, 1*(6), 37–48. https://doi.org/10.1093/schbul/1.6.37

Marzillier, J. S., & Birchwood, M. J. (1981). Behavioral treatment of cognitive disorders. In: Michelson, L., Hersen, M., & Turner, S. M. (eds.), *Future perspectives in behavior therapy.* Springer. https://doi.org/10.1007/978-1-4613-3243-5_7

Depressive Disorders 25

CORE CONCEPTS

Mood and Affect: Depression
Professional Behavior: Nursing process in the care of patients with depressive disorders
Safety
Clinical Judgment

KEY TERMS

affect
cognitive behavior therapy (CBT)
depression

melancholia
mood
persistent depressive disorder

postpartum depression
premenstrual dysphoric disorder (PMDD)
psychomotor retardation

OBJECTIVES
After reading this chapter, the student will be able to:

1. Recount historical perspectives of depression.
2. Discuss epidemiological statistics related to depression.
3. Describe various types of depressive disorders.
4. Identify predisposing factors in the development of depression.
5. Discuss implications of depression related to developmental stage.
6. Identify symptomatology associated with depression and use this information in patient assessment.
7. Formulate nursing diagnoses and goals of care for patients with depression.
8. Identify topics for patient and family teaching relevant to depression.
9. Describe appropriate nursing interventions for behaviors associated with depression.
10. Describe relevant criteria for evaluating nursing care of patients with depression.
11. Discuss various modalities used to treat depression.

Depression is likely the oldest and still one of the most frequently diagnosed psychiatric illnesses. Symptoms of depression have been described almost as far back as there is evidence of written documentation.

An occasional bout with the "blues," a feeling of sadness or downheartedness, is common among healthy people and considered a normal response to life's everyday disappointments. These episodes are short-lived as the individual adapts to losses, change, or failures (real or imagined). Pathological depression occurs when adaptation is ineffective and the symptoms are significant enough to impair functioning.

CORE CONCEPT

Mood and Affect

Mood is a pervasive and sustained emotion that may have a profound influence on a person's perception of the world. Examples of moods include depression, joy, elation, anger, and anxiety. **Affect** is described as the external, observable emotional reaction associated with an experience. A *flat affect* describes someone who lacks emotional expression and is often seen in severely depressed people.

This chapter focuses on the different manifestations of depressive illness and implications for nursing intervention. A historical perspective and epidemiological statistics related to depression are presented. Predisposing factors that have been implicated in the etiology of depression provide a framework for studying the dynamics of the disorder. Similarities and differences between depressive disorders and grief also are discussed. Depressive illnesses specific to individuals at various developmental stages are reviewed. An explanation of the symptomatology is presented as background knowledge for assessing the person with depression. Nursing care is described in the context of the six steps of the nursing process. Various medical treatment modalities are explored.

CORE CONCEPT

Depression

Depression is defined as an alteration in mood expressed by feelings of sadness, despair, and pessimism. In clinically significant depression there is a loss of interest in usual activities, and somatic symptoms may be evident. Changes in appetite, sleep patterns, and cognition are common.

Historical Perspective

Many ancient cultures (e.g., Babylonian, Egyptian, Hebrew) believed in the supernatural or divine origin of mental disorders. The Old Testament states in the Book of Samuel that King Saul was inflicted by an "evil spirit" sent from God to "torment" him.

A clearly nondivine point of view regarding depression was held by the Greek medical community from the 5 BCE through 3 AD. This perspective represented the thinking of Hippocrates, Celsus, and Galen, among others. They strongly rejected the idea of divine origin and considered the brain the seat of all emotional states. Hippocrates believed that melancholia was caused by the effect of excess black bile, a heavily toxic substance produced in the spleen or intestine, on the brain. **Melancholia** is currently used to describe a severe form of major depressive disorder (MDD) in which symptoms are exaggerated and interest or pleasure in virtually all activities is lost.

During the Renaissance, several new theories evolved. Depression was viewed by some as being the result of obstructed air circulation, excessive brooding, or situations beyond the individual's control. Depression was reflected in major literary works of the time, including Shakespeare's *King Lear, Macbeth,* and *Hamlet.*

Contemporary thinking has been substantially shaped by the works of Sigmund Freud, Emil Kraepelin, and Adolf Meyer. Having evolved from these early 20th-century models, current thinking about mood disorders generally encompasses the intrapsychic, behavioral, and biological perspectives. These perspectives support the notion of multiple causation in the development of mood disorders.

Epidemiology

MDD is one of the leading causes of disability in the United States. In addition to the disability posed by the disorder itself, recent research links depression to an increased risk for coronary artery disease (another leading cause of death), especially in women younger than age 65 (Jiang et al., 2016). In a national survey (Hasin et al., 2018) the lifetime prevalence of MDD was found to be 20.6% and commonly associated with comorbid disorders, making it not only highly prevalent but often disabling. Akiskal (2017) reported that as diagnostic evaluation of bipolar disorders (alternating episodes of depression and manic or hypomanic symptoms) has improved, current data suggest that up to 50% of all depression diagnoses may actually be bipolar illness.

There is evidence that the incidence of depression is increasing among American teens and young adults, particularly adolescent girls. In 2020, an estimated 4.1 million adolescents aged 12 to 17 in the United States had at least one major depressive episode (National Institute of Mental Health [NIMH], 2022). This number represented 17.0% of the U.S. population aged 12 to 17, and over 70% of those had at least one major depressive episode with severe impairment in the past year (over double the percentages reported in 2006). The reasons for these increases are unclear, but there is a correlation between these statistics and the increasing suicide rates among teens, and suicide is recognized as a major public health issue.

Age and Sex

The prevalence of depression is higher among women than men, generally by almost two to one. Boland and Verduin (2022) reported that this finding is "an almost universal observation, independent of country or culture" (p. 394). In 2020, the prevalence of major depressive episodes was higher among adult females (10.5%) compared with males (6.2%) and highest among individuals aged 18 to 25 (17.0%) (NIMH, 2022). Many biological explanations have been suggested, including that women have higher concentrations of monoamine oxidase (a neurotransmitter associated with depression); are more susceptible to thyroid dysfunctions; and are influenced by the hormonal changes that occur during the menstrual cycle, postpartum, and at menopause (Akiskal, 2017). Psychosocial factors contributing to depression in women may include unequal power and status (and their association with self-esteem issues), work overload, and history of sexual or physical abuse (Mayo Clinic, 2022b). However, gender-related increased risk for depression is influenced by many factors in complex interactions that are not yet clearly understood.

Socioeconomic Factors

Historically, depression was viewed as a "disease of affluence," but Ridley and associates (2020) found that the evidence supports a bicausal relationship between poverty and mental illness (particularly depression and anxiety). That is, mental illness may present economic burdens culminating in poverty, and conversely economic hardship can contribute to mental illness. Merikangas and Rihmer (2017) cited that depression is three times more prevalent among those who are unemployed. Whether these findings are related to lack of access to resources and early treatment, difficulty managing multiple stressors associated with socioeconomic well-being, or a combination of many factors requires more research.

Race and Culture

Studies have not identified a consistent association between race and affective disorder. One problem encountered in studying racial comparisons involves the multiple variables that contribute to depression in minority groups such as access to health resources and accurate diagnosis, U.S. region at birth, immigrant versus nonimmigrant nativity, and discrimination (Akincigil et al., 2012; Budhwani et al., 2015; Chang et al., 2016). In other words, some factors contributing to depression may be matters of public policy rather than biological factors associated with one's race. Boland and Verduin (2022) added that racial and ethnic differences are also challenging to measure because they are highly dependent on the methods and approaches used.

Marital Status

A number of studies have suggested that marriage has a positive effect on psychological well-being compared with those who are single or do not have a close relationship with another person (Liu et al., 2010; Marcussen, 2005; Uecker, 2012). Other studies have suggested that marital status alone is not a valid indicator of risk for depression (Lapate et al., 2014). Some of those studies have identified age as an important variable in risk for depression among married and single individuals. Lapate and associates (2014) reported that marital *stress* was associated with increased risk for depression, suggesting that social stress may also be an important variable to consider.

In a broader context, it may be that lack of social connectedness rather than marital status is associated with a higher incidence of depression. Holt-Lundstat et al. (2017) cited studies that associate lack of social connections (including high divorce rates, among others) with morbidity for many diseases (including cardiovascular disease, which has been associated with depression) and mortality. These authors suggested that there are so many factors that influence lack of social connectedness and illness that it is difficult to pinpoint one of those (such as marital status) as a singular cause.

Seasonality

Studies exploring whether seasonality is a cause of depression have yielded varying results. The *Diagnostic and Statistical Manual of Mental Disorders, Fifth Edition, Text Revision (DSM-5-TR)* (American Psychiatric Association [APA], 2022) uses the term *seasonal pattern* to describe and specify any depressive disorder that occurs at "characteristic times of the year" (p. 214). The authors noted that episodes are most common in fall or winter, but some individuals have recurrent summer episodes. Authors of one large study reported that prevalence rates of depression with seasonal patterns have varied from 1% to 12%, but in their study of 5,549 patients from primary care settings, there was no evidence of seasonal patterns for MDD (Winthorst et al., 2011). In another study, Cobb and associates (2014) found that a small but significant peak in depression symptoms occurred in winter months, but over 20 years of following those individuals, the winter seasonal pattern was not stable. Seasonal affective disorder (SAD) continues to be popularly referred to as a separate condition, although the *DSM-5-TR* does not list it as a distinct diagnosis. The reported benefits of light therapy seem to support a seasonal cause for depression during winter months when there may be less exposure to natural sunlight, but in a meta-analysis of the research on benefits of bright white light in treating depression the authors found that the evidence was not consistent or conclusive (Mårtensson et al., 2015). More recent studies have supported the benefit of bright light therapy as a short-term treatment for both seasonal disorders (Campbell et al., 2017; Maruani & Geoffroy, 2019; Pjrek et al., 2020) and nonseasonal affective disorders (Cunningham et al., 2019; Lam et al., 2015; Maruani & Geoffroy, 2019; Sikkens et al., 2019).

Types of Depressive Disorders

Major Depressive Disorder

MDD is characterized by depressed mood or loss of interest or pleasure in usual activities, impaired social and occupational functioning that has existed for at least 2 weeks, no history of manic behavior, and symptoms that cannot be attributed to use of substances or a general medical condition. Additionally, the diagnosis of MDD is specified according to whether it is a *single episode* (the individual's first encounter with a major depressive episode) or *recurrent* (the individual has a history of previous major depressive episodes). The diagnosis will also identify the degree of severity of symptoms (mild, moderate, or severe) and whether there is evidence of psychotic, catatonic, or melancholic features. The presence of anxiety and severity of suicide risk may also be noted. MDD is differentiated from schizoaffective disorder, a condition in which the individual expresses symptoms of a mood disorder as well as symptoms of schizophrenia. Read Josh's story on his experience with depression and an eventual diagnosis of schizoaffective disorder in the "Real People, Real Stories" feature. The *DSM-5-TR* (APA, 2022) diagnostic criteria for major depressive episode are presented in Box 25–1.

Persistent Depressive Disorder

Characteristics of **persistent depressive disorder** are similar to, if somewhat milder than, those ascribed to MDD. Individuals with this mood disturbance describe their mood as sad or "down in the dumps." There is no evidence of psychotic symptoms. The essential feature is a chronically depressed mood (or possibly an irritable mood in children or adolescents) for most of the day, more days than not, for at

---

Real People, Real Stories: Josh's Experience With Depression and Schizoaffective Disorder

(This individual preferred to remain anonymous, so his name has been changed.)

Consider reflecting on factors that may contribute to Josh's perceptions about his illness and his perceptions about the contributions of health-care providers to his recovery process.

Karyn: Tell me about the time when you first became aware that you had a mood disorder. [Josh had told me he had depression. I was unaware when we began the interview that his actual diagnosis was schizoaffective disorder.]

Josh: I was in senior high school and was doing well. I was in advanced placement (AP) courses, and suddenly I got an F in AP English. Nothing like that had ever happened before. I started becoming more withdrawn. I was smoking pot with my friends, and I wonder now if that had an impact. I graduated high school, then attended college for 2 years until the symptoms really surfaced. I was cut from the soccer team, so there were some disappointments, but I became very withdrawn and depressed. I had suicide ideas and a plan. I had to take a break from school, and I just wasn't doing anything; I was just very withdrawn. Four years later I was diagnosed with schizoaffective disorder.

Karyn: What did you think about that diagnosis?

Josh: I thought it was wrong. I did have some difficulty tracking objects with my eyes, and I still do when I don't get enough sleep. I guess now that I think of it, there was a time in college when I thought my roommates were talking about me, and then I started thinking people in the next room were talking about me. I would read into things a lot. Sometimes I thought I saw something out of the corner of my eye, and sometimes I heard voices.

Karyn: It seems like that would be difficult, maybe even frightening, to have these symptoms and get this diagnosis. What was that like for you?

Josh: Yeah, it was, but I was glad to get a diagnosis because then I knew what I had to deal with. At the same time, though, I thought it was too quickly made and they were too quick to prescribe pills. If I had it to do over, I would have just trusted the doctors, but I rebelled against the drugs several times—sometimes because I was having side effects like tardive dyskinesia; one time because I was convinced the meds were holding me back and even hurting me; and one time because I just gave up, since I didn't have any of the things I wanted, like marriage, a college degree, or a career. Sometimes I thought, "I can just be smarter than this, and I'll get over it." But I was very disorganized and incoherent. Each time I didn't take the pills, I became withdrawn, depressed, and hearing voices, and eventually I just couldn't find anything else to blame it on. I tried to hide the fact that I had stopped taking the pills, but it always became evident eventually. I stay on the medications now because I know I have to.

Karyn: You've come so far since then!

Josh: (smiles) Yeah, it took me 8 years to finish my college degree, but now I have a good job in information technology at a large hospital system, and I live on my own. I was engaged, and although it didn't work out, I'm dating again and hopeful about pursuing a committed relationship.

Karyn: What do you think has been most important in supporting your recovery?

Josh: My parents supported me through all of it. They were my only support, and I didn't want other people to know my "stuff." I was able to stay with my parents until I got

Real People, Real Stories: Josh's Experience With Depression and Schizoaffective Disorder—cont'd

back on my feet, and that was really important. The last time I stopped taking my meds, I'd have to consult court records to remember everything that happened, but I know there were trespassing charges. I had run-ins with the police. I also had run-ins with my parents, who eventually called in a crisis team, and I was hospitalized against my will. I was in the hospital for around 30 days, and I saw people who were homeless and had no one supporting them, and they were really doing poorly. Knowing I had some place to live really helped me. Also, I had a job and some successes at work, so that gave me focus. My job is largely mathematical and doesn't require a lot of social skills challenges. That was helpful for me because, while some people may be self-taught with social skills, I've always struggled with that. My job allows me to develop great insights, be quirky, and not have to try to figure people out.

Karyn: What are your thoughts about the impact of the health-care providers with whom you've interacted?

Josh: I work in a hospital, so I have a great appreciation for their hard work. I saw an NP [nurse practitioner] who gave me good advice and was very supportive. She asked some probing questions and confronted me at times, and that was challenging, but she was just doing her job and I was trying to hide from my illness.

She told me the medications might end up being less effective if I didn't take them or stay on them early in my illness, so that may have encouraged me to keep taking them.

I had good community health services—a case worker, a psychiatrist, and a behavioral health specialist that I found to be particularly supportive because we talked about spiritual things, and that made it okay to explore other issues. In the hospital, the nurses mostly worked at the station, and that was probably better for their safety, but still I could talk to them and they made it seem like it was okay that I was there. That was important because I wasn't sure what was happening to me, and they just talked about normal, everyday stuff. They seemed more like warm people than cold or clinical. I go to NAMI [National Alliance on Mental Illness] meetings now because I want to share the message with people who have a mental illness (and with their family members) that the professionals could see things I was unable to see at the time I was symptomatic, so it's important to trust the process. I also want families to know that having ongoing support from family members was a lifeline for me even when we were having run-ins and they were facilitating hospitalization against my will.

BOX 25-1 Diagnostic Criteria for Major Depressive Disorder

A. Five (or more) of the following symptoms have been present during the same 2-week period and represent a change from previous functioning; at least one of the symptoms is either (1) depressed mood or (2) loss of interest or pleasure. **Note:** Do not include symptoms that are clearly due to another medical condition.

1. Depressed mood most of the day, nearly every day, as indicated by either subjective report (e.g., feels sad, empty, or hopeless) or observation made by others (e.g., appears tearful). **Note:** In children and adolescents, can be irritable mood

2. Markedly diminished interest or pleasure in all, or almost all, activities most of the day, nearly every day (as indicated by either subjective account or observation)

3. Significant weight loss when not dieting or weight gain (e.g., a change of more than 5% of body weight in a month) or decrease or increase in appetite nearly every day. **Note:** In children, consider failure to make expected weight gain

4. Insomnia or hypersomnia nearly every day

5. Psychomotor agitation or retardation nearly every day (observable by others, not merely subjective feelings of restlessness or being slowed down)

6. Fatigue or loss of energy nearly every day

7. Feelings of worthlessness or excessive or inappropriate guilt (which may be delusional) nearly every day (not merely self-reproach or guilt about being sick)

8. Diminished ability to think or concentrate, or indecisiveness, nearly every day (either by subjective account or as observed by others)

9. Recurrent thoughts of death (not just fear of dying), recurrent suicidal ideation without a specific plan, a specific suicide plan, or a suicide attempt.

B. The symptoms cause clinically significant distress or impairment in social, occupation, or other important areas of functioning.

C. The episode is not attributable to the physiological effects of a substance or another medical condition.

Note: Criteria A–C represent a major depressive episode.

Note: Responses to a significant loss (e.g., bereavement, financial ruin, losses from a natural disaster, a serious medical illness or disability) may include the feelings of intense sadness, rumination about the loss, insomnia, poor appetite, and weight loss noted in Criterion A, which may resemble a depressive episode. Although such symptoms may be understandable or considered appropriate to the loss, the presence of a major depressive episode in addition to the normal response to a significant loss should also

Continued

BOX 25–1 **Diagnostic Criteria for Major Depressive Disorder–cont'd**	
be carefully considered. This decision inevitably requires the exercise of clinical judgment based on the individual's history and the cultural norms for the expression of distress in the context of loss. D. At least one major depressive episode is not better explained by schizoaffective disorder and is not super-imposed on schizophrenia, schizophreniform disorder, delusional disorder, or other specified or unspecified schizophrenia spectrum and other psychotic disorders. E. There has never been a manic episode or a hypomanic episode.	Specify: With anxious distress With mixed features With melancholic features With atypical features With mood-congruent psychotic features With mood-incongruent psychotic features With catatonia With peripartum onset With seasonal pattern

Reprinted with permission from the Diagnostic and Statistical Manual of Mental Disorders, Fifth Edition, Text Revision (DSM-5-TR) *(2022). American Psychiatric Association.*

least 2 years (1 year for children and adolescents). The diagnosis is identified as *early onset* (occurring before age 21 years) or *late onset* (occurring at age 21 years or older). The *DSM-5-TR* diagnostic criteria for persistent depressive disorder (dysthymia) are presented in Box 25–2.

Premenstrual Dysphoric Disorder

The essential features of **premenstrual dysphoric disorder (PMDD)** include markedly depressed mood, excessive anxiety, mood swings, and decreased interest in activities during the week before menses, improving shortly after the onset of menstruation, and becoming minimal or absent in the week after menses (APA, 2022). The major difference between the diagnosis of PMDD and the premenstrual mood changes that many women experience is a matter of intensity and frequency of symptoms. The symptoms of PMDD are severe enough to interfere with one's ability to function socially, at work, or school and they are recurrent for the majority of menstrual cycles over the course of a year.

Substance/Medication-Induced Depressive Disorder

The symptoms associated with a substance/medication-induced depressive disorder are considered the direct result of physiological effects of a substance (e.g., a drug of abuse, a medication, or toxin exposure). This disorder causes clinically significant distress or impairment in social, occupational, or other important areas of functioning. The depressed mood is associated with *intoxication* or *withdrawal* from substances such as alcohol, amphetamines, cocaine, hallucinogens, opioids, phencyclidine-like substances, sedatives, hypnotics, or anxiolytics and the symptoms meet the full criteria for a relevant depressive disorder (APA, 2022).

Many medications have been known to evoke mood symptoms. Classifications include anesthetics, analgesics, anticholinergics, anticonvulsants, antihypertensives, antiparkinsonian agents, antiulcer agents, cardiac medications, oral contraceptives, psychotropic medications, muscle relaxants, steroids, and sulfonamides. Some specific examples are included in the discussion of predisposing factors to depressive disorders.

Depressive Disorder Due to Another Medical Condition

This disorder is characterized by symptoms associated with a major depressive episode that are the direct physiological consequence of another medical condition (APA, 2022). The depression causes clinically significant distress or impairment in social, occupational, or other important areas of functioning. Examples of medical conditions that influence depression include stroke, traumatic brain injuries, thyroid disorders, Cushing's disease, Huntington's disease, Parkinson's disease, and multiple sclerosis.

Predisposing Factors

The etiology of depression is unclear. No single theory or hypothesis has been postulated that substantiates a clear-cut explanation for the disease. Evidence continues to mount in support of multiple causations, recognizing the combined effects of genetic, biochemical, and psychosocial influences on an individual's susceptibility to depression. Some theoretical postulates are presented here.

Biological Theories
Genetics

Affective illness has been the subject of considerable research on the relevance of hereditary factors.

BOX 25–2 Diagnostic Criteria for Persistent Depressive Disorder (Dysthymia)

A. Depressed mood for most of the day, for more days than not, as indicated by either subjective account or observation by others, for at least 2 years. **Note:** In children and adolescents, mood can be irritable and duration must be at least 1 year.

B. Presence, while depressed, of two (or more) of the following:
   1. Poor appetite or overeating
   2. Insomnia or hypersomnia
   3. Low energy or fatigue
   4. Low self-esteem
   5. Poor concentration or difficulty making decisions
   6. Feelings of hopelessness

C. During the 2-year period (1 year for children or adolescents) of the disturbance, the individual has never been without the symptoms in Criteria A and B for more than 2 months at a time.

D. Criteria for a major depressive disorder may be continuously present for 2 years.

E. There has never been a manic episode or a hypomanic episode.

F. The disturbance is not better explained by a persistent schizoaffective disorder, schizophrenia, delusional disorder, or other specified or unspecified schizophrenia spectrum and other psychotic disorder.

G. The symptoms are not attributable to the physiological effects of a substance (e.g., a drug of abuse, a medication) or another medical condition (e.g., hypothyroidism).

H. The symptoms cause clinically significant distress or impairment in social, occupational, or other important areas of functioning.

Note: If criteria are sufficient for a diagnosis of a major depressive episode at any time during the 2-year period of depressed mood, then a separate diagnosis of major depression should be made in addition to the diagnosis of persistent depressive disorder along with the relevant specifier (e.g., with intermittent major depressive episodes, with current episode).

Specify if:

With anxious distress

Specify if:

In partial remission
In full remission

With atypical features
With peripartum onset

Specify if (For most recent 2 years of persistent depressive disorder):

With pure dysthymic syndrome: Full criteria for major depressive episode have not been met in at least the preceding 2 years

With persistent major depressive episode: Full criteria for a major depressive episode have been met throughout the preceding 2-year period.

With intermittent major depressive episodes, with current episode: Full criteria for a major depressive episode are currently met, but there have been periods of at least 8 weeks in at least the preceding 2 years with symptoms below the threshold for full major depressive episode.

With intermittent major depressive episodes, with current episode: Full criteria for a major depressive episode are not currently met, but there has been one or more major depressive episodes in at least the preceding 2 years.

Specify if:

Early onset (If onset is before age 21 years)

Late onset (If onset is at age 21 years or older)

Specify current severity:

Mild
Moderate

Severe

A genetic link has been suggested in numerous studies; however, a definitive mode of genetic transmission has yet to be demonstrated. First-degree relatives of individuals with MDD have a two- to fourfold higher risk for the disorder than that of the general population (APA, 2022). Recent studies have focused on genetic variants that are associated with depression (Lipp et al., 2020). For example, one genetic variant (an *MTHFR C677T* gene mutation) has been associated with impaired folate metabolism that may lead to decreased synthesis of neurotransmitters.

Twin Studies

Twin studies suggest a strong genetic factor in the etiology of affective illness, including depressive disorders and bipolar disorders. Compared with dizygotic twins, monozygotic twins have a two to four times greater incidence of depression; *between* monozygotic twins, there is a 70% to 80% chance of both twins having the illness (Kelsoe & Greenwood, 2017). These findings suggest that although twin studies do identify a significant genetic risk, genetics does not explain all depressions. Environmental risks are not only an important variable but they are uniquely individual.

Family Studies

Family studies have shown that major depression is seven times more common among first-degree biological relatives of people with the disorder than among the general population (Kelsoe & Greenwood, 2017). The evidence to support an increased risk of depressive disorder in individuals with positive family history is compelling. It is unlikely that random environmental factors could cause the concentration of illness that is seen within families.

Adoption Studies

Further support for heritability as an etiological influence in depression comes from studies of the adopted offspring of affectively ill biological parents. These studies indicate that biological children of parents with mood disorders are at increased risk of developing a mood disorder, even when they are reared by adoptive parents who do not have the disorder (Kelsoe & Greenwood, 2017). Conversely, adoption studies have also been used to look at the effects of being reared by an adoptive parent (particularly the maternal parent) with depression and the risks for depression in nongenetically similar children. Interestingly, these studies have demonstrated an increased risk of depression (as well as oppositional defiant disorder and conduct disorder) in adopted children that cannot be explained by genetics (Natsuaki et al., 2014). Again, this finding suggests that environmental factors also play a role in the etiology of depressive illnesses.

Biochemical Influences

Biogenic Amines

It has been hypothesized that depressive illness may be related to a deficiency of the neurotransmitters norepinephrine, serotonin, and dopamine at functionally important receptor sites in the brain. Historically, the biogenic amine hypothesis of mood disorders grew out of the observation that reserpine, an antihypertensive drug that depletes the brain of amines such as norepinephrine, was associated with the development of a depressive syndrome. The catecholamine norepinephrine has been identified as a key component in the mobilization of the body to deal with stressful situations. Neurons that contain serotonin are critically involved in the regulation of many psychobiological functions, such as mood,

anxiety, arousal, vigilance, irritability, thinking, cognition, appetite, aggression, sleep–wakefulness cycles, eating, and intestinal motility. Tryptophan, the amino acid precursor of serotonin, has been shown to enhance the efficacy of antidepressant medications and on occasion to be effective as an antidepressant itself. The level of dopamine in the mesolimbic system of the brain is thought to exert a strong influence over human mood and behavior. A diminished supply of these biogenic amines inhibits the transmission of impulses from one neuronal fiber to another, causing a failure of the cells to fire or become charged (Figure 25–1).

Abnormal levels of acetylcholine, glutamate, glycine, and gamma-aminobutyric acid (GABA) have also been associated with depression. Because cholinergic agents have profound effects on mood, electroencephalograms, sleep, and neuroendocrine function, it has been suggested that the problem in depression and mania may be an imbalance between the biogenic amines and acetylcholine. Glutamate and glycine bind at *N*-methyl-D-aspartate (NMDA) receptors, and recent evidence suggests that drugs that antagonize NMDA receptors have antidepressant effects (Boland & Verduin, 2022). Reductions in GABA appear in depression, and antidepressants upregulate GABA receptors.

The precise role that neurotransmitters play in the etiology of depression is unknown because these chemicals cannot be measured in the brain. It has been theorized that because selective serotonin reuptake inhibitors (SSRIs) elevate serotonin levels, low serotonin levels in the brain must be responsible for depression. However, SSRIs also seem to be beneficial in the treatment of anxiety, leading to the hypothesis that low serotonin levels are responsible for anxiety. Further, *too much* serotonin has also been implicated in anxiety states and in schizophrenia. Boland and Verduin (2022) stated:

> It is unclear to what extent serotonin acts as a true synaptic or "private" neurotransmitter versus action as a local endocrine hormone or "social transmitter" or whether its roles differ depending on the fiber type from which it is released. (p. 955)

Newer antidepressants that act on both serotonergic and noradrenergic receptors suggest that the dysregulation of biogenic amines in depression is far more complex than can be explained by single-neurotransmitter hypotheses (Akiskal, 2017). The effectiveness of ketamine as an adjunct to antidepressant therapy has led to an additional hypothesis that modulation of excess glutamate is influential in reversing depressive symptoms. Ongoing research will hopefully clarify what are, at present, only hypotheses about the etiology of depression.

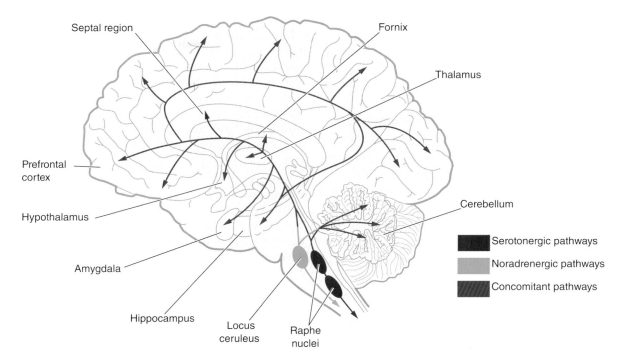

FIGURE 25–1   Neurobiology of depression.

NEUROTRANSMITTERS

Although other neurotransmitters have also been implicated in the pathophysiology of depression, disturbances in serotonin and norepinephrine have been the most extensively scrutinized.

Cell bodies of origin for the serotonin pathways lie within the raphe nuclei located in the brainstem. Those for norepinephrine originate in the locus ceruleus. Projections for both neurotransmitters extend throughout the forebrain, prefrontal cortex, cerebellum, and limbic system.

AREAS OF THE BRAIN AFFECTED

Areas of the brain affected by depression and the symptoms that they mediate include the following:
• Hippocampus: Memory impairments, feelings of worthlessness, hopelessness, and guilt
• Amygdala: Anhedonia, anxiety, reduced motivation
• Hypothalamus: Increased or decreased sleep and appetite; decreased energy and libido
• Other limbic structures: Emotional alterations
• Frontal cortex: Depressed mood; problems concentrating
• Cerebellum: Psychomotor retardation/agitation

MEDICATIONS AND THEIR EFFECTS ON THE BRAIN

All medications that increase serotonin, norepinephrine, or both can improve the emotional and vegetative symptoms of depression. Medications that produce these effects include those that block the presynaptic reuptake of the neurotransmitters or block receptors at nerve endings (tricyclics; SSRIs; SNRIs) and those that inhibit monoamine oxidase, an enzyme that is involved in the metabolism of the monoamines serotonin, norepinephrine, and dopamine (MAOIs). Novel antidepressants such as ketamine act as NMDA receptor antagonists thus blocking excitatory glutamate signaling and increasing activity in the prefrontal cortex (Shin & Kim, 2020).

Side effects of these medications relate to their specific neurotransmitter receptor–blocking action. Tricyclic (e.g., imipramine, amitriptyline) and tetracyclic (e.g., mirtazapine, maprotiline) medications block reuptake and/or receptors for serotonin, norepinephrine, acetylcholine, and histamine. SSRIs are selective serotonin reuptake inhibitors. Others, such as bupropion, venlafaxine, and duloxetine, block serotonin and norepinephrine reuptake, and also are weak inhibitors of dopamine.

Blockade of norepinephrine reuptake results in side effects of tremors, cardiac arrhythmias, sexual dysfunction, and hypertension. Blockade of serotonin reuptake results in side effects of gastrointestinal disturbances, increased agitation, and sexual dysfunction. Blockade of dopamine reuptake results in side effects of psychomotor activation. Blockade of acetylcholine reuptake results in dry mouth, blurred vision, constipation, and urinary retention. Blockade of histamine reuptake results in sedation, weight gain, and hypotension. Ketamine is associated with transient elevation in blood pressure.

Neuroendocrine Disturbances

Neuroendocrine disturbances may play a role in the pathogenesis or persistence of depressive illness. This notion has arisen in view of the marked disturbances in mood observed with the administration of certain hormones or in the presence of spontaneously occurring endocrine disease.

Hypothalamic-Pituitary-Adrenocortical Axis

In people who are depressed, the normal system of hormonal inhibition fails, resulting in hypersecretion of cortisol. Elevated serum cortisol is the basis for the dexamethasone suppression test that is sometimes used to determine whether an individual has somatically treatable depression.

Hypothalamic-Pituitary-Thyroid Axis

Thyrotropin-releasing factor (TRF) from the hypothalamus stimulates the release of thyroid-stimulating hormone (TSH) from the anterior pituitary gland. In turn, TSH stimulates the thyroid gland. Diminished TSH response to administered TRF is observed in approximately 20% to 30% of depressed people and appears to be associated with increased risk for relapse despite treatment with antidepressants (Boland & Verduin, 2022). Individuals with hypothyroidism often manifest with signs of depression (in addition to other symptoms), and nearly 20 million people in the United States (women are five to eight times more likely than men) have thyroid conditions (American Thyroid Association, 2022). Laboratory testing to evaluate TSH is relevant to distinguish between depressive disorders and thyroid disorders, because in thyroid disorders the symptoms of depression are treated with hormone replacement rather than antidepressants.

Although there is no single diagnostic test for depression, several findings from tests that may indicate depression but are nonspecific, such as increased corticotropin-releasing factor in cerebrospinal fluid, steroid overproduction (evidenced by the dexamethasone suppression test), and thyroid dysregulation (evidenced by thyrotropin challenge tests). These findings have led Akiskal (2017) to conclude that there is clear evidence of midbrain disturbance (and thus, evidence of a legitimate disease process) in clinical depression.

Physiological Influences

Depressive symptoms that occur as a consequence of a nonmood disorder or as an adverse effect of certain medications are called *secondary* depression. Secondary depression may be related to medication side effects, neurological disorders, electrolyte or hormonal disturbances, nutritional deficiencies, and other physiological or psychological conditions.

Medication Side Effects

Many drugs, either alone or in combination with other medications, can produce a depressive syndrome. Most common are those that have a direct effect on the central nervous system, such as anxiolytics, antipsychotics, sedative-hypnotics (including barbiturates and opioids), and anticonvulsant mood stabilizers. Many drugs used to treat general medical conditions have also been associated with inducing depression and several are listed here:

- Antibacterial agents, antifungal agents, and antiviral agents
- Anticonvulsants
- Antihypertensives (including beta blockers and calcium blockers)
- Antimalarials (including mefloquine)
- Antineoplastics (including vincristine and zidovudine)
- Dermatologics (including isotretinoin and finasteride)
- Hormones (including contraceptives)
- Nonnucleoside reverse transcriptase inhibitors (HIV medications)
- Respiratory agents (leukotriene inhibitors)
- Smoking cessation agents (varenicline)
- Statins
- Steroids

Neurological Disorders

An individual who has had a cerebrovascular accident (CVA) may experience despondency unrelated to the severity of the CVA. These are true mood disorders, and antidepressant drug therapy may be indicated. Brain tumors, particularly in the area of the temporal lobe, often cause symptoms of depression. Agitated depression may be part of the clinical picture associated with Alzheimer's disease, Parkinson's disease, and Huntington's disease. Agitation and restlessness may also represent underlying depression in the individual with multiple sclerosis.

Electrolyte Disturbances

Excessive levels of sodium bicarbonate or calcium can produce symptoms of depression, as can deficits in magnesium and sodium. Interestingly, hyponatremia is a side effect of serotonergic antidepressants and is especially problematic in the elderly. Potassium is also implicated in the syndrome of depression. Symptoms have been observed with excesses of potassium in the body as well as in instances of potassium depletion.

Hormonal Disturbances

Depression is associated with dysfunction of the adrenal cortex and is commonly observed in both Addison's disease and Cushing's syndrome. Other endocrine conditions that may result in symptoms of depression include hypoparathyroidism, hyperparathyroidism, hypothyroidism, and hyperthyroidism.

An imbalance of the hormones estrogen and progesterone has been implicated in the predisposition to PMDD, although the exact etiology is unknown. The interaction of these hormonal changes also has an effect on serotonin levels, which may contribute to the depression associated with this disorder. It is also noted that individuals with PMDD often have underlying depression and anxiety, so it is possible that the hormone changes are exacerbating an already existing condition (Burnett, 2021).

Nutritional Deficiencies

Deficiencies in proteins, carbohydrates, vitamin B_1 (thiamine), vitamin B_2 (riboflavin), vitamin B_6 (pyridoxine), B_9 (folate), vitamin B_{12}, iron, zinc, calcium, chromium, iodine, lithium, selenium, and potassium have all been associated with producing symptoms of depression (Kubala, 2021; Sathyanarayana et al., 2008). One large study also found that vitamin D deficiency was linked to depressive symptoms (Shin et al., 2016), although another study concluded that vitamin D_3 *supplementation* did not change the incidence or recurrence of depressive symptoms (Okereke et al., 2020). Individuals with anorexia nervosa, who have significant nutritional deficiencies, commonly have comorbid depression.

Other Physiological Conditions

Other conditions that have been associated with secondary depression include collagen disorders, such as systemic lupus erythematosus and polyarteritis nodosa; cardiovascular disease, such as cardiomyopathy, congestive heart failure, and myocardial infarction; infections, such as encephalitis, hepatitis, mononucleosis, pneumonia, and syphilis; and metabolic disorders, such as diabetes mellitus and porphyria.

The Role of Inflammation

The role of inflammation in the development of depression is an area of current research. The function of the immune system in the development of disease is being explored with regard to a host of illnesses, including cancer, autoimmune disorders, and several psychiatric disorders. Not all patients with depression have signs of inflammation, but individuals with treatment-resistant depression have been found to have high levels of C-reactive protein (CRP) and tumor necrosis factor (TNF), which are biomarkers of inflammation (Miller, 2018). Cytokines, which play a role in the inflammatory response, have specific activities in the brain and affect neurotransmitters associated with depression (monoamines) and dopamine.

Stress, another inflammatory process, has been shown to increase the permeability of the blood–brain barrier and consequently may have an effect on the development of depression when inflammatory responses in the brain trigger chemical changes. Recent research (Slezak, 2021) demonstrated, through state-of- the-art imaging, that chronic stress creates permanent changes in the brain, particularly dysregulated astrocyte metabolism, and that this is a major hallmark of depression.

Does depression trigger inflammation or is inflammation one potential cause of depression? More research is needed to answer this question, but current evidence suggests that elevated inflammation biomarkers can predict a patient's response to conventional antidepressants, psychotherapy, ketamine, and anticytokine immunotherapy (Miller, 2018). Beurel and associates (2020), in their extensive review, concluded that the relationship between depression and inflammation is bidirectional; the immune system regulates mood and dysregulation of the immune system that occurs in depressed patients hinders prognosis and response to treatment.

Psychosocial Theories

Psychoanalytical Theory

Freud (1957) presented his classic paper "Mourning and Melancholia" in 1917. He defined the distinguishing features of melancholia as

> a profoundly painful dejection, cessation of interest in the outside world, loss of the capacity to love, inhibition of all activity, and a lowering of the self-regarding feelings to a degree that finds utterances in self-reproaches and self-revilings, and culminates in a delusional expectation of punishment. (p. 242)

He observed that melancholia occurs after the loss of a loved object, either actually by death or emotionally by rejection, or the loss of some other abstraction of value to the individual. Freud indicated that in melancholia, the depressed patient's rage is internally directed because of identification with the lost object.

Learning Theory

The model of "learned helplessness" arises from Seligman's (1973) experiments with dogs. The animals were exposed to electrical stimulation from which they could not escape. Later, when they were given the opportunity to avoid the traumatic experience, they reacted with helplessness and made no attempt to escape. A similar state of helplessness exists in humans who have experienced numerous failures (either real or perceived). The individual abandons any further attempt to succeed. Seligman theorized that learned helplessness predisposes individuals to depression by imposing a feeling of lack of control over their life situations. They become depressed because they feel helpless; they have learned that whatever they do is futile. Learned helplessness can be especially damaging very early in life because the sense of mastery over one's environment is an important foundation for future emotional development.

Object Loss Theory

The theory of object loss suggests that depressive illness occurs as a result of having been abandoned by or otherwise separated from a significant other during the first 6 months of life. Because the mother represents the child's main source of security during this period, she is considered the "object." This absence of attachment, which may be either physical or emotional, leads to feelings of helplessness and despair that contribute to lifelong patterns of depression in response to loss.

Cognitive Theory

Beck and colleagues (1979) proposed a theory suggesting that the primary disturbance in depression is cognitive rather than affective. The underlying cause of the depression is cognitive distortion that results in negative, defeated attitudes. Beck and colleagues identified three cognitive distortions that they believe serve as the basis for depression:

1. Negative expectations of the environment
2. Negative expectations of the self
3. Negative expectations of the future

These cognitive distortions arise out of a defect in cognitive development, and the individual feels inadequate, worthless, and rejected by others. Outlook for the future is one of pessimism and hopelessness.

Cognitive theorists believe that depression is the product of negative thinking. This theory is in contrast to other theories, which suggest that negative thinking occurs when an individual is depressed. **Cognitive behavior therapy (CBT)** focuses on helping the individual alter mood by changing the way they think. The individual is taught to control negative thought distortions that lead to pessimism, lethargy, procrastination, indecisiveness, and low self-esteem (see Chapter 18, "Cognitive Behavior Therapy").

The Transactional Model

No single theory or hypothesis exists to substantiate a clear-cut explanation for depressive disorder. Evidence continues to mount in support of multiple causation. The transactional model recognizes the combined effects of genetic, biochemical, and psychosocial influences on an individual's susceptibility to depression. The dynamics of depression using the transactional model of stress and adaptation are presented in Figure 25–2.

Developmental Implications

Childhood

Only in recent years has a consensus developed among investigators identifying MDD as an entity in children and adolescents that can be identified using criteria similar to those used for adults. It is not uncommon, however, for the symptoms of depression to be manifested differently in childhood. In addition to some of the classic symptoms of depression (mood, appetite, sleep and energy changes, and withdrawal), children may present with irritable mood, excessive self-reproach, and excessive clinging to parents (Anxiety and Depression Association of America, 2021; Boland & Verduin, 2022). In school-age children, changes in grades, getting into trouble at school, refusal to go to school, and school phobias may be symptomatic of depression.

Other symptoms of childhood depression may include hyperactivity, delinquency, school problems, psychosomatic complaints, sleeping and eating disturbances, social isolation, delusional thinking, and suicidal thoughts or actions. Wagner and Brent (2017) noted that youth with depression are more often irritable rather than dysphoric and consequently less likely to identify themselves as depressed. Additionally, they cite that anywhere from 40% to 90% of youth with depression have other comorbid psychiatric conditions, so comprehensive assessment is essential.

The APA (2022) has included a diagnostic category in the "Depressive Disorders" chapter of the *DSM-5-TR* that relates specifically to children. This childhood disorder is called *disruptive mood dysregulation disorder.* The diagnostic criteria for disruptive mood dysregulation disorder are presented in Box 25–3.

Children may become depressed for various reasons. In many depressed children, there is a genetic predisposition toward the condition, which is then precipitated by a stressful situation. Common precipitating factors include physical or emotional detachment by the primary caregiver, parental separation or divorce, death of a loved one (person or pet), a move, academic failure, or physical illness. In any event, the common denominator is loss.

The focus of therapy with depressed children is to alleviate the child's symptoms and strengthen their coping and adaptive skills to help prevent future psychological problems. Some studies have shown that untreated childhood depression may lead to subsequent problems in adolescence and adult life. Most children are treated on an outpatient basis. Hospitalization of the depressed child usually occurs if they are actively suicidal, when the home environment precludes adherence to

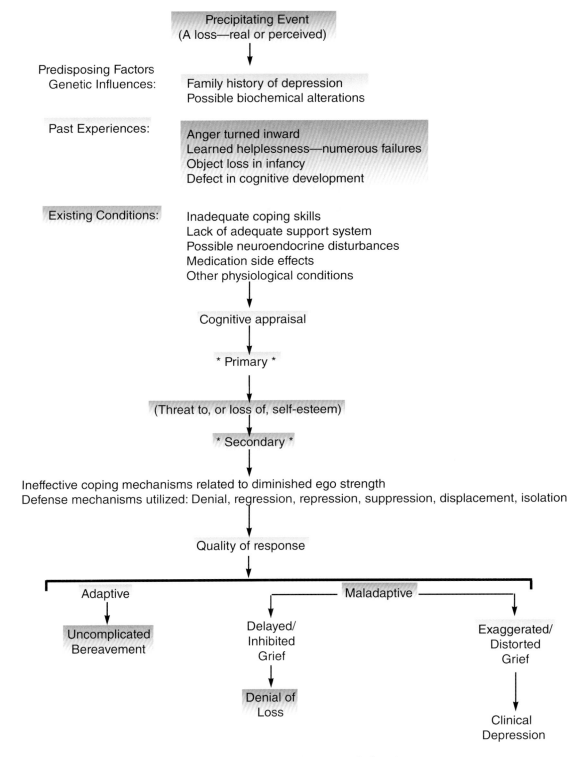

FIGURE 25–2   The dynamics of depression using the transactional model of stress and adaptation.

a treatment regimen, or if the child needs to be separated from the home because of psychosocial deprivation.

Parental and family therapy are commonly used to help the younger depressed child. Recovery is facilitated by emotional support and guidance to family members.

Children older than age 8 usually participate in family therapy. In some situations, individual treatment may be appropriate for older children. Medications such as antidepressants can be important in the treatment of children, especially for the more serious and recurrent forms of depression. The SSRIs have been used with

---

BOX 25–3 Diagnostic Criteria for Disruptive Mood Dysregulation Disorder

A. Severe recurrent temper outbursts manifested verbally (e.g., verbal rages) and/or behaviorally (e.g., physical aggression toward people or property) that are grossly out of proportion in intensity or duration to the situation or provocation.

B. The temper outbursts are inconsistent with developmental level.

C. The temper outbursts occur, on average, three or more times per week.

D. The mood between temper outbursts is persistently irritable or angry most of the day, nearly every day, and is observable by others (e.g., parents, teachers, peers).

E. Criteria A–D have been present for 12 or more months. Throughout that time, the individual has not had a period lasting 3 or more consecutive months without all of the symptoms of Criteria A–D.

F. Criteria A and D are present in at least two of three settings (i.e., at home, at school, with peers) and are severe in at least one of these.

G. The diagnosis should not be made for the first time before age 6 or after age 18 years.

H. By history or observation, the age at onset of Criteria A–E is before 10 years.

I. There has never been a distinct period lasting more than 1 day during which the full symptom criteria, except duration, for a manic or hypomanic episode have been met. **Note:** Developmentally appropriate mood elevation, such as occurs in the context of a highly positive event or its anticipation, should not be considered as a symptom of mania or hypomania.

J. The behaviors do not occur exclusively during an episode of major depressive disorder and are not better explained by another mental disorder (e.g., autism spectrum disorder, posttraumatic stress disorder, separation anxiety disorder, persistent depressive disorder).

Note: This diagnosis cannot coexist with oppositional defiant disorder, intermittent explosive disorder, or bipolar disorder, though it can coexist with others, including major depressive disorder, attention deficit-hyperactivity disorder, conduct disorder, and substance use disorders. Individuals whose symptoms meet criteria for both disruptive mood dysregulation disorder and oppositional defiant disorder should only be given the diagnosis of disruptive mood dysregulation disorder. If an individual has ever experienced a manic or hypomanic episode, the diagnosis of disruptive mood dysregulation disorder should not be assigned.

K. The symptoms are not attributable to the physiological effects of a substance or to another medical or neurological condition.

Reprinted with permission from the Diagnostic and Statistical Manual of Mental Disorders, Fifth Edition, Text Revision (DSM-5-TR) *(2022). American Psychiatric Association.*

---

success, particularly in combination with psychosocial therapies. However, because there has been some concern that the use of antidepressant medications may cause suicidal behavior in young people, the U.S. Food and Drug Administration (FDA) has applied a *boxed warning* to all antidepressant medications. The NIMH (2018) stated:

> In some cases, children, teenagers, and young adults under 25 may experience an increase in suicidal thoughts or behavior when taking antidepressants, especially in the first few weeks after starting or when the dose is changed. This warning from the FDA also says that patients of all ages taking antidepressants should be watched closely, especially during the first few weeks of treatment.

Adolescence

Depression may be even harder to recognize in an adolescent than in a younger child. Feelings of sadness, loneliness, anxiety, and hopelessness associated with depression may be perceived as the normal emotional stresses of growing up. Therefore, many young people whose symptoms are attributed to the "normal adjustments" of adolescence do not get the help they need. Depression is a major cause of suicide among teens, and suicide has been the second-leading cause of death in the 15- to 24-year-old age-group for several years (although 1999 through 2020 saw an increase in homicides, moving suicide to the third leading cause of death for that time frame) (National Center for Health Statistics, 2022).

Common symptoms of depression in the adolescent are inappropriately expressed anger, aggressiveness, running away, delinquency, social withdrawal, sexual acting out, substance misuse, restlessness, and apathy. Loss of self-esteem, sleeping and eating disturbances, and psychosomatic complaints are also common.

What, then, differentiates mood disorder from the typical stormy behavior of adolescence? A visible manifestation of *behavioral change that lasts for several weeks* is the best clue for a mood disorder. Examples include the normally outgoing and extroverted adolescent who has become withdrawn and isolated, the good student who previously received consistently high marks but is now failing and skipping classes, and the usually self-confident teenager who is now inappropriately irritable and defensive with others.

Adolescents become depressed for all the same reasons discussed under childhood depression.

In adolescence, however, depression is a common manifestation of the stress and independence conflicts associated with the normal maturation process. Depression may also be the response to death of a parent, other relative, or friend, or to a breakup with a significant other. This perception of abandonment by parents or the closest peer relationship is thought to be the most frequent immediate precipitant to adolescent suicide.

Treatment of the depressed adolescent is often conducted on an outpatient basis. Hospitalization may be required in cases of severe depression or threat of imminent suicide, when a family situation is such that treatment cannot be carried out in the home, when the physical condition precludes self-care of biological needs, or when the adolescent has indicated possible harm to self or others in the family.

In addition to supportive psychosocial intervention, antidepressant therapy may be part of the treatment of adolescent mood disorders. However, as mentioned previously, the FDA has issued a public health advisory warning the public about the increased risk of suicidal thoughts and behavior in children and adolescents treated with antidepressant medications. The advisory language does not prohibit the use of antidepressants in children and adolescents. Rather, it warns of the increased risk of suicidal ideation and encourages prescribers to balance this risk with clinical need.

Fluoxetine (Prozac) has been approved by the FDA to treat depression in children age 8 and older, and escitalopram (Lexapro) was approved in 2009 for treatment of MDD in adolescents age 12 and older. Other SSRI medications, such as sertraline, citalopram, and paroxetine, and the serotonin-norepinephrine reuptake inhibitor (SNRI) antidepressants duloxetine, venlafaxine, and desvenlafaxine, have not been approved for treatment of depression in children or adolescents, although they have been prescribed to children by physicians in "off-label use"—a use other than the FDA-approved use. In June 2003 the FDA recommended that paroxetine not be used in children and adolescents for the treatment of MDD. The FDA analysis of antidepressant medications, as reported by the Mayo Clinic (2022a), identified that a small number of adolescents taking antidepressants had an increase in suicidal thoughts and that none of the children in the study actually took their own life. Nonetheless, the potential risk is considered significant enough to carefully evaluate risks versus benefits before prescribing antidepressants to children and adolescents.

Senescence

Depression (along with dementia) is one of the most common psychiatric disorders among older adults. Estimates are that about 1% to 5% of older adults living in the community have depression but that incidence increases to 13.5% for those requiring home health care and 11.5% for older adults who are hospitalized (Centers for Disease Control and Prevention [CDC], 2021). Depression is also more common in older adults with other medical conditions, such as heart disease and those with functional limitations.

Depression among the older adult may be influenced by the value our society places on youth, vigor, and uninterrupted productivity. These societal attitudes reinforce feelings of low self-esteem, helplessness, and hopelessness that become more pervasive and intensive with advanced age. Further, the aging individual's adaptive coping strategies may be seriously challenged by major stressors, such as financial problems, physical illness, changes in body functioning, and an increasing awareness of approaching death. The problem is often intensified by the numerous losses individuals experience during this period in life, such as a spouse, friends, children, home, and independence. A phenomenon called *bereavement overload* occurs when individuals experience so many losses in their lives that they are not able to resolve one grief response before another begins. Bereavement overload predisposes older adult individuals to depressive illness.

Although they make up only about 14.5% of the population, the older adult population accounts for a proportionately larger percentage of suicides in the United States. For all ages and races, including older adults, the highest percentage of suicides is among white men at almost four times the national rate.

Some symptoms of depression in the older adult are similar to those in younger adults. However, depressive syndromes are often confused by other illnesses associated with the aging process. Symptoms of depression are often misdiagnosed as neurocognitive disorder (NCD) when in fact the memory loss, confused thinking, or apathy symptomatic of NCD actually may be the result of depression. This condition is often referred to as *pseudodementia*. The early awakening and reduced appetite typical of depression are common among many older people who are not depressed. Compounding this situation is that many medical conditions, such as endocrinological, neurological, nutritional, and metabolic disorders, often present with classic symptoms of depression. Many medications commonly prescribed to older adults, such as antihypertensives, corticosteroids, and analgesics, can also produce a depressant effect.

Depression accompanies many illnesses that are common among older people, such as Parkinson's disease, cancer, arthritis, and the early stages of

Alzheimer's disease. Treating depression in these situations can reduce unnecessary suffering and help individuals cope with their medical problems.

The most effective treatment of depression in the older adult individual is thought to be a combination of psychosocial and biological approaches. Antidepressant medications are administered with consideration for age-related physiological changes in absorption, distribution, elimination, and brain receptor sensitivity. Because of these changes, plasma concentrations of these medications can reach very high levels despite moderate oral doses. Anticholinergic side effects associated with tricyclic antidepressants can be problematic for older adults, and SSRIs have been associated with inducing significant hyponatremia in this population. Careful evaluation of side effects and dosage monitoring are essential.

Electroconvulsive therapy (ECT) is an important alternative for treatment of major depression in the geriatric population, especially considering the problematic side effects of antidepressants in this population. The response to ECT appears to be slower with advancing age and the therapeutic effects are of limited duration, but in a systematic review researchers concluded that use of ECT in the geriatric population is "highly effective, safe, and well tolerated" (Geduldig & Kellner, 2016). It may be considered the treatment of choice for the older adult individual who is an acute suicidal risk or is unable to tolerate antidepressant medications. Confusion, a side effect of ECT that typically lasts a few minutes to several hours, is generally more pronounced in older adults (Mayo Clinic, 2022c).

Other therapeutic approaches include interpersonal, behavioral, cognitive, group, and family psychotherapies. Appropriate treatment of the depressed older adult individual can bring relief from suffering and offer a new lease on life with a feeling of renewed productivity.

Postpartum Depression

The severity of depression in the postpartum period varies from a feeling of the "blues," to moderate depression, and finally to severe depression with psychotic features. About 50% of these episodes actually begin before delivery (APA, 2022), and the onset of symptoms during pregnancy, including the "baby blues," increases risk for major depression in the postpartum period. Major depression with psychotic features occurs in about 1 or 2 out of 1,000 postpartum women.

Symptoms of the baby blues include worry, sadness, and fatigue after having a baby. These symptoms affect about 80% of mothers and usually subside on their own within a week or two (NIMH, n.d.).

Symptoms of moderate **postpartum depression** have been described as depressed mood varying from day to day, with more bad days than good, worsening toward evening and associated with fatigue, irritability, loss of appetite, sleep disturbances, and loss of libido. In addition, the new mother expresses a great deal of concern about her inability to care for her baby. These symptoms begin somewhat later than those attributable to the baby blues and take from a few weeks to several months to abate.

Postpartum depression with psychotic features is characterized by depressed mood, agitation, indecision, lack of concentration, guilt, and an abnormal attitude toward bodily functions. The symptoms can be severe and incapacitating. There may be a lack of interest in or rejection of the baby or a morbid fear that the baby may be harmed, accompanied by delusions and hallucinations. Risks of suicide and infanticide should not be overlooked. There is a 30% to 50% likelihood of postpartum psychosis recurring with subsequent pregnancies (APA, 2022).

The etiology of postpartum depression remains unclear. Baby blues may be associated with hormonal changes, tryptophan metabolism, or alterations in membrane transport during the early postpartum period. Women with moderate to severe symptoms may have an increased risk for depression related to heredity, upbringing, early life experiences, personality, or social circumstances. Women who have had perinatal depression (occurring during or after the pregnancy) with previous pregnancies or who have a personal or family history of depression or bipolar disorder are at greater risk for developing postpartum depression (NIMH, n.d.). Family history of other psychiatric disorders, including schizophrenia, also increase risk (Bauer et al., 2018). The etiology of postpartum depression is likely a combination of hormonal, metabolic, and psychosocial influences.

Treatment of postpartum depression varies with the severity of the illness. Psychotic depression may be treated with antidepressant medication along with supportive psychotherapy, group therapy, and possibly family therapy. In 2019 the FDA approved the first novel drug for the treatment of postpartum depression. Brexanolone (Zulresso) is administered in an intravenous infusion over 2.5 days and is only available through a restricted distribution program in a certified health agency. In addition, because there is a risk of severe side effects, including excessive sedation and sudden loss of consciousness, this drug requires a Risk Evaluation and Mitigation Strategy (REMS). Pulse oximetry must be continuously monitored, and patients must be accompanied during interactions with children while receiving the infusion (FDA, 2019b).

Moderate depression may be relieved with supportive psychotherapy and continuing assistance with home management until the symptoms subside. The individual experiencing "baby blues" usually needs no treatment beyond reassurance from the physician or nurse that these feelings are common and will soon pass. Support and comfort from significant others also are important.

Application of the Nursing Process

Background Assessment Data

Symptomatology of depression can be viewed on a continuum from transient symptoms to severe depression according to the severity of the illness. All individuals become depressed from time to time, and these symptoms tend to be transient. Severe depression, however, is marked by significant distress that interferes with social, occupational, cognitive, and emotional functioning.

The individual who is severely depressed may demonstrate a loss of contact with reality. **Psychomotor retardation**, a slowing down of thought processes and physical movement, is a common symptom in MDD. Severe depression is associated with a complete lack of pleasure in all activities (anhedonia), and ruminations about suicide are common. MDD is an example of severe depression. A continuum of depression is presented in Figure 25–3.

A number of assessment rating scales are available for measuring the severity of depressive symptoms. Some are meant to be clinician-administered, whereas others may be self-administered. Examples of self-rating scales include the Zung Self-Rating Depression Scale and the Beck Depression Inventory. One of the most widely used clinician-administered scales is the Hamilton Depression Rating Scale (HDRS). It has been reviewed and revised over the years and exists today in several versions. The original version (Box 25–4) contains 17 items and is designed to measure mood, guilty feelings, suicidal ideation, sleep disturbances, anxiety levels, and weight loss.

Symptoms of depression can be described as alterations in four spheres of human functioning: (1) affective, (2) behavioral, (3) cognitive, and (4) physiological. Alterations within these spheres differ according to the degree of severity of symptomatology.

Transient Depression

Symptoms at this level of the continuum are not necessarily dysfunctional; in fact, they may be considered part of the broad range of typical human emotional responses that accompany everyday disappointments in life. Transient depression subsides quickly, and the individual is able to refocus on other goals and achievements. Alterations include the following:

■ **Affective:** Sadness, dejection, feeling down-hearted, having the blues
■ **Behavioral:** Some crying
■ **Cognitive:** Some difficulty getting mind off of one's disappointment
■ **Physiological:** Feeling tired and listless

Mild Depression

Symptoms at the mild level of depression are like those associated with uncomplicated grieving. Alterations at the mild level include the following:

■ **Affective:** Denial of feelings, anger, anxiety, guilt, helplessness, hopelessness, sadness, despondency
■ **Behavioral:** Tearfulness, regression, restlessness, agitation, withdrawal
■ **Cognitive:** Preoccupation with the loss, self-blame, ambivalence, blaming others
■ **Physiological:** Anorexia or overeating, insomnia or hypersomnia, headache, backache, chest pain, or other symptoms associated with the loss of a significant other

Moderate Depression

Dysthymia (also called persistent depressive disorder) is an example of moderate depression and represents a more chronic disturbance, which, according to the *DSM-5-TR*, is characterized by symptoms endure for

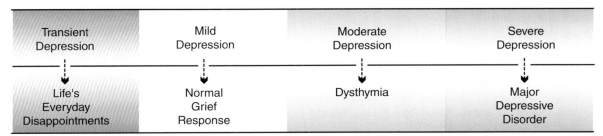

Transient Depression	Mild Depression	Moderate Depression	Severe Depression
Life's Everyday Disappointments	Normal Grief Response	Dysthymia	Major Depressive Disorder

FIGURE 25–3 A continuum of depression.

BOX 25–4 Hamilton Depression Rating Scale (HDRS)

Instructions: For each item, circle the number to select the one "cue" that best characterizes the patient.

1. **Depressed Mood (sadness, hopeless, helpless, worthless)**
   0 = Absent
   1 = These feeling states indicated only on questioning
   2 = These feeling states spontaneously reported verbally
   3 = Communicates feeling states nonverbally, i.e., through facial expression, posture, voice, tendency to weep
   4 = Patient reports virtually only these feeling states in spontaneous verbal and nonverbal communication

2. **Feelings of Guilt**
   0 = Absent
   1 = Self-reproach; feels he/she have let people down
   2 = Ideas of guilt or rumination over past errors or sinful deeds
   3 = Present illness is a punishment. Delusions of guilt
   4 = Hears accusatory or denunciatory voices and/or experiences threatening visual hallucinations

3. **Suicide**
   0 = Absent
   1 = Feels life is not worth living
   2 = Wishes he/she were dead or any thoughts of possible death to self
   3 = Suicidal ideas or gesture
   4 = Attempts at suicide (any serious attempt rates 4)

4. **Insomnia: Early in the Night**
   0 = No difficulty falling asleep
   1 = Complains of occasional difficulty falling asleep, i.e., more than 1/2 hour
   2 = Complains of nightly difficulty falling asleep

5. **Insomnia: Middle of the Night**
   0 = No difficulty
   1 = Complains of being restless and disturbed during the night
   2 = Waking during the night—any getting out of bed rates 2 (except for purposes of voiding)

6. **Insomnia: Early Hours of the Morning**
   0 = No difficulty
   1 = Waking in early hours of the morning, but goes back to sleep
   2 = Unable to fall asleep again if he/she get out of bed

7. **Work and Activities**
   0 = No difficulty
   1 = Thoughts and feelings of incapacity, fatigue, or weakness related to activities, work, or hobbies
   2 = Loss of interest in activity, hobbies, or work—either directly reported by patient, or indirectly in listlessness, indecision, and vacillation (feels he/she have to push self to work or activities)

3 = Decrease in actual time spent in activities or decrease in productivity. Rate 3 if patient does not spend at least 3 hours a day in activities (job or hobbies), excluding routine chores
   4 = Stopped working because of present illness. Rate 4 if patient engages in no activities except routine chose, or if does not perform routine chores unassisted

8. **Psychomotor Retardation (slowness of thought and speech, impaired ability to concentrate, decreased motor activity)**
   0 = Normal speech and thought
   1 = Slight retardation during the interview
   2 = Obvious retardation during the interview
   3 = Interview difficult
   4 = Complete stupor

9. **Agitation**
   0 = None
   1 = Fidgetiness
   2 = Playing with hands, hair, etc.
   3 = Moving about, can't sit still
   4 = Hand wringing, nail biting, hair pulling, biting of lips

10. **Anxiety (Psychic)**
    0 = No difficulty
    1 = Subjective tension and irritability
    2 = Worrying about minor matters
    3 = Apprehensive attitude apparent in face or speech
    4 = Fears expressed without questioning

11. **Anxiety (Somatic):** Physiological concomitants of anxiety (e.g., dry mouth, indigestion, diarrhea, cramps, belching, palpitations, headache, tremor, hyperventilation, sighing, urinary frequency, sweating, flushing)
    0 = Absent
    1 = Mild
    2 = Moderate
    3 = Severe
    4 = Incapacitating

12. **Somatic Symptoms (Gastrointestinal)**
    0 = None
    1 = Loss of appetite, but eating without encouragement. Heavy feelings in abdomen
    2 = Difficulty eating without urging from others. Requests or requires medication for constipation or gastrointestinal symptoms

13. **Somatic Symptoms (General)**
    0 = None
    1 = Heaviness in limbs, back, or head. Backaches, headache, muscle aches. Loss of energy and fatigability
    2 = Any clear-cut symptom rates 2

BOX 25–4 Hamilton Depression Rating Scale (HDRS)—cont'd

14. **Genital Symptoms** (e.g., loss of libido, impaired sexual performance, menstrual disturbances)

0 = Absent

1 = Mild

2 = Severe

15. **Hypochondriasis**

0 = Not present

1 = Self-absorption (bodily)

2 = Preoccupation with health

3 = Frequent complaints, requests for help, etc.

4 = Hypochondriacal delusions

16. **Loss of Weight (Rate *either* A *or* B)**

A. According to subjective patient history:

0 = No weight loss

1 = Probably weight loss associated with present illness

2 = Definite weight loss associated with present illness

B. According to objective weekly measurements:

0 = Less than 1-lb weight loss in week

1 = Greater than 1-lb weight loss in week

2 = Greater than 2-lb weight loss in week

17. **Insight**

0 = Acknowledges being depressed and ill

1 = Acknowledges illness but attributes cause to bad food, climate, overwork, virus, need for rest, etc.

2 = Denies being ill at all

SCORING:

0–6 = No evidence of depressive illness

7–17 = Mild depression

18–24 = Moderate depression

>24 = Severe depression

TOTAL SCORE _____

Hamilton, M. (1960). A rating scale for depression. Journal of Neurology, Neurosurgery, & Psychiatry, 23, 56–62. The HDRS is in the public domain.

at least 2 years (APA, 2022). Symptoms associated with this disorder include the following:

■ **Affective:** Feelings of sadness, dejection, helplessness, powerlessness, hopelessness; gloomy and pessimistic outlook; low self-esteem; difficulty experiencing pleasure in activities

■ **Behavioral:** Sluggish physical movements (i.e., psychomotor retardation); slumped posture; slowed speech; limited verbalizations, possibly consisting of ruminations about life's failures or regrets; social isolation with a focus on the self; increased use of substances possible; self-destructive behavior possible; decreased interest in personal hygiene and grooming

■ **Cognitive:** Slowed thinking processes; difficulty concentrating and directing attention; obsessive and repetitive thoughts, generally portraying pessimism and negativism; verbalizations and behavior reflecting suicidal ideation

■ **Physiological:** Anorexia or overeating; insomnia or hypersomnia; sleep disturbances; amenorrhea; decreased libido; headaches; backaches; chest pain; abdominal pain; low energy level; fatigue and listlessness.

Severe Depression

Severe depression (also called major depressive disorder) is characterized by an intensification of the symptoms described for moderate depression (see Box 25–2). Symptoms at the severe level of depression include the following:

■ **Affective:** Feelings of total despair, hopelessness, and worthlessness; flat (unchanging) affect, appearing devoid of emotional tone; prevalent feelings of nothingness and emptiness; apathy; loneliness; sadness; inability to feel pleasure

■ **Behavioral:** Psychomotor retardation so severe that physical movement may completely stop, or psychomotor behavior manifested by rapid, agitated, purposeless movements; slumped posture; sitting in a curled-up position; walking slowly and rigidly; virtually nonexistent communication (when verbalizations do occur, they may reflect delusional thinking); no personal hygiene and grooming; social isolation, with virtually no inclination toward interaction with others

■ **Cognitive:** Prevalent delusional thinking, with delusions of persecution and somatic delusions being most common; confusion, indecisiveness, and an inability to concentrate; hallucinations reflecting misinterpretations of the environment; excessive self-deprecation, self-blame, and thoughts of suicide

NOTE: Because of the low energy level and slow thought processes, the individual may be unable to follow through on suicidal ideas. However, the desire is strong at this level.

■ **Physiological:** A general slowdown of the entire body, reflected in sluggish digestion, constipation, and urinary retention; amenorrhea; impotence; diminished libido; anorexia; weight loss or weight gain associated with appetite changes; changes in sleep patterns, including difficulty falling asleep and awakening very early in the morning; feeling worse early in the morning and somewhat better as the day progresses (this may reflect the diurnal variation in the level of neurotransmitters that affect mood and activity); pain syndromes

Diagnosis and Outcome Identification

Using information collected during the assessment, the nurse completes the patient database from which the selection of appropriate nursing diagnoses is determined. Table 25–1 presents a list of patient behaviors and the NANDA-I nursing diagnoses (Herdman et al., 2021) that correspond to those behaviors, which may be used in planning care for the depressed patient.

Outcome Criteria

The following criteria may be used for measurement of outcomes in the care of the depressed patient.

The patient:

- Has experienced no physical harm to self
- Discusses feelings with staff and family members
- Expresses hopefulness
- Sets realistic goals for self
- Is no longer afraid to attempt new activities
- Is able to identify aspects of self-control over life situation
- Expresses personal satisfaction and support from spiritual practices
- Interacts willingly and appropriately with others
- Is able to maintain reality orientation
- Is able to concentrate, reason, solve problems, and make decisions
- Eats a well-balanced diet with snacks, to prevent weight loss and maintain nutritional status
- Sleeps 6 to 8 hours per night and reports feeling well rested
- Bathes, washes and combs hair, and dresses in clean clothing without assistance

Planning and Implementation

The following section presents a group of selected nursing diagnoses, with short- and long-term goals and nursing interventions for each.

Some institutions use a case management model to coordinate care (see Chapter 8, "The Nursing

TABLE 25–1 Assigning Nursing Diagnoses to Behaviors Commonly Associated with Depression	
BEHAVIORS	**NURSING DIAGNOSES**
Depressed mood; feelings of hopelessness and worthlessness; anger turned inward in the self; misinterpretations of reality; suicidal ideation, plan, and available means	Risk for suicidal behavior
Depression, preoccupation with thoughts of loss, self-blame, grief avoidance, inappropriate expression of anger, decreased functioning in life roles	Maladaptive grieving
Expressions of helplessness, uselessness, guilt, and shame; hypersensitivity to slight or criticism; negative, pessimistic outlook; lack of eye contact; self-negating verbalizations	Low self-esteem
Apathy, verbal expressions of having no control, dependence on others to fulfill needs	Powerlessness
Expresses anger toward God, expresses lack of meaning in life, sudden changes in spiritual practices, refuses interactions with significant others or with spiritual leaders	Spiritual distress
Withdrawn, uncommunicative, seeks to be alone, dysfunctional interaction with others, discomfort in social situations	Social isolation/Impaired social interaction
Inappropriate thinking, confusion, difficulty concentrating, impaired problem-solving ability, inaccurate interpretation of environment, memory deficit	Disturbed thought processes
Weight loss, poor muscle tone, pale conjunctiva and mucous membranes, poor skin turgor, weakness	Imbalanced nutrition: Less than body requirements
Difficulty falling asleep, difficulty staying asleep, lack of energy, difficulty concentrating, verbal reports of not feeling well rested	Insomnia
Uncombed hair, disheveled clothing, offensive body odor	Self-care deficit (hygiene, grooming)

Process in Psychiatric-Mental Health Nursing," for more detailed explanation). In case management models, the plan of care may take the form of a critical pathway.

Risk for Suicidal Behavior

Risk for suicidal behavior is defined as "susceptible to self-injurious acts associated with some intent to die" (Herdman et al., 2021, p. 523). For additional information on interventions for this diagnosis see Chapter 16, "Suicide Prevention."

Patient Goals

Outcome criteria include short- and long-term goals. Timelines are individually determined.

Short-term goals

- Patient will seek out staff when feeling an urge to harm self.
- Patient will not harm self.

Long-term goal

- Patient will not harm self.

Interventions

- Create a safe environment for the patient. Remove all potentially harmful objects from patient's access (sharp objects, straps, belts, ties, glass items, alcohol). Supervise closely during meals and medication administration. Perform room searches as deemed necessary.

> **CLINICAL PEARL** Ask the patient directly, "Have you thought about killing yourself?" or "Have you thought about harming yourself in any way?" "If so, what do you plan to do? Do you have the means to carry out this plan?" "How strong are your intentions to die?" The risk of suicide is greatly increased if the patient has developed a plan, has strong intentions, and especially if means exist for the patient to execute the plan.

- Assess frequently for the presence and lethality risk of suicidal ideation. The intensity of suicide ideation can change over hours or days, so it is important to assess subjective and objective data to evaluate current risk. Discussion of suicidal feelings with a trusted individual provides some relief to the patient.
- Convey an attitude of unconditional acceptance of the patient as a worthwhile individual.
- Encourage the patient to actively participate in establishing a safety plan. (See Chapter 16, "Suicide Prevention," for guidelines on establishing safety plans.) Suicidal patients are often ambivalent about their feelings. Discussion of strategies for maintaining safety with a trusted individual may provide assistance before the patient experiences a crisis.

> **CLINICAL PEARL** Be direct. Talk openly and matter-of-factly about suicide. Listen actively and encourage expression of feelings, including anger. Accept the patient's feelings in a nonjudgmental manner.

- Maintain close observation of the patient. Depending on the level of suicide precaution, provide one-to-one contact, constant visual observation, or checks at least every 15 minutes conducted at irregular intervals. Place the patient in a room close to the nurse's station; do not assign to a private room. Accompany the patient to off-ward activities if attendance is indicated and, if necessary, to the bathroom. Close observation is necessary to ensure that the patient does not harm self in any way. Being alert for suicidal and escape attempts facilitates being able to prevent or interrupt harmful behavior.
- Maintain special care in administering medications to prevent the patient from saving up to overdose or discarding and not taking.
- Make rounds at frequent, *irregular* intervals (especially at night, toward early morning, at change of shift, or other predictably busy times for staff). Irregular patient checks prevent staff surveillance from becoming predictable. Awareness of patient's location is important, especially when staff is busy, unavailable, or less observable.
- Encourage verbalizations of honest feelings. Through exploration and discussion, help the patient identify symbols of hope in their life.
- Encourage the patient to express angry feelings within appropriate limits. Provide a safe method of hostility release. Help the patient identify the true source of anger and work on adaptive coping skills for use outside the treatment setting. Depression and suicidal behaviors may be viewed as anger turned inward on the self. If this anger can be verbalized in a nonthreatening environment, the patient may be able to eventually resolve these feelings.
- Identify community resources that the patient may use as a support system and from whom they may request help if feeling suicidal once discharged from the hospital. Having a concrete plan for seeking assistance during a crisis may discourage or prevent self-destructive behaviors.
- Orient the patient to reality, as required. Point out sensory misperceptions or misinterpretations of the environment. Take care not to belittle the patient's fears or indicate disapproval of verbal expressions.
- Most important, spend time with patient. Spending time provides a feeling of safety and security while also conveying the message, "I want to spend time with you because I think you are a worthwhile person."

Maladaptive Grieving

Maladaptive grieving is defined as "a disorder that occurs after the death of a significant other [or any other loss of significance to the individual], in which the experience of distress accompanying bereavement fails to follow sociocultural expectations" (Herdman et al., 2021, p. 421). Table 25–2 presents this nursing diagnosis in care plan format.

Patient Goals

Outcome criteria include short- and long-term goals. Timelines are individually determined.

Short-term goals

■ Patient will express anger about the loss.
■ Patient will identify coping strategies and rational thought patterns in response to loss.

Long-term goal

■ Patient will be able to recognize their own position in the grief process while progressing at own pace toward resolution.

Interventions

■ Determine the stage of grief in which the patient is fixed. Identify behaviors associated with this stage. It is important to obtain accurate baseline assessment data to effectively plan care for the grieving patient.
■ Develop a trusting relationship. Show empathy, concern, and unconditional positive regard. Be honest and keep all promises. Convey an accepting attitude and encourage the patient to express feelings openly.
■ Encourage the patient to express anger within appropriate limits. Do not become defensive if the

---

Table 25–2 | CARE PLAN FOR THE DEPRESSED PATIENT

NURSING DIAGNOSIS: MALADAPTIVE GRIEVING

RELATED TO: Real or perceived loss, bereavement overload

EVIDENCED BY: Denial of loss, inappropriate expression of anger, idealization of or obsession with lost object, inability to carry out activities of daily living

OUTCOME CRITERIA	NURSING INTERVENTIONS	RATIONALE
Short-Term Goals: ■ Patient expresses anger about the loss. ■ Patient verbalizes behaviors associated with normal grieving. **Long-Term Goal:** ■ Patient is able to recognize their own position in the grief process while progressing at own pace toward resolution.	1. Determine the stage of grief in which the patient is fixed. Identify behaviors associated with this stage.	1. Accurate baseline assessment data are necessary to effectively plan care for the grieving patient.
	2. Develop a trusting relationship with the patient. Show empathy, concern, and unconditional positive regard. Be honest and keep all promises.	2. Trust is the basis for a therapeutic relationship.
	3. Convey an accepting attitude, and enable the patient to express feelings openly.	3. An accepting attitude conveys to patient that you believe they are a worthwhile person. Trust is enhanced.
	4. Encourage the patient to express anger. Do not become defensive if the initial expression of anger is displaced on the nurse or therapist. Help the patient explore angry feelings so that they may be directed toward the actual intended person or situation.	4. Verbalization of feelings in a nonthreatening environment may help the patient come to terms with unresolved issues.
	5. Help the patient to discharge pent-up anger through participation in large motor activities (e.g., brisk walks, jogging, physical exercises, volleyball, exercise bike).	5. Physical exercise provides a safe and effective method for discharging pent-up tension.

Table 25–2 | CARE PLAN FOR THE DEPRESSED PATIENT—cont'd

OUTCOME CRITERIA	NURSING INTERVENTIONS	RATIONALE
	6. Teach the normal stages of grief and behaviors associated with each stage. Help the patient to understand that feelings such as guilt and anger toward the lost concept are appropriate and acceptable during the grief process and should be expressed rather than held inside.	6. Knowledge of acceptability of the feelings associated with normal grieving may help to relieve some of the guilt that these responses generate.
	7. Encourage the patient to review the relationship with the lost concept. With support and sensitivity, point out the reality of the situation in areas where misrepresentations are expressed.	7. Patients must give up an idealized perception and be able to accept both positive and negative aspects about the lost concept before the grief process is complete.
	8. Communicate to the patient that crying is acceptable. Use of touch may also be therapeutic.	8. Some cultures believe it is important to remain stoic and refrain from crying openly. Individuals from certain cultures are uncomfortable with touch. It is important to be aware of cultural influences before employing these interventions.
	9. Encourage the patient to reach out for spiritual support during this time in whatever form is desirable to them. Assess spiritual needs of the patient, and assist as necessary in the fulfillment of those needs.	9. Patients may find comfort in religious rituals with which they are familiar.

initial expression of anger is displaced on the nurse or therapist. Help the patient explore angry feelings so that the feelings may be directed toward the actual intended person or situation.

■ Help the patient to discharge pent-up anger through participation in large motor activities (e.g., brisk walks, jogging, physical exercises, volleyball, exercise bike). Physical exercise provides a safe and effective method for discharging pent-up tension.

■ Teach the stages of grief and behaviors associated with each stage. Help the patient understand that feelings such as guilt and anger toward the lost concept/entity are appropriate and acceptable during the grief process and should be expressed rather than held inside. Knowledge of acceptability of the feelings associated with grieving may

help relieve some of the guilt that these responses generate.

■ Encourage the patient to review the relationship with the lost concept/entity. With support and sensitivity, point out the reality of the situation in areas where misrepresentations are expressed. The patient must give up an idealized perception and be able to accept both positive and negative aspects about the lost concept/entity before the grief process is complete.

■ Communicate to the patient that crying is acceptable by verbal reassurance and, in some cases, with caring touch. Use of touch must also consider cultural influences and trauma history before including this as part of the intervention.

■ Assist the patient in problem-solving as they attempt to determine methods for more adaptive coping with the experienced loss. Provide positive feedback for strategies identified and decisions made.

■ Encourage the patient to reach out for spiritual support during this time in whatever form is desirable to them. Assess spiritual needs of the patient and assist as necessary in the fulfillment of those needs. (See Chapter 11, "Psychosocial Interventions and Spiritual Care," for more information about spiritual assessment and interventions.)

■ Encourage the patient to attend a support group of individuals who are experiencing life situations similar to their own and assist the patient to locate a group of this type.

Low Self-Esteem/Self-Care Deficit

Low self-esteem is defined as "negative perception of self-worth, self-acceptance, self-respect, competence, and attitude toward self" either long-standing or in response to a current situation (Herdman et al., 2021, pp. 348–353). *Self-care deficit* is defined as "inability to independently complete [activities of daily living (ADLs)]" (Herdman et al., 2021, pp. 317–319).

Patient Goals

Short-term goals

■ Patient will verbalize attributes they like about themselves.

■ Patient will participate in activities of daily living (ADLs) with assistance from health-care provider.

Long-term goals

■ By time of discharge from treatment, the patient will exhibit increased feelings of self-worth as evidenced by verbal expression of positive aspects of self, past accomplishments, and future prospects.

■ By time of discharge from treatment, the patient will exhibit increased feelings of self-worth by setting realistic goals and trying to reach them, thereby demonstrating a decrease in fear of failure.

■ By time of discharge from treatment, the patient will satisfactorily accomplish ADLs independently.

Interventions

■ Be accepting of the patient and spend time with them even though pessimism and negativism may seem objectionable. Focus on strengths and accomplishments and minimize failures.

■ Promote attendance in therapy groups that offer the patient simple methods of accomplishment. Encourage the patient to be as independent as possible.

■ Encourage the patient to recognize areas of change and provide assistance toward this effort.

■ Teach assertiveness techniques: the ability to recognize the differences among passive, assertive, and aggressive behaviors and the importance of respecting the human rights of others while protecting one's own basic human rights. Self-esteem is enhanced by the ability to interact with others in an assertive manner. (See Chapter 13, "Assertiveness Training" and Chapter 14, "Promoting Self-Esteem."

■ Teach effective communication skills, such as "I" messages, as a means to avoid making judgmental statements.

■ Encourage independence in the performance of ADLs but intervene when the patient is unable to perform them.

> **CLINICAL PEARL** Offer recognition and positive reinforcement for independent accomplishments. (Example: "Mrs. J., I see you have put on a clean dress and combed your hair.")

■ Show the patient how to perform activities with which they are having difficulty. When a patient is depressed, they may require simple, concrete demonstrations of activities that would be performed without difficulty under normal conditions.

■ Keep strict records of food and fluid intake. Offer nutritious snacks and fluids between meals. The patient may be unable to tolerate large amounts of food at mealtimes and may therefore require additional nourishment at other times during the day to receive adequate nutrition.

■ Before bedtime, provide nursing measures that promote sleep, such as back rub; warm bath; warm, nonstimulating drinks; soft music; and relaxation exercises.

Powerlessness

Powerlessness is defined as "A state of actual or perceived loss of control or influence over factors or events that affect one's well-being, personal life, or the society (adapted from American Psychology Association)" (Herdman et al., 2021, p. 426).

Patient Goals

Short-term goal

■ Patient will participate in decision making regarding own care within 5 days.

Long-term goal

■ Patient will be able to effectively problem solve ways to take control of their life situation by time of discharge from treatment, thereby decreasing feelings of powerlessness.

Interventions

- Encourage the patient to take as much responsibility as possible for their own self-care practices. In the most acute stage of severe depression, patients may have extreme difficulty making decisions. At this point, it may be more helpful to use *active communication* to help the patient accomplish even basic ADLs. For example, "It's time to eat lunch," rather than, "Would you like to eat lunch now?" Ongoing assessment is important so that the patient can be encouraged to make choices as soon as possible. Providing the patient with choices whenever possible will increase feelings of control. For example,
  - Include the patient in setting the goals of care they wish to achieve.
  - Allow the patient to establish their own schedule for self-care activities.
  - Provide the patient with privacy as need is determined.
  - Provide positive feedback for decisions made. Respect the patient's right to make those decisions independently, and refrain from attempting to influence them toward those that may seem more logical.
- Help the patient set realistic goals. Unrealistic goals set the patient up for failure and reinforce feelings of powerlessness.
- Help the patient identify areas of their life situation that can be controlled. The patient's emotional condition interferes with their ability to solve problems. Assistance is required to perceive the benefits and consequences of available alternatives accurately.
- Discuss with the patient areas of life that are not within their ability to control. Encourage verbalization of feelings related to this inability to deal with unresolved issues and accept what cannot be changed.

Concept Care Mapping

The concept map care plan is an approach to planning and organizing nursing care (see Chapter 8, "The Nursing Process in Psychiatric-Mental Health Nursing") that allows visualization of interrelationships between medical diagnoses, nursing diagnoses, assessment data, and treatments. An example of a concept map care plan for a patient with depression is presented in Figure 25–4.

Patient and Family Education

The role of patient teacher is important in the psychiatric area, as it is in all areas of nursing. A list of topics for patient and family education relevant to depression is presented in Box 25–5.

Evaluation of Care for the Depressed Patient

In the final step of the nursing process, a reassessment is conducted to determine whether the nursing actions have been successful in achieving the objectives of care. Evaluation of the nursing actions for the depressed patient may be facilitated by gathering information using the following types of questions:

- Has self-harm to the individual been avoided?
- Have suicidal ideations subsided?
- Does the individual know where to seek assistance outside the hospital when suicidal thoughts occur?
- Has the patient discussed the recent loss with staff and family members?
- Is the patient able to verbalize feelings and behaviors associated with each stage of the grieving process and recognize their position in the process?
- Has obsession with and idealization of the lost object subsided?
- Is anger toward the lost object expressed appropriately?
- Does the patient set realistic goals for self?
- Is the patient able to verbalize positive aspects about self, past accomplishments, and future prospects, including a desire to live?
- Can the patient identify areas of their life situation over which they have control?
- Is the patient able to participate in usual religious practices and feel satisfaction and support from them?
- Is the patient seeking interaction with others in an appropriate manner?
- Does the patient maintain reality orientation with no evidence of delusional thinking?
- Is the patient able to concentrate and make decisions concerning own self-care?
- Is the patient selecting and consuming foods sufficiently high in nutrients and calories to maintain weight and nutritional status?
- Does the patient sleep without difficulty and wake feeling rested?
- Does the patient attend to personal hygiene and grooming?
- Have somatic complaints subsided?

Quality and Safety Education for Nurses (QSEN)

Health Professions Education: A Bridge to Quality (Institute of Medicine, 2003; now the National Academy of Medicine) challenged faculties of medicine,

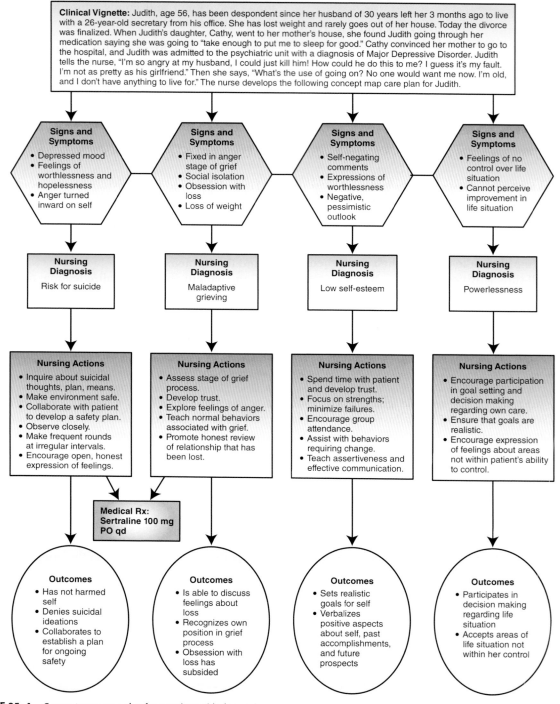

Clinical Vignette: Judith, age 56, has been despondent since her husband of 30 years left her 3 months ago to live with a 26-year-old secretary from his office. She has lost weight and rarely goes out of her house. Today the divorce was finalized. When Judith's daughter, Cathy, went to her mother's house, she found Judith going through her medication saying she was going to "take enough to put me to sleep for good." Cathy convinced her mother to go to the hospital, and Judith was admitted to the psychiatric unit with a diagnosis of Major Depressive Disorder. Judith tells the nurse, "I'm so angry at my husband, I could just kill him! How could he do this to me? I guess it's my fault. I'm not as pretty as his girlfriend." Then she says, "What's the use of going on? No one would want me now. I'm old, and I don't have anything to live for." The nurse develops the following concept map care plan for Judith.

Signs and Symptoms
- Depressed mood
- Feelings of worthlessness and hopelessness
- Anger turned inward on self

Signs and Symptoms
- Fixed in anger stage of grief
- Social isolation
- Obsession with loss
- Loss of weight

Signs and Symptoms
- Self-negating comments
- Expressions of worthlessness
- Negative, pessimistic outlook

Signs and Symptoms
- Feelings of no control over life situation
- Cannot perceive improvement in life situation

Nursing Diagnosis

Risk for suicide

Nursing Diagnosis

Maladaptive grieving

Nursing Diagnosis

Low self-esteem

Nursing Diagnosis

Powerlessness

Nursing Actions
- Inquire about suicidal thoughts, plan, means.
- Make environment safe.
- Collaborate with patient to develop a safety plan.
- Observe closely.
- Make frequent rounds at irregular intervals.
- Encourage open, honest expression of feelings.

Nursing Actions
- Assess stage of grief process.
- Develop trust.
- Explore feelings of anger.
- Teach normal behaviors associated with grief.
- Promote honest review of relationship that has been lost.

Nursing Actions
- Spend time with patient and develop trust.
- Focus on strengths; minimize failures.
- Encourage group attendance.
- Assist with behaviors requiring change.
- Teach assertiveness and effective communication.

Nursing Actions
- Encourage participation in goal setting and decision making regarding own care.
- Ensure that goals are realistic.
- Encourage expression of feelings about areas not within patient's ability to control.

Medical Rx: Sertraline 100 mg PO qd

Outcomes
- Has not harmed self
- Denies suicidal ideations
- Collaborates to establish a plan for ongoing safety

Outcomes
- Is able to discuss feelings about loss
- Recognizes own position in grief process
- Obsession with loss has subsided

Outcomes
- Sets realistic goals for self
- Verbalizes positive aspects about self, past accomplishments, and future prospects

Outcomes
- Participates in decision making regarding life situation
- Accepts areas of life situation not within her control

FIGURE 25–4 Concept map care plan for a patient with depression.

nursing, and other health professions to ensure that their graduates have achieved a core set of competencies to meet the needs of the 21st-century health-care system. These competencies include *providing patient-centered care, working in interdisciplinary teams, maintaining safety, employing evidence-based practice, applying quality improvement,* and *utilizing informatics.*

 Safety is a key issue when caring for the patient with depression. The risk for suicide is high in this population and thorough assessment of risks and warning signs should be conducted for all individuals presenting with depression. In addition, the self-care deficits that are common in this population place the patient at risk for injury. Close or continuous monitoring may be necessary.

BOX 25–5 Topics for Patient and Family Education Related to Depression

NATURE OF THE ILLNESS
1. Stages of grief and symptoms associated with each stage
2. What is depression?
3. Why do people get depressed?
4. What are the symptoms of depression?

MANAGEMENT OF THE ILLNESS
1. Medication management
   a. Nuisance side effects
   b. Side effects to report to physician
   c. Importance of taking medications regularly
   d. Length of time to take effect
   e. Diet (related to monoamine oxidase inhibitors)
2. Assertiveness techniques
3. Stress-management techniques
4. Ways to increase self-esteem
5. Electroconvulsive therapy

SUPPORT SERVICES
1. Suicide hotline
2. Support groups
3. Legal and/or financial assistance

Real Nurses, Real Advice

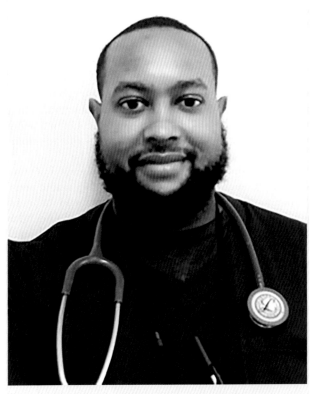

"The anhedonia, psychomotor retardation, and anergia in acute depression can make assessment a challenge. It's important to offer hope to a client who may be uncertain about how to navigate their present state of deep depression and to remain diligent while not making the patient feel pressured to speak. Paraphrasing what the patient has said to you conveys understanding and provides validation. Open-ended questions encourage the patient to elaborate rather than just answer 'yes' or 'no.'"

—Larry Johnson, RN

Treatment Modalities for Depression

Individual Psychotherapy

Research has documented both the importance of close and satisfactory attachments in the prevention of depression and the role of disrupted attachments in the development of depression (Teo et al., 2013). With this concept in mind, interpersonal psychotherapy focuses on the client's current interpersonal relations. Interpersonal psychotherapy with the depressed person proceeds through three phases and interventions.

Phase I

During the first phase, the client is assessed to determine the extent of the illness, education about depression is provided, and a therapeutic contract is negotiated

Phase II

Treatment at this phase focuses on helping the client resolve maladaptive grief reactions. This may include resolving the ambivalence with a lost relationship and assistance with establishing new relationships. Other areas of treatment focus may include interpersonal disputes between the client and a significant other, difficult role transitions at various developmental life cycles, and correction of interpersonal deficits that may interfere with the client's ability to initiate or sustain interpersonal relationships.

Phase III

During the final phase of interpersonal psychotherapy, the therapeutic alliance is terminated. The expected outcome is that through reassurance, clarification of emotional states, improvement of interpersonal communication, testing of perceptions, and performance in interpersonal settings, the individual with depression has improved relationship skills and social functioning.

Group Therapy

Group therapy forms an important dimension of multimodal treatment for the depressed client. Once an acute phase of the illness has passed, groups can provide an atmosphere in which individuals may discuss issues in their lives that cause, maintain, or arise from having a serious affective disorder. The element of peer support provides a feeling of security, as troublesome or embarrassing issues are discussed and resolved. Some groups have other specific purposes, such as helping to monitor medication-related issues or serving as an avenue for promoting education related to the affective disorder and its treatment. Therapy groups help members gain a sense of perspective on their condition and encourage them to link up with others who have common problems. A sense of hope is conveyed when the individual is able to see that they are not alone or unique in experiencing affective illness.

Self-help groups offer another avenue of support for the depressed client. These groups are usually peer-led and are not meant to substitute for or compete with professional therapy. Rather, they offer supplementary support that frequently enhances compliance with the medical regimen. Examples of self-help groups are the Depression and Bipolar Support Alliance (DBSA), Depressives Anonymous, Recovery International, and GriefShare (grief recovery support groups). Although self-help groups are not psychotherapy groups, they do provide important adjunctive support experiences, which often have therapeutic benefit for participants.

Family Therapy

The ultimate objectives in working with families of clients with mood disorders are to resolve the symptoms and initiate or restore adaptive family functioning. Similar to group therapy, the most effective approach appears to be a combination of psychotherapeutic and pharmacotherapeutic treatments. Boland and Verduin (2022) stated that family therapy is indicated:

> if the disorder jeopardizes the patient's marriage or family functioning or if the mood disorder is promoted or maintained by the family situation. Family therapy examines the role of the mood-disordered member in the overall psychological well-being of the whole family; it also examines the role of the entire family in the maintenance of the patient's symptoms. (p. 393)

Cognitive Behavior Therapy

In CBT, the individual is taught to control thought distortions that are a factor in the development and maintenance of mood disorders. In the cognitive model, depression is characterized by a triad of negative distortions related to expectations of the environment, self, and future. The environment and activities within it are viewed as unsatisfying, the self is unrealistically devalued, and the future is perceived as hopeless.

The general goals in CBT are to obtain symptom relief as quickly as possible, assist the client in identifying dysfunctional patterns of thinking and behaving, and guide the client to evidence and logic that effectively tests the validity of the dysfunctional thinking (see Chapter 18, "Cognitive Behavior Therapy"). Therapy focuses on changing "automatic thoughts" that occur spontaneously and contribute to the distorted affect. Following are examples of automatic thoughts that may be common cognitive distortions in depression:

- **Personalizing:** "I'm the only one who failed."
- **All or nothing:** "I'm a complete failure."
- **Mind reading:** "He thinks I'm foolish."
- **Discounting positives:** "The other questions were so easy. Any dummy could have gotten them right."

The client is asked to describe evidence that both supports and disputes the automatic thought. The logic underlying the inferences is then reviewed with the client. Another technique involves evaluating what would most likely happen if the client's automatic thoughts were true. Implications of the consequences are then discussed.

Clients should not become discouraged if one technique seems not to be working. No single technique works with all clients. They should be reassured that many techniques may be used, and both therapist and client may explore these possibilities.

CBT has offered encouraging results in the treatment of depression. The results of several studies with depressed clients show that in some cases CBT is equally or more effective than antidepressant medication (Amick et al., 2015; Gautam et al., 2020; Grosse Holtforth et al., 2019).

Electroconvulsive Therapy

ECT is the induction of a grand mal (generalized) seizure through the application of electrical current to the brain. ECT is effective with clients who are acutely suicidal and in the treatment of severe depression, particularly in those clients who are also experiencing psychotic symptoms and those with psychomotor retardation and neurovegetative changes, such as disturbances in sleep, appetite, and energy. It is typically considered for treatment only after trials of therapy with antidepressant medication have proven ineffective (see Chapter 19, "Electroconvulsive Therapy," for a detailed discussion of ECT).

Repetitive Transcranial Magnetic Stimulation

Repetitive transcranial magnetic stimulation (rTMS) is a procedure that is used to treat depression by stimulating nerve cells in the brain. This procedure uses very short pulses of magnetic energy to stimulate nerve cells at localized areas in the cerebral cortex, similar to the electrical activity observed with ECT. However, unlike with ECT, the electrical waves generated by rTMS do not result in generalized seizure activity (George et al., 2013). The waves are passed through a coil placed on the scalp to areas of the brain involved in mood regulation. It is noninvasive and considered generally safe. High-frequency waves are used to stimulate the left prefrontal cortex, and low-frequency waves are used to stimulate the right prefrontal cortex. This combination has been shown most effective in treating depression (Sharma et al., 2018). A typical course of treatment consists of 40-minute sessions, three to five times a week for 4 to 6 weeks (Raposelli, 2015). In rare instances, seizures have been triggered with the use of rTMS therapy, particularly with high-frequency rTMS, but more common adverse effects include tinnitus, headache, or facial twitching (Sharma et al., 2018).

Gaynes and associates (2014) conducted a meta-analysis demonstrating that rTMS had a remission rate of 30%. Effectiveness ratings for ECT have varied from 17% to 70%. Although the effectiveness ratings may seem small or highly variable, both treatments provide an option for patients who are otherwise treatment-resistant. Magnezi and associates (2016) compared ECT to rTMS and found that although ECT was more effective than rTMS and additionally relieved anxiety symptoms, ECT had a much higher incidence (60%) of adverse effects, mostly related to memory loss. From the client's perspective, rTMS was still deemed preferable to ECT (if it was covered by insurance), which may be related to the stigma associated with ECT. George and associates (2013) stated:

> Since FDA approval, TMS has been generally safe and well tolerated with a low incidence of treatment discontinuation, and the therapeutic effects once obtained appear at least as durable as other antidepressant treatments. TMS also shows promise in several other psychiatric disorders, particularly treating acute and chronic pain. (p. 17)

More recently, researchers compared rTMS to pharmacotherapy and found both to be effective but identified rTMS as more cost-effective (Raposelli, 2015). Currently, not all insurance companies cover this treatment, so from the client's standpoint, it may be a more expensive alternative. Raposelli reported that up to 40% of clients with MDD do not respond to pharmacotherapy; therefore alternatives such as ECT and TMS may offer hope of recovery for treatment-resistant conditions.

Vagus Nerve Stimulation and Deep Brain Stimulation

During studies for the treatment of epilepsy, vagus nerve stimulation (VNS) was found to improve mood. This treatment involves implanting an electronic device in the skin to stimulate the vagus nerve. Chronic stimulation of these nerve fibers changes activity in the brainstem nuclei that alters serotonin activity and has anticonvulsant effects (Boland & Verduin, 2022). Positron emission tomography studies performed during treatment demonstrate metabolic changes in areas of the brain associated with mood disorders (Sharma et al., 2018), including the amygdala, hippocampus, and cingulate gyrus. Response rates vary from 13% to 40%, with remission rates around 13%. Success rates are lower than those for ECT (Boland & Verduin, 2022), but it provides an alternative for those individuals who have not responded to less invasive treatments.

A novel approach is deep brain stimulation (DBS), which is a form of psychosurgery. In this procedure, as in VNS, an electrode is implanted with the intent of stimulating brain function. The implant is deeper than that used in VNS and requires a craniotomy. DBS has been well studied to determine its safety and effectiveness for other conditions, and controlled trials are ongoing. The procedure is reversible, and stimulation levels can easily be adjusted (Sharma et al., 2018). There is no consensus on the best area of the brain for implantation, but studies have reported improvement regardless of the site of electrode placement (Sharma et al., 2018). Berlim and associates (2014) conducted a systematic review of several studies using DBS and determined a response rate of approximately 40% and a remission rate of approximately 26%. Currently, DBS is reserved for clients with severe, incapacitating depression or obsessive-compulsive disorder who have not responded to any more conservative treatments.

Bright Light Therapy

The prevalence of depression with a seasonal pattern is reported to be up to 10% but varies on the basis of geographic location (Kurlansik & Ibay, 2013). The *DSM-5-TR* identifies this disorder as Major Depressive Disorder, Recurrent, With Seasonal Pattern. It has commonly been known as SAD.

One theory suggests that SAD is related to fluctuations in levels of the hormone melatonin (Cotterell, 2010), which is produced by the pineal gland. Melatonin plays a role in the regulation of biological rhythms for sleep and activation. It is produced during the cycle of darkness, and its production ceases during daylight hours. During the months of longer darkness hours, production of melatonin increases, which seems to trigger the symptoms of SAD in susceptible people. Other research has pointed to seasonal serotonin transporter fluctuations associated with variation in exposure to daylight (McMahon et al., 2016).

Bright light therapy, or exposure to light, has been shown in several studies to be an effective short-term treatment for SAD (Campbell et al., 2017; Pjrek et al., 2020; Maruani & Geoffroy, 2019). The light therapy is administered by a 10,000-lux light box, which contains white fluorescent light tubes covered with a plastic screen that blocks ultraviolet rays. The individual sits in front of the box with eyes open (although one should not look directly into the light). Therapy usually begins with 10- to 15-minute sessions and gradually progresses to 30 to 45 minutes. The mechanism of action is believed to be related to retinal stimulation, which triggers a reduction of melatonin and an increase in serotonin in the brain (Rodriguez, 2015). Studies have demonstrated benefits of bright light therapy in nonseasonal affective disorders as well (Cunningham et al., 2019; Lam et al., 2015; Maruani & Geoffroy, 2019; Sikkens et al., 2019). Some people notice improvement rapidly, within a few days, whereas others may take several weeks to feel better. Side effects appear to be dosage related and include headache, eyestrain, nausea, irritability, photophobia (eye sensitivity to light), or insomnia (when light therapy is used late in the day), and (rarely) hypomania, but these effects are usually mild and short-lived (Kurlansik & Ibay, 2013).

Light therapy and antidepressants have shown comparable efficacy in studies of SAD treatment. One study compared the efficacy of light therapy to daily treatment with 20 mg of fluoxetine (Lam et al., 2015). The authors concluded that bright light therapy alone and in combination were efficacious in the treatment MDD. Sikkens and associates (2019), noting that depression is often accompanied by sleep disorders, used bright light therapy to reset the study subjects' circadian rhythm. The individuals were maintained on antidepressant medication as well, and overall response was around 35%. Although improvement is often noted within 2 weeks, most people relapse in the short term. Therefore, treatment should be continued until an expected time of spontaneous remission, such as the change in

season to spring or summer (Kurlansik & Ibay, 2013). More recent studies have demonstrated that CBT is as effective as light therapy with the added benefit of preventing recurrences over time (Rohan et al., 2016).

Physical Exercise

Physical exercise has long been recognized as beneficial in reducing symptoms of depression. Al-Qahtania and associates (2018), while recognizing that antidepressant therapy is considered first-line treatment, conducted a narrative review and reported on the evidence base and the underlying mechanisms supporting physical exercise as an important treatment strategy. There were 112 studies cited that consistently demonstrated that physical exercise had a positive effect of reducing symptoms of depression. Some studies focused on the effect of exercise in increasing availability of neurotransmitters and consistently demonstrated positive effects. Other studies focused on the strongly supported evidence of inflammation as a contributory factor in depression; these studies demonstrated that aerobic exercise decreased the proinflammatory factors that are associated with depression. Studies on the role of cortisol found that although acute exercise may increase cortisol levels, regular exercise demonstrated neuroprotective effects by promoting neuroplasticity, thereby improving cognition, ability to cope with stress, and a reduction in symptoms of depression. Additional evidence supported the benefits of exercise on stimulating the endocannabinoid system and growth factor secretion, two mechanisms associated with antidepressant effects.

Psychopharmacology

Antidepressant medication is generally considered first-line treatment for severe clinical depression and is used in the treatment of other depressive disorders. These include tricyclics, tetracyclics, monoamine oxidase inhibitors (MAOIs), SSRIs, SNRIs, and SSRI/SNRI combination drugs. Examples of commonly used antidepressant medications are presented in Table 25–3. A detailed description of these medications can be found in Chapter 4, "Psychopharmacology." In addition to the side effects and safety issues addressed in Chapter 4, it is important to highlight that antidepressant medication can be lethal in overdose. Depressed, suicidal patients must be observed closely and suicide risk assessed frequently in the use of this treatment modality.

Atypical antipsychotics have been advanced as an add-on treatment for patients who are not responding to antidepressant medication. Antipsychotics carry

TABLE 25–3 Selected Medications Used in the Treatment of Depression

CHEMICAL CLASS	GENERIC (TRADE) NAME	DAILY ADULT DOSAGE RANGE (mg)
TRICYCLICS	Amitriptyline	50–300
	Amoxapine	50–300
	Clomipramine (Anafranil)	25–250
	Desipramine (Norpramin)	25–300
	Doxepin	25–300
	Imipramine (Tofranil)	30–300
	Nortriptyline (Aventyl; Pamelor)	30–100
	Protriptyline (Vivactil)	15–60
	Trimipramine (Surmontil)	50–300
SELECTIVE SEROTONIN REUPTAKE INHIBITORS (SSRIs)	Citalopram (Celexa)	20–40
	Escitalopram (Lexapro)	10–20
	Fluoxetine (Prozac; Serafem)	20–80
	Fluvoxamine (Luvox)	50–300
	Paroxetine (Paxil)	10–50 (CR: 12.5–75)
	Sertraline (Zoloft)	25–200
	Vilazodone (Viibryd) (also acts as a partial serotonergic agonist)	40
	Vortioxetine (Brintellix)	10–20
MONOAMINE OXIDASE INHIBITORS	Isocarboxazid (Marplan)	20–60
	Phenelzine (Nardil)	45–90
	Tranylcypromine (Parnate)	30–60
	Selegiline Transdermal System (Emsam)	6/24 hr–12/24 hr patch
ATYPICAL ANTIDEPRESSANTS	Bupropion (Wellbutrin)	200–450
	Mirtazapine (Remeron)	15–45
	Nefazodone	200–600
	Trazodone	150–600
SEROTONIN-NOREPINEPHRINE REUPTAKE INHIBITORS (SNRIs)	Desvenlafaxine (Pristiq)	50–400
	Duloxetine (Cymbalta)	40–60
	Levomilnacipran (Fetzima)	20–120
	Venlafaxine (Effexor)	75–375
PSYCHOTHERAPEUTIC COMBINATIONS	Olanzapine and fluoxetine (Symbyax)	6/25–12/50
	Chlordiazepoxide and fluoxetine (Limbitrol)	20/50–40/100
	Perphenazine and amitriptyline (Etrafon)	6/30–16/200
CORTICOSTEROID, GABA-A RECEPTOR MODULATOR	Brexanolone (Zulresso) (for postpartum depression)	(IV) Infusion over 60 hours: 30 mcg/kg/hr for 4 hr, then ↑ to 60 mcg/kg/hr for 20 hr, then ↑ to 90 mcg/kg/hr for 28 hr, then ↓ to 60 mcg/kg/hr for 4 hr, then↓ to 30 mcg/kg/hr for 4 hr, then discontinue. Total duration of infusion = 60 hr.
NMDA RECEPTOR ANTAGONIST	Esketamine (Spravato) Schedule III	(Nasal) 56 mg (2 sprays) – 84 mg (3 sprays) maintenance dose is weekly or every other week

a *boxed warning* for risk of sudden death in elderly patients with NCDs, and a recent population-based cohort study identified that there is a similar increased risk of mortality in middle-aged adults (Gerhard et al., 2020). The risk was determined to be higher in the 55- to 64-year-old age group and among women. The researchers report that although the causes of increased mortality are not clear, cardiac and infectious causes are likely. Their findings suggest that atypical antipsychotics should only be added in treatment-resistant cases and after careful evaluation of risks versus benefits.

In 2019 the FDA approved a nasal spray formulation of esketamine (Spravato) for limited distribution (certified doctor's offices and clinics) to treat patients with refractory (treatment-resistant) depression. Early clinical trials of intranasal esketamine reported improved depression and suicide symptoms within 4 hours, which is a revolutionary claim (Canuso et al., 2018). More recent studies have indicated that some benefits are seen within 2 days of treatment (FDA, 2019a). This option is particularly attractive considering the substantial lag period in the therapeutic effect of other antidepressants. It is intended for use along with an oral antidepressant. Concerns that will need continued evaluation include side effects of sedation, dissociation, and addiction potential associated with the use of ketamine preparations. But there is hope that its use will provide an option for individuals with treatment-resistant depression and recurrent suicide risk. Other ketamine-like medications are being investigated in clinical trials.

The most recent research has focused on the potential benefits of classic psychedelic drugs, such as psilocybin and LSD, in treating MDD (Holoyda, 2021). These drugs activate the serotonin 5-HT$_2$A receptors. Previous research has demonstrated the benefits of psilocybin for cancer treatment among patients with depression and for treatment-resistant depression (Davis et al., 2020). Davis and associates' research supported that two sessions with psilocybin administration demonstrated efficacy in treating MDD. Research is ongoing.

CLINICAL PEARL All antidepressants carry an FDA *boxed warning* for increased risk of suicidality in children, adolescents, and young adults.

CLINICAL PEARL As antidepressant drugs take effect and mood begins to lift, the individual may have increased energy with which to implement a suicide plan. Suicide potential often increases as the level of depression decreases. The nurse should be particularly alert to sudden lifts in mood.

Patient and Family Education Related to Antidepressants

The patient should:

■ Continue to take the medication even though symptoms have not subsided. The therapeutic effect may not be seen for as long as 4 weeks. If after this time no improvement is noted, the physician may prescribe a different medication.

■ Use caution when driving or operating dangerous machinery. Drowsiness and dizziness can occur. If these side effects become persistent or interfere with ADLs, the patient should report them to the physician. Dosage adjustment may be necessary.

■ Not discontinue use of the drug abruptly. To do so might produce withdrawal symptoms, such as nausea, vertigo, insomnia, headache, malaise, nightmares, and return of symptoms for which the medication was prescribed.

■ Use sunscreen and wear protective clothing when spending time outdoors. The skin may be sensitive to sunburn.

■ Report occurrence of any of the following symptoms to the physician immediately: sore throat, fever, malaise, yellowish skin, unusual bleeding, easy bruising, persistent nausea/vomiting, severe headache, rapid heart rate, difficulty urinating, anorexia/weight loss, seizure activity, stiff or sore neck, and chest pain.

■ Rise slowly from a sitting or lying position to prevent a sudden drop in blood pressure.

■ Take frequent sips of water, chew sugarless gum, or suck on hard candy if dry mouth is a problem. Good oral care (frequent brushing and flossing) is very important.

■ Not consume the following foods or medications while taking MAOIs: aged cheese, wine (especially Chianti), beer, chocolate, colas, coffee, tea, sour cream, smoked and processed meats, beef or chicken liver, canned figs, soy sauce, overripe and fermented foods, pickled herring, raisins, caviar, yogurt, yeast products, broad beans, cold remedies, or diet pills. To do so could cause a life-threatening hypertensive crisis.

■ Avoid smoking while receiving tricyclic therapy. Smoking increases the metabolism of tricyclics, requiring an adjustment in dosage to achieve the therapeutic effect.

■ Avoid drinking alcohol while taking antidepressant therapy. These drugs potentiate the effects of each other.

■ Avoid use of other medications (including over-the-counter medications) without a physician's approval while receiving antidepressant therapy. Many medications contain substances that could precipitate a life-threatening hypertensive crisis in combination with antidepressant medication.

■ Notify the physician immediately if inappropriate or prolonged penile erections occur while taking trazodone. If the erection persists longer than 1 hour, seek emergency department treatment. This condition is rare but has occurred in some men who have taken trazodone. If measures are not instituted immediately, impotence can result.

- Not "double up" on medication if a dose of bupropion (Wellbutrin) is missed unless advised to do so by the physician. Taking bupropion in divided doses will decrease the risk of seizures and other adverse effects.
- Follow the correct procedure for applying the selegiline transdermal patch:
  - Apply to dry, intact skin on upper torso, upper thigh, or outer surface of upper arm.
  - Apply approximately same time each day to a new spot on the skin after removing and discarding old patch.
  - Wash hands thoroughly after applying the patch.
  - Avoid exposing application site to direct heat (e.g., heating pads, electric blankets, heat lamps, hot tub, or prolonged direct sunlight).
  - If patch falls off, apply new patch to a new site and resume previous schedule.
- Be aware of possible risks of taking antidepressants during pregnancy. Safe use during pregnancy and lactation has not been fully established. These drugs are believed to readily cross the placental barrier; if so, the fetus could experience adverse effects of the drug. Consult the physician immediately if pregnancy occurs, is suspected, or is planned to identify risks versus benefits of continuing antidepressant therapy.
- Be aware of the side effects of antidepressants. Refer to written materials furnished by health-care providers for safe self-administration.
- Carry a card or other identification at all times describing the medications being taken.

Pharmacogenomics

Recent genetic studies have demonstrated that variations in genes can predict whether a person will respond to SSRIs (van Schaik et al., 2020). This finding is important because, as van Schaik and associates noted, between 30% and 50% of people do not respond to the first antidepressant they are prescribed. Patients and family members often express frustration as medications and dosages are changed to find the right antidepressant and dosage that will be effective for the individual. Genotyping has also demonstrated benefits in identifying which individuals may be more prone to certain side effects. One study cited by Lee (2015) demonstrated that Asian populations with a specific genotype were at increased risk for sexual dysfunction side effects associated with SSRIs. This information could be useful because sexual dysfunction is a primary reason that many people choose to stop taking these medications.

Although there continue to be differences of opinion about the usefulness of genetic testing, a recent meta-analysis of studies conducted between 2013 and 2019 concluded that individuals who had pharmacogenetic-guided therapy were 1.71 times more likely to achieve symptom remission compared with those who had treatment as usual (Bousman et al., 2019). Some issues of controversy include questions about cost-effectiveness, the lack of clinical practice guidelines, and what types of tests are most beneficial.

CLINICAL JUDGMENT IN ACTION: CASE STUDY AND SAMPLE CARE PLAN

NURSING HISTORY AND ASSESSMENT

Recognizing cues: The nurse must demonstrate ability to recognize what information is most important to making an assessment (National Council of State Boards of Nursing [NCSBN], 2021). This information is italicized in the following.

Seth is a 45-year-old white male admitted to the psychiatric unit of a general medical center by his family physician, Dr. Jones, who reported that Seth had become **increasingly despondent over the past month.** His wife reported that he had made statements such as, **"Life is not worth living,"** and **"I think I could just take all those pills Dr. Jones prescribed at one time; then it would all be over."** Seth says he loves his wife and children and does not want to hurt them but feels they no longer need him. He states, **"They would probably be better off without me."** His wife appears to be very concerned about his condition, although in his despondency, he seems oblivious to her feelings. His mother (a widow) lives in a neighboring state, and he sees her infrequently. His **father had a substance use disorder and physically abused Seth and his siblings.** He admits that he is somewhat bitter toward his mother for allowing him and his siblings to "suffer from the physical and emotional brutality of their father." His siblings and their families live in distant states, and he sees them rarely, during holiday gatherings.

Seth earned a college degree while working full time at night to pay his way. He is employed in the administration department of a large corporation. Over the past 12 years, Seth has watched while a number of his peers were promoted to management positions. Seth has been considered for several of these positions but has never been selected. Last month, a management position became available for which Seth felt he was qualified. He applied for this

Continued

CLINICAL JUDGMENT IN ACTION: CASE STUDY AND SAMPLE CARE PLAN—cont'd

position, believing he had a good chance of being promoted. However, his wife reports that when the announcement was made that the position had been given to a younger man who had been with the company only 5 years, Seth initially expressed anger and then seemed to accept the decision. But **over the past few weeks, he has become increasingly withdrawn.** He speaks to very few people at the office and is **falling behind in his work.** At home, he **eats very little, talks to family members only when they ask a direct question, withdraws to his bedroom very early in the evening, and does not come out until time to leave for work the next morning.** Today, he refused to get out of bed or to go to work, and he **told his wife he has nothing to live for.** His wife convinced him to talk to their family doctor, who admitted him to the hospital after hearing **Seth acknowledge that he desires to end his life.** The referring psychiatrist diagnosed Seth with Major Depressive Disorder.

> **Analyzing cues: The nurse must be able to interpret the information** (NCSBN, 2021).

The nurse interprets that Seth has been experiencing progressive symptoms of depression and currently is experiencing suicidal ideation. The nurse also interprets that Seth's history of trauma suggests that trauma-informed care will be important in all nursing interventions.

> **Prioritize hypotheses: The nurse must be able to identify the client's most important needs** (NCSBN, 2021).

The priority concern is maintaining patient safety as Seth manifests warning signs of suicidal behavior. His recent disappointments at work and dysfunctional family relationships suggest maladaptive grieving as an additional concern.

NURSING DIAGNOSES AND OUTCOME IDENTIFICATION

Generate solutions: The nurse must be able to connect their prioritized understanding of client needs to a course of action or plan of care (NCSBN, 2021).

From the assessment data, the nurse develops the following nursing diagnoses for Seth:

1. Risk for suicidal behavior related to depressed mood and expressions of having nothing to live for.
   a. Short-Term Goals:
      ■ Seth will discuss suicide ideation and intentions with staff.
      ■ Seth will collaborate with the nurse to identify a plan for maintaining safety.
   b. Long-Term Goal:
      ■ Seth will not harm himself during his hospitalization.
2. Maladaptive grieving related to unresolved losses (job promotion and unsatisfactory parent-child relationships)

evidenced by expressed anger over loss of a job opportunity and desire to end his life.
   a. Short-Term Goal:
      ■ Seth will discuss anger toward boss and parents within 1 week.
   b. Long-Term Goal:
      ■ Seth will verbalize his position in the grief process and begin to progress toward resolution by time of discharge from treatment.

PLANNING AND IMPLEMENTATION

RISK FOR SUICIDAL BEHAVIOR

Take Action: The nurse must be able to identify what actions need to be taken and how they will be implemented (NCSBN, 2021).

The following nursing interventions have been identified for Seth's care:

1. Develop a trusting relationship with Seth that facilitates open, nonjudgmental discussion of suicidal ideation and related thoughts and feelings.
2. Ask Seth directly, "Have you thought about killing yourself? If so, what do you plan to do? Do you have the means to carry out this plan? How strong are your intentions to die?"
3. Create a safe environment. Remove all potentially harmful objects from immediate access (sharp objects, straps, belts, ties, glass items).
4. Assess suicide risk each shift and identify any changes in level of hopelessness. Encourage verbalizations of honest feelings. Through exploration and discussion, help Seth to identify symbols of hope in his life (participating in activities he finds satisfying outside of his job).
5. Allow Seth to express angry feelings within appropriate limits. Encourage use of the exercise room and other activities for releasing energy appropriately. Help him identify the true source of his anger, and work on adaptive coping skills for use outside the hospital (e.g., jogging, exercise club available to employees of his company).
6. Identify community resources that he may use as a support system and from whom he may request help if feeling suicidal (e.g., suicidal or crisis hotline; psychiatrist or social worker at community mental health center; hospital HELP line).
7. Introduce Seth to support and education groups for adult children of alcoholics (ACoA).
8. Spend time with Seth. Spending time with him will help him to feel safe and secure while conveying the message that he is a worthwhile person.

MALADAPTIVE GRIEVING

The following nursing interventions have been identified for Seth:

1. Discuss with Seth the stages in the grief process and encourage him to explore his feelings so that he may come to realize the connection between grief and his anger.

CLINICAL JUDGMENT IN ACTION: CASE STUDY AND SAMPLE CARE PLAN—cont'd

2. Develop a trusting relationship with Seth. Show empathy and caring. Be honest and keep all promises.

3. Convey an accepting attitude—one in which Seth is not afraid to express his feelings openly.

4. Allow him to verbalize feelings of anger. The initial expression of anger may be displaced onto the health-care provider. Do not become defensive if this should occur. Have Seth write letters (not to be mailed) to his boss and to his parents stating his true feelings toward them. Discuss these feelings with him, then destroy the letters.

5. Assist Seth to discharge pent-up anger through participation in large motor activities (brisk walks, jogging, physical exercises, volleyball, exercise bike, or other equipment).

6. Help Seth to understand that feelings such as guilt and anger toward his boss and parents are appropriate and acceptable during the grieving process. Help him also to understand that he must work through these feelings and move past this stage to eventually feel better. Knowledge of acceptability of the feelings associated with normal grieving may help to relieve some of the guilt that these responses generate. Knowing why he is experiencing these feelings may also help to resolve them.

7. Encourage Seth to review the relationship with his parents. Educate Seth about common roles and behaviors of members in an alcoholic family. Encourage Seth to identify his roles and behaviors within his family of origin. Assist Seth in problem-solving as he attempts to determine methods for more adaptive coping.

Suggest alternatives to automatic negative thinking (e.g., thought-stopping techniques). Provide positive feedback for strategies identified and decisions made.

8. Encourage Seth to reach out for spiritual support during this time in whatever form is desirable to him. Assess spiritual needs (see Chapter 11, "Psychosocial Interventions and Spiritual Care"), and assist as necessary in the fulfillment of those needs. Seth may find comfort in religious rituals with which he is familiar.

EVALUATION

Evaluate outcomes: The nurse must be able to evaluate actions taken and determine whether they have had a positive, neutral, or negative impact (NCSBN, 2021).

The outcome criteria identified for Seth have been met. He sought out staff when feelings of suicide surfaced and has identified a safety plan with which he reports willingness to engage. He has not harmed himself in any way. He verbalizes no further thoughts of suicide and expresses hope for the future. He is able to verbalize names of resources outside the hospital from whom he may request help if thoughts of suicide return. Seth is able to verbalize normal stages of the grief process and behaviors associated with each stage. He is able to identify his own position in the grief process and express honest feelings related to the loss of his job promotion and satisfactory parent-child relationships. He expresses willingness to continue exploring behaviors and coping mechanisms through a local ACoA meeting.

Summary and Key Points

■ Depression is one of the oldest recognized psychiatric illnesses that is still highly prevalent today.

■ The cause of depressive disorders is not entirely known. Several factors, including genetics, biochemical influences, and psychosocial experiences, likely enter into the development of the disorder.

■ Secondary depression occurs in response to other physiological disorders and may be induced by a variety of substances or medications.

■ Symptoms of depression occur along a continuum according to the degree of severity from transient to severe. Severe depression is diagnostically referred to as major depressive disorder.

■ The disorder occurs in all developmental levels, including childhood, adolescence, adulthood, senescence, and during the postpartum period.

■ Treatment of depression includes individual therapy, group and family therapy, cognitive therapy, electroconvulsive therapy, bright light therapy, repetitive transcranial magnetic stimulation, vagus nerve and deep brain stimulation, physical exercise, and psychopharmacology.

■ Nursing care of the depressed patient is provided using the six steps of the nursing process.

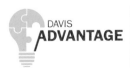

DAVIS
ADVANTAGE   Go to **Davis Advantage** to complete your learning: strengthen understanding, apply your knowledge, and prepare for the Next Gen NCLEX®.

Review Questions

1. A client, age 68, is a widow of 6 months. Over the last month she has become socially withdrawn, has lost weight, and told her sister today that she "doesn't have anything more to live for." She has been hospitalized with major depressive disorder. The *priority* nursing diagnosis for this client would be:
   a. Imbalanced nutrition: less than body requirements.
   b. Maladaptive grieving.
   c. Risk for suicidal behavior.
   d. Social isolation.

2. The goal of cognitive behavior therapy with depressed clients is to:
   a. Identify and change dysfunctional patterns of thinking.
   b. Resolve the symptoms and initiate or restore adaptive family functioning.
   c. Alter the neurotransmitters that are creating the depressed mood.
   d. Provide feedback from peers who are having similar experiences.

3. A client expresses interest in alternative treatments for depression with seasonal variations and asks the nurse about bright light therapy. Which of the following are evidence-based teaching points that the nurse may share with the client? (Select all that apply.)
   a. Light therapy has demonstrated effectiveness that is comparable to antidepressants.
   b. Light therapy should be used regularly until the season changes.
   c. Light therapy should be used only when electroconvulsive therapy has proven to be ineffective.
   d. Side effects such as headache, nausea, or agitation, when they occur, are usually mild and transient.
   e. Light therapy causes sedation, so the best time to use it is before bedtime.

4. A client has just been admitted to the psychiatric unit with a diagnosis of major depressive disorder. Which of the following behavioral manifestations might the nurse expect to assess? (Select all that apply)
   a. Slumped posture
   b. Hallucinations
   c. Feelings of despair
   d. Appears to have boundless energy
   e. Anorexia

5. A client with depression asks the nurse, "Why would they be checking my thyroid function when I clearly have depression and I'm not overweight?" Which of these is an accurate response?
   a. An underactive thyroid gland can manifest as depression.
   b. Depression has been proven to be a hormonal illness.
   c. Thyroid hormone replacement is a first-line treatment for most clients with depression.
   d. All of the above.

6. An acutely depressed client isolates themselves in their room on the psychiatric unit and just sits, staring into space. Which of these is the best example of an active communication approach with this client?
   a. "Do you like exercise?"
   b. "Come with me. I will go with you to group therapy."
   c. "Would you like to go to group therapy, stay in bed, or come out to the day lounge for some activities?"
   d. "Why do you stay in your room all the time?"

Clinical Judgment Questions

7. A client who has been taking sertraline (Zoloft) 50 mg PO bid for depression tells the nurse, "I've been on this medication for almost a week and I don't feel a bit better." What is the most appropriate response by the nurse?
   a. "Cheer up. You have so much to be happy about."
   b. "Sometimes it takes several weeks for the medicine to bring about an improvement in symptoms."
   c. "I'll report that to the physician. Maybe he will order something different."
   d. "Try not to dwell on your symptoms. Why don't you join the others down in the dayroom?"

8. A client reports to the mental health clinic with complaints of feeling more depressed over the last few weeks. The patient's score on the Hamilton Depression Rating Scale is 40. What is the priority nursing action at this finding?
   a. Assess the client's history of treatment for depression.
   b. Encourage the client to keep weekly follow-up appointments at the clinic.
   c. Educate the client about treatment options for mild, moderate, and severe depression.
   d. Assess the client's current risk for suicide.

9. A client whose husband died 6 months ago is given a diagnosis of major depressive disorder. She says to the nurse, "I start feeling angry that Harold died and left me all alone; he should have stopped smoking years ago! But then I start feeling guilty for feeling that way." What is an appropriate response by the nurse?
   a. "Yes, he should have stopped smoking. Then he probably wouldn't have gotten lung cancer."
   b. "I can understand how you must feel."
   c. "Those feelings are a normal part of the grief response."
   d. "Just think about the good times that you had while he was alive."

10. A client is admitted to the hospital with major depressive disorder and repeatedly makes self-negative statements. Which of the following interventions are identified as those that will promote positive self-esteem in the client? (Select all that apply)
    a. Teach assertive communication skills.
    b. Make observations to the client when they complete a goal or task.
    c. Instruct the client that you will not talk with them unless they stop talking negatively about themselves.
    d. Offer to spend time with the client using a nonjudgmental, accepting approach.

IMPLICATIONS OF RESEARCH FOR EVIDENCE-BASED PRACTICE

Kauffman, K., Davey, C. H., Dolata, J., Figueroa, M., Gunzler, D., Huml, A., Pencak, J., Sajatovic, M., & Sehgal, A. R. (2021). Changes in self-reported depressive symptoms among adults in the United States from 2005 to 2016. *Journal of the American Psychiatric Nurses Association, 27*(2), 148–155.

DESCRIPTION OF THE STUDY: The aim of this study was to evaluate national trends in self-reported depressive symptoms over an 11-year period. Interview data from the National Health and Nutrition Examination Survey, Patient Health Questionnaire (PHQ-9) were examined to identify trends in depressive symptomatology (n = 31,191).

RESULTS OF THE STUDY: The authors found that the proportion of individuals with clinically significant PHQ-9 scores increased from 6.2% to 8.1% over the period being studied. The odds of having a PHQ-9 score that indicated greater severity of depression increased by 27%. The associated symptoms demonstrating the greatest increases include anhedonia, guilt/worthlessness, changes in appetite, and changes in activity levels.

IMPLICATIONS FOR NURSING PRACTICE: The reasons for the increases in self-reported depressive symptoms were not clarified in this study, but the finding that self-reported depressive symptoms are increasing and demonstrating greater severity highlights the importance of screening for depression in all health-care settings and making appropriate referrals to mental health services as needed.

TEST YOUR CLINICAL REASONING AND CLINICAL JUDGMENT SKILLS

Emma is a 17-year-old high school senior. She will graduate in 1 month and has plans to attend the state university a few hours from her home. Emma has always made good grades in school, has participated in many activities, and is a pep squad cheerleader. She had been dating the star quarterback, Alan, since last summer, and they had spoken many times about going to the senior prom together. About a month before the prom, Alan broke up with Emma and began dating Salima, whom he subsequently took to the prom. Since that time, Emma has become despondent. She does not go out with her friends, she dropped out of the pep squad, her grades have fallen, and she has lost 10 pounds. She attends classes most of the time, but evenings and weekends she spends in her room alone listening to music, crying, and sleeping. Her parents have become very concerned and contacted the family physician, who has had Emma admitted to the psychiatric unit of the local hospital. The admitting psychiatrist has made the diagnosis of Major Depressive Disorder. Emma tells the nurse, "Sometimes I drive around and try to find Alan and Salima. I don't know why he broke up with me. I hate myself! I just want to die!"

Answer the following questions related to Emma:

1. What is the primary nursing diagnosis that is identified for Emma?
2. To determine the seriousness of this problem, what are important nursing assessments that must be made?
3. What medication might the physician order for Emma?
4. What concern has the FDA identified that is associated with this medication?

Communication Exercises

1. Carrie, age 75, is a patient on the psychiatric unit with a diagnosis of Major Depressive Disorder. She says to the nurse, "I never knew my life would end up like this. I've lost my husband, all my friends, and my home."

   How would the nurse respond appropriately to this statement by Carrie?

2. "I have spent my whole life taking care of others. Now someone else has to take care of me. I feel so useless."

   How would the nurse respond appropriately to this statement by Carrie?

3. "I don't know why anyone would want to bother taking care of me. I really have nothing left to live for."

   How would the nurse respond appropriately to this statement by Carrie?

 MOVIE CONNECTIONS

Prozac Nation (depression) • *The Butcher Boy* (depression) • *Night, Mother* (depression) • *The Prince of Tides* (depression/suicide) • *The Perks of Being a Wallflower* (depression/suicide) • *The Beaver* (depression) • *I'm Here, Too* (depression)

References

Akincigil, A., Olfson, M., Siegel, M., Zurlo, K. A., Walkup, J. T., & Crystal, S. (2012). Racial and ethnic disparities in depression care in community-dwelling elderly in the United States. *American Journal of Public Health.* doi:10.2105/AJPH.2011.300349

Akiskal, H. S. (2017). Mood disorders: Historical introduction and conceptual overview. In Sadock, B. J., Sadock, V. A., & Ruiz, P. (Eds.), *Comprehensive textbook of psychiatry* (10th ed., pp. 1599–1603). Wolters Kluwer.

Al-Qahtania, A. M., Shaikh, M. A., & Shaikh, I. A. (2018). Exercise as a treatment modality for depression: A narrative review. *Alexandria Journal of Medicine, 54*(4), 429–435. https://doi.org/10.1016/j.ajme.2018.05.004

American Psychiatric Association (APA). (2022). *Diagnostic and statistical manual of mental disorders, fifth edition, text revision (DSM-5-TR).* American Psychiatric Association.

American Thyroid Association. (2022). *Prevalence and impact of thyroid disease.* https://www.thyroid.org/media-main/press-room/#:~:text = Prevalence%20and%20Impact%20of%20Thyroid,are%20unaware%20of%20their%20condition

Amick, H. R., Gartlehner, G., Gaynes, B. N., Forneris, C., Asher, G. N., Morgan, L. C., Coker-Schwimmer, E., Boland, E., Lux, L. J., Gaylord, S., Bann, C., Pierl, C. B., & Lohr, K. N. (2015). Comparative benefits and harms of second generation antidepressants and cognitive behavioral therapies in initial treatment of major depressive disorder: Systematic review and meta-analysis. *British Medical Journal, 351,* h6019. doi:http://dx.doi.org/10.1136/bmj.h6019

Anxiety and Depression Association of America. (2021). *Anxiety and depression in children.* https://adaa.org/find-help/by-demographics/children/anxiety-and-depression

Bauer, A. E., Maegbaek, M. L., Liu, X., Wray, N. R., Sullivan, P. F., Miller, W. C., Meltzer-Brody, S., & Munk-Olsen, T. (2018). Familiality of psychiatric disorders and risk of postpartum psychiatric episodes: A population-based cohort study. *American Journal of Psychiatry.* doi:10.1176/appi.ajp.2018.17111184

Berlim, M. T., McGirr, A., Van den Eynde, F., Fleck, M. P., & Giacobbe, P. (2014). Effectiveness and acceptability of deep brain stimulation (DBS) of the subgenual cingulate cortex for treatment-resistant depression: A systematic review and exploratory meta-analysis. *Journal of Affective Disorders, 15,* 31–38. doi:10.1016/j.jad.2014.02.016

Beurel, E., Toups, M., & Nemeroff, C. B. (2020). The bidirectional relationship of depression and inflammation: Double trouble. *Neuron, 107*(2), 234–256. https://doi.org/10.1016/j.neuron.2020.06.002

Boland, R., & Verduin, M. L. (2022). *Kaplan & Sadock's synopsis of psychiatry* (P. Ruiz, Ed.). (12th ed.). Wolters Kluwer.

Bousman, C. A., Arandjelovic, K., Mancuso, S. G., Eyre, H. A., & Dunlop, B. W. (2019). Pharmacogenetic tests and depressive symptom remission: A meta-analysis of randomized controlled trials. *Pharmacogenomics 20*(1), 37–47. doi:10.2217/pgs-2018-0142

Budhwani, H., Hearld, K. R., & Chavez-Yenter, D. (2015). Depression in racial and ethnic minorities: The impact of nativity and discrimination. *Journal of Racial and Ethnic Health Disparities, 2*(1), 34–42.

Burnett, T. (2021). *Premenstrual dysphoric disorder: Different from PMS?* Mayo Clinic. http://www.mayoclinic.org/diseases-conditions/premenstrual-syndrome expert-answers/pmdd/faq-20058315

Campbell, P. D., Miller, A. M., & Woesner, M. E. (2017). Bright light therapy: Seasonal affective disorder and beyond. *The Einstein Journal of Biology and Medicine, 32,* E13–E25.

Canuso, C. M., Singh, J. B., Fedgchin, M., Alphs, L., Lane, R., Lim, P., Pinter C., Hough, D., Sanacora, G., Husseini, M., & Drevets, W. C. (2018). Efficacy and safety of intranasal esketamine for the rapid reduction of symptoms of depression and suicidality in patients at imminent risk for suicide: Results of a double-blind, randomized, placebo-controlled study. *American Journal of Psychiatry, 175*(7), 620–630. doi:10.1176/appi.ajp.2018.17060720

Centers for Disease Control and Prevention (CDC). (2021). *Depression is not a normal part of growing older.* https://www.cdc.gov/aging/mentalhealth/depression.htm

Chang, S. C., Wang, W., Pan, A., Jones, R. N., Kawachi, I., & Okereki, O. (2016). Racial variation in depression risk factors and symptom trajectories among older women. *American Journal of Geriatric Psychiatry, 24*(11), 1051–1062. https://doi.org/10.1016/j.jagp.2016.07.008

Cobb, B. S., Coryell, W. H., Cavanough, J., Keller, M., Solomon, D., Endicott, J., & Fiedorowicz, J. G. (2014). Seasonal variation of depressive symptoms in unipolar major depressive disorder. *Comprehensive Psychiatry, 55*(8), 1891–1899. doi:10.1016/j.comppsych.2014.07.021

Cotterell, D. (2010). Pathogenesis and management of seasonal affective disorder. *Progress in Neurology and Psychiatry, 14*(5), 18–25. doi:10.1002/pnp.173

Cunningham, J. E. A., Stamp, J. A., & Shapiro, C. M. (2019). Sleep and major depressive disorder: A review of nonpharmacological chronotherapeutic treatments for unipolar depression. *Sleep Medicine, 61,* 6–18. https://doi.org/10.1016/j.sleep.2019.04.012

Davis, A. K., Barrett, F. S., May, D. G., Cosimano, M. P., Sepeda, N. D., Johnson, M. W., Finan, P. H., & Griffiths, R. R. (2020).

Effects of psilocybin-assisted therapy on major depressive disorder: A randomized clinical trial. *JAMA Psychiatry, 78*(5), 1–9. https://doi.org/10.1001/jamapsychiatry.2020.3285

Food and Drug Administration. (2019a). *FDA approves new nasal spray medication for treatment-resistant depression; available only at a certified doctor's office or clinic [Press release].* https://www.fda.gov/news-events/press-announcements/fda-approves-new-nasal-spray-medication-treatment-resistant-depression-available-only-certified

Food and Drug Administration. (2019b). *Zulresso (brexanolone): Highlights of prescribing information.* https://www.accessdata.fda.gov/drugsatfda_docs/label/2019/211371lbl.pdf

Gautam, M., Tripathi, A., Deshmukh, D., & Gaur, M. (2020). Cognitive behavioral therapy for depression. *Indian Journal of Psychiatry, 62*(Suppl 2), S223–S229. https://doi.org/10.4103/psychiatry.IndianJPsychiatry_772_19

Gaynes, B. N., Lloyd, S. W., Lux, L., Gartlehner, G., Hansen, R.A., Brode, S., Jonas, D. E., Swinson Evans, T., Viswanathan, M., & Lohr, K. N. (2014). Repetitive transcranial magnetic stimulation for treatment-resistant depression. *Journal of Clinical Psychiatry, 75*(5), 477–489.

Geduldig, E. T., & Kellner, C. H. (2016). Electroconvulsive therapy in the elderly: New findings in geriatric depression. *Current Psychiatry Reports, 18,* 40. https://doi.org/10.1007/s11920-016-0674-5

George, M. S., Taylor, J. J., & Short, E. B. (2013). The expanding evidence base for rTMS treatment of depression. *Current Opinion in Psychiatry, 26*(1), 13–18. doi:10.1097/YCO.0b013e32835ab46d

Gerhard, T., Stroup, T. S., Correll, C. U., Setoguchi, S., Strom, B. L., Huang, C., Tan, Z., Crystal, S., & Olfson, M. (2020). Mortality risk of antipsychotic augmentation for adult depression. *PLoS ONE, 15*(9), e0239206. https://journals.plos.org/plosone/article?id = 10.1371/journal.pone.0239206

Grosse Holtforth, M., Krieger, T., Zimmermann, J., Altenstein-Yamanaka, D., Dörig, N., Meisch, L., & Hayes, A. M. (2019). A randomized-controlled trial of cognitive-behavioral therapy for depression with integrated techniques from emotion-focused and exposure therapies. *Psychotherapy Research, 29*(1), 30–44. https://doi.org/10.1080/10503307.2017.1397796

Hasin, D. S., Sarvet, A. L., Meyers, J. L., Saha, T. D., Ruan, W. J., Stohl, M., & Grant, B. F. (2018). Epidemiology of adult DSM-5 major depressive disorder and its specifiers in the United States. *JAMA Psychiatry, 75*(4), 336–346. https://doi.org/10.1001/jamapsychiatry.2017.4602

Herdman, T. H., Kamitsuru, S., & Lopes, C. T. (Eds.). (2021). *NANDA-I, Inc. nursing diagnoses: Definitions and classification, 2021–2023.* Theime.

Holoyda, B. (2021). The rebirth of psychedelic psychiatry. *Current Psychiatry, 20*(1), 13–19.

Institute of Medicine. (2003). *Health professions education: A bridge to quality.* National Academies Press.

Holt-Lundstat, J., Robles, T. F., & Sbarra, D. A. (2017). Advancing social connection as a public health priority in the United States. *American Psychologist, 72*(6), 517–530. doi.org/10.1037/amp0000103

Jiang, X., Asmaro, R., O'Sullivan, D. O., Budnik, E., & Schnatz, P. F. (2016). Depression may be one of the strongest risk factors for coronary artery disease in women aged <65 years: A 10-year prospective longitudinal study. Abstract S-17. Presented at NAMS 2016 Annual Meeting; October 5–8, 2016; Orlando, FL.

Kauffman, K., Davey, C. H., Dolata, J., Figueroa, M., Gunzler, D., Huml, A., Pencak, J., Sajatovic, M., & Sehgal, A. R. (2021). Changes in self-reported depressive symptoms among adults in the United States from 2005 to 2016. *Journal of the American Psychiatric Nurses Association, 27*(2), 148–155.

Kelsoe, J. R., & Greenwood, T. A. (2017). Mood disorders: Genetics. In Sadock, B. J., Sadock, V. A., & Ruiz, P. (Eds.), *Comprehensive textbook of psychiatry* (10th ed., pp. 1619–1630). Wolters Kluwer.

Kubala, J. (2021). 11 herbs, vitamins, and supplements to help fight depression. *Healthline.* https://www.healthline.com/health/depression/herbs-vitamins-supplements

Kurlansik, S. L., & Ibay, A. D. (2013). Seasonal affective disorder. *Indian Journal of Clinical Practice, 24*(7), 607–610.

Lam, R. W., Levitt, A. J., Levitan, R. D., Michelak, E., Morehouse, R., Rammasubbu, R., & Tam, E. M. (2015). Efficacy of bright light treatment, fluoxetine, and the combination in patients with nonseasonal major depressive disorder: A randomized clinical trial. *JAMA Psychiatry, 73*(1), 56–63. doi:10.1001/jamapsychiatry.2015.2235

Lapate, R. C., Van Reekum, C. M., Schaefer, S. M., Greischar, L. L., Norris, C. J., Bachhuber, D., & Davidson, R. J. (2014). Prolonged marital stress is associated with short-lived responses to positive stimuli. *Psychophysiology, 51*(6), 499–509. doi:10.1111/psyp.12203

Lee, K. C. (2015). Using pharmacogenomics to aid antidepressant prescribing. *Psychiatry Advisor.* www.psychiatryadvisor.com/mood-disorders/using-pharmacogenomics-to-aid-antidepressant-prescribing/article/394244/2

Lipp, M., Pasternak, A., & Ward, K. (2020). Impact of the MTHFR C677T variant on depression. *Current Psychiatry, 19*(10), 41–53.

Liu, H., Elliott, S., & Umberson, D. J. (2010). Marriage in young adulthood. In Grant J. E., & Potenza, M. N. (Eds.), *Young adult mental health* (pp. 169–180). Oxford University Press.

Magnezi, R., Aminov, E., Shmuel, D., Dreifuss, M., & Dannon, P. (2016). Comparison between neurostimulation techniques repetitive transcranial magnetic stimulation vs electroconvulsive therapy for the treatment of resistant depression: Patient preference and cost-effectiveness. *Patient Preference and Adherence, 10,* 1481–1487. doi:10.2147/PPA.S105654

Marcussen, K. (2005). Explaining differences in mental health between married and cohabiting individuals. *Social Psychology Quarterly, 68,* 239–257.

Mårtensson, B., Pettersson, A., Berglund, L., & Ekselius, L. (2015). Bright white light therapy in depression: A critical review of the evidence. *Journal of Affective Disorders, 182,* 1–7. doi:10.1016/j.jad.2015.04.013

Maruani, J., & Geoffroy, P. A. (2019). Bright light as a personalized precision treatment of mood disorders. *Frontiers in Psychiatry, 10,* 85. doi:10.3389/fpsyt.2019.00085

Mayo Clinic. (2022a). *Antidepressants for children and teens.* www.mayoclinic.org/diseases-conditions/teen-depression/in-depth/antidepressants/art-20047502

Mayo Clinic (2022b). *Depression in women: Understanding the gender gap.* https://www.mayoclinic.org/diseases-conditions/depression/in-depth/depression/art-20047725

Mayo Clinic. (2022c). *Electroconvulsive therapy.* https://www.mayoclinic.org/tests-procedures/electroconvulsive-therapy/about/pac-20393894

McMahon, B., Andersen, S. B., Madsen, M. K., Hjordt, L. V., Hageman, I., Dam, H., Svarer, C., Cunha-Bang, S., Baaré, W., Madsen, J., Hasholt, L., Holst, K., Frokjaer, V. G., & Knudsen, G. M. (2016). Seasonal difference in brain serotonin transporter binding predicts symptom severity in patients with seasonal affective disorder. *Brain, 139*(Pt 5), 1605–1614. doi:10.1093/brain/aww043

Merikangas, K. R., & Rihmer, Z. (2017). Mood disorders: Epidemiology. In Sadock, B. J., Sadock, V. A., & Ruiz, P. (Eds.), *Comprehensive textbook of psychiatry* (10th ed., pp. 1614–1619). Wolters Kluwer.

Miller, A. H. (2018). *Five things to know about inflammation and depression.* https://www.psychiatrictimes.com/view/five-things-know-about-inflammation-and-depression

National Center for Health Statistics (NCHS). (2022). *Faststats: Adolescent health.* https://www.cdc.gov/nchs/fastats/adolescent-health.htm

National Council of State Boards of Nursing (NCSBN). (2021). *Next generation NCLEX®: Comparison between case studies and stand-alone items.* https://www.ncsbn.org/public-files/NGN_Fall21_English_Final.pdf

National Institute of Mental Health (NIMH). (n.d.). *Postpartum depression facts.* https://www.nimh.nih.gov/health/publications/postpartum-depression-facts/index.shtml

National Institute of Mental Health (NIMH). (2022). *Major depression.* https://www.nimh.nih.gov/health/statistics/major-depression

National Institute of Mental Health (NIMH). (2018). *Depression.* https://www.nimh.nih.gov/health/topics/depression/index.shtml

Natsuaki, M. N., Shaw, D. S., Neiderhiser, J. M, Ganiban, J., Gordon, H. T., Reiss, D., & Leve, L. D. (2014). Raised by depressed parents: Is it an environmental risk? *Clinical Child and Family Psychology Review, 17*(4), 357–367. doi:10.1007/s10567-014-0169-z

Okereke, O., Reynolds, C., Mischoulon, D., Chang, G., Vyas, C. M., Cook, N., Weinberg, A., Bubes, V., Copeland, T., Friedenberg, G., Lee, M., Buring, J., & Manson, J. E. (2020). Effect of long-term vitamin D3 supplementation vs placebo on risk of depression or clinically relevant depressive symptoms and on change in mood scores: A randomized clinical trial. *JAMA, 324*(5), 471–480. https://doi.org/10.1001/jama.2020.10224

Pjrek, E., Friedrich, M. E., Cambioli, L., Dold, M., Jäger, F., Komorowski, A., Lanzenberger, R., Kasper, S., & Winkler, D. (2020). The efficacy of light therapy in the treatment of seasonal affective disorder: A meta-analysis of randomized controlled trials. *Psychotherapy and Psychosomatics, 89,* 17–24. doi:10.1159/000502891

Raposelli, D. (2015). Is TMS cost effective? *Psychiatric Times.* https://www.psychiatrictimes.com/view/tms-cost-effective

Ridley, M., Rao, G., Schilbach, F., & Patel, V. (2020). Poverty, depression, and anxiety: Causal evidence and mechanisms. *Science, 370*(6522). https://doi.org/10.1126/science.aay0214

Rodriguez, T. (2015). Using bright light therapy beyond seasonal affective disorder. *Psychiatry Advisor.* www.psychiatryadvisor.com/mood-disorders/depression-mood-winter-season-light-sad-antidepressant/article/457643

Rohan, K. J., Mahon, J. N., Evans, M., Ho, S.-Y., Meyerhoff, J., Postolache, T. T., & Vacek, P. M. (2016). Outcomes one and two winters following cognitive-behavioral therapy or light therapy for seasonal affective disorder. *American Journal of Psychiatry, 173,* 244–251.

Sathyanarayana Rao, T. S., Asha, M. R., Ramsh, B. M., & Jagannatha Rao, K. S. (2008). Understanding nutrition, depression, and mental illness. *Indian Journal of Psychiatry, 50*(2), 77–82. doi:10.4103/0019-5545.42391

Sharma, M. S., Ang-Rabeanes, M., Selek, S., Gajwani, P., & Soares, J. C. (2018). Neuromodulatory options for treatment-resistant depression. *Current Psychiatry, 17*(3), 26–37.

Shin, C., & Kim, Y. K. (2020). Ketamine in major depressive disorder: mechanisms and future perspectives. *Psychiatry Investigation, 17*(3), 181–192. https://doi.org/10.30773/pi.2019.0236

Shin, Y. C., Jung, C. H., Kim, H. J., Kim, E. J., &, Lim, S. W. (2016). The associations among vitamin D deficiency, C-reactive protein, and depressive symptoms. *Journal of Psychosomatic Research, 90,* 98–104. doi:http://dx.doi.org/10.1016/j.jpsychores.2016.10.001

Sikkens, D., Riemersma-Van der Lek, R. F., Meesters, Y., Schoevers, R. A., & Haarman, B. C. M. (2019). Combined sleep deprivation and light therapy: Clinical treatment outcomes in patients with complex unipolar and bipolar depression. *Journal of Affective Disorders, 246,* 727–730. https://doi.org/10.1016/j.jad.2018.12.117.

Slezak, M. (2021). Studying depression at a molecular level. *Psychiatric Times.* https://www.psy chiatrictimes.com/view/studying-depression-molecular-level

Teo, A. R., Choi, H., & Valenstein, M. (2013). Social relationships and depression: Ten-year follow-up from a nationally representative study. *PLoS ONE, 8*(4), e62396. https://doi.org/10.1371/journal.pone.0062396

Uecker, J. E. (2012). Marriage and mental health among young adults. *Journal of Health and Social Behavior, 53*(1), 67–83. https://doi.org/10.1177/0022146511419206

van Schaik, R. H. N., Müller, D. J., Serretti, A. & Ingelman-Sundberg, M. (2020). Pharmacogenetics in psychiatry: An update on clinical usability. *Frontiers in Pharmacology, 11,* 575540. doi: 10.3389/fphar.2020.575540

Wagner, K. D., & Brent, D. A. (2017). Mood disorders in children and adolescents: Depressive disorders and suicide. In Sadock, B. J., Sadock, V. A, & Ruiz, P. (Eds.), *Comprehensive textbook of psychiatry* (10th ed., pp. 3674–3685). Philadelphia, PA: Wolters Kluwer.

Winthorst, W., Post, W., Meesters, Y., Penninx, B., & Nolen, W. A. (2011). Seasonality in depressive and anxiety symptoms among primary care patients and in patients with depressive and anxiety disorders; results from the Netherlands Study of Depression and Anxiety. *BMC Psychiatry, 11*(1), 1–18. doi:10.1186/1471-244X-11-198

Classical References

Beck, A. T., Rush, A. J., Shaw, B. F., & Emery, G. (1979). *Cognitive theory of depression.* Guilford Press.

Freud, S. (1957). *Mourning and melancholia,* vol. 14 (standard ed.). Hogarth Press. (Original work published 1917.)

Hamilton, M. (1960). A rating scale for depression. *Journal of Neurology, Neurosurgery, & Psychiatry, 23,* 56–62.

Seligman, M. E. P. (1973). Fall into helplessness. *Psychology Today, 7,* 43–48.

Bipolar and Related Disorders 26

CORE CONCEPTS

Mood and Affect: Mania

Professional Behavior: Nursing process in the care of patients with bipolar and related disorders

Safety

Clinical Judgment

KEY TERMS

bipolar disorder

cyclothymic disorder

delirious mania

flight of ideas

hypomanic episode

manic episode

pressured speech

OBJECTIVES
After reading this chapter, the student will be able to:

1. Recount historical perspectives of bipolar disorder.
2. Discuss epidemiological statistics related to bipolar disorder.
3. Describe various types of bipolar disorders.
4. Identify predisposing factors in the development of bipolar disorder.
5. Discuss implications of bipolar disorder related to developmental stage.
6. Identify symptomatology associated with bipolar disorder and use this information in patient assessment.
7. Formulate nursing diagnoses and goals of care for patients experiencing a manic episode.
8. Identify topics for patient and family teaching relevant to bipolar disorder.
9. Describe appropriate nursing interventions for patients experiencing a manic episode.
10. Describe relevant criteria for evaluating nursing care of patients experiencing a manic episode.
11. Discuss various modalities relevant to the treatment of bipolar disorder.

Mood was defined in Chapter 25, "Depressive Disorders," as a pervasive and sustained emotion that may have a profound influence on a person's perception of the world. Examples of mood include depression, joy, elation, anger, and anxiety. *Affect* is described as the external, observable emotional reaction associated with an experience.

The previous chapter focused on the consequences of maladaptive grieving as it is manifested in depressive disorders. This chapter addresses mood disorders as they are manifested in cycles of manic episodes and depression—called **bipolar disorder.** A historical perspective and epidemiological statistics related to bipolar disorder are presented. Predisposing factors implicated in the etiology of bipolar disorder provide a framework for studying the dynamics of the disorder.

The implications of bipolar disorder relevant to children and adolescents are discussed. An explanation of the symptomatology is presented as background knowledge for assessing the person with bipolar disorder. Nursing care is described in the context of the six steps of the nursing process. Various medical treatment modalities also are explored.

CORE CONCEPT

Mania

An alteration in mood that may be expressed by feelings of elation, inflated self-esteem, grandiosity, hyperactivity, agitation, racing thoughts, and accelerated speech. A manic episode can occur as part of the psychiatric disorder bipolar disorder, as part of some other medical conditions, or in response to some substances.

Historical Perspective

Documentation of the symptoms associated with bipolar disorder dates back to around the second century in ancient Greece. Aretaeus of Cappadocia, a Greek physician, is credited with associating these extremes of mood with the same illness. He described patients who could at times laugh and play all night and day but at other times appeared "torpid, dull, and sorrowful" (Burton, 2012). His view that these mood swings were part of the same illness did not gain acceptance until much later.

In early writings, "mania" was categorized with all forms of "severe madness." In 1025, the Persian physician Avicenna wrote *The Canon of Medicine* in which he described mania as "bestial madness characterized by rapid onset and remission, with agitation and irritability."

The modern concept of manic-depressive illness began to emerge in the 19th century. In 1854 Jules Baillarger presented information to the French Imperial Academy of Medicine in which he used the term *dual-form insanity* to describe the illness. In the same year, Jean-Pierre Falret described the same disorder, one with alternating periods of depression and manic excitation, with the term *circular insanity* (Burton, 2012). Falret also noted that this disorder appeared to have genetic underpinnings, a belief that is adhered to today (Krans, 2019).

Contemporary thinking about bipolar disorder has been shaped by the works of Emil Kraepelin, who first coined the term *manic-depressive* in 1913. He added that this disorder was characterized by acute episodes followed by relatively symptom-free periods.

In 1980 the American Psychiatric Association (APA) adopted the term *bipolar disorder* as the diagnostic category for manic-depressive illness in the third edition of the *Diagnostic and Statistical Manual of Mental Disorders*. This term identified a period of mood elevation and excitation as a defining characteristic of the disorder that distinguishes it from other mood or psychotic disorders. In addition, it replaced the term *mania* because descriptions of people as "maniacs" were considered stigmatizing (Krans, 2019). The words "mania" and "manic," however, are still used to describe an abnormal mood state of elation with symptoms that include agitation, insomnia, grandiose delusions, racing thoughts, boundless energy, and increased libido, among others.

Epidemiology

Bipolar disorder affects approximately 4.4% of American adults at some point in their lives and 82.9% of cases are considered severe (National Institute of Mental Health [NIMH], n.d.). The incidence of bipolar disorder is roughly equal between men and women. The average age of onset for bipolar disorder is 25 years, and after the first manic episode, the disorder tends to be recurrent. Bipolar disorder is associated with increased mortality in general and particularly with death by suicide (Merikangas & Rihmer, 2017).

Unlike depressive disorders, bipolar disorder appears to occur more frequently among the higher socioeconomic classes with an overrepresentation among socially active, creative individuals (Merikangas & Rihmer, 2017). Bipolar disorder is the sixth-leading cause of disability in the middle-age group, but for those who respond to lithium treatment (about 33% of those treated with lithium), bipolar disorder is completely treatable, with no further episodes. Unfortunately, many individuals go for years without an accurate diagnosis or treatment, and for some the consequences can be devastating.

Types of Bipolar Disorders

A bipolar disorder is characterized by mood swings from profound depression to extreme euphoria (mania), with intervening periods of normalcy. Delusions or hallucinations may or may not be part of the clinical picture, and onset of symptoms may reflect a seasonal pattern.

During a **manic episode**, the mood is elevated, expansive, or irritable. The disturbance is sufficiently severe to cause marked impairment in occupational functioning or in usual social activities or relationships with others, or to require hospitalization to prevent harm to self or others. Motor activity is excessive and frenzied. Psychotic features may be present. The *Diagnostic and Statistical Manual of Mental Disorders, Fifth Edition, Text Revision (DSM-5-TR)* (APA, 2022) diagnostic criteria for a manic episode are presented in Box 26–1.

A somewhat milder degree of this clinical symptom picture is a hypomanic episode. A **hypomanic episode** is not severe enough to cause marked impairment in social or occupational functioning or to require hospitalization, and it does not include psychotic features. The *DSM-5-TR* diagnostic criteria for a hypomanic episode are presented in Box 26–2.

The diagnostic picture for depression associated with bipolar disorder is similar to that described for major depressive disorder (MDD), with one major distinction: the individual must have a history of one or more manic episodes. When the presentation includes co-occurring symptoms of both depression and mania, the diagnosis is further specified as *with mixed features.*

Bipolar I Disorder

Bipolar I disorder is the diagnosis given to an individual who is experiencing a manic episode or has a history of one or more manic episodes. The person may also have experienced episodes of depression. This diagnosis is further specified by the current or most recent behavioral episode experienced. For example, the specifier might be *single manic episode* (to describe individuals having a first episode of mania) or *current* (or most recent) *episode manic, hypomanic, mixed,* or *depressed* (to describe individuals who have had recurrent mood episodes). Psychotic or catatonic features may also be noted. Although the length of manic episodes (and depressive episodes) is variable, when an individual has more than four manic and depressive episodes in a year, they are referred to as having *rapid cycling* bipolar disorder.

Bipolar II Disorder

The bipolar II disorder diagnostic category is characterized by recurrent bouts of major depression with episodic occurrence of hypomania. The individual who is assigned this diagnosis may present with symptoms (or history) of depression or hypomania. The person has never experienced a full manic episode, and the hypomanic episode is "not severe enough to cause marked impairment in social or occupational functioning or to necessitate hospitalization" (APA, 2022, p. 151). However, the major depressive episodes can cause significant impairment in functioning and increase risk for suicide attempts. The diagnosis may specify whether the current or most recent episode is hypomanic, depressed, or with mixed features.

Cyclothymic Disorder

The essential feature of **cyclothymic disorder** is a chronic mood disturbance of at least 2 years'

BOX 26–1 Diagnostic Criteria for a Manic Episode

A. A distinct period of abnormally and persistently elevated, expansive, or irritable mood, and abnormally and persistently increased activity or energy, lasting at least 1 week and present most of the day, nearly every day (or any duration if hospitalization is necessary).

B. During the period of mood disturbance and increased energy or activity, three (or more) of the following symptoms (four if the mood is only irritable) are present to a significant degree, and represent a noticeable change from usual behavior:
1. Inflated self-esteem or grandiosity.
2. Decreased need for sleep (e.g., feels rested after only 3 hours of sleep).
3. More talkative than usual or pressure to keep talking.
4. Flight of ideas or subjective experience that thoughts are racing.
5. Distractibility (i.e., attention too easily drawn to unimportant or irrelevant external stimuli), as reported or observed.
6. Increase in goal-directed activity (either socially, at work or school, or sexually) or psychomotor agitation (i.e., purposeless non–goal-directed activity).
7. Excessive involvement in activities that have a high potential for painful consequences (e.g., engaging in unrestrained buying sprees, sexual indiscretions, or foolish business investments).

C. The mood disturbance is sufficiently severe to cause marked impairment in social or occupational functioning or to necessitate hospitalization to prevent harm to self or others, or there are psychotic features.

D. The episode is not attributable to the physiological effects of a substance (e.g., a drug of abuse, a medication, or other treatment) or to another medical condition. **Note:** A full manic episode that emerges during antidepressant treatment (e.g., medication, electroconvulsive therapy) but persists at a fully syndromal level beyond the physiological effect of that treatment is sufficient evidence for a manic episode and, therefore, a bipolar I diagnosis.

BOX 26–2 Diagnostic Criteria for a Hypomanic Episode

A. A distinct period of abnormally and persistently elevated, expansive, or irritable mood and abnormally and persistently increased activity or energy, lasting at least 4 consecutive days and present most of the day, nearly every day.

B. During the period of mood disturbance and increased energy and activity, three (or more) of the following symptoms (four if the mood is only irritable) have persisted, represent a noticeable change from usual behavior, and have been present to a significant degree:

   1. Inflated self-esteem or grandiosity.

   2. Decreased need for sleep (e.g., feels rested after only 3 hours of sleep).

   3. More talkative than usual or pressure to keep talking.

   4. Flight of ideas or subjective experience that thoughts are racing.

   5. Distractibility (i.e., attention too easily drawn to unimportant or irrelevant external stimuli), as reported or observed.

   6. Increase in goal-directed activity (either socially, at work or school, or sexually) or psychomotor agitation.

   7. Excessive involvement in pleasurable activities that have a high potential for painful consequences (e.g., engaging in unrestrained buying sprees, sexual indiscretions, or foolish business investments).

C. The episode is associated with an unequivocal change in functioning that is uncharacteristic of the individual when not symptomatic.

D. The disturbance in mood and the change in functioning are observable by others.

E. The episode is not severe enough to cause marked impairment in social or occupational functioning or to necessitate hospitalization. If there are psychotic features, the episode is, by definition, manic.

F. The episode is not attributable to the physiological effects of a substance (e.g., a drug of abuse, a medication, or other treatment).

   Note: A full hypomanic episode that emerges during antidepressant treatment (medication, electroconvulsive therapy) but persists at a fully syndromal level beyond the physiological effect of that treatment is sufficient evidence for a hypomanic episode diagnosis. However, caution is indicated so that one or two symptoms (particularly increased irritability, edginess, or agitation after antidepressant use) are not taken as sufficient for diagnosis of a hypomanic episode, nor necessarily indicative of a bipolar diathesis.

Reprinted with permission from the *Diagnostic and Statistical Manual of Mental Disorders, Fifth Edition, Text Revision (DSM-5-TR)* (2022). American Psychiatric Association.

duration, involving numerous periods of elevated mood that do not meet the criteria for a hypomanic episode, and numerous periods of depressed mood of insufficient severity or duration to meet the criteria for major depressive episode. *DSM-5-TR* criteria specify that symptoms must be present for at least half the time (over the 2-year period) and the individual is never without the symptoms for more than 2 months (APA, 2022).

Substance/Medication-Induced Bipolar Disorder

The disturbance of mood associated with this disorder is considered to be the direct result of physiological effects of a substance (e.g., ingestion of or withdrawal from a drug of abuse or a medication). The mood disturbance may involve elevated, expansive, or irritable mood with inflated self-esteem, decreased need for sleep, and distractibility. The disorder causes clinically significant distress or impairment in social, occupational, or other important areas of functioning.

Mood disturbances are associated with *intoxication* from substances such as alcohol, amphetamines, cocaine, hallucinogens, inhalants, opioids, phencyclidine, sedatives, hypnotics, and anxiolytics. Symptoms

can also occur during *withdrawal* from substances such as alcohol, amphetamines, cocaine, sedatives, hypnotics, and anxiolytics.

Many medications have been known to evoke mood symptoms. Classifications include anesthetics, analgesics, anticholinergics, anticonvulsants, antihypertensives, antiparkinsonian agents, antiulcer agents, cardiac medications, oral contraceptives, psychotropic medications, muscle relaxants, steroids, and sulfonamides. Some specific examples are included in the discussion of predisposing factors associated with bipolar disorders.

Bipolar Disorder Due to Another Medical Condition

This disorder is characterized by an abnormally and persistently elevated, expansive, or irritable mood and excessive activity or energy judged to be the direct physiological consequence of another medical condition (APA, 2022). The mood disturbance causes clinically significant distress or impairment in social, occupational, or other important areas of functioning. Types of medical conditions that are associated with bipolar symptoms include thyroid disorders, stroke, traumatic brain injury, multiple sclerosis, systemic lupus erythematosus, AIDS, and others.

Predisposing Factors

The exact etiology of bipolar disorder has yet to be determined. Scientific evidence supports a chemical imbalance in the brain, although the cause of the imbalance remains unclear. Theories that consider a combination of hereditary factors and environmental triggers (stressful life events) appear to hold the most credibility.

Biological Theories

Genetics

Research suggests that bipolar disorder strongly reflects an underlying genetic vulnerability. Evidence from family, twin, and adoption studies exists to support this observation. Studies of genetic variants have found common genetic variations that correlate significantly with attention deficit-hyperactivity disorder (ADHD), bipolar disorder, MDD, and schizophrenia (The Brainstorm Consortium et al., 2018).

Twin Studies

Twin studies have indicated a concordance rate for bipolar disorder among monozygotic twins at 60% to 80%, compared with 10% to 20% in dizygotic twins. Because monozygotic twins have identical genes and dizygotic twins share approximately one-half their genes, this concordance rate is strong evidence that genes play a major role in the etiology. However, because both identical twins do not always develop the illness, other factors may also play a role. It is likely that many different genes, as well as environmental factors, are involved, although researchers do not yet know how these factors interact to cause bipolar disorder.

Family Studies

Although the pattern of inheritance for bipolar disorder is not completely understood, the risk is greatest among first-degree relatives (MedlinePlus, 2021). Boland and Verduin (2022) reported that a family history of bipolar disorder conveys a higher risk for mood disorders in general and a threefold increase in the rate of bipolar disorder; first-degree relatives have a 10-fold risk of developing the disorder. This increased risk is also present in children born to parents with bipolar disorder who were adopted at birth and reared by adoptive parents without evidence of the disorder.

Other Genetic Studies

Soreff (2022) stated that bipolar disorder, and especially bipolar I disorder, has a major genetic component with *ANK3*, *CACNA1C*, and *CLOCK* genes, and these genetic roles take several forms.

The *ANK3* protein, located on the first part of the axon, is involved in making the determination of whether a neuron will fire. Studies have shown that lithium carbonate, the most common medication used to prevent manic episodes, reduces expression of *ANK3* (Leussis et al., 2013). The *CACNA1C* protein regulates the influx and outflow of calcium from cells and is the site of action of the calcium channel blockers sometimes used in the treatment of bipolar disorder. The CLOCK gene is associated with circadian rhythm regulation, and sleep–wake cycles are known to be significantly disrupted in patients with bipolar disorder.

Research looking specifically at factors associated with lithium's effectiveness identified "a number of candidate genes related to neurotransmitters, intracellular signaling, neuroprotection, circadian rhythms, and other pathogenic mechanisms of bipolar disorder [that] were found to be associated with lithium's prophylactic response" (Rybakowski, 2014, p. 353). Evidence from another study identified common gene sets that demonstrated altered expression in patients with schizophrenia, bipolar disorder, and depression (Darby et al., 2016). Specifically, ribosomal genes were overexpressed, and those involved with neuronal connections, such as gamma-aminobutyric acid (GABA) signaling, were underexpressed. The researchers suggested that this finding may lead the way to RNA processing and protein synthesis as targets for therapeutic intervention. Ongoing genetic research will continue to shed light on the genetic influences in the development of bipolar disorder and the genetic factors that affect treatment response.

Biochemical Influences

Biogenic Amines

Early studies associated symptoms of mania with a functional excess of norepinephrine and dopamine. The level of the neurotransmitter serotonin is believed to remain low in both depression and mania, but the exact mechanisms and biochemical influences are complex and not yet completely understood. For example, although low levels of serotonin are thought to play a role in both depression and manic states, selective serotonin reuptake inhibitors (SSRIs) sometimes trigger manic episodes and rapid cycling of mood swings in people with bipolar disorders. It is likely that multiple factors influence serotonin's role in this illness. Acetylcholine is another neurotransmitter believed to be related to symptoms of bipolar disorder. Excessive levels of glutamate, an excitatory neurotransmitter, have been associated with bipolar disorder. Many of the mood stabilizers used to treat bipolar disorder inhibit the actions of glutamate. The primary support for neurotransmitter hypotheses is the effects that neuroleptic drugs have on the levels of these biogenic amines and the resulting reduction in symptoms of the disorder. Although several neurotransmitters have been implicated in influencing symptoms, the cause of bipolar disorder remains unknown.

Physiological Influences

Neuroanatomical Factors

Neuroanatomical changes have been correlated with dysfunction in the prefrontal cortex, basal ganglia, temporal and frontal lobes of the forebrain, and parts of the limbic system including the amygdala, thalamus, and striatum. The different symptoms in bipolar disorder may be correlated to those specific areas of dysfunction or may be evidence of downregulation of specific circuits in response to abnormal activity in other circuits (Boland & Verduin, 2022). Akiskal (2017) added that circadian disturbances seen in both depression and manic episodes can be conceptualized as dysfunction in the limbic system. Although causality of bipolar disorder cannot be defined as solely a neuroanatomical disorder, these findings suggest that mood disorders, including bipolar disorder, involve pathology in the brain.

Medication Side Effects

Certain medications used to treat somatic illnesses have been known to trigger manic responses. The most common of these are the steroids frequently used to treat chronic illnesses, such as multiple sclerosis and systemic lupus erythematosus. Some individuals whose first episode of mania occurred during steroid therapy have reported spontaneous recurrence of manic symptoms years later. Amphetamines, antidepressants, and high doses of anticonvulsants and narcotics also have the potential for initiating a manic episode.

Psychosocial Theories

Interest in psychosocial theories has declined in recent years with the focus of research on genetic and biochemical predisposing factors. Consequently, conditions such as schizophrenia and bipolar disorder are currently viewed as diseases of the brain with biological etiologies. However, several studies have confirmed a link between childhood trauma (emotional, physical, and sexual abuse) and the development of bipolar disorder (Aas et al., 2016; Janiri et al., 2015; Quidé et al., 2020; Watson et al., 2013). Aas and associates (2016) identified that the experience of childhood trauma incites changes in genes along several different pathways. These genetic changes may be linked not only to an increased risk for bipolar disorder but also earlier onset, more severe symptoms, substance use, and suicide risk. Research efforts continue to focus on this apparent interaction of genetics and psychosocial stressors. More research is needed to translate these connections into practical applications for treatment or prevention.

The Transactional Model of Stress and Adaptation

Bipolar disorder clearly results from an interaction between genetic, biological, and psychosocial determinants. The transactional model takes into consideration these etiological influences as well as those associated with past experiences, existing conditions, and the individual's perception of the event. Figure 26–1 depicts the dynamics of bipolar mania using the transactional model of stress and adaptation.

Developmental Implications

Childhood and Adolescence

The lifetime prevalence of adolescent bipolar disorders is estimated to be about 1%; in younger children, the incidence is rare, but children and adolescents are often difficult to diagnose. In the past decade, diagnosis of bipolar I disorder in youth has rapidly increased, which prompted researchers to look more closely at factors contributing to this trend. More recent studies have shown that in 63% to 69% of diagnoses, bipolar disorder actually began before age 19 years, and about 25% had an onset at or before 13 years of age (Post et al., 2020). A connection is thought to exist between ADHD and the development of bipolar disorder in youth. A recent study found that a diagnosis of ADHD conferred a 10-fold increase in the risk for later development of bipolar disorder compared with children without the diagnosis (Meier et al., 2018). ADHD is the most common comorbidity in children and adolescents with bipolar disorder with studies reporting anywhere from 60% to 90% comorbidity of the two conditions and there is overlap in both genetics and symptoms (particularly irritability, hyperactivity, accelerated speech, and distractability) (Kowatch, 2016). Osser (2021) noted that when ADHD and bipolar disorder are comorbid, the course of the disease is more severe than either diagnosis alone and there is an increased risk of suicide attempts.

For youth that manifest with a host of *atypical* symptoms, including nondiscrete mood episodes,

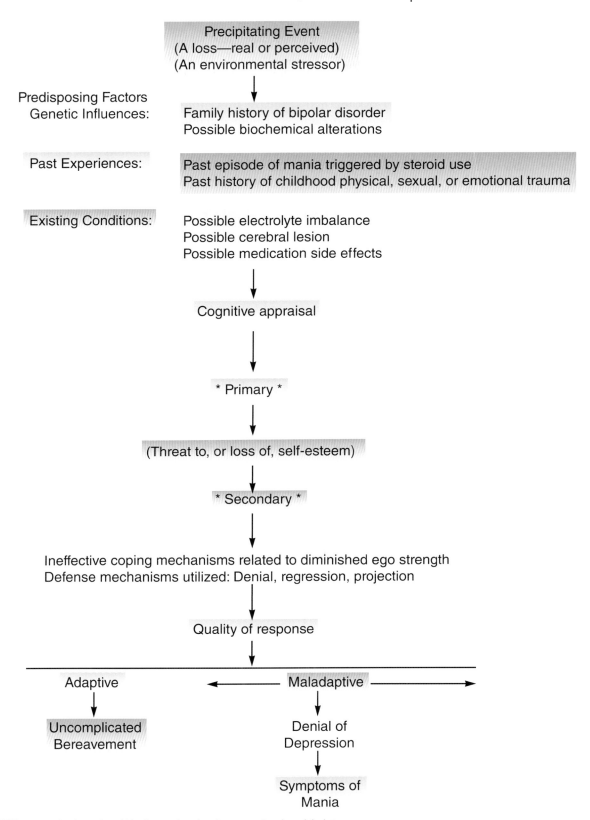

FIGURE 26–1 The dynamics of bipolar mania using the transactional model of stress.

chronic irritability, and temper tantrums, the *DSM-5-TR* incorporated a diagnosis, *disruptive mood dysregulation disorder*, that more aptly describes this symptom profile. A longitudinal study of children with nonepisodic irritability, however, found that although these children had a higher risk for anxiety and depression, they were not typically at higher risk for developing bipolar disorder (Stringaris, 2010).

Because family studies show a familial risk for bipolar disorder, whenever a child is exhibiting mood-related symptoms (including depression) and particularly when there is a family history of bipolar disorders, the possibility for a developing bipolar disorder should be carefully evaluated. True bipolar disorder in adolescents, as with adults, is considered a chronic illness (much like diabetes) and medication treatment is typically lifelong.

Treatment Strategies for Children and Adolescents

Psychopharmacology

Medications approved by the U.S. Food and Drug Administration (FDA) for treatment of acute mania in children and adolescents include lithium, risperidone, aripiprazole, quetiapine, olanzapine, and asenapine. Only two medications are approved for the treatment of bipolar depression: olanzapine/fluoxetine combination drugs and lurasidone. Nonpharmacological interventions, including mood charting, managing stress and sleep cycles, maintaining healthy diet and exercise, and avoiding alcohol and drugs, should be considered as well in this population. Nurses can play a primary role in offering such education and interventions.

Because ADHD has been identified as the most common comorbid condition in children and adolescents with bipolar disorder and stimulants can exacerbate mania, it is suggested that medication for ADHD be initiated only after bipolar symptoms have been controlled with a mood-stabilizing agent (Jain & Jain, 2014). Nonstimulant medications indicated for ADHD (e.g., atomoxetine, bupropion, the tricyclic antidepressants) may also induce switches to mania or hypomania. Bipolar disorder in children and adolescents appears to be a chronic condition with a high risk of relapse. Maintenance therapy incorporates the same medications used to treat acute symptoms, although few research studies exist that deal with long-term maintenance of bipolar disorder in children.

Family Interventions

Although pharmacological treatment is acknowledged as the primary method of stabilizing acute symptoms, a combination of medications with psychosocial interventions has been recognized as playing an important role in preventing relapses and improving adjustment. Treatment adherence must be emphasized as an essential component of relapse prevention.

Family dynamics and attitudes can influence the outcome of a person's recovery. Interventions with family members must include education that promotes understanding that at least some of the individual's negative behaviors are attributable to an illness that must be managed and are not deliberate or under their control.

Studies show that psychoeducational family-focused focused therapy (FFT) is an effective method of reducing relapses and increasing medication adherence in people with bipolar disorder (Miklowitz & Chung, 2016). In addition, Miklowitz and Chung found that individuals involved in FFT who demonstrated a high risk for developing bipolar disorder (those with depressive symptoms and a first-degree relative with bipolar disorder) recovered more quickly than those who were provided only educational sessions. FFT includes psychoeducation about bipolar disorder (e.g., symptoms, early recognition, etiology, treatment, self-management), communication training, and problem-solving skills training. Teaching the person and family about early warning signs and how to respond provides the individual with a needed support system and the family with tools to provide that support.

Application of the Nursing Process to Bipolar Disorder (Mania)

Background Assessment Data

Symptoms of manic states can be described according to three stages: hypomania, acute mania, and delirious mania. Symptoms of mood, cognition and perception, and activity and behavior are presented for each stage.

Stage I: Hypomania

At this stage, the disturbance is not sufficiently severe to cause marked impairment in social or occupational functioning or to require hospitalization and there are no psychotic features (APA, 2022).

Mood

The mood of the person with hypomania is cheerful and expansive, but an underlying irritability surfaces rapidly when the person's wishes and desires go unfulfilled. The nature of the hypomanic person is volatile and fluctuating. The disturbances in mood and change in functioning are noticed by others as different from when the individual was asymptomatic (APA, 2022).

Cognition and Perception

Perceptions of the self are exalted—the individual has ideas of great worth and ability. Flight of ideas may be present and the individual may perceive that their thoughts are racing. Perception of the environment is heightened, but the individual is easily distracted by irrelevant stimuli.

Activity and Behavior

Individuals with hypomania exhibit increased motor activity or psychomotor agitation and demonstrate an increase in goal-directed activity. They may appear extroverted and sociable and thus attract numerous acquaintances but typically these relationships are superficial. They may be hypertalkative, loud, and sometimes inappropriate in conversation. Increased libido is common and may lead to excessive pleasure seeking without attention to potential consequences. Some individuals experience anorexia and weight loss. The exalted self-perception may lead the individual to engage in grandiose behaviors, such as phoning the president of the United States or running up debt on a credit card without having the resources to pay.

Stage II: Acute Mania

Symptoms of acute mania may progress in intensification from those experienced in hypomania, or they may be manifested directly. Most individuals experience marked impairment in functioning and require hospitalization (see Box 26–1).

Mood

Acute mania is characterized by euphoria and elation. The person appears to be on a continuous "high." However, the mood is always subject to frequent variation, easily changing to irritability and anger or even to sadness and crying.

Cognition and Perception

Cognition and perception become fragmented and often psychotic in acute mania. Accelerated thinking proceeds to racing thoughts; overconnection of ideas; and rapid, abrupt movement from one thought to another, which is termed **flight of ideas**, and may be manifested by **pressured speech**, a continuous flow of accelerated speaking or loquaciousness, to the point that conversing with this individual may be extremely difficult. When flight of ideas is severe, speech may be disorganized and incoherent. Distractibility becomes all-pervasive. Attention can be diverted by even the smallest of stimuli. Hallucinations and delusions (usually paranoid and grandiose) are common.

Activity and Behavior

Psychomotor activity is excessive. Sexual interest is increased. There is poor impulse control and low frustration tolerance. The individual who is normally discreet may become socially and sexually uninhibited. Excessive spending is common. In acute mania, the individual typically has little insight into their behavior and communication. This lack of insight manifests at times as unreliable reporting of events and denial of problems when confronted by friends or family, which may be interpreted as lying. Energy seems inexhaustible, and the need for sleep is diminished. An individual experiencing acute mania may go for many days without sleep and still not feel tired. Hygiene and grooming may be neglected. Dress may be disorganized, flamboyant, or bizarre, and the use of excessive makeup or jewelry is common.

Stage III: Delirious Mania

Delirious mania is a serious form of the manic stage of bipolar disorder characterized by severe clouding of consciousness and an intensification of the symptoms associated with acute mania. This condition has become relatively rare since the availability of antipsychotic medication.

Mood

The mood of the delirious person is very labile. They may exhibit feelings of despair, quickly converting to unrestrained merriment and ecstasy or becoming irritable or totally indifferent to the environment. Panic-level anxiety may be evident.

Cognition and Perception

Cognition and perception are characterized by a clouding of consciousness, with accompanying confusion, disorientation, and sometimes stupor. Other common manifestations include religiosity, delusions of grandeur or persecution, and auditory or visual hallucinations. The individual is extremely distractible and incoherent.

Activity and Behavior

Psychomotor activity is frenzied and characterized by agitated, purposeless movements. The safety of the individual is at stake unless this activity is curtailed. Exhaustion, injury to self or others, and eventually death could occur without intervention.

Diagnosis and Outcome Identification

Using information collected during the assessment, the nurse completes the patient database, from which the selection of appropriate nursing diagnoses is determined. Table 26–1 presents a list of patient behaviors and the NANDA International nursing

TABLE 26–1	Assigning Nursing Diagnoses to Behaviors Commonly Exhibited by Individuals Experiencing a Manic Episode	
BEHAVIORS	**NURSING DIAGNOSES**
Extreme hyperactivity; increased agitation and lack of control over purposeless and potentially injurious movements	Risk for injury
Manic excitement, delusional thinking, hallucinations, impulsivity	Risk for violence: Self-directed or other-directed
Loss of weight, amenorrhea, refusal or inability to sit still long enough to eat	Imbalanced nutrition: Less than body requirements
Delusions of grandeur and persecution; inaccurate interpretation of the environment	Disturbed thought processes
Auditory and visual hallucinations; disorientation	Disturbed sensory-perception*
Inability to develop satisfying relationships, manipulation of others for own desires, use of unsuccessful social interaction behaviors	Impaired social interaction
Difficulty falling asleep, sleeping only short periods	Insomnia

*This diagnoses has been resigned from the NANDA-I list of approved diagnoses. It is used in this instance because it is most compatible with the identified behaviors.

diagnoses (Herdman et al., 2021) that correspond to those behaviors, which may be used in planning care for the patient experiencing a manic episode.

Outcome Criteria

The following criteria may be used for measuring outcomes in the care of the patient experiencing a manic episode.

The patient:

■ Exhibits no evidence of physical injury
■ Has not harmed self or others
■ Is no longer exhibiting signs of physical agitation
■ Eats a well-balanced diet with snacks to prevent weight loss and maintain nutritional status
■ Verbalizes an accurate interpretation of the environment
■ Verbalizes that hallucinatory activity has ceased and demonstrates no outward behavior indicating hallucinations
■ Accepts responsibility for own behaviors
■ Does not manipulate others for gratification of own needs
■ Interacts appropriately with others
■ Is able to fall asleep within 30 minutes of retiring
■ Is able to sleep 6 to 8 hours per night without medication

Planning and Implementation

The following section presents a group of selected nursing diagnoses, with short- and long-term goals and nursing interventions for each. Some institutions

use a case management model to coordinate care (see Chapter 8, "The Nursing Process in Psychiatric-Mental Health Nursing," for a more detailed explanation). In case-management models, the plan of care may take the form of a critical pathway.

Risk for Violence: Self-Directed or Other-Directed

Risk for self- or other-directed violence is defined as "susceptible to behaviors in which an individual demonstrates that he or she can be physically, emotionally, and/or sexually harmful to [self or to others]" (Herdman et al., 2021, pp. 522–523).

Patient Goals

Outcome criteria include short- and long-term goals. Timelines are individually determined.

Short-term goals

■ Within [a specified time], patient will recognize signs of increasing anxiety and agitation and report to staff (or other care provider) for assistance with intervention.
■ Patient will not harm self or others.

Long-term goal

■ Patient will not harm self or others.

Interventions

■ Maintain a low level of stimuli in the patient's environment (low lighting, few people, simple decor, low noise level). The anxiety level rises in a stimulating environment. A suspicious, agitated patient may perceive individuals as threatening.

■ Assess for concurrent substance use issues. There is a high incidence of comorbid substance use disorders in patients with bipolar disorder. Substance use issues can increase the patient's risk for harm to self or others. The use of mood-altering chemicals in addition to those prescribed also can make the evaluation of pharmacotherapy more difficult. (See Chapter 23, "Substance-Related and Addictive Disorders," for more information on substance use disorders and relevant nursing interventions.)

■ Observe the patient's behavior frequently. Do this while performing routine activities to avoid creating suspiciousness in the individual. Close observation is necessary so that intervention can occur if required to ensure patient (and others') safety.

■ Remove all dangerous objects from the patient's environment so the patient may not use them to harm self or others while in an agitated, confused state.

 ■ Intervene at the first sign of increased anxiety, agitation, or verbal or behavioral aggression. Offer empathetic responses to patient's feelings: "You seem anxious (or frustrated, or angry) about this situation. How can I help?" Validation of the patient's feelings conveys a caring attitude, and offering assistance reinforces trust. Because the patient may be highly distractible, providing a distraction can aid in diffusing anxiety and agitation as well.

■ Maintain a calm attitude toward the patient. As the patient's anxiety increases, offer some alternatives: participating in a physical activity (e.g., walking or other physical exercise), talking about the situation, and taking antianxiety medication. Offering alternatives to the patient empowers them to have a sense of control over the situation.

■ Have sufficient staff available to safely redirect the patient if it becomes necessary. This provides physical security for staff and patients.

■ If the patient is not calmed by "talking down" or by medication, and the behavior is such that it poses imminent harm to the patient or others, use of mechanical restraints may be necessary.

> **CLINICAL PEARL** The "least restrictive alternative" must be selected when planning interventions for a violent patient. Restraints should be used only as a last resort, after all other interventions have been unsuccessful and the patient is clearly at risk of harm to self or others.

■ If restraint is deemed necessary, ensure that sufficient staff is available to assist. Follow protocol established by the institution.

■ As agitation decreases, assess the patient's readiness for restraint removal or reduction. Remove one restraint at a time while assessing the patient's response. This approach minimizes the risk of injury to patient and staff.

Impaired Social Interaction

Impaired social interaction is defined as "insufficient or excessive quantity or ineffective quality of social exchange" (Herdman et al., 2021, p. 384). Table 26–2 presents this nursing diagnosis in care plan format.

Imbalanced Nutrition: Less Than Body Requirements and Insomnia

Imbalanced nutrition: Less than body requirements is defined as "intake of nutrients insufficient to meet metabolic needs" (Herdman et al., 2021, p. 213). *Insomnia* is defined as "inability to initiate or maintain sleep, which impairs functioning" (p. 274).

Patient Goals

Outcome criteria include short- and long-term goals. Timelines are individually determined.

Short-term goals

■ Patient will consume sufficient food and between-meal snacks to meet recommended daily allowances of nutrients.

■ Within 3 days, with the aid of a sleeping medication, patient will sleep 4 to 6 hours without awakening.

Long-term goals

■ Patient will exhibit no signs or symptoms of malnutrition.

■ By time of discharge from treatment, patient will be able to acquire 6 to 8 hours of uninterrupted sleep without medication.

Interventions

■ In collaboration with the dietitian, determine the number of calories required to provide adequate nutrition for maintenance or realistic (according to body structure and height) weight gain. Determine the patient's likes and dislikes and collaborate with the dietitian to provide favorite foods if possible. The patient is more likely to eat foods that they particularly enjoy.

■ Provide the patient with high-protein, high-calorie, nutritious finger foods and drinks that can be consumed "on the run." Because of the hyperactive state, the patient may have difficulty sitting still long enough to eat a meal. They are more likely to consume food and drinks that can be carried around and eaten with little effort. Have juice and snacks available on the unit at all times. Regular nutritious intake is required to compensate for increased caloric requirements of hyperactivity.

Table 26–2 | CARE PLAN FOR THE PATIENT EXPERIENCING A MANIC EPISODE

NURSING DIAGNOSIS: IMPAIRED SOCIAL INTERACTION
RELATED TO: Delusional thought processes (grandeur and/or persecution); underdeveloped ego and low self-esteem
EVIDENCED BY: Inability to develop satisfying relationships and manipulation of others for own desires

OUTCOME CRITERIA	NURSING INTERVENTIONS	RATIONALE
Short-Term Goal: ■ Patient verbalizes which of their interaction behaviors are appropriate and which are inappropriate within 1 week. **Long-Term Goal:** ■ Patient demonstrates use of appropriate interaction skills as evidenced by lack of, or marked decrease in, manipulation of others to fulfill own desires.	1. Recognize the purpose manipulative behaviors serve for patient: to reduce feelings of insecurity by increasing feelings of power and control. 2. Set limits on manipulative behaviors. Explain to the patient what is expected and what the consequences are if limits are violated. Terms of the limitations must be agreed on by all staff who will be working with the patient. 3. Do not argue, bargain, or try to reason with the patient. Merely state the limits and expectations. Confront the patient as soon as possible when interactions with others are manipulative or exploitative. Follow through with established consequences for unacceptable behavior. 4. Provide positive reinforcement for nonmanipulative behaviors. Explore feelings and help the patient seek more appropriate ways of dealing with them. 5. Help the patient recognize that they must accept the consequences of their own behaviors and refrain from attributing them to others. 6. Help the patient identify positive aspects about self, recognize accomplishments, and feel good about them.	1. Understanding the motivation behind the manipulation may facilitate acceptance of the individual and their behavior. 2. When the patient is unable to establish their own limits, limitations must be clearly defined for them. Establishing consequences for violation of established limits promotes extinguishing the behavior. 3. Because the patient may be vulnerable to impulsive, reckless, or pleasure-seeking behavior without considering consequences, they should receive immediate feedback when behavior is unacceptable. Consistency in enforcing the consequences is essential if positive outcomes are to be achieved. Inconsistency creates confusion and encourages testing of limits. 4. Positive reinforcement enhances self-esteem and promotes repetition of desirable behaviors. 5. The patient must accept responsibility for their own behaviors before adaptive change can occur. 6. As self-esteem is increased, the patient will feel less need to manipulate others for own gratification.

■ Maintain an accurate record of intake, output, and calorie count. Weigh the patient daily. Administer vitamin and mineral supplements as ordered by the physician. Monitor laboratory values and report significant changes to the physician. It is important to carefully monitor data that provide an objective assessment of the patient's nutritional status.

■ Assess the patient's activity level. They may ignore or be unaware of feelings of fatigue. Observe for signs such as increasing restlessness; fine tremors; slurred speech; and puffy, dark circles under eyes. The patient could collapse from exhaustion if hyperactivity is not interrupted and rest is not achieved.

■ Monitor sleep patterns. Provide a structured schedule of activities that includes established times for naps or rest. Accurate baseline data are important in planning care to help the patient with this problem. A structured schedule, including time for short naps, will help the hyperactive patient achieve much-needed rest.

■ Patient should avoid intake of caffeinated drinks, such as tea, coffee, and colas. Caffeine is a central nervous system (CNS) stimulant and may interfere with the patient's achievement of rest and sleep.

■ Before bedtime, provide nursing measures that promote sleep, such as back rub; warm bath; warm, nonstimulating drinks; soft music; and relaxation exercises.

■ Administer sedative medications as ordered to help the patient achieve sleep until a normal sleep pattern is restored.

Concept Care Mapping

The concept map care plan (see Chapter 8, "The Nursing Process in Psychiatric-Mental Health Nursing") is a diagrammatic teaching and learning strategy that allows visualization of interrelationships between medical diagnoses, nursing diagnoses, assessment data, and treatments. An example of a concept map care plan for a patient experiencing a manic episode is presented in Figure 26–2.

Patient and Family Education

The role of patient teacher is important in the psychiatric area, as it is in all areas of nursing. A list of topics for patient and family education relevant to bipolar disorder is presented in Box 26–3.

Evaluation of Care for the Patient Experiencing a Manic Episode

In the final step of the nursing process, a reassessment is conducted to determine whether the nursing actions have been successful in achieving the objectives of care. Evaluation of the nursing actions for the patient experiencing a manic episode may be facilitated by gathering information using the following types of questions.

■ Has the individual avoided personal injury?
■ Has violence to the patient or others been prevented?
■ Has agitation subsided?
■ Have nutritional status and weight been stabilized? Is the patient able to select foods to maintain adequate nutrition?
■ Have delusions and hallucinations ceased? Is the patient able to interpret the environment correctly?
■ Is the patient able to make decisions about own self-care? Has hygiene and grooming improved?
■ Is behavior socially acceptable? Is patient able to interact with others in a satisfactory manner? Has the patient stopped manipulating others to fulfill their own desires?
■ Is the patient able to sleep 6 to 8 hours per night and awaken feeling rested?
■ Does the patient understand the importance of maintenance medication therapy? Does the patient understand that symptoms may return if medication is discontinued?
■ Can the patient taking lithium verbalize early signs of lithium toxicity? Does the patient understand the necessity for monthly blood level checks?

Treatment Modalities for Bipolar Disorder (Mania)

Individual Psychotherapy

In a review of the evidence on psychotherapy for clients with bipolar disorder, Swartz and Swanson (2014) concluded that bipolar-specific psychotherapies in conjunction with medication treatment have better outcomes than medication alone. Evidence supports the benefits of psychoeducation, cognitive behavior therapy (CBT), FFT, interpersonal and social rhythm therapy (IPSRT), and integrated care management (Strakowski, 2016).

IPSRT is a type of therapy specifically designed for bipolar clients. Developed by Frank (2005), IPSRT focuses on helping clients regulate social rhythms or daily activities such as the sleep–wakefulness cycle and exercise routines that may otherwise disrupt underlying biological rhythms and contribute to mood disturbances. In combination with this strategy, IPSRT also engages principles of interpersonal therapy to help clients address relationship problems.

Group Therapy

Once an acute phase of the illness has passed, groups can provide an atmosphere in which individuals may

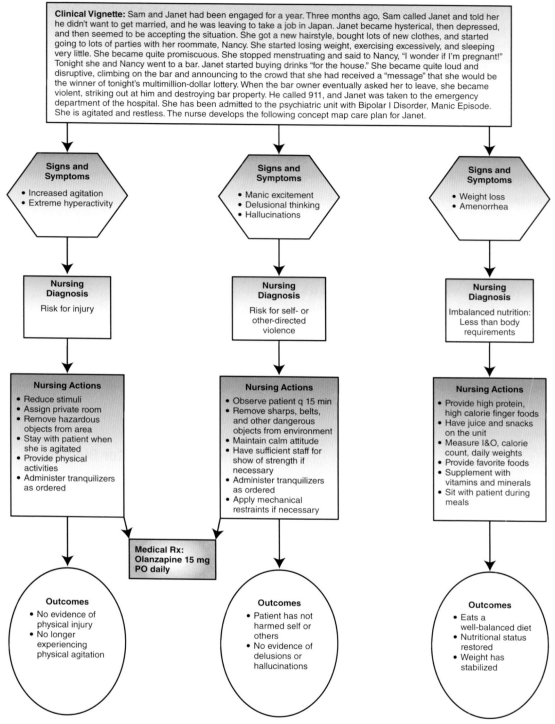

Clinical Vignette: Sam and Janet had been engaged for a year. Three months ago, Sam called Janet and told her he didn't want to get married, and he was leaving to take a job in Japan. Janet became hysterical, then depressed, and then seemed to be accepting the situation. She got a new hairstyle, bought lots of new clothes, and started going to lots of parties with her roommate, Nancy. She started losing weight, exercising excessively, and sleeping very little. She became quite promiscuous. She stopped menstruating and said to Nancy, "I wonder if I'm pregnant!" Tonight she and Nancy went to a bar. Janet started buying drinks "for the house." She became quite loud and disruptive, climbing on the bar and announcing to the crowd that she had received a "message" that she would be the winner of tonight's multimillion-dollar lottery. When the bar owner eventually asked her to leave, she became violent, striking out at him and destroying bar property. He called 911, and Janet was taken to the emergency department of the hospital. She has been admitted to the psychiatric unit with Bipolar I Disorder, Manic Episode. She is agitated and restless. The nurse develops the following concept map care plan for Janet.

FIGURE 26–2   Concept map care plan for a patient with bipolar disorder, manic episode.

discuss issues in their lives that cause, maintain, or arise from having a serious affective disorder. Both group psychoeducation and group CBT have demonstrated benefits for this population (Swartz & Swanson, 2014). The element of peer support may provide a feeling of security, as troublesome or embarrassing

issues are discussed and resolved. Some groups have other specific purposes, such as helping to monitor medication-related issues or promoting education related to the affective disorder and its treatment.

Support groups help members gain a sense of perspective on their condition and tangibly encourage

BOX 26–3 Topics for Patient and Family Education Related to Bipolar Disorder

NATURE OF THE ILLNESS
1. Causes of bipolar disorder
2. Cyclic nature of the illness
3. Symptoms of depression
4. Symptoms of mania

MANAGEMENT OF THE ILLNESS
1. Medication management
   a. Lithium
   b. Others
      1) Carbamazepine
      2) Valproic acid
      3) Clonazepam
      4) Verapamil
      5) Lamotrigine
      6) Gabapentin
      7) Topiramate
      8) Oxcarbazepine
      9) Olanzapine
      10) Risperidone
      11) Chlorpromazine
      12) Aripiprazole
      13) Quetiapine
      14) Ziprasidone
      15) Asenapine
   c. Side effects
   d. Symptoms of lithium toxicity
   e. Importance of regular blood tests
   f. Adverse effects
   g. Importance of not stopping medication, even when feeling well
2. Assertive techniques
3. Anger management
4. Strategies for illness symptom management

SUPPORT SERVICES
1. Crisis hotline
2. Support groups
3. Individual psychotherapy
4. Legal and/or financial assistance

them to connect with others who have common problems. A sense of hope is conveyed when the individual sees that they are not alone or unique in experiencing affective illness.

Self-help groups offer another avenue of support for the individual with bipolar disorder. These groups are usually peer-led and are not meant to substitute for or compete with professional therapy. They offer supplementary support that frequently enhances compliance with the medical regimen. Examples of self-help groups are the Depression and Bipolar Support Alliance (DBSA) and the Child and Adolescent Bipolar Foundation. These organizations have online resources to put individuals in touch with local support groups. Although self-help groups are not psychotherapy groups, they do provide important adjunctive support experiences that often have therapeutic benefit for participants.

Family Therapy

The ultimate objectives of working with families of clients with mood disorders are to resolve the symptoms and initiate or restore adaptive family functioning. Some studies focusing on bipolar disorder have shown that behavioral family treatment combined with medication substantially reduces relapse rates compared with medication therapy alone. Boland and Verduin (2022) suggested that efficacious family therapy may include education about the disorder, relapse prevention plans that are agreed upon by the whole family, and communication and problem-solving skills training.

Family functioning and marital relationships are often disrupted in clients with bipolar disorder, especially when symptoms are contributing to disloyalty in the marriage and financial problems related to the client's excessive spending behaviors. Whether intervention occurs in the form of family education, support, formal therapy, or a combination of these approaches, it is clear that families need to be involved in treatment whenever possible.

Cognitive Behavior Therapy

CBT is supported in evidence as an adjunctive treatment in all stages of the bipolar disorder except acute mania (Özdel et al., 2021). It has demonstrated effectiveness for decreasing the relapse rate, improving depressive symptoms and mania severity, and psychosocial functioning (Chiang et al., 2017). In CBT, the individual is taught to control thought distortions that are considered a factor in the development and maintenance of mood disorders. In the cognitive model, depression is characterized by a triad of negative distortions related to expectations of the environment, self, and future. The environment and activities within it are viewed as unsatisfying, the self is unrealistically devalued, and the future is perceived as hopeless. In the same model, mania is characterized by exaggeratedly positive cognitions and perceptions. The individual perceives the self as highly valued and powerful. Life is experienced with overstated self-assurance, and the future is viewed with unrealistic optimism.

The general goals in CBT are to obtain symptom relief as quickly as possible, assist the client in identifying dysfunctional patterns of thinking and behaving, and guide the individual to evidence and logic that effectively tests the validity of the dysfunctional thinking (see Chapter 18, "Cognitive Behavior

Therapy"). Therapy focuses on changing "automatic thoughts" that occur spontaneously and contribute to the distorted affect. Examples of automatic thoughts in bipolar mania include the following:

- **Personalizing:** "I'm the only reason my husband is a successful businessman."
- **All or nothing:** "Everything I do is great."
- **Mind reading:** "She thinks I'm wonderful."
- **Discounting negatives:** "None of those mistakes are really important."

The client is asked to describe evidence that both supports and disputes the automatic thought. The logic underlying the inferences is then reviewed with the client. Another technique involves evaluating what would most likely happen if the client's automatic thoughts were true. Implications of the consequences are then discussed.

Clients should not become discouraged if one technique does not seem to be working. No single technique works with all clients. Clients should be reassured that many techniques may be used, and both therapist and client may explore these possibilities.

The Recovery Model

Research provides support for recovery as an obtainable objective for individuals with bipolar disorder. See "Real, People, Real Stories" to learn more about Bridget's recovery journey. Conceptual models of recovery from mental illness are presented in Chapter 20, "The Recovery Model." The recovery model has been used primarily in caring for individuals with serious mental illness, such as schizophrenia and bipolar disorder. However, the concepts have utility for all individuals experiencing emotional conditions with which they require assistance and who have a desire to take control and manage their lives more independently.

Real People, Real Stories

BRIDGET'S STORY

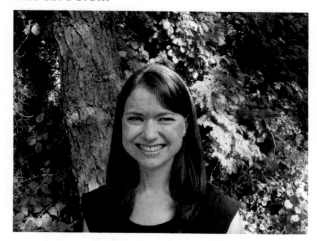

Bridget is a PhD, advanced practice registered nurse with bipolar disorder. Her story highlights the progression of her illness, her insights about illness management, and her courageous efforts to advocate for herself and others.

Karyn: I really appreciate you sharing your insights with other health-care professionals. So tell me about your history with bipolar disorder.

Bridget: I was diagnosed with depression at the age of 13, was on medication for that, and was stable until about 24 years of age. At that time I was working on night shift as a labor and delivery nurse. I remember having a very stressful night and some ethical disagreements with some others and I couldn't sleep for a couple of nights. It threw me into a manic episode. I took melatonin and Nyquil and had a bad reaction. I was having visual hallucinations of interconnecting lights. I have heard other people say that Nyquil can trigger that.

Karyn: I have also read of accounts of people having hallucinations in reaction to dextromethorphan. What happened next?

Bridget: I didn't sleep for days. It was acute and recognizable; very uncomfortable and very scary. I was too sick to return to work and still very upset about ongoing disagreements about patient care issues, so when I returned to work it was at a different hospital that rotated shifts. Rotating working the night and day shift worked better for my health. I would work 2 weeks of the night shift and then rotate to working 4 weeks of the day shift. Although not as ideal as working straight day shifts, this month of day shifts allowed me to catch up and stabilize my sleep.

I got accepted into a midwifery program and between the stresses of work, moving, and school, I had a second episode; first manic then depressive. I was concerned that I would have to drop out of school because I couldn't manage graduate school classes along with my recovery. In addition, I read about the importance of regulating sleep patterns in managing this illness and a midwife's schedule requires very irregular sleep patterns. Babies are not born nine to five. However, I couldn't drop out or even go part-time or else I would lose my health insurance. My professors really helped me work out arrangements and accommodations so I could remain a student and keep my insurance and continue working on my degree in midwifery.

The next couple of years I was stable but it was frightening; I never knew how well I would recover from episodes. I had a counselor tell me I might have to cut back my expectations for my life. I went to support groups and felt like they brought me down more; there was a lot of complaining and one person told me I would probably only be able to work part-time. I had different expectations for what I wanted to do.

Karyn: How long does an acute episode typically last?

Bridget: The manic episodes seem to be sudden in onset then it "gets dark" and then it's a slow return. The worst episode has been for 2 months but I would say full recovery takes around 9 months to 1 year. After that I'm able to get back into the swing of things.

Karyn: What do you mean when you say it "gets dark"?

Bridget: It's very frightening. There is a sense of loss of control. I lose weight quickly and people think I'm anorexic but it's just that my metabolism gets really fast. Not being able to sleep adds to the traumatization. Then there's the depression and suicidal thoughts. That's when it gets really dark. But I was stable for a 2–3-year period before I had a third episode. That was the worst one. I was going through another stressful period but some of it was positive stress; graduating from school, in a new relationship, accepted to a prestigious program for doctoral nursing study, and I was going through some medication changes. It seemed like any treatment was just "putting a bottle cap on a tidal wave." I was hospitalized three times, was having symptoms of psychosis, and it took about a year to get back on track. It's been 6 years since that last episode.

Karyn: What do you think has been most helpful in moving toward this recovery?

Bridget: Having a supportive family. My family has knowledge and history with mental illnesses and that has been a blessing. In my family, recovery is the expectation and chronic illness is the exception. Also, I have long-term friends that stuck with me and never gave up on me; even my doctor said I have amazing friends. The medications are important even though I have a love-hate relationship with them. The only time I refused medication it was because I thought I was having a bad reaction, but people thought I was just not recognizing I was sick. It's still a blurry line ... the judgments were snap ... in fairness, I was a lot to handle ... but it was scary. I was being told I had to take something I felt was hurting me so I was uncooperative. Now I recognize they were well-intentioned people doing the best they could.

Also I found work I love; as a childbirth educator. I got married and that has been a stabilizing factor. The medications seem to be working. I had been taking Trileptal but I stopped taking that so I wouldn't have to worry about its effects when I got pregnant, and my workplace has been accommodating.

Karyn: Accommodating?

Bridget: Well, I had been in circumstances before my current job; like once I was shoved by a coworker and I threw milk at her. The coworker maintained they were justified. In another circumstance when a coworker found out I had bipolar disorder she told my supervisor I should not be able to work there. I was very scared and felt like I had to become a strong advocate for myself. The truth is my illness requires little accommodation most of the time. When I am well, I am very well and a fairly high functioning person. I get sick fairly infrequently and when I do, I just need some time to recover, just like any other illness. It does help to have understanding and compassion from my superiors. When I've been able to garner support from them, I've been able to pursue recovery and my life goals.

There was a journal editor and a mentor I connected with after grad school that was so encouraging in terms of me pursuing my PhD. At the time, I had so much shame and guilt about having bipolar disorder, but she extended compassion to me that I wasn't even able to extend to myself. She saw and encouraged me to work to my full potential.

Karyn: What are the most important things that you want nurses to know about providing care for patients with bipolar disorder, particularly in an acute manic episode?

Bridget: Number one: Better listening is key. Even if the patient does not seem to be making sense, there most likely is a kernel of truth in what they are saying. Be patient. Listen and look for that kernel of truth. I remember trying to talk to my psychiatrist about wanting lithium but we never got to discuss that because he was yelling at me that I was being uncooperative with the hospital treatment plan. I signed out AMA because ... it felt safer. That's a whole other story.

Number two: A little compassion goes a long way. Patients can tell right away who is there to help them and who is just there for the paycheck.

Number three: Look patients in the eye and call them by their name. Many people, when they are in an acute episode of illness, feel very lost and confused; talking to them directly and personally is really grounding. It helps people reclaim their dignity. Remember, being sick is hard: whether it's cancer or diabetes or bipolar disorder. It takes a lot to manage. Trust that people are truly doing the best that they can with the resources they are given. The mental health system can be very difficult to navigate, especially when someone is acutely ill. It makes it hard to get stabilized and get better. The more you can treat people with dignity, respect their requests when possible, listen, and offer compassion, the better they will do.

In a systematic review of qualitative research on patient perspectives with regard to their support needs from health-care professionals (Beentjes et al., 2020), individuals with severe mental illness identified that empowering them in their self-management (recovery) efforts requires five elements: information support, emotional support, acknowledgment (validation that symptoms are part of their illness, that they are not stupid, to be taken seriously, and to be given time to talk), encouragement, and guidance.

In bipolar disorder, recovery is a continuous process. The individual identifies goals based on personal values or what they define as giving meaning and purpose to life. The clinician and client work together to develop a treatment plan that is in alignment with the goals set forth by the client. In the recovery process, the individual may continue to experience symptoms but collaborates with clinicians to develop a management strategy. Management strategies include the following:

- Developing self-awareness
- Becoming an expert on the disorder
- Taking medications regularly
- Avoiding drugs and alcohol
- Recognizing earliest symptoms
- Identifying and reducing sources of stress
- Knowing when to seek help
- Developing a personal support system
- Managing lifestyle factors such as sleep time and exercise
- Developing a plan for emergencies

Throughout the ongoing recovery process, individuals actively work on the strategies they have identified to keep themselves well. The clinician serves as a support person to help the individual take the necessary steps to achieve the goals they had previously set forth.

Although there is no cure for bipolar disorder, there are effective treatments and interventions. Recovery is possible when the client is empowered and actively engaged in a multifaceted illness management approach.

Electroconvulsive Therapy

Episodes of acute mania are occasionally treated with electroconvulsive therapy (ECT), particularly when the client does not tolerate or fails to respond to lithium or other drug treatment or when life is threatened by dangerous behavior or exhaustion. See Chapter 19, "Electroconvulsive Therapy," for a detailed discussion of ECT.

One recent study (McGirr et al., 2021) explored the use of intermittent transcranial magnetic stimulation (which has been used for the treatment of major depression) for patients with acute bipolar depression. However, the study was terminated when they found it to be ineffective, and in some cases, to increase risk for triggering a hypomanic episode.

Bright Light Therapy

Bright light therapy (BLT) may have benefits for patients with bipolar depression. Circadian rhythm dysregulation has been linked to the disorder itself and to several symptoms common in bipolar disorder, including sleep disturbances and metabolic changes (Nasr et al., 2018). Although the mechanism of action is unclear, it is hypothesized that BLT may "reset" areas of the brain associated with circadian rhythm regulation. Current evidence supports that BLT improves symptoms of bipolar depression and is not associated with mood shifts toward a manic episode (Sit et al., 2017; Tseng et al., 2016; Zhou et al., 2018).

Psychopharmacology With Mood-Stabilizing Agents

For many years, the drug of choice for treatment and management of bipolar *mania* was lithium carbonate. However, in recent years many investigators and clinicians in practice have more often used other medications, including antipsychotic drugs and anticonvulsant drugs that have a mood-stabilizing effect, either alone or in combination with lithium. Laski and associates (2022) promoted that lithium should continue to be a first-line treatment for bipolar disorder based on research demonstrating lithium's superior effectiveness in reducing suicides and evidence suggesting that lithium may afford some level of protection against dementia. (See Chapter 4, "Psychopharmacology," for a detailed discussion of indications, actions, contraindications, and other safety issues related to mood-stabilizing agents.)

Both lithium and other mood stabilizers also demonstrate effectiveness in managing bipolar *depression*. Five antipsychotic medications are currently approved by the FDA for managing depressive episodes in bipolar disorder: olanzapine/fluoxetine combinations, quetiapine/quetiapine XR, lurasidone, cariprazine, and lumateperone (Meyer, 2022). More recently, Lybalvi, a combination drug of olanzapine and samidorphan (an opioid antagonist), has been approved for bipolar I disorder (and schizophrenia) with research that demonstrated significantly less weight gain than treatment with olanzapine alone (Citrome, 2022). Calabrese (2022) noted that antidepressants as monotherapy should be used with caution and perhaps avoided altogether if the patient has mood switching (from depression to hypomanic or manic episodes), rapid cycling without antidepressant therapy, or mixed symptoms. Strakowski (2016) identified that antidepressants carry as high as a 40% risk of potentially triggering a switch from depression to mania in individuals with bipolar disorder.

People who respond to lithium can be virtually symptom-free over the long term. Because only about 33% of people treated with lithium respond positively (Rybakowski, 2014), the availability of other pharmacological treatments is important in the treatment of this illness. Because bipolar disorder is a chronic, episodic illness, most people will remain on medication throughout their lives. See Table 26–3 for a list of commonly used medications in the treatment of bipolar disorder. Lithium, like other medications, has side effects. Most notably, when the therapeutic range (0.6–1.2 mEq/L) is exceeded, toxic side effects and death can occur.

Calcium channel blockers, a class of medications used to treat hypertension and cardiac arrhythmias, have been used off-label as a treatment for bipolar disorder based on evidence (D'Onofrio et al., 2017) that a calcium signaling dysfunction may be occurring in people with bipolar disorder (lithium carbonate has also been shown to down-regulate Ca^{2+} activity). To date, though, it has not become an established or common therapeutic approach.

Patient and Family Education for Lithium

The patient should:

■ Take medication regularly, even when feeling well. Discontinuation can result in the return of symptoms.
■ Not drive or operate dangerous machinery until lithium levels are stabilized. Drowsiness and dizziness can occur.
■ Maintain an adequate dietary sodium intake. Eat a variety of healthy foods, avoid "junk" foods, drink six to eight large glasses of water each day and avoid excessive use of beverages containing caffeine (coffee, tea, colas), which promote increased urine output.
■ Notify the physician if vomiting or diarrhea occurs. These symptoms can result in sodium loss and an increased risk of lithium toxicity.
■ Carry a card or other identification noting that they are taking lithium.
■ Be aware of appropriate diet should weight gain become a problem. Include adequate sodium and other nutrients while decreasing number of calories.
■ Be aware of risks of becoming pregnant while receiving lithium therapy. Notify the physician as soon as possible if pregnancy is suspected or planned.
■ Be aware of side effects and symptoms associated with toxicity. Notify the physician if any of the following symptoms occur: persistent nausea and vomiting, severe diarrhea, ataxia, blurred vision, tinnitus, excessive urine output, increasing tremors, or mental confusion.
■ Refer to written materials furnished by healthcare providers while receiving self-administered maintenance therapy. Keep appointments for outpatient follow-up; have serum lithium level checked every 1 to 2 months or as advised by physician.

TABLE 26–3 Selected Medications for the Treatment of Bipolar Disorder

CLASSIFICATION: GENERIC (TRADE)	CONTRAINDICATIONS/PRECAUTIONS	DAILY ADULT DOSAGE RANGE
ANTIMANIC		
Lithium carbonate (Eskalith, Lithobid)	Hypersensitivity Cardiac or renal disease, dehydration, sodium depletion, brain damage, pregnancy and lactation Caution with thyroid disorders, diabetes, urinary retention, history of seizures, and the elderly	Acute mania: 1,800–2,400 mg Maintenance: 900–1,200 mg Therapeutic range: 0.6–1.2 mEq/L
ANTICONVULSANTS		
Carbamazepine (Tegretol)	Hypersensitivity With MAOIs, lactation Caution with elderly; liver, renal, cardiac disease; pregnancy	200–1,600 mg Therapeutic range: 4–12 mcg/mL
Clonazepam (Klonopin)	Hypersensitivity, glaucoma, liver disease, lactation Caution in elderly; liver, renal disease; pregnancy	0.5–20 mg Therapeutic range: 0.02–0.08 mcg/mL
Valproic acid (Depakene; Depakote [also contains sodium valproate])	Hypersensitivity, liver disease Caution in elderly; renal, cardiac diseases; pregnancy and lactation	5 mg/kg–60 mg/kg Therapeutic range: 50–150 mcg/mL

Continued

TABLE 26–3 Selected Medications for the Treatment of Bipolar Disorder—cont'd

CLASSIFICATION: GENERIC (TRADE)	CONTRAINDICATIONS/PRECAUTIONS	DAILY ADULT DOSAGE RANGE
Lamotrigine (Lamictal)	Hypersensitivity Caution in renal and hepatic insufficiency, pregnancy, lactation, and children <16 years old	100–200 mg
Gabapentin (Neurontin)	Hypersensitivity and children <3 years Caution in renal insufficiency, pregnancy, lactation, children, and the elderly	900–1,800 mg
Topiramate (Topamax)	Hypersensitivity Caution in renal and hepatic impairment, pregnancy, lactation, children, and the elderly	50–400 mg
Oxcarbazepine (Trileptal)	Hypersensitivity Caution in renal and hepatic impairment, pregnancy, lactation, children, and the elderly	600–2,400 mg
ANTIPSYCHOTICS		
Olanzapine (Zyprexa) Olanzapine-samidorphan (Lybalvi) *Also FDA approved for the treatment of bipolar depression	Hypersensitivity, children, lactation Caution with hepatic or cardiovascular disease, history of seizures, coma or other CNS depression, prostatic hypertrophy, narrow-angle glaucoma, diabetes or risk factors for diabetes, pregnancy, elderly and debilitated patients, history of suicide attempts Olanzapine-samidorphan is contraindicated in patients using opioids or undergoing acute opioid withdrawal	10–20 mg 5 mg/10 mg–20 mg/ 10 mg
Olanzapine and fluoxetine (Symbyax)		6/25–12/50 mg/
Aripiprazole (Abilify) (Abilify Maintenance)		10–30 mg 300 mg–400 mg (IM once monthly)
Lurasidone (Latuda) *Also FDA approved for the treatment of bipolar depression		20–120 mg
Cariprazine (Vraylar) *Also FDA approved for the treatment of bipolar depression		1.5 mg–6 mg
Quetiapine (Seroquel) Quetiapine XR		100–800 mg
Risperidone (Risperdal)		1–6 mg
Ziprasidone (Geodon)		40–160 mg
Asenapine (Saphris)		10–20 mg
Lumateperone (Caplyta) *Also FDA approved for the treatment of bipolar depression		42 mg 21 mg when there is moderate or severe hepatic impairment

CNS, Central nervous system, IM, intramuscular; MAOI, monoamine oxidase inhibitor.

Patient and Family Education for Anticonvulsant Mood Stabilizers

The patient should:

- Refrain from discontinuing the drug abruptly. Physician will administer orders for tapering the drug when therapy is to be discontinued.
- Report the following symptoms to the physician immediately: skin rash, unusual bleeding, spontaneous bruising, sore throat, fever, malaise, dark urine, and yellow skin or eyes.
- Not drive or operate dangerous machinery until reaction to the medication has been established.
- Avoid consuming alcoholic beverages and nonprescription medications without approval from physician.
- Carry a card at all times identifying the name of medications being taken.

CLINICAL PEARL The FDA requires that all antiepileptic (anticonvulsant) drugs carry a warning label indicating that use of the drugs increases risk for suicidal thoughts and behaviors. Patients being treated with these medications should be monitored for the emergence or worsening of depression, suicidal thoughts or behavior, or any unusual changes in mood or behavior.

Patient and Family Education for Calcium Channel Blockers

The patient should:

- Take medication with meals if gastrointestinal upset occurs.
- Use caution when driving or when operating dangerous machinery. Dizziness, drowsiness, and blurred vision can occur.
- Refrain from discontinuing the drug abruptly. To do so may precipitate cardiovascular problems. Physician will administer orders for tapering the drug when therapy is to be discontinued.
- Report occurrence of any of the following symptoms to physician immediately: irregular heartbeat, shortness of breath, swelling of the hands and feet, pronounced dizziness, chest pain, profound mood swings, severe and persistent headache.
- Rise slowly from a sitting or lying position to prevent a sudden drop in blood pressure.
- Avoid taking other medications (including over-the-counter [OTC] medications) without a physician's approval.
- Carry a card at all times describing medications being taken.

Patient and Family Education for Antipsychotics

The patient should:

- Use caution when driving or operating dangerous machinery. Drowsiness and dizziness can occur.

- Refrain from discontinuing the drug abruptly after long-term use. To do so might produce withdrawal symptoms, such as nausea, vomiting, dizziness, gastritis, headache, tachycardia, insomnia, and tremulousness. The physician will administer orders for tapering the drug when therapy is to be discontinued.
- Use sunblock lotion and wear protective clothing when spending time outdoors. Skin is more susceptible to sunburn, which can occur in as little as 30 minutes.
- Report the occurrence of any of the following symptoms to the physician immediately: sore throat, fever, malaise, unusual bleeding, easy bruising, persistent nausea and vomiting, severe headache, rapid heart rate, difficulty urinating, muscle twitching, tremors, dark-colored urine, excessive urination, excessive thirst, excessive hunger, weakness, pale stools, yellow skin or eyes, muscular incoordination, or skin rash.
- Rise slowly from a sitting or lying position to prevent a sudden drop in blood pressure.
- Take frequent sips of water, chew sugarless gum, or suck on hard candy if dry mouth is a problem. Good oral care (frequent brushing, flossing) is very important.
- Consult the physician regarding smoking while on antipsychotic therapy. Smoking increases the metabolism of these drugs, requiring an adjustment in dosage to achieve a therapeutic effect.
- Dress warmly in cold weather and avoid extended exposure to very high or low temperatures. Body temperature is harder to maintain with this medication.
- Avoid drinking alcohol while on antipsychotic therapy. These substances potentiate each other's effects.
- Avoid taking other medications (including OTC products) without the physician's approval. Many medications contain substances that interact with antipsychotic medications in a way that may be harmful.
- Be aware of possible risks of taking antipsychotics during pregnancy. Antipsychotics are thought to readily cross the placenta and may cause adverse fetal effects. Inform the physician immediately if pregnancy occurs, is suspected, or is planned.
- Be aware of side effects of antipsychotic medications. Refer to written materials furnished by health-care providers for safe self-administration.
- Continue to take the medication even if feeling well. Symptoms may return if medication is discontinued.
- Carry a card or other identification at all times describing medications being taken.

CLINICAL JUDGMENT IN ACTION: CASE STUDY AND SAMPLE CARE PLAN

NURSING HISTORY AND ASSESSMENT

Recognizing cues: The nurse must demonstrate ability to recognize what information is most important to making an assessment (National Council of State Boards of Nursing [NCSBN], 2021). This information is italicized in the following.

Candace, age 32, recently moved to New York City from Omaha, Nebraska, where she had been working as a television reporter. She felt that Omaha had become "too boring" and wanted to experience the big city life. Candace *has a history of bipolar I disorder* and has been maintained *on lithium since she was 23 years old.* Since she arrived in New York City, she has *run out of her medication and has not found a doctor to have her prescription renewed.* She has been staying in an inexpensive apartment and living on savings. She has been seeking employment in her chosen line of work, but it has been *2 months now,* and she has been *unable to find a job.* She is *becoming anxious as her savings have depleted.* She has *lost 15 lbs. and has trouble sleeping.*

Today, *after two failed interviews, Candace went to a bar and began drinking.* She *ordered several rounds of drinks for everyone in the bar and told the bartender to "put it on my tab."* The bartender called the police when Candace *refused to pay her tab and became loud and belligerent.* He said she began *shouting that she knew the mayor, and he was going to help her find a job, and if they didn't leave her alone, she would tell the mayor how they were treating her.* She took out her cell phone and said she was calling the mayor. When others in the room began laughing at her, she began cursing and *saying that they "would be sorry one day that they laughed at her."* When the police arrived, Candace *was resistant and had to be physically restrained.* The police took Candace to the emergency department of the community hospital, where she was admitted with a **diagnosis of Bipolar I Disorder, current episode manic.** The psychiatrist ordered olanzapine 10 mg IM STAT, olanzapine 10 mg PO daily, lithium carbonate 600 mg PO bid, and vitamin supplement daily and ordered her lithium level to be tested before administration of the first dose of lithium.

Analyzing cues: The nurse must be able to interpret the information (NCSBN, 2021).

The nurse interprets that Candace, after having been without medication for 2 months, is experiencing a relapse of bipolar disorder. The symptoms are interfering with her physical well-being as evidenced by weight loss and trouble sleeping. Her false belief about her connection to the mayor and her purchasing drinks for people without money to pay for them suggests grandiose ideation and her threats toward patrons warrants further assessment

for risk of other-directed violence. Her drinking behavior in response to disappointments may suggest the need for further assessment r/t substance misuse.

Prioritize hypotheses: The nurse must be able to identify the client's most important needs (NCSBN, 2021).

The nurse prioritizes safety needs, the two most pressing of which are Candace's significant weight loss in the last 2 months and her risk for violence toward others or self-injury while she is in an agitated state. The most immediate of these protecting her safety from self- or other-directed violence.

NURSING DIAGNOSES AND OUTCOME IDENTIFICATION

Generate solutions: The nurse must be able to connect their prioritized understanding of client needs to a course of action or plan of care (NCSBN, 2021).

From the assessment data, the admitting nurse develops the following nursing diagnoses for Candace:

1. Risk for self- or other-directed violence related to manic hyperactivity, delusional thinking, impulsivity
   a. Short-Term Goal:
      ■ Agitation and hyperactivity will be maintained at a manageable level with the administration of tranquilizing medication.
   b. Long-Term Goal:
      ■ Candace will not harm self or others during hospitalization.
2. Imbalanced nutrition: Less than body requirements related to lack of appetite and excessive physical agitation, evidenced by loss of weight.
   a. Short-Term Goal:
      ■ Candace will consume sufficient finger foods and between-meal snacks to meet recommended daily allowances of nutrients.
   b. Long-Term Goal:
      ■ Candace will begin to regain weight and exhibit no signs or symptoms of malnutrition.

PLANNING AND IMPLEMENTATION

Take Action: The nurse must be able to identify what actions need to be taken and how they will be implemented (NCSBN, 2021).

RISK FOR SELF- OR OTHER-DIRECTED VIOLENCE

The following nursing interventions have been identified for Candace:

1. Place Candace in a private room near the nurse's station. Observe her behavior frequently.
2. Remove all dangerous objects from her environment.
3. Plan some physical activities for Candace (e.g., treadmill, exercise bike) and regular rest periods during the day.

CLINICAL JUDGMENT IN ACTION: CASE STUDY AND SAMPLE CARE PLAN—cont'd

4. Administer tranquilizing medication as ordered by physician.
5. Monitor lithium levels three times during the first week of therapy. Monitor for signs and symptoms of toxicity (e.g., ataxia, blurred vision, severe diarrhea, persistent nausea and vomiting, tinnitus).
6. Ensure that sufficient staff is available to intervene should Candace become agitated and aggressive.

IMBALANCED NUTRITION: LESS THAN BODY REQUIREMENTS

The following nursing interventions have been identified for Candace:

1. Consult dietitian to determine appropriate diet for Candace to restore nutrition and gain weight. Ensure that her diet includes foods that she particularly likes.
2. Ensure that Candace has access to finger foods and between-meal snacks if she cannot or will not sit still to eat off a meal tray.
3. Maintain an accurate record of intake, output, and calorie count.
4. Obtain daily weights.
5. Administer vitamin supplement, as ordered by physician.
6. Sit with Candace during mealtime.

EVALUATION

Evaluate outcomes: The nurse must be able to evaluate actions taken and determine whether they have had a positive, neutral, or negative effect (NCSBN, 2021).

The outcome criteria identified for Candace have been met. She has not harmed herself or others in any way. She is able to verbalize names of resources outside the hospital from whom she may request help if needed. With help from the social worker, she has applied for unemployment assistance and will begin receiving help within 2 weeks. She has gained 3 pounds in the hospital and verbalizes understanding of the importance of maintaining good nutrition. She is taking her medication regularly and has a follow-up appointment with the psychiatric nurse practitioner, who will see Candace biweekly to evaluate adherence with medication and laboratory requirements. Candace verbalizes understanding of the importance of taking her medication continuously. She has a hopeful but realistic attitude about finding work in New York City and states that she will give herself a deadline after which she plans to return to her home in Omaha where she will be near family and friends.

Summary and Key Points

■ Bipolar disorder is manifested by mood swings from profound depression to extreme elation and euphoria.

■ Genetic influences have been strongly implicated in the development of bipolar disorder. Various physiological factors, such as biochemical and electrolyte alterations, as well as cerebral structural changes, have been implicated. Side effects of certain medications may also induce symptoms of mania. No single theory can explain the etiology of bipolar disorder, and it is likely that the illness is caused by a combination of factors.

■ Symptoms of mania may be observed on a continuum of three phases, each identified by the degree of severity: phase I, hypomania; phase II, acute mania; and phase III, delirious mania.

■ The symptoms of bipolar disorder may occur in children and adolescents as well as in adults.

■ Treatment of bipolar disorder may include individual therapy, group and family therapy, cognitive therapy, ECT, BLT, and psychopharmacology. For the majority of people, the most effective treatment appears to be a combination of psychotropic medication and psychosocial therapy.

■ Some clinicians choose a course of therapy based on a model of recovery similar to that used for many years to treat addiction. The basic premise of a recovery model is empowerment of the client; it is designed to allow people primary control over decisions about their care and to enable a person with a mental health problem to live a meaningful life in a community of choice while striving to achieve their full potential.

■ For many years, the pharmacological treatment of choice for bipolar mania was lithium carbonate. Several other medications are now being used with satisfactory results, including anticonvulsants and antipsychotics.

■ There is a narrow margin between the therapeutic and toxic levels of lithium. Serum lithium levels must be monitored regularly while on maintenance therapy.

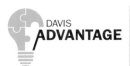
DAVIS ADVANTAGE

Go to **Davis Advantage** to complete your learning: strengthen understanding, apply your knowledge, and prepare for the Next Gen NCLEX®.

Review Questions

1. One way to promote adequate nutritional intake for a client in an acute manic episode who is not eating is to:
   a. Sit with the client during meals to reinforce the importance of eating everything on the tray.
   b. Have family members bring food from home so the client will have only favorite foods.
   c. Provide high-calorie, nutritious finger foods and snacks that can be eaten "on the run."
   d. Restrict the client to their room until they begin to gain weight.

2. The physician orders lithium carbonate 600 mg tid for a newly diagnosed patient with bipolar I disorder. There is a narrow margin between the therapeutic and toxic levels of lithium. The therapeutic range for *acute* mania is:
   a. .6–1.2 mEq/L
   b. .1–5 mEq/L
   c. Above 1.2 mEq/L
   d. 6–12 mEq/L

3. Although historically lithium has been the medication of choice for mania, several others have been used with good results. Which of the following are used in the treatment of bipolar disorder? (Select all that apply.)
   a. Olanzapine (Zyprexa)
   b. Oxycodone (OxyContin)
   c. Carbamazepine (Tegretol)
   d. Gabapentin (Neurontin)
   e. Tranylcypromine (Parnate)

4. A client who is experiencing a manic episode is admitted to the psychiatric unit after being brought to the emergency department by a family member. The client yells, "I need to get out of here because the interplanetary council has elected me president of the universe." This behavior is an example of:
   a. A delusion of grandeur
   b. A delusion of persecution
   c. An auditory hallucination
   d. Lithium toxicity

5. Which is the most common comorbid condition in children with bipolar disorder?
   a. Schizophrenia
   b. Substance disorders
   c. Oppositional defiant disorder
   d. Attention deficit-hyperactivity disorder

6. A nurse is educating a patient about their lithium therapy and explaining the signs and symptoms of lithium toxicity. Which of the following would she instruct the patient to be on the alert for?
   a. Fever, sore throat, malaise
   b. Tinnitus, severe diarrhea, ataxia
   c. Occipital headache, palpitations, chest pain
   d. Skin rash, marked rise in blood pressure, bradycardia

Clinical Judgment Questions

7. A client is brought to the emergency department by a family member who reports that the client stopped taking mood stabilizer medication a few months ago and is now agitated, pacing, demanding, and speaking very loudly. The family member reports that the client eats very little, is losing weight, and almost never sleep. What is the *priority* nursing diagnosis?
   a. Imbalanced nutrition: Less than body requirements related to not eating
   b. Risk for injury related to hyperactivity
   c. Disturbed sleep pattern related to agitation
   d. Ineffective coping related to denial of depression

8. A female client experiencing a manic episode enters the milieu area dressed in a provocative and physically revealing outfit. Which of the following is the most appropriate intervention by the nurse?
   a. Tell her, in front of the other patients, that she cannot dress like a whore while she is in the hospital.
   b. Do nothing and allow her to learn from the responses of her peers.
   c. Quietly walk with her back to her room and help her change into something more appropriate.
   d. Explain to her that if she wears this outfit, she must remain in her room.

9. The nurse is providing medication education to a client on lithium. Which of the following are important points to include? (Select all that apply.)
   a. Significant reductions in sodium intake increase the risk for lithium toxicity.
   b. Weight loss is a common side effect of lithium.
   c. Serum lithium levels will need to be checked at regular intervals throughout treatment.
   d. Lithium therapy should be continued even during periods when the patient feels well.

10. A client admitted to the inpatient psychiatric unit with bipolar disorder tells the nurse, "I need to sit in on change-of-shift report because I have been appointed director of this unit." Which action by the nurse demonstrates the best clinical judgment at this point?
    a. Invite the client to sit in on the change-of-shift report, but do not share any confidential client information.
    b. Instruct the client that this is not permitted and redirect the client to other unit activities that are available.
    c. Tell the client that she is delusional but that these symptoms will go away with medication.
    d. Place the client in seclusion for protection of self and others.

IMPLICATIONS OF RESEARCH FOR EVIDENCE-BASED PRACTICE

Zimmerman, M., Balling, C., Dalrymple, K., & Chelminski, I. (2019). Screening for borderline personality disorder in psychiatric outpatients with major depressive disorder and bipolar disorder. *Journal of Clinical Psychiatry, 80*(1), 18m12257. https://doi.org/10.4088/JCP.18m12257

DESCRIPTION OF THE STUDY: Bipolar disorder is often confused with borderline personality disorder because of several mood symptoms that appear to overlap between the two disorders. In addition, borderline personality disorder and bipolar disorder are sometimes comorbid conditions. Noting that borderline personality disorder is a serious illness and frequently underdiagnosed, the researchers used a semistructured, DSM-criteria interview to attempt to differentiate borderline personality disorder from bipolar disorder and from MDD (n = 3764).

RESULTS OF THE STUDY: The researchers' findings supported that screening for affective instability was highly predictive of borderline personality disorder (greater than 90% sensitivity) in patients with MDD, bipolar disorder, and other diagnoses.

IMPLICATIONS FOR NURSING PRACTICE: Affective instability, one of the *DSM-5-TR* criteria for diagnosing borderline personality disorder, is related to "a marked reactivity of mood (e.g., intense episodic dysphoria, irritability, or anxiety usually lasting a few hours and rarely more than a few days" (APA, 2022, p. 753). This is unlike the mood swings from depression to elation that are seen in bipolar disorder in that the mood changes in borderline personality disorder are rapid, shorter lived, difficult to regulate, and often triggered by interpersonal events in the environment. Nurses should recognize the potential for confusion between symptoms of bipolar disorder and borderline personality disorder and consider screening for evidence of affective instability to determine whether a treatment plan for borderline personality disorder, in addition to bipolar disorder, is appropriate. This may be accomplished by incorporating established screening tools such as the Affective Lability Scale or the Affective Intensity Scale and through semistructured interview questions.

TEST YOUR CLINICAL REASONING AND CLINICAL JUDGMENT SKILLS

Allie, age 29, had been working in the typing pool of a large corporation for 6 years. Her immediate supervisor recently retired, and Allie was promoted to supervisor, in charge of 20 people in the department. She was flattered by the promotion but anxious about the additional responsibility of the position. Shortly after the promotion, she overheard two of her former coworkers saying, "Why in the world did they choose her? She's not the best one for the job. I know *I* certainly won't be able to respect her as a boss!" Hearing these comments added to Allie's anxiety and self-doubt.

Shortly after Allie began her new duties, her friends and coworkers noticed a change. She had a great deal of energy and worked long hours on her job. She began to speak very loudly and rapidly. Her roommate noticed that Allie slept very little yet seldom appeared tired. Every night she would go out to bars and dances. Sometimes she brought men she had just met home to the apartment, something she had never done before. She bought lots of clothes and makeup and had her hair restyled in a more youthful look. She failed to pay her share of the rent and bills but came home with a brand new convertible. She lost her temper and screamed at her roommate, "Mind your own business!" when asked to pay her share.

She became irritable at work, and several of her subordinates reported her behavior to the corporate manager. When the manager confronted Allie about her behavior, she lost control, shouting, cursing, and striking out at anyone and anything that happened to be within her reach. The security officers restrained her and took her to the emergency department of the hospital, where she was admitted to the psychiatric unit. She had no previous history of psychiatric illness.

The psychiatrist assigned a diagnosis of bipolar I disorder and wrote orders for olanzapine (Zyprexa) 10 mg IM STAT, olanzapine 15 mg PO daily, and lithium carbonate 600 mg tid.

Answer the following questions related to Allie:

1. What are the most important considerations for the nurse who is taking care of Allie?
2. Why was Allie given the diagnosis of bipolar I disorder?
3. The doctor should order a lithium level drawn after 4 to 6 days. For what symptoms should the nurse be on alert?
4. Why did the physician order olanzapine in addition to the lithium carbonate?

Communication Exercises

1. Kyle, a newly admitted patient diagnosed with bipolar disorder, states to the nurse, "I was looking at the sky, blue is the color of my eyes, too. I went to Florida on a plane."

   How might the nurse respond to this patient's statement?

2. Darcy, who is in a manic phase of bipolar disorder, is jumping from chair to chair in the patient lounge during visiting hours, loudly proclaiming to the visitors that she is a famous gymnast. She begins doing somersaults, nearly tripping a visitor.

   How might the nurse respond to the patient at this point?

 MOVIE CONNECTIONS

Lust for Life (bipolar disorder) • *Call Me Anna* (bipolar disorder) • *Blue Sky* (bipolar disorder) • *A Woman Under the Influence* (bipolar disorder) • *Mr. Jones* (bipolar disorder) • *Frances* (bipolar disorder) • *The Whole Wide World* (bipolar disorder) • *Pollock* (bipolar disorder) • *Silver Linings Playbook* (bipolar disorder) • *Touched With Fire* (bipolar disorder)

References

Aas, M., Henry, C., Andreassen, O. A., Bellivier, F., Melle, I., & Etain, B. (2016). The role of childhood trauma in bipolar disorders. *International Journal of Bipolar Disorders, 4*(2), 1–10. doi:10.1186/s40345-015-0042-0

Akiskal, H. S. (2017). Mood disorders: Historical introduction and conceptual overview. In Sadock, B. J., Sadock, V. A., & Ruiz, P. (Eds.), *Comprehensive textbook of psychiatry* (10th ed., pp. 1599–1603). Wolters Kluwer.

American Psychiatric Association (APA). (2022). *Diagnostic and statistical manual of mental disorders, fifth edition, text revision (DSM-5-TR).* American Psychiatric Association.

Beentjes, T. A. A., van Gaal, B. G. I., van Achterberg, T., & Goossens, P. J. J. (2020). Self-management support needs from the perspective of individuals with severe mental illness: A systematic review and thematic synthesis of qualitative research. *Journal of the American Psychiatric Nurses Association, 265,* 464–479.

Boland, R., & Verduin, M. L. (2022). *Kaplan & Sadock's synopsis of psychiatry* (P. Ruiz, Ed.). (12th ed.). Wolters Kluwer.

Burton, N. (2012). *A short history of bipolar disorder.* https://www.psychologytoday.com/blog/hide-and-seek/201206/short-history-bipolar-disorder

Calabrese, J. R. (2022). Management of bipolar depression: Where we are, where we are going. *Current Psychiatry (supplement), 21*(3), 3–8.

Chiang, K. J., Tsai, J. C., Liu, D., Lin, C. H., Chiu, H. L., & Chou, K. R. (2017). Efficacy of cognitive-behavioral therapy in patients with bipolar disorder: A meta-analysis of randomized controlled trials. *PLoS One, 12*(5), e0176849. https://doi.org/10.1371/journal.pone.0176849

Citrome, L. (2022). Olanzapine-samidorphan combination for schizophrenia or bipolar I disorder. *Current Psychiatry, 21*(1), 35–40.

Darby, M. M., Yolken, R. H., & Sabunciyan, S. (2016). Consistently altered expression of gene sets in postmortem brains of individuals with major psychiatric disorders. *Translational Psychiatry, 6*(9), e890. doi:10.1038/tp.2016.173

D'Onofrio, S., Mahaffey, S., & Garcia-Rill, E. (2017). Role of calcium channels in bipolar disorder. *Current Psychopharmacology, 6*(2), 122–135. https://doi.org/10.2174/2211556006666171024141949

Frank, E. (2005). *Treating bipolar disorder: A clinician's guide to interpersonal and social rhythm therapy.* Guilford Press.

Herdman, T. H., Kamitsuru, S., & Lopes, C. T. (Eds.). (2021). *NANDA-I, Inc. nursing diagnoses: Definitions and classification, 2021–2023.* Thieme.

Jain, R., & Jain, S. (2014). *Facing the diagnostic challenge of comorbid bipolar disorder and ADHD.* www.psychiatryadvisor.com/adhd/facing-the-diagnostic-challenge-of-comorbid-bipolar-disorder-and-adhd/article/370068

Janiri, D., Sani, G., Danese, E., Simonetti, A., Ambrosi, E., Angeletti, G., Erbuto, D., Caltagirone, C., Girardi, P., & Spalletta, G. (2015). Childhood traumatic experiences of patients with bipolar disorder type I and type II. *Journal of Affective Disorders, 175*(8), 92–97. doi:http://dx.doi.org/10.1016/j.jad.2014.12.055

Kowatch, R. A. (2016). Diagnosis, phenomenology, differential diagnosis, and comorbidity of pediatric bipolar disorder. *The Journal of Clinical Psychiatry, 77,* Suppl E1:e1. doi: 10.4088/JCP.15017su1c.01

Krans, B. (2019). *The history of bipolar disorder.* www.healthline.com/health/bipolar-disorder/history-bipolar#1

Laski, M., Foreman, R., Hancock, H., & Tavakoli, H. R. (2022). Lithium: An underutilized element. *Current Psychiatry, 20*(12), 27–34.

Leussis, M. P., Berry-Scott, E. M., Saito, M., Jhuang, H., Haan, G., Alkan, O., Luce, C. J., Madison, J. M., Sklar, P., Serre, T., Root, D. E., & Petryshen, T. L. (2013).The *ANK3* bipolar disorder gene regulates psychiatric-related behaviors that are modulated by lithium and stress. *Biological Psychiatry, 73*(7), 683–696. doi:10.1016/j.biopsych.2012.10.016

McGirr, A., Vila-Rodriguez, F., Cole, J., Torres, I. J., Arumugham, S. S., Keramatian, K., Saraf, G., Lam, R. W., Chakrabarty, T., & Yatham, L. N. (2021). Efficacy of active vs sham intermittent theta burst transcranial magnetic stimulation for patients with bipolar depression: A randomized clinical trial. *JAMA Network Open, 4*(3), e210963. https://doi.org/10.1001/jamanetworkopen.2021.0963

MedlinePlus. (2021). Bipolar disorder. *MedlinePlus.* https://medlineplus.gov/genetics/condition/bipolar-disorder/#inheritance

Meier, S. M., Pavlova, B., Dalsgaard, S., Nordentoft, M., Mors, O., Mortensen, P. B., & Uher, R. (2018). Attention-deficit hyperactivity disorder and anxiety disorders as precursors of bipolar disorder onset in adulthood. *British Journal of Psychiatry, 3*(3), 555–560. https://doi.org/10.1192/bjp.2018.111

Merikangas, K. R., & Rihmer, Z. (2017). Mood disorders: Epidemiology. In Sadock, B. J., Sadock, V. A., & Ruiz, P. (Eds.), *Comprehensive textbook of psychiatry* (10th ed., pp. 1614–1619). Wolters Kluwer.

Meyer, J. M. (2022). Lumateperone for major depressive episodes in bipolar I or bipolar II disorder. *Current Psychiatry, 21*(3), 44–51. doi:10.12788/cp.0227

Miklowitz, D. J., & Chung, B. (2016). Family focused therapy for bipolar disorder: Reflections on 30 years of research. *Family Process, 55*(3), 483–499. doi:10.1111/famp.12237

Nasr, S. J., Elmaadawi, A. Z., & Patel, R. (2018). Bright light therapy for bipolar depression. *Current Psychiatry, 17*(11), 28–32.

National Council of State Boards of Nursing (NCSBN). (2021). *Next generation NCLEX®: comparison between case studies and stand-alone items.* https://www.ncsbn.org/public-files/NGN_Fall21_English_Final.pdf

National Institute of Mental Health (NIMH). (n.d.). *Prevalence of bipolar disorder among adults.* www.nimh.nih.gov/health/statistics/prevalence/bipolar-disorder-among-adults.shtml

Özdel, K., Kart, A., & Türkçapar, M. H. (2021). Cognitive behavioral therapy in treatment of bipolar disorder. *Noro Psikiyatri Arsivi, 58*(Suppl 1), S66–S76. https://doi.org/10.29399/npa.27419

Osser, D. (2021). ADHD in patients with bipolar disorder: Genetics, diagnosis, and treatment. *Psychiatric Times, 38*(1).

https://www.psychiatrictimes.com/view/adhd-bipolar-genetics-diagnosis-treatment

Post, R. M., Goldstein, B. I., Birmaher, B., Findling, R. L., Frey, B. N., DelBello, M. P., & Miklowitz, D. J. (2020). Toward prevention of bipolar disorder in at-risk children: Potential strategies ahead of the data. *Journal of Affective Disorders, 1*(272), 508–520. doi: 10.1016/j.jad.2020.03.025.

Quidé, Y., Tozzi, L., Corcoran, M., Cannon, D. M., & Dauvermann, M. R. (2020). The impact of childhood trauma on developing bipolar disorder: Current understanding and ensuring continued progress. *Neuropsychiatric Disease and Treatment, 16,* 3095–3115. https://doi.org/10.2147/NDT.S285540

Rybakowski, J. (2014). Factors associated with lithium efficacy in bipolar disorder *Harvard Review of Psychiatry, 22*(6), 353–357. doi:10.1097/HRP.0000000000000006

Sit, D. K., McGowan, J., Wiltrout, C., Diler, R. S., Dills, J., Luther, J., Yang, A., Ciolino J. D., Seltman, H., Wisniewski, S. R., Terman, M., & Wisner, K. (2017). Adjunctive bright light therapy for bipolar depression: A randomized double-blind placebo-controlled trial. *American Journal of Psychiatry, 175*(2), 133–139. https://doi.org/10.1176/appi.ajp.2017.16101200

Soreff, S. (2022). Bipolar disorder. *Medscape.* http://emedicine.medscape.com/article/286342-overview

Strakowski, S. (2016). A guide to treating unipolar and bipolar depression. www.medscape.com/viewarticle/871539#vp_6

Stringaris, A., Baroni, A., Haimm, C., Brotman, M., Lowe, C. H., Myers, F., Rustgi, E., Wheeler, W., Kayser, R., Towbin, K., & Leibenluft, E. (2010). Pediatric bipolar disorder versus severe mood dysregulation: Risk for manic episodes on follow-up. *Journal of the American Academy of Child and Adolescent Psychiatry, 49*(4), 397–405.

Swartz, H., & Swanson, J. (2014). Psychotherapy for bipolar disorder in adults: A review of the evidence. *American Psychiatric Publishing, 12*(3), 251–266. doi:10.1176/appi.focus.12.3.251

The Brainstorm Consortium, Anttila, V., Bulik-Sullivan, B., Finucane, H. K., Walters, R. K., Duncan, J. B., Escott-Price, V., Falcone, G. J., & Neale, B. M. (2018). Analysis of shared heritability in common disorders of the brain. *Science, 360*(6395). doi:10.1126/science.aap8757

Tseng, P. T., Chen, Y. W., Tu, K. Y., Chung, W., Wang, H. Y., Wu, C. K., & Lin, P. Y. (2016). Light therapy in the treatment of patients with bipolar depression: A meta-analytic study. *European Neuropsychopharmacology, 26*(6), 1037–1047.

Watson, S., Gallagher, P., Dougall, D., Porter, R., Moncrieff, J., Ferrier, I. N., & Young, A. H. (2013). Childhood trauma in bipolar disorder. *Australian and New Zealand Journal of Psychiatry, 48*(6), 564–570. doi:10.1177/0004867413516681

Zhou, T. H., Dang, W. M., Ma, Y. T., Hu, C. Q., Wang, N., Zhang, G. Y., Wang, G., Shi, C., Zhang, H., Guo, B., Zhou, S. Z., Feng, L., Geng, S. X., Tong, Y. Z., Tang, G. W., He, Z. K., Zhen, L., & Yu, X. (2018). Clinical efficacy, onset time and safety of bright light therapy in acute bipolar depression as an adjunctive therapy: A randomized controlled trial. *Journal of Affective Disorders, 227,* 90–96. doi:10.1016/j.jad.2017.09.038

Zimmerman, M., Balling, C., Dalrymple, K., & Chelminski, I. (2019). Screening for borderline personality disorder in psychiatric outpatients with major depressive disorder and bipolar disorder. *Journal of Clinical Psychiatry, 80*(1), 18m12257. https://doi.org/10.4088/JCP.18m12257

27

Anxiety, Obsessive-Compulsive, and Related Disorders

KEY TERMS

agoraphobia

anxiety

body dysmorphic disorder

compulsions

fear

generalized anxiety disorder
  (GAD)

habit-reversal training (HRT)

hoarding disorder

implosion therapy (flooding)

obsessions

obsessive-compulsive
  disorders (OCDs)

panic disorder

phobia

social anxiety disorder (SAD)

specific phobia

stress

systematic desensitization

trichotillomania

OBJECTIVES
After reading this chapter, the student will be able to:

1. Differentiate between stress, anxiety, and fear.
2. Discuss historical aspects and epidemiological statistics related to anxiety, obsessive-compulsive, and related disorders.
3. Differentiate between normal anxiety and psychoneurotic anxiety.
4. Describe types of anxiety, obsessive-compulsive, and related disorders, and identify symptomatology associated with each. Use this information in patient assessment.
5. Identify predisposing factors in the development of anxiety, obsessive-compulsive, and related disorders.

6. Formulate nursing diagnoses and outcome criteria for patients with anxiety, obsessive-compulsive, and related disorders.
7. Describe appropriate nursing interventions for behaviors associated with anxiety, obsessive-compulsive, and related disorders.
8. Identify topics for patient and family teaching relevant to anxiety, obsessive-compulsive, and related disorders.
9. Evaluate nursing care of patients with anxiety, obsessive-compulsive, and related disorders.
10. Discuss various modalities relevant to treatment of anxiety, obsessive-compulsive, and related disorders.

Prince Harry, of the British Royal Family, shared in an interview that he had incapacitating panic attacks after the death of his mother, Princess Diana (Sykes, 2017). In the interview he described these attacks as follows:

> "In my case, every single time I was in any room with loads of people, which is quite often, I was just pouring with sweat, my heart beating—boom, boom, boom, boom—literally, just like a washing machine. I was like, 'Oh my God, get me out of here now. Oh, hang on, I can't get out of here, I have got to just hide it."

He reports having struggled with these attacks for several years before recognizing he needed professional help and learned that the panic attacks were linked to unresolved grief over the death of his mother more than a decade earlier. His story highlights not only the effect that anxiety disorders can have on one's functioning but also that treatment can be successful and improve one's quality of life.

CORE CONCEPT

Anxiety
A feeling of discomfort, apprehension, or dread related to anticipation of danger, the source of which is often nonspecific or unknown is termed **anxiety**. Anxiety is considered a disorder (or pathological) when fears and anxieties are excessive (in a cultural context), and there are associated behavioral disturbances such as interference with social and occupational functioning (American Psychiatric Association [APA], 2022).

Individuals face anxiety on a daily basis. Anxiety provides the motivation for achievement and is a necessary force for survival. The term *anxiety* is often used interchangeably with the word *stress;* however, they are not the same. **Stress,** or more properly, a *stressor,* is an external pressure that is brought to bear on the individual. Anxiety is the subjective emotional response to that stressor. (See Chapter 2, "Mental Health and Mental Illness: Historical and Theoretical Concepts," for an overview of anxiety as a psychological response to stress.)

Anxiety may be distinguished from fear in that the former is an internal emotional process, whereas **fear** is an emotion related to a cognitive sense of danger. In other words, fear involves the intellectual appraisal of a stimulus perceived to be threatening; anxiety is an emotional response of internal tension and worry that may be diffuse and not directly related to an external cause.

This chapter focuses on disorders that are characterized by exaggerated and often disabling anxiety reactions. Historical aspects and epidemiology are presented. Predisposing factors that have been implicated in the etiology of these disorders provide a framework for studying the dynamics of phobias, obsessive-compulsive disorders, generalized anxiety disorder, panic disorder, and other anxiety disorders. Various theories of causation are presented, although it is most likely that a combination of factors contributes to the etiology of these disorders. The neurobiology of anxiety disorders is presented in Figure 27–1.

An explanation of the symptomatology is presented as background knowledge for assessing the patient with an anxiety or OCD. Nursing care is described in the context of the nursing process. Various treatment modalities are explored.

Historical Aspects

Individuals have experienced anxiety throughout the ages. Yet anxiety, like fear, was not clearly defined or isolated as a separate entity by psychiatrists or psychologists until the 19th and 20th centuries. In fact, what we now know as anxiety was once solely identified by its physiological symptoms, focusing largely on the cardiovascular system.

Freud first introduced the term *anxiety neurosis* in 1895. He wrote, "I call this syndrome 'anxiety neurosis' because all its components can be grouped round the chief symptom of anxiety" (Freud, 1959). Although Freud attempted to negate the previous concept of the problem as strictly physical, it was some time before physicians of internal medicine were ready to accept psychological implications of anxiety symptoms. It was not until World War II that the psychological dimensions of various functional heart conditions were recognized.

For many years, anxiety disorders were viewed as purely psychological or purely biological in nature. Researchers now focus on the interrelatedness of mind and body, and anxiety disorders provide an excellent example of this complex relationship. It is likely that various factors, including genetic, developmental, environmental, and psychological, play a role in the etiology of anxiety disorders.

Epidemiology

Anxiety disorders are the most common of all psychiatric illnesses and result in considerable functional impairment and distress (Anxiety and Depression Association of America [ADAA], 2022). Statistics vary widely, but anxiety disorders appear to be more common in women than in men. Social anxiety and OCDs are exceptions, as they occur equally among men and women. Prevalence rates (ADAA, 2022) for

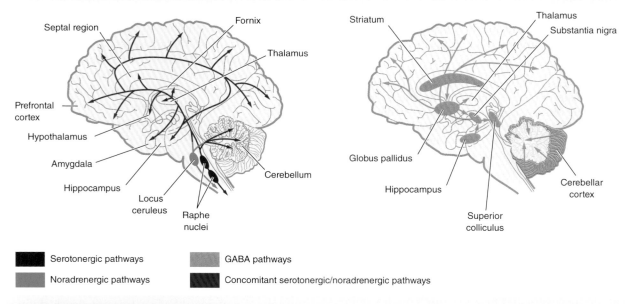

FIGURE 27-1 Neurobiology of anxiety disorders.

NEUROTRANSMITTERS

Although other neurotransmitters have also been implicated in the pathophysiology of anxiety disorders, disturbances in serotonin, norepinephrine, and gamma-aminobutyric acid (GABA) appear to be most significant.

Cell bodies of origin for the serotonin pathways lie within the raphe nuclei located in the brainstem. Serotonin is thought to be decreased in anxiety disorders (based on the efficacy of SSRIs in the treatment of anxiety disorders), but some studies suggest that serotonin may have a modulating effect in response to intense emotions in general. Cell bodies for norepinephrine originate in the locus ceruleus. Norepinephrine is thought to be increased in anxiety disorders. GABA is the major inhibitory neurotransmitter in the brain, involved in the reduction and slowing of cellular activity. It is synthesized from glutamic acid, with vitamin B_6 as a cofactor. It is found in almost every region of the brain. GABA is thought to be decreased in anxiety disorders (allowing for increased cellular excitability).

AREAS OF THE BRAIN AFFECTED

Areas of the brain affected by anxiety disorders and the symptoms that they mediate include the following:
• Amygdala: Fear; particularly important in panic and phobic disorders
• Hippocampus: Associated with memory related to fear responses
• Locus ceruleus: Arousal
• Brainstem: Respiratory activation; heart rate
• Hypothalamus: Activation of stress response
• Frontal cortex: Cognitive interpretations
• Thalamus: Integration of sensory stimuli
• Basal ganglia: Tremor

Anxiolytic Agent	Action	Side Effects
Benzodiazepines	Increases the affinity of the GABA$_A$ receptor for GABA	Sedation, dizziness, weakness, ataxia, decreased motor performance, dependence, withdrawal
Selective serotonin reuptake inhibitors (SSRIs)	Block reuptake of serotonin into the presynaptic nerve terminal, increasing synaptic concentration of serotonin	Nausea, diarrhea, headache, insomnia, somnolence, sexual dysfunction
Selective norepinephrine reuptake inhibitors (SNRIs)	Inhibit reuptake of neuronal serotonin and norepinephrine; mild reuptake of dopamine	Headache, dry mouth, nausea, somnolence, dizziness, insomnia, asthenia, constipation, diarrhea
Noradrenergic agents (e.g., propranolol, clonidine)	Propranolol: Blocks beta-adrenergic receptor activity Clonidine: Stimulates alpha-adrenergic receptors	Propranolol: Bradycardia, hypotension, weakness, fatigue, impotence, gastrointestinal upset, bronchospasm Clonidine: Dry mouth, sedation, fatigue, hypotension
Barbiturates	Central nervous system (CNS) depression. Also produces effects in the hepatic and cardiovascular systems	Somnolence, agitation, confusion, ataxia, dizziness, bradycardia, hypotension, constipation
Buspirone	Partial agonist of 5-HT$_1$A receptor	Dizziness, drowsiness, dry mouth, headache, nervousness, nausea, insomnia

anxiety disorders within the general population are identified as follows:

Specific phobias: 9.1%
Social anxiety disorder: 7.1%
Post-traumatic stress disorder (PTSD): 3.6%
Generalized anxiety disorder: 3.1%
Panic disorder: 2.7%
Obsessive compulsive disorder: 1.2%

The lifetime prevalence for any anxiety disorder is estimated at 31.1% for adults and 31.9% for adolescents (National Institute of Mental Health [NIMH], n.d.). Common comorbidities include another anxiety disorder, depression, and substance use disorders. Vulnerability to comorbidities include parental psychiatric history, childhood trauma, and negative life events, but regardless of the contributing factors, comorbidities are associated with poorer outcomes, higher health-care utilization, and greater impairment in functioning. In general, studies support a moderate genetic vulnerability, and gene-environment studies support the influence of early developmental trauma and stressful life events in anxiety disorders (Gottschalk & Domschke, 2017).

How Much Is Too Much?

Anxiety is usually considered a normal reaction to a realistic danger or threat to biological integrity or self-concept. Normal anxiety dissipates when the danger or threat is no longer present.

It is difficult to draw a precise line between normal and abnormal anxiety. Normality is determined by societal standards; what is considered normal in Chicago, Illinois, may not be so in Cairo, Egypt. There may even be regional differences within a country or cultural differences within a region. The following criteria can be used to determine whether an individual's anxious response is abnormal or pathological.

1. *It is out of proportion to the situation that is creating it.*

Example

Mrs. K. witnessed a serious automobile accident 4 weeks ago when she was out driving in her car, and since that time, she refuses to drive even to the grocery store a few miles from her house. When he is available, her husband must take her wherever she needs to go.

2. *The anxiety interferes with social, occupational, or other important areas of functioning.*

Example

Because of the anxiety associated with driving her car, Mrs. K. has been forced to quit her job in a downtown bank for lack of transportation.

It is clear that when anxiety becomes excessive and persistent, humans respond in a variety of ways that are likely a complex interaction of genetic vulnerability, biochemical influences, and environmental factors. Various manifestations of pathological anxiety are discussed in the following section.

Application of the Nursing Process—Assessment

CORE CONCEPT

Panic
A sudden, overwhelming feeling of terror or impending doom. This most severe form of emotional anxiety is usually accompanied by behavioral, cognitive, and physiological signs and symptoms considered extremely intense and frightening.

Panic Disorder

Background Assessment Data

Panic disorder is characterized by recurrent, unexpected panic attacks accompanied by either persistent worry about additional panic attacks, significant maladaptive behavior changes, or both. The *Diagnostic and Statistical Manual of Mental Disorders, Fifth Edition, Text Revision (DSM-5-TR)* (APA, 2022) states that at least four of the following symptoms must be present to identify the presence of a panic attack.

- Palpitations, pounding heart, or accelerated heart rate
- Sweating
- Trembling or shaking
- Sensations of shortness of breath or smothering
- Feelings of choking
- Chest pain or discomfort
- Nausea or abdominal distress
- Feeling dizzy, unsteady, lightheaded, or faint
- Chills or heat sensations
- Paresthesias (numbness or tingling sensations)
- Derealization (feelings of unreality) or depersonalization (feelings of being detached from oneself)
- Fear of losing control or going crazy
- Fear of dying

The attacks usually last minutes or, more rarely, hours. The individual often experiences varying degrees of nervousness and apprehension between attacks. Symptoms of depression are common.

The average age of onset of panic disorder is in the late 20s. Frequency and severity of the panic attacks vary widely. Some individuals may have attacks of moderate severity weekly; others may have less severe or limited symptom attacks several times a week. Still others may experience panic attacks separated by weeks or months. The disorder may last for a few weeks or months or for several years. Sometimes the individual experiences periods of remission and exacerbation. Limited-symptom attacks ("fearful spells" that do not meet criteria for panic attacks) may be a risk factor for later panic attacks and panic disorder. Genetic vulnerability, a predisposition for negative emotions, history of trauma, respiratory disturbances such as asthma, and smoking have also been identified as risk factors (APA, 2022).

Generalized Anxiety Disorder
Background Assessment Data

Generalized anxiety disorder (GAD) is characterized by persistent, unrealistic, and excessive anxiety and worry that have occurred more days than not for at least 6 months and cannot be attributed to specific organic factors, such as caffeine intoxication or hyperthyroidism. The anxiety and worry are associated with three or more of the following symptoms: "restlessness or feeling keyed up or on edge, being easily fatigued, difficulty concentrating or mind going blank, irritability, muscle tension, and sleep disturbance" (APA, 2022, p. 250). These symptoms are like those often associated with anxiety in the general population, but unlike the typical experience of anxiety, the symptoms in GAD are intense enough to cause clinically significant impairment in social, occupational, or other important areas of functioning. The individual often avoids activities or events that may result in negative outcomes or spends considerable time and effort preparing for such activities. Anxiety and worry often result in procrastination in behavior or decision making, and the individual repeatedly seeks reassurance from others.

The disorder may begin in childhood or adolescence, but onset is more common after age 20. Depressive symptoms are common, and numerous somatic complaints may also be a part of the clinical picture. GAD tends to be chronic, with frequent stress-related exacerbations and fluctuations in the course of the illness.

Theories of Etiology Related to Panic and Generalized Anxiety Disorders
Psychodynamic Theory

The psychodynamic view focuses on the inability of the ego to intervene when conflict occurs between the id and the superego, producing anxiety. For various reasons (unsatisfactory parent-child relationship, conditional love or provisional gratification), ego development is delayed. When developmental defects in ego functions compromise the capacity to

modulate anxiety, the individual resorts to unconscious mechanisms to resolve the conflict. Use of defense mechanisms rather than coping and management skills results in maladaptive responses to anxiety.

Cognitive Theory

The main thesis of the cognitive view is that faulty, distorted, or counterproductive thinking patterns accompany or precede maladaptive behaviors and emotional disorders. A disturbance in this central mechanism of cognition results in a disturbance in feeling and behavior. Because of distorted thinking, anxiety is maintained by an erroneous or dysfunctional appraisal of a situation. There is a loss of ability to reason regarding the problem, whether it is physical or interpersonal. The individual feels vulnerable in a given situation, and the distorted thinking results in an irrational appraisal, fostering a negative outcome.

Biological Aspects

Research into the psychobiological correlation of panic and generalized anxiety disorders have implicated several possible biological causes.

Genetics Genetic studies have identified variations on specific genes that may be associated with anxiety disorders (including panic disorder and OCD), and twin studies estimate the heritability to range from 30% to 50% (Smoller, 2020). However, as Smoller points out, genetic findings are indicative of risk rather than determinants of illness, and many genetic studies are yielding more insights about the effect of environmental factors in interaction with genes rather than the effect of genetic influences alone (Gottschalk & Domschke, 2017).

Neuroanatomical Structural brain imaging studies in people with panic disorder have implicated pathological involvement in the temporal lobes, particularly the hippocampus and the amygdala (Boland & Verduin, 2022). Dysfunctions in the limbic system (often referred to as "the emotional brain") and the frontal cerebral cortex have also been noted in individuals with anxiety disorders.

Biochemical Abnormal elevations of blood lactate have been noted in people with panic disorder. Likewise, infusion of sodium lactate into individuals with anxiety produced symptoms of panic disorder. Studies have suggested that people with panic disorders may be more sensitive to hypercapnia (which increases lactate levels), and carbon dioxide (CO_2) challenge tests have supported this sensitivity (Amaral et al., 2013). Additionally, studies of various medications and treatments such as cognitive behavior therapy (CBT) have demonstrated decreased sensitivity to CO_2 inhalation after treatment, suggesting a relationship between lactate levels and anxiety reduction.

Neurochemical Strong evidence exists for the involvement of the neurotransmitter norepinephrine in the etiology of panic disorder. Norepinephrine is known to mediate arousal and causes hyperarousal and anxiety. This fact has been demonstrated by a notable increase in anxiety after the administration of substances, such as yohimbine, which increase the synaptic availability of norepinephrine. The neurotransmitters serotonin and gamma-aminobutyric acid (GABA) are thought to be decreased in anxiety disorders. These hypotheses are related to the efficacy of benzodiazepines, which enhance the activity of GABA, and the efficacy of selective serotonin reuptake inhibitors (SSRIs), which enhance the activity of serotonin. Similarly, deep-breathing exercises have been shown to elevate thalamic GABA levels through stimulation of vagal nerve pathways with a subsequent reduction in heart rate and improvement in emotional regulation and stress responses (Gerbarg & Brown, 2016).

Although levels of neurochemicals such as serotonin and GABA undoubtedly play a role in anxiety disorders, low levels are inadequate in describing what is more likely a complex interaction of many factors. As Chandra (2020) noted, some anxiety disorders, such as SAD, are marked by high not low levels of serotonin and some patients experience temporary anxiety when they begin taking SSRI and serotonin and norepinephrine reuptake inhibitor (SNRI) medications. Abell and El-Mallakh (2021) described serotonin's role as "biphasic," and they identified that a specific type of "serotonin-mediated anxiety" is associated with particularly high levels of 5-hydroxytryptamine (5-HT) (serotonin) (p. 38).

CORE CONCEPT

Phobia

A **phobia** is an irrational fear of a specific object or situation resulting in an intense aversion toward the feared stimulus. Exposure to the feared object or situation is typically accompanied by intense anxiety or panic attacks.

Two common phobia disorders are agoraphobia and SAD (formerly called social phobia). The estimated lifetime prevalence of agoraphobia among U.S. adults is 1.3%, and approximately 40% of those cases are considered severe (NIMH, n.d.). SAD is more common, with an estimated lifetime prevalence of 12.1% (NIMH, n.d.), and the prevalence is increasing in the United States and East Asian countries (APA, 2022). A specific phobia, in which a person has an exaggerated fear response to a specific object or situation, is estimated to affect 8% to 12% of the U.S. adult population (APA, 2022).

Agoraphobia

Background Assessment Data

The literal Greek translation of the word *agoraphobia* is "fear of the marketplace." **Agoraphobia** is the fear of being in open public places, but more specifically, is defined as the fear of being vulnerable and unable to get help or escape the setting (Kimmel & Roy-Burn, 2017) should panic symptoms occur. The individual may have experienced the symptoms in the past and is preoccupied with fears of their recurrence. The *DSM-5-TR* diagnostic criteria for agoraphobia are presented in Box 27–1.

The onset of symptoms most commonly occurs in individuals in their 20s and 30s and persists for many years. It is diagnosed more commonly in women than in men. Impairment can be severe. In extreme cases, the individual is unable to leave their home without being accompanied by a friend or relative. If this is not possible, the person may become completely confined to their home.

Social Anxiety Disorder

Background Assessment Data

Social anxiety disorder (SAD) is an excessive fear of situations in which a person might do something embarrassing or be evaluated negatively by others. The individual has extreme concerns about being exposed to possible scrutiny by others and fears social or performance situations in which embarrassment may occur (APA, 2022). In some instances, the fear may be quite defined, such as the fear of speaking or eating in a public place, fear of using a public restroom, or fear of writing in the presence of others. In other cases, the social phobia may involve general social situations, such as saying things or answering questions in a manner that would provoke laughter on the part of others. Exposure to the phobic situation usually results in feelings of panic anxiety, with sweating, tachycardia, and dyspnea.

Onset of symptoms often occurs in late childhood or early adolescence and runs a chronic, sometimes lifelong, course. It appears to be more common in women than in men (Kimmel & Roy-Burn, 2017). Impairment interferes with social or occupational functioning and causes marked distress. The *DSM-5-TR* diagnostic criteria for SAD are presented in Box 27–2.

BOX 27–1 Diagnostic Criteria for Agoraphobia

A. Marked fear or anxiety about two (or more) of the following five situations:
   1. Using public transportation (e.g., automobiles, buses, trains, ships, planes)
   2. Being in open spaces (e.g., parking lots, marketplaces, bridges)
   3. Being in enclosed places (e.g., shops, theaters, cinemas)
   4. Standing in line or being in a crowd
   5. Being outside of the home alone
B. The individual fears these situations because of thoughts that escape might be difficult or help might not be available in the event of panic-like symptoms or other incapacitating or embarrassing symptoms (e.g., fear of falling in the elderly, fear of incontinence).
C. The agoraphobic situations almost always provoke fear or anxiety.
D. The agoraphobic situations are actively avoided, require the presence of a companion, or are endured with intense fear or anxiety.
E. The fear or anxiety is out of proportion to the actual danger posed by the agoraphobic situations and to the sociocultural context.

F. The fear, anxiety, or avoidance is persistent, typically lasting 6 months or more.
G. The fear, anxiety, or avoidance causes clinically significant distress or impairment in social, occupational, or other important areas of functioning.
H. If another medical condition (e.g., inflammatory bowel disease, Parkinson's disease) is present, the fear, anxiety, or avoidance is clearly excessive.
I. The fear, anxiety, or avoidance is not better explained by the symptoms of another mental disorder—for example, the symptoms are not confined to specific phobia, situational type; do not involve only social situations (as in social anxiety disorder); and are not related exclusively to obsessions (as in obsessive-compulsive disorder), perceived defects or flaws in physical appearance (as in body dysmorphic disorder), reminders of traumatic events (as in post-traumatic stress disorder), or fear of separation (as in separation anxiety disorder).

Note: Agoraphobia is diagnosed irrespective of the presence of panic disorder. If an individual's presentation meets criteria for panic disorder and agoraphobia, both diagnoses should be assigned.

BOX 27–2 Diagnostic Criteria for Social Anxiety Disorder (Social Phobia)

A. Marked fear or anxiety about one or more social situations in which the individual is exposed to possible scrutiny by others. Examples include social interactions (e.g., having a conversation, meeting unfamiliar people), being observed (e.g., eating or drinking), and performing in front of others (e.g., giving a speech). **Note:** In children, the anxiety must occur in peer settings and not just during interactions with adults.
B. The individual fears that he or she will act in a way or show anxiety symptoms that will be negatively evaluated (i.e., will be humiliating or embarrassing; will lead to rejection or offend others).
C. The social situations almost always provoke fear or anxiety. **Note:** In children, the fear or anxiety may be expressed by crying, tantrums, freezing, clinging, shrinking, or failing to speak in social situations.
D. The social situations are avoided or endured with intense fear or anxiety.
E. The fear or anxiety is out of proportion to the actual threat posed by the social situation and to the sociocultural context.

F. The fear, anxiety, or avoidance is persistent, typically lasting 6 months or more.
G. The fear, anxiety, or avoidance causes clinically significant distress or impairment in social, occupation, or other important areas of functioning.
H. The fear, anxiety, or avoidance is not attributable to the physiological effects of a substance (e.g., a drug of abuse, a medication) or another medical condition.
I. The fear, anxiety, or avoidance is not better explained by the symptoms of another mental disorder, such as panic disorder, body dysmorphic disorder, or autism spectrum disorder.
J. If another medical condition (e.g., Parkinson's disease, obesity, disfigurement from burns or injury) is present, the fear, anxiety, or avoidance is clearly unrelated or is excessive.

Specify if:

Performance only: If the fear is restricted to speaking or performing in public

Specific Phobia

Background Assessment Data

Specific phobia is identified by a fear of specific objects or situations that could conceivably cause harm (e.g., snakes, heights), but the person's reaction to them is excessive, unreasonable, and inappropriate.

Specific phobias are often identified when other anxiety disorders have become a focus of clinical attention. Treatment is generally aimed at the primary diagnosis because it usually produces the greatest distress and interferes with functioning more so than does a specific phobia. A diagnosis of specific phobia is made only when the irrational fear restricts the individual's activities and interferes with their daily living.

The phobic person may be no more (or less) anxious than anyone else until exposed to the phobic object or situation. Exposure to the phobic stimulus produces overwhelming symptoms of panic, including palpitations, sweating, dizziness, and difficulty breathing. In fact, these symptoms may occur in response to the individual merely *thinking* about the phobic stimulus. Invariably, the person recognizes that their fear is excessive or unreasonable but is powerless to change, even though they may occasionally endure the phobic stimulus when experiencing intense anxiety.

Phobias may begin at almost any age. Those that begin in childhood often disappear without treatment, but those that begin or persist into adulthood usually require assistance with therapy. The disorder is diagnosed more often in women than in men.

Although the disorder is relatively common among the general population, people seldom seek treatment unless the phobia interferes with the ability to function. The individual who has a fear of snakes but who lives on the 23rd floor of an urban, high-rise apartment building is not likely to be bothered by the phobia unless they decide to move to an area where snakes are prevalent. On the other hand, a fear of elevators may interfere with this individual's daily functioning.

Specific phobias are classified according to the phobic stimulus. A list of some of the identified phobias appears in Table 27–1. This list is by no means inclusive. People can become phobic about almost any object or situation, and anyone with a little knowledge of Greek or Latin can produce a phobia classification, thereby making possibilities for the list almost infinite.

Theories of Etiology Related to Phobias

The cause of phobias is unknown. However, various theories exist that may offer insight into the etiology.

TABLE 27–1 **Classification of Specific Phobias**	
CLASSIFICATION	**FEAR**
Acrophobia	Height
Ailurophobia	Cats
Algophobia	Pain
Anthophobia	Flowers
Anthropophobia	People
Aquaphobia	Water
Arachnophobia	Spiders
Astraphobia	Lightning
Belonephobia	Needles
Brontophobia	Thunder
Claustrophobia	Closed spaces
Cynophobia	Dogs
Dementophobia	Insanity
Equinophobia	Horses
Gamophobia	Marriage
Herpetophobia	Lizards, reptiles
Homophobia	Homosexuality
Murophobia	Mice
Mysophobia	Dirt, germs, contamination
Numerophobia	Numbers
Nyctophobia	Darkness
Ochophobia	Riding in a car
Ophidiophobia	Snakes
Pyrophobia	Fire
Scoleciphobia	Worms
Siderodromophobia	Railroads or train travel
Taphophobia	Being buried alive
Thanatophobia	Death
Trichophobia	Hair
Triskaidekaphobia	The number 13
Xenophobia	Strangers
Zoophobia	Animals

Psychoanalytic Theory

Modern psychoanalysts believe that unconscious fears may be expressed symbolically as phobias. For example, a female child who was sexually abused by an adult male family friend when he was taking her for a ride in his boat grew up with an intense, irrational fear of all water vessels. Psychoanalytic theory postulates that fear of the man was repressed and displaced onto boats. Boats became an unconscious symbol for the feared person, but one that the young girl viewed as safer because her fear of boats prevented her from having to confront the real fear.

Learning Theory

Classic conditioning in the case of phobias may be explained as follows: a stressful stimulus produces an "unconditioned" response of fear. When the stressful stimulus is repeatedly paired with a harmless object, eventually the harmless object alone produces a "conditioned" response: fear. The fear becomes a phobia when the individual consciously avoids the harmless object to escape fear.

Some learning theorists contend that fears are conditioned responses and thus are learned by imposing rewards for certain behaviors. In the instance of phobias, when the individual avoids the phobic object, they escape fear, which is indeed a powerful reward.

Phobias also may be acquired by direct learning or imitation (modeling). For example, a mother who exhibits fear toward an object will provide a model for the child, who may also develop a phobia of the same object.

Cognitive Theory

Cognitive theorists espouse that anxiety is the product of faulty cognitions or anxiety-inducing self-instructions. Two types of faulty thinking have been investigated: negative self-statements and irrational beliefs. Cognitive theorists believe that some individuals engage in negative and irrational thinking that produces anxiety reactions. The individual begins to engage in avoidance behaviors to prevent the anxiety reactions, and phobias result.

Related to the cognitive theory is the involvement of locus of control. Johnson and Sarason (1978) proposed that one's locus of control orientation may be an important variable in the development of phobias. They further suggested that individuals with an internal locus of control (those who perceive they have control over outcomes in life) and those with an external locus of control (those who rely on chance or other people to control outcomes) might respond differently to life change. Individuals with an external control orientation experiencing anxiety attacks in a stressful period are likely to mislabel the anxiety and attribute it to external sources (e.g., crowded areas) or to a disease (e.g., heart attack). They may perceive the experienced anxiety as outside of their control. Figure 27–2 depicts a graphic model of the relationship between locus of control and the development of phobias.

Although internal locus of control orientation has generally been accepted as beneficial in managing stressors, a recent study (Reknes et al., 2019) found the opposite to be true when the stressor was bullying. For example, the target of bullying may experience more stress with failed attempts to control bullying situations. Their findings suggest that although locus of control, as a personality trait, is a variable in the development of phobias, some stressors may have a different effect on one's locus of control orientation than others.

Biological Aspects

Neuroanatomical Specific areas in the prefrontal cortex and the amygdala play a role in storing and recalling information about threatening or potentially deadly events. Similar future events can trigger these memories, after which the amygdala triggers the release of fight-or-flight hormones and the individual experiences heightened stress and fear as though the original threat was happening again (Brazier, 2020). Other researchers (Dias & Ressler, 2014) have found that parental traumatic exposure creates gene "memories" that are passed down to subsequent generations via parental gametes, which are then expressed as phobias in their offspring. Kimmel and Roy-Burn (2017) noted that

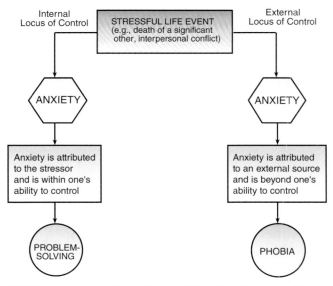

FIGURE 27–2 Locus of control as a variable in the etiology of phobias.

although there may be a genetic vulnerability to phobias, environmental factors such as trauma play a more central role.

Temperament Children experience fears as a part of normal development. Most infants are afraid of loud noises. Common fears of toddlers and preschoolers include strangers, animals, darkness, and fears of being separated from parents or attachment figures. School-age children are afraid of death and experience anxiety about school achievement. Fear of social rejection and sexual anxieties are common among adolescents.

Innate fears represent a part of the overall characteristics or tendencies one is born with that influence how one responds to specific situations. Innate fears usually do not reach phobic intensity but may have the capacity for such development if reinforced by events in later life. For example, a 4-year-old girl is afraid of dogs. By age 5, however, she has overcome her fear and plays with her own dog and the neighbors' dogs without fear. Then, when she is 19, she is bitten by a stray dog and develops a phobia of dogs.

Life Experiences

Certain early experiences may set the stage for phobic reactions later in life. Some researchers believe that phobias, particularly specific phobias, are symbolic of original anxiety-producing objects or situations that have been repressed. For example:

- A child who is punished by being locked in a closet develops a phobia of elevators or other enclosed places.
- A child who falls down a flight of stairs develops a phobia of high places.
- A young adult who survived a plane crash during childhood in which both parents were killed has a phobia of airplanes.

Anxiety Disorder Due to Another Medical Condition and Substance/Medication-Induced Anxiety Disorder

Background Assessment Data

The symptoms associated with these disorders are the direct physiological consequence of another medical condition, substance intoxication or withdrawal, or exposure to a medication. Several medical conditions are associated with the development of anxiety symptoms. Some of these include cardiac conditions, such as myocardial infarction, congestive heart failure, and mitral valve prolapse; endocrine conditions, such as hypoglycemia, hypothyroidism or hyperthyroidism, and pheochromocytoma; respiratory conditions, such as chronic obstructive pulmonary disease

and hyperventilation; and neurological conditions, such as complex partial seizures, neoplasms, and encephalitis.

Nursing care of patients with this disorder must take into consideration the underlying cause of the anxiety. Holistic nursing care is essential to ensure that the patient's physiological and psychosocial needs are met. Nursing actions appropriate for the specific medical condition must also be considered.

The diagnosis of substance-induced anxiety disorder is made only if the anxiety symptoms are in excess of those usually associated with the intoxication or withdrawal syndrome and warrant independent clinical attention. Evidence of intoxication or withdrawal must be available from the history, physical examination, or laboratory findings to substantiate the diagnosis. Substance-induced anxiety disorder may be associated with use of the following substances: alcohol, amphetamines, cocaine, inhalants, opioids, hallucinogens, sedatives, hypnotics, anxiolytics, caffeine, cannabis, or other substances (APA, 2022). Nursing care of the patient with substance-induced anxiety disorder must take into consideration the nature of the substance and the context in which the symptoms occur; that is, intoxication or withdrawal.

CORE CONCEPT

Obsessions

Intrusive thoughts that are recurrent and stressful are termed **obsessions**. Although they are recognized by the individual as irrational, they continue to be repetitive and cannot be ignored.

CORE CONCEPT

Compulsions

Repetitive ritualistic behaviors or mental acts an individual feels driven to perform according to rigidly applied rules that are intended to reduce the anxiety associated with obsessive thoughts are termed **compulsions** (APA, 2022).

Obsessive-Compulsive Disorder

Background Assessment Data

The manifestations of **obsessive-compulsive disorder (OCD)** include the presence of obsessions, compulsions, or both, the severity of which is significant enough to cause distress or impairment in social, occupational, or other important areas of functioning (APA, 2022). The individual recognizes that the behavior is excessive or unreasonable, but because of the feeling of relief from discomfort that it promotes, is compelled to continue the act. Common compulsions include hand washing, ordering, checking, praying, counting, and repeating words silently.

The disorder is equally common among men and women. It may begin in childhood but more often begins in adolescence or early adulthood. The course is usually chronic and may be complicated by depression or substance use disorders. The *DSM-5-TR* diagnostic criteria for OCD are presented in Box 27–3.

Body Dysmorphic Disorder

Background Assessment Data

Body dysmorphic disorder is characterized by the exaggerated belief that one's body is deformed or defective in some specific way. The most common complaints involve flaws of the face or head, such as wrinkles or scars, the shape of the nose, excessive facial hair, and facial asymmetry, that are slight or not observable by others (Stein & Lochner, 2017). However, any body part can be the focus of distorted beliefs, including eyes, lips, teeth, stomach, genitals, or body weight. In some instances a true defect is present. The significance of the defect is unrealistically exaggerated, however, and the person's concern is grossly excessive. These beliefs are differentiated from delusions in that individuals with body dysmorphic disorder are aware that their beliefs are exaggerated. In some cases, however, people with body dysmorphic disorder also develop psychotic disorders.

BOX 27–3 Diagnostic Criteria for Obsessive-Compulsive Disorder

A. Presence of obsessions, compulsions, or both:

Obsessions are defined by (1) and (2)

1. Recurrent and persistent thoughts, urges, or images that are experienced, at some time during the disturbance, as intrusive and unwanted, and that in most individuals cause marked anxiety or distress.
2. The individual attempts to ignore or suppress such thoughts, urges, or images, or to neutralize them with some other thought or action (i.e., by performing a compulsion).

Compulsions are defined by (1) and (2):

1. Repetitive behaviors (e.g., hand washing, ordering, checking) or mental acts (e.g., praying, counting, repeating words silently) that the person feels driven to perform in response to an obsession or according to rules that must be applied rigidly.
2. The behaviors or mental acts are aimed at preventing or reducing anxiety or distress, or preventing some dreaded event or situation; however, these behaviors or mental acts either are not connected in a realistic way with what they are designed to neutralize or prevent or are clearly excessive. **Note:** Young children may not be able to articulate the aims of these behaviors or mental acts.

B. The obsessions or compulsions are time-consuming (e.g., take more than 1 hour a day) or cause clinically significant distress or impairment in social, occupational, or other important areas of functioning.

C. The obsessive-compulsive symptoms are not attributable to the direct physiological effects of a substance (e.g., a drug of abuse, a medication) or another medical condition.

D. The disturbance is not better explained by the symptoms of another mental disorder (e.g., excessive worries, as in generalized anxiety disorder; preoccupation with appearance, as in body dysmorphic disorder; difficulty discarding or parting with possessions, as in hoarding disorder; hair pulling, as in trichotillomania [hair-pulling disorder]; skin picking, as in excoriation [skin-picking] disorder; stereotypies, as in stereotypic movement disorder; ritualized eating behavior, as in eating disorders; preoccupation with substances or gambling, as in substance-related and addictive disorders; preoccupation with having an illness, as in illness anxiety disorder; sexual urges or fantasies, as in paraphilic disorders; impulses, as in disruptive, impulse-control, and conduct disorders; guilty ruminations, as in major depressive disorder; thought insertion or delusional preoccupations, as in schizophrenia spectrum and other psychotic disorders; or repetitive patterns of behavior, as in autism spectrum disorder).

Specify if:

With good or fair insight: The individual recognizes that obsessive-compulsive disorder beliefs are definitely or probably not true or that they may or may not be true.

With poor insight: The individual thinks obsessive-compulsive disorder beliefs are probably true.

With absent insight/delusional beliefs: The individual is completely convinced that obsessive-compulsive disorder beliefs are true.

Specify if:

Tic-related: The individual has a current or past history of a tic disorder.

People with body dysmorphic disorder often have other comorbid mental disorders. The most frequent comorbidity is depression, with a lifetime prevalence rate of 75%; other less common comorbidities include OCD, panic attacks, and substance use disorders (Boland & Verduin, 2022). Social and occupational impairment may occur because of the excessive anxiety experienced by the individual about the imagined defect. The person's medical history may reflect numerous visits to plastic surgeons and dermatologists in an unrelenting drive to correct the imagined defect. The individual may undergo unnecessary surgical procedures toward this effort. The *DSM-5-TR* diagnostic criteria for body dysmorphic disorder are presented in Box 27–4.

Trichotillomania (Hair-Pulling Disorder)

Background Assessment Data

The *DSM-5-TR* defines **trichotillomania** as the recurrent pulling out of one's hair that results in hair loss (APA, 2022). The impulse is preceded by an increasing sense of tension and results in a sense of release or gratification from pulling out the hair. The most common sites for hair pulling are the scalp, eyebrows, and eyelashes, but it may occur in any area of the body on which hair grows. The areas of hair loss are often found on the opposite side of the body from the dominant hand. Pain is seldom reported as accompanying the hair pulling, although tingling and pruritus in the area are not uncommon. Comorbid psychiatric disorders are common with hair-pulling disorder; the most common are mood and other anxiety disorders (Stein & Lochner, 2017). Some children under 6 years of age have been reported to have mild symptoms of hair-pulling disorder, usually in response to a significant loss or other anxiety-producing event (such as family issues, school issues, physical appearance, or concurrent illness) (Chandran et al., 2015). More significant trichotillomania typically begins in adolescence or early adulthood with a variable course. It may be accompanied by nail-biting, head banging, scratching, biting, or other acts of self-mutilation. Because the repetitive behavior of hair pulling is intended to decrease anxiety, it may be considered within the spectrum of OCDs. This phenomenon occurs more often in women than in men, and prevalence estimates vary widely from 1% to 13.4% (Pond, 2020).

Hoarding Disorder

Background Assessment Data

The *DSM-5-TR* defines the essential feature of **hoarding disorder** as "persistent difficulties discarding or parting with possessions, regardless of their actual value" (APA, 2022, p. 277). Additionally, the diagnosis may be specified as *with excessive acquisition*, which identifies the excessive need for continual acquiring of items (either by buying them or by other means).

BOX 27–4 Diagnostic Criteria for Body Dysmorphic Disorder

A. Preoccupation with one or more perceived defects or flaws in physical appearance that are not observable or appear slight to others.

B. At some point during the course of the disorder, the individual has performed repetitive behaviors (e.g., mirror checking, excessive grooming, skin picking, reassurance seeking) or mental acts (e.g., comparing his or her appearance with that of others) in response to the appearance concerns.

C. The preoccupation causes clinically significant distress or impairment in social, occupational, or other important areas of functioning.

D. The appearance preoccupation is not better explained by concerns with body fat or weight in an individual whose symptoms meet diagnostic criteria for an eating disorder.

Specify if:

With muscle dysmorphia: The individual is preoccupied with the idea that his or her body build is too small or insufficiently muscular. This specifier is used even if the individual is preoccupied with other body areas, which is often the case.

Specify if:

Indicate degree of insight regarding body dysmorphic disorder beliefs (e.g., "I look ugly" or "I look deformed").

With good or fair insight: The individual recognizes that the body dysmorphic disorder beliefs are definitely or probably not true or that they may or may not be true.

With poor insight: The individual thinks that the body dysmorphic disorder beliefs are probably true.

With absent insight/delusional beliefs: The individual is completely convinced that the body dysmorphic disorder beliefs are true.

In previous editions of the *DSM*, hoarding was considered a symptom of OCD. However, in the *DSM-5-TR*, it is classified as a distinct disorder.

Individuals with hoarding disorder collect items until virtually all surfaces within the home are covered. There may be only narrow pathways winding through stacks of clutter. Some individuals also hoard food and animals, keeping dozens or hundreds of pets, often in unsanitary conditions (Mayo Clinic, 2022).

Community surveys estimate the prevalence of clinically significant hoarding in the United States and Europe to range from 1.5% to 6% (APA, 2022). More men than women are diagnosed with the disorder, and it is almost three times more prevalent in adults older than 65 years of age than in younger adults (ages 30 to 40) (APA, 2022). The symptoms, regardless of when they begin, appear to become more severe with each decade of life. Associated symptoms include perfectionism, indecisiveness, anxiety, depression, distractibility, and difficulty planning and organizing tasks (APA, 2022). In addition to OCD, hoarding is associated with high comorbidity for dependent, avoidant, schizotypal, and paranoid personality disorders (Boland & Verduin, 2022). Research has shown that hoarding disorder runs in families and there may be a genetic vulnerability (Dozier & Ayers, 2017).

Treatment of hoarding disorder has been met with mixed results. It is often difficult to convince individuals with the disorder that they are actually ill. Change is slow, and the relapse rate is high; when possessions or animals are taken away, they are often quickly replaced to provide emotional comfort (Mayo Clinic, 2022). Psychoeducation about the disorder is almost always the initial intervention, and the primary treatment is CBT. Psychopharmacology with SSRIs may be added, particularly when there is evidence of comorbid anxiety or depression. Families and friends may misinterpret hoarding behavior as laziness or uncleanliness. Psychoeducation that includes the patient's identified support system assists the patient in a recovery plan. Some experts have identified unresolved grief issues as associated with hoarding behavior, which may provide another avenue for psychological intervention (Meyers, 2016).

Theories of Etiology in Obsessive-Compulsive and Related Disorders

Psychoanalytic Theory

Psychoanalytic theorists propose that individuals with OCD have underdeveloped egos (for any of a variety of reasons: unsatisfactory parent-child relationship, conditional love, or provisional gratification). The psychoanalytical concept views people with OCD as having regressed to earlier developmental stages of the infantile superego—the harsh, exacting, punitive characteristics that now reappear as part of the psychopathology. Regression and use of defense mechanisms (isolation, undoing, displacement, reaction formation) produce the clinical symptoms of obsessions and compulsions.

Learning Theory

Learning theorists explain obsessive-compulsive behavior as a conditioned response to a traumatic event. The traumatic event produces anxiety and discomfort, and the individual learns to prevent the anxiety and discomfort by avoiding the situation with which they are associated. This type of learning is called *passive avoidance* (staying away from the source). When passive avoidance is not possible, the individual learns to engage in behaviors that provide relief from the anxiety and discomfort associated with the traumatic situation. This type of learning is called *active avoidance* and describes the behavior pattern of the individual with OCD.

According to this classic conditioning interpretation, a traumatic event should mark the beginning of the obsessive-compulsive behaviors. However, in a significant number of cases, the onset of the behavior is gradual, and people relate the onset of their problems to life stress in general rather than to one or more traumatic events.

Psychosocial Influences

The onset of trichotillomania can be related to stressful situations in more than one-quarter of cases. Additional factors that have been implicated include disturbances in the mother-child relationship, fear of abandonment, and recent object loss. Trichotillomania has at times been connected to childhood trauma, but Woods (as cited by Kaplan, 2012) indicated that only 5% of patients have comorbid trichotillomania and PTSD. Hoarding disorder has been associated with unmanaged stress after the sudden loss of a loved one, divorce, or other significant life stressors (Mayo Clinic, 2022).

Biological Aspects

Genetics Twin studies and family studies support a genetic susceptibility for OCD, especially in childhood-onset OCD (Stein & Lochner, 2017). Trichotillomania has commonly been associated with OCDs among first-degree relatives, leading researchers to conclude that the disorder has a possible hereditary or familial predisposition. Structural abnormalities in various areas of the brain and alterations in the serotonin and endogenous opioid systems have also been noted.

Genetics also may play a role in the development of hoarding disorder. Family and twin studies indicate that approximately 50% of individuals who hoard report having a relative who also hoards (APA, 2022).

Neuroanatomy Recent findings suggest that neurobiological disturbances may play a role in the pathogenesis and maintenance of OCD. Abnormalities in various regions of the brain have been implicated in the neurobiology of OCD. Neuroimaging and neurocognitive assessment have identified an impairment in motor inhibition responses (the ability to stop an action once initiated) in patients with OCD and trichotillomania (Kaplan, 2012). In individuals with hoarding disorder, neuroimaging studies have indicated blunted activity in the cingulate cortex (particularly the insula), the area of the brain that connects the emotional part of the brain with the parts that control higher-level thinking and overactivity in the insular and anterior cingulate cortex during possession-related choices (Stevens et al., 2020).

Biochemical Factors Dopaminergic, serotonergic, and glutamate systems have all been implicated in the etiology of obsessive-compulsive behaviors. Drugs that have been used successfully in alleviating the symptoms of OCD are clomipramine and the SSRIs, all of which are believed to block the neuronal reuptake of serotonin, thereby potentiating serotoninergic activity in the central nervous system (see Figure 27–1). The serotonergic system may also be a factor in the etiology of body dysmorphic disorder. This relationship between OCD and serotonin levels is suggested by the high incidence of comorbidity with major mood disorder and anxiety disorder and the positive responsiveness of the condition to the serotonin-specific drugs.

Genome studies have implicated glutamate function in OCD, but more research is needed (Stein & Lochner, 2017). Glutamate has also been implicated in the etiology of several other disorders including Parkinson's disease, Alzheimer's dementia, and schizophrenia (Karthik et al., 2020), which may be relevant in the common risks for and comorbidities among these disorders. Support for the involvement of glutamate in OCD is the evidence that medications like lamotrigine, topiramate, and riluzole, which mainly reduce glutamate transmission overall, have been observed to reduce compulsions specifically in a subset of patients (Karthik et al., 2020).

Transactional Model of Stress and Adaptation

Anxiety, obsessive-compulsive, and related disorders are most likely caused by multiple factors. In Figure 27–3, a graphic depiction of this theory of multiple causation is presented in the transactional model of stress and adaptation.

Assessment Scales

Several assessment rating scales are available for measuring severity of anxiety symptoms. Some are meant to be administered by the clinician, whereas others may be self-administered. Examples of self-rating scales include the Beck Anxiety Inventory and the Zung Self-Rated Anxiety Scale. One of the most widely used clinician-administered scales is the Hamilton Anxiety Rating Scale (HAM-A), which is used in both clinical and research settings. The scale consists of 14 items and measures both psychic and somatic anxiety symptoms (psychological distress and physical complaints associated with anxiety). The HAM-A is presented in Box 27–5.

Diagnosis and Outcome Identification

Nursing diagnoses are formulated from the data gathered during the assessment phase and with background knowledge regarding predisposing factors to the disorder. Table 27–2 lists patient behaviors and the NANDA International (NANDA-I) nursing diagnoses (Herdman et al., 2021) that correspond to those behaviors, which may be used in planning care for patients with anxiety, obsessive-compulsive, and related disorders.

Outcome Criteria

The following criteria may be used for measurement of outcomes in the care of the patient with anxiety disorders.

The patient:

■ Is able to recognize signs of escalating anxiety and intervene before reaching panic level *(panic and GADs)*
■ Is able to maintain anxiety at a manageable level and make independent decisions about life situations *(panic and GADs)*
■ Functions adaptively in the presence of the phobic object or situation without experiencing panic anxiety *(phobic disorder)*
■ Verbalizes a plan of action for responding in the presence of the phobic object or situation without developing panic anxiety *(phobic disorder)*
■ Is able to maintain anxiety at a manageable level without resorting to the use of ritualistic behavior *(OCD)*

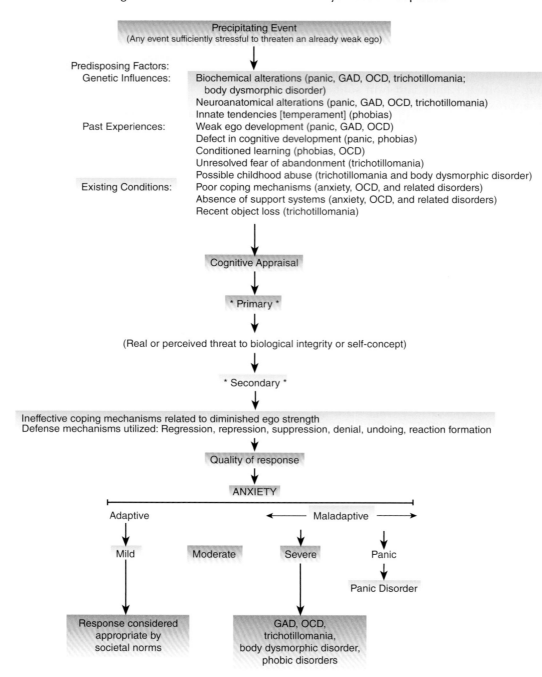

FIGURE 27–3 The dynamics of anxiety, obsessive-compulsive, and related disorders using the transactional model of stress and adaptation.

■ Demonstrates adaptive coping strategies for dealing with anxiety instead of ritualistic behaviors *(OCD)*

■ Verbalizes a realistic perception of their appearance and expresses feelings that reflect a positive body image *(body dysmorphic disorder)*

■ Verbalizes and demonstrates more adaptive strategies for coping with stressful situations *(trichotillomania)*

Planning and Implementation

Care Plan for the Patient With Anxiety, OCD, and Related Disorders

The following section presents a group of selected nursing diagnoses, with short- and long-term goals and nursing interventions for each. Rationales for interventions are included in italics.

BOX 27–5 Hamilton Anxiety Rating Scale (HAM-A)

The following are descriptions of symptoms commonly associated with anxiety. Assign the client the rating between 0 and 4 (for each of the 14 items) that best describes the extent to which he/she has these symptoms.

0 = Not present   **1 = Mild**   **2 = Moderate**   **3 = Severe**   **4 = Very severe**

Rating

1. Anxious mood

_____

Worries, anticipation of the worst, fearful anticipation, irritability

2. Tension

_____

Feelings of tension, fatigability, startle response, moved to tears easily, trembling, feelings of restlessness, inability to relax

3. Fears

_____

Of dark, of strangers, of being left alone, of animals, of traffic, of crowds

4. Insomnia

_____

Difficulty in falling asleep, broken sleep, unsatisfying sleep and fatigue on waking, dreams, nightmares, night terrors

5. Intellectual

_____

Difficulty in concentration, poor memory

6. Depressed mood

_____

Loss of interest, lack of pleasure in hobbies, depression, early waking, diurnal swing

7. Somatic (muscular)

_____

Pains and aches, twitching, stiffness, myoclonic jerks, grinding of teeth, unsteady voice, increased muscular tone

Rating

8. Somatic (sensory)

_____

Tinnitus, blurred vision, hot/cold flushes, feelings of weakness, tingling sensation

9. Cardiovascular symptoms

_____

Tachycardia, palpitations, pain in chest, throbbing of vessels, feeling faint

10. Respiratory symptoms

_____

Pressure or constriction in chest, choking feelings, sighing, dyspnea

11. Gastrointestinal symptoms

_____

Difficulty swallowing, flatulence, abdominal pain and fullness, burning sensations, nausea/vomiting, borborygmi, diarrhea, constipation, weight loss

12. Genitourinary symptoms

_____

Urinary frequency, urinary urgency, amenorrhea, menorrhagia, loss of libido, premature ejaculation, impotence

13. Autonomic symptoms

_____

Dry mouth, flushing, pallor, tendency to sweat, giddiness, tension headache

14. Behavior at interview

_____

Fidgeting, restlessness or pacing, tremor of hands, furrowed brow, strained face, sighing or rapid respiration, facial pallor, swallowing, clearing throat

Client's Total Score _____

SCORING:

14–17 = Mild anxiety

18–24 = Moderate anxiety

25–30 = Severe anxiety

Source: Hamilton, M. (1959). The assessment of anxiety states by rating. *British Journal of Medical Psychology, 32*(1), 50–55. The HAM-A is in the public domain.

Some institutions use a case management model to coordinate care (see Chapter 8, "The Nursing Process in Psychiatric-Mental Health Nursing," for a more detailed explanation). In case management models, the plan of care may take the form of a critical pathway.

Anxiety (Severe or Panic)

Anxiety is defined as a "An emotional response to a diffuse threat in which the individual anticipates nonspecific impending danger, catastrophe, or misfortune" (Herdman et al., 2021, p. 405). Table 27–3 presents this nursing diagnosis in care plan format.

Patient Goals

Outcome criteria include short- and long-term goals. Timelines are individually determined.

Short-term goal

■ The patient will verbalize ways to intervene in escalating anxiety within 1 week.

TABLE 27–2 **Assigning Nursing Diagnoses to Behaviors Commonly Associated With Anxiety, Obsessive-Compulsive, and Related Disorders**	
BEHAVIORS	**NURSING DIAGNOSES**
Palpitations, trembling, sweating, chest pain, shortness of breath, fear of going crazy, fear of dying *(panic disorder)*; excessive worry, difficulty concentrating, sleep disturbance *(generalized anxiety disorder)*	**Anxiety (severe/panic)**
Verbal expressions of having no control over life situation; nonparticipation in decision making related to own care or life situation; expressions of doubt regarding role performance *(panic and generalized anxiety disorders)*	**Powerlessness**
Behavior directed toward avoidance of a feared object or situation *(phobic disorder)*	**Fear**
Stays at home alone, afraid to venture out alone *(agoraphobia)*	**Social isolation**
Ritualistic behavior; obsessive thoughts, inability to meet basic needs; severe level of anxiety *(OCD)*	**Ineffective coping**
Inability to fulfill usual patterns of responsibility because of need to perform rituals *(OCD)*	**Ineffective role performance**
Preoccupation with an imagined defect; verbalizations that are out of proportion to any actual physical abnormality that may exist; numerous visits to plastic surgeons or dermatologists seeking relief *(body dysmorphic disorder)*	**Disturbed body image**
Repetitive and impulsive pulling out of one's hair *(trichotillomania)*	**Ineffective impulse control**

Table 27–3 | **CARE PLAN FOR THE PATIENT WITH ANXIETY, OBSESSIVE-COMPULSIVE, AND RELATED DISORDERS**		

NURSING DIAGNOSIS: PANIC ANXIETY

RELATED TO: Real or perceived threat to biological integrity or self-concept

EVIDENCED BY: Any or all of the physical symptoms identified by the ***DSM-5-TR***

OUTCOME CRITERIA	NURSING INTERVENTIONS	RATIONALE
Short-Term Goal: ■ The patient verbalizes ways to intervene in escalating anxiety within 1 week. **Long-Term Goal:** ■ By time of discharge from treatment, the patient is able to recognize onset of anxiety symptoms and intervene before reaching panic level.	1. Stay with the patient and offer reassurance of safety and security. Do not leave the patient in panic anxiety alone. 2. Maintain a calm, nonthreatening, matter-of-fact approach. 3. Use simple words and brief messages, spoken calmly and clearly, to explain hospital experiences.	1. The patient may fear for their life. Presence of a trusted individual provides a feeling of security and assurance of personal safety. 2. Anxiety may be transferred from staff to patient or vice versa. Patients develop a feeling of security in the presence of a calm staff person. 3. In an intensely anxious situation, patients are unable to comprehend anything but the most elemental communication.

Table 27–3 | CARE PLAN FOR THE PATIENT WITH ANXIETY, OBSESSIVE-COMPULSIVE, AND RELATED DISORDERS—cont'd

OUTCOME CRITERIA	NURSING INTERVENTIONS	RATIONALE
	4. If hyperventilation occurs, help the patient breathe into a small paper bag held over the mouth and nose. Six to 12 natural breaths should be taken, alternating with short periods of diaphragmatic breathing.	4. Hyperventilation may occur during periods of extreme anxiety. Hyperventilation causes the amount of carbon dioxide in the blood to decrease, possibly resulting in lightheadedness, rapid heart rate, shortness of breath, numbness or tingling in the hands or feet, and syncope. Hyperventilation may result in injury to the patient, and patient safety is a nursing priority. The technique here should not be used with patients who have coronary or respiratory disorders, such as coronary artery disease, asthma, or chronic obstructive pulmonary disease.
	5. Keep immediate surroundings low in stimuli (dim lighting, few people, simple decor).	5. A stimulating environment may increase level of anxiety.
	6. Administer tranquilizing medication, as ordered by the physician. Assess for effectiveness and side effects.	6. Antianxiety medication provides relief from the immobilizing effects of anxiety.
	7. When level of anxiety has been reduced, explore possible reasons for occurrence.	7. Recognition of precipitating factor(s) is the first step in teaching patient to interrupt escalation of anxiety.
	8. Teach signs and symptoms of escalating anxiety, and ways to interrupt its progression (relaxation techniques, such as deep-breathing exercises and meditation, or physical exercise, such as brisk walks and jogging).	8. Relaxation techniques result in a physiological response opposite that of the anxiety response. Physical activities discharge excess energy in a healthful manner.

Long-term goal

■ By the time of discharge from treatment, the patient will be able to recognize symptoms of onset of anxiety and intervene before reaching panic stage.

Interventions

■ Stay with the patient who is experiencing panic anxiety and offer reassurance of safety and security. *At this level of anxiety, patients often express a fear of dying or of "going crazy." They need the presence of and assurance of their safety from a trusted individual.*

■ Maintain a calm, nonthreatening, matter-of-fact approach. *Anxiety can be transferred from staff to patient or vice versa. The presence of a calm person provides a feeling of security to an anxious patient.*

■ Use simple words and brief messages, spoken calmly and clearly, to explain hospital experiences to the patient. *In an intensely anxious situation, the patient is able to comprehend only the most elementary communication.*

■ If hyperventilation occurs, help the patient breathe into a small paper bag held over the mouth and nose. Six to 12 natural breaths should be taken, alternating with short periods of diaphragmatic breathing. *Hyperventilation may occur during periods of extreme anxiety. Hyperventilation causes the amount* *of CO_2 in the blood to decrease, possibly resulting in lightheadedness, rapid heart rate, shortness of breath, numbness or tingling in the hands or feet, and syncope. This technique should not be used with patients who have coronary or respiratory disorders, such as coronary artery disease, asthma, or chronic obstructive pulmonary disease.*

■ Keep the immediate surroundings low in stimuli (dim lighting, few people, simple decor). *A stimulating environment may increase the level of anxiety.*

■ Administer antianxiety medications as ordered by the physician. Assess the medication for effectiveness and adverse side effects.

■ When the level of anxiety has been reduced, explore with the patient possible reasons for its occurrence. *If the patient is going to learn to interrupt escalating anxiety, they must first learn to recognize the factors that precipitate its onset.*

■ Teach the patient the signs and symptoms of escalating anxiety. Discuss ways to interrupt its progression, such as relaxation techniques, deep-breathing exercises, physical exercises, brisk walks, jogging, and meditation. Encourage the patient to identify which method they feel is most appropriate for them. *Relaxation techniques result in a physiological response opposite to that of the anxiety response, and physical activities discharge excess energy in a healthful manner.*

Fear

Fear is defined as the "Basic, intense emotional response aroused by the detection of imminent threat, involving an immediate alarm reaction (American Psychological Association)" (Herdman et al., 2021, p. 419).

Patient Goals

Outcome criteria include short- and long-term goals. Timelines are individually determined.

Short-term goal

■ Patient will discuss the phobic object or situation with the health-care provider within (time specified).

Long-term goal

■ By time of discharge from treatment, patient will be able to function in the presence of the phobic object or situation without experiencing panic anxiety.

Interventions

■ Explore the patient's perception of threat to physical integrity or threat to self-concept. Reassure the patient of their safety and security. *It is important to understand the patient's perception of the phobic object or situation to assist with the desensitization process.*

■ Discuss the reality of the situation with the patient to recognize aspects that can be changed and those that cannot. *The patient must accept the reality of the situation (aspects that cannot change) before the work of reducing the fear can progress. For example, a man who has a fear of flying and whose employment position requires long-distance air travel must accept that he needs to conquer the fear of flying if he is going to stay in this particular job.*

■ Include the patient in making decisions related to the selection of alternative coping strategies. For example, the patient may choose to either avoid the phobic stimulus or attempt to eliminate the fear associated with it. *Encouraging the patient to make choices promotes feelings of empowerment and serves to increase feelings of self-worth.*

■ If the patient elects to work on elimination of the fear, referral to treatment for systematic desensitization or implosion therapy may be recommended. (See the explanation of these techniques under "Treatment Modalities" at the end of this chapter.) *Systematic desensitization is a plan of behavior modification designed to expose the individual gradually to the situation or object (either in reality or through fantasizing) until the fear is no longer experienced. With implosion therapy, the individual is "flooded" with stimuli related to the phobic situation or object (rather than in gradual steps) until anxiety associated with the object or situation is no longer experienced. Fear is decreased as the physical and psychological sensations diminish in response to repeated exposure to the phobic stimulus under nonthreatening conditions.*

■ Encourage the patient to explore underlying feelings that may be contributing to irrational fears and to face them rather than suppress them. *Exploring underlying feelings may help the patient confront unresolved conflicts and develop more adaptive coping abilities.*

Ineffective Coping

Ineffective coping is defined as "a pattern of invalid appraisal of the stressors, with cognitive and/or behavioral efforts, that fails to manage demands related to well-being" (Herdman et al., 2021, p. 408).

Patient Goals

Outcome criteria include short- and long-term goals. Timelines are individually determined.

Short-term goal

■ Within 1 week, the patient will decrease participation in ritualistic behavior by one-half.

Long-term goal

■ By the time of discharge from treatment, the patient will demonstrate the ability to cope effectively without resorting to obsessive-compulsive behaviors or increased dependency.

Interventions

■ Work with the patient to determine the types of situations that increase anxiety and result in ritualistic behaviors. *If the patient is going to learn to interrupt escalating anxiety, they must first learn to recognize the factors that precipitate its onset.*

■ Initially meet the patient's dependency needs as required. To suddenly eliminate all avenues for dependency would create intense anxiety on the part of the patient. Encourage independence and give positive reinforcement for independent behaviors. *Positive reinforcement enhances self-esteem and promotes repetition of the desired behaviors.*

■ In the beginning of treatment, allow plenty of time for rituals. Do not be judgmental or verbalize disapproval of the behavior. *To deny the patient this activity may precipitate a panic level of anxiety. Also, low levels of anxiety provide a better foundation for exploring thoughts, feelings, and associated behaviors, and mild anxiety is most beneficial for teaching and learning.*

■ Support the patient's efforts to explore the meaning and purpose of the behavior. They are most likely unaware of the relationship between emotional problems and compulsive behaviors. *Knowledge and recognition of this fact are important before change can occur.*

■ Provide a structured schedule of activities for the patient, including adequate time for the completion of rituals. *The anxious individual needs a great deal of structure in their life. Assistance is needed with decision making, and structure provides a sense of security and comfort to deal with activities of daily living.*

■ Gradually begin to limit the amount of time allotted for ritualistic behavior as the patient becomes more involved in other activities. *Anxiety is minimized when the patient is able to replace ritualistic behaviors with more adaptive ones. Give positive reinforcement for nonritualistic behaviors.*

■ Help the patient learn ways to interrupt obsessive thoughts and ritualistic behavior with techniques such as thought-stopping (see Chapter 18, "Cognitive Behavior Therapy") and relaxation techniques, including physical exercise or other constructive activity with which the patient feels comfortable. *Knowledge and practice of coping techniques that are more adaptive will help the patient change and let go of maladaptive responses to anxiety.*

Disturbed Body Image

Disturbed body image is defined as the "negative mental picture of one's physical self" (Herdman et al., 2021, p. 355).

Patient Goals

Outcome criteria include short- and long-term goals. Timelines are individually determined.

Short-term goal

■ Patient will verbalize understanding that changes in bodily structure or function are exaggerated out of proportion to the change that actually exists. (Time frame for this goal must be determined according to individual patient's situation.)

Long-term goal

■ Patient will verbalize perception of own body that is realistic to actual structure or function by time of discharge from treatment.

Interventions

■ Assess the patient's perception of their body image. Keep in mind that this image is real to the patient even though they may recognize it as an exaggeration. *Assessment information is necessary to develop an accurate plan of care. Denial of the patient's feelings impedes the development of a trusting, therapeutic relationship.*

■ Help the patient see that their body image is distorted or out of proportion in relation to the significance of an actual physical anomaly. *Recognition that a misperception exists is necessary before the patient can accept reality and reduce the significance of the imagined defect.*

■ Encourage verbalization of fears and anxieties associated with identified stressful life situations. Discuss alternative adaptive coping strategies. *Verbalization of feelings with a trusted individual may help the patient come to terms with unresolved issues. Knowledge of alternative coping strategies may help the patient respond to stress more adaptively in the future.*

■ Involve the patient in activities that reinforce a positive sense of self not based on appearance. *When the patient is able to develop self-satisfaction based on accomplishments and unconditional acceptance, significance of the imagined defect or minor physical anomaly will diminish.*

■ Refer the patient to support groups for individuals with similar histories (e.g., Adult Children of Alcoholics [ACOA], Victims of Incest, Survivors of Suicide [SOS], Adults Abused as Children).

Ineffective Impulse Control (as seen in trichotillomania)

Ineffective impulse control is defined as "a pattern of performing rapid, unplanned reactions to internal or external stimuli without regard for the negative consequences of these reactions to the impulsive individual or to others" (Herdman et al., 2021, p. 330).

Patient Goals

Outcome criteria include short- and long-term goals. Timelines are individually determined.

Short-term goal

■ Patient will verbalize adaptive ways to cope with stress by means other than pulling out hair (time dimension to be individually determined).

Long-term goal

■ Patient will be able to demonstrate adaptive coping strategies in response to stress and a discontinuation of pulling out own hair (time dimension to be individually determined).

Interventions

■ Support the patient in their effort to stop hair pulling. Help the patient understand that it is possible to discontinue the behavior. The patient realizes that the behavior is maladaptive but feels helpless to stop. Support from the nurse builds trust.

■ Ensure that a nonjudgmental attitude is conveyed and criticism of the behavior is avoided. An attitude of acceptance promotes feelings of dignity and self-worth.

■ Assist the patient with **habit-reversal training (HRT)**, which has been shown to be an effective tool in treatment of hair-pulling disorder. HRT involves three components:

  1. **Awareness training:** Help the patient become aware of times when the hair pulling most often occurs (e.g., the patient learns to recognize urges, thoughts, or sensations that precede the behavior; the therapist points out to the patient each time the behavior occurs). Awareness helps the patient identify situations in which the behavior occurs or is most likely to occur and gives the patient a feeling of increased self-control.

  2. **Competing response training:** In this step, the patient learns to substitute another response to the urge to pull their hair. For example, when a patient experiences a hair-pulling urge, suggest that the individual ball up their hands into fists, tightening arm muscles, and "locking" their arms to make hair pulling impossible at that moment. Substituting an incompatible behavior may help to extinguish the undesirable behavior.

  3. **Social support:** Encourage family members to participate in the therapy process and offer positive feedback for attempts at habit reversal. Positive feedback enhances self-esteem and increases the patient's desire to continue with the therapy. It also provides cues for family members to use in their attempts to help the patient in treatment.

■ Once the patient has become aware of hair-pulling times, reinforce that occupying the hands, when hair pulling is anticipated, can help to prevent automatic behaviors from occurring.

■ Practice stress management techniques: deep breathing, meditation, stretching, physical exercise, listening to soft music. Hair pulling is thought to occur at times of increased anxiety.

■ Offer support and encouragement when setbacks occur. Help the patient to understand the importance of not quitting when it seems that change is not happening as quickly as they would like. Although some people see a decrease in the behavior within a few days, most take several months to notice the greatest change.

Concept Care Mapping

The concept map care plan (see Chapter 8, "The Nursing Process in Psychiatric-Mental Health Nursing") is a diagrammatic teaching and learning strategy that allows visualization of interrelationships between medical diagnoses, nursing diagnoses, assessment data, and treatments. An example of a concept map care plan for the patient with an anxiety disorder is presented in Figure 27–4.

Patient and Family Education

The role of patient teacher is important in the psychiatric area, as it is in all areas of nursing. A list of topics for patient and family education relevant to anxiety disorders is presented in Box 27–6.

Evaluation

In the final step of the nursing process, a reassessment is conducted to determine whether the nursing actions have been successful in achieving the objectives of care. Evaluation of the nursing actions for the patient with an anxiety disorder, OCD, or a related disorder may be facilitated by assessing whether the patient can do the following:

■ Recognize signs and symptoms of escalating anxiety

■ Use learned skills to interrupt the escalating anxiety before it reaches the panic level

■ Demonstrate the activities (e.g., relaxation techniques, physical exercise) most appropriate for them that can be used to maintain anxiety at a manageable level

■ Maintain anxiety at a manageable level without medication

■ Verbalize a long-term plan for preventing panic anxiety in the face of a stressful situation

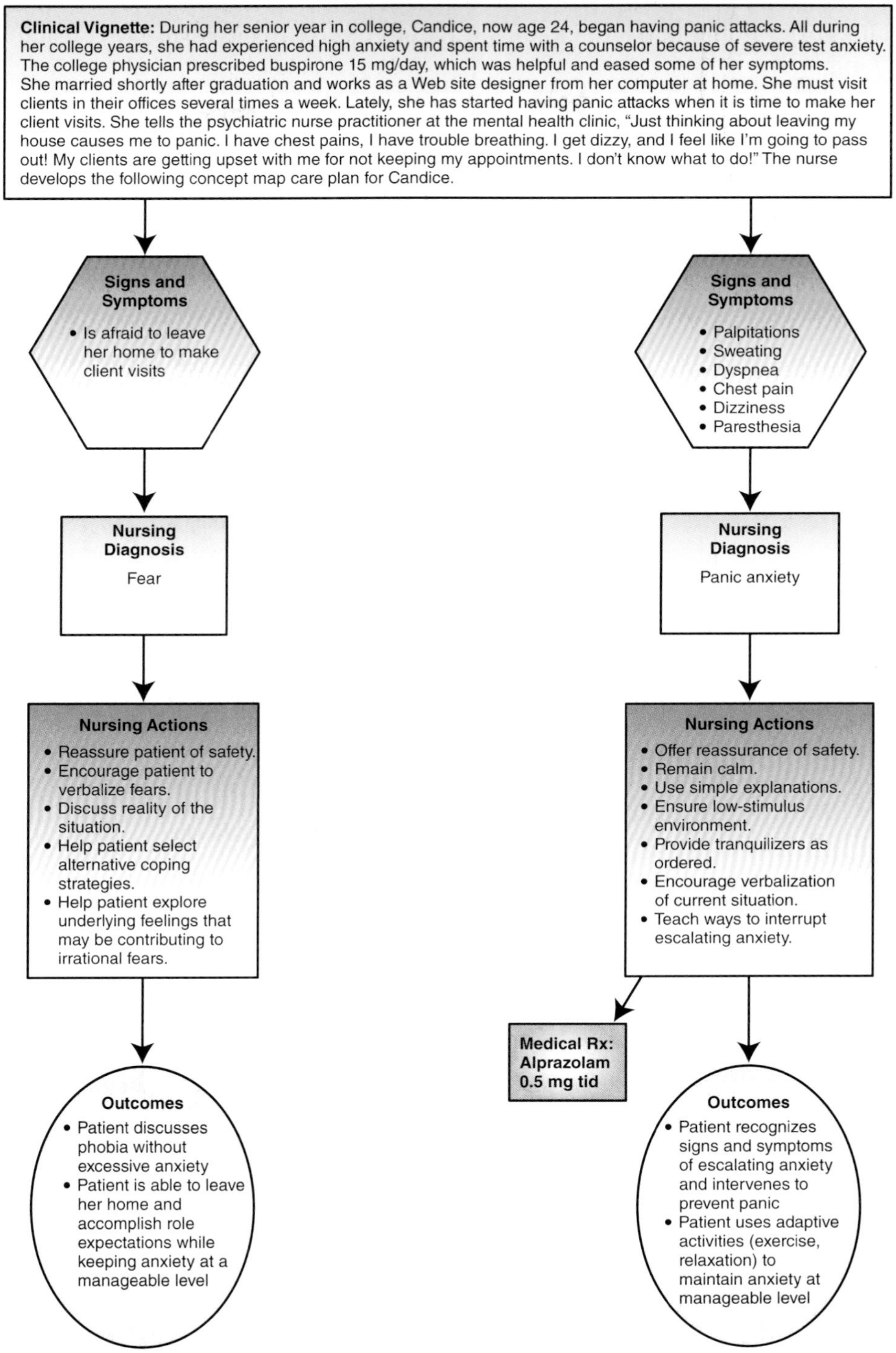

Clinical Vignette: During her senior year in college, Candice, now age 24, began having panic attacks. All during her college years, she had experienced high anxiety and spent time with a counselor because of severe test anxiety. The college physician prescribed buspirone 15 mg/day, which was helpful and eased some of her symptoms. She married shortly after graduation and works as a Web site designer from her computer at home. She must visit clients in their offices several times a week. Lately, she has started having panic attacks when it is time to make her client visits. She tells the psychiatric nurse practitioner at the mental health clinic, "Just thinking about leaving my house causes me to panic. I have chest pains, I have trouble breathing. I get dizzy, and I feel like I'm going to pass out! My clients are getting upset with me for not keeping my appointments. I don't know what to do!" The nurse develops the following concept map care plan for Candice.

Signs and Symptoms
- Is afraid to leave her home to make client visits

Signs and Symptoms
- Palpitations
- Sweating
- Dyspnea
- Chest pain
- Dizziness
- Paresthesia

Nursing Diagnosis
Fear

Nursing Diagnosis
Panic anxiety

Nursing Actions
- Reassure patient of safety.
- Encourage patient to verbalize fears.
- Discuss reality of the situation.
- Help patient select alternative coping strategies.
- Help patient explore underlying feelings that may be contributing to irrational fears.

Nursing Actions
- Offer reassurance of safety.
- Remain calm.
- Use simple explanations.
- Ensure low-stimulus environment.
- Provide tranquilizers as ordered.
- Encourage verbalization of current situation.
- Teach ways to interrupt escalating anxiety.

Medical Rx: Alprazolam 0.5 mg tid

Outcomes
- Patient discusses phobia without excessive anxiety
- Patient is able to leave her home and accomplish role expectations while keeping anxiety at a manageable level

Outcomes
- Patient recognizes signs and symptoms of escalating anxiety and intervenes to prevent panic
- Patient uses adaptive activities (exercise, relaxation) to maintain anxiety at manageable level

FIGURE 27–4 Concept map care plan for a patient with agoraphobia.

- Discuss the phobic object or situation without becoming anxious
- Function in the presence of the phobic object or situation without experiencing panic anxiety
- Refrain from performing rituals when anxiety level rises
- Demonstrate substitute behaviors to maintain anxiety at a manageable level
- Recognize the relationship between escalating anxiety and the dependence on ritualistic behaviors for relief
- Refrain from hair pulling (for patients with trichotillomania)
- Successfully substitute a more adaptive behavior when urges to pull hair occur (for patients with trichotillomania)

BOX 27–6 Topics for Patient and Family Education Related to Anxiety, Obsessive-Compulsive, and Related Disorders

NATURE OF THE ILLNESS
1. What is anxiety?
2. To what might it be related?
3. What is OCD?
4. What is body dysmorphic disorder?
5. What is trichotillomania?
6. Symptoms of anxiety disorders.

MANAGEMENT OF THE ILLNESS
1. Medication management:
   • Possible adverse effects
   • Length of time to take effect
   • What to expect from the medication
   a. For panic disorder and generalized anxiety disorder
      (1) Benzodiazepines
      (2) Buspirone (BuSpar)
      (3) Tricyclics
      (4) SSRIs
      (5) SNRIs
      (6) Propranolol
      (7) Clonidine
   b. For phobic disorders
      (1) Benzodiazepines
      (2) Tricyclics
      (3) Propranolol
      (4) SSRIs
   c. For OCD
      (1) SSRIs
      (2) Clomipramine

   d. For body dysmorphic disorder
      (1) Clomipramine
      (2) Fluoxetine
   e. For hair-pulling disorder (trichotillomania)
      (1) Chlorpromazine
      (2) Amitriptyline
      (3) Lithium carbonate
      (4) SSRIs/pimozide
      (5) Olanzapine
2. Stress management (Complementary therapies)
   a. Teach ways to interrupt escalating anxiety
      (1) Relaxation techniques
         (a) Progressive muscle relaxation
         (b) Imagery
         (c) Music therapy
         (d) Meditation
         (e) Yoga
         (f) Physical exercise
      (2) Massage therapy or aromatherapy massage
      (3) Pet therapy
      (4) Qigong
      (5) Auricular acupressure
      (6) Reiki touch therapy

SUPPORT SERVICES
1. Crisis hotline
2. Support groups
3. Individual psychotherapy

■ Verbalize a realistic perception and satisfactory acceptance of personal appearance (for patients with body dysmorphic disorder)

Treatment Modalities

Individual Psychotherapy

Most clients experience a marked lessening of anxiety when allowed to discuss their difficulties with a concerned and sympathetic therapist. Supportive psychotherapy is designed to help clients identify their personal strengths and explore adaptive coping mechanisms. Insight-oriented psychotherapy, which is rooted in Freudian psychology, is designed to help clients identify, explore, and resolve internal psychological conflicts that are contributing to anxiety.

The psychotherapist also can use logical and rational explanations to increase the client's understanding of various situations that create anxiety in their life. Psychoeducational information may also be presented in individual psychotherapy.

Cognitive Behavior Therapy

The cognitive model relates how individuals respond in stressful situations to their subjective cognitive appraisal of the event. Anxiety is experienced when the cognitive appraisal is one of danger with which the individual perceives that they are unable to cope. Impaired cognition can contribute to anxiety and related disorders when the individual's appraisals are chronically negative. Automatic negative appraisals provoke self-doubts, negative evaluations, and negative predictions. Anxiety is maintained by this dysfunctional appraisal of a situation.

CBT strives to assist the individual to reduce anxiety responses by altering cognitive distortions. Anxiety is described as being the result of exaggerated, *automatic* thinking.

CBT for anxiety is brief and time-limited, usually lasting from 5 to 20 sessions. Brief therapy discourages the client's dependency on the therapist, which is prevalent in anxiety disorders, and encourages the client's self-sufficiency.

A sound therapeutic relationship is a necessary condition for effective CBT. For the therapeutic process to occur, the client must be able to talk openly about fears and feelings. A major part of treatment consists of encouraging the client to face frightening situations to be able to view them realistically and talking about them is one way of achieving this goal. Treatment is a collaborative effort between client and therapist.

Rather than offering suggestions and explanations, the therapist uses questions to encourage the client to correct their anxiety-producing thoughts. The client is encouraged to become aware of the thoughts, examine them for cognitive distortions, substitute more balanced thoughts, and eventually develop new patterns of thinking.

CBT is structured and orderly, which is important for the client with an anxiety or related disorder who is often confused and lacks self-assurance. The focus is on solving current problems. Together, the client and therapist work to identify and correct maladaptive thoughts and behaviors that maintain a problem and block its solution.

CBT is based on educating the client that one develops anxiety because one has learned inappropriate ways of thinking about and responding to life experiences. The belief is that, with practice, individuals can learn more effective ways of responding to these experiences through cognitive reframing. Homework assignments, a central feature of CBT, provide an experimental, problem-solving approach to overcoming long-held anxieties. Through fulfillment of these personal "experiments," the effectiveness of specific strategies and techniques is determined.

Behavior Therapy

Behavior modification has been used to treat trichotillomania. Various techniques have been tried, including covert desensitization and HRT. These may include a system of positive and negative reinforcements to modify the hair-pulling behaviors. With HRT, in an attempt to extinguish the unwanted behavior, the individual learns to become more aware of the hair pulling, identify times of occurrence, and substitute a more adaptive coping strategy. (See interventions listed under the nursing diagnosis "Ineffective Impulse Control.")

Other forms of behavior therapy include systematic desensitization and implosion therapy, or flooding. They are commonly used to treat clients with phobic disorders and modify the stereotyped behavior of clients with OCD. They have also been shown to be effective in a variety of other anxiety-producing situations.

Systematic Desensitization

In **systematic desensitization**, the client is gradually exposed to the phobic stimulus in either a real or imagined situation. The concept was introduced by Joseph Wolpe in 1958 and is based on behavioral conditioning principles. Emphasis is placed on reciprocal inhibition or counterconditioning.

Reciprocal inhibition is the restriction of anxiety before the effort of reducing avoidance behavior. The rationale behind this concept is that because relaxation is antagonistic to anxiety, individuals cannot be anxious and relaxed at the same time.

Systematic desensitization with reciprocal inhibition involves two main elements:

1. Training in relaxation techniques
2. Progressive exposure to a hierarchy of fear stimuli while in the relaxed state

The individual is instructed to use relaxation techniques that are most effective for them (e.g., progressive relaxation, mental imagery, tense and relax, meditation). When the individual has mastered the relaxation technique, exposure to the phobic stimulus is initiated. They are asked to present a hierarchal arrangement of situations pertaining to the phobic stimulus in order from most disturbing to least disturbing. While in a state of maximum relaxation, the client may be asked to imagine the phobic stimulus. Initial exposure is focused on a concept of the phobic stimulus that produces the least amount of fear or anxiety. In subsequent sessions, the individual is gradually exposed to stimuli that are more fearful. Sessions may be executed in fantasy, in real-life (in vivo) situations, or sometimes in a combination of both. Following is a case study describing systematic desensitization.

Implosion Therapy (Flooding)

Implosion therapy (flooding), is a therapeutic process in which the client must imagine, for a prolonged period, situations or participate in real-life situations that they find extremely frightening. Relaxation training is not part of this technique. Plenty of time must be allowed for these sessions because brief periods may be ineffective or even harmful. A session is terminated when the client responds with considerably less anxiety than at the beginning of the session.

In implosion therapy, the therapist "floods" the client with information concerning situations that trigger anxiety in them. The therapist describes anxiety-provoking situations in vivid detail and is guided by the client's response; the more anxiety provoked, the more expedient is the therapeutic endeavor. The same theme is continued as long as it arouses anxiety. The therapy is continued until a topic no longer elicits inappropriate anxiety on the part of the client.

CASE STUDY: SYSTEMATIC DESENSITIZATION

Carlos was afraid to ride on elevators. He had been known to climb 24 flights of stairs in an office building to avoid riding the elevator. Carlos's office had plans for moving the company to a high-rise building soon, with offices on the 32nd floor. Carlos sought assistance from a therapist for help to treat this fear. He was taught to achieve a sense of calmness and well-being by using a combination of mental imagery and progressive relaxation techniques. In the relaxed state, Carlos was initially instructed to imagine the entry level of his office building, with a clear image of the bank of elevators. In subsequent sessions, and always in the relaxed state, Carlos progressed to images of walking onto an elevator, having the

elevator door close after he had entered, riding the elevator to the 32nd floor, and emerging from the elevator once the doors were opened. The progression included being accompanied in the activities by the therapist and eventually accomplishing them alone.

Therapy for Carlos also included in vivo sessions in which he was exposed to the phobic stimulus in real-life situations (always after achieving a state of relaxation). This technique, combining imagined and in vivo procedures, proved successful for Carlos, and his employment in the high-rise complex was no longer in jeopardy because of his fear of elevators.

Complementary Therapies/Integrative Health Strategies

Many complementary therapies are available that may be used alone or integrated with medication and other treatments for anxiety. Nonpharmacological approaches are important treatment strategies particularly because many antianxiety agents are only recommended for short-term treatment related to their potential for dependence.

Sagarwala and Nasrallah (2018) reviewed complementary approaches that were supported in evidence for both reducing anxiety measurements and showing biological evidence of effectiveness via reduced cortisol levels. Those that were supported by this evidence in randomized controlled trials were:

- Acupuncture
- Aromatherapy massage
- Auricular acupressure
- Massage therapy
- Music therapy
- Pet therapy
- Qigong (rhythmic movement and posturing)
- Relaxation exercises
- Reiki touch therapy
- Yoga

See Chapter 11 "Psychosocial Interventions and Spiritual Care" for further discussion of relaxation exercises and online Chapter 40, "Complementary Therapies and Integrative Health," for further discussion of integrative health strategies.

Psychopharmacology
Antianxiety Agents

Antianxiety drugs are also called *anxiolytics* and historically were referred to as *minor tranquilizers*. Antianxiety agents are used in the treatment of anxiety

disorders, anxiety symptoms, acute alcohol withdrawal, skeletal muscle spasms, convulsive disorders, status epilepticus, and preoperative sedation. Their use and efficacy for periods greater than 4 months have not been evaluated. Benzodiazepines have been the traditional medication treatment for acute anxiety states and are an important adjunct in treatment because a reduction in anxiety is essential for learning and adaptation. However, because they also have the potential for dependence, they are typically a short-term intervention. They also pose certain risks for some patients, including those who are pregnant, the elderly, those who have current or past substance use disorders, current users of prescribed opioids (risk of respiratory depression and death), and patients with chronic obstructive pulmonary disease (Weber & Duchemin, 2018).

Buspirone and other SSRIs have demonstrated efficacy in treating anxiety disorders as well and are not addictive. (See Chapter 4, "Psychopharmacology," for a detailed description of contraindications, precautions, and other safety issues related to this class of drugs.)

Several drugs can be used off-label to treat anxiety, including atypical antipsychotics, mirtazapine (a tetracyclic antidepressant), gabapentin or pregabalin (analgesic and mood stabilizer that also carry risk for dependence), antihistamines such as diphenhydramine, and other anticonvulsants such as lamotrigine and topiramate (Weber & Duchemin, 2018). Selected antianxiety agents are presented in Table 27–4.

Medications for Specific Disorders
For Panic and Generalized Anxiety Disorders

Anxiolytics Benzodiazepines have been used with success in the acute treatment of GAD. They can

TABLE 27–4 **Antianxiety Agents**			
CLASSIFICATION: GENERIC (TRADE) NAME	**CONTROLLED CATEGORIES**	**DAILY ADULT DOSAGE RANGE (mg)**	**COMMON SIDE EFFECTS OF ANTIANXIETY AGENTS**
ANTIHISTAMINE: Hydroxyzine (Vistaril)		100–400	■ Drowsiness, confusion, lethargy. ■ Tolerance; physical and psychological dependence (does not apply to buspirone). Patient should be tapered off long-term use.
BENZODIAZEPINES: Alprazolam (Xanax, Niravam)	CIV	0.75–4	
Chlordiazepoxide (Librium)	CIV	15–100	■ Potentiates the effects of other CNS depressants. Patient should not take alcohol or other CNS depressants with the medication.
Clonazepam (Klonopin)	CIV	1.5–20	
Clorazepate (Tranxene)	CIV	15–60	■ May aggravate symptoms of depression.
Diazepam (Valium, Diastat)	CIV	4–40	■ Orthostatic hypotension. Patient should rise slowly from a lying or sitting position.
Lorazepam (Ativan)	CIV	2–6	■ Paradoxical excitement. If symptoms opposite to the desired effect occur, notify physician immediately.
Oxazepam (Serax)	CIV	30–120	
Midazolam (Versed)*	CIV	5	■ Dry mouth. ■ Nausea and vomiting. May be taken with food or milk.
CARBAMATE DERIVATIVE: Meprobamate (Miltown, Equanil)	CIV	400–1,600	■ Blood dyscrasias. Symptoms of sore throat, fever, malaise, easy bruising, or unusual bleeding should be reported to the physician immediately.
AZASPIRODECANEDIONE Buspirone		15–60	■ Delayed onset (with buspirone). Lag time of 10–14 days for anxiety symptoms to diminish with buspirone. Buspirone is not recommended for prn administration.

*Primarily used for preoperative sedation, antianxiety, and conscious sedation.
CNS, Central nervous system.
Note: Antidepressants (which are also used in the treatment of anxiety disorders) are listed in Chapter 25, "Depressive Disorders."

be prescribed on an as-needed basis when the patient is feeling particularly anxious. Alprazolam, lorazepam, and clonazepam have been particularly effective in the treatment of panic disorder. The major risks with benzodiazepine therapy are physical dependence and tolerance, which may encourage abuse. Because withdrawal symptoms can be life-threatening, people must be warned against abrupt discontinuation of the drug and should be tapered off the medication at the end of therapy. Because of this addiction potential, their use as a first-line treatment has been surpassed in favor by the SSRIs, SNRIs, and buspirone.

The antianxiety agent buspirone is effective for the treatment of GAD (Boland & Verduin, 2022). One disadvantage of buspirone is its lag period (similar to antidepressants) in alleviating symptoms. However, the lack of risk for physical dependence or tolerance may make buspirone the drug of choice in the treatment of GAD.

Antidepressants Several antidepressants are effective as major antianxiety agents. The tricyclics clomipramine and imipramine have been used with success in people experiencing panic disorder. However, since the advent of SSRIs, the tricyclics are less widely used because of their tendency to produce severe side effects at the high doses required to relieve symptoms of panic disorder.

The SSRIs have been effective in the treatment of panic disorder. Paroxetine, fluoxetine, and sertraline have been approved by the U.S. Food and Drug Administration (FDA) for this purpose. Venlafaxine, an SNRI, is also approved by the FDA for treatment of panic disorder. Patients with panic disorder appear to be sensitive to treatment with antidepressants, so doses are lower initially and titrated slowly.

SSRIs and SNRIs are considered first-line treatments for GAD. The FDA has approved paroxetine (Paxil), escitalopram (Lexapro), duloxetine (Cymbalta), and extended-release venlafaxine (Effexor

XR) in the treatment of GAD. Atypical antidepressants such as nefazodone (Serzone) and mirtazapine (Remeron), although not approved by the FDA for anxiety disorder treatment, have also been identified as beneficial (Bhatt, 2019).

Antihypertensive Agents Several studies have called attention to the effectiveness of beta blockers (e.g., propranolol) and alpha-2-receptor agonists (e.g., clonidine) in the amelioration of anxiety symptoms (Bhatt, 2019). Propranolol has potent effects on the somatic manifestations of anxiety (e.g., palpitations, tremors), with less dramatic effects on the psychic component of anxiety. It appears to be most effective in the treatment of acute situational anxiety (e.g., performance anxiety; test anxiety), but it is not the first-line drug of choice in the treatment of panic disorder and GAD. Propranolol also demonstrated effectiveness in reducing hyperarousal states for up to 1 week after patients with PTSD had a flashback (Bhatt, 2019).

Clonidine is effective in blocking the acute anxiety effects in conditions such as opioid and nicotine withdrawal. However, its usefulness is limited in the long-term treatment of panic and GADs, particularly because of the development of tolerance to its antianxiety effects.

Anticonvulsants Pregabalin (Lyrica), which is a GABA derivative, may have benefits in treating anxiety disorders, but it is a schedule V controlled substance and therefore may pose a risk for dependence or drug diversion (Bhatt, 2019).

For Phobic Disorders

Anxiolytics Benzodiazepines have been successful in the treatment of SAD. They are well tolerated and have a rapid onset of action. However, because of their potential for misuse and dependence, they are not considered a first-line choice of treatment.

Antidepressants In recent years, SSRIs have become the first-line treatment of choice for SAD, and paroxetine and sertraline have been approved by the FDA for this purpose. Several other SSRIs and SNRIs have been used off-label to treat SAD, including fluoxetine, escitalopram, fluvoxamine, duloxetine, and venlafaxine (Garakani et al., 2021). Specific phobias generally are not treated with medication unless panic attacks accompany the phobia.

Antihypertensive Agents The beta blockers propranolol and atenolol have been used with success in people experiencing anticipatory performance anxiety or "stage fright." This type of phobic response produces symptoms such as sweaty palms, racing pulse, trembling hands, dry mouth, labored breathing, nausea, and memory loss. The beta blockers appear to be effective in reducing these symptoms in some individuals.

Novel Treatments Controlled trials for novel anxiety pharmacotherapy, including neuropeptides, glutamatergic agents (such as ketamine and d-cycloserine), and cannabinoids (including cannabidiol), primarily in GAD or SAD have had largely negative results, with only some promise for kava (although there is risk of liver toxicity) and an inhaled neurosteroid (which modulates GABA and glutamate receptors) (Garakani et al., 2021). The researchers noted that:

> cannabidiol and nabilone are the most promising cannabinoids in the treatment of anxiety disorders, but the level of evidence for these drugs is still very low. Overall, THC, THC-CBD and dronabinol seem to be ineffective and potentially harmful for subjects with anxiety disorders (p. 234).

Melatonin receptor agonists and hallucinogens such as psilocybin and LSD have also been studied for potential anxiolytic benefits but more research is needed. Garakani and associates (2021) added that about 33% of patients with anxiety disorders are treatment resistant and currently little is known about effective treatments for this population.

For Obsessive-Compulsive Disorder

Antidepressants The SSRIs fluoxetine (Prozac), paroxetine (Paxil), sertraline (Zoloft), and fluvoxamine (Luvox) have been approved by the FDA for the treatment of OCD. Dosages greater than those used for treating depression may be required for OCD. Common side effects include sleep disturbances, headache, and restlessness. These effects are often transient and are less troublesome than those of the tricyclics.

The tricyclic antidepressant clomipramine (Anafranil) was the first drug approved by the FDA in the treatment of OCD. Clomipramine is more selective for serotonin reuptake than any of the other tricyclics. Its efficacy in the treatment of OCD is well established, although the adverse effects, such as those associated with all the tricyclics, may make it less desirable than the SSRIs.

For Body Dysmorphic Disorder

Antidepressants SSRIs are effective in treating body dysmorphic disorder but the effective doses are higher than those used to treat depression and the duration of treatment is longer (Boland & Verduin, 2022).

For Trichotillomania (Hair-Pulling Disorder)

No medications have demonstrated consistent benefits for people with trichotillomania, but SSRIs have yielded moderate results for some individuals with this condition. *N*-acetylcysteine (an amino acid) may also have some benefits (Elston, 2019).

CLINICAL JUDGMENT IN ACTION: CASE STUDY AND SAMPLE CARE PLAN

NURSING HISTORY AND ASSESSMENT

Recognizing cues: The nurse must demonstrate the ability to recognize what information is most important to making an assessment (National Council of State Boards of Nursing [NCSBN], 2021). This information is italicized in the following.

Stephanie is a 34-year-old mother of a 7-year-old girl named April. Stephanie's husband, Chris, brought her to the emergency department when she began **complaining of chest pain and shortness of breath. Diagnostic testing ruled out cardiac problems,** and Stephanie was referred for psychiatric evaluation. Chris was present at the admission interview. He explained to the nurse that Stephanie **has become increasingly "nervous and high-strung" over the past few years.** Four years ago, April, then 3 years old, was attending nursery school 2 days a week. April became sick with a severe case of influenza that developed into **pneumonia.** She was hospitalized, and her **prognosis was questionable for a short while,** although she **eventually made a complete recovery.** Since that time, however, Stephanie has been **extremely anxious about her family's health. She is fastidious about housekeeping and scrubs her floors three times a week. She launders the bedclothes daily and uses bleach on all the countertops and door handles several times a day. She washes the woodwork twice a week. She washes her hands incessantly, and they are red and noticeably chapped.** Chris explained that Stephanie **becomes very upset if she is not able to perform all of her cleaning chores according to her self-assigned schedule.** This afternoon, April came home from school with a note from the teacher saying that **a child in April's class had been diagnosed with a case of meningitis. Chris told the nurse, "Stephanie just lost it. She got all upset and started crying and had trouble breathing. Then she got those pains in her chest.** That's when I brought her to the hospital." Stephanie is admitted to the psychiatric unit with a **diagnosis of Obsessive-Compulsive Disorder.** The physician orders alprazolam 0.5 mg tid and paroxetine 20 mg every morning.

The night nurse finds her **up at 2 a.m. scrubbing the shower with a hand towel. She refuses to sleep in the bed, stating that it must certainly be contaminated. When the day nurse makes morning rounds, she finds Stephanie in the bathroom washing her hands.**

Analyzing cues: The nurse must be able to interpret the information (NCSBN, 2021).

The nurse analyzes that although there has been anxiety associated with a previous illness, Stephanie's current behavior is disproportional to any current threats. The patient's recurrent anxiety is interpreted as evidence of an obsession and her strong need to repetitively clean things is interpreted as a compulsion.

Prioritize hypotheses: The nurse must be able to identify the client's most important needs (NCSBN, 2021).

The nurse identifies anxiety and maladaptive coping as the priority concerns because the patient's anxiety and maladaptive behaviors are interfering with basic needs such as sleep and skin integrity and the anxiety has been severe enough to culminate in panic attacks.

NURSING DIAGNOSES AND OUTCOME IDENTIFICATION

Generate solutions: The nurse must be able to connect their prioritized understanding of client needs to a course of action or plan of care (NCSBN, 2021).

From the assessment data, the nurse develops the following nursing diagnoses for Stephanie:

1. Panic anxiety related to the perceived threat to biological integrity evidenced by chest pain and shortness of breath.
   a. Short-term goal:
      ■ Patient will be able to relax with effects of medication.
   b. Long-term goal:
      ■ Patient will be able to maintain anxiety at manageable level.
2. Ineffective coping related to panic anxiety and weak ego strength evidenced by compulsive cleaning and washing hands.
   a. Short-term goal:
      ■ Patient will reduce amount of time performing rituals within 3 days.
   b. Long-term goal:
      ■ Patient will demonstrate ability to cope effectively without resorting to ritualistic behavior.

PLANNING AND IMPLEMENTATION

Take Action: The nurse must be able to identify what actions need to be taken and how they will be implemented (NCSBN, 2021).

PANIC ANXIETY

The following nursing interventions have been identified for Stephanie:

1. Stay with Stephanie and reassure her that she is safe and that she is not going to die.
2. Maintain a calm, nonthreatening manner.
3. Speak very clearly and calmly and use simple words and messages.
4. Keep the lights low, the noise level down as much as possible, and as few people in her environment as is necessary.

Continued

CLINICAL JUDGMENT IN ACTION: CASE STUDY AND SAMPLE CARE PLAN—cont'd

5. Administer the alprazolam and paroxetine as ordered by the physician. Monitor for effectiveness and side effects.
6. After several days, when the anxiety has subsided, discuss with Stephane the causes that precipitated this attack.
7. Teach her the signs that indicate her anxiety level is rising.
8. Teach strategies that she may employ to interrupt the escalation of the anxiety. She may choose which is best for her: relaxation exercises, physical exercise, meditation.

INEFFECTIVE COPING
The following nursing interventions have been identified for Stephanie:

1. Initially, allow Stephanie all the time she needs to wash her hands, straighten up her room, change her own sheets, and so on. To deny her these rituals would result in panic anxiety.
2. Initiate discussions with Stephanie about her behavior. She ultimately must come to understand that these rituals are her way of keeping her anxiety under control.
3. Within a couple of days, begin to limit the amount of time Stephanie may spend on her rituals. Assign her to groups and activities that take up her time and distract her from her obsessions.
4. Explore with Stephanie the types of situations that cause her anxiety to rise. Help her to correlate these times of increased anxiety to initiation of the ritualistic behavior.
5. Help her with problem-solving and with making decisions about more adaptive ways to respond to situations that cause her anxiety to rise.

6. Explore her fears surrounding the health of her daughter. Help her to recognize which fears are legitimate and which are irrational.
7. Discuss possible activities in which she may participate that may distract from obsessions about contamination. Make suggestions and encourage her to follow through. Examples may include enrollment in classes at the local community college, volunteer work at the local hospital, or part-time employment.
8. Explain to her that she will likely be discharged from the hospital with a prescription for paroxetine. Teach her about the medication, how it should be taken, possible side effects, and what to report to the physician.
9. Suggest that she may benefit from attendance in an anxiety disorder support group. If she is interested, help locate one that would be convenient and appropriate for her.

EVALUATION
Evaluate outcomes: The nurse must be able to evaluate actions taken and determine whether they have had a positive, neutral, or negative effect (NCSBN, 2021).

The outcome criteria for Stephanie have been met. She has remained calm during her hospital stay with the use of the medication. The use of ritualistic behavior in the hospital setting diminished rapidly. She has discussed situations that she knows cause her anxiety to rise. She has learned relaxation exercises and practices them daily. She plans to start jogging and has the phone number for an anxiety support group that she plans to call. She says that she hopes the support group will help her maintain rationality about her daughter's health. She states that she understands about the need to take paroxetine and plans to take it every morning.

Summary and Key Points

■ Anxiety is a necessary force for survival and has been experienced by humanity throughout the ages.

■ Anxiety was first described as a physiological disorder and identified by its physical symptoms, particularly the cardiac symptoms. The psychological implications for the symptoms were not recognized until the early 1900s.

■ Anxiety is considered a normal reaction to a realistic danger or threat to biological integrity or self-concept.

■ The normality of the anxiety experienced in response to a stressor is defined by societal and cultural standards.

■ Anxiety disorders are more common in women than in men by at least two to one.

■ Studies of familial patterns suggest that a familial predisposition to anxiety disorders probably exists.

■ The *DSM-5-TR* identifies several broad categories of anxiety and related disorders. They include panic and generalized anxiety disorders, phobic disorders, and obsessive-compulsive disorder and related disorders, such as body dysmorphic disorder and trichotillomania. Anxiety disorders may also be the result of other medical conditions and intoxication or withdrawal from substances.

■ Panic disorder is characterized by recurrent panic attacks, the onset of which are unpredictable and manifested by intense apprehension, fear, and physical discomfort.

■ Generalized anxiety disorder is characterized by chronic, unrealistic, and excessive anxiety and worry.

■ Social anxiety disorder is an excessive fear of situations in which a person might do something embarrassing or be evaluated negatively by others.

■ Specific phobia is a marked, persistent, and excessive or unreasonable fear when in the presence of or when anticipating an encounter with a specific object or situation.

■ Agoraphobia is a fear of being in places or situations from which escape might be difficult or in which help might not be available if the person becomes anxious.

■ Obsessive-compulsive disorder involves recurrent obsessions or compulsions that are severe enough to interfere with social and occupational functioning.

■ Body dysmorphic disorder is an exaggerated belief that the body is deformed or defective in some specific way.

■ Trichotillomania (also known as hair-pulling disorder) is a disorder of impulse characterized by the recurrent pulling out of one's own hair that results in noticeable hair loss.

■ Hoarding disorder is defined by the persistent difficulty in discarding or parting with possessions, regardless of their actual value.

■ Several elements, including psychosocial factors, biological influences, and learning experiences, most likely contribute to the development of these disorders.

■ Treatment of anxiety and related disorders includes individual psychotherapy, cognitive behavior therapy, behavior therapy (including implosion therapy, systematic desensitization, and HRT), complementary therapies, and psychopharmacology.

■ Nurses can help patients with anxiety and related disorders gain insight and increase self-awareness about their illness.

■ Intervention focuses on assisting patients to learn techniques with which they may interrupt the escalation of anxiety before it reaches unmanageable proportions and to replace maladaptive behavior patterns with new, more adaptive, coping skills.

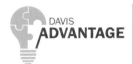

Go to **Davis Advantage** to complete your learning: strengthen understanding, apply your knowledge, and prepare for the Next Gen NCLEX®.

Review Questions

1. A client has been diagnosed with agoraphobia. Which behavior would be most characteristic of this disorder?
   a. The client experiences panic anxiety when she encounters snakes.
   b. The client refuses to fly in an airplane.
   c. The client will not eat in a public place.
   d. The client stays at home for fear of being in a place from which they cannot escape.

2. Which of the following is the most appropriate therapy for a client with agoraphobia?
   a. 10 mg Valium qid
   b. Group therapy with other people with agoraphobia
   c. Facing the fear in gradual step progression
   d. Hypnosis

3. With implosion therapy, a client with phobic anxiety would be:
   a. Taught relaxation exercises.
   b. Subjected to graded intensities of the fear.
   c. Instructed to stop the therapeutic session as soon as anxiety is experienced.
   d. Presented with intense exposure to a variety of stimuli associated with the phobic object or situation.

4. A client with OCD spends many hours each day washing their hands. Which is the most likely reason for such frequent hand washing?
   a. Relieve anxiety
   b. Reduce the probability of infection
   c. Reduce delusions
   d. Improve self-concept

5. A client is receiving treatment at the mental health clinic with habit-reversal training. Which of the following elements would be included in this therapy? (Select all that apply.)
   a. Awareness training
   b. Competing response training
   c. Social support
   d. Hypnotherapy
   e. Aversive therapy

Clinical Judgment Questions

6. The *initial* care plan for a client with OCD who washes their hands obsessively would include which of the following nursing interventions?
   a. Keep the client's bathroom locked so they cannot wash their hands all the time.
   b. Structure the client's schedule so they have plenty of time for hand washing.
   c. Place the client in isolation until they promise to stop washing their hands so much.
   d. Explain the client's behavior to them, because they are probably unaware that it is maladaptive.

7. A client with OCD says to the nurse, "I've been here 4 days now, and I'm feeling better. I feel comfortable on this unit, and I'm not ill-at-ease with the staff or other patients anymore." In light of this change, which nursing intervention is most appropriate?
   a. Give attention to the ritualistic behaviors each time they occur and point out their inappropriateness.
   b. Ignore the ritualistic behaviors, and they will be eliminated for lack of reinforcement.
   c. Set limits on the amount of time the client may engage in the ritualistic behavior.
   d. Allow the client all the time they want to carry out the ritualistic behavior.

8. A new client at the mental health clinic is diagnosed with body dysmorphic disorder. Which of the following nursing interventions is a priority?
   a. Support the client's efforts to seek corrective surgery.
   b. Recommend the client see a physician for treatment with antipsychotic medication.
   c. Encourage the client to describe reasons for seeking treatment.
   d. Reinforce to the client that their body is perfectly normal.

9. A client who is experiencing a panic attack has just arrived at the emergency department. Which is the *priority* nursing intervention for this client?
   a. Stay with the client and reassure them of their safety.
   b. Administer a dose of diazepam.
   c. Leave the client alone in a quiet room so they can calm down.
   d. Encourage the client to talk about what triggered the attack.

10. A client with generalized anxiety disorder who has been prescribed buspirone 15 mg daily, says to the nurse, "Why do I have to take this every day? My friend's doctor ordered Xanax for him, and he only takes it when he is feeling anxious." Which of the following would be an appropriate response by the nurse?
    a. "Xanax is not effective for generalized anxiety disorder."
    b. "Buspirone must be taken daily in order to be effective."
    c. "I will ask the doctor if he will change your dose of buspirone to prn so that you don't have to take it every day."
    d. "Your friend really should be taking the Xanax every day."

IMPLICATIONS OF RESEARCH FOR EVIDENCE-BASED PRACTICE

Teismann, T., Lukaschek, K., Hiller, T. S., Breitbart, J., Brettschneider, C., Schumacher, U., Margraf, J., Gensichen, J., & the Jena Paradies Study Group. (2018) Suicidal ideation in primary care patients suffering from panic disorder with or without agoraphobia. *BMC Psychiatry, 18,* 305. https://doi.org/10.1186/s12888-018-1894-5

DESCRIPTION OF THE STUDY: Recognizing that suicide ideation is common among individuals with panic disorder, the researchers investigated primary care patients with panic disorder (n = 296) to better understand the rates and risk factors for suicide ideation.

RESULTS OF THE STUDY: Suicidal ideation was experienced by 25% of the respondents. In a logistic regression analysis, depression diagnosis and depression severity emerged as significant risk factors for suicidal ideation.

Anxiety measures were not associated with suicidal ideation.

IMPLICATIONS FOR NURSING PRACTICE: Suicide is a major health problem in the United States, and the increase in incidence has prompted researchers to explore variables that are most associated with suicide risk. The findings in this study highlight the importance of assessing for symptoms of depression and suicidal ideation in individuals with anxiety disorders. (See Chapter 16, "Suicide Prevention," for a more thorough discussion of current assessment tools and interventions associated with risks for suicide.) Current research on the topic of suicide is rapidly expanding the evidence base related to this health concern, and nurses in any practice setting need to remain informed of the latest research to improve safety and quality care for this population.

TEST YOUR CLINICAL REASONING AND CLINICAL JUDGMENT SKILLS

Sarah, age 25, was taken to the emergency department by her friends. They were at a dinner party when Sarah suddenly clasped her chest and started having difficulty breathing. She complained of nausea and was perspiring profusely. She had calmed down some by the time they reached the hospital. She denied any pain, and electrocardiogram and laboratory results were unremarkable.

Sarah told the admitting nurse that she had a history of these "attacks." She began having them in her sophomore year of college. She knew her parents had expectations that she should follow in their footsteps and become an attorney. They also expected her to earn grades that would promote acceptance by a top Ivy League university. Sarah experienced her first attack when she made a B in English during her third semester of college. Since that time, she has experienced these symptoms sporadically, often in conjunction with her perception of the need to excel. She graduated with top honors from Harvard.

Last week, Sarah was promoted within her law firm. She was assigned her first solo case of representing a couple whose baby had died at birth and who were suing the physician for malpractice. She has experienced these panic symptoms daily for the past week, stating, "I feel like I'm going crazy!"

Sarah is transferred to the psychiatric unit. The psychiatrist diagnoses panic disorder.

Answer the following questions related to Sarah:

1. What would be the priority nursing diagnosis for Sarah?
2. What is the priority nursing intervention with Sarah?
3. What medical treatment might you expect the physician to prescribe?

Communication Exercises

1. John, who was just admitted to the psychiatric unit with panic disorder, approaches the nurse with complaints of numbness in his fingers and shortness of breath.

   What would be some appropriate responses by the nurse?
2. After attending a group that discussed irrational thinking patterns, John asks the nurse, "How does this cognitive behavior therapy work?"

   What would be some appropriate responses to John's question?

MOVIE CONNECTIONS

As Good As It Gets (OCD) • *The Aviator* (OCD) • *What About Bob?* (phobias) • *Copycat* (agoraphobia) • *Analyze This* (panic disorder) • *Vertigo* (specific phobia) • *Dirty, Filthy Love* (trichotillomania and other anxiety disorders) • *Sparrow's Dance* (agoraphobia)

References

Abell, S. R., & El-Mallakh, R. S. (2021). Serotonin-mediated anxiety: How to recognize and treat it. *Current Psychiatry, 20*(11), 37–40. doi:10.12788/cp.0168

Amaral, J. M., Spadaro, P. T., Pereira, V. M., Oliveira e Silva, A. C., & Nardi, A. E. (2013). The carbon dioxide challenge test in panic disorder: A systematic review of preclinical and clinical research. *Revista Brasileira de Psiquiatria, 35*(3), 318–331. doi:http://dx.doi.org/10.1590/1516-4446-2012-1045

American Psychiatric Association (APA). (2022). *Diagnostic and statistical manual of mental disorders, fifth edition, text revision (DSM-5-TR).* American Psychiatric Association.

Anxiety and Depression Association of America (ADAA). (2022). *Facts and statistics.* https://adaa.org/understanding-anxiety/facts-statistics

Bhatt, N. (2019). *Anxiety disorders.* http://emedicine.medscape.com/article/286227-overview#a2

Boland, R., & Verduin, M. L. (2022). *Kaplan & Sadock's synopsis of psychiatry* (P. Ruiz, Ed.). (12th ed.). Wolters Kluwer.

Brazier, Y. (2020). Everything you need to know about phobias. *Medical News Today.* https://www.medicalnewstoday.com/articles/249347

Chandra, S. (2020). *Anxiety: It's not just serotonin.* https://www.chandramd.com/blog/anxiety-its-not-just-serotonin

Chandran, N. S., Novak, J., Iorizzo, M., Grimalt, R., & Oranje, A. P. (2015). Trichotillomania in children. *Skin Appendage Disorders, 1*(1), 18–24. https://doi.org/10.1159/000371809

Dias, B. G., & Ressler, K. J. (2014). Parental olfactory experience influences behavior and neural structure in subsequent generations. *Nature Neuroscience, 17*, 86–96. doi:10.1038/nn.3594

Dozier, M. E., & Ayers, C. R. (2017). The etiology of hoarding disorder: A review. *Psychopathology, 50*(5), 291–296. https://doi.org/10.1159/000479235

Elston, D. M. (2019). *Trichotillomania.* http://emedicine.medscape.com/article/1071854-overview#a3

Garakani, A., Murrough, J. W., Freire, R. C., Thom, R. P., Larkin, K., Buono, F. D., & Iosifescu, D. V. (2021). Pharmacotherapy of anxiety disorders: Current and emerging treatment options. *Focus, 19*(2), 222–242. https://doi.org/10.1176/appi.focus.19203

Gerbarg, P. L., & Brown, R. P. (2016). Neurobiology and neurophysiology of breath practices in psychiatric care. *Psychiatric Times.* https://www.psychiatrictimes.com/view/neurobiology-and-neurophysiology-breath-practices-psychiatric-care

Gottschalk, M. G., & Domschke, K. (2017). Genetics of generalized anxiety disorder and related traits. *Dialogues in Clinical Neuroscience, 19*(2), 159–168. https://doi.org/10.31887/DCNS.2017.19.2/kdomschke

Herdman, T. H., Kamitsuru, S., & Lopes, C. T. (Eds.). (2021). *NANDA-I, Inc. nursing diagnoses: Definitions and classification, 2021–2023.* Thieme.

Kaplan, A. (2012). Update on trichotillomania. *Psychiatric Times.* https://www.psychiatrictimes.com/view/update-trichotillomania

Karthik, S., Sharma, L. P., & Narayanaswamy, J. C. (2020). Investigating the role of glutamate in obsessive-compulsive disorder: Current perspectives. *Neuropsychiatric Disease and Treatment, 16*, 1003–1013. https://doi.org/10.2147/NDT.S211703

Kimmel, R. J., & Roy-Burn, P. (2017). Clinical features of the anxiety disorders. In Sadock, B. J., Sadock, V. A., & Ruiz, P. (Eds.), *Comprehensive textbook of psychiatry* (10th ed., pp. 1723–1730). Wolters Kluwer.

Mayo Clinic. (2022). *Hoarding.* https://www.mayoclinic.org/diseases-conditions/hoarding-disorder/symptoms-causes/syc-20356056

Meyers, L. (2016). *Help for those who hoard.* https://ct.counseling.org/tag/hoarding/

National Council of State Boards of Nursing (NCSBN). (2021). *Next generation NCLEX®: comparison between case studies and stand-alone items.* https://www.ncsbn.org/public-files/NGN_Fall21_English_Final.pdf

National Institute of Mental Health (NIMH). (n.d.). *Statistics: Any anxiety disorder.* https://www.nimh.nih.gov/health/statistics/any-anxiety-disorder

Pond, E. (2020). *Trichotillomania: Diagnosis, treatment, and prognosis of a complex psychiatric disorder.* https://www.psychiatryadvisor.com/home/topics/anxiety/obsessive-compulsive-and-related-disorders/hair-pulling-review/

Reknes, I., Visockaite, G., Liefooghe, A., Lovakov, A., & Einarsen, S. V. (2019). Locus of control moderates the relationship between exposure to bullying behaviors and psychological strain. *Frontiers in Psychology, 10*, 1323. https://doi.org/10.3389/fpsyg.2019.01323

Smoller, J.W. (2020). Anxiety genetics goes genomic. *The American Journal of Psychiatry, 177*(3), 190–194. https://doi.org/10.1176/appi.ajp.2020.20010038

Sagarwala, R., & Nasrallah, H. (2018). Complementary treatments for anxiety: Beyond pharmacotherapy and psychotherapy. *Current Psychiatry, 17*(7), 29–36.

Stein, D. J., & Lochner, C. (2017). Obsessive-compulsive and related disorders. In Sadock, B. J., Sadock, V. A., & Ruiz, P. (Eds.), *Comprehensive textbook of psychiatry* (10th ed., pp. 1785–1798). Wolters Kluwer.

Stevens, M. C., Levy, H. C., Hallion, L. S., Wootton, B. M., & Tolin, D. F. (2020). Functional neuroimaging test of an emerging neurobiological model of hoarding disorder. *Biological Psychiatry: Cognitive Neuroscience and Neuroimaging, 5*(1), 68–75. https://doi.org/10.1016/j.bpsc.2019.08.010

Sykes, T. (2017). Prince Harry on his panic attacks: "We're all mental." *The Daily Beast.* https://www.thedailybeast.com/prince-harry-on-panic-attacks-were-all-mental

Teismann, T., Lukaschek, K., Hiller, T. S., Breitbart, J., Brettschneider, C., Schumacher, U., Margraf, J., Gensichen, J., & the Jena Paradies Study Group. (2018). Suicidal ideation in primary care patients suffering from panic disorder with or without agoraphobia. *BMC Psychiatry, 18*, 305. https://doi.org/10.1186/s12888-018-1894-5

Weber, S. R., & Duchemin, A. M. (2018). Benzodiazepines: Sensible prescribing in light of the risks. *Current Psychiatry, 17*(2), 23–27.

Classical References

Freud, S. (1959). On the grounds for detaching a particular syndrome from neurasthenia under the description "anxiety neurosis." In *The standard edition of the complete psychological works of Sigmund Freud* (Vol. 3). Hogarth Press.

Hamilton, M. (1959). The assessment of anxiety states by rating. *British Journal of Medical Psychology, 32*(1), 50–55. doi:10.1111/j.2044-8341.1959.tb00467.x

Johnson, J. H., & Sarason, I. B. (1978). Life stress, depression and anxiety: Internal-external control as moderator variable. *Journal of Psychosomatic Research, 22*(3), 205–208. doi:http://dx.doi.org/10.1016/0022-3999(78)90025-9

Trauma- and Stressor-Related Disorders

28

CORE CONCEPTS

Stress and Coping: Trauma

Professional Behavior: Nursing process in the care of patients with trauma- and stressor-related disorders

Safety

Clinical Judgment

KEY TERMS

acute stress disorder (ASD)

adjustment disorder

post-traumatic stress disorder (PTSD)

prolonged grief disorder

trauma-informed care

OBJECTIVES

After reading this chapter, the student will be able to:

1. Discuss historical and epidemiological aspects related to trauma- and stressor-related disorders.
2. Describe various types of trauma- and stressor-related disorders and identify symptomatology associated with each; use this information in patient assessment.
3. Identify predisposing factors in the development of trauma- and stressor-related disorders.
4. Formulate nursing diagnoses and goals of care for patients with trauma- and stressor-related disorders.

5. Describe the concepts and principles associated with trauma-informed care.
6. Describe appropriate nursing interventions for behaviors associated with trauma- and stressor-related disorders.
7. Evaluate the nursing care of patients with trauma- and stressor-related disorders.
8. Discuss various modalities relevant to treatment of trauma- and stressor-related disorders.

In 2011 a massive earthquake and tsunami claimed the lives of thousands and destroyed communities in eastern Japan. Yuri Sato, a public health nurse charged with helping survivors, shared her courageous experience (Frances, 2015):

As public health nurses, our immediate task was to treat the injured and sick; collect and dispense medicines; and respond to the desperate conditions of the townspeople. We launched and managed an aid station and a welfare evacuation site for those in need of urgent nursing care; established countermeasures against infectious disorders; and arranged for emergency food supplies and sanitation. ... With the entire town disaster-stricken, I was overcome with a sense of doubt and anxiety. Questions continually spun around in my mind: "What is mental health care when all of us have suffered so greatly?" But with everyone in mourning, we were single-mindedly focused on not losing any more lives to suicide or accident. ... People continued to be unable to accept the deaths of family members, relatives and friends—and the fact that so many were still missing. I often heard "I should have died," "Why did I survive?" or "I want my time to come soon." I also felt this way, but had too much work to do to linger on my own losses and feelings about them.

Traumas such as these test the very fiber of our human spirit and emotional well-being. Anyone hearing Ms. Sato's recollections would agree that the events were (and are) painfully traumatic. For some, the stress associated with trauma continues to cause enduring, significant distress and interference with their ability to function, leading to conditions called trauma- and stressor-related disorders.

The *Diagnostic and Statistical Manual of Mental Disorders, Fifth Edition, Text Revision (DSM-5-TR)* (American Psychiatric Association [APA], 2022) chapter on "Trauma- and Stressor-Related Disorders" includes disorders in which "exposure to a traumatic or stressful event is listed specifically as a diagnostic criterion" (p. 295). Four of the diagnostic categories are the focus of this chapter: adjustment disorders, acute stress disorders, post-traumatic stress disorder (PTSD), and prolonged grief disorder. Two additional disorders (reactive attachment disorder and disinhibited social engagement disorder) are also included in the *DSM-5-TR* chapter on trauma- and stressor-related disorders and are identified as childhood disorders associated with absence of adequate caregiving during childhood (social neglect). Chapter 28 focuses on disorders that occur after exposure to an identifiable stressor or an extremely traumatic event. Epidemiology is presented, and predisposing factors associated with the etiology of these disorders are discussed. An explanation of the symptomatology is presented as background knowledge for assessing people with trauma- and stressor-related disorders. Nursing care is described in the context of the nursing process. Various treatment modalities are explored.

Historical and Epidemiological Aspects

The concept of a post-trauma response has been referred to as *shell shock, battle fatigue, accident neurosis,* and *post-traumatic neurosis.* Reports of symptoms and syndromes with PTSD-like features have existed in writing throughout the centuries. In the early part of the 20th century, traumatic neurosis was viewed as the ego's inability to master the degree of disorganization brought about by a traumatic experience. Very little was written about post-traumatic neurosis between 1950 and 1970. This absence was followed in the 1970s and 1980s with expansive research and writing on the subject. Many of the papers written during this time were about Vietnam veterans.

Although the renewed interest in PTSD was linked to the psychological casualties of war, it is well recognized that any experience of significant trauma may be associated with the development of this disorder.

The diagnostic category of PTSD did not appear until the third edition of the *DSM* in 1980, after a need was indicated by increasing numbers of trauma-related stress disorders among Vietnam veterans and victims of multiple disasters. The *DSM-5-TR* (APA, 2022) describes the trauma that precedes PTSD as an event that is either directly experienced or witnessed, occurring in a close family member or close friend, or involves repeated exposure to aversive details about a traumatic event. Examples of such events include (but are not limited to) threatened or actual sexual violence, exposure to war, threatened or actual physical attack, torture, natural or man-made disasters, and severe motor vehicle accidents.

About 60% of men and 50% of women are exposed to a traumatic event in their lifetimes (Department of Veterans Affairs, 2022). Women are more likely to experience sexual assault and childhood sexual abuse, whereas men are more likely to experience accidents, physical assaults, combat, or proximity to death or injury. About 12 million adults in the United States experience PTSD in a given year, which is a small portion of those who have experienced a trauma, and the disorder is twice as common in women as men (Department of Veteran Affairs, 2022).

Historically, as previously stated, individuals who experienced stress reactions that followed exposure to an extremely traumatic event were given the diagnosis of PTSD. Accordingly, stress reactions from "normal" daily events (e.g., divorce, failure, rejection) were characterized as adjustment disorders (Friedman, 1996). Currently, the definition of an adjustment disorder is broader in spectrum and may involve single, multiple, recurrent, or continuous stressors. It is primarily differentiated from PTSD and ASDs by the time of onset and duration of symptoms (APA, 2022).

A number of studies have indicated that adjustment disorders are probably quite common, although prevalence rates range from 5% to 50% depending on the population being studied (Frank, 2021). The *DSM-5-TR* (APA, 2022) reports that, in hospital psychiatric consultation services, adjustment disorder has often been the most common diagnosis, frequently reaching 50%.

Other studies have found higher rates among specific high-risk groups including those recently unemployed (27%) and bereaved individuals (18%) (O'Donnell et al., 2019). General examples of other situations that commonly result in adjustment disorders include enduring a stressful experience such as a major life change or medical illness, giving birth to a stillborn child, being a victim of bullying or harassment, or being incarcerated (Katzman & Geppert, 2017).

Application of the Nursing Process— Trauma-Related Disorders

CORE CONCEPT
Trauma
An extremely distressing experience that causes severe emotional shock and may have long-lasting psychological effects.

Trauma-Informed Care

Experts highlight the importance of trauma-informed care as essential to improving the quality of care for clients both in and outside of behavioral health-care settings (Hopper et al., 2010; Substance Abuse and Mental Health Services Administration [SAMHSA], 2022). **Trauma-informed care** generally describes a philosophical approach that values awareness and understanding of trauma when assessing, planning, and implementing care. SAMHSA (2014) advances the following principles (4Rs) in defining this approach. Trauma-informed care:

■ **R**ealizes the widespread effect of trauma and various paths for recovery.
■ **R**ecognizes the signs and symptoms of trauma in clients, families, staff, and all those involved with the system.
■ **R**esponds by fully integrating knowledge about trauma in policies, procedures, and practices.
■ Seeks to actively resist **r**etraumatization.

Hopper and associates (2010) discussed applying this approach with the homeless population (a significant problem for people with severe mental illness). The authors described the many traumatic experiences that culminate in homelessness and the often co-occurring illnesses such as depression, substance abuse, and severe mental illness. To ignore the significance of trauma or to provide uninformed care leaves this population vulnerable to revictimization and "further complicates their service needs" (p. 81). These authors advanced the following definition of trauma-informed care:

> Trauma-informed care is a strength-based framework that is grounded in understanding of and responsiveness to the effect of trauma that emphasizes physical, psychological, and emotional safety

for both providers and survivors to rebuild a sense of control and empowerment. (p. 82)

Inherent in this definition is the importance of health-care providers being aware of the effect of trauma on themselves, as it may have an effect on their effectiveness in providing care to patients.

 Interventions that are considered trauma-informed highlight the importance of respect for the client, collaboration and connection, providing information about the connections between trauma and other health concerns, instilling hope, and empowering the trauma survivor to guide and direct their recovery plan (the essence of patient-centered care).

Childhood trauma, including physical, emotional, and sexual abuse, is also often identified as significant in the development of behavioral problems, eating disorders, some personality disorders, depression, and substance abuse.

Health-care providers, if they do not fully understand the effect of previous trauma on the client's current health concerns, may unwittingly retraumatize clients. Interventions such as seclusion and restraint, which are designed to protect the client's safety when they are at imminent risk of harm to themselves or others, may be retraumatizing to a client with a history of trauma. Much attention has been given to the importance of trauma-informed care in behavioral health-care settings because of the recognition that trauma history may be associated with other mental illnesses. However, nurses in every practice setting must incorporate this approach in assessment and care provision because trauma history can affect any patient's response to care. See the "Real People, Real Stories" feature in Chapter 34, "Survivors of Abuse or Neglect," for Diana's perspective on how previous traumas affect her response in general health-care settings.

Post-Traumatic Stress Disorder and Acute Stress Disorder

Background Assessment Data

Post-traumatic stress disorder (PTSD) is described as a multisymptom response triggered by an extremely traumatic event. These symptoms are not related to common experiences such as uncomplicated bereavement, marital conflict, or chronic illness but are associated with events that would be markedly distressing to almost anyone. The individual may experience or witness the trauma alone or in the presence of others. Characteristic symptoms include reexperiencing the traumatic event, a sustained high level of anxiety or arousal, or a general numbing of responsiveness. Intrusive recollections or nightmares of the event are common. Some individuals may be unable to remember certain aspects of the trauma.

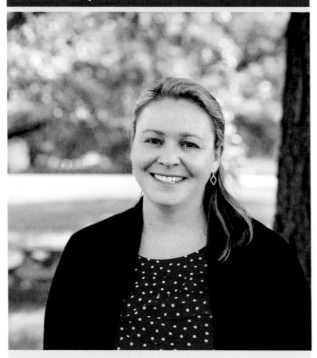

Real Nurses, Real Advice

"Everyone has a story to tell and trauma manifests in a variety of ways. When you conduct a nursing assessment it is helpful to lay the foundation for trauma-informed care by letting the patient know that we ask the same assessment questions of everyone, but some of them may be more difficult for some patients and this is a safe space to discuss any concerns. Then don't be afraid to address uncomfortable topics with questions or statements such as 'Do you have a history of trauma?,' 'Tell me your story,' and 'What happened to you?' Using a trauma-informed care approach will help you gain rapport with your patients."

–Jennifer Graber, Nurse Educator, EdD, APRN, PMHCNS-BC

Symptoms of depression are common with this disorder and may be severe enough to warrant a diagnosis of a depressive disorder in addition to PTSD. In the case of a life-threatening trauma shared with others, survivors often describe painful guilt feelings about surviving when others lost their lives. They may also express trauma and guilt feelings about the things they had to do to survive. Substance abuse, anger and aggressive behavior, and relationship problems are common. The full symptom picture must be present for more than 1 month and cause significant interference with social, occupational, and other areas of functioning. The disorder can occur at any age. Symptoms may begin within the first 3 months after the trauma, or there may be a delay of several months or even years.

The *DSM-5-TR* diagnostic criteria for PTSD are presented in Box 28–1.

The *DSM-5-TR* describes a disorder similar to PTSD called **acute stress disorder (ASD)**. There are similarities between the two disorders in terms of precipitating traumatic events and symptomatology, but in ASD the symptoms are time-limited, lasting up to 1 month after the trauma. By definition, if the symptoms last longer than 1 month, the diagnosis would be PTSD. The *DSM-5-TR* diagnostic criteria for ASD are presented in Box 28–2.

Predisposing Factors for PTSD and ASD
Psychosocial Theory

The widely accepted psychosocial model seeks to explain why some people exposed to massive trauma develop trauma-related disorders and others do not. Variables include characteristics that relate to (1) the traumatic experience, (2) the individual, and (3) the recovery environment.

The Traumatic Experience

Specific characteristics of the trauma have been identified as crucial in the determination of an individual's long-term response to stress:

■ Severity and duration of the stressor
■ Extent of anticipatory preparation for the event
■ Exposure to death
■ Numbers affected by life threat
■ Amount of control over recurrence
■ Location where the trauma was experienced (e.g., familiar surroundings, at home, in a foreign country)

The Individual

Variables that are considered important in determining an individual's response to trauma include the following:

■ Degree of ego-strength
■ Effectiveness of coping resources
■ Presence of preexisting psychopathology
■ Outcomes of previous experiences with stress and trauma
■ Behavioral tendencies (temperament)
■ Current psychosocial developmental stage
■ Demographic factors (e.g., age, socioeconomic status, education)

The Recovery Environment

The quality of the environment in which the individual attempts to work through the traumatic experience is correlated with the outcome. Environmental variables include the following:

■ Availability of social supports
■ The cohesiveness and protectiveness of family and friends

BOX 28–1 **Diagnostic Criteria for Post-Traumatic Stress Disorder**

Note: The following criteria apply to adults, adolescents, and children older than 6 years.

A. Exposure to actual or threatened death, serious injury, or sexual violence, in one (or more) of the following ways:
   1. Directly experiencing the traumatic event(s).
   2. Witnessing, in person, the event(s) as it occurred to others.
   3. Learning that the traumatic event(s) occurred to a close family member or close friend. In cases of actual or threatened death of a family member or friend, the event(s) must have been violent or accidental.
   4. Experiencing repeated or extreme exposure to aversive details of the traumatic event(s) (e.g., first responders collecting human remains; police officers repeatedly exposed to details of child abuse). **Note:** Criterion A4 does not apply to exposure through electronic media, television, movies, or pictures, unless this exposure is work related.

B. Presence of one (or more) of the following intrusion symptoms associated with the traumatic event(s), beginning after the traumatic event(s) occurred:
   1. Recurrent, involuntary, and intrusive distressing memories of the traumatic event(s). **Note:** In children older than 6 years, repetitive play may occur in which themes or aspects of the traumatic event(s) are expressed.
   2. Recurrent distressing dreams in which the content and/or effect of the dream is related to the traumatic event(s). **Note:** In children, there may be frightening dreams without recognizable content.
   3. Dissociative reactions (e.g., flashbacks) in which the individual feels or acts as if the traumatic event(s) were recurring. (Such reactions may occur on a continuum, with the most extreme expression being a complete loss of awareness of present surroundings.) **Note:** In children, trauma-specific reenactment may occur in play.
   4. Intense or prolonged psychological distress at exposure to internal or external cues that symbolize or resemble an aspect of the traumatic event(s).
   5. Marked physiological reactions to internal or external cues that symbolize or resemble an aspect of the traumatic event(s).

C. Persistent avoidance of stimuli associated with the traumatic event(s) beginning after the traumatic event(s) occurred, as evidenced by one or both of the following:
   1. Avoidance of or efforts to avoid distressing memories, thoughts, or feelings about or closely associated with the traumatic event(s).
   2. Avoidance of or efforts to avoid external reminders (people, places, conversations, activities, objects, situations) that arouse distressing memories, thoughts, or feelings about or closely associated with the traumatic event(s).

D. Negative alterations in cognitions and mood associated with the traumatic event(s), beginning or worsening after the traumatic event(s) occurred, as evidenced by two or more of the following:
   1. Inability to remember an important aspect of the traumatic event(s) (typically due to dissociative amnesia and not to other factors such as head injury, alcohol, or drugs).
   2. Persistent and exaggerated negative beliefs or expectations about oneself, others, or the world (e.g., "I am bad," "No one can be trusted," "The world is completely dangerous," "My whole nervous system is permanently ruined").
   3. Persistent, distorted cognitions about the cause or consequences of the traumatic event(s) that lead the individual to blame himself/herself or others.
   4. Persistent negative emotional state (e.g., fear, horror, anger, guilt, or shame).
   5. Markedly diminished interest or participation in significant activities.
   6. Feelings of detachment or estrangement from others.
   7. Persistent inability to experience positive emotions (e.g., inability to experience happiness, satisfaction, or loving feelings).

E. Marked alterations in arousal and reactivity associated with the traumatic event(s), beginning or worsening after the traumatic event(s) occurred, as evidenced by two or more of the following:
   1. Irritable behavior and angry outbursts (with little or no provocation) typically expressed as verbal or physical aggression toward people or objects.
   2. Reckless or self-destructive behavior.
   3. Hypervigilance.
   4. Exaggerated startle response.
   5. Problems with concentration.
   6. Sleep disturbance (e.g., difficulty falling or staying asleep or restless sleep).

F. Duration of the disturbance (Criteria B, C, D, and E) is more than 1 month.

G. The disturbance causes clinically significant distress or impairment in social, occupation, or other important areas of functioning.

H. The disturbance is not attributable to the physiological effects of a substance (e.g., medication, alcohol) or another medical condition.

Specify whether:

With dissociative symptoms: The individual's symptoms meet the criteria for posttraumatic stress disorder; and in addition, in response to the stressor, the individual experiences persistent or recurrent symptoms of either of the following:
   1. Depersonalization: Persistent or recurrent experiences of feeling detached from, and as if one were

Continued

BOX 28–1 Diagnostic Criteria for Post-Traumatic Stress Disorder—cont'd

an outside observer of, one's mental processes or body (e.g., feeling as though one were in a dream; feeling a sense of unreality of self or body, or of time moving slowly).

2. Derealization: Persistent or recurrent experiences of unreality of surroundings (e.g., the world around

the individual is experienced as unreal, dreamlike, distant, or distorted).

With delayed expression: If the full diagnostic criteria are not met until at least 6 months after the event (although the onset and expression of some symptoms may be immediate)

Reprinted with permission from the *Diagnostic and Statistical Manual of Mental Disorders, Fifth Edition, Text Revision (DSM-5-TR)*. (2022). American Psychiatric Association.

BOX 28–2 Diagnostic Criteria for Acute Stress Disorder

A. Exposure to actual or threatened death, serious injury, or sexual violation, in one (or more) of the following ways:
   1. Directly experiencing the traumatic event(s).
   2. Witnessing, in person, the event(s) as it occurred to others.
   3. Learning that the event(s) occurred to a close family member or close friend. **Note:** In cases of actual or threatened death of a family member or friend, the event(s) must have been violent or accidental.
   4. Experiencing repeated or extreme exposure to aversive details of the traumatic event(s) (e.g., first responders collecting human remains, police officers repeatedly exposed to details of child abuse). **Note:** This does not apply to exposure through electronic media, television, movies, or pictures, unless this exposure is work related.
B. Presence of nine (or more) of the following symptoms from any of the five categories of intrusion, negative mood, dissociation, avoidance, and arousal, beginning or worsening after the traumatic event(s) occurred:

INTRUSION SYMPTOMS
   1. Recurrent, involuntary, and intrusive distressing memories of the traumatic event(s). **Note:** In children, repetitive play may occur in which themes or aspects of the traumatic event(s) are expressed.
   2. Recurrent distressing dreams in which the content and/or effect of the dream are related to the event(s). **Note:** In children, there may be frightening dreams without recognizable content.
   3. Dissociative reactions (e.g., flashbacks) in which the individual feels or acts as if the traumatic event(s) were recurring. (Such reactions may occur on a continuum, with the most extreme expression being a complete loss of awareness of present surroundings.) **Note:** In children, trauma-specific reenactment may occur in play.
   4. Intense or prolonged psychological distress or marked physiological reactions in response to internal or external cues that symbolize or resemble an aspect of the traumatic event(s).

NEGATIVE MOOD
   5. Persistent inability to experience positive emotions (e.g., inability to experience happiness, satisfaction, or loving feelings).

DISSOCIATIVE SYMPTOMS
   6. An altered sense of the reality of one's surroundings or oneself (e.g., seeing oneself from another's perspective, being in a daze, time slowing).
   7. Inability to remember an important aspect of the traumatic event(s) (typically due to dissociative amnesia and not to other factors such as head injury, alcohol, or drugs).

AVOIDANCE SYMPTOMS
   8. Efforts to avoid distressing memories, thoughts, or feelings about or closely associated with the traumatic event(s).
   9. Efforts to avoid external reminders (people, places, conversations, activities, objects, situations) that arouse distressing memories, thoughts, or feelings about or closely associated with the traumatic event(s).

AROUSAL SYMPTOMS
   10. Sleep disturbance (e.g., difficulty falling or staying asleep, or restless sleep).
   11. Irritable behavior and angry outbursts (with little or no provocation), typically expressed as verbal or physical aggression toward people or objects.
   12. Hypervigilance.
   13. Problems with concentration.
   14. Exaggerated startle response.
C. Duration of the disturbance (symptoms in Criteria B) is 3 days to 1 month after trauma exposure. **Note:** Symptoms typically begin immediately after the trauma, but persistence for at least 3 days and up to a month is needed to meet disorder criteria.
D. The disturbance causes clinically significant distress or impairment in social, occupational, or other important areas of functioning.
E. The disturbance is not attributable to the direct physiological effects of a substance (e.g., medication or alcohol) or another medical condition (e.g., mild traumatic brain injury), and is not better explained by brief psychotic disorder.

Reprinted with permission from the *Diagnostic and Statistical Manual of Mental Disorders, Fifth Edition, Text Revision (DSM-5-TR)*. (2022). American Psychiatric Association.

■ The attitudes of society regarding the experience
■ Cultural and subcultural influences

In a longitudinal study of Vietnam veterans, it was shown that the best predictors of war-related PTSD were "African American race, lower education level, negative homecoming reception, lower current social support, and greater past-year stress" in the recovery environment (Steenkamp et al., 2017, p. 711). Further, it was found that these factors can predict PTSD symptom severity and symptom change up to 40 years postdeployment.

Learning Theory

Learning theory holds that trauma-related disorders are related to aversive learning experiences. In PTSD, for example, the individual associates the traumatic event with fear which culminates in a conditioned fear to stimuli associated with the event and "more general overreactivity—or failure to adapt—to intense, novel, or fear-related stimuli" (Lissek & van Meurs, 2015).

Cognitive Theory

These models take into consideration the cognitive appraisal of an event and focus on assumptions that an individual makes about the world. Epstein's (1991) classic model outlined three fundamental beliefs that most people construct within a personal view of reality:

1. The world is benevolent and a source of joy.
2. The world is meaningful and controllable.
3. The self is worthy (e.g., lovable, good, and competent).

Park and associates' (2012) research added support to the cognitive theory in their finding that the extent to which an individual's appraisal of an event violates their beliefs about themselves and the world damages their beliefs and is strongly related to the development and maintenance of PTSD over time.

As life situations occur, some disequilibrium is expected until accommodation for the changed circumstance has been made and it becomes assimilated into one's personal view of reality. An individual is vulnerable to trauma-related disorders when fundamental beliefs are invalidated by a trauma that cannot be comprehended, and a sense of helplessness and hopelessness prevail.

Biological Aspects

Exposure to trauma has been associated with hyperarousal of the sympathetic nervous system, excessive amygdala activity, and decreased hippocampus volume, all of which are neurobiological reactions to heightened stress. Dysfunctions in the hypothalamic-pituitary-adrenal (HPA) axis, either from chronic stress or exposure to an extreme stressor, have been linked to many psychiatric illnesses, including PTSD, depression, Alzheimer's disease, and substance abuse, and to medical conditions such as inflammatory disorders and cardiovascular disease (Valentino & Van Bockstaele, 2015). These links are evident in the comorbidity or increased risk for developing one or more of the previously mentioned disorders among individuals with PTSD. For example, a recent meta-analysis (Günak et al., 2020) found that PTSD is associated with a significant risk for all causes of dementia. Substance use disorders and depression are commonly diagnosed comorbidities with PTSD. Adverse childhood experiences (ACEs), traumas occurring before the age of 18, have been linked to several chronic health conditions, risky health behaviors, substance abuse, and early death (Centers for Disease Control and Prevention [CDC], 2021).

Neuroendocrine abnormalities, including serotonin, glutamate, thyroid, and endogenous opioids (among others), have also been associated with stress responses and PTSD. Valentino and Van Bockstaele (2015) identified that the activation of endogenous opioids both reduces stress and mimics the stress response depending on which opioid receptors are activated. Studies have shown that opioids administered shortly after exposure to a trauma reduced the incidence of PTSD, suggesting a protective effect. Chronic activation, however, may sensitize neurons in a way that increases vulnerability to stress-induced relapse. Lanius and associates (2014) discussed the effects of repeated activation of opioid receptors, including the effect of increasing one's addiction potential to other drugs or even to the learned experience of relief when traumatic stress is reexperienced. He identified that opiate antagonists such as naltrexone have demonstrated effectiveness in treatment.

Other biological systems have also been implicated in the symptomatology of PTSD. Norepinephrine, dopamine, and benzodiazepine receptors are other neurotransmitters believed to be dysregulated in individuals with PTSD. Lower concentrations of neuropeptide Y (NPY), an anxiolytic peptide, have been shown to increase susceptibility to PTSD in combat veterans, and catechol-O-methyltransferase (COMT) gene variants have been linked to deficits in stress responses and emotional resilience (Togay & El-Mallakh, 2020).

A large-scale genome study (Stein et al., 2021) of over 250,000 veterans identified specific genes associated with PTSD and related mood symptoms of anxiety and depression. Their research supports a biological and, specifically, genetic influence in the development of this disorder. Whether these factors are suggestive of vulnerability to PTSD or whether these changes result from the brain's efforts to process trauma remains unclear. As with other disorders, it is likely that a complex dynamic of biological, social, and psychological factors is involved.

Diagnosis and Outcome Identification

Nursing diagnoses are formulated from the data gathered during the assessment phase and with background knowledge regarding predisposing factors to the disorder. Following are some common nursing diagnoses for patients with trauma-related disorders:

■ Post-trauma syndrome related to distressing events outside the range of usual human experience, evidenced by flashbacks, intrusive recollections, nightmares, psychological numbness related to the event, dissociation, or amnesia

■ Maladaptive grieving related to loss of self as perceived before the trauma or other actual or perceived losses incurred during or after the event, evidenced by irritability and explosiveness, self-destructiveness, substance abuse, verbalization of survival guilt, or guilt about behavior required for survival

The following criteria may be used for measurement of outcomes in the care of the patient with a trauma-related disorder.

The patient:

■ Can acknowledge the traumatic event and the effect it has had on their life

■ Is experiencing fewer flashbacks, intrusive recollections, and nightmares than they had on admission (or at the beginning of therapy)

■ Can demonstrate adaptive coping strategies (e.g., relaxation techniques, mental imagery, music, art)

■ Can concentrate and has made realistic goals for the future

■ Includes significant others in the recovery process and willingly accepts their support

■ Verbalizes no ideas or intent of self-harm

■ Has worked through feelings of survivor's guilt

■ Gets enough sleep to avoid risk of injury

■ Verbalizes community resources from which they may seek assistance in times of stress

■ Attends support group of individuals who have recovered or are recovering from similar traumatic experiences

■ Verbalizes desire to put the trauma in the past and progress with their life

Planning and Implementation

The following section presents a group of selected nursing diagnoses with short- and long-term goals and nursing interventions for each. Rationales for interventions are italicized. Table 28–1 presents the nursing diagnosis of post-trauma syndrome in care plan format.

See the "Real People, Real Stories" feature in Chapter 37, "Military Families," to learn more about Sean's postmilitary experience with PTSD and the importance of compassionate nursing intervention in his trauma recovery.

Table 28–1 | CARE PLAN FOR THE PATIENT WITH A TRAUMA-RELATED DISORDER

NURSING DIAGNOSIS: POST-TRAUMA SYNDROME

RELATED TO: Distressing event considered to be outside the range of usual human experience

EVIDENCED BY: Flashbacks, intrusive recollections, nightmares, psychological numbness related to the event, dissociation, or amnesia

OUTCOME CRITERIA	NURSING INTERVENTIONS	RATIONALE
Short-Term Goals: ■ Patient will begin a healthy grief resolution, initiating the process of psychological healing (within time frame specific to individual). ■ Patient will demonstrate ability to deal with emotional reactions in an individually appropriate manner.	1. a. Assign the same staff as often as possible. b. Use a nonthreatening, matter-of-fact, but friendly approach. c. Respect the patient's wishes regarding discomfort interacting with some individuals (especially important if the trauma was rape).	1. A post-trauma patient may be suspicious of others in their environment. All of these interventions serve to facilitate a trusting relationship.

Table 28–1 | CARE PLAN FOR THE PATIENT WITH A TRAUMA-RELATED DISORDER—cont'd

OUTCOME CRITERIA	NURSING INTERVENTIONS	RATIONALE
Long-Term Goal: ■ Patient will integrate the traumatic experience into their personal view of reality, renew significant relationships, and establish meaningful goals for the future.	d. Be consistent; keep all promises; convey acceptance; spend time with the patient. 2. Stay with patient during periods of flashbacks and nightmares. Offer reassurance of safety and security and that these symptoms are not uncommon after a trauma of the magnitude they have experienced. 3. Obtain accurate history from significant others about the trauma and the patient's specific response. 4. Encourage the patient to talk about the *trauma at their own pace.* Provide a nonthreatening, private environment, and include a significant other if the patient wishes. Acknowledge and validate the patient's feelings as they are expressed. 5. Discuss coping strategies used in response to the trauma, as well as those used during stressful situations in the past. Determine those that have been most helpful and discuss alternative strategies for the future. Include available support systems, including religious and cultural influences. Identify maladaptive coping strategies (e.g., substance use, psychosomatic responses) and practice more adaptive coping strategies for possible future post-trauma responses. 6. Assist the patient to try to comprehend the trauma if possible. Discuss feelings of vulnerability and the individual's "place" in the world after the trauma.	2. Presence of a trusted individual may calm fears for personal safety and reassure the patient that they are not in danger. 3. Various types of traumas elicit different responses in patients (e.g., human-engendered traumas often generate a greater degree of humiliation and guilt in victims than trauma associated with natural disasters). 4. This debriefing process is the first step in the progression toward resolution. 5. Resolution of the post-trauma response is largely dependent on the effectiveness of the coping strategies employed. 6. Post-trauma response is largely a function of the shattering of basic beliefs the victim holds about self and world. Assimilation of the event into one's personal view of reality requires that some degree of meaning associated with the event be incorporated into the basic beliefs, which will affect how the individual eventually comes to reappraise self and world (Epstein, 1991).

Post-Trauma Syndrome

Post-trauma syndrome is defined as "a sustained maladaptive response to a traumatic, overwhelming event" (Herdman et al., 2021, p.396).

Patient Goals

Outcome criteria include short- and long-term goals. Timelines are individually determined.

Short-term goals

- The patient will begin to move toward a healthy resolution of grief, initiating the process of psychological healing (within a time frame specific to the individual).
- The patient will demonstrate ability to deal with emotional reactions in an individually appropriate manner.

Long-term goal

- The patient will integrate the traumatic experience into their persona, renew significant relationships, and establish meaningful goals for the future.

Interventions

- Establishing a trusting relationship with this individual is essential before care can be given. To promote trust, assign the same staff members as often as possible. Use a nonthreatening, matter-of-fact, but friendly approach. Ask for permission before using touch as an intervention. Respect the patient's wishes regarding interaction with individuals of opposite sex at this time (especially important if the trauma was rape). Be consistent, keep all promises, and convey an attitude of unconditional acceptance. *A post-trauma patient may be suspicious of others in their environment.*
- Stay with the patient during periods of flashbacks and nightmares. Offer reassurance of safety and security and that these symptoms are not uncommon after a trauma of the magnitude they have experienced. *The presence of a trusted individual may help to calm fears for personal safety and reassure the anxious patient that they are not in danger.*
- Obtain an accurate history from significant others about the trauma and the patient's specific response. *Various types of traumas elicit different responses in patients. For example, human-engendered traumas often generate a greater degree of humiliation and guilt in victims than does trauma associated with natural disasters.*
- Encourage the patient to talk about the trauma *at their own pace.* Provide a nonthreatening, private environment and include a significant other if the patient wishes. Acknowledge and validate the patient's feelings as they are expressed. *This debriefing process is the first step in the progression toward resolution.*
- Discuss coping strategies used in response to the trauma, as well as those used during stressful situations in the past. Determine those that have been most helpful and discuss alternative strategies for the future. *Patients who have experienced multiple or sustained traumas may find longer-term PTSD-focused therapy to be beneficial.* Include available support systems, including religious and cultural influences. Identify maladaptive coping strategies, such as substance use or psychosomatic responses, and practice more adaptive coping strategies for possible future post-trauma responses. *Resolution of the post-trauma response is largely dependent on the effectiveness of the coping strategies employed.*
- Assist the individual to comprehend the trauma if possible. Discuss feelings of vulnerability and the individual's "place" in the world after the trauma. *Post-trauma response is associated with the shattering of basic beliefs the survivor holds about self and world. Assimilation of the event into one's persona requires incorporating some degree of meaning associated with the event into one's basic beliefs, which will affect how the individual eventually comes to reappraise self and world (Epstein, 1991).*

Maladaptive Grieving

Maladaptive grieving is defined as "a disorder that occurs after the death of a significant other [or any other loss of significance to the individual], in which the experience of distress accompanying bereavement fails to follow sociocultural expectation" (Herdman et al., 2021, p. 421).

Patient Goals

Outcome criteria include short- and long-term goals. Timelines are individually determined.

Short-term goal

- Patient will verbalize feelings (guilt, anger, self-blame, hopelessness) associated with the trauma.

Long-term goal

- Patient will demonstrate progress in dealing with stages of grief and will verbalize a sense of optimism and hope for the future.

Interventions

- Acknowledge feelings of guilt or self-blame the patient may express. Guilt at having survived a trauma in which others died is common. *The patient needs to discuss these feelings and recognize that they are not responsible for what happened but must take responsibility for their own recovery.*

■ Assess stage of grief in which the patient is fixed. Discuss normalcy of feelings and behaviors related to stages of grief. *Knowledge of grief stages is necessary for accurate intervention. Guilt may be generated if patient believes it is unacceptable to have these feelings. Knowing these feelings are part of the normal grief response can provide a sense of relief.*

■ Assess effect of the trauma on the patient's ability to resume regular activities of daily living. Consider employment, marital relationship, and sleep patterns. *After a trauma, individuals are at high risk for physical injury because of disruption in the ability to concentrate and problem solve and lack of sufficient sleep. Isolation and avoidance behaviors may interfere with interpersonal relatedness.*

■ Assess for self-destructive ideas and behavior. *The trauma may result in feelings of hopelessness and worthlessness, leading to an increased risk for suicide.*

■ Assess for maladaptive coping strategies such as substance abuse. *These behaviors interfere with and delay the recovery process.*

■ Identify available community resources from which the individual may seek assistance if problems with complicated grieving persist. Support groups for victims of various types of trauma exist within most communities. *The presence of support systems in the recovery environment is associated with the successful recovery from trauma.*

Evaluation

Reassessment is conducted to determine whether the nursing actions have been successful in achieving the objectives of care. The following criteria may be used for measurement of outcomes in the care of the patient with a trauma-related disorder. The patient:

■ Can acknowledge the traumatic event and the effect it has had on their life.

■ Is experiencing fewer flashbacks, intrusive recollections, and nightmares than on admission (or at the beginning of therapy).

■ Can demonstrate adaptive coping strategies (e.g., relaxation techniques, mental imagery, music, art).

■ Can concentrate and has made realistic goals for the future.

■ Includes significant others in the recovery process and willingly accepts their support.

■ Verbalizes no ideas or intent of self-harm.

■ Has worked through feelings of survivor's guilt.

■ Gets enough sleep to avoid risk of injury.

■ Verbalizes community resources from which to seek assistance in times of stress.

■ Attends support group of individuals who have recovered or are recovering from similar traumatic experiences.

■ Identifies a plan of action for dealing with symptoms should they recur.

Application of the Nursing Process— Stressor-Related Disorders

In the latest edition of the *DSM-5-TR* a distinct syndrome, prolonged grief disorder, was added (APA, 2022). Although symptoms of bereavement (beyond normal bereavement) may occur in adjustment disorders, **prolonged grief disorder** is diagnosed when the stressor is specifically the death of a person who was close to the bereaved individual and clinically significant distress or impairment in functioning endures beyond a year of the associated death. See Chapter 36 "The Bereaved Individual" for further discussion of grief-related issues.

Adjustment Disorders—Background Assessment Data

CORE CONCEPT

Stress

A state of disequilibrium and tension that occurs when there is disharmony between demands occurring within an individual's internal or external environment and their ability to cope with those demands.

An **adjustment disorder** is characterized by a maladaptive reaction to an identifiable stressor or stressors that result in the development of clinically significant emotional or behavioral symptoms (APA, 2022). The response occurs within 3 months after onset of the stressor and persists for no longer than 6 months after the stressor or its consequences have ended.

The individual shows impairment in social and occupational functioning or exhibits symptoms that are more than an expected reaction to the stressor. The symptoms are expected to remit soon after the stressor is relieved or, if the stressor persists, when a new level of adaptation is achieved.

The stressor itself can be almost anything, but an individual's response to a particular stressor cannot be predicted. If an individual is highly predisposed or vulnerable to maladaptive responses, a severe form of the disorder may follow what most people would consider only a mild or moderate stressor. On the other hand, a less vulnerable individual may develop only a mild form of the disorder in response to what others might consider a severe stressor.

A number of clinical presentations are associated with adjustment disorders. The following categories, identified by the *DSM-5-TR* (APA, 2022), are distinguished by the predominant features of the maladaptive response.

Adjustment Disorder With Depressed Mood

This category is the most commonly diagnosed adjustment disorder. The clinical presentation is one of predominant mood disturbance, although less pronounced than that of major depressive disorder. The symptoms, such as depressed mood, tearfulness, and feelings of hopelessness, exceed the expected or normative response to an identified stressor.

Adjustment Disorder With Anxiety

This category denotes a maladaptive response to a stressor in which the predominant manifestation is anxiety. For example, the symptoms may reveal nervousness, worry, and jitteriness. The clinician must differentiate this diagnosis from those of anxiety disorders.

Adjustment Disorder With Mixed Anxiety and Depressed Mood

The predominant features of this category include disturbances in mood (depression, feelings of hopelessness and sadness) and manifestations of anxiety (nervousness, worry, jitteriness) that are more intense than what would be expected or considered a normative response to an identified stressor.

Adjustment Disorder With Disturbance of Conduct

This category is characterized by conduct in which there is violation of the rights of others or of major age-appropriate societal norms and rules. Examples include truancy, vandalism, reckless driving, fighting, and defaulting on legal responsibilities. Differential diagnosis must be made from conduct disorder or antisocial personality disorder, both of which are of longer duration and pervasive responses to a variety of situations.

Adjustment Disorder With Mixed Disturbance of Emotions and Conduct

The predominant features of this category include emotional disturbances (e.g., anxiety or depression) as well as disturbances of conduct in which there is violation of the rights of others or of major age-appropriate societal norms and rules (e.g., truancy, vandalism, fighting).

Adjustment Disorder Unspecified

This subtype is used when the maladaptive reaction is not consistent with any of the other categories. The individual may have physical complaints, withdraw from relationships, or exhibit impaired work or academic performance, but without significant disturbance in emotions or conduct.

Predisposing Factors for Adjustment Disorders

Biological Aspects

Chronic disorders, such as neurocognitive or intellectual developmental disorders, are thought to impair the ability of an individual to adapt to stress, causing increased vulnerability to an adjustment disorder. Genetic factors also may influence individual risks for maladaptive response to stress.

Psychosocial Theories

Some proponents of psychoanalytic theory view adjustment disorder as a maladaptive response to stress caused by early childhood trauma, increased dependency, and retarded ego development. Other psychoanalysts put considerable weight on birth characteristics that contribute to how individuals respond to stress. In many instances, adjustment disorder is precipitated by a specific, meaningful stressor connecting with a point of vulnerability in an individual of otherwise adequate ego strength.

Predisposition to adjustment disorder has also been associated with lack of achievement of developmental stage tasks, low self-esteem, and lack of available support systems. When a stressor occurs and the individual does not have the developmental maturity, attachment to or available support systems, or adequate coping strategies to adapt, normal functioning is disrupted, resulting in psychological or somatic symptoms.

Transactional Model of Stress and Adaptation

Why are some individuals able to confront stressful situations adaptively and even gain strength from the experience, while others not only fail to cope adaptively but may even encounter psychopathological dysfunction? The transactional model of stress and adaptation takes into consideration the interaction between the individual and the environment.

The type of stressor that one experiences may influence one's adaptation. *Sudden shock* stressors occur without warning, and *continuous stressors* are those an individual is exposed to over an extended period. Although many studies have focused on individuals' responses to sudden shock stressors, continuous stressors have been more commonly cited as precipitants to maladaptive functioning.

Both situational and intrapersonal factors most likely contribute to an individual's stress response. Situational factors include personal and general economic conditions; occupational and recreational opportunities; and the availability of social supports such as family, friends, neighbors, and cultural or religious support groups.

Preexisting personality and behavioral traits may also predispose an individual to an adjustment disorder and other stress-related disorders. The most common comorbidities are personality disorders and substance use disorders (Casey, 2013). Studies have found that personality traits (including rigidity, perfectionism, cautiousness, and slow adaptation to change) are related to the development of many emotional disorders (Lynch, 2018). Other factors that might influence one's ability to adjust to life changes include social skills, coping strategies, the presence of psychiatric illness, and level of intelligence.

Diagnosis and Outcome Identification

Nursing diagnoses are formulated from the data gathered during the assessment phase and with background knowledge regarding predisposing factors to the disorder. Nursing diagnoses that may be used for the patient with an adjustment disorder include the following:

■ Maladaptive grieving related to real or perceived loss of any concept of value to the individual, evidenced by interference with life functioning, developmental regression, or somatic complaints

■ Risk-prone health behavior related to change in health status requiring modification in lifestyle (e.g., chronic illness, physical disability), evidenced by inability to problem solve or set realistic goals for the future (appropriate diagnosis for the person with adjustment disorder if the precipitating stressor was a change in health status)

■ Anxiety (moderate to severe) related to situational or maturational crisis evidenced by restlessness, increased helplessness, and diminished productivity

Outcome Criteria

The following criteria may be used for measurement of outcomes in the care of the patient with an adjustment disorder.

The patient:

■ Verbalizes acceptable behaviors associated with each stage of the grief process

■ Demonstrates a reinvestment in the environment

■ Accomplishes activities of daily living independently

■ Demonstrates ability for adequate occupational and social functioning

■ Verbalizes awareness of change in health status and the effect it will have on lifestyle

■ Solves problems and sets realistic goals for the future

■ Demonstrates ability to cope effectively with change in lifestyle

Planning and Implementation

The following section presents a group of selected nursing diagnoses, with short- and long-term goals and nursing interventions for each. Rationales for interventions are italicized.

Maladaptive Grieving

Maladaptive grieving is defined as "a disorder that occurs after the death of a significant other [or any other loss of significance to the individual], in which the experience of distress accompanying bereavement fails to follow sociocultural expectations" (Herdman et al., 2021, p. 421).

Patient Goals

Outcome criteria include short- and long-term goals. Timelines are individually determined.

Short-term goal

■ By the end of 1 week, the patient will express anger toward the lost entity.

Long-term goal

■ The patient will be able to verbalize behaviors associated with the normal stages of grief and identify own position in grief process, while progressing at own pace toward resolution.

Interventions

■ Determine the stage of grief in which patient is fixed. Identify behaviors associated with this stage. *Accurate baseline assessment data are necessary to plan effective care for the grieving patient.*

■ Develop a trusting relationship. Show empathy and caring. Be honest and keep all promises. *Trust is the basis for a therapeutic relationship.*

■ Convey an accepting attitude to encourage the patient to express feelings openly. *An accepting attitude conveys that you believe the patient is a worthwhile person. Trust is enhanced.*

■ Allow the patient to express anger. Do not become defensive if the initial expression of anger is displaced on the nurse or therapist. Help the patient explore angry feelings so that they may be directed toward the intended object or person. *Verbalization of feelings in a nonthreatening environment may help the patient come to terms with unresolved issues.*

■ Assist the patient to discharge pent-up anger through participation in large motor activities (e.g., brisk walks, jogging, physical exercises, volleyball, exercise bike). *Physical exercise provides a safe and effective method for discharging pent-up tension.*

■ Explain the normal stages of grief and the behaviors associated with each stage. Help the patient to understand that feelings such as guilt and anger toward the lost entity or concept are natural and acceptable during the grief process. *Knowledge of the acceptability of the feelings associated with normal grieving may help the patient to explore their own grief process.*

■ Encourage the patient to review their perception of the loss or change. With support and sensitivity, point out the reality of the situation in areas where misrepresentations are expressed. *The patient must give up an idealized perception and be able to accept both positive and negative aspects about the painful life change before the grief process is complete.*

■ Communicate to the patient that crying is acceptable. *Normalizing the patient's expression of emotions facilitates establishing rapport.*

■ Help the patient explore problem-solving as they attempt to determine methods for more adaptive coping with the stressor. Provide positive feedback for strategies identified and decisions made. *Positive reinforcement enhances self-esteem and encourages repetition of desirable behaviors.*

■ Encourage the patient to reach out for spiritual support during this time in whatever form is desirable. Assess patient's spiritual needs and assist as necessary in the fulfillment of those needs. *For some individuals, spiritual support can enhance successful adaptation to painful life experiences.*

Risk-Prone Health Behavior

Risk-prone health behavior is defined as "impaired ability to modify lifestyle and/or actions in a manner that improves the level of wellness" (Herdman et al., 2021, p. 198).

Patient Goals

Outcome criteria include short- and long-term goals. Timelines are individually determined.

Short-term goals

■ The patient and primary nurse will discuss the kinds of lifestyle changes that will occur because of the change in health status.

■ With the help of the primary nurse, the patient will formulate a plan of action for incorporating these changes into their lifestyle.

■ The patient will demonstrate movement toward independence, considering the change in health status.

Long-term goal

■ The patient will demonstrate competence to function independently to their optimal ability,

considering the change in health status, by the time of discharge from treatment.

Interventions

■ Encourage the patient to talk about their lifestyle before the change in health status. Discuss coping mechanisms that were used at stressful times in the past. *It is important to identify the patient's strengths so that they may be used to facilitate adaptation to the change or loss that has occurred.*

■ Encourage the patient to discuss the change or loss and to express anger associated with it. *Anger is a normal stage in the grieving process and, if not released appropriately, may be turned inward on the self, leading to pathological depression.*

■ Encourage the patient to express fears associated with lifestyle alterations imposed by the chronic illness, physical disability, or other change in health status. *Change often creates a feeling of disequilibrium, and the individual may respond with fears that are irrational or unfounded. The patient may benefit from feedback that corrects misperceptions about how life will be with the change in health status.*

■ Assess the patient's risk for suicidal behavior. *Adjustment disorders have been associated with increased risk for suicide.*

■ Assist with activities of daily living as required but encourage independence to the extent that the patient's ability allows. Give positive feedback for activities accomplished independently. *Independent accomplishments and positive feedback enhance self-esteem and encourage repetition of desired behaviors. Successes also provide hope that adaptive functioning is possible and decrease feelings of powerlessness.*

■ Help the patient with decision making regarding incorporation of the change or loss into their lifestyle. Identify problems the change or loss is likely to create. Discuss alternative solutions, weighing potential benefits and consequences of each alternative. Support the patient's decision in the selection of an alternative. *The significant anxiety that usually accompanies a major lifestyle change often interferes with an individual's ability to solve problems and to make appropriate decisions. The patient may need assistance with this process to progress toward successful adaptation.*

■ Use role-playing to practice new behavioral responses to stressful situations that might occur concerning the health status change. *Role-playing decreases anxiety and provides a feeling of security by developing a plan of action for responding appropriately when a stressful situation occurs.*

■ Ensure that the patient and family are fully knowledgeable regarding the physiology of the change in health status and understand the necessity of such knowledge for optimal wellness. Encourage them to ask questions and provide printed material with additional explanation. *Knowing what to expect regarding the change or loss decreases anxiety and enhances the capacity for wellness.*

■ Ensure that the patient can identify resources within the community from which they may seek assistance in adapting to the change in health status. Examples include self-help or support groups and public health nurses, counselors, or social workers. Encourage the patient to keep follow-up appointments with their physician and to call the physician's office before the follow-up date if problems or concerns arise. Support services provide a feeling of security that one is not alone and a means to prevent decompensation when stress becomes intolerable.

Evaluation

Reassessment is conducted to determine whether the nursing actions have been successful in achieving the objectives of care. Evaluation of the nursing actions for the patient with an adjustment disorder may be facilitated by gathering information using the following types of questions:

Does the patient:

■ Verbalize understanding of the grief process and their position in the process?

■ Recognize their adaptive and maladaptive behaviors associated with the grief response?

■ Demonstrate evidence of progression along the grief response?

■ Accomplish activities of daily living independently?

■ Demonstrate the ability to perform occupational and social activities adequately?

■ Discuss the change in health status and modification of lifestyle it will affect?

■ Demonstrate acceptance of the modification?

■ Participate in decision making and problem-solving for their future?

■ Set realistic goals for the future?

■ Demonstrate new adaptive coping strategies for dealing with the change in lifestyle?

■ Identify available resources to whom they may go for support or assistance should it be necessary?

Patient and Family Education

The role of patient teacher is important in the psychiatric area, as it is in all areas of nursing. A list of topics for patient and family education relevant to trauma- and stressor-related disorders is presented in Box 28–3.

BOX 28–3 Topics for Patient and Family Education Related to Trauma- and Stressor-Related Disorders

NATURE OF PTSD AND STRESSOR-RELATED DISORDERS

Definitions of trauma and stressor-related disorders

Long-term effects of trauma on physical and mental health

Common comorbidities such as depression, anxiety, and substance use disorders

MANAGEMENT OF PTSD

Medication management options: SSRIs, anxiolytics, ketamine

Psychotherapies: trauma-focused psychotherapy, CBT, DBT, prolonged exposure therapy, eye movement desensitization therapy

Community resources: trauma-focused support groups, meditation groups

---

CBT, Cognitive behavior therapy; DBT, dialectical behavior therapy; PTSD, post-traumatic stress disorder; SSRIs, selective serotonin reuptake inhibitors.

Treatment Modalities

Trauma-Related Disorders

Cognitive Behavior Therapy

Cognitive behavior therapy (CBT) for PTSD and ASD strives to help the individual recognize and modify trauma-related thoughts and beliefs. The individual learns to modify the relationships between thoughts and feelings and to identify and challenge inaccurate or extreme automatic negative thoughts. The goal is to replace these negative thoughts with more accurate and less distressing thoughts and to cope more effectively with feelings such as anger, guilt, and fear. The individual learns to modify the appraisal of self and the world as it has been affected by the trauma and to regain hope and optimism about safety, trust, power and control, self-esteem, and intimacy.

Stress inoculation therapy (SIT) is a type of CBT that focuses on learning new ways of coping with stressful events through education and practicing alternative responses such as meditation, deep breathing, and other relaxation exercises. Recent research (Bohus et al., 2020) supports the effectiveness of dialectical behavior therapy (DBT) (a therapy with several features common to CBT) in patients with complex PTSD associated with severe childhood abuse.

Prolonged Exposure Therapy

Prolonged exposure (PE) therapy is a type of behavioral therapy similar to implosion therapy (flooding) (see Chapter 27, "Anxiety, Obsessive-Compulsive, and Related Disorders," for a discussion of implosion therapy). It can be conducted in an imagined or real (in vivo) situation. In the imagined situation, the individual is exposed to repeated and prolonged mental recounting of the traumatic experience. In vivo exposure involves systematic confrontation, within safe limits, of trauma-related situations that are feared and avoided. This intense emotional processing of the traumatic event serves to neutralize the memories so that they no longer result in anxious arousal or escape and avoidance behaviors. PE has four main parts: (1) education about the treatment, (2) breathing retraining for relaxation, (3) imagined exposure through repeated discussion about the trauma with a therapist, and (4) exposure to real-world situations related to the trauma.

Group and Family Therapy

Group therapy has demonstrated efficacy for people with PTSD and especially with military veterans and survivors of catastrophic disasters (Boland & Verduin, 2022). The importance of being able to share their experiences with empathetic fellow veterans, talk about problems in social adaptation, and discuss options for managing aggression toward others has been emphasized. Some PTSD groups are informal and leaderless, such as self-help or support groups, and some are led by experienced group therapists who may have had some firsthand experience with trauma. Some groups involve family members, recognizing that they may also be severely affected by symptoms of PTSD. For example, family members of military veterans sometimes develop PTSD symptoms as a result of exposure to their loved one's PTSD (see Chapter 37, "Military Families," for further discussion of this topic).

Eye Movement Desensitization and Reprocessing

Eye movement desensitization and reprocessing (EMDR) is a type of psychotherapy that was developed in 1989 by psychologist Francine Shapiro. It "has evolved from a simple technique into an integrative psychotherapy approach with a theoretical model that emphasizes the brain's information processing system and memories of disturbing experiences as the basis of pathology" (Shapiro, 2007, p. 3). EMDR has been shown to be an effective therapy for PTSD and other trauma-related disorders (Maxfield & Hyer, 2002; Rothbaum et al., 2005; Valiente-Gómez et al., 2017). It has

been used experimentally in the treatment of other disorders, including depression, adjustment disorder, phobias, addictions, generalized anxiety disorder, and panic disorder. Clinical practice guidelines from the International Society for Traumatic Stress Studies (ISTSS), the APA, and the National Institute for Health Care Excellence (NICE) all support the effectiveness of EMDR for PTSD, although different organizations vary in the strength of their recommendations (Dominguez & Lee, 2019). The World Health Organization (WHO, 2013) supports the use of CBT and EMDR as advanced treatments for patients with PTSD.

The exact biological mechanisms by which EMDR achieves its therapeutic effects are unknown. Some studies have indicated that eye movements cause a decrease in imagery vividness and distress and an increase in memory access. The process involves rapid eye movements while processing painful emotions. The EMDR International Association (2022a) clarified that therapy is not focused on talking in detail about the distressing issue or trying to change associated emotions, thoughts, and behaviors; instead, the process allows the brain to resolve unprocessed traumatic memories and "resume its natural healing process."

While concentrating on a particular emotion or physical sensation surrounding the traumatic event, the individual is asked to focus eye movements on the therapist's fingers as the therapist moves them from left to right and back again. Later the person is asked to focus on a positive belief to replace the negative, disturbing belief again while tracking the therapist's fingers. Although some individuals report rapid results with this therapy, research has indicated that from 5 to 12 sessions are required to achieve lasting treatment effects. Special precautions may be needed when using EMDR in people with neurological impairments (e.g., seizure disorders), severe dissociative disorders, or unstable substance abuse and those who are suicidal or experiencing psychosis (UPMC, Center for Integrative Medicine, 2022).

Clients often feel rapid relief with EMDR. However, to achieve lasting results, it is important that each of the eight phases is completed. Treatment is not complete until "EMDR therapy has focused on the past memories that are contributing to the problem, the present situations that are disturbing, and what skills the client may need for the future" (EMDR International Association, 2022b).

Digital Therapeutics

In 2020, the U.S. Food and Drug Administration (FDA) approved a prescription Apple Watch application designed to improve sleep quality in adults with PTSD-related nightmares (FDA, 2020). The watch's sensors detect heart rate abnormalities that might be related to nightmares and then it vibrates, reportedly to interrupt the dream without disturbing sleep. It is currently undergoing additional trials but may be available with a physician's recommendation.

Psychopharmacology

Trauma-focused psychotherapy is considered the first-line treatment for PTSD (Jeffreys, 2021); however, many medications have demonstrated benefits as well.

Antidepressants

Selective serotonin reuptake inhibitors (SSRIs) are now considered first-line treatments for PTSD because of their efficacy, tolerability, and safety ratings. Paroxetine and sertraline have been approved by the FDA for this purpose. Additionally, fluoxetine and the selective norepinephrine reuptake inhibitor venlafaxine, although not FDA approved for PTSD, have demonstrated effectiveness (Jeffreys, 2022). The tricyclic antidepressants amitriptyline (Elavil) and imipramine (Tofranil) have been supported by several well-controlled studies and may be used as an alternative medication if the patient is not responding to an SSRI. The monoamine oxidase inhibitor phenelzine has also demonstrated efficacy in the treatment of PTSD.

Anxiolytics

Alprazolam has been prescribed for PTSD patients for its antidepressant and antipanic effects despite the absence of controlled studies demonstrating its efficacy in PTSD. Jeffreys (2022) recommended against using benzodiazepines in PTSD based on a meta-analysis finding that they worsened patients' PTSD symptoms. In addition, their addictive properties make them less desirable than some of the other medications in the treatment of post-trauma patients.

Buspirone, which has serotonergic properties similar to those of SSRIs, may be useful for treating anxiety in PTSD, and these drugs also have less addiction potential than benzodiazepines. Animal studies (Malikowska-Racia et al., 2020) supported the benefit of buspirone in treating people with PTSD, but more controlled trials with this drug are needed.

Antihypertensives

Beta blockers reduce both central and peripheral manifestations of hyperarousal and may reduce aggression as well; although there has been great interest in using these drugs to prevent PTSD, the evidence does not support this (Jeffreys, 2022).

Other Medications

Ketamine, an anesthetic agent that has demonstrated benefits in treatment of depression and obsessive-compulsive disorder, was found in clinical trials (Feder et al., 2021) to benefit some patients with PTSD. It modulates glutaminergic activity at N-methyl-D-aspartate (NMDA) receptors and serotonergic activity at 5-HT_1 receptors and is thought to disrupt the fear associated with trauma. Currently, ketamine is not FDA approved for this use but is prescribed as an off-label use. It is administered intravenously at subanesthetic doses and usually involves a series of treatments. Jeffreys (2021) cautioned that its effects are short term and there is potential for addiction. 3,4-Methylenedioxymethamphetamine (MDMA) is also in clinical trials for the treatment of PTSD, and early findings suggest that MDMA-assisted psychotherapy may be beneficial in helping reduce fear and facilitate processing of traumatic memories (Mitchell et al., 2021).

The endocannabinoid system may be another avenue for treatment, as decreased levels of endogenous cannabinoids have been found in PTSD patients (Jeffreys, 2022). Although direct stimulation of this pathway has demonstrated negative effects on PTSD and potential for addiction, indirect stimulation of this pathway might provide some additional treatment options. Early trials with fatty acid amide hydrolase (FAAH) inhibitors, which block the breakdown of endocannabinoids, showed promise in helping participants to develop fear-extinction memories (Mayo et al., 2019). More research is needed to confirm these benefits.

The alpha-1 antagonist prazosin (Minipress) has demonstrated benefit in reducing nightmares and enhancing normal dreaming patterns in people with PTSD. However, Veterans Health Administration clinical practice guidelines now recommend against its use in PTSD based on a large trial that found no difference between prazosin and placebo (Jeffreys, 2022). Finally, there is interest in glucocorticoids because several actions, including potentiating glutamate at NMDA receptors, may influence decreased retrieval of fear memories (Jeffreys, 2022).

Adjustment Disorders

Various treatments are used for clients with adjustment disorders. The primary focus of intervention is to maximize the potential for adaptation.

Individual Psychotherapy

Individual psychotherapy is the most common treatment for adjustment disorder. Individual psychotherapy allows the client to examine the stressor that is causing the problem, possibly assign personal meaning to the stressor, and confront unresolved issues that may be exacerbating this crisis. Treatment works to remove these blocks to adaptation so that normal developmental progression can resume. Techniques are used to clarify links between the current stressor and past experiences and assist with the development of more adaptive coping strategies.

Family Therapy

The focus of treatment is shifted from the individual to the system of relationships in which the individual is involved. The maladaptive response of the identified client is viewed as symptomatic of a dysfunctional family system. All family members are included in the therapy, and treatment serves to improve the functioning within the family network. Emphasis is placed on communication, family rules, and interaction patterns among the family members.

Behavior Therapy

The goal of behavior therapy is to replace ineffective response patterns with more adaptive ones. The situations that promote ineffective responses are identified, and carefully designed reinforcement schedules along with role modeling and coaching are used to alter the maladaptive response patterns. This type of treatment is very effective when implemented in an inpatient setting where the client's behavior and its consequences may be more readily controlled.

Self-Help Groups

Group experiences, with or without a professional facilitator, provide an arena in which members may consider and compare their responses to individuals with similar life experiences. Members benefit from learning that they are not alone in their painful experiences. Hope is derived from knowing that others have survived and even grown from similar traumas. Members of the group exchange advice, share coping strategies, and provide support and encouragement for each other.

Crisis Intervention

Crisis intervention (or emergency intervention) is sometimes warranted, particularly if the patient is demonstrating or at risk for suicidal behavior. Crisis intervention is short term and focused on resolving the immediate crisis and maintaining client safety. The ultimate goal of crisis intervention in the treatment of adjustment disorder (or generally) is to restore adaptive functioning and promote personal growth.

Psychopharmacology

Adjustment disorder is not commonly treated with medications because (1) their effect may be temporary and only mask the real problem, interfering with the possibility of finding a more permanent solution; and (2) some psychoactive drugs carry the potential for physiological and psychological dependence.

When the client with adjustment disorder has symptoms of anxiety or depression, the physician may prescribe antianxiety or antidepressant medication. These medications are considered only adjuncts to psychotherapy and should not be given as primary therapy. They are given to alleviate symptoms so that the individual may more effectively cope while attempting to adapt to the stressful situation.

CLINICAL JUDGMENT IN ACTION: CASE STUDY AND SAMPLE CARE PLAN

NURSING HISTORY AND ASSESSMENT

Recognizing cues: The nurse must demonstrate ability to recognize what information is most important to making an assessment (National Council of State Boards of Nursing [NCSBN], 2021). This information is italicized in the following.

Marissa, age 22, was born in a small town in Oklahoma. She lived there her whole life, even living at home while she attended a nearby college to earn a baccalaureate degree in education. She is an only child, and her parents were in their 40s when she was born. She was engaged throughout her college years to her high school sweetheart, Dave, who graduated 6 months ago from the state university with a degree in aeronautical engineering.

Upon his graduation, he accepted a position with NASA at Kennedy Space Center in Florida. Marissa and Dave were married 5 months ago and **recently moved** to a small apartment in Cape Canaveral, where Dave began his work with NASA. The plan was for Marissa to seek employment upon their arrival, but she has been **unable to move ahead** with those plans. She **stays in the apartment most days, talking on the phone to her parents and crying about how much she misses them and her home in Oklahoma.** She has **met very few people and has no desire to do so.** She **sleeps a lot and has lost 5 pounds in the last 3 weeks.** She has been having **severe headaches.** Her husband has become very concerned about her and made an appointment for her with a private physician. After a complete and **unremarkable physical examination,** the physician referred Marissa to the mental health clinic, where she was admitted to the day treatment center with a diagnosis of adjustment disorder with **depressed mood.**

CLINICAL JUDGMENT IN ACTION: CASE STUDY AND SAMPLE CARE PLAN—cont'd

Analyzing cues: The nurse must be able to interpret the information (NCSBN, 2021).

The nurse identifies that several of Marissa's symptoms (isolating in her apartment with no desire for social interaction, frequent crying, weight loss, and hypersomnia) are associated with depression. In addition, Marissa's focus on missing her parents and her home in Oklahoma represent anxiety associated with a significant loss. Noting that depression may be associated with increased risk for suicide, the nurse conducts a thorough suicide risk assessment. Marissa does not demonstrate risk for suicide. The nurse further interprets that Marissa's weight loss, although possibly symptomatic, is not profound.

Prioritize hypotheses: The nurse must be able to identify the client's most important needs (NCSBN, 2021).

Having ruled out immediate risk for suicide and immediate concerns over her weight loss, the nurse prioritizes focusing on Marissa's depression and anxiety associated with recent losses.

NURSING DIAGNOSES AND OUTCOME IDENTIFICATION

Generate solutions: The nurse must be able to connect their prioritized understanding of client needs to a course of action or plan of care (NCSBN, 2021).

From the assessment data, the nurse develops the following nursing diagnoses for Marissa:

1. Maladaptive grieving related to feelings of loss associated with leaving her parents and her lifetime home.
   a. Short-term goal:
      ■ Within 1 week, Marissa will express anger about the loss associated with her move.
   b. Long-term goal:
      ■ Marissa will be able to verbalize behaviors associated with the normal stages of grief and identify her position in the grief process while progressing at her own pace toward resolution.
2. Relocation stress syndrome related to moving away from parents and familiar environment in which she had spent her whole life.
   a. Short-term goal:
      ■ Within 1 week, Marissa will verbalize at least one positive aspect regarding relocation to her new environment.
   b. Long-term goal:
      ■ Within 1 month, Marissa will demonstrate positive adaptation to her new environment as evidenced by involvement in activities, expression of satisfaction with new acquaintances, and elimination of previously evident physical and psychological symptoms associated with the relocation.

PLANNING AND IMPLEMENTATION

Take Action: The nurse must be able to identify what actions need to be taken and how they will be implemented (NCSBN, 2021).

MALADAPTIVE GRIEVING

The following nursing interventions have been identified for Marissa:

1. Determine the stage of grief in which Marissa is fixed. Identify behaviors associated with this stage.
2. Develop a trusting relationship with Marissa. Show empathy and caring. Be honest and keep all promises.
3. Convey an accepting attitude so that Marissa is not afraid to express her feelings openly.
4. Allow Marissa to express her anger. Do not become defensive if the initial expression of anger is displaced on nurse or therapist. Help Marissa explore angry feelings so that they may be directed toward the intended object or situation.
5. Help Marissa discharge pent-up anger through participation in large motor activities (e.g., brisk walks, jogging, physical exercises, or activity of her choice).
6. Explain to Marissa the normal stages of grief and the behaviors associated with each stage. Help her to understand that these feelings are normal and acceptable during a grief process.
7. Encourage Marissa to review her personal perception of the move. With support and sensitivity, point out the reality of the situation in areas where misrepresentations are expressed.
8. Help Marissa solve problems as she attempts to determine methods for more adaptive coping with her life change. Provide positive feedback for strategies identified and decisions made.
9. Encourage Marissa to reach out for spiritual support during this time in whatever form is desirable to her. Assess her spiritual needs and assist as necessary in the fulfillment of those needs.

RELOCATION STRESS SYNDROME

The following nursing interventions have been identified for Marissa:

1. Encourage Marissa to discuss feelings (concerns, fears, anger) regarding this relocation.
2. Encourage Marissa to discuss how the change will affect her life. Ensure that Marissa is involved in decision making and problem-solving regarding the move.
3. Help Marissa identify positive aspects about the move.
4. Help Marissa identify resources within the new community from which assistance with various types of services may be obtained.

Continued

CLINICAL JUDGMENT IN ACTION: CASE STUDY AND SAMPLE CARE PLAN—cont'd

5. Identify groups within the community that specialize in helping individuals adapt to relocation. Examples include Newcomers' Club, Welcome Wagon International, and school and church organizations.
6. Refer Marissa to a support group (e.g., Depression and Bipolar Support Alliance [DBSA]).

EVALUATION

Evaluate outcomes: The nurse must be able to evaluate actions taken and determine whether they have had a positive, neutral, or negative effect (NCSBN, 2021).

The outcome criteria for Marissa have been met. She is no longer having headaches and has regained some of her weight. She has joined a chapter of DBSA and has made some new acquaintances. She has applied to become a substitute teacher in the local school district, and she and Dave have joined the local Methodist church, where they have started to socialize with several couples their age. They have also adopted Molly, a 2-year-old mutt from the local shelter, who showers Marissa with love and keeps her company when no one else is around. They take daily walks together. Marissa still talks to her parents on the phone daily but no longer has feelings of despair about living so far away from them. Her parents provide encouragement and give her positive feedback for achieving a satisfactory adaptation to her new environment. They are planning a visit to see Marissa and Dave in the near future.

Summary and Key Points

■ Post-traumatic stress disorder (PTSD) is the development of characteristic symptoms after exposure to an extreme traumatic stressor involving a personal threat to physical integrity or to the integrity of others. Symptoms may begin within the first 3 months after the trauma or there may be a delay of several months or even years.

■ The symptoms of PTSD are associated with events that would be markedly distressing to almost anyone and include reexperiencing the trauma, a sustained high level of anxiety or arousal, or a general numbing of responsiveness.

■ Acute stress disorder (ASD) is similar to PTSD in symptomatology and its precipitation by traumatic events. In ASD, the symptoms are time-limited, lasting up to 1 month after the trauma. When the symptoms last longer than 1 month, the diagnosis is PTSD.

■ Predisposing factors to trauma-related disorders include psychosocial, learning, cognitive, and biological influences.

■ Adjustment disorders are relatively common. Some studies indicate they are the most commonly ascribed psychiatric diagnoses in patients hospitalized for medical and surgical problems.

■ Clinical symptoms associated with adjustment disorders include inability to function socially or occupationally in response to an identifiable stressor.

■ Adjustment disorder is distinguished by the predominant features of the maladaptive response. These include depression, anxiety, mixed anxiety and depression, disturbance of conduct, and mixed disturbance of emotions and conduct.

■ Of the two types of stressors discussed (i.e., sudden shock and continuous stressors), more individuals respond with maladaptive behaviors to long-term continuous stressors.

■ Treatment modalities for PTSD include cognitive behavior therapy (CBT), PE therapy, group and family therapy, eye movement desensitization and reprocessing (EMDR), digital therapeutics, and psychopharmacology.

■ Treatment modalities for adjustment disorders include individual psychotherapy, family therapy, behavior therapy, self-help groups, crisis intervention, and medications to treat anxiety or depression.

■ Nursing care of individuals with trauma- and stressor-related disorders is accomplished using the steps of the nursing process.

■ Trauma-informed care identifies and considers the effect of previous trauma when developing a care plan for clients in any setting because this client is vulnerable to retraumatization.

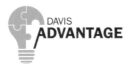

Go to **Davis Advantage** to complete your learning: strengthen understanding, apply your knowledge, and prepare for the Next Gen NCLEX®.

Review Questions

1. A client, who is a veteran of the war in Iraq, is diagnosed with PTSD. The client says to the nurse, "I can't figure out why God took my buddy instead of me." From this statement, the nurse assesses which of the following in the client?
   a. Repressed anger
   b. Survivor's guilt
   c. Intrusive thoughts
   d. Spiritual distress

2. Which of the following treatment regimens would most appropriately be ordered for a client with PTSD?
   a. Paroxetine and group therapy
   b. Diazepam and implosion therapy
   c. Alprazolam and behavior therapy
   d. Carbamazepine and cognitive behavior therapy

3. Which of the following may be influential in the predisposition to PTSD?
   a. Resilient personality traits
   b. Ketamine deficiency
   c. History of dementia
   d. Severity of the stressor and availability of support systems

4. Which of the following is true regarding the diagnosis of adjustment disorder?
   a. The client will require long-term psychotherapy to achieve relief.
   b. The client likely inherited a genetic tendency for the disorder.
   c. Symptoms will likely remit once the client has accepted the changes that precipitated the difficulties with adjustment.
   d. Adjustment disorders are not typically related to an identified stressor.

5. The physician orders sertraline (Zoloft) for a client who is hospitalized with adjustment disorder with depressed mood. This medication is intended to:
   a. Increase energy and elevate mood.
   b. Increase suicidal ideation.
   c. Prevent psychotic symptoms.
   d. Help the client adjust to change.

6. Trauma-informed care is a philosophical approach that includes which of the following principles? (Select all that apply.)
   a. Nurses need to be aware of the potential for trauma in any client and provide care that minimizes the risk of revictimization or retraumatization.
   b. Medications need to be given before any other interventions are considered.
   c. Trauma-informed care highlights the importance of providing care that protects the physical, psychological, and emotional safety of the client.
   d. Trauma-informed care is based on the principle that traumas are not correlated with depression or increased risk for suicide.

Clinical Judgment Questions

7. A client experiences a nightmare during their first night in the hospital and explains to the nurse that they were dreaming about gunfire all around and people being killed. The nurse's most appropriate initial intervention is to:
   a. Administer alprazolam as ordered prn for anxiety.
   b. Call the physician and report the incident.
   c. Stay with the client and reassure them of their safety.
   d. Have the client listen to a tape of relaxation exercises.

8. A client who recently divorced after 10 years of marriage is admitted to the hospital with a diagnosis of adjustment disorder with depressed mood. The client acknowledges difficulty adjusting to an independent lifestyle and having thoughts of taking an overdose of acetaminophen. Which is the priority nursing diagnosis for this client?
   a. Social isolation
   b. Maladaptive grieving
   c. Ineffective communication
   d. Risk for suicidal behavior

9. A client, who is depressed following the breakup of a very stormy marriage, says to the nurse, "I feel so bad. I thought I would feel better once I left, but I feel worse!" Which is the best response by the nurse?
   a. "Cheer up. You have a lot to be happy about."
   b. "You are grieving the loss of your marriage. It's natural for you to feel bad."
   c. "Try not to dwell on how you feel. If you don't think about it, you'll feel better."
   d. "You did the right thing. Knowing that should make you feel better."

10. A client, age 16, has recently been diagnosed with diabetes mellitus. The client must watch their diet and take an oral hypoglycemic medication daily. The client has become very depressed, and the client's mother reports that they refuse to change their diet and often skips their medication. The client has been hospitalized for stabilization of their blood glucose level. The psychiatric nurse practitioner has been called in as a consultant. Which nursing diagnosis by the psychiatric nurse would be a priority for the client at this time?
    a. Anxiety related to hospitalization, evidenced by nonadherence
    b. Low self-esteem related to feeling different from their peers, evidenced by social isolation
    c. Risk for suicide related to new diagnosis of diabetes mellitus
    d. Risk-prone health behavior related to denial of the seriousness of their illness, evidenced by refusal to follow diet and take medication

TEST YOUR CLINICAL REASONING AND CLINICAL JUDGMENT SKILLS

Alice, age 48, underwent a mastectomy of the right breast after a mammogram revealed a lump that was found to be malignant when biopsied. Since her surgery 6 weeks ago, Alice has refused to see any of her friends. She stays in her bedroom, speaks to her husband only when he speaks first, is having difficulty sleeping, and eats very little. She refuses to look at the mastectomy scar and has refused to see the Reach to Recovery representative who has tried several times to help fit her with a prosthesis. Her husband has become very worried about her and spoke to the family doctor, who recommended a psychiatrist. She has been admitted to the psychiatric unit with a diagnosis of adjustment disorder with depressed mood.

Answer the following questions about Alice:

1. What would be the primary nursing diagnosis for Alice?
2. Describe a short-term goal and a long-term goal for Alice.
3. Discuss a priority nursing intervention in working with Alice.

🎬 MOVIE CONNECTIONS

The Deer Hunter (PTSD) • *Hell and Back Again* (PTSD) • *Jackknife* (PTSD) • *Brothers* (PTSD) • *The War at Home* (PTSD) • *Fearless* (PTSD) • *The Fisher King* (PTSD) • *The Changeover* (PTSD and comorbid mental health issues) • The Perks of Being a Wallflower (PTSD) • *A Private War* (PTSD)

References

American Psychiatric Association (APA). (2022) *Diagnostic and statistical manual of mental disorders, fifth edition, text revision.* American Psychiatric Association.

Bohus, M., Kleindiens, N., Hahn, C., Müller-Engelmann, M., Ludäscher, P., Steil, R., Fydrich, T., Kuehner, C., Resick, P. A., Stiglmayr, C., Schmahl, C., & Priebe, K. (2020). Dialectical behavior therapy for posttraumatic stress disorder (DBT-PTSD) compared with cognitive processing therapy (CPT) in complex presentations of PTSD in women survivors of childhood abuse: A randomized clinical trial. *JAMA Psychiatry, 77*(12), 1235–1245. https://doi.org/10.1001/jamapsychiatry.2020.2148

Boland, R., & Verduin, M. L. (2022). *Kaplan & Sadock's synopsis of psychiatry* (P. Ruiz, Ed.). (12th ed.). Wolters Kluwer.

Casey, P. (2013). Adjustment disorders: Diagnosis and treatment. *Psychiatric times.* https://www.psychiatrictimes.com/view/adjustment-disorders-diagnostic-and-treatment-issues

Centers for Disease Control and Prevention (CDC). (2021). *Adverse childhood experiences.* https://www.cdc.gov/violenceprevention/aces/

Department of Veterans Affairs. (2022). *How common is PTSD in adults?* https://www.ptsd.va.gov/understand/common/common_adults.asp

Dominguez, S., & Lee, C. (2019). Differences in international guidelines regarding EMDR for posttraumatic stress disorder: Why they diverge and suggestions for future research. *Journal of EMDR Practice and Research, 13*(4), 247–260.

EMDR International Association. (2022a). *About EMDR therapy.* https://www.emdria.org/about-emdr-therapy/

EMDR International Association. (2022b). *Experiencing EMDR therapy.* https://www.emdria.org/about-emdr-therapy/experiencing-emdr-therapy/

Feder, A., Costi, S., Rutter, S. B., Collins, A. B., Govindarajulu, U., Jha, M. W. K., Horn, S. R., Kautz, M., Corniquel, M., Collins, K. A.,

Bevilacqua, L., Glasgow, A. M., Brallier, J., Pietrzak, R. H., Murrough, J. W., & Charney, D. S. (2021). A randomized controlled trial of repeated ketamine administration for chronic posttraumatic stress disorder. *American Journal of Psychiatry, 178*(2), 193–202. https://doi.org/10.1176/appi.ajp.2020.20050596

Frances, A. (2015). "We should live"—Surviving after catastrophic death. *Psychiatric Times.* https://www.psychiatrictimes.com/view/we-should-live-surviving-after-catastrophic-death

Frank, J. B. (2021). Adjustment disorders. *Medscape.* https://emedicine.medscape.com/article/2192631-overview

Günak, M., Billings, J., Carratu, E., Marchant, N., Favarato, G., & Orgeta, V. (2020). Post-traumatic stress disorder as a risk factor for dementia: Systematic review and meta-analysis. *The British Journal of Psychiatry, 217*(5), 600–608. https://doi.org/10.1192/bjp.2020.150

Herdman, T. H., Kamitsuru, S., & Lopes, C. T. (Eds.). (2021). *NANDA-I, Inc. nursing diagnoses: Definitions and classification, 2021–2023.* Thieme.

Hopper, E. K., Bassuk, E. L., & Olivet, J. (2010). Shelter from the storm: Trauma-informed care in homelessness services settings. *The Open Health Services and Policy Journal, 3*(2), 80–100. doi:10.2174/1874924001003010080

Jeffreys, M. (2022). *Clinician's guide to medications for PTSD.* https://www.ptsd.va.gov/professional/treat/txessentials/clinician_guide_meds.asp

Katzman, J. W., & Geppert, C. M. (2017). Adjustment disorders. In Sadock, B. J., Sadock, V. A., & Ruiz, P. (Eds.), *Comprehensive textbook of psychiatry* (10th ed., pp. 2116–2125). Wolters Kluwer.

Lanius, U. F., Paulson, S. L., & Corrigan, F. M. (Eds.). (2014). *Neurobiology and treatment of traumatic dissociation: Toward an embodied self.* Springer.

Lissek, S., & van Meurs, B. (2015). Learning models of PTSD: Theoretical accounts and psychobiological evidence. *International Journal of Psychophysiology, 98*(3 Pt 2), 594–605. doi: 10.1016/j.ijpsycho.2014.11.006

Lynch, T. R. (2018). *Radically open dialectical behavior therapy: Theory and practice for treating disorders of overcontrol.* Context Press.

Malikowska-Racia, N., Popik, P., & Salat, K. (2020). Behavioral effects of buspirone in a mouse model of posttraumatic stress disorder. *Behavioural Brain Research, 381.* https://doi.org/10.1016/j.bbr.2019.112380

Maxfield, L., & Hyer, L. (2002). The relationship between efficacy and methodology in studies investigating EMDR treatment of PTSD. *Journal of Clinical Psychology, 58*(1), 23–41.

Mayo, L. M., Asratian, A., Linde, J., Moreno, M., Haataja, R., Hammar, V., Augier, G., Hill, M. N., & Heilig, M. (2019). Elevated anandamide, enhanced recall of fear extinction, and attenuated stress responses following inhibition of fatty acid amide hydrolase: A randomized, controlled experimental medicine trial. *Biological Psychiatry, 87*(6), 538–547. https://doi.org/10.1016/j.biopsych.2019.07.034

Mitchell, J. M., Bogenschutz, M., Lilienstein, A., Harrison, C., Kleiman, S., Parker-Guilbert, K., Ot'alora, G. M., Garas, W., Paleos, C., Gorman, I., Nicholas, C., Mithoefer, M., Carlin, S., Poulter, B., Mithoefer, A., Quevedo, S., Wells, G., Klaire, S. S., van der Kolk, B., Tzarfaty, K., Amiaz, R., ... Doblin, R. (2021). MDMA-assisted therapy for severe PTSD: A randomized, double-blind, placebo-controlled phase 3 study. *Nature Medicine, 27*(6), 1025–1033. https://doi.org/10.1038/s41591-021-01336-3

National Council of State Boards of Nursing (NCSBN). (2021). *Next generation NCLEX®: comparison between case studies and stand-alone items.* https://www.ncsbn.org/public-files/NGN_Fall21_English_Final.pdf

O'Donnell, M. L., Agathos, J. A., Metcalf, O., Gibson, K., & Lau, W. (2019). Adjustment disorder: Current developments and future directions. International *Journal of Environmental Research and Public Health, 16*(14), 2537. https://doi.org/10.3390/ijerph16142537

Park, C. L., Mills, M. A., & Edmondson, D. (2012). PTSD as meaning violation: Testing a cognitive worldview perspective. *Psychological Trauma: Theory, Research, Practice and Policy, 4*(1), 66–73. https://doi.org/10.1037/a0018792

Rothbaum, B. O., Astin, M. C., & Marsteller, F. (2005). Prolonged exposure versus and reprocessing (EMDR) for PTSD rape victims. *Journal of Traumatic Stress, 18*(6), 607–616.

Shapiro, F. (2007). EMDR and case conceptualization from an adaptive information processing perspective. In Shapiro, F., Kaslow, F. W., & Maxfield, L. (Eds.), *Handbook of EMDR and family therapy processes* (pp. 3–34). Wiley.

Steenkamp, M. M., Schlenger, W. E., Corry, N., Henn-Haase C., Qian, M., Li, M., Horesh, D., Karstoft, K. I., Williams, C., Ho, C. L., Shalev, A., Kulka, R., & Marmar, C. (2017). Predictors of PTSD 40 years after combat: Findings from the National Vietnam Veterans longitudinal study. *Depression and Anxiety, 34*(8), 711–722. https://doi.org/10.1002/da.22628

Stein, M. B., Levey, D. F., Cheng, Z., Wendt, F. R., Harrington, K., Pathak, G. A., Cho, K., Quaden, R., Radhakrishnan, K., Girgenti, M. J., Ho, Y. A., Posner, D., Aslan, M., Duman, R. S., Zhao, H., Department of Veterans Affairs Cooperative Studies Program (no. 575B); VA Million Veteran Program, Polimanti, R., Concato, J., & Gelernter J. (2021). Genome-wide association analyses of post-traumatic stress disorder and its symptom subdomains in the Million Veteran Program. *Nature Genetics, 53*(2), 174–184. https://doi.org/10.1038/s41588-02000767-

Substance Abuse and Mental Health Services Administration. (2014). *TIP 57: Trauma-Informed Care in Behavioral Health Services.* https://www.samhsa.gov/resource/ebp/tip-57-trauma-informed-care-behavioral-health-services

Substance Abuse and Mental Health Services Administration. (2022). *Trauma and violence.* https://www.samhsa.gov/trauma-violence

Togay, B., & El-Mallakh, R. S. (2020). Posttraumatic stress disorder: From pathophysiology to pharmacology. *Current Psychiatry, 19*(5), 33–37.

UPMC, Center for Integrative Medicine. (2022). *Eye movement desensitization and reprocessing.* http://www.upmc.com/Services/integrative-medicine/services/Pages/eye-movement.aspx

U.S. Food and Drug Administration. (2020). *FDA permits marketing of new device designed to reduce sleep disturbance related to nightmares in certain adults* [Press release]. https://www.fda.gov/news-events/press-announcements/fda-permits-marketing-new-device-designed-reduce-sleep-disturbance-related-nightmares-certain-adults

Valentino, R. J., & Van Bockstaele, E. (2015). Endogenous opioids: The downside to opposing stress. *Neurobiology of Stress, 1,* 23–32. doi:http://dx.doi.org/10.1016/j.ynstr.2014.09.006

Valiente-Gómez, A., Moreno-Alcázar, A., Treen, D., Cedrón, C., Colom, F., Pérez, V., & Amann, B. L. (2017). EMDR beyond PTSD: A systematic literature review. *Frontiers in Psychiatry, 8.* https://doi.org/10.3389/fpsyg.2017.01668

World Health Organization (WHO). (2013). *WHO releases guidance on mental health care after trauma* [Press release]. https://www.who.int/news/item/06-08-2013-who-releases-guidance-on-mental-health-care-after-trauma

Classical References

Epstein, S. (1991). Beliefs and symptoms in maladaptive resolutions of the traumatic neurosis. In Ozer, D., Healy, Jr., J. M., & Stewart, A. J. (Eds.), *Perspectives on personality* (Vol. 3). Jessica Kingsley.

Friedman, M. J. (1996). PTSD diagnosis and treatment for mental health clinicians. *Community Mental Health Journal, 32*(2), 173–189. doi:10.1007/BF02249755

29

Somatic Symptom and Dissociative Disorders

CORE CONCEPTS

Stress and Coping:
Amnesia, dissociation, and somatic symptoms

Professional Behavior:
Nursing process in the care of patients with somatic symptom and dissociative disorders

Safety

Clinical Judgment

KEY TERMS

abreaction	fugue	secondary gain
anosmia	generalized amnesia	selective amnesia
aphonia	integration	somatization
depersonalization	localized amnesia	tertiary gain
derealization	primary gain	
factitious disorder	pseudocyesis	

OBJECTIVES

After reading this chapter, the student will be able to:

1. Discuss historical aspects and epidemiology related to somatic symptom and dissociative disorders.
2. Describe various types of somatic symptom and dissociative disorders and identify symptomatology associated with each; use this information in patient assessment.
3. Identify predisposing factors in the development of somatic symptom and dissociative disorders.
4. Formulate nursing diagnoses and goals of care for patients with somatic symptom and dissociative disorders.
5. Describe appropriate nursing interventions for behaviors associated with somatic symptom and dissociative disorders.
6. Evaluate the nursing care of patients with somatic symptom and dissociative disorders.
7. Discuss modalities relevant to treatment of somatic symptom and dissociative disorders.

Disorders with primarily somatic symptoms are characterized by physical symptoms suggesting medical disease but without demonstrable organic pathology. For this reason, most people with a somatic symptom and related disorders are seen in primary care and hospital settings rather than in mental health-care settings. It is important to note that an inability to attribute a pathophysiological cause to an individual's symptoms is not sufficient to diagnose them with a mental illness. Somatic symptom and related disorders are classified as mental disorders by the *Diagnostic and Statistical Manual of Mental Disorders,*

Fifth Edition, Text Revision (DSM-5-TR) when an individual's excessive focus on somatic symptoms is beyond any medical explanation *and* the symptoms cause significant distress and impairment in their functioning (American Psychiatric Association [APA], 2022).

The *DSM-5-TR* identifies a specific disorder called *somatic symptom disorder* and several related disorders including *illness anxiety disorder, conversion disorder, factitious disorders, psychological factors affecting other medical conditions,* and others (APA, 2022). The common focus of these diagnoses is distress and impairment secondary to somatic symptoms, as described previously. The prevalence of somatic symptom disorder in primary care settings has been estimated to be as high as 11% and hypochondriasis (no longer a diagnostic category in the *DSM-5-TR* but similar to illness anxiety disorder) from 1.3% to 10% (APA, 2022). Studies have estimated the incidence of conversion symptoms (somatic symptoms that can't be medically explained) among patients in general hospital settings to be as high as 20% to 25%, with 5% meeting the full criteria for a conversion disorder (Ali et al., 2015). The wide variation of these estimates highlights the lack of consensus in diagnosing and reporting these conditions.

Dissociative disorders are defined by a disruption in psychobiological functions that would otherwise be integrated aspects of experience and cognition, including memory, identity, consciousness, perception, behavior, emotion, body representation, and motor control. Dissociative responses occur when anxiety becomes overwhelming and the personality becomes disorganized. Defense mechanisms that normally govern consciousness, identity, and memory break down, and behavior occurs with little or no participation on the part of the conscious personality. Types of dissociative disorders described by the *DSM-5-TR* include *depersonalization/derealization disorder, dissociative amnesia, dissociative identity disorder (DID),* and others.

This chapter focuses on disorders characterized by severe repressed anxiety that manifests as physical symptoms, fear of illness, and dissociative behaviors. Historical aspects and epidemiology are presented. Predisposing factors that have been implicated in the etiology of these responses provide a framework for studying the dynamics of somatic symptom and dissociative disorders. An explanation of the symptomatology of these disorders is presented as background knowledge for assessing the patient, and nursing care is described in the context of the nursing process. Additional treatment modalities are explored.

Historical Aspects

Historically, somatic symptom disorders were identified as hysterical neuroses. The concept of hysteria is at least 4,000 years old and probably originated in Egypt. The term has been in use since the time of Hippocrates. In its original use, hysteria referred to a condition of emotional excitability that affected psychological, sensory, vasomotor, and visceral functions.

Over the years, symptoms of hysterical neuroses have been associated with witchcraft, demonology, and sorcery; dysfunction of the nervous system; and unexpressed emotions. They have also historically been viewed as primarily an affliction of women. Critics have argued that the depiction of women as prone to hysteria not only is sexist but has interfered with women receiving adequate medical evaluation for symptoms.

Somatic symptom disorders are thought to occur in response to repressed severe anxiety. Freud (1962) observed that under hypnosis, patients with hysterical neurosis could recall memories and emotional experiences that would relieve their symptoms. This observation led to his proposal that unexpressed emotion can be "converted" into physical symptoms.

CORE CONCEPT

Dissociation

An unconscious defense mechanism in which there is separation of normally related mental processes such as identity, memory, and cognition from affect; the detachment of ideas and memories from events or experiences.

Freud (1962) viewed dissociation as a type of repression, an active defense mechanism used to remove threatening or unacceptable mental contents from conscious awareness. He also described the defense of ego-splitting in the management of incompatible mental contents. Although the study of dissociative processes dates back to the 19th century, scientists still know remarkably little about the phenomena. Questions remain unanswered: Are dissociative disorders psychopathological processes or ego-protective devices? Are dissociative processes under voluntary control, or are they a totally unconscious effort? In either case, they may serve to reduce a person's awareness and anxiety associated with events that are perceived as extremely stressful.

Although symptoms such as dissociation are considered an unconscious defense mechanism, some individuals consciously fabricate symptoms. The syndrome of fabricating symptoms for emotional gain was first described by Richard Asher in 1951. He described a pattern of behavior in which individuals fabricated or embellished their histories and signs and symptoms of illness. He termed this condition *Munchausen syndrome* after Baron Friedrich Hieronymus Freiherr von Munchhausen, a German cavalry officer and nobleman, who was known for his fabricated stories and fanciful exaggerations about himself (Asher, 1951). Currently the *DSM-5-TR* describes this syndrome as **factitious disorder.** These include *factitious disorder imposed on self,* or when someone deceptively induces injury or illness in another person, *factitious disorder imposed on another.*

Epidemiology

The prevalence of somatic symptom disorder is estimated to be 5% to 7% (Yates, 2019). Although historically this disorder has been thought to be more prevalent in women, the *DSM-5-TR* (APA, 2022) suggests that the higher reported female prevalence may be related to the fact that women tend to report somatic symptoms more often than males do.

Lifetime prevalence rates of conversion disorder vary widely. Statistics within the general population have ranged from 5% to 30% (Ali, 2015). The disorder occurs more frequently in women than in men and more frequently in adolescents and young adults than in other age groups.

The prevalence of illness anxiety disorder, which along with somatic symptom disorder was similar to the diagnosis of hypochondriasis in the *DSM-5-TR,* is especially difficult to establish. The best estimate is based on data about the prevalence of hypochondriasis, estimated at between 3% and 8% (APA, 2022). Some people previously diagnosed with hypochondriasis might better meet diagnostic criteria for somatic symptom disorder under this new classification. There are similarities between these two disorders, but in somatic symptom disorder, the primary symptom is significant somatic sensations, whereas in illness anxiety disorder, there are few to no somatic symptoms, but anxiety or fear about having or acquiring an illness is a primary concern. Kahn (2018) noted that preoccupation with illness is not uncommon because 10% to 20% of people who are healthy and 45% of people without a major psychiatric disorder have intermittent unfounded worries about illness. More research is needed to better understand the epidemiology of each of these disorders.

Hypochondriasis was relabeled as illness anxiety disorder, at least in part, to eliminate myths and stigmas associated with the former diagnosis (Dimsdale, 2020). Illness anxiety disorder is equally common among men and women, and onset most commonly occurs in early adulthood. Data on the prevalence of factitious disorder are unknown. Estimates based on samples of hospital patients identify that about 1% meet criteria for factitious disorder (APA, 2022). Factitious disorder imposed on another is most often perpetrated by mothers against infants but accounts for less than 0.04% of reported cases of child abuse in the United States (Boland & Verduin, 2022).

Dissociative syndromes, although often portrayed in fictional media, are statistically quite rare. However, when they do occur, they may present dramatic clinical pictures of severe disturbance in normal personality functioning. Dissociative amnesia occurs most frequently under conditions of war or during natural disasters. In recent years, the number of reported cases has increased, possibly attributable to increased awareness of the phenomenon and subsequent identification of cases that were previously undiagnosed. It appears to be equally common in men and women. Dissociative amnesia can occur at any age but is difficult to diagnose in children because it is easily confused with inattention or oppositional behavior.

Estimates of the prevalence of DID, previously called *multiple personality disorder,* also vary. In early childhood the ratio of female to male DID cases is 1 to 1 but increases steadily to approximately 8 to 1 by late adolesc ence (Boland & Verduin, 2022). Onset likely occurs in childhood, although manifestations of the disorder may not be recognized until late adolescence or early adulthood.

The prevalence of severe episodes of depersonalization/derealization disorder is unknown. Single brief episodes may occur in as many as one-half of all adults, particularly when under severe psychosocial stress; when sleep deprived; during travel to unfamiliar places; or when intoxicated with hallucinogens, marijuana, or alcohol. Symptoms usually begin in adolescence or early adulthood. The disorder is chronic, with periods of remission and exacerbation. The incidence of depersonalization/derealization disorder is high under conditions of sustained traumatization, such as in military combat or prisoner-of-war camps. It has also been reported in many individuals who endure near-death experiences.

Application of the Nursing Process

Background Assessment Data: Types of Somatic Symptom Disorders
Somatic Symptom Disorder

Somatic symptom disorder is a syndrome of multiple somatic symptoms that cannot be explained medically and are associated with psychosocial distress and frequent visits to health-care professionals to seek assistance. Symptoms may be vague, dramatized, or exaggerated in presentation, and an excessive amount of time and energy is devoted to worry and concern about the symptoms. Individuals with somatic symptom disorder are so convinced that their symptoms are related to organic pathology that they adamantly reject and are often irritated by any implication that stress or psychosocial factors play a role in their conditions.

One study (van den Houte et al., 2017 as cited by Dimsdale, 2017) found that participants who had difficulty identifying feelings (a component of the personality trait *alexithymia*, which is characterized by marked dysfunction in emotional awareness and social attachment) reported more somatic symptoms than healthy controls. Their findings suggested that alexithymia may be an important construct in the development of somatic symptom disorders. The disorder is chronic, with symptoms beginning before age 30. Anxiety and depression are frequent comorbidities, and consequently, there is an increased risk for suicide attempts (Yates, 2019).

Somatic symptom disorder usually runs a fluctuating course, with periods of remission and exacerbation. Patients often receive medical care from several physicians, sometimes concurrently, leading to the possibility of dangerous treatment combinations. They tend to seek relief through overmedicating with prescribed analgesics or antianxiety agents. Substance use disorders are common comorbidities with somatic symptom disorder. The *DSM-5-TR* diagnostic criteria for somatic symptom disorder are presented in Box 29–1.

Illness Anxiety Disorder

Illness anxiety disorder is defined as an unrealistic or inaccurate interpretation of physical symptoms or sensations, leading to a preoccupation with and fear of having a serious disease. The fear becomes disabling and persists despite appropriate reassurance that no organic pathology can be detected. Symptoms may be minimal or absent, but the individual is highly anxious about and suspicious of the presence of an undiagnosed, serious medical illness (APA, 2022).

Individuals with illness anxiety disorder are extremely conscious of bodily sensations and changes and may become convinced that a rapid heart rate indicates they have heart disease or that a small sore is skin cancer. They are profoundly preoccupied with their bodies and are keenly aware of even the slightest change in feeling or sensation. The response to these small changes, however, is usually unrealistic and exaggerated.

Some individuals with illness anxiety disorder have a long history of "doctor shopping" and are convinced that they are not receiving the proper medical care. Others avoid seeking medical assistance because to do so would increase their anxiety to intolerable levels.

BOX 29–1 Diagnostic Criteria for Somatic Symptom Disorder

A. One or more somatic symptoms that are distressing or result in significant disruption in daily life.

B. Excessive thoughts, feelings, or behaviors related to the somatic symptoms or associated health concerns as manifested by at least one of the following:
1. Disproportionate and persistent thoughts about the seriousness of one's symptoms.
2. Persistently high level of anxiety about health or symptoms.
3. Excessive time and energy devoted to these symptoms or health concerns.

C. Although any one symptom may not be continuously present, the state of being symptomatic is persistent (typically more than 6 months).

Specify if:

With predominant pain (the somatic symptoms predominantly involve pain)

Persistent (a persistent course is characterized by severe symptoms, marked impairment, and long duration [more than 6 months])

Specify current severity:

Mild (only one of the symptoms specified in Criterion B is fulfilled)

Moderate (two or more of the symptoms specified in Criterion B are fulfilled)

Severe (two or more of the symptoms specified in Criterion B are fulfilled, plus there are multiple somatic complaints [or one very severe somatic symptom])

Collaboration and ongoing communication with other clinicians are essential to "minimize inconsistent or conflicting messages and potentially reduce splitting" (Joshi, 2020, p. 54) in the care of patients with an illness anxiety disorder. Teamwork and collaboration form one of the six essential competencies identified by the Institute of Medicine (now the National Academy of Medicine) (2003) and adopted as a Quality and Safety Education for Nurses (QSEN) competency (QSEN Institute, 2020) for improving quality in healthcare education and practice.

Psychiatric comorbidities are common, including generalized anxiety disorder, depression, somatization disorder, and panic disorder; in addition, patients with illness anxiety disorder are three times more likely to have a concurrent personality disorder (Soreff, 2018). Preoccupation with the fear of serious disease may interfere with social or occupational functioning. Some individuals are able to function appropriately on the job, limiting their physical complaints to nonwork time.

Individuals with illness anxiety disorder are so apprehensive and fearful that they become alarmed at the slightest intimation of serious illness. Even reading about a disease or hearing that someone they know has been diagnosed with an illness precipitates alarm. Both somatic symptom disorder and illness anxiety disorder have similar features to what was previously called hypochondriasis, but the *DSM-5-TR* identifies two separate disorders to distinguish between individuals who are primarily preoccupied with perceived physical symptoms (somatic symptom disorder) and those who are primarily focused on fear of illness in general (illness anxiety disorder). The *DSM-5-TR* diagnostic criteria for illness anxiety disorder are presented in Box 29–2.

Functional Neurological Symptom Disorder (Conversion Disorder)

Functional neurological symptom disorder (previously called conversion disorder) is a loss of or change in body function that cannot be explained by any known medical disorder or pathophysiological mechanism. Although there is a psychological component involved in the initiation, exacerbation, or perpetuation of the symptom, it may or may not be obvious or easily identifiable.

Conversion symptoms affect voluntary motor or sensory functioning suggestive of neurological disease. Examples include paralysis, **aphonia** (inability to produce voice), seizures, coordination disturbance, difficulty swallowing, urinary retention, akinesia, blindness, deafness, double vision, **anosmia** (inability to perceive smell), loss of pain sensation, and hallucinations. Abnormal limb shaking with impaired or loss of consciousness that resembles epileptic seizures is another type of conversion disorder symptom, referred to as *psychogenic* or *nonepileptic seizures*. **Pseudocyesis** (false pregnancy) is a conversion symptom and may represent a strong desire to be pregnant.

The *DSM-5-TR* clarifies that although the diagnosis of functional neurological symptom disorder requires that the symptom is not explained by neurological disease, it should not be made simply because results from investigations are normal or because the symptom is "bizarre." "The diagnosis rests on clinical

---

BOX 29–2 Diagnostic Criteria for Illness Anxiety Disorder

A. Preoccupation with having or acquiring a serious illness.

B. Somatic symptoms are not present or, if present, are only mild in intensity. If another medical condition is present or there is a high risk for developing a medical condition (e.g., strong family history is present), the preoccupation is clearly excessive or disproportionate.

C. There is a high level of anxiety about health, and the individual is easily alarmed about personal health status.

D. The individual performs excessive health-related behaviors (e.g., repeatedly checks his or her body for signs of illness) or exhibits maladaptive avoidance (e.g., avoids doctors' appointments and hospitals).

E. Illness preoccupation has been present for at least 6 months, but the specific illness that is feared may change over that period of time.

F. The illness-related preoccupation is not better explained by another mental disorder, such as somatic symptom disorder, panic disorder, generalized anxiety disorder, body dysmorphic disorder, obsessive-compulsive disorder, or delusional disorder, somatic type.

Specify whether:

Care-seeking type: Medical care, including physician visits or undergoing tests and procedures, is frequently used.

Care-avoidant type: Medical care is rarely used.

Reprinted with permission from the *Diagnostic and Statistical Manual of Mental Disorders, Fifth Edition, Text Revision (DSM-5-TR)* (2022). American Psychiatric Association.

findings showing clear evidence of incompatibility with recognized neurological disease" (APA, 2022, p. 361). For example, if a patient appears to be having a seizure but the electroencephalogram (EEG) is normal, the eyes are closed and resist opening, and there is no urinary incontinence, functional neurological symptom disorder may be diagnosed. It is likely that multiple factors play a role in the etiology.

Although not diagnostic of a functional neurological symptom disorder, some people display an apparent indifference to symptoms that seem very serious to others; for example, an individual who finds themselves suddenly unable to walk but appears unconcerned about this dramatic change. This feature is coined *la belle indifference* (beautiful ignorance). Most symptoms of conversion disorder resolve within a few weeks. About 20% of individuals with the diagnosis have a relapse within 1 year. The *DSM-5-TR* states the prognosis is better when the symptoms are of short duration, when the client accepts the diagnosis, when comorbid physical disease is absent, and when there are no identified maladaptive personality traits (APA, 2022). The *DSM-5-TR* diagnostic criteria for conversion disorder are presented in Box 29–3.

Psychological Factors Affecting Other Medical Conditions

Psychological factors play a role in virtually all medical conditions. However, in this disorder, it is evident that psychological or behavioral factors are clearly implicated in the development, exacerbation, or delayed recovery from a medical condition.

Factitious Disorder

Factitious disorder involves conscious, intentional feigning of physical or psychological symptoms. Individuals with factitious disorder pretend to be ill to receive emotional care and support commonly associated with the role of "patient." Even though the behaviors are deliberate and intentional, there may be an associated compulsive element that diminishes personal control. Individuals with this disorder characteristically become so skilled at presenting their "symptoms" that they successfully gain admission to hospitals and treatment centers. To accomplish this, they may aggravate existing symptoms, induce new ones, or even inflict painful injuries on themselves. The disorder has also been identified as *Munchausen*

BOX 29–3 Diagnostic Criteria for Functional Neurological Symptom Disorder (Conversion Disorder)

A. One or more symptoms of altered voluntary motor or sensory function.
B. Clinical findings provide evidence of incompatibility between the symptom and recognized neurological or medical conditions.
C. The symptom or deficit is not better explained by another medical or mental disorder.
D. The symptom or deficit causes clinically significant distress or impairment in social, occupational, or other important areas of functioning or warrants medical evaluation.

Specify symptom type:

With weakness or paralysis
With abnormal movement (e.g., tremor, dystonia, myoclonus, gait disorder)
With swallowing symptoms
With speech symptom (e.g., dysphonia, slurred speech)
With attacks or seizures
With anesthesia or sensory loss
With special sensory symptom (e.g., visual, olfactory, or hearing disturbance)
With mixed symptoms

Specify if:

Acute episode: Symptoms present for less than 6 months.
Persistent: Symptoms occurring for 6 months or more.

Specify if:

With psychological stressor (specify stressor)
Without psychological stressor

syndrome, and feigned symptoms may be psychological, physical, or a combination of both.

Factitious disorder imposed on another (previously called *factitious disorder by proxy*) describes a condition in which physical or psychological symptoms are falsified or induced in another person. Diagnosis of factitious disorder can be difficult, as individuals become very inventive in their quest to produce symptoms. "The most common case of factitious disorder by proxy involves a mother who deceives medical personnel into believing her child is ill" (Boland & Verduin, 2022, p. 457). This may be accomplished by lying about the child's medical history, manipulating data such as by contaminating laboratory samples, and inducing illness or injury in their child through use of substances or other physical assaults.

Predisposing Factors Associated With Somatic Symptom and Related Disorders

Genetic

Escobar and Dimsdale (2017) reported that somatic symptom and related disorders should be conceptualized as a complex interaction of genetic vulnerabilities; history of trauma; learning; and environmental, psychological, and behavioral influences. Although the specific genetic vulnerabilities are not well understood, the authors reported that there is no evidence of familial aggregation in somatic symptom disorder.

Biochemical

Although biochemical factors of somatic symptom disorder are not clearly understood, decreased levels of serotonin and endorphins may play a role in the sensation of pain.

Neuroanatomical

Magnetic resonance imaging (MRI) studies of patients with a variety of somatoform disorders found that these patients had volume reductions in the hypothalamus, left fusiform gyrus, right cuneus, left inferior frontal gyrus, left posterior cingulate, and right amygdala (Delvecchio et al., 2019). The authors concluded that these findings suggest selective impairments in specific corticolimbic regions associated with two overlapping circuits, the neuromatrix of pain and the emotion regulation system.

Psychodynamic

Psychodynamic theorists view illness anxiety disorder (and factitious disorder) as an ego defense mechanism. Physical complaints are the expression of low self-esteem and feelings of worthlessness because it is easier to feel something is wrong with the body than to feel something is wrong with the self. Another psychodynamic view of illness anxiety disorder (as well as somatic symptom disorder, predominantly pain) is related to a defense against guilt. The individual views the self as "bad," based on real or imagined past misconduct, and considers physical suffering the deserved punishment required for atonement.

Another view suggests that individuals with factitious disorders were victims of child abuse or neglect. Frequent childhood hospitalizations provided a reprieve from the traumatic home situation and a loving and caring environment that was absent in the child's family. This theory proposes that the individual with factitious disorder is attempting to recapture the only positive support they may have known by seeking out the environment in which it was received as a child. Regarding factitious disorder imposed on another, Boland and Verduin (2022) have stated: "One apparent purpose of the behavior is for the caretaker to indirectly assume the sick role; another is to be relieved of the caretaking role by having the child hospitalized" (p. 457).

The psychodynamic theory of conversion disorder proposes that emotions associated with a traumatic event that the individual cannot express because of moral or ethical unacceptability are "converted" into physical symptoms. The unacceptable emotions are repressed and converted to a somatic symptom that is symbolic in some way of the original emotional trauma.

Escobar and Dimsdale (2017) reported that up to two-thirds of patients in primary care settings complain of symptoms for which no disease entity can be identified, and up to two-thirds of those patients meet criteria for a major psychiatric disorder. The authors suggested that this finding reinforces the belief that individuals with psychiatric disorders more typically present with physical rather than psychological complaints in primary care settings.

Family Dynamics

Another view suggests that in families who have difficulty resolving conflicts, a child's illness creates a shift in focus from the unresolved conflicts to the child's illness. This shift provides a reprieve from the instability posed by issues that the family cannot confront openly, and the child, in turn, receives positive reinforcement for the illness. **Somatization,** a focus on physical symptoms, becomes reinforced as a way to shift the focus away from family issues and discord. The stabilization of the family achieved by somatizing is referred to as a tertiary gain.

Learning Theory

Somatic complaints are often reinforced when the sick role relieves the individual from the need to deal with a stressful situation, whether it be within society or within the family. The sick person learns that there are emotional gains conferred by staying in the sick role. For example, they may be able to avoid stressful obligations, postpone unwelcome challenges, or be excused from troublesome duties (**primary gain**). They may become the prominent focus of attention because of the illness (**secondary gain**) or being in the sick role relieves conflict within the family as concern is shifted to the ill person and away from the real issue (**tertiary gain**). These types of positive reinforcement virtually guarantee repetition of the response.

Past experience with serious or life-threatening physical illness, either personal or that of close family members, can predispose an individual to illness anxiety disorder. Once an individual has experienced a threat to biological integrity, they may develop a fear of recurrence. As a result, the individual responds to minor physical changes in an exaggerated way, leading to excessive anxiety and health concerns.

Background Assessment Data for Dissociative Disorders

Dissociative Amnesia

CORE CONCEPT

Amnesia
Partial or total loss of memory. Memory loss may be temporary or permanent.

Amnesia may be caused by a host of medical conditions, including stroke, encephalitis, degenerative brain diseases (such as Alzheimer's disease), chronic alcohol abuse, brain tumors, seizures, and some medications. Dissociative amnesia stems from extreme emotional or physical trauma and is described in the *DM-5-TR* as an inability to recall important personal information, usually of a traumatic or stressful nature, that is too extensive to be explained by ordinary forgetfulness and is not due to the direct effects of substance use or a neurological or other medical condition (APA, 2022). The *DSM-5-TR* states that the most common types of dissociative amnesia are localized, selective, and generalized. Localized and selective amnesia are related to a specific stressful event. For example, the individual with **localized amnesia** is unable to recall all incidents associated with a stressful period. It may be broader than just a single event, such as the inability to remember months or years of child abuse (APA, 2022). In **selective amnesia,** the individual can recall only certain incidents associated with a stressful

event for a specific period after the event. In **generalized amnesia,** the individual has amnesia for both identity and total life history.

The individual with amnesia usually appears alert and may not indicate to observers that anything is wrong, although some people may present with alterations in consciousness, with conversion symptoms, or in trance states. Individuals with amnesia are often brought to general hospital emergency departments by police who have found them wandering confusedly around the streets.

The onset of an amnestic episode usually follows severe psychosocial stress. Termination is typically abrupt and followed by complete recovery. Recurrences are unusual. A specific subtype of dissociative amnesia is *with dissociative fugue.* Dissociative **fugue** is characterized by sudden, unexpected travel away from customary places or by bewildered wandering, with the inability to recall some or all of one's past. An individual in a fugue state may not be able to recall personal identity and sometimes assumes a new identity.

The *DSM-5-TR* diagnostic criteria for dissociative amnesia are presented in Box 29–4.

Dissociative Identity Disorder

DID was formerly called *multiple personality disorder* and is characterized by the existence of two or more personality states in a single individual. These different personality states are sometimes referred to as *alter identities* or just *alters.* Only one of the personalities is evident at any given moment, and one of them is dominant most of the time over the course of the disorder. Each personality is unique and composed of a complex set of memories, behavior patterns, and social relationships that surface at different times. Transition from one personality state to another may be sudden or gradual and is sometimes quite dramatic. Boland and Verduin (2022) stated: "Patients often describe a profound sense of concretized internal division or personified internal conflicts between parts of themselves … these parts may have proper names or be designated by their predominant affect or function, for example, 'the angry one' or 'the wife'" (p. 443).

DID has been a controversial disorder since it gained attention after the 1976 movie *Sybil,* which portrayed the presumed true story of a woman who reported having 16 different personalities. Diagnosis of DID increased significantly in the years after the movie, and in 1980 the APA formally recognized the disorder as a psychiatric illness (Haberman, 2014). Since then, critics have reported that both the patient "Sybil" and her psychiatrist acknowledged her case as fabrication. Dr. David Speigel, a psychiatrist who was

---

BOX 29–4 Diagnostic Criteria for Dissociative Amnesia

A. An inability to recall important autobiographical information, usually of a traumatic or stressful nature, that is inconsistent with ordinary forgetting. *Note:* Dissociative amnesia most often consists of localized or selective amnesia for a specific event or events; or generalized amnesia for identity and life history.
B. The symptoms cause clinically significant distress or impairment in social, occupational, or other important areas of functioning.
C. The disturbance is not attributable to the physiological effects of a substance (e.g., alcohol or other drug of abuse, a medication) or a neurological or other medical condition (e.g., partial complex seizures, transient global amnesia, sequelae of a closed head injury/traumatic brain injury, other neurological condition).
D. The disturbance is not better explained by dissociative identity disorder, post-traumatic stress disorder, acute stress disorder, somatic symptom disorder, or major or mild neurocognitive disorder.

Specify if:

With dissociative fugue (apparently purposeful travel or bewildered wandering that is associated with amnesia for identity or for other important autobiographical information)

Reprinted with permission from the *Diagnostic and Statistical Manual of Mental Disorders, Fifth Edition, Text Revision (DSM-5-TR)* (2022). American Psychiatric Association.

---

involved in promoting the APA's adoption of DID as the preferred term for this condition, is quoted in Haberman's review (2014) as saying "[the term] multiple personality carries with it the implication that they really have more than one personality. The problem is fragmentation of identity, not that you really are 12 people … that you have not more than one but less than one personality."

Although questions persist about whether this disorder has been over-diagnosed, there are certainly individuals who present with fragmented identity. Most have been victims of severe childhood physical and sexual abuse. It is not uncommon for patients with DID to also manifest with symptoms of other dissociative disorders such as amnesia, fugue states, depersonalization, and derealization (Boland & Verduin, 2022). Generally, there is amnesia for the events that took place when another personality was being manifested, and patients report "gaps" in autobiographical histories, "lost time," or "blackouts." They may "wake up" in unfamiliar situations with no idea where they are, how they got there, or the identities of the people around them. They may be accused of lying when they deny remembering or being responsible for events or actions.

DID is not always incapacitating. Some individuals with DID maintain responsible positions, complete graduate degrees, and are successful spouses and parents before diagnosis and while in treatment. Before they are diagnosed with DID, many individuals are misdiagnosed with depression, borderline and antisocial personality disorders, schizophrenia, epilepsy, or bipolar disorder. The *DSM-5-TR* diagnostic criteria for DID are presented in Box 29–5.

BOX 29–5 Diagnostic Criteria for Dissociative Identity Disorder

A. Disruption of identity characterized by two or more distinct personality states, which may be described in some cultures as an experience of possession. The disruption in identity involves marked discontinuity in sense of self and sense of agency, accompanied by related alterations in affect, behavior, consciousness, memory, perception, cognition, and/or sensory-motor functioning. These signs and symptoms may be observed by others or reported by the individual.
B. Recurrent gaps in the recall of everyday events, important personal information, and/or traumatic events that are inconsistent with ordinary forgetting.
C. The symptoms cause clinically significant distress or impairment in social, occupational, or other important areas of functioning.
D. The disturbance is not a normal part of a broadly accepted cultural or religious practice. *Note:* In children, the symptoms are not better explained by imaginary playmates or other fantasy play.
E. The symptoms are not attributable to the physiological effects of a substance (e.g., blackouts or chaotic behavior during alcohol intoxication) or another medical condition (e.g., complex partial seizures).

Reprinted with permission from the *Diagnostic and Statistical Manual of Mental Disorders, Fifth Edition, Text Revision (DSM-5-TR)* (2022). American Psychiatric Association.

Depersonalization-Derealization Disorder

Depersonalization-derealization disorder is characterized by a temporary change in the quality of self-awareness, which often takes the form of feelings of unreality, changes in body image, feelings of detachment from the environment, or a sense of observing oneself from outside the body. For example, a soldier in recalling an experience in combat describes observing himself from a distance and wondering what he would do if he were in that situation. **Depersonalization** (a disturbance in the perception of oneself) is differentiated from **derealization**, which describes an alteration in the perception of the external environment. Both of these phenomena also occur in a variety of psychiatric illnesses such as schizophrenia, depression, anxiety states, and neurocognitive disorders. As previously stated, the symptoms of depersonalization and derealization are very common. It is estimated that approximately 50% of all adults have experienced transient episodes of these symptoms. They are also identified as the third most common reported psychiatric symptoms after depression and anxiety (Boland & Verduin, 2022). Diagnosis of the disorder is only made if the symptoms cause significant distress or impairment in functioning.

The *DSM-5-TR* describes this disorder as persistent or recurrent episodes of depersonalization, derealization, or both (APA, 2022). There may be a mechanical or dreamlike feeling or a belief that the body's physical characteristics have changed. If derealization is present, objects in the environment are perceived as altered in size or shape. Other people in the environment may seem automated or mechanical.

These distorted perceptions are experienced as disturbing and often accompanied by anxiety, depression, fear of going insane, obsessive thoughts, somatic complaints, and an alteration in the subjective sense of time.

The *DSM 5-TR-* diagnostic criteria for depersonalization-derealization disorder are presented in Box 29–6.

Predisposing Factors Associated With Dissociative Disorders

Genetics

The overwhelming majority of adults with DID (85% to 97%) have a history of physical and sexual abuse, and although genetic factors may illuminate the interaction of the individual with environmental stress, current research does not show evidence of a significant genetic contribution (Sar et al., 2017).

Neurobiological

Sar and associates (2017) reported that there are both structural and functional neuroimaging findings that demonstrate differences between patients with DID and nonclinical populations. Areas of the brain that have been associated with memory include the hippocampus, amygdala, fornix, mammillary bodies, thalamus, and frontal cortex. One study found that hippocampal volume was significantly smaller in individuals with DID and it was correlated to a higher severity of childhood trauma and dissociative symptoms (Chalavi et al., 2015).

Various studies have implicated the N-methyl-D-aspartate (NMDA) glutamate receptor, neuropeptide Y, norepinephrine, serotonin, and the opioid system in depersonalization (Boland & Verduin, 2022). Dissociative experiences have been reported in patients with temporal lobe epilepsy and severe migraine headaches (Özdemir et al., 2016). EEG abnormalities have been observed in some people with DID.

BOX 29–6 Diagnostic Criteria for Depersonalization-Derealization Disorder

A. The presence of persistent or recurrent depersonalization, derealization, or both:
  1. Depersonalization: Experiences of unreality, detachment, or being an outside observer with respect to one's thoughts, feelings, sensations, body, or actions (e.g., perceptual alterations, distorted sense of time, unreal or absent self, emotional and/or physical numbing).
  2. Derealization: Experiences of unreality or detachment with respect to surroundings (e.g., individuals or objects are experienced as unreal, dreamlike, foggy, lifeless, or visually distorted).
B. During the depersonalization or derealization experiences, reality testing remains intact.
C. The symptoms cause clinically significant distress or impairment in social, occupational, or other important areas of functioning.
D. The disturbance is not attributable to the physiological effects of a substance (e.g., a drug of abuse, medication) or another medical condition (e.g., seizures).
E. The disturbance is not better explained by another mental disorder, such as schizophrenia, panic disorder, major depressive disorder, acute stress disorder, post-traumatic stress disorder, or another dissociative disorder.

Reprinted with permission from the *Diagnostic and Statistical Manual of Mental Disorders, Fifth Edition, Text Revision (DSM-5-TR)* (2022). American Psychiatric Association.

Psychodynamic Theory

Freud (1962) believed that dissociative behaviors occurred when individuals repressed distressing mental contents from conscious awareness. He believed that the unconscious was a dynamic entity in which repressed mental contents were stored and unavailable to conscious recall. Current psychodynamic explanations of dissociation are based on Freud's concepts. The repression of mental contents is believed to protect the individual from extreme emotional pain triggered by either disturbing external circumstances or anxiety-provoking internal urges and feelings. In the case of depersonalization and derealization, the pain and anxiety are expressed as feelings of unreality or detachment from the environment of the painful situation.

Psychological Trauma

Several studies support the etiology of dissociative disorders as a response to traumatic experiences that overwhelm the individual's capacity to cope by any means other than dissociation (Irwin, 1999; Muller, 2014; Chalavi et al., 2015). In DID, these experiences are most often physical, sexual, or psychological abuse by a parent or significant other in the child's life. The most widely accepted explanation for DID is that it begins as a survival strategy to help children cope with severe sexual, physical, or psychological abuse and evolves into a fragmented identity as the victim struggles to integrate conflicting aspects of personality into a cohesive whole. Dissociative amnesia is frequently related to acute and extreme trauma but may also develop in the clinical presentation of DID. Dissociative amnesia is also often noted in response to combat trauma during wartime.

Transactional Model of Stress and Adaptation

The etiology of dissociative disorders is likely influenced by multiple factors. In Figure 29–1, a graphic depiction of this theory of multiple causation is presented in the transactional model of stress and adaptation.

Diagnosis and Outcome Identification

Nursing diagnoses are formulated from the data gathered during the assessment phase and with background knowledge regarding predisposing factors to the disorder. Table 29–1 presents a list of patient behaviors and the NANDA-I nursing diagnoses (Herdman et al., 2021) that correspond to those behaviors, which may be used in planning care for patients with somatic symptom and dissociative disorders.

Outcome Criteria

The following criteria may be used for measurement of outcomes in the care of the patient with somatic symptom and dissociative disorders.

The patient:

■ Effectively uses adaptive coping strategies during stressful situations without resorting to physical symptoms (*somatic symptom disorder*)
■ Interprets bodily sensations rationally, verbalizes understanding of the significance of the irrational fear, and has decreased the number and frequency of physical complaints (*illness anxiety disorder and somatic symptom disorder*)
■ Is free of physical disability and is able to verbalize understanding of the possible correlation between the loss of or alteration in function and extreme emotional stress (*conversion disorder*)
■ Can recall events associated with a traumatic or stressful situation (*dissociative amnesia*)
■ Can verbalize the extreme anxiety that precipitated the dissociation (*depersonalization-derealization disorder*)
■ Can demonstrate adaptive coping strategies to avert dissociative behaviors in the face of severe anxiety (*depersonalization-derealization disorder*)
■ Verbalizes understanding of the existence of multiple personality states and the purposes they serve (*DID*)
■ Is able to maintain a sense of reality during stressful situations (*depersonalization-derealization disorder*)

Planning and Implementation

The following section presents a group of selected nursing diagnoses, with short- and long-term goals and nursing interventions for each. Rationales for nursing interventions are italicized. Trauma-informed care should be a foundation for all interventions for this population.

Ineffective Coping

Ineffective coping is defined as "a pattern of invalid appraisal of the stressors, with cognitive and/or behavioral responses that fails to manage demands related to well-being" (Herdman et al., 2021, p. 408). This nursing diagnosis may be relevant to any somatic symptom and related disorders as well as to patients with dissociative disorders.

Patient Goals

Outcome criteria include short- and long-term goals. Timelines are individually determined.

Short-term goal

■ Within (specified time), the patient will verbalize understanding of the correlation between physical symptoms and psychological problems.

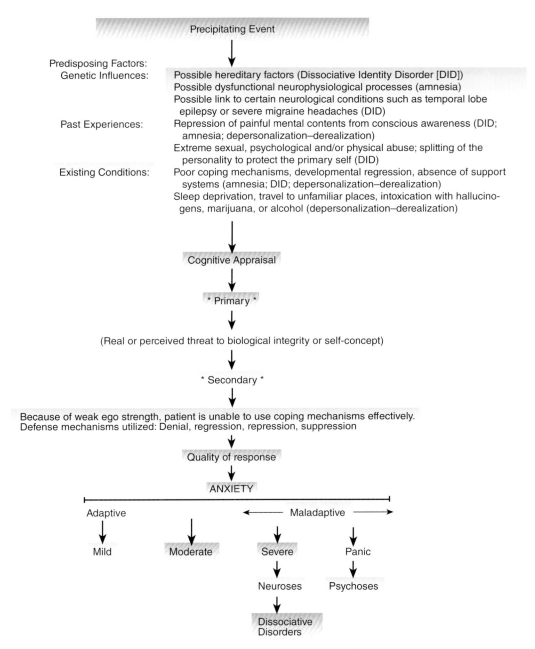

FIGURE 29–1   The dynamics of a dissociative using the transactional model of stress and adaptation.

Long-term goal

■ By time of discharge from treatment, the patient will demonstrate the ability to cope with stress by means other than preoccupation with physical symptoms.

Interventions

■ Monitor the physician's ongoing assessments, laboratory reports, and other data to maintain assurance that the possibility of organic pathology is clearly ruled out. Review findings with the patient. *Accurate medical assessment is vital for the provision of adequate and appropriate care. Honest explanation may help the patient understand the psychological implications.*

■ Recognize and accept that the physical complaint is real to the patient even though no organic etiology can be identified. *Denial of the patient's feelings is nontherapeutic and interferes with establishment of a trusting relationship.*

■ Provide pain medication as prescribed by physician. *Patient comfort and safety are nursing priorities.*

■ Identify gains that the physical symptoms are providing for the patient: increased dependency,

TABLE 29–1	Assigning Nursing Diagnoses to Behaviors Commonly Associated With Somatic Symptom and Dissociative Disorders	
BEHAVIORS	**NURSING DIAGNOSES**
Verbalization of numerous physical complaints in the absence of any pathophysiological evidence; focus on the self and physical symptoms *(somatic symptom disorder)*	Ineffective coping; chronic pain
History of "doctor shopping" for evidence of organic pathology to substantiate physical symptoms; statements such as, "I don't know why the doctor put me on the psychiatric unit. I have a physical problem" *(somatic symptom disorder)*	Deficient knowledge (psychological causes for physical symptoms)
Preoccupation with and unrealistic interpretation of bodily signs and sensations *(illness anxiety disorder)*	Fear (of having a serious disease)
Loss or alteration in physical functioning without evidence of organic pathology *(conversion disorder)*	Disturbed sensory perception*
Alteration in the perception or experience of the self or the environment *(depersonalization/derealization disorder)*	Self-care deficit
Need for assistance to carry out self-care activities such as eating, dressing, maintaining hygiene, and toileting due to alteration in physical functioning *(conversion disorder)*	Deficient knowledge (psychological factors affecting medical condition)
History of numerous exacerbations of physical illness; inappropriate or exaggerated behaviors; denial of emotional problems *(psychological factors affecting other medical conditions)*	Denial
Loss of memory *(dissociative amnesia)*	Impaired memory
Verbalizations of frustration over lack of control and dependence on others *(dissociative amnesia)*	Powerlessness
Unresolved grief; depression; self-blame associated with childhood abuse *(dissociative identity disorder [DID])*	Risk for suicidal behavior
Presence of more than one personality within the individual *(DID)*	Disturbed personality identity
Feigning of physical or psychological symptoms to gain attention *(factitious disorder)*	Ineffective coping

*This diagnosis has been resigned from the NANDA-I list of approved diagnoses. It is used in this instance because it is most compatible with the identified behaviors.

attention, and distraction from other problems. *Identification of underlying motivation is important in assisting the patient with problem resolution.*

■ Initially, fulfill the patient's most urgent dependency needs, but gradually withdraw attention to physical symptoms. Minimize time given in response to physical complaints. *Anxiety and maladaptive behaviors will increase if dependency needs are ignored initially. Gradual withdrawal of positive reinforcement will discourage repetition of maladaptive behaviors.*

■ Explain to the patient that any new physical complaints will be referred to the physician and give no further attention to them. Follow up on the physician's assessment of the complaint. The possibility of organic pathology must always be considered. Failure to do so could jeopardize patient safety.

■ Encourage the patient to verbalize fears and anxieties. Explain that attention will be withdrawn if rumination about physical complaints begins and follow through with this intention. *Without consistency of limit setting, change is unlikely.*

■ Help the patient recognize that physical symptoms often occur because of, or are exacerbated by, specific stressors. Discuss alternative coping strategies that patient may use in response to stress (e.g., relaxation exercises, physical activities, assertiveness skills). *The patient may need help with problem-solving.* Give positive reinforcement for adaptive coping strategies.

■ Have the patient keep a diary of appearance, duration, and intensity of physical symptoms. A separate record of situations that the patient finds especially stressful should also be kept. *Comparison of these records may provide objective data from which to observe the relationship between physical symptoms and stress.*

■ Help the patient identify ways to achieve recognition from others without resorting to physical symptoms. *Positive recognition from others enhances self-esteem and minimizes the need for attention through maladaptive behaviors.*

■ Provide instruction in relaxation techniques and assertiveness skills. *These approaches decrease anxiety and increase self-esteem, which facilitate adaptive responses to stressful situations.*

Fear (of Having a Serious Disease)

Fear is defined as the "Basic, intense emotional response aroused by the detection of imminent threat, involving an immediate alarm reaction (American Psychological Association)" (Herdman et al., 2021, p. 419). This nursing diagnosis is particularly relevant to patients with illness anxiety disorder but may pertain also to patients with somatic symptom disorder and some dissociative disorders.

Patient Goals

Outcome criteria include short- and long-term goals. Timelines are individually determined.

Short-term goal

■ Patient will verbalize that fears associated with bodily sensations are irrational (within time limit deemed appropriate for specific individual).

Long-term goal

■ Patient interprets bodily sensations correctly.

Interventions

■ Monitor the physician's ongoing assessments and laboratory reports. *Organic pathology must be clearly ruled out.*

■ Refer all new physical complaints to the physician. *To ignore all physical complaints could place the patient's safety in jeopardy.*

■ Assess the function the patient's illness is fulfilling for them (e.g., unfulfilled needs for dependency, nurturing, caring, attention, or control). *This information may provide insight into reasons for maladaptive behavior and provide direction for planning patient care.*

■ Identify times during which the preoccupation with physical symptoms worsens. Determine the extent of correlation of physical complaints with times of increased anxiety. *The patient may be unaware of the psychosocial implications of the physical complaints. Knowledge of the relationship is the first step in the process of creating change.*

■ Convey empathy. Let the patient know that you understand how a specific symptom may conjure up fears of previous life-threatening illness. *Unconditional acceptance and empathy promote a therapeutic nurse–patient relationship.*

■ Initially allow the patient a limited amount of time (e.g., 10 minutes each hour) to discuss physical symptoms. *Because preoccupation with physical symptoms has been their primary method of coping, complete prohibition of this activity would likely raise the patient's anxiety level significantly, further exacerbating the behavior.*

■ Help the patient determine what techniques may be most useful for them to implement when fear and anxiety are exacerbated (e.g., relaxation techniques, mental imagery, thought-stopping techniques, physical exercise). *All of these techniques are effective in reducing anxiety and may assist the patient in the transition from focusing on fear of physical illness to the discussion of honest feelings.*

■ Gradually increase the limit on the amount of time spent each hour in discussing physical symptoms. If the patient violates the limits, withdraw attention. *Lack of positive reinforcement may help to extinguish the maladaptive behavior.*

■ Encourage the patient to discuss *feelings* associated with fear of serious illness. Verbalization of feelings in a nonthreatening environment facilitates expression and resolution of disturbing emotional issues. *When the patient can express feelings directly, there is less need to express them through physical symptoms.*

■ Role-play the patient's plan for dealing with the fear the next time it assumes control and before anxiety becomes disabling. *Anxiety and fears are minimized when the patient has achieved a degree of comfort through practicing a plan for dealing with stressful situations in the future.*

Disturbed Sensory Perception

Disturbed sensory perception, no longer identified as a NANDA-I diagnosis, is retained here and may be defined as an impaired or exaggerated sensory perception. This may include an exaggerated sensation of pain, impairment of function or mobility without medical basis, other somatic sensations, and distorted perception of the self (depersonalization) or distorted perception of the environment (derealization). The nursing diagnosis of disturbed sensory perception is relevant to patients with somatic symptom disorders, conversion disorder symptoms, and depersonalization derealization disorder. Table 29–2 presents this nursing diagnosis in care plan format.

Patient Goals

Outcome criteria include short- and long-term goals. Timelines are individually determined.

Table 29–2 | CARE PLAN FOR THE PATIENT WITH A FUNCTIONAL NEUROLOGICAL SYMPTOM DISORDER (CONVERSION DISORDER)

NURSING DIAGNOSIS: DISTURBED SENSORY PERCEPTION
RELATED TO: Repressed severe anxiety
EVIDENCED BY: Loss or alteration in physical functioning, without evidence of organic pathology

OUTCOME CRITERIA	NURSING INTERVENTIONS	RATIONALE
Short-Term Goal ■ Patient will verbalize understanding of emotional problems as a contributing factor to the alteration in physical functioning (within time limit appropriate for specific individual). **Long-Term Goal** ■ Patient will demonstrate recovery of lost or altered function.	1. Monitor physician's ongoing assessments, laboratory reports, and other data to ensure that possibility of organic pathology is clearly ruled out.	1. Failure to do so may jeopardize patient safety.
	2. Identify primary or secondary gains that the physical symptom may be providing for the patient (e.g., increased dependency, attention, protection from experiencing a stressful event).	2. Primary and secondary gains are often etiological factors and may be used to assist in problem resolution.
	3. Do not focus on the disability and encourage the patient to be as independent as possible. Intervene only when the patient requires assistance.	3. Positive reinforcement would encourage continual use of the maladaptive response for secondary gains, such as dependency.
	4. Maintain nonjudgmental attitude when providing assistance to the patient. The physical symptom is not within the patient's conscious control and is very real to them.	4. A judgmental attitude interferes with the nurse's ability to provide therapeutic care for the patient.
	5. Do not reinforce the patient's attempts to use the disability as a manipulative tool to avoid participation in therapeutic activities. Withdraw attention if the patient continues to focus on physical limitation.	5. Lack of reinforcement may help to extinguish the maladaptive response.
	6. Encourage the patient to verbalize fears and anxieties. Help identify physical symptoms as a coping mechanism that is used in times of extreme stress.	6. Patients with conversion disorder are usually unaware of the psychological implications of their illness.
	7. Help the patient identify coping mechanisms that they could use when faced with stressful situations rather than retreating from reality with a physical disability.	7. Patients need assistance with problem-solving at this severe level of anxiety.
	8. Give positive reinforcement for identification or demonstration of alternative, more adaptive coping strategies.	8. Positive reinforcement enhances self-esteem and encourages repetition of desirable behaviors.

Short-term goal

■ The patient will verbalize understanding of emotional problems as a contributing factor to the alteration in sensory perceptions (within time limit appropriate for specific individual).

Long-term goal

■ The patient will demonstrate recovery of lost or altered function.

Interventions

■ Monitor the physician's ongoing assessments, laboratory reports, and other data to ensure that the possibility of organic pathology is clearly ruled out. *Failure to do so may jeopardize the patient's safety.*

■ Identify primary or secondary gains that the physical symptom is providing for the patient (e.g., increased dependency, attention, protection from experiencing a stressful event). *These are considered to be etiological factors and may be used to assist in problem resolution.*

■ Do not focus on the disability and encourage the patient to be as independent as possible. Intervene only when the patient requires assistance. *Positive reinforcement encourages continued use of the maladaptive response for secondary gains, such as dependency.*

■ Maintain a nonjudgmental attitude when providing assistance with self-care activities to the patient. *The physical symptom is not within the patient's conscious control and is very real to them.*

■ Do not reinforce the patient's use of the disability as a manipulative tool to avoid participating in therapeutic activities. Withdraw attention if the patient continues to focus on the physical limitation. *Lack of reinforcement may help to extinguish the maladaptive response.*

■ Encourage the patient to verbalize fears and anxieties. Help identify physical symptoms as a coping mechanism that is used in times of extreme stress. *Patients with conversion disorder are usually unaware of the psychological implications of their illness.*

■ Help the patient identify coping mechanisms that they could use when faced with stressful situations rather than retreating from reality with a physical disability. *The patient needs assistance with problem-solving at this severe level of anxiety.*

■ Give positive reinforcement for identification or demonstration of alternative, more adaptive coping strategies.

■ Discuss ways the patient may more adaptively respond to stress and use role-play to practice using these new methods. *Having practiced through role-play helps to prepare the patient to face stressful situations by using these new behaviors when they occur in real life.*

■ For patients experiencing depersonalization, also use the following interventions:
  ■ Provide support and encouragement during times of depersonalization. Patients manifesting these symptoms may express fear and anxiety. They do not understand the response and may express a fear of going insane. *Support and encouragement from a trusted individual provide a feeling of security when fears and anxieties are manifested.*

■ Explain the depersonalization behaviors and the purpose they usually serve for the patient. This knowledge may help to minimize fears and anxieties associated with their occurrence. Help relate these behaviors to times of severe psychological stress that the patient has experienced. *The patient may be unaware that the occurrence of depersonalization behaviors is related to severe anxiety. Knowledge of this relationship is the first step in the process of behavioral change.*

Deficient Knowledge (Psychological Factors Affecting Medical Condition)

Deficient knowledge is defined as "absence of cognitive information related to a specific topic or its acquisition" (Herdman et al., 2021, p. 331). This nursing diagnosis may be relevant to patients with any somatic or related disorder as well as to patients with dissociative disorders.

Patient Goals

Outcome criteria include short- and long-term goals. Timelines are individually determined.

Short-term goal

■ Patient will cooperate with plan for teaching provided by primary nurse.

Long-term goal

■ By time of discharge from treatment, patient will be able to verbalize psychological factors affecting their physical condition.

Interventions

■ Assess the patient's level of knowledge regarding the effects of psychological problems on the body. *An adequate database is necessary for the development of an effective teaching plan.*

■ Assess the patient's level of anxiety and readiness to learn. *Learning is inhibited beyond the moderate level of anxiety.*

■ Discuss results of physical examinations and laboratory tests. Explain the purpose and results of each. *Fear of the unknown may contribute to an elevated level of anxiety. The patient has the right to know about and accept or refuse any medical treatment.*

■ Explore the patient's feelings and fears as the patient demonstrates readiness. Go slowly. These feelings may have been suppressed or repressed for so long that their disclosure may be a very painful experience. Be supportive. *Expression of feelings in the presence of a trusted individual and in a nonthreatening environment may encourage the individual to confront unresolved issues.*

■ Have the patient keep a diary of appearance, duration, and intensity of physical symptoms. A separate record of situations the patient finds especially stressful should also be kept. *Comparison of these records may provide objective data from which to observe the relationship between physical symptoms and stress.*

■ Help the patient identify needs that are being met through the sick role. Together, formulate more adaptive means for fulfilling these needs. Practice by role-playing. *Repetition through practice serves to reduce discomfort in the actual situation.*

■ Provide instruction in assertiveness techniques, especially the ability to recognize the differences among passive, assertive, and aggressive behaviors and the importance of respecting the rights of others while protecting one's own basic rights. *These skills promote preservation of the patient's self-esteem while also improving their ability to form satisfactory interpersonal relationships.*

■ Discuss adaptive methods of stress management, such as relaxation techniques, physical exercise, meditation, and breathing exercises. *Use of these adaptive techniques may decrease appearance of physical symptoms in response to stress.*

Impaired Memory

Impaired memory is defined as a "persistent inability to remember or recall bits of information or skills while maintaining the capacity to independently perform activities of daily living" (Herdman et al., 2021, p. 333). This nursing diagnosis is particularly relevant in patients with dissociative disorders such as dissociative amnesia.

Patient Goals

Outcome criteria include short- and long-term goals. Timelines are individually determined.

Short-term goal

■ The patient will verbalize understanding that the loss of memory is related to a stressful situation and begin discussing the stressful situation with nurse or therapist.

Long-term goal

■ The patient will recover deficits in memory and develop more adaptive coping mechanisms to deal with stressful situations.

Interventions

■ Obtain as much information as possible about the patient from family and significant others if possible. Consider likes, dislikes, important people, activities, music, and pets. *A comprehensive baseline assessment is necessary for the development of an effective plan of care.*

■ Do not confront the patient with information they do not appear to remember. *Individuals who are exposed to painful information from which the amnesia is providing protection may decompensate even further into a psychotic state.*

■ Instead, expose the patient to stimuli that represent pleasant experiences from the past, such as smells associated with enjoyable activities, beloved pets, and music the patient enjoys. As memory begins to return, engage the patient in activities that may provide additional stimulation. *Recall often occurs during activities that simulate life experiences.*

■ Listen empathically when the patient discusses situations that have been especially stressful and explore the feelings associated with those times. *Verbalization of feelings in a nonthreatening environment may help the patient come to terms with unresolved issues that may be contributing to the dissociative process.*

■ Identify specific conflicts that remain unresolved and help the patient identify possible solutions. Provide instruction regarding more adaptive ways to respond to anxiety. *Unless these underlying conflicts are resolved, any improvement in coping behaviors must be viewed as temporary.*

■ Provide positive feedback for decisions made. Respect the patient's right to make those decisions independently and refrain from attempting to influence them toward those that may seem more logical. *Independent choice provides a feeling of control, decreases feelings of powerlessness, and increases self-esteem.*

Disturbed Personal Identity

Disturbed personal identity is defined as the "inability to maintain an integrated and complete perception of self" (Herdman et al., 2021, p. 345). This nursing diagnosis is particularly relevant for the patient with DID.

Patient Goals

Outcome criteria include short- and long-term goals. Timelines are individually determined.

Short-term goals

■ The patient will verbalize understanding about the existence of multiple personality states within the self.

■ The patient will be able to recognize stressful situations that precipitate transition from one personality to another.

Long-term goals

■ The patient will verbalize understanding of the reasons for fragmented identity.
■ The patient will enter into and cooperate with long-term therapy, with the ultimate goal of integration into one personality.

Interventions

■ The nurse must develop a trusting relationship with the patient. Trust is the basis of a therapeutic relationship. Listen nonjudgmentally when the patient transitions from one personality state to another. Help the patient understand the existence of the subpersonalities and the need each serves in the personal identity of the individual. The patient may initially be unaware of the dissociative response. *Knowledge of the needs each personality fulfills is the first step in the integration process and the patient's ability to face unresolved issues without dissociation.*
■ Help the patient identify stressful situations that precipitate transition from one personality to another. Carefully observe and record these transitions. *Identification of stressors is required to assist the patient in responding more adaptively and eliminate the need for transition to another personality.*
■ Use nursing interventions necessary to deal with maladaptive behaviors associated with individual subpersonalities. For example, if one personality is suicidal, precautions must be taken to guard against the patient's self-harm. If another personality displays physical hostility, precautions must be taken to protect others.

> **CLINICAL PEARL** It may be possible to seek assistance from one of the subpersonalities. For example, a strong-willed personality may help to control the behaviors of a suicidal personality. "Helping the identities to be aware of one another as legitimate parts of the self and to negotiate and resolve their conflicts is at the very core of the therapeutic process" (International Society for the Study of Trauma and Dissociation, 2011, p. 132).

■ Help subpersonalities understand that their "being" will not be destroyed, but rather integrated into a unified identity within the individual. *Because the subpersonalities function as separate entities, the idea of total elimination generates fear and defensiveness.*
■ Provide support during disclosure of painful experiences and reassurance when the patient becomes discouraged with lengthy treatment.

Concept Care Mapping

The concept map care plan (see Chapter 8, "The Nursing Process in Psychiatric-Mental Health Nursing") is a diagrammatic teaching and learning strategy that allows visualization of interrelationships between medical diagnoses, nursing diagnoses, assessment data, and treatments. Examples of concept map care plans for patients with somatic symptom and dissociative disorders are presented in Figures 29–2 and 29–3.

Patient and Family Education

The role of patient teacher is important in the psychiatric area, as it is in all areas of nursing. For patients with dissociative disorders, the patient and family need to be educated about various treatment options that are focused on trauma treatment. Family therapy may be recommended and is often crucial for long-term stabilization (Boland & Verduin, 2022). For patients with somatic symptom disorders, it is important to educate about the benefits of cognitive behavior therapy (CBT), but Boland and Verduin (2022) noted that patients may respond better to recommendations for exercise, yoga, meditation, and massage because some people may not be open to psychological explanations for their symptoms.

Evaluation

Reassessment is conducted to determine whether the nursing actions have been successful in achieving the objectives of care. Evaluation of the nursing actions for the patient with a somatic symptom disorder may be facilitated by gathering information using the following types of questions:

Does the patient:

■ Recognize signs and symptoms of escalating anxiety?
■ Intervene with adaptive coping strategies to interrupt the escalating anxiety before physical symptoms are exacerbated?
■ Verbalize an understanding of the correlation between physical symptoms and times of escalating anxiety?
■ Identify a plan for dealing with increased stress to prevent exacerbation of physical symptoms?
■ Demonstrate a decrease in ruminations about physical symptoms?
■ Express that fears of serious illness have diminished?
■ Demonstrate full recovery from previous loss or alteration of physical functioning?

Evaluation of the nursing actions for the patient with a dissociative disorder may be facilitated by gathering information using the following types of questions:

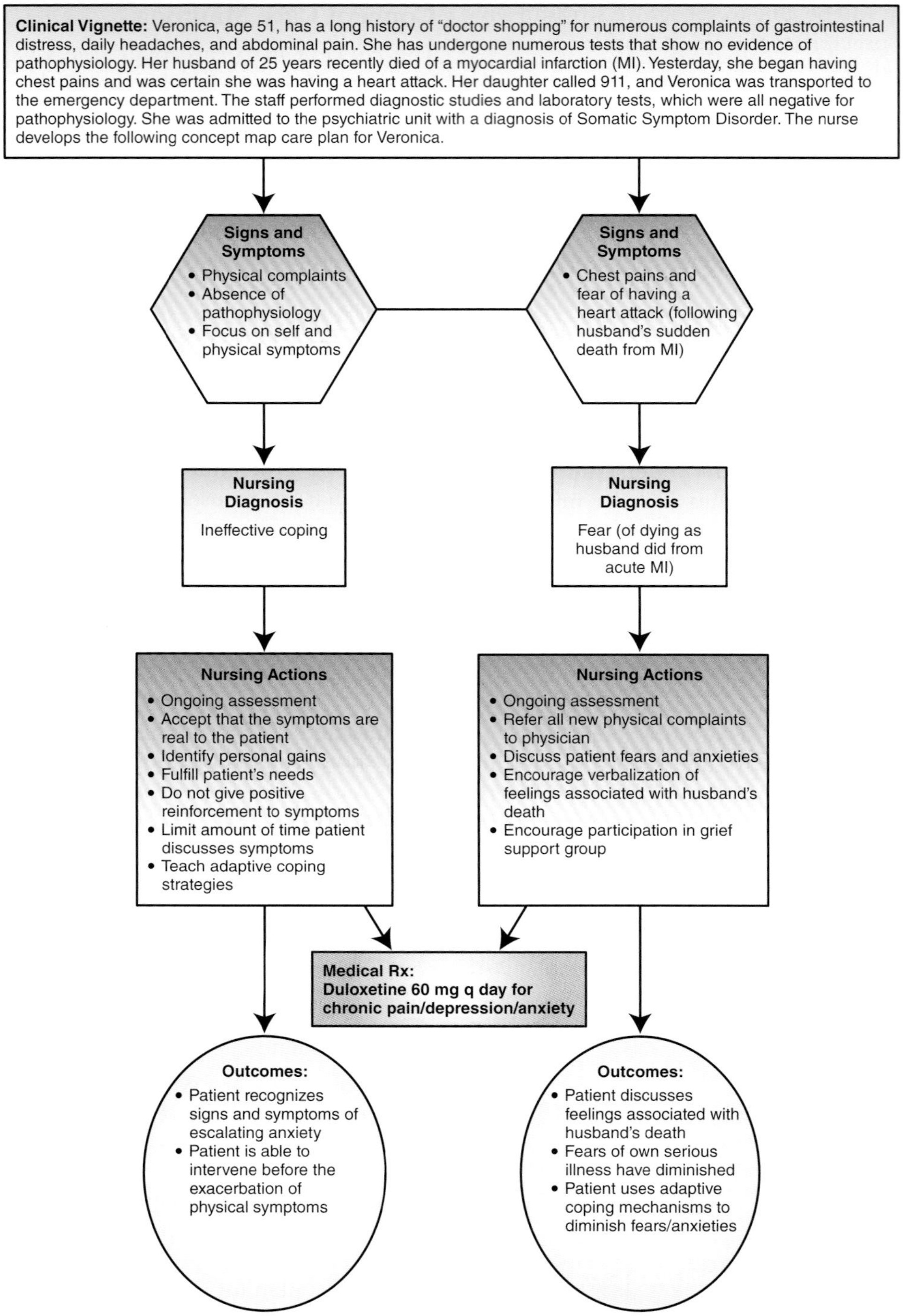

Clinical Vignette: Veronica, age 51, has a long history of "doctor shopping" for numerous complaints of gastrointestinal distress, daily headaches, and abdominal pain. She has undergone numerous tests that show no evidence of pathophysiology. Her husband of 25 years recently died of a myocardial infarction (MI). Yesterday, she began having chest pains and was certain she was having a heart attack. Her daughter called 911, and Veronica was transported to the emergency department. The staff performed diagnostic studies and laboratory tests, which were all negative for pathophysiology. She was admitted to the psychiatric unit with a diagnosis of Somatic Symptom Disorder. The nurse develops the following concept map care plan for Veronica.

Signs and Symptoms
- Physical complaints
- Absence of pathophysiology
- Focus on self and physical symptoms

Signs and Symptoms
- Chest pains and fear of having a heart attack (following husband's sudden death from MI)

Nursing Diagnosis

Ineffective coping

Nursing Diagnosis

Fear (of dying as husband did from acute MI)

Nursing Actions
- Ongoing assessment
- Accept that the symptoms are real to the patient
- Identify personal gains
- Fulfill patient's needs
- Do not give positive reinforcement to symptoms
- Limit amount of time patient discusses symptoms
- Teach adaptive coping strategies

Nursing Actions
- Ongoing assessment
- Refer all new physical complaints to physician
- Discuss patient fears and anxieties
- Encourage verbalization of feelings associated with husband's death
- Encourage participation in grief support group

Medical Rx:
Duloxetine 60 mg q day for chronic pain/depression/anxiety

Outcomes:
- Patient recognizes signs and symptoms of escalating anxiety
- Patient is able to intervene before the exacerbation of physical symptoms

Outcomes:
- Patient discusses feelings associated with husband's death
- Fears of own serious illness have diminished
- Patient uses adaptive coping mechanisms to diminish fears/anxieties

FIGURE 29–2 Concept map care plan for a patient with somatic symptom disorder.

Does the patient:

- Recall memories accurately?
- Connect occurrence of psychological stress to loss of memory?
- Discuss fears and anxieties with members of the staff in an effort toward resolution?
- Discuss the presence of various identities within the self?
- Verbalize situations that precipitate transition from one identity to another?
- Maintain a sense of reality during stressful situations?
- Verbalize a correlation between stressful situations and the onset of depersonalization behaviors?
- Demonstrate more adaptive coping strategies for dealing with stress without resorting to dissociation?

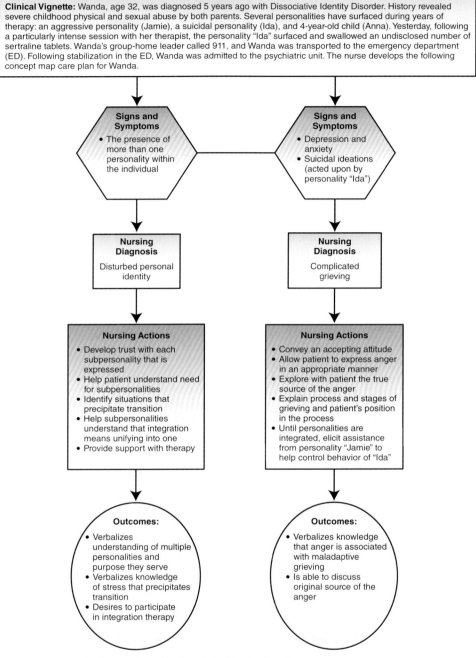

Clinical Vignette: Wanda, age 32, was diagnosed 5 years ago with Dissociative Identity Disorder. History revealed severe childhood physical and sexual abuse by both parents. Several personalities have surfaced during years of therapy: an aggressive personality (Jamie), a suicidal personality (Ida), and 4-year-old child (Anna). Yesterday, following a particularly intense session with her therapist, the personality "Ida" surfaced and swallowed an undisclosed number of sertraline tablets. Wanda's group-home leader called 911, and Wanda was transported to the emergency department (ED). Following stabilization in the ED, Wanda was admitted to the psychiatric unit. The nurse develops the following concept map care plan for Wanda.

Signs and Symptoms
• The presence of more than one personality within the individual

Signs and Symptoms
• Depression and anxiety
• Suicidal ideations (acted upon by personality "Ida")

Nursing Diagnosis
Disturbed personal identity

Nursing Diagnosis
Complicated grieving

Nursing Actions
• Develop trust with each subpersonality that is expressed
• Help patient understand need for subpersonalities
• Identify situations that precipitate transition
• Help subpersonalities understand that integration means unifying into one
• Provide support with therapy

Nursing Actions
• Convey an accepting attitude
• Allow patient to express anger in an appropriate manner
• Explore with patient the true source of the anger
• Explain process and stages of grieving and patient's position in the process
• Until personalities are integrated, elicit assistance from personality "Jamie" to help control behavior of "Ida"

Outcomes:
• Verbalizes understanding of multiple personalities and purpose they serve
• Verbalizes knowledge of stress that precipitates transition
• Desires to participate in integration therapy

Outcomes:
• Verbalizes knowledge that anger is associated with maladaptive grieving
• Is able to discuss original source of the anger

FIGURE 29–3 Concept map care plan for a patient with dissociative identity disorder.

Treatment Modalities

Somatic Symptom Disorders
Individual Psychotherapy

The goal of psychotherapy is to help clients develop healthy and adaptive behaviors, encourage them to move beyond their somatization, and enable them to manage their lives more effectively. The focus is on personal and social difficulties that the client experiences in daily life as well as the achievement of practical solutions for these difficulties.

Treatment is initiated with a complete physical examination to rule out organic pathology. Clients may be more amenable to psychotherapeutic treatment, particularly stress management, when it is conducted in a medical setting. Regular noninvasive medical assessments are recommended to reassure clients that their concerns are being heard (Yates, 2019). In addition, regular assessment may limit health-care seeking behavior and provide an ongoing opportunity for education and stress management.

Group Psychotherapy

Group therapy may be helpful for somatic symptom disorders because it provides a setting where clients can share their experiences of illness, learn to verbalize thoughts and feelings, and be confronted by group members and leaders when they reject responsibility for maladaptive behaviors. It is the treatment of choice for both somatic symptom disorder and illness anxiety disorder, in part because it provides the social support and anxiety reduction that these clients need.

Cognitive Behavior Therapy and Psychoeducation

Escobar and Dimsdale (2017) reported that several studies support CBT as an effective strategy for reducing symptoms in clients with somatic diseases. Evidence supports that CBT is particularly effective in reducing depressive symptoms in clients with somatic disorders (Yates, 2019). Psychoeducation includes teaching the individual that the symptoms may be related to or exacerbated by stress and anxiety. This teaching should be done in the context of a trusting relationship between the health-care provider and the client because the client may resist the suggestion that physical symptoms could have a psychological foundation. Psychoeducation for family members and other support persons focuses on teaching these individuals to reward the client's autonomy, self-sufficiency, and independence while taking care not to reinforce passivity and dependence associated with the sick role. This process becomes more difficult when the client is very regressed and the sick role is well established. In conversion disorder, symptoms usually abate spontaneously, but behavior therapy may be beneficial.

Psychopharmacology

Although studies have shown CBT to have the highest efficacy in people with somatic symptom and related disorders, antidepressants (and particularly first generation tricyclics) have demonstrated benefit for pain syndromes (Boland & Verduin, 2022). Anxiety may be treated in the short term with antianxiety agents, but long-term use should be avoided because of the potential for physical dependence. Benzodiazepines should be used cautiously in patients with dissociative disorders because they can also exacerbate dissociation (Gentile et al., 2014). In the treatment of conversion disorders, parenteral amobarbital or lorazepam may be helpful in revealing historical information related to trauma.

Dissociative Amnesia

Many cases of dissociative amnesia resolve spontaneously when the individual is removed from the stressful situation. For more refractory conditions, intravenous administration of amobarbital is useful in the retrieval of lost memories. Most clinicians recommend supportive psychotherapy to reinforce adjustment to the psychological effect of the retrieved memories and associated emotions.

In some instances, psychotherapy is used as the primary treatment. Techniques of persuasion and free or directed association are used to help the client remember. In other cases, hypnosis may be required to mobilize the memories. Hypnosis is sometimes facilitated by the use of pharmacological agents, such as sodium amobarbital. Supportive psychotherapy, group psychotherapy, and cognitive therapy may be employed once the memories have been obtained through hypnosis to help the client integrate the memories into their conscious state. CBT has an added benefit that when clients begin to correct cognitive distortions about the associated trauma, they may develop better recall of details about traumatic events (Boland & Verduin, 2022).

Dissociative Identity Disorder

The goal of therapy for the client with DID is to optimize the client's function and potential. The achievement of **integration** (a blending of all the subpersonalities into a unified whole) is usually considered desirable, but some clients choose not to pursue this lengthy therapeutic regimen. In these cases, resolution, or a smooth collaboration among the subpersonalities, may be all that is realistic.

Intensive, long-term psychotherapy with the DID client is directed toward uncovering the underlying psychological conflicts, helping them gain insight into these conflicts, and striving to synthesize the various identities into one integrated personality. The therapist who engages in psychotherapy with this client must be skilled in various approaches, including insight-oriented psychotherapy, CBT, and especially trauma-informed and post-traumatic stress disorder (PTSD) treatment approaches. Clients are assisted in recalling past traumas in detail. They must mentally reexperience the abuse that caused their illness. This process, called **abreaction,** or "remembering with feeling," is so painful that clients may actually cry, scream, and feel the pain that they felt at the time of the abuse.

During therapy, each subpersonality is actively explored and encouraged to become aware of the others across previously amnestic barriers. Traumatic memories associated with the different personality manifestations, especially those related to childhood abuse, are examined. The course of treatment is often difficult and anxiety-provoking to client and therapist alike, especially when aggressive or suicidal personalities dominate. In these instances, brief periods of hospitalization may be necessary as an interim supportive measure. Escobar and Dimsdale (2017) identified that the standard of care for clients with DID (and dissociative amnesia) is a three-phase process: (1) stabilization, in which the focus is on safety and symptom control; (2) intensive focus on trauma issues; and (3) reintegration of the personality and a moving away from a framework of traumatization and victimization.

When integration is achieved, the individual is able to integrate all the feelings, experiences, memories, skills, and talents that were previously in the command of the various personalities. The individual learns how to function effectively without the necessity of creating separate identities to cope with life. Integration is possible only after years of intense psychotherapy, and even then, recovery is often incomplete.

Depersonalization-Derealization Disorder

Information about the treatment of depersonalization-derealization disorder is sparse and inconclusive. Various psychiatric medications have been tried, both singly and in combination: antidepressants, mood stabilizers, anticonvulsants, and antipsychotics. Results have been sporadic at best. If other psychiatric disorders, such as schizophrenia, are evident, they too may be treated pharmacologically. For clients with evident intrapsychic conflict, analytically oriented insight psychotherapy may be useful. Some clients with depersonalization-derealization disorders have benefited from hypnotherapy or CBT.

CLINICAL JUDGMENT IN ACTION: CASE STUDY AND SAMPLE CARE PLAN

NURSING HISTORY AND ASSESSMENT

Recognizing cues: The nurse must demonstrate ability to recognize what information is most important to making an assessment (National Council of State Boards of Nursing [NCSBN], 2021). This information is italicized in the following.

Jake is a 54-year-old patient of the psychiatric outpatient department of the VA Medical Center. At age 42, Jake was diagnosed with colon cancer and **underwent a colon resection.** Since that time, he has had regular follow-up examinations, with **no recurrence of the cancer** and **no residual effects.** He did not require follow-up chemotherapy or radiation therapy. For 10 years, Jake has had yearly physical and laboratory examinations. He regularly complains to his family physician of mild abdominal pain, sensations of "fullness," "bowel rumblings," and what he calls a "firm mass," which he says he can sometimes feel in his lower left quadrant. The physician has performed x-rays of the entire gastrointestinal (GI) tract, an esophagoscopy, gastroscopy, and colonoscopy. **All results were negative for organic pathology.** Rather than being relieved, Jake appears **resentful and disappointed that the physician has not been able to reveal a pathological problem.** Jake's job is in jeopardy because of his **excessive use of sick leave.** The family physician has referred Jake for **psychiatric evaluation.** Jake was admitted as an outpatient with the **diagnosis of Illness Anxiety Disorder.** He has been assigned to Lisa, a psychiatric nurse practitioner.

Analyzing cues: The nurse must be able to interpret the information (NCSBN, 2021).

Lisa notes that after thorough evaluation, physical causes for Jake's complaints have been ruled out yet Jake remains anxious that there is something physically wrong. Lisa prioritizes that further psychosocial assessment is needed. In her assessment, Lisa learns that Jake has lived much of his adult life in isolation. He was never close to his parents, who worked and seldom had time for Jake or his sister. Jake told Lisa, "My parents really didn't care about me. They were too busy taking care of the farm. I think they only had kids so they would have some help on the farm. When I left home, they really didn't care if they ever saw me again. In fact, they never called me at all until after I got sick." He has never been married nor had a serious relationship. "Women don't like me much. I spend most of my time alone. I guess I don't really like people, and they don't really like me." Jake denies suicide ideation. He states, "I would never do that. I don't want to die but I feel like something is very wrong with me physically." Lisa interprets that social isolation is related to low self-esteem and Jake agrees with this assessment but acknowledges that his fear of illness is his most important concern at present.

Prioritize hypotheses: The nurse must be able to identify the client's most important needs (NCSBN, 2021).

Having ruled out emergent safety concerns Lisa discusses anxiety management with Jake and they agree to the following plan.

Generate solutions: The nurse must be able to connect their prioritized understanding of client needs to a course of action or plan of care (NCSBN, 2021).

NURSING DIAGNOSES AND OUTCOME IDENTIFICATION

The following nursing diagnoses have been prioritized for Jake:

1. Fear (of cancer recurrence) related to history of colon cancer evidenced by numerous complaints of the

Continued

CLINICAL JUDGMENT IN ACTION: CASE STUDY AND SAMPLE CARE PLAN—cont'd

GI tract and insistence that something is wrong despite objective tests that rule out pathophysiology.

  a. Short-term goal:

- Patient will verbalize that fears associated with bodily sensations are irrational.

  b. Long-term goal:

- Patient interprets bodily sensations correctly.

2. Chronic low self-esteem related to unfulfilled needs for nurturing and caring evidenced by patient's statements that parents don't care and people don't like him; social isolation.

  a. Short-term goal:

- Within 2 weeks, the patient will verbalize aspects about self that he likes.

  b. Long-term goal:

- By discharge from treatment, the patient will demonstrate acceptance of self as a person of worth, as evidenced by setting realistic goals, limiting physical complaints and hostility toward others, and verbalizing positive prospects for the future.

PLANNING AND IMPLEMENTATION

Take action: The nurse must be able to identify what actions need to be taken and how they will be implemented (NCSBN, 2021).

FEAR (OF CANCER RECURRENCE)

The following nursing interventions have been identified for Jake:

1. Monitor the physician's ongoing assessments and laboratory reports to ensure that pathology is ruled out.
2. Refer any new physical complaints to the physician.
3. Assess what function these physical complaints are fulfilling for Jake. Is it a way for him to get the attention that he cannot get in any other way?
4. Show empathy for his feelings. Empathize with his fears that GI symptoms may raise anxiety about the colon cancer recurring.
5. Encourage Jake to talk about his fears of cancer recurrence. What feelings did he have when it was first diagnosed? How did he deal with those feelings? What are his fears at this time?
6. Have Jake keep a diary of the appearance of the symptoms. In a separate diary, have Jake keep a record of situations that create stress for him. Compare these two records. Correlate whether symptoms appear at times of increased anxiety.
7. Help Jake determine techniques that may be useful for him to implement when fear and anxiety are exacerbated (e.g., relaxation techniques; mental imagery; thought-stopping techniques; physical exercise).
8. Offer positive feedback when Jake responds to stressful situations with coping strategies other than physical complaints.

CHRONIC LOW SELF-ESTEEM

The following nursing interventions have been identified for Jake:

1. Convey acceptance and unconditional positive regard and remain nonjudgmental at all times.
2. Encourage Jake to participate in decision making regarding his care and life situations.
3. Help Jake to recognize and focus on strengths and accomplishments. Minimize attention given to past (real or perceived) failures.
4. Encourage Jake to talk about feelings related to his unsatisfactory relationship with his parents.
5. Discuss things in his life that Jake would like to change. Help him determine what *can* be changed and what changes are not realistic.
6. Encourage participation in group activities and in therapy groups that offer simple methods of achievement. Give recognition and positive feedback for actual accomplishments.
7. Teach assertiveness techniques and effective communication techniques.
8. Offer positive feedback for appropriate social interactions with others. Role-play with Jake situations that he finds particularly stressful. Identify strategies for communicating with others that focus on topics other than physical symptoms.
9. Help Jake to set realistic goals for his future.

EVALUATION

Evaluate outcomes: The nurse must be able to evaluate actions taken and determine whether they have had a positive, neutral, or negative effect (NCSBN, 2021).

Some of the outcome criteria for Jake have been met, and some are ongoing. He has come to realize that the fears about his "symptoms" are not rational. He understands that the physician has performed adequate diagnostic procedures to rule out illness. He still has fears of cancer occurrence and discusses these fears with the nurse practitioner weekly. He has kept his symptoms and stressful situations diaries and has correlated the appearance of some of the symptoms to times of increased anxiety. He has started running and tries to use this as a strategy to keep the anxiety from escalating out of proportion and bringing on new physical symptoms. He continues to discuss feelings associated with his childhood, and the nurse has helped him see that he has had numerous accomplishments in his life, even though they were not recognized by his parents or others. He has joined a support group for depressed persons and states that he "has made a few friends." He has made a long-term goal of joining a church with the hope of meeting new people. He is missing fewer workdays because of illness, and his job is no longer in jeopardy.

Summary and Key Points

- Somatic symptom and related disorders and dissociative disorders are associated with anxiety that occurs at a severe level. The anxiety is repressed and manifested in the form of symptoms and behaviors associated with these disorders.

- Somatic symptom and related disorders affect about 5% to 7% of the general population. Types of somatic disorders include somatic symptom disorder, illness anxiety disorder, conversion disorder, psychological factors affecting other medical conditions, factitious disorder, and other specified or unspecified somatic symptom and related disorders.

- Somatic symptom disorder is manifested by physical symptoms that may be vague, dramatized, or exaggerated in presentation. No evidence of organic pathology can be identified.

- Illness anxiety disorder is an unrealistic preoccupation with fear of having a serious illness. This disorder may follow a personal experience or the experience of a close family member with a serious or life-threatening illness.

- The individual with a functional neurological symptom disorder (conversion disorder) experiences a loss of or alteration in bodily functioning, unsubstantiated by medical or pathophysiological explanation. Psychological factors may be evident by the primary or secondary gains the individual achieves from experiencing the physiological manifestation.

- With the diagnosis of psychological factors affecting medical condition, psychological or behavioral factors have been implicated in the development, exacerbation, or delayed recovery from a medical condition.

- In factitious disorder, the individual falsifies physical or psychological signs or symptoms or induces injury to the self or another person to receive attention from medical personnel.

- A dissociative response has been described as a defense mechanism to protect the ego in the face of overwhelming anxiety.

- Dissociative responses result in an alteration in the normally integrative functions of identity, memory, or consciousness.

- Classification of dissociative disorders includes dissociative amnesia, dissociative identity disorder (DID), depersonalization/derealization disorder, and other specified or unspecified dissociative disorders.

- The individual with dissociative amnesia is unable to recall important personal information that is too extensive to be explained by ordinary forgetfulness.

- The prominent feature of DID is the existence of two or more personality states within a single individual. An individual may have many personality states, each of which allows them to endure painful stimuli that the identity is too fragmented to integrate as one whole personality.

- Depersonalization/derealization disorder is characterized by an alteration in the perception of oneself or the environment. Depersonalization is described as a feeling of unreality or detachment from one's body. Derealization is an experience of unreality or detachment from one's surroundings.

- Individuals with somatic symptom and dissociative disorders often receive initial health care in areas other than psychiatry.

- Nurses can assist patients with these disorders by helping them understand the role of anxiety in symptom development and identify and establish new, more adaptive cognitive and behavior patterns. Nurses should provide trauma-informed care and be aware of resources for referral to specialists in trauma care and PTSD treatment.

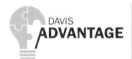

Go to **Davis Advantage** to complete your learning: strengthen understanding, apply your knowledge, and prepare for the Next Gen NCLEX®.

Review Questions

1. Which symptom profiles would be expected when assessing a client with somatic symptom disorder?
   a. Multiple somatic symptoms in several body systems
   b. Fear of having a serious disease
   c. Loss or alteration in sensorimotor functioning
   d. Belief that their body is deformed or defective in some way

2. Which of the following ego defense mechanisms describes the underlying psychodynamics of somatic symptom disorder?
   a. Denial of depression
   b. Repression of anxiety
   c. Suppression of grief
   d. Displacement of anger

3. Nursing care for a client with somatic symptom disorder should focus on helping the client to:
   a. Eliminate stressors.
   b. Discontinue focusing on numerous physical complaints.
   c. Take medication only as prescribed.
   d. Learn more adaptive coping strategies.

4. A client diagnosed with somatic symptom disorder states, "My doctor thinks I should see a psychiatrist. I can't imagine why he would make such a suggestion." What is the most common basis for the client's statement?
   a. Lack of trust in the physician
   b. Lack of understanding about the correlation of symptoms and stress
   c. Lack of understanding about the role of a psychiatrist
   d. Lack of financial resources

5. What is the ultimate goal of therapy for a client with dissociative identity disorder?
   a. Integration of the identities into one cohesive personality
   b. The ability to switch from one identity to another voluntarily
   c. The ability to select one personality as the dominant self
   d. Recognition that the various identities exist

6. The ultimate goal of therapy for a client with dissociative identity disorder is most likely achieved through:
   a. Crisis intervention and directed association.
   b. Psychotherapy and hypnosis.
   c. Psychoanalysis and free association.
   d. Insight psychotherapy and dextroamphetamines.

7. Which of the following symptoms is consistent with a diagnosis of illness anxiety disorder?
   a. Complains of a multitude of incapacitating physical symptoms
   b. Manifests with pseudoseizures or pseudocyesis
   c. Takes substances to induce vomiting to convince the nurse that she needs treatment
   d. Expresses persistent fears of having life-threatening disease

Clinical Judgment Questions

Questions 8 through 10 refer to the following case study:

The client, previously diagnosed with dissociative identity disorder, has been involved in individual and group therapy for the last 6 years. The client reports to the nurse at the mental health clinic that they have had trouble sleeping in the last 2 weeks and had a panic attack the prior evening. Their reason for coming to the mental health clinic was that they "are beginning to recall frightening memories of being abused as a child and they are afraid to be alone at present."

8. Which of these is a priority response by the nurse?
    a. Ask the client to describe their memories in detail.
    b. Conduct an assessment of the client's sleep patterns.
    c. Offer to stay with the client and listen empathically.
    d. Encourage the client not to discuss these memories to avoid retraumatization.

9. During assessment the client reveals that the anxiety has become unmanageable, begins talking like a small child that appears to be a different identity, and states "Janie wants to kill herself." What is the priority nursing diagnosis for this client?
    a. Disturbed personal identity related to childhood abuse
    b. Disturbed sensory perception related to repressed anxiety
    c. Impaired memory related to disturbed thought processes
    d. Risk for suicidal behavior related to maladaptive grief

10. In establishing trust with this client, the nurse should:
    a. Respond as if the client did not have multiple personalities.
    b. Listen nonjudgmentally and respond empathically when the client transitions to different personality states.
    c. Ignore behaviors that the client attributes to other subpersonalities.
    d. Explain to the client that they must remain in their primary identity state while communicating with the nurse.
    e. All of the above

IMPLICATIONS OF RESEARCH FOR EVIDENCE-BASED PRACTICE

Lebel, S., Mutsaers, B., Tomei, C., Leclair, C. S., Jones, G., Petricone-Westwood, D., Rutkowski, N., Ta, V., Trudel, G., Laflamme, S. Z., Lavigne, A-A., & Dinkel, A. (2020). Health anxiety and illness-related fears across diverse chronic illnesses: A systematic review on conceptualization, measurement, prevalence, course, and correlates. *PLoS ONE, 15*(7), e0234124. https://doi.org/10.1371/journal.pone.0234124

DESCRIPTION OF THE STUDY: The authors, noting that health-related fears are common among patients with chronic illnesses, conducted a systematic review of 401 articles to investigate the conceptual, theoretical, and measurement overlap, and differences between distinct perspectives on management of illness-related fears in various chronic illnesses and to clarify the prevalence, course, and correlates of these fears.

RESULTS OF THE STUDY: The review found that across different conceptualizations of illness anxiety, there were three commonalities: a high level of clinically significant levels of fear, a stable course over time, and a deleterious effect on the quality of life. Although there appeared to

be applicability of *DSM-5-TR* disorders to the experience of fear in patients with chronic illnesses, only a minority of the reviewed articles employed a psychiatric perspective. The authors recommend conceptualizing health anxiety (HA) on a continuum from mild and transient to severe. They further identify the need to conceptualize HA as having affective, cognitive, behavioral, and perceptual features.

IMPLICATIONS FOR NURSING PRACTICE: The setting, patient population, and perspectives of different health-care professionals can all be influential in how nurses respond to the needs of a patient with illness anxiety. The authors' research underscores the importance of systematic review to clarify and unify conceptualizations with the goal of ensuring that, across settings and across populations of patients with chronic illnesses, illness anxiety is recognized as not only a significant concern but also one that affects an individual's mood, cognition, behavior, and perceptions. Nurses in any practice setting should be attentive to assessing for the severity of illness or health anxiety and consider interventions that address mood, cognitive, perceptual, and behavioral symptoms.

TEST YOUR CLINICAL REASONING AND CLINICAL JUDGMENT SKILLS

Tom was admitted to the psychiatric unit from the emergency department of a general hospital in the Midwest. The owner of a local bar called the police when Tom suddenly seemed to "lose control. He just went ballistic." The police reported that Tom did not know where he was or how he got there. He kept saying, "My name is John Brown, and I live in Philadelphia." When the police ran an identity check on Tom, they found that he was indeed John Brown from Philadelphia, and his wife had reported him missing a month ago. Mrs. Brown explained that about 12 months before his disappearance, her husband, who was a shop foreman at a large manufacturing plant, had been having considerable difficulty at work. He had been passed over for a promotion, and his supervisor was very critical of his work. Several of his staff had left the company for other jobs, and without enough help, Tom had been unable to meet shop deadlines. Work stress made him very difficult to live with at home. Previously an easygoing, extroverted individual, he became withdrawn and extremely critical of his wife and children. Immediately preceding his disappearance, he had had a violent argument with his 18-year-old son, who called Tom a "loser" and stormed out of the house to stay with some friends. It was the day after this argument that Tom disappeared. The psychiatrist assigns a diagnosis of Dissociative Amnesia, with dissociative fugue.

Answer the following questions related to Tom:

1. Describe the *priority* nursing intervention with Tom as he is admitted to the psychiatric unit.
2. What approach should be taken to help Tom with his problem?
3. What is the long-term goal of therapy for Tom?

 MOVIE CONNECTIONS

Bandits (illness anxiety disorder) • *Hannah and Her Sisters* (illness anxiety disorder) • *Send Me No Flowers* (illness anxiety disorder) • *Dead Again* (amnesia) • *Mirage* (amnesia) • *Suddenly Last Summer* (amnesia) • *Sybil* (DID) • *The Three Faces of Eve* (DID) • *Identity* (DID)

References

Ali, S., Jabeen, S., Pate, R. J., Shahid, M., Chinala, S., Nathani, M., & Shah, R. (2015). Conversion disorder—mind versus body: A review. *Innovations in Clinical Neuroscience, 12*(5–6), 27–33.

American Psychiatric Association (APA). (2022). *Diagnostic and statistical manual of mental disorders, fifth edition, text revision (DSM-5-TR)*. American Psychiatric Association.

Boland, R., & Verduin, M. L. (2022). *Kaplan & Sadock's synopsis of psychiatry* (P. Ruiz, Ed.). (12th ed.). Wolters Kluwer.

Chalavi, S., Vissia, E. M., Giesen, M. E., Nijenhuis, E. R. S., Draijer, N., Cole, J. H., Dazzan, P., Pariante, C. M., Madsen, S. K., Rajagopalan, P., Thompson, P. M., Toga, A. W., Veltman, D. J.,

& Reinders, A. T. (2015). Abnormal hippocampal morphology in dissociative identity disorder and post-traumatic stress disorder correlates with childhood trauma and dissociative symptoms. *Human Brain Mapping, 36*, 1692–1704.

Delvecchio, G., Rossetti, M. G., Caletti, E., Arighi, A., Galimberti, D., Basilico, P., Mercurio, M., Paoli, R., Cinnante, C., Triulzi, F., Altamura, A. C., Scarpini, E., & Brambilla, P. (2019). The neuroanatomy of somatoform disorders: A magnetic resonance imaging study. *Psychosomatics, 60*(3), 278–288. https://doi.org/10.1016/j.psym.2018.07.005

Dimsdale, J. (2020). Illness anxiety disorder. *Merck Manual: Professional Version.* http://www.merckmanuals.com/professional/psychiatric-disorders/somatic-symptom-and-related-disorders/illness-anxiety-disorder

Dimsdale J. E. (2017). Research on somatization and somatic symptom disorders: Ars longa, vita brevis. *Psychosomatic Medicine, 79*(9), 971–973. https://doi.org/10.1097/PSY.0000000000000533

Escobar, J. I., & Dimsdale, J. E. (2017). Somatic symptom and related disorders. In Sadock, B. J., Sadock, V. A., & Ruiz, P. (Eds.), *Comprehensive textbook of psychiatry* (10th ed., pp. 1827–1845). Wolters Kluwer.

Gentile, J. P., Snyder, M., & Gillig, P. M. (2014). Stress and trauma: Psychotherapy and pharmacotherapy for depersonalization/derealization disorder. *Innovations in Clinical Neuroscience, 11*(7–8), 37–41.

Haberman, C. (2014). Debate persists over diagnosing mental disorders, long after "Sybil." *New York Times.* https://www.nytimes.com/search?query=Debate+persists+over+diagnosing+mental+disorders%2C+long+after+%E2%80%9CSybil.%E2%80%9D+

Herdman, T. H., Kamitsuru, S., Lopes, C. T. (Eds.). (2021). *NANDA-I Inc. nursing diagnoses: Definitions and classification, 2021–2023.* Thieme.

Institute of Medicine. (2003). *Health professions education: A bridge to quality.* National Academies Press.

International Society for the Study of Trauma and Dissociation. (2011). Guidelines for treating dissociative identity disorder in adults, third revision. *Journal of Trauma & Dissociation, 12*(2), 115–187. http://dx.doi.org/10.1080/15299732.2011.537247

Joshi, K. G. (2020). Strategies for treating patients with health anxiety. *Current Psychiatry, 19*(4), 54–60.

Kahn, D. (2018). *Illness anxiety disorder (formerly hypochondriasis).* https://emedicine.medscape.com/article/290955-overview#a6

Lebel, S., Mutsaers, B., Tomei, C., Leclair, C. S., Jones, G., Petricone-Westwood, D., Rutkowski, N., Ta, V., Trudel, G., Laflamme, S. Z., Lavigne, A-A., & Dinkel, A. (2020). Health anxiety and illness-related fears across diverse chronic illnesses: A systematic review on conceptualization, measurement, prevalence, course, and correlates. *PLoS ONE, 15*(7), e0234124. https://doi.org/10.1371/journal.pone

Muller, M. (2014). Fragmented child: Disorganized attachment and dissociation. *Psychology Today.* https://www.psychologytoday.com/us/blog/talking-about-trauma/201406/fragmented-child-disorganized-attachment-and-dissociation

National Council of State Boards of Nursing (NCSBN). (2021). *Next generation NCLEX®: comparison between case studies and stand-alone items.* https://www.ncsbn.org/public-files/NGN_Fall21_English_Final.pdf

Özdemir, O., Cilingir, V., Özdemir, P. G., Milanlioglu, A., Hamamci, M., & Yilmaz, E. (2016). Dissociative experiences in patients with epilepsy. *Arquivos de Neuro-Psiquiatria, 74*(3), 189–194. https://doi.org/10.1590/0004-282X20160045

QSEN Institute. (2020). *Competencies.* http://qsen.org/competencies/

Sar, V., Dorahy, M. J., & Krüger, C. (2017). Revisiting the etiological aspects of dissociative identity disorder: A biopsychosocial perspective. *Psychology Research and Behavior Management, 10,* 137–146. https://doi.org/10.2147/PRBM.S113743

Soreff, S. (2018). Fast five quiz: Are you prepared to treat patients with illness anxiety disorder? https://reference.medscape.com/viewarticle/895692_2

Van den Houte, M., Bogaerts, K., Van Diest, I., De, J., Persoons, P., Van Oudenhove, L., & Van den Bergh, O. (2017). Inducing somatic symptoms in functional syndrome patients: Effects of manipulating state negative affect. *Psychosomatic Medicine, 79*(9), 1000–1007. https://doi.org/10.1097/PSY.0000000000000527

Yates, W. (2019). Somatic symptom disorders. *Medscape.* http://emedicine.medscape.com/article/294908-overview

Classical References

Asher, R. (1951). Munchausen's syndrome. *The Lancet, 257*(6650), 339–341.

Freud, S. (1962). The neuro-psychoses of defense. In Strachey, J. (Ed.), *Standard edition of the complete psychological works of Sigmund Freud,* vol. 3. Hogarth Press. (Original work published 1894.)

Irwin, H. J. (1999). Pathological and nonpathological dissociation: The relevance of childhood trauma. *The Journal of Psychology, 133*(2), 157–164.

30 Eating Disorders

KEY TERMS

amenorrhea

anorexia nervosa (AN)

binge-eating disorder (BED)

binging

bulimia nervosa (BN)

emaciated

lanugo

obesity

purging

refeeding syndrome

OBJECTIVES

After reading this chapter, the student will be able to:

1. Identify and differentiate among several eating disorders.
2. Discuss epidemiological statistics related to eating disorders.
3. Describe symptomatology associated with anorexia nervosa, bulimia nervosa, and obesity, and use the information in patient assessment.
4. Identify predisposing factors in the development of eating disorders.
5. Formulate nursing diagnoses and outcomes of care for patients with eating disorders.
6. Describe appropriate interventions for behaviors associated with eating disorders.
7. Identify topics for patient and family teaching relevant to eating disorders.
8. Evaluate the nursing care of patients with eating disorders.
9. Discuss various modalities relevant to the treatment of eating disorders.

Nutrition is required to sustain life, and most individuals acquire nutrients from eating food; however, nutrition and life sustenance are not the only reasons most people eat food. Indeed, in an affluent culture, life sustenance may not even be a consideration. It is sometimes difficult to remember that many people in the affluent American culture, as well as all over the world, are starving from lack of food.

The hypothalamus contains the appetite regulation center within the brain. This complex neural system regulates the body's ability to recognize when it is hungry and when it has been sated. Studies have shown evidence of serotonin and dopamine dysfunction in individuals with eating disorders (Frank et al., 2021; Pruccoli et al., 2021; Riva, 2016). These neurotransmitters play a role in regulating eating behavior in the hypothalamus.

Society and culture also have a substantial influence on eating behaviors. Eating is a social activity. Seldom does an event of any social significance occur without the presence of food. Yet society and culture also influence how people, especially women, should look. History reveals a regularity of fluctuations in what society has considered desirable in the human female body. Archives and historical paintings from the 16th and 17th centuries reveal that plump, full-figured women were considered fashionable and desirable. In the Victorian era, beauty was characterized by a slender, wan appearance that continued through the flapper era of the 1920s. During the Depression era and World War II, the full-bodied woman was again admired, only to be superseded in the late 1960s by images of super thin models propagated by the media, which remains the ideal of today. It's been said that "a woman can't be too rich or too thin." Eating disorders, as we know them, can refute this concept.

This chapter explores the disorders associated with undereating and overeating. Because psychological or behavioral factors play a potential role in the presentation of these disorders, they fall well within the realm of psychiatry and psychiatric nursing. Epidemiology and predisposing factors in anorexia nervosa, bulimia nervosa, and binge-eating disorder are presented. An explanation of the symptomatology is presented as background knowledge for assessing the patient with an eating disorder. Nursing care is described in the context of the nursing process. Various treatment modalities are explored.

Epidemiology

The prevalence of AN has increased since the mid-20th century, both in the United States and in Western Europe. Epidemiological studies have found that across all ages and genders, the lifetime prevalence for an episode of AN is 00.6% to 0.80%% (Boland & Verduin, 2022). Once thought to be rare among males, more recent research suggests that 1 in 3 individuals with an eating disorder is male (Kumar, 2021) and the incidence is on the rise as well as underreported (Sangha et al., 2019). See "Real People, Real Stories" for more about Vic's experience with an eating disorder.

Real People, Real Stories: Living With an Eating Disorder

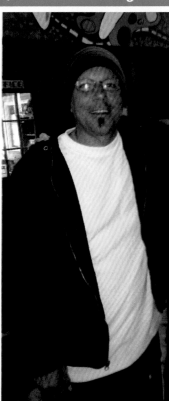

(Following is an excerpt of our conversation.)

Karyn: First of all, I appreciate your willingness to share your story.

Vic: I want to talk about this because there is such a stigma associated with being a guy and having an eating disorder. And it's hard for guys to find a support group of people who really "get it."

Karyn: What has your experience been with encountering stigma?

Vic: Well, my weight has sometimes been really high and sometimes very low. I fluctuate between anorexia and bulimia. So when my weight is really low, people have presumed I have AIDS. And in general, because eating disorders are presumed to be a female disorder, people have assumed I was gay. In high school, I was very heavy, and the guys on the football team teased me a lot. I talked to my girlfriend at the time, and she suggested I try purging. I was using food and alcohol for comfort, but then I had to purge. I started working out a lot, and when I started getting compliments on my appearance, I began binging and purging every day and drinking alcohol. It was a stress relief for a while, but then it just wasn't working anymore, and I still hated my appearance. To this day, there's not one thing I like about my appearance even though my physician is happy with my current weight. I was hiding it from my family for some time: wearing baggy clothes and two sets of clothes so people wouldn't see my flaws. The behaviors are very isolating. When I tried to talk to my dad. he just told

Continued

Real People, Real Stories: Living With an Eating Disorder—cont'd

me to be a man … but there was a lot of physical and emotional abuse from him, so I didn't get support there.

Karyn: Where have you found support?

Vic: My mom and my fiancée are my biggest supports, but it's a struggle to find support with other guys who have eating disorders, and I feel like they would really understand. I tried to start a support group on Facebook, and no one responded. I have an individual counselor who knows a lot about eating disorders, and I have a family practice physician, and they are both helpful. It's just not the same as having the support of others who are having the same experiences that you are.

Karyn: Have you ever been engaged in group treatment specifically for eating disorders?

Vic: I tried, at one point, but most insurances don't cover eating disorder treatment, or the treatment program doesn't take insurance. I went into treatment in 2009 for alcohol rehabilitation, and they didn't address the eating disorder. In fact, they kind of force you to eat and tell you that you'll probably gain weight as you go through rehab, so the bulimia kicked in again for me because I didn't want to get fat like the other people in recovery. But I've been sober since 2009, and I take Vivitrol injections (to manage alcohol dependence) once a month; it blocks the pleasure centers.

Karyn: And has that been effective?

Vic: Oh yes, definitely. And my AA buddies are very supportive, but they don't see food as a similar issue to alcohol, so they don't really see a need to discuss that. Plus, you can't abstain from food like you can from alcohol. And society itself can be a trigger: television, all the messages that you need to be a certain way, picnics, going out to eat, grocery stores, talking about food, et cetera. And I think I have an element of "people pleasing" in my personality, so I'm always worried about what other people are thinking about me.

Karyn: It's not uncommon for people with eating disorders to also have depression and sometimes have suicide thoughts. Have you ever been in that place?

Vic: Yeah, once last year I took an overdose of pills with some alcohol, but I called some friends, and they got me in to get help.

Karyn: Do you still have times when you have those thoughts?

Vic: No. I'm doing really well right now. I still dabble from time to time with "the behavior" [Vic described this as his term for binging/purging or calorie restriction, stating that sometimes using the words can be a trigger for him], but not like before when I was taking up to 20 laxatives a day and my whole day was preoccupied with planning "the behaviors." I'm working in a setting that treats dual diagnosis clients, and I am hopeful that there may be opportunities to establish peer support groups for men with eating disorders, much like what exists in AA for alcohol recovery. As a guy, you just can't go to a group that is all women and talk about this stuff, especially what's going on with your body. And I don't want to be accused of "thirteen-steppin."

Karyn: "'Thirteen-steppin'?"

Vic: Yeah, that's the "thirteenth step" in the twelve-step program. It's the guys that go to AA meetings to pick up girls who are in recovery because they know they are more vulnerable when they're trying to stay sober. [Chuckles]

Karyn: [Chuckles] I didn't know that was a thing. But I understand what you're saying about the difficulty of finding support with other men who understand and are willing to acknowledge their eating disorder. I hope the peer support group works out, and in the meantime, I'm glad to hear that you are accessing resources to support your health.

Social interests may also play a role in the prevalence of eating disorders. Ballet, modeling, wrestling, and other careers and sports that focus on weight restriction may lead to preoccupation with one's body and increase the risk for AN. It was once believed that AN was more prevalent in the higher socioeconomic classes, but evidence is lacking to support this hypothesis. The lifetime prevalence of BN is 0.28% to 1% (American Psychiatric Association [APA], 2022). Onset of BN typically occurs in late adolescence or early adulthood and is more prevalent in women than in men.

Binge-eating disorder (BED) is defined in the *Diagnostic and Statistical Manual of Mental Disorders, Fifth Edition, Text Revision (DSM-5-TR)* as recurrent episodes of eating significantly more than most people would eat in a similar period under similar circumstances, and these episodes occur at least once a week for 3 months (APA, 2022). It is the most common eating disorder and affects women almost twice as often as men (Boland & Verduin, 2022). The lifetime prevalence of BED ranges from 0.85% to 2.8% of the U.S. population (APA, 2022). Weight gain and obesity are major health risks associated with this disorder, and rates of BED are particularly high in obese and overweight individuals (Boland & Verduin, 2022).

Obesity has been defined as a body mass index (BMI) (weight/height^2) of 30 or greater. In the United States, the prevalence of obesity has increased since 1999 from 30.5% to 41.9% in 2020 (Centers for Disease Control and Prevention [CDC], 2022). This percentage is higher among non-Hispanic black

(49.9%) and Hispanic (45.6%) populations (CDC, 2022). The association between socioeconomics and obesity is complex, with variations based on level of education (higher education was associated with less obesity), sex, and race/ethnicity (among men, obesity prevalence was lower in the lowest and highest income groups compared with the middle-income group but higher in the highest income bracket among non-Hispanic black men) (CDC, 2022). Interestingly, the *DSM-5-TR* does not include obesity as a mental health disorder with the rationale that "a range of genetic, physiological, behavioral, and environmental factors that vary across individuals contributes to the development of obesity; thus, obesity is not considered a mental disorder" (APA, 2022, p. 371). The *DSM-5-TR* also notes, however, that obesity is a significant problem in several mental disorders (at least in part related to side effects of psychotropic medications) and that obesity may be a risk factor for the development of illnesses such as depression. BED, which *is* identified as a mental illness, carries a high risk for weight gain and obesity.

Application of the Nursing Process

Background Assessment Data: Anorexia Nervosa

> **CORE CONCEPT**
> **Anorexia**
> Prolonged loss of appetite.

> **CORE CONCEPT**
> **Body Image**
> A subjective concept of one's physical appearance based on the personal perceptions of self and the reactions of others.

Anorexia nervosa (AN) is characterized by a morbid fear of obesity. Symptoms include gross distortion of body image, preoccupation with food, and refusal to eat. The term *anorexia* is actually a misnomer. It was initially believed that individuals with AN did not experience sensations of hunger. However, research indicates that they do indeed feel hunger (Giordano, 2021), and it is only with food intake of fewer than 200 calories per day that hunger sensations cease.

The distorted body image is manifested by the individual's perception of being "fat" when they are obviously underweight or even **emaciated** (excessively thin). Weight loss is usually accomplished by a reduction in food intake and often extensive exercising. Self-induced vomiting and the abuse of laxatives or diuretics may occur. The *DSM-5-TR* further specifies that some individuals with AN lose weight exclusively by restricting intake, whereas others have binging and purging episodes (APA, 2022).

Weight loss is excessive, with some individuals who present for health-care services weighing less than 85% of expected weight. In spite of a weight that is "less than minimally expected" or "less than minimally normal," behaviors to interfere with weight gain persist. Other signs include hypothermia, bradycardia, hypotension with orthostatic changes, peripheral edema, **lanugo** (fine, neonatal-like hair growth), bone fractures, acrocyanosis (bluish color to hands and feet related to poor circulation), and a variety of metabolic changes. **Amenorrhea** (absence of menstruation) usually follows severe weight loss, but sometimes it happens early in the disorder before severe weight loss has occurred. Associated symptoms include cold intolerance, dizziness, chest pain, abdominal bloating, pain or discomfort, constipation, weakness, decreased concentration, and poor memory.

Individuals with AN may be obsessed with food. For example, they may hoard or conceal food, talk about food and recipes at great length, or prepare elaborate meals for others, only to restrict themselves to limited low-calorie food intake. Compulsive behaviors, such as hand washing, may also be present.

Age at onset is usually early to late adolescence, and psychosexual development is often delayed. Feelings of depression and anxiety or irritability often accompany the disorder. Depression is strongly correlated with eating disorders, some of which may be secondary to malnutrition. In general though, common comorbidities with AN include bipolar disorder, depression, anxiety (often reported as occurring before the onset of AN), obsessive-compulsive disorder (especially among those with the restrictive eating type of AN), and substance use disorders (especially among those with the binge-eating/purging type of AN) (APA, 2022). Box 30–1 outlines the *DSM-5-TR* diagnostic criteria for AN.

Background Assessment Data: Bulimia Nervosa

> **CORE CONCEPT**
> **Bulimia**
> Excessive, insatiable appetite.

Bulimia nervosa (BN) is an episodic, uncontrolled, compulsive, rapid ingestion of large quantities of food

---

BOX 30-1 Diagnostic Criteria for Anorexia Nervosa

A. Restriction of energy intake relative to requirements leading to a significantly low body weight in the context of age, sex, developmental trajectory, and physical health. *Significantly low weight* is defined as a weight that is less than minimally normal, or, for children and adolescents, less than that minimally expected.

B. Intense fear of gaining weight or becoming fat, or persistent behavior that interferes with weight gain, even though at a significantly low weight.

C. Disturbance in the way in which one's body weight or shape is experienced, undue influence of body weight or shape on self-evaluation, or persistent lack of recognition of the seriousness of the current low body weight.

Specify whether:

Restricting type: During the last 3 months, the individual has not engaged in recurrent episodes of binge eating or purging behavior (i.e., self-induced vomiting or the misuse of laxatives, diuretics, or enemas). This subtype describes presentations in which weight loss is accomplished primarily through dieting, fasting, and/or excessive exercise.

Binge-eating/purging type: During the last 3 months, the individual has engaged in recurrent episodes of binge eating or purging behavior (i.e., self-induced vomiting or the misuse of laxatives, diuretics, or enemas).

Specify if:

In partial remission: After full criteria for anorexia nervosa were previously met, Criterion A (low body weight) has not been met for a sustained period, but either Criterion B (intense fear of gaining weight or becoming fat, or behavior that interferes with weight gain) or Criterion C (disturbances in self-perception of weight and shape) is still met.

In full remission: After full criteria for anorexia nervosa were previously met, none of the criteria have been met for a sustained period of time.

Specify current severity:

The minimum level of severity is based, for adults, on current body mass index (BMI; see below) or, for children and adolescents, on BMI percentile. The ranges below are derived from World Health Organization categories for thinness in adults; for children and adolescents, corresponding BMI percentiles should be used. The level of severity may be increased to reflect clinical symptoms, the degree of functional disability, and the need for supervision.

Mild: BMI ≥17 kg/m²   Severe: BMI 15–15.99 kg/m²

Moderate: BMI 16–16.99 kg/m²   Extreme: BMI <15 kg/m²

Reprinted with permission from the *Diagnostic and Statistical Manual of Mental Disorders, Fifth Edition, Text Revision (DSM-5-TR)* (2022). American Psychiatric Association.

---

over a short period of time, termed **binging,** followed by inappropriate compensatory behaviors to rid the body of the excess calories. The food consumed during a binge often has a high caloric content, a sweet taste, and a soft or smooth texture that can be eaten rapidly, sometimes even without being chewed (Boland & Verduin, 2022). The binging episodes often occur in secret and are usually terminated only by abdominal discomfort, sleep, social interruption, or self-induced vomiting. Although the eating binges may bring pleasure while they are occurring, self-degradation and depressed mood commonly follow.

To rid the body of the excessive calories, the individual engages in **purging** behaviors (self-induced vomiting or the misuse of laxatives, diuretics, or enemas) or other inappropriate compensatory behaviors, such as fasting or excessive exercise. Among these individuals, there is a persistent overconcern with personal appearance, particularly regarding how they believe others perceive them. Weight fluctuations are common because of the alternating binges and fasts. However, most individuals with bulimia are within a normal weight range—some slightly underweight, some slightly overweight.

Excessive vomiting and laxative or diuretic misuse may lead to problems with dehydration and electrolyte imbalance. Gastric acid in the vomitus also contributes to the erosion of tooth enamel. In rare instances, the individual may experience tears in the gastric or esophageal mucosa. Some individuals develop calluses on the dorsal surface of their hands, typically on knuckles, secondary to long-term self-induced vomiting. This feature is called *Russell's sign* after the British psychiatrist who first described it. It cannot be a reliable diagnostic symptom, however, because many individuals with purging behavior can induce vomiting without using their hands.

Common comorbidities include mood disorders, anxiety disorders, or substance use disorder, most frequently involving central nervous system (CNS) stimulants or alcohol. In a systematic review and meta-analysis (Serra et al., 2022), researchers found that almost

42% of patients with the restrictive type of AN presented with symptoms of binging and purging at follow-up. Patients with BN and a history of previous lifetime AN had worse decision-making ability, worse general and specific functioning, decreased bone density, more antecedents of lifetime suicide attempts, more dietary restraint, and more frequent use of laxatives (Strumila et al., 2020). The *DSM-5-TR* diagnostic criteria for BN are presented in Box 30–2.

Background Assessment Data: Binge-Eating Disorder

Individuals with BED have episodes of binge eating that may be similar to those with BN; however, BED does not include compensatory purging. As a result, this individual is at risk for substantial weight gain. The episodes of eating are considered binges when they occur over a defined period of time, usually less than 2 hours (APA, 2022). Food consumption not only is rapid but often continues to the point that the individual feels uncomfortably full. Interpersonal stressors, low self-esteem, and boredom are identified as possible triggers. Typically, clients describe their eating as out of control. There is often accompanying guilt and depression. BED is associated with significant comorbidities, particularly major depressive disorder and alcohol use disorder (APA, 2022). Another difference between BN and BED is that rates of improvement are consistently higher among individuals with BED than among those with BN (APA, 2022). The *DSM-5-TR* diagnostic criteria for BED are presented in Box 30–3.

Predisposing Factors and Theories of Etiology Associated With Anorexia Nervosa, Bulimia Nervosa, and Binge-Eating Disorder

Biological Influences

Genetics A hereditary predisposition to eating disorders has been hypothesized based on family histories and an apparent association with other disorders for which the likelihood of genetic influences exists. Some studies identify higher concordance rates in monozygotic than in dizygotic twins (Boland & Verduin, 2022). AN is more common among sisters of those with the disorder than among the general population, but social factors, such as modeling and mimicking, may influence these relationships. Childhood obesity and early onset of puberty are associated with increased risk for BN, which may also be related to genetic vulnerabilities (APA, 2022).

BOX 30–2 Diagnostic Criteria for Bulimia Nervosa

A. Recurrent episodes of binge eating. An episode of binge eating is characterized by both of the following:
  1. Eating, in a discrete period of time (e.g., within any 2-hour period) an amount of food that is definitely larger than most individuals would eat during a similar period of time and under similar circumstances.
  2. A sense of lack of control over eating during the episode (e.g., a feeling that one cannot stop eating or control what or how much one is eating).
B. Recurrent inappropriate compensatory behaviors in order to prevent weight gain, such as self-induced vomiting; misuse of laxatives, diuretics, or other medications; fasting; or excessive exercise.
C. The binge eating and inappropriate compensatory behaviors both occur, on average, at least once a week for 3 months.
D. Self-evaluation is unduly influenced by body shape and weight.
E. The disturbance does not occur exclusively during episodes of anorexia nervosa.

  Specify if:

In partial remission: After full criteria for bulimia nervosa were previously met, some, but not all, of the criteria have been met for a sustained period of time.

In full remission: After full criteria for bulimia nervosa were previously met, none of the criteria have been met for a sustained period of time.

  Specify current severity:
    The minimum level of severity is based on the frequency of inappropriate compensatory behaviors (see below). The level of severity may be increased to reflect other symptoms and the degree of functional disability.

Mild: An average of 1–3 episodes of inappropriate compensatory behaviors per week.

Moderate: An average of 4–7 episodes of inappropriate compensatory behaviors per week.

Severe: An average of 8–13 episodes of inappropriate compensatory behaviors per week.

Extreme: An average of 14 or more episodes of inappropriate compensatory behaviors per week.

BOX 30–3 Diagnostic Criteria for Binge-Eating Disorder

A. Recurrent episodes of binge eating. An episode of binge eating is characterized by both of the following:
  1. Eating, in a discrete period of time (e.g., within any 2-hour period), an amount of food that is definitely larger than what most people would eat in a similar period of time under similar circumstances
  2. A sense of lack of control over eating during the episode (e.g., a feeling that one cannot stop eating or control what or how much one is eating)
B. The binge-eating episodes are associated with three (or more) of the following:
  1. Eating much more rapidly than normal
  2. Eating until feeling uncomfortably full
  3. Eating large amounts of food when not feeling physically hungry
  4. Eating alone because of feeling embarrassed by how much one is eating
  5. Feeling disgusted with oneself, depressed, or very guilty afterward
C. Marked distress regarding binge eating is present.
D. The binge eating occurs, on average, at least once a week for 3 months.
E. The binge eating is not associated with the recurrent use of inappropriate compensatory behavior as in bulimia nervosa and does not occur exclusively during the course of bulimia nervosa or anorexia nervosa.

Specify if:

In partial remission: After full criteria for binge-eating disorder were previously met, binge eating occurs at an average frequency of less than one episode per week for a sustained period of time.

In full remission: After full criteria for binge-eating disorder were previously met, none of the criteria have been met for a sustained period of time.

Specify current severity:
  The minimum level of severity is based on the frequency of episodes of binge eating (see below). The level of severity may be increased to reflect other symptoms and the degree of functional disability.

Mild: 1–3 binge-eating episodes per week

Moderate: 4–7 binge-eating episodes per week

Severe: 8–13 binge-eating episodes per week

Extreme: 14 or more binge-eating episodes per week

Reprinted with permission from the *Diagnostic and Statistical Manual of Mental Disorders, Fifth Edition, Text Revision (DSM-5-TR)* (2022). American Psychiatric Association.

Neurochemical Influences Neurochemical influences in BN and AN may be associated with the neurotransmitters serotonin and norepinephrine. Neurobiological changes that occur in starvation, including depression and obsessional thinking, may contribute to maintaining the illness. This hypothesis has been supported by the positive response some individuals have shown to therapy with selective serotonin reuptake inhibitors (SSRIs). SSRIs (particularly fluoxetine) have demonstrated effectiveness in treating patients with BN but not those with AN (Milano & Capasso, 2019). However, SSRIs may be used to treat the depression that often accompanies AN. Individuals with BED have manifested several neurobiological disturbances, including delayed gastric emptying, enlarged stomach capacity, and decreased secretion of cholecystokinin (CCK), which is a hormone responsible for signaling satiety. Endogenous opioid peptides appear to play a key role in food and alcohol reward among individuals with AN and BN, which may be associated with the addictive components of the disorder and with denial of hunger in AN (Valbrun & Zvonarev, 2020). Some individuals with AN have been shown to gain weight when given naloxone, an opioid antagonist. Valbrun and Zvonarev (2020) identified that a combination of bupropion (an antidepressant) and naltrexone (an opioid antagonist) have been associated with weight loss and therefore may be beneficial in treating BED. The dopamine reward system has also been implicated in eating disorders. Questions remain as to whether neurochemical changes are causal or are an outcome of the body's reaction to changes in nutrition and mood.

Food restriction and binging and purging behaviors have all been associated with lower regional brain volumes or cortical thickness, which generally return to normal when normal eating and weight are reestablished (Frank, 2019). Frank also found altered functional connectivity in AN between the amygdala and the frontal cortex, which could account for poor emotion regulation.

Psychological Influences

Psychodynamic theories suggest that the development of an eating disorder is rooted in an unfulfilled sense of separation-individuation. When events occur that threaten the vulnerable ego, feelings of lack of control over one's body (self) emerge. Behaviors associated with food and eating provide feelings of control over one's life.

The psychological underpinnings in eating disorders are complex, but some commonly identified psychological predisposing factors for eating disorders include a history of low self-esteem, depression, anxiety, and obsessive-compulsive traits in childhood. More recently, a childhood history of trauma (adverse childhood experiences) has been associated with the development of eating disorders. Groth and associates (2020) reported that approximately 50% of adolescents with an eating disorder identify a history of trauma and abuse.

Family Influences

Historically, parents of children with eating disorders have been presumed to be overcontrolling and perfectionistic, causing pathology in their children. This theory has been problematic, at least in part because not all siblings in the same family develop eating disorders. There is insufficient evidence to support these claims, and they may have contributed to resistance toward seeking health care based on parents' fear that they will be judged as the cause of the problem. The American Academy for Eating Disorders (AED) published a position statement (2009) that included the following:

> The AED stands firmly against any model of eating disorders in which family influences are seen as the primary cause of eating disorders, condemns statements that blame families for their child's illness, and recommends that families be included in the treatment of younger patients, unless this is clearly ill-advised on clinical grounds.

Both perfectionistic and depressive tendencies do appear to be common in patients with AN, and conflicts certainly arise in a family when a child is starving themselves, but it has become clear that family members need to be involved in treatment rather than shunned or blamed. Family-based approaches, such as the Maudsley approach (see later in this chapter), are supported by clinical evidence (Rienecke, 2017).

Background Assessment Data: Body Mass Index

Assessment for the presence of an eating disorder is facilitated by an understanding of the measurements for BMI. The following formula is used to determine an individual's BMI:

$$\text{Body mass index} = \text{Weight (kg)}/\text{Height (m)}^2$$

The BMI range for normal weight is 18.5 to 24.9. Studies by the National Center for Health Statistics indicate that *overweight* is defined as a BMI of 25.0 to 29.9 (based on U.S. Dietary Guidelines for Americans). Based on World Health Organization criteria, *obesity* is defined as a BMI of 30.0 or greater. The average American woman has a BMI of 26, and fashion models typically have BMIs of less than 18. AN is characterized by a BMI of 17 or lower. In extreme AN, the BMI may be less than 15. Hospitalization is indicated when the median BMI is less than 75% of that expected for the individual's age and sex (Toulany & Katzman, 2022). Table 30–1 presents an example of some BMIs based on weight (in pounds) and height (in inches).

Diagnosis and Outcome Identification

Nursing diagnoses are formulated from the data gathered during the assessment phase and with background knowledge regarding predisposing factors to the disorder. Table 30–2 presents a list of patient behaviors and the NANDA-I nursing diagnoses (Herdman et al., 2021) that correspond to those behaviors, which may be used in planning care for patients with eating disorders.

Outcome Criteria

The following criteria may be used for measurement of outcomes in the care of the patient with eating disorders.

The patient:

- Has achieved and maintained an expected BMI for age with consideration for body build, weight history, and any physiological disturbances
- Has vital signs, blood pressure, and laboratory serum studies within normal limits
- Verbalizes importance of adequate nutrition
- Verbalizes knowledge regarding consequences of fluid loss caused by self-induced vomiting (or laxative/diuretic abuse) and the importance of adequate fluid intake (AN, BN)
- Verbalizes events that precipitate anxiety and demonstrates techniques for its reduction
- Verbalizes ways in which they may gain more control of the environment and thereby reduce feelings of powerlessness
- Expresses less preoccupation with own appearance (AN, BN)
- Demonstrates ability to take control of own life without resorting to maladaptive eating behaviors (AN, BN, BED)

TABLE 30–1 Body Mass Index (BMI) Chart

HEIGHT (INCHES) / BODY WEIGHT (POUNDS)

BMI	19	20	21	22	23	24	25	26	27	28	29	30	31	32	33	34	35	36	37	38	39	40
58	91	96	100	105	110	115	119	124	129	134	138	143	148	153	158	162	167	172	177	181	186	191
59	94	99	104	109	114	119	124	128	133	138	143	148	153	158	163	168	173	178	183	188	193	198
60	97	102	107	112	118	123	128	133	138	143	148	153	158	163	168	174	179	184	189	194	199	204
61	100	106	111	116	122	127	132	137	143	148	153	158	164	169	174	180	185	190	195	201	206	211
62	104	109	115	120	126	131	136	142	147	153	158	163	169	175	180	186	191	196	202	207	213	218
63	107	113	118	124	130	135	141	146	152	158	163	169	175	180	186	191	197	203	208	214	220	225
64	110	116	122	128	134	140	145	151	157	163	169	174	180	186	192	197	204	209	215	221	227	232
65	114	120	126	132	138	144	150	156	162	168	174	180	186	192	198	204	210	216	222	228	234	240
66	118	124	130	136	142	148	155	161	167	173	179	186	192	198	204	210	216	223	229	235	241	247
67	121	127	134	140	146	153	159	166	172	178	185	191	198	204	211	217	223	230	236	242	249	255
68	125	131	138	144	151	158	164	171	177	184	190	197	203	210	216	223	230	236	243	249	256	262
69	128	135	142	149	155	162	169	176	182	189	196	203	209	216	223	230	236	243	250	257	263	270
70	132	139	146	153	160	167	174	181	188	195	202	209	216	222	229	236	243	250	257	264	271	278
71	136	143	150	157	165	172	179	186	193	200	208	215	222	229	236	243	250	257	265	272	279	286
72	140	147	154	162	169	177	184	191	199	206	213	221	228	235	242	250	258	265	272	279	287	294
73	144	151	159	166	174	182	189	197	204	212	219	227	235	242	250	257	265	272	280	288	295	302
74	148	155	163	171	179	186	194	202	210	218	225	233	241	249	256	264	272	280	287	295	303	311
75	152	160	168	176	184	192	200	208	216	224	232	240	248	256	264	272	279	287	295	303	311	319
76	156	164	172	180	189	197	205	213	221	230	238	246	254	263	271	279	287	295	304	312	320	328

Source: National Heart, Lung, and Blood Institute. (n.d.). *Aim for a healthy weight: Body mass index tables.* www.nhlbi.nih.gov/guidelines/obesity/bmi_tbl.htm

TABLE 30–2 **Assigning Nursing Diagnoses to Behaviors Commonly Associated With Eating Disorders**	
BEHAVIORS	**NURSING DIAGNOSES**
Refusal to eat; abuse of laxatives, diuretics, and/or diet pills; loss of 15% of expected body weight; pale conjunctiva and mucous membranes; poor muscle tone; amenorrhea; poor skin turgor; electrolyte imbalances; hypothermia; bradycardia; hypotension; cardiac irregularities; edema	Imbalanced nutrition: Less than body requirements
Decreased fluid intake; abnormal fluid loss caused by self-induced vomiting; excessive use of laxatives, enemas, or diuretics; electrolyte imbalance; decreased urine output; increased urine concentration; elevated hematocrit; decreased blood pressure; increased pulse rate; dry skin; decreased skin turgor; weakness	Deficient fluid volume
Minimizes symptoms; unable to admit effect of disease on life pattern; does not perceive personal relevance of symptoms; does not perceive personal relevance of danger	Denial
Compulsive eating; excessive intake in relation to metabolic needs; sedentary lifestyle; weight 20% over ideal for height and frame; BMI of 30 or more	Obesity
Distorted body image; views self as fat, even in the presence of normal body weight or severe emaciation; denies that problem with low body weight exists; difficulty accepting positive reinforcement; self-destructive behavior (self-induced vomiting, abuse of laxatives or diuretics, refusal to eat); preoccupation with appearance and how others perceive it *(anorexia nervosa, bulimia nervosa)* Verbalization of negative feelings about the way they look and the desire to lose weight *(obesity)* Lack of eye contact; depressed mood *(all)*	Disturbed body image/low self-esteem
Increased tension; increased helplessness; overexcited; apprehensive; fearful; restlessness; poor eye contact; increased difficulty taking oral nourishment; inability to learn	Anxiety (moderate to severe)

■ Has established a healthy pattern of eating for weight control, and weight loss toward a desired goal is progressing (BED)
■ Verbalizes plans for maintenance of weight control and relapse prevention (BED)

Planning and Implementation

In most instances, individuals with eating disorders are treated on an outpatient basis, but in some cases, hospitalization becomes necessary. Assessment findings that may necessitate hospitalization include the following:

■ **Malnutrition:** Individuals 20% below expected weight for height require inpatient treatment; those 30% below expected weight for height are recommended for long-term intensive hospital treatment (2 to 6 months) (Boland & Verduin, 2022)
■ **Dehydration:** Assessment includes thirst, orthostatic hypotension, tachycardia, elevated sodium levels, and other symptoms
■ **Severe electrolyte imbalance:** Potassium levels below 3 mmol/L, phosphate levels below 3 mg/dL, magnesium levels below 1.4 mEq/L, calcium below 7 mg/dL
■ **Cardiac arrhythmia:** ST segment and T wave changes usually related to electrolyte imbalances
■ **Severe bradycardia:** Below 50 beats per minute

■ **Hypothermia:** Body temperature below 96.8°F
■ **Hypotension:** A pattern of low blood pressure or orthostatic hypotension (20 mm Hg or greater drop in systolic blood pressure with positional changes and pulse rate increase by 20 or more beats)
■ **Suicidal ideation:** (see Chapter 16, "Suicide Prevention," for an in-depth discussion of suicide risk assessment)

In addition to the physical assessment parameters listed previously, when an eating disorder is suspected, a general assessment includes asking patients about their eating patterns and body image, their dieting patterns, whether or not they feel driven to be thin, exercise patterns, and any use of substances including diet pills, laxatives, or diuretics. Assess where the patient is getting information about weight loss, eating behaviors, and calorie restriction methods; several Web sites have been established that teach others how to starve themselves and avoid detection. Although the individual may not be forthcoming with this information, asking the parents about their child's use of Internet resources may reveal the need for close monitoring and restrictions on Internet use. Evidence of calluses on the dorsum of the hands, parotid enlargement, mouth ulcers, dental caries, and edema may also be assessment findings in the patient with purging behaviors.

Individuals with AN should be carefully assessed for infections because studies have found an increased risk of morbidity and mortality from infectious diseases in this population (DeSarbo & DeSarbo, 2020). Factors that can complicate this assessment include delayed fever response in patients with AN. Further similar changes in laboratory values (lower lymphocyte counts, elevated inflammatory cytokines and leukocyte counts, significantly decreased T-cell counts) occur in both AN and infectious disease processes like COVID-19, which could delay diagnosis and treatment (DeSarbo & DeSarbo, 2020).

The following section presents a group of selected nursing diagnoses, with short- and long-term goals and nursing interventions for each. Rationales for selected interventions are italicized.

Imbalanced Nutrition: Less Than Body Requirements/Deficient Fluid Volume (Risk for or Actual)

Imbalanced nutrition: less than body requirements is defined as "intake of nutrients insufficient to meet metabolic needs" (Herdman et al., 2021, p. 213). *Deficient fluid volume* is defined as "decreased intravascular, interstitial, and/or intracellular fluid" (p. 244). Table 30–3 presents these nursing diagnoses in care plan format.

Patient Goals

Outcome criteria include short- and long-term goals. Timelines are individually determined.

Short-term goals

■ The patient will gain (*x*) pounds per week (amount to be established by patient, nurse, and dietitian).
■ The patient will drink (*x*) milliliters of fluid each hour during waking hours.

Long-term goal

■ By time of discharge from treatment, the patient will exhibit no signs or symptoms of malnutrition or dehydration.

Interventions

■ For the patient who is emaciated and unable or unwilling to maintain an adequate oral intake, the physician may order a liquid diet to be administered via nasogastric tube. *Without adequate nutrition, a life-threatening situation exists.* Nursing care of the individual receiving tube feedings should

---

Table 30–3 | CARE PLAN FOR PATIENT WITH EATING DISORDERS: ANOREXIA NERVOSA AND BULIMIA NERVOSA

NURSING DIAGNOSES: IMBALANCED NUTRITION: LESS THAN BODY REQUIREMENTS/DEFICIENT FLUID VOLUME (RISK FOR OR ACTUAL)

RELATED TO: Refusal to eat/drink; self-induced vomiting; abuse of laxatives/diuretics

EVIDENCED BY: Loss of weight; poor muscle tone and skin turgor; lanugo; bradycardia; hypotension; cardiac arrhythmias; pale, dry mucous membranes

OUTCOME CRITERIA	NURSING INTERVENTIONS	RATIONALE
Short-Term Goals: ■ Patient will gain x pounds per week (amount to be established by patient, nurse, and dietitian) ■ Patient will drink x milliliters of fluid each hour during waking hours. **Long-Term Goal:** ■ By time of discharge from treatment, patient will exhibit no signs or symptoms of malnutrition or dehydration.	1. For the patient who is emaciated and is unable or unwilling to maintain an adequate oral intake, the physician may order a liquid diet to be administered via nasogastric tube. Nursing care of the individual receiving tube feedings should be administered according to established hospital protocol. 2. For the patient who is willing to consume an oral diet, collaborate with the dietitian to determine the number of calories and fluids required to provide adequate nutrition and realistic weight gain.	1. Without adequate nutrition, a life-threatening situation exists. 2. Adequate calories are required to allow a weight gain of 2–3 pounds per week.

Table 30–3 | CARE PLAN FOR PATIENT WITH EATING DISORDERS: ANOREXIA NERVOSA AND BULIMIA NERVOSA—cont'd

OUTCOME CRITERIA	NURSING INTERVENTIONS	RATIONALE
	3. Monitor laboratory values for phosphate, potassium, calcium, and magnesium while nutrition is being restored.	3. Refeeding syndrome, a series of negative intracellular electrolyte shifts associated with aggressive renourishment in a malnourished patient, poses a risk for hypophosphatemia, hypokalemia, hypocalcemia, and hypomagnesemia. Cardiovascular collapse, arrhythmias, altered mental status, and death can occur in untreated refeeding syndrome. Electrolyte supplementation may be indicated.
	4. Explain to the patient that privileges and restrictions will be based on compliance with treatment and direct weight gain. Do not focus on food and eating.	4. The real issues have little to do with food or eating patterns. Focus on the control issues that have precipitated these behaviors.
	5. Weigh patient daily (without the patient observing the numbers on the scale) immediately upon arising and after first voiding. Always use the same scale, if possible. Keep strict record of intake and output. Assess skin turgor and integrity regularly. Assess moisture and color of oral mucous membranes.	5. These assessments are important measurements of nutritional status and provide guidelines for treatment.
	6. Stay with patient during established time for meals (usually 30 minutes) and for at least 1 hour after meals.	6. Lengthy mealtimes put excessive focus on food and eating and provide patient with attention and reinforcement. The hour after meals may be used to discard food stashed from tray or to engage in self-induced vomiting.
	7. If weight loss occurs, enforce restrictions.	7. Restrictions and limits must be established and carried out consistently to avoid power struggles, to encourage patient compliance with therapy, and to ensure patient safety.
	8. Ensure that the patient and family understand that if nutritional status deteriorates, tube feedings will be initiated. Feeding should be implemented in a matter-of-fact, nonpunitive way.	8. This intervention is carried out for the patient's safety and protection from a life-threatening condition.
	9. Encourage the patient to explore and identify the true feelings and fears that contribute to maladaptive eating behaviors.	9. Emotional issues must be resolved if these maladaptive responses are to be eliminated.

be administered according to established hospital procedures.

■ For the patient who is willing to consume an oral diet, collaborate with the dietitian to determine the number of calories and fluids required to provide adequate nutrition and realistic weight gain.

■ Monitor laboratory values for phosphate, potassium, calcium, and magnesium while nutrition is being restored. **Refeeding syndrome,** *a series of negative intracellular electrolyte shifts associated with aggressive renourishment in a malnourished patient, poses a risk for hypophosphatemia, hypokalemia, hypocalcemia, and hypomagnesemia. Cardiovascular collapse, arrhythmias, altered mental status, and death can occur in individuals with untreated refeeding syndrome.* Electrolyte supplementation may be indicated (Toulany & Katzman, 2022).

■ Explain the program of behavior modification to patient and family. Explain that privileges and restrictions will be based on compliance with treatment and direct weight gain.

■ Do not focus on food and eating specifically. Instead, focus on the emotional issues that have precipitated these behaviors.

■ Do not discuss food or eating with the patient once the treatment protocol has been established. Do, however, offer support and positive reinforcement for obvious improvements in eating behaviors.

■ Keep a strict record of intake and output. Weigh the patient daily immediately on arising and after first voiding. Always use the same scale, if possible. Weighing a patient in such a way that the patient cannot see the numbers on a scale may be beneficial in reducing their focus on daily weight fluctuations or evidence of weight gain.

■ Assess vital signs, including blood pressure with positional changes to evaluate for orthostatic hypotension, and pulse to evaluate for bradycardia. Bradycardia may be more pronounced at rest, so regular assessment during these times is especially important.

■ Assess skin turgor and integrity regularly. Assess moisture and color of oral mucous membranes. *The condition of the skin and mucous membranes provides valuable data regarding patient hydration.* Discourage the patient from bathing every day if the skin is very dry.

■ Sit with the patient during mealtimes for support and to observe the amount ingested. A limit (usually 30 minutes) should be imposed on the time allotted for meals. *Without a time limit, meals can become lengthy, drawn-out sessions, providing the patient with attention based on food and eating.*

■ The patient should be observed for at least 1 hour after meals. *The patient may use this time to discard food that has been stashed from the food tray or to engage in self-induced vomiting. They may need to be accompanied to the bathroom if self-induced vomiting is suspected.*

■ If weight loss occurs, enforce restrictions. *Restrictions and limits must be established and carried out consistently to avoid power struggles and encourage patient compliance with therapy.*

■ Ensure that the patient and family understand that if nutritional status deteriorates, tube feedings will be initiated. The possibility of nasogastric feeding should be explained in a matter-of-fact, nonpunitive way as a necessity for the patient's safety and protection from a life-threatening condition.

■ Encourage the patient to explore and identify the true feelings and fears that contribute to maladaptive eating behaviors. *Emotional issues must be resolved if these maladaptive responses are to be eliminated.*

Denial

Denial is defined as a "conscious or unconscious attempt to disavow the knowledge or meaning of an event to reduce anxiety and/or fear, leading to the detriment of health" (Herdman et al., 2021, p. 418).

Patient Goals

Outcome criteria include short- and long-term goals. Timelines are individually determined.

Short-term goal

■ The patient will verbalize understanding of the correlation between emotional issues and maladaptive eating behaviors (within a time frame deemed appropriate for the individual patient).

Long-term goal

■ By time of discharge from treatment, the patient will display adaptive eating behaviors and will demonstrate an ability to cope with emotional issues in a more adaptive manner.

Interventions

■ Establish a trusting relationship with the patient by being honest, accepting, and available and by keeping all promises. Convey unconditional positive regard.

■ Acknowledge the patient's anger at feelings of loss of control caused by the established eating regimen associated with the program of behavior modification. *Anger is a normal human response and should be expressed appropriately. Feelings that are not expressed remain unresolved and may complicate an already serious situation.*

■ Avoid arguing or bargaining with the patient who is resistant to treatment. State matter-of-factly which behaviors are unacceptable and how privileges will be restricted for noncompliance. It is essential that all staff members are consistent with this intervention.

■ Encourage the patient to verbalize feelings regarding their role within the family and issues related to dependence and independence, the intense need for achievement, and sexuality. Help the patient recognize how maladaptive eating behaviors may be related to these emotional issues. Discuss ways in which they can gain control over these problematic areas of life without resorting to maladaptive eating behaviors.

Obesity

Obesity is defined as "a condition in which an individual accumulates abnormal or excessive fat for age and gender that exceeds overweight" (Herdman et al., 2021, p. 26).

Patient Goals

Outcome criteria include short- and long-term goals. Timelines are individually determined.

Short-term goal

■ Patient will verbalize understanding of what must be done to lose weight.

Long-term goal

■ Patient will demonstrate a change in eating patterns that results in a steady weight loss.

Interventions

■ Encourage the patient to keep a diary of food intake. *A food diary provides the opportunity for the patient to gain a realistic picture of the amount of food ingested and provides information that can be used to tailor a dietary program.*

■ Discuss feelings and emotions associated with eating. *These discussions help identify when the patient is eating to satisfy an emotional need rather than a physiological one.*

■ With input from the patient, formulate an eating plan that includes food from the required food groups with emphasis on low-fat intake. It is helpful to keep the plan as similar as possible to the patient's usual eating pattern. The diet must eliminate calories while maintaining adequate nutrition. *The patient is more likely to stay on the eating plan if they are able to participate in its creation and it deviates as little as possible from usual types of foods.*

■ Identify realistic incremental goals for weekly weight loss. Reasonable weight loss (1 to 2 pounds per week) results in more lasting effects. Excessive,

rapid weight loss may result in fatigue and irritability and ultimately lead to failure in meeting goals for weight loss. *Motivation is more easily sustained by meeting "stair-step" goals.*

■ Plan a progressive exercise program tailored to individual goals and choice. *Exercise may enhance weight loss by burning calories and reducing appetite, increasing energy, toning muscles, and enhancing a sense of well-being and accomplishment. Walking is an excellent choice for overweight individuals.*

■ Discuss the probability of reaching plateaus when weight remains stable for extended periods. *The patient should know that plateaus are likely to happen as changes in metabolism occur. Plateaus cause frustration, and the patient may need additional support during these times to remain on the weight-loss program.*

■ Provide instruction about medications to assist with weight loss if ordered by the physician. *Appetite-suppressant drugs and others that have weight loss as a side effect may be helpful to someone who is severely overweight. They should be used for this purpose for only a short period while the individual attempts to adjust to the new pattern of eating.*

Disturbed Body Image/Low Self-Esteem

Disturbed body image is defined as "negative mental picture of one's physical self" (Herdman et al., 2021, p. 355). *Low self-esteem* is defined as "negative perception of self-worth, self-acceptance, self-respect, competence, and attitude toward self" (p. 348).

Patient Goals (For the Patient With AN or BN)

Outcome criteria include short- and long-term goals. Timelines are individually determined.

Short-term goal

■ The patient will verbally acknowledge misperception of body image as "fat" within specified time (depending on severity and chronicity of condition).

Long-term goal

■ By the time of discharge from treatment, the patient will demonstrate an increase in self-esteem as manifested by verbalizing positive aspects of self and exhibiting less preoccupation with own appearance as a more realistic body image is developed.

Patient Goals (For the Patient With BED and Associated Obesity)

Outcome criteria include short- and long-term goals. Timelines are individually determined.

Short-term goal

■ The patient will begin to accept self based on personal attributes rather than on appearance.

Long-term goal

■ The patient will pursue loss of weight as desired.

Interventions

For the patient with AN or BN:

■ Assess the patient for history of trauma (adverse childhood experiences). *Awareness of trauma history is essential to providing trauma-informed care.*

■ Help the patient develop a realistic perception of body image and relationship with food. Compare specific measurements of the patient's body with the patient's perceived calculations. *There may be a large discrepancy between the actual body size and the patient's perception of their body size. The patient needs to recognize that the misperception of body image is unhealthy and that maintaining control through maladaptive eating behaviors is dangerous—even life-threatening.*

■ Promote feelings of control within the environment through participation and independent decision making. Through positive feedback, help the patient learn to accept self as is, including weaknesses as well as strengths. *The patient must come to understand that they are a capable, autonomous individual who can perform outside the family unit and is not expected to be perfect. Control of the patient's life must be achieved in other ways besides dieting and weight loss.*

■ Help the patient realize that perfection is unrealistic and explore this need with them. *As the patient begins to feel better about self, identifies positive self-attributes, and develops the ability to accept certain personal inadequacies, the need for unrealistic achievement should diminish.*

For the patient with BED and associated obesity:

■ Assess the patient's feelings and attitudes about overeating and obesity. *Obesity and compulsive eating behaviors may have deep-rooted psychological implications, such as compensation for lack of love and nurturing or a defense against intimacy.*

■ Ensure that the patient has privacy during self-care activities. *The obese individual may be sensitive or self-conscious about their body.*

■ Have the patient recall coping patterns related to food in the family of origin, and explore how these patterns may affect the current situation. *Parents are role models for their children. Maladaptive eating behaviors may have been learned within the family system and are supported through positive reinforcement. The parent may substitute food for affection and love, and eating is associated with a feeling of satisfaction, becoming the primary defense.*

■ Determine the patient's motivation for developing healthier patterns of eating. *The individual may harbor repressed feelings of hostility that may be expressed inwardly on the self. Because of a poor self-concept, the person often has difficulty with relationships. When the motivation is to lose weight for someone else, healthier eating is less likely to be sustainable.*

■ Help the patient identify positive self-attributes. Focus on strengths and past accomplishments unrelated to physical appearance. It is important that self-esteem not be tied solely to body size. *The patient needs to recognize that obesity need not interfere with positive feelings regarding self-concept and self-worth.*

■ Refer the patient to a support or therapy group. *Support groups can provide companionship, increase motivation, decrease loneliness and social ostracism, and give practical solutions to common problems. Group therapy can help the patient deal with underlying psychological concerns.*

Concept Care Mapping

The concept map care plan (see Chapter 8, "The Nursing Process in Psychiatric-Mental Health Nursing") is a diagrammatic teaching and learning strategy that allows visualization of interrelationships between medical diagnoses, nursing diagnoses, assessment data, and treatments. Examples of concept map care plans for patients with selected eating disorders are presented in Figures 30–1 and 30–2.

Patient and Family Education

The role of patient teacher is important in the psychiatric area, as it is in all areas of nursing. It is essential to include the family in education and treatment unless there are overriding reasons not to do so. A list of topics for patient and family education relevant to eating disorders is presented in Box 30–4.

Evaluation

Evaluation of the patient with an eating disorder requires a reassessment of the behaviors for which the patient sought treatment. Behavioral change will be required on the part of both the patient and family members. The following types of questions may provide assistance in gathering data required for evaluating the effectiveness of the nursing interventions in achieving the goals of therapy.

For the patient with AN or BN

Has the patient:

■ Steadily gained 2 to 3 pounds per week to at least 80% of expected body weight for age and size?

■ Demonstrated no signs and symptoms of malnutrition and dehydration?

■ Consistently consumed adequate calories as determined by the dietitian?

Clinical Vignette: Allie, age 18, graduated from high school 6 months ago. She is 5'10" tall and had frequently been teased by her peers because of her height. She lived in a rural community and was often ridiculed for her plan to become a model after graduation. But Allie was determined, and instead of going to college, she moved to New York City to pursue her dream. However, at the first modeling agency, she was told that she would never be accepted for modeling at her weight (140 pounds) and to come back when she had lost at least 15 pounds. She was devastated but steadfast in her determination to succeed. She cut her calories to 500 a day, exercised relentlessly, took over-the-counter laxatives and diuretics, and engaged in self-induced vomiting when she ate more than she felt she should. She became weak and chronically fatigued but persisted, until yesterday when she collapsed at the gym and the owner called 911. She was admitted to the psychiatric unit weighing 118 pounds, with poor skin turgor, blood pressure 75/45, and pulse 60 and irregular. She tells the nurse, "I can't be a model unless I get thin! Everyone at home will think I'm a failure!" The nurse develops the following concept map care plan for Allie.

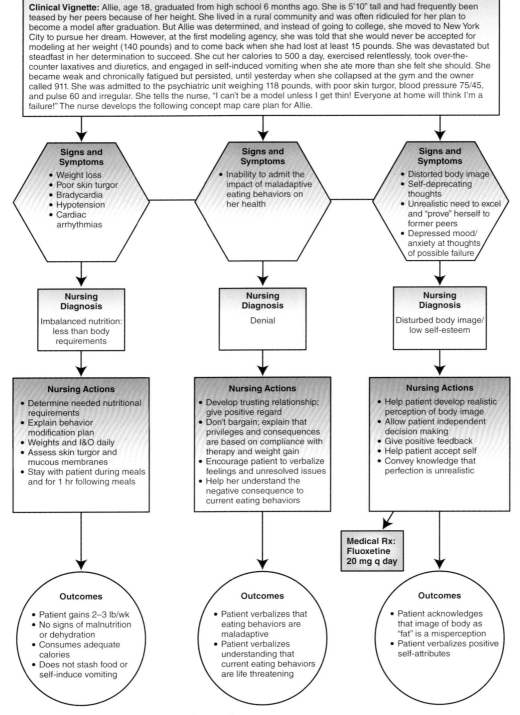

Signs and Symptoms
- Weight loss
- Poor skin turgor
- Bradycardia
- Hypotension
- Cardiac arrhythmias

Signs and Symptoms
- Inability to admit the impact of maladaptive eating behaviors on her health

Signs and Symptoms
- Distorted body image
- Self-deprecating thoughts
- Unrealistic need to excel and "prove" herself to former peers
- Depressed mood/anxiety at thoughts of possible failure

Nursing Diagnosis
Imbalanced nutrition: less than body requirements

Nursing Diagnosis
Denial

Nursing Diagnosis
Disturbed body image/low self-esteem

Nursing Actions
- Determine needed nutritional requirements
- Explain behavior modification plan
- Weights and I&O daily
- Assess skin turgor and mucous membranes
- Stay with patient during meals and for 1 hr following meals

Nursing Actions
- Develop trusting relationship; give positive regard
- Don't bargain; explain that privileges and consequences are based on compliance with therapy and weight gain
- Encourage patient to verbalize feelings and unresolved issues
- Help her understand the negative consequence to current eating behaviors

Nursing Actions
- Help patient develop realistic perception of body image
- Allow patient independent decision making
- Give positive feedback
- Help patient accept self
- Convey knowledge that perfection is unrealistic

Medical Rx: Fluoxetine 20 mg q day

Outcomes
- Patient gains 2–3 lb/wk
- No signs of malnutrition or dehydration
- Consumes adequate calories
- Does not stash food or self-induce vomiting

Outcomes
- Patient verbalizes that eating behaviors are maladaptive
- Patient verbalizes understanding that current eating behaviors are life threatening

Outcomes
- Patient acknowledges that image of body as "fat" is a misperception
- Patient verbalizes positive self-attributes

FIGURE 30–1   Concept map care plan for a patient with anorexia nervosa.

■ Attempted to stash food from the tray to discard later?

■ Attempted to self-induce vomiting?

■ Admitted that a problem exists and that eating behaviors are maladaptive?

■ Discontinued maladaptive behaviors to manipulate calorie restriction?

■ Discussed feelings related to family roles, sexuality, dependence/independence, and the need for achievement?

■ Verbalized understanding of how the use of maladaptive eating behaviors was an effort to achieve a feeling of some control over life events?

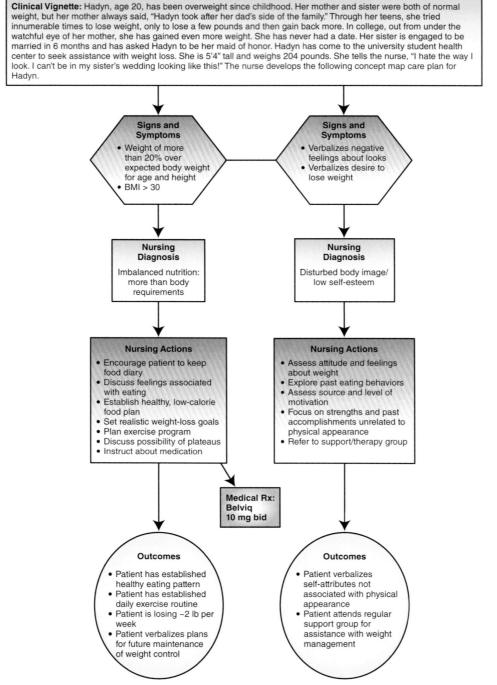

Clinical Vignette: Hadyn, age 20, has been overweight since childhood. Her mother and sister were both of normal weight, but her mother always said, "Hadyn took after her dad's side of the family." Through her teens, she tried innumerable times to lose weight, only to lose a few pounds and then gain back more. In college, out from under the watchful eye of her mother, she has gained even more weight. She has never had a date. Her sister is engaged to be married in 6 months and has asked Hadyn to be her maid of honor. Hadyn has come to the university student health center to seek assistance with weight loss. She is 5'4" tall and weighs 204 pounds. She tells the nurse, "I hate the way I look. I can't be in my sister's wedding looking like this!" The nurse develops the following concept map care plan for Hadyn.

Signs and Symptoms
• Weight of more than 20% over expected body weight for age and height
• BMI > 30

Signs and Symptoms
• Verbalizes negative feelings about looks
• Verbalizes desire to lose weight

Nursing Diagnosis
Imbalanced nutrition: more than body requirements

Nursing Diagnosis
Disturbed body image/ low self-esteem

Nursing Actions
• Encourage patient to keep food diary
• Discuss feelings associated with eating
• Establish healthy, low-calorie food plan
• Set realistic weight-loss goals
• Plan exercise program
• Discuss possibility of plateaus
• Instruct about medication

Nursing Actions
• Assess attitude and feelings about weight
• Explore past eating behaviors
• Assess source and level of motivation
• Focus on strengths and past accomplishments unrelated to physical appearance
• Refer to support/therapy group

Medical Rx:
Belviq
10 mg bid

Outcomes
• Patient has established healthy eating pattern
• Patient has established daily exercise routine
• Patient is losing ~2 lb per week
• Patient verbalizes plans for future maintenance of weight control

Outcomes
• Patient verbalizes self-attributes not associated with physical appearance
• Patient attends regular support group for assistance with weight management

FIGURE 30–2 Concept map care plan for a patient with obesity.

■ Acknowledged that perception of body image as "fat" is incorrect?

For the patient with BED and associated obesity

Has the patient:

■ Shown a steady weight loss since starting the new eating plan?
■ Verbalized a relapse prevention plan to avoid triggers and abstain from binging?

■ Verbalized positive self-attributes not associated with body size or appearance?

For the patient with AN, BN, or BED and associated obesity

Has the patient:

■ Developed a more realistic perception of body image?
■ Acknowledged that past self-expectations may have been unrealistic?

BOX 30–4 Topics for Patient/Family Education Related to Eating Disorders

NATURE OF THE ILLNESS

1. Symptoms of anorexia nervosa
2. Symptoms of bulimia nervosa
3. Symptoms of binge-eating disorder
4. What constitutes obesity
5. Causes of eating disorders
6. Effects of the illness or condition on the body
7. Behaviors that may reinforce unhealthy responses such as television and social media, peer focus on clothing sizes, eating, and weight. Internet sources have become a means for sharing information among people with anorexia about how the individual can distract parents and health-care providers from recognizing the extent of weight loss. Family members can learn more about some of these behaviors to look out for and may want to monitor their child's use of Internet and social media resources.

MANAGEMENT OF THE ILLNESS

1. Principles of nutrition (foods for maintenance of wellness)
2. Ways patient may feel in control of life (aside from eating)
3. Importance of expressing fears and feelings, rather than holding them inside
4. Alternative coping strategies (to maladaptive eating behaviors)
5. For the obese patient with obesity:
   a. How to plan a reduced-calorie, nutritious diet
   b. How to read food content labels
   c. How to establish a realistic weight loss plan
   d. How to establish a planned program of physical activity
6. Correct administration of prescribed medications
7. Indication for and side effects of prescribed medications
8. Relaxation techniques
9. Problem-solving skills
10. Discuss the Maudsley approach for treatment of anorexia nervosa as an evidence-based option for family involvement in the recovery program

SUPPORT SERVICES

1. Weight Watchers International (WW)
   www.weightwatchers.com
2. Overeaters Anonymous
   oa.org
3. National Association of Anorexia Nervosa and Associated Disorders (ANAD)
   (630) 577-1330 (helpline)
   www.anad.org
4. National Eating Disorders Association
   www.nationaleatingdisorders.org
5. National Association for Males With Eating Disorders
   (In 2019, this organization merged with NEDA)
   https://www.nationaleatingdisorders.org

■ Verbalized improvement in self-acceptance?
■ Developed adaptive coping strategies to deal with stress without resorting to maladaptive eating behaviors?

Treatment Modalities

The immediate aim of treatment in eating disorders is to restore the individual's nutritional status. Ideally, treatment of eating disorders occurs outside of the hospital setting, but hospitalization may be necessary if the condition becomes life-threatening. Complications of emaciation, dehydration, and electrolyte imbalance can lead to death. Electrolytes should be monitored daily for the first week after initiation of nutritional rehabilitation and refeeding because the greatest risk for refeeding syndrome occurs during this time (Toulany & Katzman, 2022). Once the physical condition is no longer life-threatening, other treatment modalities may be initiated.

Behavior Modification

Psychological interventions to change the maladaptive eating behaviors of clients with AN and BN have become the widely accepted treatment. Behavior modification approaches are designed to ensure that the program does not "control" the client. Issues of control are central in these disorders, so for the program to be successful, the client must be engaged in the treatment.

Successes have been observed when the client with AN is allowed to contract for privileges based on weight gain. The client has input into the care plan and can clearly see what the treatment choices are. The client has control over eating, the amount of exercise pursued, and even whether or not to induce vomiting. Goals of therapy, along with the responsibilities of each for goal achievement, are agreed on by client and staff.

Staff and client also agree on a system of rewards and privileges that can be earned by the client, who is given ultimate control. The individual has a choice of whether or not to abide by the contract, whether or not to gain weight, and whether or not to earn the desired privilege.

This method of treatment gives a great deal of autonomy to the client. It must be understood, however, that these behavior modification techniques are helpful for weight restoration only. Adjunctive individual psychotherapy and family psychoeducation may be required to prevent or reduce further morbidity.

Cognitive behavior therapy (CBT) and dialectical behavior therapy (DBT) have demonstrated benefits in clients with anorexia, bulimia, and BEDs (de Jong et al; 2018; Wisniewski & Ben-Porath, 2015). By confronting irrational thinking patterns and associated feelings, CBT and DBT strive to eliminate the emotional components associated with unhealthy eating patterns. Enhanced CBT (CBT-E), a form of CBT specifically for the treatment of eating disorders, has demonstrated benefits in both reducing psychopathology and improving BMI (Dalle Grave et al., 2019)

Family Treatment: The Maudsley Approach

The Maudsley approach is an evidence-based, family-centered program for the treatment of adolescents with AN that modifies the traditional concept of the adolescent being in control of their calorie intake. This approach actively involves the family in each step of the process. Available evidence supports the use of family-based treatment as the first line of outpatient psychological treatment for adolescents with AN (Toulany & Katzman, 2022). Evidence also supports family-based programs in the treatment of BN (Rienecke et al., 2017).

The treatment program is conducted in an intensive outpatient program and involves three phases of treatment. Phase I is focused on weight restoration, and in this phase the parents are actively engaged in establishing the rules and guidelines around eating. Parents often need substantial support during this phase because they typically encounter frequent power struggles with their child. When the client accepts parental demands for increased food intake, demonstrates steady weight gain, and there is a change in the mood of the family (e.g., relief at having taken charge of the eating disorder; both adolescents and their parents identify reduced anxiety), phase II is ready to begin (LeGrange & Lock, n.d.). In this phase, control of maintaining weight gain is returned to the adolescent. Once the client demonstrates the ability to maintain greater than 95% of ideal weight, the shift to phase III focuses on assisting the adolescent to develop a healthy self-identity. This includes incorporating CBT and DBT skills, which have demonstrated effectiveness in treating this condition.

A newer, modified version of the Maudsley approach (Maudsley Model of Anorexia Nervosa Treatment for Adults [MANTRA]), designed for treatment of adults through a manualized treatment program, incorporates principles of CBT, writing tasks to support developing emotional regulation skills, and motivational interviewing to engage the client's willingness to change. Significant others participate in some treatment sessions to discuss any associated conflicts as well as identify strategies for supporting the client in their recovery. Studies have supported stable benefits in improving eating disorder psychopathology and BMI as well as low dropout rates (Wittek et al., 2021).

Individual Therapy

Although individual psychotherapy is not the therapy of choice for eating disorders, it may be an adjunct to a comprehensive, multifaceted treatment approach when underlying comorbid psychological problems are contributing to the maladaptive behaviors. In supportive psychotherapy, the therapist encourages the client to explore unresolved conflicts and recognize the maladaptive eating behaviors as defense mechanisms to ease emotional pain. The goals are to resolve personal issues and establish more adaptive coping strategies for dealing with stressful situations.

Psychopharmacology

Research has not yet identified a medication that results in a definitive improvement of AN (Boland & Verduin, 2022). As previously mentioned, SSRIs (particularly fluoxetine) have demonstrated benefits in treating BN but not AN. SSRIs may be beneficial in the treatment of comorbid depression, but they also carry a boxed warning about risk of increasing suicide ideation in adolescents. The anticholinergic side effects of tricyclic antidepressants, including orthostatic hypotension, may be problematic for patients who are already at risk for these symptoms. It is important to recognize that depression and other mood and cognitive symptoms can be a sign of malnutrition and starvation. When nutrition is restored, those symptoms often improve.

Use of antidepressants (particularly fluoxetine) in the treatment of BN appears to have benefits for patients with and without depressive symptoms. It is possible that fluoxetine, an SSRI, may decrease the craving for carbohydrates, thereby decreasing the incidence of binge eating, which is often associated with consumption of large amounts of carbohydrates. A dosage of 60 mg to 80 mg/day (the usual antidepressant dosage) may be required. Other SSRIs, tricyclic antidepressants (particularly amitriptyline and desipramine), trazodone, and monoamine oxidase inhibitors may also be helpful (Boland & Verduin, 2022).

High-dose SSRIs have demonstrated some effectiveness in promoting weight loss for those with BED, but the weight loss was temporary (Boland & Verduin, 2022). Remember, too, that weight gain is a secondary symptom of BED. An effective medication needs to also manage the symptom of binging. Two medications, topiramate (and a combination medication of topiramate with phentermine) and lisdexamfetamine (a dopamine-norepinephrine reuptake inhibitor, originally used in the treatment of attention deficit-hyperactivity disorder) have demonstrated benefits in reducing both incidents of binge eating and weight gain in obese patients with BED (Levitan et al., 2021). Currently, lisdexamfetamine (Vyvanse) has been approved by the U.S. Food and Drug Administration (FDA) specifically for short-term treatment of BED. Most studies reveal that medication in combination with CBT is more beneficial than medication alone (Boland & Verduin, 2022). Two FDA-approved combination drugs for treatment of obesity include Qsymia (phentermine [an amphetamine-like drug] and topiramate), approved for chronic weight management in obese patients over the age of 12, and Contrave (naltrexone and bupropion). Historically, amphetamines were commonly prescribed for weight loss and are still currently prescribed with great caution, but they are less favored because of their potential for dependence, addiction, and illegal diversion on the street market.

CLINICAL JUDGMENT IN ACTION: CASE STUDY AND SAMPLE CARE PLAN

NURSING HISTORY AND ASSESSMENT

Recognizing cues: The nurse must demonstrate ability to recognize what information is most important to making an assessment (National Council of State Boards of Nursing [NCSBN], 2021).

This information is italicized in the following.

When Katie **fainted** in history class, she was taken to the university health center by her roommate, Ashley. Ashley told the nurse that Katie has been **taking a lot of over-the-counter laxatives and diuretics.** She also said that Katie often **self-induced vomiting when she felt that she had eaten too much.** After an initial physical assessment, the nurse in the university health center referred Katie to the mental health clinic.

At the mental health clinic, Katie **weighed 110 pounds and measured 5 feet 6 inches tall.** She admitted to the psychiatric nurse that she tried to keep her weight down by dieting, but sometimes she **got so hungry that she would overeat, and then she felt the need to self-induce vomiting to get rid of the calories.** "I really don't like doing it, but lots of the girls do. In fact, that is where I got the idea. I always thought I was too fat in high school, but the competition wasn't so great there. Here all the girls are so pretty—and so thin! It's the only way I can keep my weight down!"

Katie also admitted that she **hoards food** in her dorm room and that she **eats when she is feeling particularly anxious and depressed** (often during the night). She **admitted to having eaten several bags of potato chips and whole packages of cookies in a single sitting.** She sometimes drives to the local hamburger stand in the middle of the night, orders several hamburgers, fries, and milkshakes, and consumes them as she sits in her car alone. She stated that she feels so much better while she is eating these foods but then feels panicky after they have been consumed. That is when she self-induces vomiting. "Then I feel **more depressed, and the only thing that helps is eating! I feel so out of control!**"

Analyzing cues: The nurse must be able to interpret the information (NCSBN, 2021).

The nurse interprets that Katie is underweight but has developed a pattern of binging and purging related to anxiety and depression and she expresses feeling out of control.

Prioritize hypotheses: The nurse must be able to identify the client's most important needs (NCSBN, 2021).

Continued

CLINICAL JUDGMENT IN ACTION: CASE STUDY AND SAMPLE CARE PLAN—cont'd

The nurse, having ruled out the need for immediate nutritional support and based on Katie's reports of feeling out of control, collaborates with Katie to prioritize working on developing more adaptive coping strategies.

NURSING DIAGNOSES AND OUTCOME IDENTIFICATION

Generate solutions: The nurse must be able to connect their prioritized understanding of client needs to a course of action or plan of care (NCSBN, 2021).

From the assessment data, the nurse develops the following nursing diagnosis for Katie:

1. Ineffective coping related to feelings of helplessness, low self-esteem, and lack of control in life situation
   a. Short-term goal:
      ■ Patient will identify and discuss fears and anxieties with the nurse.
   b. Long-term goal:
      ■ Patient will identify adaptive coping strategies that can be realistically incorporated into her lifestyle, thereby eliminating binging and purging in response to anxiety.

PLANNING AND IMPLEMENTATION

Take Action: The nurse must be able to identify what actions need to be taken and how they will be implemented (NCSBN, 2021).

INEFFECTIVE COPING

The following nursing interventions have been identified for Katie.

1. Establish a trusting relationship with Katie. Be honest and accepting. Show unconditional positive regard.
2. Help Katie identify the situations that produce anxiety and discuss how she coped with these situations before she began binging and purging.
3. Help Katie identify the emotions that precipitate binging (e.g., fear, boredom, anger, loneliness).
4. Once these high-risk situations have been identified, help her identify alternate behaviors, such as exercise, a hobby, or a warm bath.
5. Encourage Katie to express feelings that have been suppressed because they were considered unacceptable. Help her identify healthier ways to express those feelings.
6. Use role-play with Katie to deal with feelings and experiment with new behaviors.
7. Explore the dynamics of Katie's family and encourage family involvement for support with Katie's consent.
8. Teach the concepts of good nutrition and the importance of healthy eating patterns in overall wellness.
9. Consult with the physician about a prescription for fluoxetine for Katie.
10. Help Katie find a support group for individuals with eating disorders. Encourage regular attendance in this group.

EVALUATION

Evaluate outcomes: The nurse must be able to evaluate actions taken and determine whether they have had a positive, neutral, or negative effect (NCSBN, 2021).

The outcome criteria for Katie have been met. She discussed with the nurse the feelings that triggered binging episodes and the situations that precipitated those feelings. She has joined a support group of individuals with eating disorders and now has a "buddy" who she may call (even in the middle of the night) when she is feeling like binging. She has started riding her bicycle regularly and goes to the fitness center when she is feeling especially anxious. She still sees the mental health nurse weekly and continues to discuss her fears and anxieties. The urges to binge at stressful times have not disappeared completely. However, they have decreased in frequency, and Katie is now able to choose more adaptive strategies for dealing with stress.

Summary and Key Points

- The incidence of eating disorders has continued to increase since the middle of the 20th century.
- Individuals with anorexia nervosa (AN), a disorder characterized by a morbid fear of obesity and a gross distortion of body image, literally can starve themselves to death.
- The individual with AN believes they are fat even when emaciated. The disorder is commonly accompanied by depression and anxiety.
- Bulimia nervosa (BN) is an eating disorder characterized by the consumption of large amounts of food, usually in a short period of time, and often in secret.
- With BN, tension is relieved and pleasure felt during the time of the binge, but these feelings are soon followed by guilt and depression.
- Individuals with BN "purge" themselves of the excessive intake with self-induced vomiting or the misuse of laxatives, diuretics, or enemas. They are also at risk for mood and anxiety disorders.

■ Binge-eating disorder (BED) is characterized by the consumption of large amounts of food by an individual who feels a lack of control over the eating behavior. It differs from bulimia nervosa in that the individual does not engage in behaviors to rid the body of the excess calories.

■ Compulsive eating can result in obesity, which is defined by the National Institutes of Health as a BMI of 30 or more.

■ Predisposing factors to eating disorders include genetics, physiological factors, family dynamics, and environmental and lifestyle factors.

■ Patients presenting with symptoms of any eating disorder should be assessed for history of trauma and adverse childhood experiences in order to provide trauma-informed care.

■ Treatment modalities for eating disorders include behavior modification, individual psychotherapy, cognitive behavior therapy, family treatment (such as the Maudsley approach), and psychopharmacology.

■ Refeeding syndrome, a potential outcome of aggressive nutritional restoration in malnourished clients, is associated with hypophosphatemia, hypokalemia, hypocalcemia, and hypomagnesemia. These electrolyte imbalances can result in cardiac arrhythmias, cardiovascular collapse, delirium, and death.

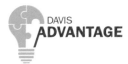 **DAVIS ADVANTAGE**   Go to **Davis Advantage** to complete your learning: strengthen understanding, apply your knowledge, and prepare for the Next Gen NCLEX®.

Review Questions

1. Some individuals with obesity take amphetamines to suppress appetite and help them lose weight. Which of the following is an adverse effect associated with the use of amphetamines that makes this practice undesirable?
   a. Bradycardia
   b. Amenorrhea
   c. Tolerance
   d. Convulsions

2. The Maudsley approach to treatment of adolescents with anorexia nervosa advances which of the following fundamental concepts?
   a. The patient's family should be actively involved in each phase of treatment.
   b. Parents should be prohibited from involvement in helping their child eat because there are often control issues.
   c. Adolescents need to work on developing healthy self-identities before they can begin to gain weight.
   d. Individual psychotherapy is the most effective treatment for adolescents with anorexia nervosa.

3. A client has sought help for their concern that they are binge eating and feels like it has "gotten out of control." The client asks the nurse what can be done to help them. Which of the following is the most accurate response?
   a. "Nothing can be done."
   b. "Some medications and psychological treatments have demonstrated effectiveness in reducing binge-eating behaviors."
   c. "The primary problem is obesity. I can help you set up a calorie-restricted diet."
   d. "Medications can help with weight loss, but there are no medications effective for reducing binge eating."

4. Which of the following physical manifestations would you expect to assess in a client suffering from anorexia nervosa?
   a. Tachycardia, hypertension, hyperthermia
   b. Bradycardia, hypertension, hyperthermia
   c. Bradycardia, hypotension, hypothermia
   d. Tachycardia, hypotension, hypothermia

5. Which medication has been used with some success in clients with bulimia nervosa?
   a. Lorcaserin (Belviq)
   b. Diazepam (Valium)
   c. Fluoxetine (Prozac)
   d. Carbamazepine (Tegretol)

6. A client is hospitalized on the psychiatric unit with a history and current diagnosis of bulimia nervosa. Which of the following symptoms would be congruent with this client's diagnosis?
   a. Binging, purging, obesity, hyperkalemia
   b. Binging, purging, normal weight, hypokalemia
   c. Binging, laxative abuse, amenorrhea, severe weight loss
   d. Binging, purging, severe weight loss, hyperkalemia

Clinical Judgment Questions

7. A 14-year-old client has just been admitted to the psychiatric unit for anorexia nervosa. The individual is emaciated and refusing to eat. What is the priority nursing diagnosis for this client?
   a. Maladaptive grieving
   b. Imbalanced nutrition: Less than body requirements.
   c. Interrupted family processes
   d. Anxiety (severe)

8. The nurse is caring for a client who has been hospitalized with anorexia nervosa and is severely malnourished. The client continues to refuse to eat. What is the most appropriate response by the nurse?
   a. "You know that if you don't eat, you will die."
   b. "If you continue to refuse to take food orally, you will be fed through a nasogastric tube."
   c. "You might as well leave if you are not going to follow your therapy regimen."
   d. "You don't have to eat if you don't want to. It is your choice."

9. A hospitalized client with bulimia nervosa is discussing their need to vomit and tells the nurse they are afraid they will gain weight. Which is the most appropriate response by the nurse?
   a. "Don't worry. The dietitian will ensure you don't get too many calories in your diet."
   b. "Don't worry about your weight. We are going to work on other problems while you are in the hospital."
   c. "I understand that you are concerned about your weight, and we will talk about the importance of good nutrition, but for now I want you to tell me about your recent invitation to join the National Honor Society. That's quite an accomplishment."
   d. "You are not fat, and the staff will ensure that you do not gain weight while you are in the hospital, because we know that is important to you."

10. A client presents in the emergency department with complaints of suicidal ideation. The following information is collected by the nurse. Which of these assessment findings suggests that bulimia nervosa might be a health problem? (Select all that apply.)
    a. Parotid glands appear enlarged.
    b. Teeth have a "moth-eaten" pattern of tooth decay.
    c. Client reports taking laxatives daily.
    d. Client's weight is within the expected range.

IMPLICATIONS OF RESEARCH FOR EVIDENCE-BASED PRACTICE

Bryant, E., Spielman, K., Le, A., Marks, P., National Eating Disorder Research Consortium, Touyz, S., & Maguire, S. (2022). Screening, assessment and diagnosis in the eating disorders: Findings from a rapid review. *Journal of Eating Disorders, 10*(78), 1–16. https://doi.org/10.1186/s40337-022-00597-8

DESCRIPTION OF THE STUDY: The authors conducted a review of literature (87 studies) to identify gaps in screening, assessment, and diagnosis of eating disorders.

RESULTS OF THE STUDY: The authors found that screening studies showed a high prevalence of screening but only modest improvements in help-seeking among those studies that followed up with individuals postscreening. In health-care settings, inadequate screening and detection of eating disorders was found to be compounded by self-stigma, and personal and health system barriers. In addition, although all groups are at risk of delayed or no diagnosis, those at particular risk include LGBTQ+ and gender diverse individuals, individuals with obesity, and males. The authors conclude that a majority of individuals with eating disorders remain undiagnosed and untreated despite a high prevalence of these conditions, and more research is needed to identify better screening and detection methods.

IMPLICATIONS FOR NURSING PRACTICE: The results of this study highlight the importance of identifying personal and health-care barriers to effective screening, detection, and treatment of the patient with an eating disorder. Nurses have an opportunity to use these findings to advocate for system and care delivery changes as well as conduct much-needed research to improve care for this population.

TEST YOUR CLINICAL REASONING AND CLINICAL JUDGMENT SKILLS

Janice, a high school sophomore, wanted desperately to become a cheerleader. She practiced endlessly before tryouts, but she was not selected. A week later, her boyfriend, Roy, broke up with her to date another girl. Janice, who was 5 feet 3 inches tall and, at that time, weighed 110 pounds, decided it was because she was too fat. She began to exercise at every possible moment. She skipped meals and tried to keep her daily consumption to no more than 300 calories. She lost a great deal of weight but became very weak. She felt cold all of the time and wore sweaters in the warm weather. She collapsed during her physical education class at school and was rushed to the emergency department. On admission, she weighed 90 pounds. She was emaciated and anemic. The physician admitted her with a diagnosis of anorexia nervosa.

Answer the following questions about Janice:

1. What will be the *primary* consideration in her care?
2. How will treatment be directed toward helping her gain weight?
3. How will the nurse know if Janice is using self-induced vomiting to rid herself of food consumed at meals?

Communication Exercises

1. Helena was admitted to the psychiatric unit with a diagnosis of severe anorexia nervosa. After completing a meal, she asks the nurse to be excused so she can use the restroom.

   How should the nurse respond to Helena's request?

2. John has been seeking counseling for a binge-eating disorder. When the nurse is weighing him, John states, "I hate myself. I should never have let myself get like this. I'm completely out of control."

   What would be the most empathic response by the nurse?

 ## MOVIE CONNECTIONS

The Best Little Girl in the World (AN) • *Kate's Secret* (BN) • *For the Love of Nancy* (AN) • *Super Size Me* (obesity) • *To the Bone* (AN) • *Sharing the Secret* (BN) • *Life Is Sweet* (BN)

References

American Academy for Eating Disorders. (2009). *Position statement: The role of the family in eating disorders.* https://www.aedweb.org/get-involved/advocacy/position-statements/role-of-the-family

American Psychiatric Association (APA). (2022). *Diagnostic and statistical manual of mental disorders, fifth edition, text revision (DSM-5-TR).* American Psychiatric Association.

Boland, R. & Verduin, M. L. (Eds.). (2022). *Kaplan & Sadock's synopsis of psychiatry* (12th ed.). Wolters Kluwer.

Bryant, E., Spielman, K., Le, A., Marks, P., National Eating Disorder Research Consortium, Touyz, S., & Maguire, S. (2022). Screening, assessment and diagnosis in the eating disorders: Findings from a rapid review. *Journal of Eating Disorders, 10*(78), 1–16. https://doi.org/10.1186/s40337-022-00597-8

Centers for Disease Control and Prevention (CDC). (2022). *Defining adult overweight and obesity.* www.cdc.gov/obesity/adult/index.html

Dalle Grave, R., Sartirana, M., & Calugi, S. (2019). Enhanced cognitive behavioral therapy for adolescents with anorexia nervosa: Outcomes and predictors of change in a real-world setting. *International Journal of Eating Disorders, 52*,1042–1046. doi:10.1002/eat.23122.

de Jong, M., Schoorl, M., & Hoek, H.W. (2018). Enhanced cognitive behavioural therapy for patients with eating disorders: a systematic review. *Current Opinion in Psychiatry, 31*(6), 436-444. doi: 10.1097/YCO.0000000000000452

DeSarbo, J. R., & DeSarbo, L. (2020). Anorexia nervosa and COVID-19. *Current Psychiatry, 19*(8), 23–27.

Frank, G. K. W. (2019). Neuroimaging and eating disorders. *Current Opinion in Psychiatry, 32*(6), 478–483. doi:10.1097/YCO.0000000000000544

Frank, G. K. W., Shott, M. E., Stoddard, J., Swindle, S., & Pryor, T. L. (2021). Reward processing across the eating disorders spectrum implicates body mass index and ventral striatal circuitry. *JAMA Psychiatry, 78*(10), 1123–1133. doi.org/10.1001/jamapsychiatry.2021.1580

Giordano, S. (2021). Secret hunger: The case of anorexia nervosa. *Topoi 40*, 545–554. https://doi.org/10.1007/s11245-020-09718-x

Groth, T., Hilsenroth, M., Boccio, D., & Gold, J. (2020). Relationship between trauma history and eating disorders in adolescents. *Journal of Childhood and Adolescent Trauma, 13*(4), 443–453. doi:10.1007/s40653-019-00275-z

Herdman, T. H., Kamitsuru, S., & Lopes, C. T. (Eds.). (2021). *NANDA-I, inc. nursing diagnoses: Definitions and classification, 2021–2023.* Thieme.

Kumar, N. (2021). *Eating disorders in men are not talked about enough — and they're on the rise.* https://www.healthline.com/health/eating-disorders/eating-disorders-in-men

LeGrange, D., & Lock, J. (n.d.). *Family based treatment of adolescent anorexia nervosa: The Maudsley approach.* www.maudsleyparents.org/whatismaudsley.html

Levitan, M. N., Papelbaum, M., Carta, M. G., Appolinario, J. C., & Nardi, A. E. (2021). Binge eating disorder: A 5-year retrospective study on experimental drugs. *Journal of Experimental Pharmacology, 13*, 33–47. https://doi.org/10.2147/JEP.S255376

Milano, W., & Capasso, A. (2019). Psychopharmacological options in the multidisciplinary and multidimensional treatment of eating disorders. *The Open Neurology Journal, 13*, 22–31. doi:10.2174/1874205X01913010022

National Council of State Boards of Nursing (NCSBN). (2021). *Next generation NCLEX®: Comparison between case studies and stand-alone items.* https://www.ncsbn.org/public-files/NGN_Fall21_English_Final.pdf

National Heart, Lung, and Blood Institute. (n.d.). *Aim for a healthy weight: Body mass index tables.* www.nhlbi.nih.gov/guidelines/obesity/bmi_tbl.htm

Pruccoli, J., Parmeggiani, A., Cordelli, D. M., & Lanari, M. (2021). The role of the noradrenergic system in eating disorders: A systematic review. *International Journal of Molecular Sciences, 22*, 11086. https://doi.org/10.3390/ijms222011086

Rienecke, R. D. (2017). Family based treatment of eating disorders in adolescents: Current insights. *Adolescent Health, Medicine and Therapeutics, 8*, 69–79. https://doi.org/10.2147/AHMT.S115775

Riva, G. (2016). Neurobiology of anorexia nervosa: Serotonin dysfunctions link self-starvation with body image disturbances through an impaired body memory. *Frontiers in Human Neuroscience, 24.* https://doi.org/10.3389/fnhum.2016.00600

Sangha, S., Oliffe, J. L., Kelly, M. T., & McCuaig, F. (2019). Eating disorders in males: How primary care providers can improve recognition, diagnosis, and treatment. *American Journal of Men's Health, 13*(3), 1557988319857424. doi:10.1177/1557988319857424

Serra, R., Di Nicolantonio, C., Di Febo, R., De Crescenzo, F., Vanderlinden, J., Vrieze, E., Bruffaerts, R., Loriedo, C., Pasquini, M., & Tarsitani, L. (2022). The transition from restrictive anorexia nervosa to binging and purging: A systematic review and meta-analysis. *Eating and Weight Disorders, 27*, 857–865. https://doi.org/10.1007/s40519-021-01226-0

Strumila, R., Nobile, B., Maimoun, L., Jaussent, I., Seneque, M., Thiebaut, S., Iceta, S., Dupuis-Maurin, K., Lefebvre, P., Courtet, P., Renard, E., & Guillaume, S. (2020). The implications of previous history of anorexia nervosa in patients with current bulimia nervosa: Alterations in daily functioning, decision-making, and bone status. *European Eating Disorders Review, 28*(1), 34–45.

Toulany, A., & Katzman, D. K. (2022). Restrictive anorexia nervosa. *Cancer Therapy Advisor.* https://www.cancertherapyadvisor.com/home/decision-support-in-medicine/pediatrics/restrictive-anorexia-nervosa/

Valbrun, L. P., & Zvonarev, V. (2020). The opioid system and food intake: Use of opiate antagonists in treatment of binge eating disorder and abnormal eating behavior. *The Journal of Clinical Medicine Research, 12*(2), 41–63. doi:https://doi.org/10.14740/jocmr4066

Wisniewski, L., & Ben-Porath, D. D. (2015). Dialectical behavior therapy and eating disorders: The use of contingency management procedures to manage dialectical dilemmas. *American Journal of Psychotherapy, 69*(2), 129–40. doi:10.1176/appi.psychotherapy.2015.69.2.129

Wittek, T., Truttmann, S., Zeiler, M., Philipp, J., Auer-Welsbach, E., Koubek, D., Ohmann, S., Werneck-Rohrer, S., Sackl-Pammer, P., Schöfbeck, G., Mairhofer, D., Kahlenberg, L., Schmidt, U., Karwautz, A. F. K., & Wagner, G. (2021). The Maudsley model of anorexia nervosa treatment for adolescents and young adults (MANTRa): A study protocol for a multicenter cohort study. *Journal of Eating Disorders, 9*(1), 33. doi:10.1186/s40337-021-00387-8

Personality Disorders

31

CORE CONCEPTS

Stress and Coping

Professionalism:
  Nursing process in
  the care of patients
  with personality
  disorders

Safety

Clinical Judgment

KEY TERMS

antisocial personality disorder

avoidant personality disorder

borderline personality disorder (BPD)

dependent personality disorder

histrionic personality disorder

narcissistic personality disorder

object constancy

obsessive-compulsive personality disorder

paranoid personality disorder

personality

schizoid personality disorder

schizotypal personality disorder

splitting

OBJECTIVES
After reading this chapter, the student will be able to:

1. Define *personality*.
2. Compare stages of personality development according to Sullivan, Erikson, and Mahler.
3. Identify various types of personality disorders.
4. Discuss historical and epidemiological statistics related to various personality disorders.
5. Describe symptomatology associated with borderline personality disorder and antisocial personality disorder and use these data in patient assessment.
6. Identify predisposing factors for borderline personality disorder and antisocial personality disorder.

7. Formulate nursing diagnoses and goals of care for patients with borderline personality disorder and antisocial personality disorder.
8. Describe appropriate nursing interventions for behaviors associated with borderline personality disorder and antisocial personality disorder.
9. Evaluate nursing care of patients with borderline personality disorder and antisocial personality disorder.
10. Discuss various modalities relevant to treatment of personality disorders.

CORE CONCEPT

Personality

Personality is defined as the totality of emotional and behavioral characteristics that are particular to a specific person and that remain somewhat stable and predictable over time.

The word *personality* is derived from the Greek term *persona*. It was originally used to describe the theatrical mask worn by some dramatic actors at the time. Over the years, it has lost its connotation of pretense and illusion and has come to represent the person behind the mask—the "real" person.

Personality *traits* may be defined as characteristics with which an individual is born or develops early in life. They influence the way the individual perceives and relates to the environment and are quite stable over time. Personality *disorders* occur when these traits deviate markedly from the expectations of the individual's culture, become pervasive and inflexible, contribute to maladaptive patterns of behavior or impairment in functioning, and lead to distress (American Psychiatric Association [APA], 2022). One of the most common symptoms occurring in personality disorders is disrupted interpersonal relationships. Other symptoms include cognitive and affective disturbances and difficulty with impulse control. Cognitive symptoms may appear more prominently in schizotypal and paranoid personality disorders. In borderline personality and antisocial personality disorders, interpersonal dysfunctions may be more prominent. Virtually all individuals exhibit some behaviors associated with

the various personality disorders from time to time. Boland & Verduin (2022) noted that personality disorders are characterized as *ego-syntonic* (the individual is not troubled by behavior that is maladaptive) and *alloplastic* (the individual tries to adapt by changing the environment rather than themselves). As previously stated, the diagnosis of personality disorder is made only when significant functional impairment occurs in response to these personality characteristics.

Personality development occurs in response to a number of biological and psychological influences. These variables include (but are not limited to) heredity, temperament, experiential learning, and social interaction. Functional brain imaging and person-centered analysis have confirmed a model for human temperaments and character traits that is consistent among people from various cultures (Cloninger & Svrakic, 2017) and rooted in biological underpinnings (Bierzynska et al., 2019). These advances provide a firmer foundation for treatment of personality disorders based on a thorough assessment that includes laboratory findings, mental status, and clinical history.

Many theorists have attempted to organize information about personality development. Most suggest that it occurs in an orderly, stepwise fashion. These stages overlap, however, as maturation occurs at different rates in different individuals. The theories of Sullivan (1953), Erikson (1963), and Mahler and associates (1975) are presented at length in online Chapter 38, "Theoretical Models of Personality Development." The stages of personality development according to these three theorists are compared in Table 31–1. It is important for the nurse

TABLE 31–1 **Comparison of Personality Development–Sullivan, Erikson, and Mahler**		
MAJOR DEVELOPMENTAL TASKS AND DESIGNATED AGES		
SULLIVAN	**ERIKSON**	**MAHLER**
BIRTH TO 2 YEARS		
Birth to 18 months: Relief from anxiety through oral gratification of needs	Birth to 18 months: To develop a basic trust in the mothering figure and be able to generalize it to others	Birth to 1 month: Fulfillment of basic needs for survival and comfort
		1 to 5 months: Developing awareness of external sources of need fulfillment
		5 to 10 months: Commencement of a primary recognition of separateness from the mothering figure
		10 to 16 months: Increased independence through locomotor functioning; increased sense of separateness of self

TABLE 31–1 Comparison of Personality Development–Sullivan, Erikson, and Mahler–cont'd		
MAJOR DEVELOPMENTAL TASKS AND DESIGNATED AGES		
SULLIVAN	**ERIKSON**	**MAHLER**
CHILDHOOD		
18 months to 6 years: Learning to experience a delay in personal gratification without undue anxiety	18 months to 3 years: To gain some self-control and independence within the environment	16 to 24 months: Acute awareness of separateness of self; learning to seek "emotional refueling" from mothering figure to maintain feeling of security
6 to 9 years: Learning to form satisfactory peer relationships	3 to 6 years: To develop a sense of purpose and the ability to initiate and direct own activities	24 to 36 months: Sense of separateness established; on the way to object constancy: able to internalize a sustained image of loved object/person when it is out of sight; resolution of separation anxiety
9 to 12 years: Learning to form satisfactory relationships with persons of the same gender; the initiation of feelings of affection for another person	6 to 12 years: To achieve a sense of self-confidence by learning, competing, performing successfully, and receiving recognition from significant others, peers, and acquaintances	
ADOLESCENCE		
12 to 14 years: Learning to form satisfactory relationships with persons of the opposite gender; developing a sense of identity	12 to 20 years: To integrate the tasks mastered in the previous stages into a secure sense of self	14 to 21 years: Establishing self-identity; experiences satisfying relationships; working to develop a lasting, intimate opposite-gender relationship
ADULTHOOD		
	20 to 30 years: To form an intense, lasting relationship or a commitment to another person, a cause, an institution, or a creative effort	
	30 to 65 years: To achieve the life goals established for oneself, while also considering the welfare of future generations	
	65 years to death To review one's life and derive meaning from both positive and negative events, while achieving a positive sense of self-worth. In late, older adulthood (80 years and beyond) an additional stage of development, *transcendence,* refers to a period in which one develops a broader sense of one's meaning and spirituality that transcends themselves.	

to understand "normal" personality development before learning what is considered maladaptive.

Historical and epidemiological aspects of personality disorders are discussed in this chapter. Predisposing factors that have been implicated in the etiology of personality disorders are presented. Symptomatology is explained to provide background knowledge for assessing clients with personality disorders.

Individuals with personality disorders as their primary diagnosis often are not treated in acute care settings. However, many patients with other psychiatric and medical diagnoses manifest symptoms of personality disorders. Nurses are likely to encounter patients with these personality characteristics in all healthcare settings.

Nurses working in *psychiatric* settings are likely to encounter patients with borderline and antisocial personality characteristics. The behavior of patients with borderline personality disorder (BPD) is usually unstable, and hospitalization is often required as a result of attempts at self-injury. The patient with antisocial personality disorder may enter psychiatric care as a result of judicially ordered evaluation. Psychiatric intervention may be an alternative to imprisonment for antisocial behavior if it is deemed potentially helpful.

Historical aspects and epidemiology of personality disorders are discussed in this chapter. Predisposing factors that have been implicated in the etiology of personality disorders are presented, and symptomatology is explained to provide background knowledge for assessing patients with personality disorders. Nursing care of patients with BPD or antisocial personality disorder is presented in this chapter in the context of the nursing process. Various medical treatment modalities for personality disorders are explored.

Historical Aspects

In 4th century BC, Hippocrates concluded that all disease resulted from an excess of or imbalance in four bodily humors: yellow bile, black bile, blood, and phlegm. Hippocrates identified four fundamental personality styles that he concluded stemmed from excesses in the four humors: the irritable and hostile choleric (yellow bile), the pessimistic melancholic (black bile), the overly optimistic and extraverted sanguine (blood), and the apathetic phlegmatic (phlegm).

In 1801, the medical profession first recognized that personality disorders, apart from psychosis, were cause for special concern with the realization that an individual can behave irrationally even when the powers of intellect are intact. Nineteenth-century psychiatrists embraced the term *moral insanity,* the concept of which defines what we know today as personality disorders.

Historically, individuals with personality disorders have been labeled as "bad" or "immoral" and as deviants in the range of normal personality dimensions. The events and sequences that result in pathology of the personality are complicated and difficult to unravel. Continued study is needed to facilitate understanding of this complex behavioral phenomenon.

A major difficulty for psychiatrists has been the classification of personality disorders. Ten specific types of personality disorders are identified in the *Diagnostic and Statistical Manual of Mental Disorders, Fifth Edition, Text Revision (DSM-5-TR)* (APA, 2022). The APA has proposed a new, complex diagnostic system to identify impairments in personality functioning specifically related to the dimensions of *self* and *interpersonal relations* and personality *trait domains and facets.* This system addresses symptoms that may differ not only among personality disorders but also among individuals with the same personality disorder. This trait-specific diagnostic methodology is described in the *DSM-5-TR* as an alternative approach to diagnosis of personality disorder and is recommended for further study.

The current diagnostic system classifies personality disorders into three clusters according to descriptions of personality traits. These include the following:

1. **Cluster A:** Behaviors described as odd or eccentric
   a. Paranoid personality disorder
   b. Schizoid personality disorder
   c. Schizotypal personality disorder
2. **Cluster B:** Behaviors described as dramatic, emotional, or erratic
   a. Antisocial personality disorder
   b. Borderline personality disorder
   c. Histrionic personality disorder
   d. Narcissistic personality disorder
3. **Cluster C:** Behaviors described as anxious or fearful
   a. Avoidant personality disorder
   b. Dependent personality disorder
   c. Obsessive-compulsive personality disorder

Types of Personality Disorders

Paranoid Personality Disorder
Definition and Epidemiology

Paranoid personality disorder is defined as a pattern of pervasive mistrust and suspiciousness of others, and misinterpretation of others' motives as malevolent (APA, 2022). This pattern begins by early adulthood and remains present in a variety of contexts. Prevalence has been estimated at 1% to 4% of the general population. Symptoms are generally mild but interfere with occupational and social functioning. The disorder is more common in men than in women.

Clinical Picture

Individuals with paranoid personality disorder are constantly on guard, hypervigilant, and ready for any real or imagined threat. They appear tense and irritable. They have developed a hard exterior and become immune or insensitive to the feelings of others. They avoid interactions with other people lest they are forced to relinquish some of their power. They always feel that others plan to take advantage of them and any perceived slights, injuries, or insults become long-held grudges.

They are extremely oversensitive and tend to misinterpret even minute cues within the environment, magnifying and distorting them into thoughts of trickery and deception. Because they trust no one, they are constantly "testing" the honesty of others. The suspicions are without sufficient evidence but remain as doubts about the loyalty of friends, family, and spouses. Their intimidating manner provokes exasperation and anger in those with whom they come in contact.

Individuals with paranoid personality disorder maintain their self-esteem by attributing their shortcomings to others. They do not accept responsibility for their behaviors and feelings and project this responsibility onto others. They are envious and hostile toward those who are highly successful and believe the only reason they are not as successful is that they have been treated unfairly. Any real or imagined threat can release hostility and anger fueled by animosities from the past. The desire for reprisal and vindication is so intense that a possible loss of control can result in aggression and violence. These outbursts are usually brief, and the paranoid person soon regains external control, rationalizes the behavior, and reconstructs the defenses central to their personality pattern.

Predisposing Factors

Research has indicated a possible hereditary link in paranoid personality disorder. Studies have revealed a higher incidence of paranoid personality disorder among relatives of individuals with schizophrenia than among control subjects (Boland & Verduin, 2022).

Psychological predisposing factors, as is the case with many personality disorders, include a history of childhood trauma, including neglect. People with paranoid personality disorder may have been subjected to parental antagonism and harassment. They learned to perceive the world as harsh and unkind, a place calling for protective vigilance and mistrust. They developed a "chip-on-the-shoulder" attitude and were met with many rebuffs and rejection from others. Anticipating humiliation and betrayal by others, they learned to defend themselves by attacking first.

Schizoid Personality Disorder
Definition and Epidemiology

Schizoid personality disorder is characterized primarily by a profound defect in the ability to form personal relationships, and individuals with this disorder are often seen by others as eccentric, isolated, aloof, or lonely. These individuals display a lifelong pattern of social withdrawal, and their discomfort with human interaction is apparent. The prevalence of schizoid personality disorder is difficult to determine because, as with many other personality disorders, it may go undiagnosed unless it is recognized when the individual seeks health care for other reasons. Estimates of its prevalence within the general population vary between 3% and 5%. Significant numbers of people with the disorder are never observed in a clinical setting. Diagnosis of this disorder is more common in men than in women.

Clinical Picture

People with schizoid personality disorder appear cold, aloof, and indifferent to others. They typically have a long-standing history of engaging in primarily solitary activities or engaging more with animals than people. They prefer to work in isolation and are unsociable, with little need or desire for emotional ties. They are able to invest enormous affective energy in intellectual pursuits. They may appear withdrawn, anxious, or uneasy in social situations and have difficulty being jovial. Their behavior and conversation exhibit little or no spontaneity and their affect is commonly bland and constricted.

The *DSM-5-TR* identifies schizoid personality disorder as a "pervasive pattern of detachment from social relationships and a restricted range of expression of emotions in interpersonal settings" (APA, 2022, p. 741).

Predisposing Factors

Although the role of heredity in the etiology of schizoid personality disorder is unclear, introversion appears to be a highly inheritable characteristic. It is more common in individuals with relatives who have schizophrenia or schizotypal personality disorder.

Psychosocially, the development of schizoid personality is probably influenced by early interactional patterns that the person found cold and unsatisfying. The childhoods of these individuals have often been characterized as bleak, cold, and lacking empathy and nurturing. A child brought up with this type of parenting may develop schizoid personality traits if that child possesses a temperamental disposition that is shy, anxious, and introverted.

Schizotypal Personality Disorder
Definition and Epidemiology

Individuals with **schizotypal personality disorder** present with behavior that is odd and eccentric but does not decompensate to the level of schizophrenia. Schizotypal personality is marked by symptoms that are closer to those of schizophrenia than those in schizoid personality and, as such, show significant peculiarities in thinking, behavior, and appearance. Studies indicate that schizotypal personality disorder has a prevalence of around 4%. Symptoms of depression and anxiety are common and often it is these symptoms that lead the individual to seek treatment (APA, 2022).

Clinical Picture

Individuals with schizotypal personality disorder are aloof and isolated and behave in a bland and apathetic manner. Magical thinking, ideas of reference, illusions, and depersonalization are part of their everyday world. Examples include superstitions; belief in clairvoyance, telepathy, or "sixth sense"; and beliefs that "others can feel my feelings."

Speech patterns are sometimes bizarre. People with this disorder often cannot orient their thoughts logically and become lost in personal irrelevancies and tangential asides that seem vague and digress from the topic at hand. This feature only further alienates them from others.

Individuals with schizotypal personality disorder are distinguished from those with schizophrenia by the absence of psychosis. Under stress, these individuals may decompensate and demonstrate psychotic symptoms, such as delusional thoughts, hallucinations, or bizarre behaviors, but they are usually of brief duration (Boland & Verduin, 2022). They often talk or gesture to themselves, as if "living in their own world." Their affect is bland or inappropriate, such as laughing at their own problems or at a situation that most people would consider sad.

Predisposing Factors

Evidence suggests that schizotypal personality disorder is more common among the first-degree biological relatives of people with schizophrenia than among the general population and, although a personality disorder, it is also included as one of the schizophrenia spectrum disorders in the *DSM-5-TR* (APA, 2022). Twin studies reveal a higher incidence in monozygotic twins than dizygotic twins (Boland & Verduin, 2022).

Psychological and environmental factors may also interact with genetic vulnerability in the development of schizotypal personality traits. For children who manifest with schizotypal personality traits, affective blandness, peculiar behaviors, and discomfort with interpersonal relationships may provoke other children to avoid relationships with them, or worse, engage in bullying, which reinforces their withdrawal from others. Having failed repeatedly to cope with these adversities, they withdraw and reduce contact with individuals and situations that evoked sadness and humiliation. Their new inner world provides them with a more significant and potentially rewarding existence than the one experienced in reality.

Antisocial Personality Disorder
Definition and Epidemiology

Antisocial personality disorder is a pattern of socially irresponsible, exploitative, and guiltless behavior that reflects a general disregard for the rights of others. Individuals with this disorder exploit and manipulate others for personal gain and are unconcerned with obeying the law. They have difficulty sustaining consistent employment and developing stable relationships. This personality disorder has been extensively studied and has been included in all editions of the *DSM*. In the United States, prevalence is estimated to be about 3.6% and the highest prevalence (greater than 70%) is among those with substance use disorders and those in prisons or other forensic settings (APA, 2022). It is more common in men than in women and may be higher in samples affected by poverty or sociocultural factors such as migration (APA, 2022). The *DSM-5-TR* currently identifies antisocial personality and psychopathy as synonymous terms, but other sources suggest that they are better understood as distinct disorders (Junewicz & Billick, 2021). Substance use disorder is commonly identified as a comorbid disorder.

Note: The clinical picture, predisposing factors, nursing diagnoses, and interventions for care of patients with antisocial personality disorder are presented later in this chapter.

Borderline Personality Disorder
Definition and Epidemiology

Borderline personality disorder (BPD) is characterized by a pattern of intense and chaotic relationships, with affective instability (emotional dysregulation) and fluctuating attitudes toward other people. Individuals with this disorder are impulsive, directly and indirectly self-destructive, and lack a clear sense of identity.

Prevalence of borderline personality is estimated at 1% to 2% of the population. Separation or divorce are common and intense fear of abandonment may lead to impulsive actions including self-mutilating or suicidal behaviors (APA, 2022). It is generally estimated to be more common in women than men, and more common in younger persons, suggesting a tendency toward maturation and remission (Boland & Verduin, 2022).

> **Note:** The clinical picture, predisposing factors, nursing diagnoses, and interventions for care of patients with BPD are presented later in this chapter.

Histrionic Personality Disorder

Definition and Epidemiology

Histrionic personality disorder is characterized by colorful, dramatic, and extroverted behavior in excitable, emotional people. They have difficulty maintaining long-lasting relationships, although they require constant affirmation of approval and acceptance from others. They often engage in seductive, flirtatious behavior to reassure themselves of their attractiveness and gain approval. The disorder has a prevalence of about 2% and tends to run in families; some researchers have identified a genetic link between histrionic personality disorder, antisocial personality disorder, and alcohol use disorder (Boland & Verduin, 2022).

Clinical Picture

People with histrionic personality disorder tend to be self-dramatizing, attention-seeking, overly gregarious, and seductive. They use manipulative and exhibitionistic behaviors in their demands to be the center of attention. People with histrionic personality disorder often demonstrate, to an extreme, what our society tends to foster and admire in its members: to be well liked, successful, popular, extroverted, attractive, and sociable. However, beneath these surface characteristics is a driven quality—an all-consuming need for approval and a desperate striving to be conspicuous and evoke affection or attract attention at all costs. Failure to evoke the attention and approval they seek often results in feelings of dejection and anxiety.

Individuals with this disorder are highly distractible and flighty by nature. They have difficulty paying attention to detail. They can portray themselves as carefree and sophisticated on the one hand and as inhibited and naive on the other. They tend to be highly suggestible, impressionable, and easily influenced by others. They are strongly dependent.

Interpersonal relationships are fleeting and superficial. Interaction with others tends to be provocative or sexually inappropriate. The person with histrionic personality disorder, having failed throughout life to develop the richness of inner feelings and without resources from which to draw, lacks the ability to provide another with genuinely sustained affection. They tend to misinterpret relationships as more intimate than they truly are. Somatic complaints are not uncommon in these individuals, and fleeting episodes of psychosis may occur during periods of extreme stress.

The *DSM-5-TR* summarizes histrionic personality disorder as "a pervasive pattern of excessive emotionality and attention-seeking" (APA, 2022, p. 757).

Predisposing Factors

Heredity may be a factor because the disorder is more common among first-degree biological relatives of people with the disorder than in the general population. Some traits may be inherited, whereas others are related to a combination of genetic predisposition and childhood experiences. At present, however, the exact cause is unknown.

From a psychosocial perspective, learning experiences may contribute to the development of histrionic personality disorder. The child may have learned that positive reinforcement was contingent on the ability to perform parentally approved and admired behaviors.

Narcissistic Personality Disorder

Definition and Epidemiology

People with **narcissistic personality disorder** have an exaggerated sense of self-worth. They lack empathy and are hypersensitive to the evaluation of others. They believe that they have the inalienable right to receive special consideration and that their desire is sufficient justification for possessing whatever they seek.

This diagnosis appeared for the first time in the third edition of the *DSM*. However, the concept of narcissism has its roots in the 19th century. It was viewed by early psychoanalysts as a normal phase of psychosexual development. The prevalence of narcissistic personality disorder is estimated at 1% to 6%. It is diagnosed more often in men than in women.

Clinical Picture

Individuals with narcissistic personality disorder appear to lack humility, be overly self-centered, and exploit others to fulfill their own desires. They often do not perceive their behavior as being inappropriate or objectionable. Because they view themselves as "superior" beings, they believe they are entitled to special rights and privileges.

Although often grounded in grandiose distortions of reality, their moods are usually optimistic, relaxed, cheerful, and carefree. Their mood can easily change, however, because of fragile self-esteem. If they do not meet self-expectations, do not receive the positive feedback they expect from others, or if they draw criticism from others, they may respond with rage, shame, humiliation, or dejection. They may turn inward and fantasize rationalizations that convince them of their continued stature and perfection.

The exploitation of others for self-gratification results in impaired interpersonal relationships. In selecting a mate, narcissistic individuals frequently choose a person who will provide them with the praise and positive feedback that they require and who will not ask much from their partner in return.

The *DSM-5-TR* identifies the various behaviors in narcissistic personality disorder as a "pervasive pattern of grandiosity (in fantasy or behavior), need for admiration and lack of empathy" (APA, 2022, p. 760).

Predisposing Factors

Although the causes are unknown, psychodynamic theories have suggested that narcissistic personality disorder evolves from a parent-child dynamic of excessive adoration or excessive criticism that is poorly attuned with the child's experience (Mayo Clinic, 2022). Children may then grow to project an image of invulnerability and self-sufficiency that conceals their true sense of emptiness and contributes to their inability to feel deep emotion.

Genetics and environment may both have a role in the development of narcissistic personality disorder. Having an innately oversensitive temperament may be an associated factor. In addition, research has identified a decreased volume of gray matter in areas of the brain responsible for empathy, emotional regulation, compassion, and cognitive functions (Gregory & Soriano, 2022).

Avoidant Personality Disorder
Definition and Epidemiology

The individual with **avoidant personality disorder** is extremely sensitive to rejection and thus may lead a very socially withdrawn life. It is not that they are asocial; in fact, there may be a strong desire for companionship. The extreme shyness and fear of rejection, however, create the need for unusually strong assurances of unconditional acceptance. Prevalence of the disorder in the general population is about 2% to 3%, and it appears to be equally common in men and women.

Clinical Picture

Individuals with this disorder are awkward and uncomfortable in social situations. From a distance, others may perceive them as timid, withdrawn, or perhaps cold and strange. Those who have closer relationships with them, however, soon learn of their sensitivities, touchiness, evasiveness, and mistrustful qualities.

Their speech is usually slow and constrained, with frequent hesitations, fragmentary thought sequences, and occasional confused and irrelevant digressions. They are often lonely and express feelings of being unwanted. They view others as critical, betraying, and humiliating. They desire to have close relationships but avoid connecting with others because of their fear of being rejected. Depression, anxiety, and anger at oneself for failing to develop social relations are commonly experienced.

The *DSM-5-TR* describes the various manifestations of avoidant personality disorder as "a pervasive pattern of social inhibition, feelings of inadequacy, and hypersensitivity to negative evaluation" (APA, 2022, p. 764).

Predisposing Factors

There is no clear cause of avoidant personality disorder. Contributing factors are most likely a combination of biological, genetic, and psychosocial influences. Some infants who exhibit traits of hyper-irritability, crankiness, tension, and withdrawal behaviors may possess a temperamental disposition toward an avoidant pattern later in life.

Psychosocial influences may include childhood trauma or neglect, leading to fears of abandonment or views of the world as a hostile and dangerous place.

Dependent Personality Disorder
Definition and Epidemiology

Dependent personality disorder is characterized by lack of self-confidence and extreme reliance on others to take responsibility for them, sometimes to the point of intense discomfort with being alone for even brief periods. Individuals with this disorder tend to allow others to make decisions, feel helpless when alone, act submissively, subordinate needs to others, tolerate mistreatment by others, demean oneself to gain acceptance, and fail to function adequately in situations that require assertive or dominant behavior.

Clinical Picture

Individuals with dependent personality disorder have a notable lack of self-confidence that is often apparent in their posture, voice, and mannerisms. They are typically passive and acquiescent to the desires of others. They are overly generous and thoughtful and underplay their own attractiveness and achievements. They may appear to others to "see the world through rose-colored glasses." But when alone, they may feel pessimistic, discouraged, and dejected, and they hide those feelings from others.

Individuals with dependent personality disorder assume the passive and submissive role in relationships even to the point of allowing others to make important decisions for them. Should a dependent relationship end, they feel fearful and vulnerable because they lack confidence in their ability to care for themselves. They may hastily and indiscriminately attempt to establish another relationship with someone they believe can provide them with the nurturance and guidance they need.

They avoid positions of responsibility and become anxious when forced into them. They have feelings of low self-worth and are easily hurt by criticism and disapproval. They will do almost anything, even if it is unpleasant or demeaning, to earn the acceptance of others.

The *DSM-5-TR* describes the manifestations of dependent personality disorder as "a pervasive and excessive need to be taken care of that leads to submissive and clinging behaviors and fears of separation" (APA, 2022, p. 768).

Predisposing Factors

An infant may be genetically predisposed to a dependent temperament. Twin studies measuring submissiveness have shown a higher correlation between identical twins than fraternal twins, but predisposition to dependent personality disorder is likely a combination of genetic and environmental vulnerabilities.

Psychosocially, dependency is fostered in infancy when stimulation and nurturance are experienced exclusively from one source. The infant becomes attached to one source to the exclusion of all others. If this exclusive attachment continues as the child grows, the dependency is nurtured. A problem may arise when parents become overprotective and discourage independent behaviors on the part of the child. Parents who make new experiences unnecessarily easy for the child and refuse to allow them to learn by experience encourage their child to give up efforts at achieving autonomy. Dependent behaviors may be subtly rewarded in this environment, and the child may come to fear a loss of love or attachment from the parental figure if independent behaviors are attempted.

Obsessive-Compulsive Personality Disorder
Definition and Epidemiology

Individuals with **obsessive-compulsive personality disorder** tend to have a serious and formal demeanor and have difficulty expressing emotions. They are overly disciplined, perfectionistic, and preoccupied with rules. They are inflexible about the way in which things must be done and have a devotion to productivity to the exclusion of personal pleasure.

An intense fear of making mistakes leads to difficulty with decision making. The disorder is relatively common and occurs more often in men than in women. Within the family constellation, it appears to be most common in oldest children. Recurrent obsessions and compulsions are absent in this personality disorder; if the client presents with such symptoms, they are diagnosed with obsessive-compulsive *disorder* rather than obsessive-compulsive *personality* disorder. Prevalence is estimated at anywhere from 2% to 8%.

Clinical Picture

Individuals with obsessive-compulsive personality disorder are inflexible and lack spontaneity. They are meticulous and work diligently and patiently at tasks that require accuracy and discipline. They are especially concerned with matters of organization and efficiency and tend to be rigid and unbending about rules and procedures.

Social behavior tends to be polite and formal. They are very "rank conscious," a characteristic that is reflected in their contrasting behaviors with "superiors" as opposed to "inferiors." They tend to be solicitous to and ingratiating with authority figures. With subordinates, however, the compulsive person can become quite autocratic and condemnatory, often appearing pompous and self-righteous.

People with obsessive-compulsive personality disorder typify the "bureaucratic personality." They see themselves as conscientious, loyal, dependable, and responsible and are contemptuous of people whose behavior they consider frivolous and impulsive. Emotional behavior is considered immature and irresponsible.

Although on the surface these individuals appear to be calm and controlled, underneath this exterior lies a great deal of ambivalence, conflict, and hostility. Individuals with this disorder commonly use the defense mechanism of reaction formation. Not daring to expose their true feelings of defiance and anger, they withhold these feelings so strongly that the opposite feelings come forth. The defense mechanisms of isolation, intellectualization, rationalization, and undoing are also commonly evident.

The *DSM-5-TR* diagnostic criteria for obsessive-compulsive personality disorder are presented in Box 31–1. These criteria can be compared and contrasted to the diagnostic criteria for obsessive-compulsive disorder presented in Chapter 27, "Anxiety, Obsessive-Compulsive, and Related Disorders."

Predisposing Factors

Genetic vulnerability may be a predisposing factor because this disorder occurs more frequently in first-degree biological relatives than in the general

---

BOX 31–1 Diagnostic Criteria for Obsessive-Compulsive Personality Disorder

A. A pervasive pattern of preoccupation with orderliness, perfectionism, and mental and interpersonal control, at the expense of flexibility, openness, and efficiency, beginning by early adulthood and present in a variety of contexts, as indicated by four (or more) of the following:

1. Is preoccupied with details, rules, lists, order, organization, or schedules to the extent that the major point of the activity is lost
2. Shows perfectionism that interferes with task completion (e.g., is unable to complete a project because their own overly strict standards are not met)
3. Is excessively devoted to work and productivity to the exclusion of leisure activities and friendships (not accounted for by obvious economic necessity)
4. Is overconscientious, scrupulous, and inflexible about matters of morality, ethics, or values (not accounted for by cultural or religious identification)
5. Is unable to discard worn-out or worthless objects even when they have no sentimental value
6. Is reluctant to delegate tasks or to work with others unless they submit to exactly his or her way of doing things
7. Adopts a miserly spending style toward both self and others; money is viewed as something to be hoarded for future catastrophes
8. Shows rigidity and stubbornness

Reprinted with permission from the *Diagnostic and Statistical Manual of Mental Disorders, Fifth Edition, Text Revision (DSM-5-TR)*. (Copyright 2022). *American Psychiatric Association.*

---

population (Boland & Verduin, 2022). The psychoanalytical view posits that the individual with obsessive-compulsive personality disorder was reared in an overly controlled environment. These parents expect their children to live up to imposed standards of conduct and condemn them if they do not. Praise for positive behaviors is bestowed on the child less frequently than punishment is for undesirable behaviors. In this environment, individuals become experts in learning what they must *not* do to avoid punishment and condemnation rather than what they *can* do to achieve attention and praise. They learn to heed rigid restrictions and rules. Positive achievements are expected, taken for granted, and only occasionally acknowledged by their parents, whose comments and judgments are limited to pointing out transgressions and infractions of rules.

Application of the Nursing Process

Borderline Personality Disorder (Background Assessment Data)

Historically, there have been patients who did not classically conform to the standard categories of neuroses or psychoses. The designation "borderline" was introduced to identify patients who seem to fall on the border between the two categories. Other terms that have been used to identify this disorder include *ambulatory schizophrenia, pseudoneurotic schizophrenia,* and *emotionally unstable personality.* When the term *borderline* was first proposed for inclusion in the third edition of the *DSM*, some psychiatrists feared it might be used as a "wastebasket" diagnosis for

difficult-to-treat patients. However, a specific set of criteria, listed in Box 31–2, has been established for diagnosing what has been described as "a consistent and stable course of unstable behavior."

Clinical Picture

Individuals with BPD always seem to be in a state of crisis and have frequent mood swings (although there may also be comorbid bipolar disorder). Their affect is one of extreme intensity, and their behavior reflects frequent changeability, within days, hours, or even minutes. They are sometimes described as "thriving on chaos," because they frequently generate chaos, particularly in interpersonal relationships. Often these individuals exhibit a single, dominant affective tone, such as depression, which may give way periodically to anxious agitation or inappropriate outbursts of anger.

Chronic Depression

Depression is so common in this disorder that before the inclusion of BPD in the *DSM*, many of these patients were diagnosed with depressive disorder. Depression may be rooted in feelings of abandonment by the mother in early childhood (see "Predisposing Factors to Borderline Personality Disorder"). Underlying the depression is a sense of rage that is sporadically turned inward on the self and externally on the environment. Seldom is the individual aware of the true source of these feelings until well into long-term therapy.

Bipolar Disorder

Much has been written about the common comorbidity of BPD with bipolar disorder and the overlap

BOX 31–2 **Diagnostic Criteria for Borderline Personality Disorder**

A pervasive pattern of instability of interpersonal relationships, self-image, and affects, and marked impulsivity beginning by early adulthood and present in a variety of contexts, as indicated by five (or more) of the following:

1. Frantic efforts to avoid real or imagined abandonment (Note: Do not include suicidal or self-mutilating behavior covered in criterion 5.)
2. A pattern of unstable and intense interpersonal relationships characterized by alternating between extremes of idealization and devaluation
3. Identity disturbance: markedly and persistently unstable self-image or sense of self
4. Impulsivity in at least two areas that are potentially self-damaging (e.g., spending, sex, substance abuse, reckless driving, binge eating) (Note: Do not include suicidal or self-mutilating behavior covered in criterion 5.)
5. Recurrent suicidal behavior, gestures, or threats, or self-mutilating behavior
6. Affective instability due to marked reactivity of mood (e.g., intense episodic dysphoria, irritability, or anxiety, usually lasting a few hours and only rarely more than a few days)
7. Chronic feelings of emptiness
8. Inappropriate, intense anger or difficulty controlling anger (e.g., frequent displays of temper, constant anger, recurrent physical fights)
9. Transient, stress-related paranoid ideation or severe dissociative symptoms

Reprinted with permission from the *Diagnostic and Statistical Manual of Mental Disorders, Fifth Edition, Text Revision (DSM-5-TR).* (Copyright 2022). American Psychiatric Association.

of features. These common features have led some to suggest that BPD should be considered a disorder along a bipolar spectrum, but most current reviews conclude that they are distinct disorders (Zimmerman, 2019). Supporting the concept that these two illnesses, although distinct, are very similar are the findings that both illnesses have a shared genetic variance, childhood parent loss, early trauma, and dysfunctional family environment as predisposing factors (Ditrich et al., 2021; Rodriguez, 2017). Affective instability is considered a core symptom in BPD and includes mood shifts from depression to irritability, anxiety, or anger.

Inability to Be Alone

Because of their chronic fear of abandonment, individuals with BPD have little tolerance for being alone. They prefer a frantic search for companionship, no matter how unsatisfactory, to sitting with feelings of loneliness, emptiness, and boredom (Boland & Verduin, 2022).

Patterns of Interaction

Clinging and Distancing

The individual with BPD commonly exhibits a pattern of interaction with others characterized by clinging and distancing behaviors. When clinging to another individual, they may exhibit helpless, dependent, or even childlike behaviors. They want to spend all their time with this person and express a frequent need to talk with and often seek constant reassurance from them. Impulsive behaviors, even self-mutilation, may result when they cannot

be with this chosen individual. Distancing behaviors are characterized by hostility, anger, and devaluation of others, arising from a feeling of discomfort with closeness. Distancing behaviors also occur in response to separations, confrontations, or attempts to limit certain behaviors. Devaluation of others is manifested by discrediting or undermining their strengths and personal significance.

Splitting

Splitting is a primitive ego defense mechanism common in people with BPD that arises from their lack of achievement of **object constancy** (the ability to maintain and feel secure about relationships) and is manifested by an inability to integrate and accept both positive and negative feelings. In their view, people—including themselves—and life situations are either all good or all bad. For example, a nurse–patient relationship may be perceived as intense and overvalued (e.g., "no one else in the world can help me the way you do"). This perception persists until the individual with BPD feels threatened in some way, which could be as simple as the nurse looking at the person with a different facial expression or not being immediately available to spend time with the person. Because this individual also struggles with emotional regulation, suddenly the nurse is devalued, valuing is shifted to another nurse, and the image of the former nurse changes from beneficent caregiver to hateful and cruel persecutor. These shifting allegiances and valuing/devaluing responses can generate conflict, anger, and frustration in staff members (or in any interpersonal relationships) unless this dynamic is clearly understood and managed appropriately.

Manipulation

In their efforts to prevent the separation they so desperately fear, individuals with this disorder become adept at manipulation. Virtually any behavior becomes an acceptable means of achieving the desired result: relief from separation anxiety. Pitting one individual against another is a common ploy to allay these fears of abandonment.

Self-Destructive Behaviors

Repetitive self-mutilating behaviors are classic manifestations of BPD. Suicide ideation and acts of self-harm are common and about 10% of individuals with BPD die by suicide (Paris, 2019). Although these acts can be fatal, more commonly they are manipulative gestures designed to elicit a rescue response from significant others. Suicide attempts are quite common and result from feelings of abandonment after separation from a significant other. The endeavor is often attempted, however, with a measure of "safety," (e.g., such as swallowing pills in an area where the person will be discovered by others or swallowing pills and making a phone call to report the deed to someone).

Other types of destructive behaviors include cutting, scratching, and burning. Various theories have been suggested about why these individuals can inflict pain on themselves. One hypothesis suggests they may have higher levels of endorphins in their bodies than most people, thereby increasing their threshold for pain. Another theory relates to the individual's personal identity disturbance. It proposes that because many of the self-mutilating behaviors take place when the individual is in a state of depersonalization and derealization, they do not initially feel the pain. The mutilation continues until pain is felt in an attempt to counteract the feelings of unreality. Some individuals with BPD have reported that "to feel pain is better than to feel nothing." The pain validates their existence.

Impulsivity

Individuals with BPD have poor impulse control. Impulsive behaviors associated with BPD include substance abuse, gambling, promiscuity, reckless driving, binging and purging, and acts of self-harm. Often, these behaviors occur in response to real or perceived feelings of abandonment.

Predisposing Factors to Borderline Personality Disorder

Biological Influences

BPD, once thought to be an entirely psychodynamic illness, has been the focus of much research, revealing a wealth of information about the neurobiological underpinnings of this illness. Research supports that BPD evolves through a complex interplay of environmental factors, brain anatomy and function, genetics, and epigenetics.

Biochemical Clients with BPD have a high incidence of major depressive episodes, and antidepressants have demonstrated benefits in some cases (Boland & Verduin, 2022). Several studies indicate that childhood trauma is associated with disruptions in glutaminergic, serotonergic, dopaminergic, and noradrenergic transmission (Cattane et al., 2017). The recognition of childhood trauma as a key predisposing factor in BPD has led to the deduction that BPD is the result of alterations in several interacting neurotransmitter systems. As stated elsewhere, questions remain about whether these dysfunctions contribute to the development of such disorders or whether they are a neurochemical response to intense emotional states.

Genetic An increased prevalence of major depression, antisocial personality disorder, and substance use disorders in first-degree relatives of individuals with borderline personality suggest that there are complex genetic vulnerabilities as well as environmental influences (Boland & Verduin, 2022). Many studies have shown personality traits (such as impulsivity, affect lability, and neuroticism) to be heritable, and one study (Zwir, 2020) concluded that self-regulatory personality traits are a function of complex interactions among more than 700 genes which modulate specific molecular processes in brain.

Epigenetic studies have identified changes to the oxytocin system as associated with decreased empathy (which is a core symptom in BPD), and women with BPD have been observed to have lower oxytocin levels (Saeed & Kallis, 2021). Further, a study using intranasal oxytocin found that patients with BPD had significantly higher affective empathy after administration (Domes et al., 2019).

Neurobiological Volumetric reductions have been observed in the corpus callosum, hippocampus, and prefrontal cortex as well as some abnormalities in the amygdala (particularly in females with BPD who have had traumatic experiences in childhood) (Bozzatello et al., 2021).

Psychosocial Influences

Childhood Trauma In up to 90% of individuals with BPD there is a history of abuse and neglect in childhood (Bozzatello et al., 2021). This trauma is believed to influence object constancy disruptions and attachment issues that are characteristic in BPD. In a review of research within the last 20 years (Bozzatello et al., 2021), the authors concluded that childhood trauma in interaction with temperamental traits (impulsive aggression and negative affectivity), environmental factors (abuse, neglect, childhood bullying victimization, and dysfunctional family environment), and specific polymorphisms of genes characterize the individual at risk for BPD.

Developmental Factors

Theory of Object Relations According to Mahler's theory of object relations (Mahler et al., 1975), infants pass through six phases from birth to 36 months, when a sense of separateness from the parenting figure is finally established. Between the ages of 16 and 24 months (phase 5, the rapprochement phase), children become acutely aware of their separateness. Because this separation is frightening, they look to the mother for "emotional refueling" and to maintain a sense of security while beginning to explore their separateness and independence. (See Table 31–1 for a more detailed outline of Mahler's theory.)

According to object relations theorists, the individual with BPD becomes fixed in the rapprochement phase of development. This fixation occurs when the child shows increasing separation and autonomy. The mother, who feels secure in the relationship as long as the child is dependent, begins to feel threatened by the child's increasing independence. The mother may be experiencing her own fears of abandonment. In response to separation behaviors, the mother withdraws the emotional support or "refueling" that is so vitally needed during this phase for the child to feel secure. Instead, the mother rewards clinging, dependent behaviors and punishes (withholding emotional support) independent behaviors. With the child's sense of emotional survival at stake, the child learns to behave in a manner that satisfies the parental wishes. The child develops an internal conflict based on fear of abandonment. They want to achieve independence common to this stage of development but fear that the mother will withdraw emotional support as a result. This unresolved fear of abandonment remains with the child into adulthood. Unresolved grief for the nurturing they failed to receive results in internalized rage that manifests in the depression so common in people with BPD.

Diagnosis and Outcome Identification

Nursing diagnoses are formulated from the data gathered during the assessment phase and with background knowledge regarding predisposing factors to the disorder. Table 31–2 presents a list of patient behaviors and the NANDA-I nursing diagnoses that correspond to these behaviors, which may be used in planning care for patients with BPD.

Outcome Criteria

The following criteria may be used for measurement of outcomes in the care of patients with BPD.

TABLE 31–2 Assigning Nursing Diagnoses to Behaviors Commonly Associated With Borderline Personality Disorder

BEHAVIORS	NURSING DIAGNOSES
Risk factors: History of self-injurious behavior; history of inability to plan solutions; impulsivity; irresistible urge to damage self; feels threatened with loss of significant relationships	Risk for self-mutilation
Risk factors: History of suicide attempts; suicidal ideation; suicidal plan; impulsiveness; childhood abuse; fears of abandonment; internalized rage	Risk for self-directed violence Risk for suicidal behavior
Risk factors: Body language (e.g., rigid posture, clenching of fists and jaw, hyperactivity, pacing, breathlessness, threatening stances); history of childhood abuse; impulsivity; transient psychotic symptomatology	Risk for other-directed violence
Depression; persistent emotional distress; rumination; separation distress; traumatic distress; verbalizes feeling empty; inappropriate expression of anger	Maladaptive grieving
Alternating clinging and distancing behaviors; staff splitting; manipulation	Impaired social interaction
Feelings of depersonalization and derealization	Disturbed personal identity
Transient psychotic symptoms (disorganized thinking; misinterpretation of the environment); increased tension; decreased perceptual field	Anxiety (severe to panic)
Dependent on others; excessively seeks reassurance; manipulation of others; inability to tolerate being alone	Chronic low self-esteem

The patient:

■ Has not harmed self
■ Seeks out staff when desire for self-mutilation is strong
■ Is able to identify true source of anger
■ Expresses anger appropriately
■ Relates to more than one staff member
■ Completes activities of daily living independently
■ Does not manipulate one staff member against the other to fulfill own desires

Planning and Implementation

The patient with BPD is at high risk for stigmatization, even among health-care professionals. Patient behaviors, such as manipulating, lying, and splitting, may violate the nurse's sense of success in establishing a trusting relationship with this individual and may culminate in negative or distancing behaviors from the nurse. The following guidelines may help decrease negative attitudes and stigmatization of this patient:

■ Understand the disorder and the effect of childhood trauma on the dynamics of the patient's behavior to develop an approach of compassion and convey hopefulness that this condition is treatable.
■ Recognize that even brief encounters with a patient during short hospital stays provide an opportunity to convey connectedness and a sense that they are valued. These encounters are particularly important because the patient with BPD is interpersonally hypersensitive, fears abandonment, and has had a history of instability in interpersonal relationships
■ Frequently reflect on your feelings in response to patient behavior. For example, self-harming behaviors by the patient frequently generate feelings of anger and frustration in nurses when the behavior seems to be manipulative rather than a sign of true distress. These feelings may culminate in the nurse distancing themselves from the patient. Indeed, self-harming behaviors may be used as a tool for manipulating others *and* they are a sign of true distress.
■ Develop a clear model of communication and intervention with team members for the hospitalized patient with BPD. Consistency in intervention helps to model healthy interpersonal skills for the patient and may minimize successful efforts at splitting staff members. In addition, when health-care team members develop strong communication skills with each other, it provides a foundation for discussing and confronting negative attitudes toward the patient and promotes culture change. For example, McNee and associates (2014) developed

a commitment among team members that they would avoid using phrases like "acting out" or "attention-seeking" because these reinforced a culture of negativity toward the patient.

The following section presents a group of selected nursing diagnoses common to patients with BPD, with short- and long-term goals and nursing interventions for each. Rationales for nursing interventions are italicized.

Risk for Self-Mutilation/Risk for Self-Directed or Other-Directed Violence

Risk for self-mutilation is defined as "susceptible to deliberate self-injurious behavior causing tissue damage with the intent of causing nonfatal injury to attain relief of tension" (Herdman et al., 2021, p. 526). *Risk for self-directed or other-directed violence* is defined as "susceptible to behaviors in which an individual demonstrates that he or she can be physically, emotionally, and/or sexually harmful to self or others" (pp. 522–523).

Patient Goals

Outcome criteria include short- and long-term goals. Timelines are individually determined.

Short-term goals

■ The patient will seek out a staff member if feelings of harming self or others emerge.
■ The patient will not harm self or others.

Long-term goal

■ The patient will not harm self or others.

Interventions

■ Observe the patient's behavior frequently. Do this through routine activities and interactions; avoid appearing watchful and suspicious. *Close observation is required so that intervention can occur if required to ensure the patient's (and others') safety.*
■ Encourage the patient to seek out a staff member when the urge for self-mutilation is experienced. *Discussing feelings of self-harm with a trusted individual provides some relief to the patient. An attitude of acceptance of the patient as a worthwhile individual supports the therapeutic relationship.*
■ If self-mutilation occurs, care for the patient's wounds in a matter-of-fact manner. Do not give positive reinforcement for this behavior by offering sympathy or additional attention. *Lack of attention to the maladaptive behavior may decrease repetition of its use.*
■ Encourage the patient to talk about feelings they were having just before this behavior occurred. *To problem solve the situation with the patient, knowledge of the precipitating factors is important.*

■ Act as a role model for the appropriate expression of angry feelings and give positive reinforcement to the patient when attempts to appropriately express anger are made. *It is vital that the patient expresses angry feelings because suicide and other self-destructive behaviors are often viewed as a result of anger turned inward on the self.*

■ Remove dangerous objects from the patient's environment so that they may not purposefully or inadvertently use them to inflict harm to self or others. *Patient safety is a priority.*

■ Try to redirect violent behavior with physical outlets for the patient's anxiety (e.g., walking, jogging). *Physical exercise is a safe and effective way of relieving pent-up tension.*

■ Administer sedative medications as ordered by the physician or obtain an order if necessary. Monitor the patient for effectiveness of the medication and adverse side effects and to ensure that the patient is not hoarding medication. *Close monitoring is important because impulsivity is a common symptom in BPD and may increase the risk for an overdose attempt. Tranquilizing medications such as anxiolytics or antipsychotics may have a calming effect on the patient and thus prevent aggressive behaviors, but an important precaution is that studies have found a positive correlation between sedative use and increased emotional dysregulation as well as a vulnerability to substance use disorders* (Richmond et al., 2020)

■ If the patient is not calmed by "talking down" or by medication, use of mechanical restraints may be necessary. The "least restrictive alternative" must be applied when planning interventions for a violent patient. *Restraints should be used only as a last resort, after all other interventions have been unsuccessful, and the patient is clearly at risk of harm to self or others. Trauma-informed care should always be the foundation for decisions about appropriate intervention.*

■ Ensure that sufficient staff is available to control the patient if it becomes necessary due to imminent threats of violence. *This promotes safety for the patient, staff, and others.*

■ As agitation decreases, assess the patient's readiness for restraint removal or reduction. Remove one restraint at a time while assessing the patient's response. *This minimizes the risk of injury to patient and staff.*

■ If warranted by high acuity of the situation, staff may need to be assigned on a one-to-one basis. *Because of their extreme fear of abandonment, patients with BPD should not be left alone at a stressful time, as it may cause an acute rise in anxiety and agitation levels.*

Maladaptive Grieving

Maladaptive grieving is defined as "a disorder that occurs after the death of a significant other [or any other loss of significance to the individual], in which the experience of distress accompanying bereavement fails to follow sociocultural expectations" (Herdman et al., 2021, p. 421). Table 31–3 presents this nursing diagnosis in care plan format.

Patient Goals

Outcome criteria include short- and long-term goals. Timelines are individually determined.

Short-term goal

■ Within 5 days, the patient will discuss maladaptive patterns of expressing anger with nurse or therapist.

Long-term goal

■ By the time of discharge from treatment, the patient will be able to identify the true source of angry feelings, accept ownership of these feelings, and express them in a socially acceptable manner, and thus demonstrate satisfactorily progress through the grieving process.

Interventions

■ Convey an accepting attitude—one that creates a nonthreatening environment for the patient to express feelings. Be honest and keep all promises. *An accepting attitude conveys to the patient that you believe they are a worthwhile person and promotes trust within the therapeutic relationship.*

■ Identify the function that anger, frustration, and rage serve for the patient. Allow them to express these feelings within reason. *Verbalization of feelings in a nonthreatening environment may help the patient come to terms with unresolved issues.*

■ Encourage the patient to discharge pent-up anger through participation in large motor activities (e.g., brisk walks, jogging, physical exercises, volleyball, exercise bike). *Physical exercise provides a safe and effective method for discharging pent-up tension.*

■ Explore the true source of anger with the patient. This activity may be painful and often leads to regression as the patient confronts feelings of early abandonment or abuse. It may seem that the patient must "get worse before they can get better." *Reconciliation of the feelings associated with this stage is necessary before progression through the grieving process can continue.*

■ As anger is displaced onto the nurse or therapist, caution must be taken to guard against the negative effects of countertransference. *These behaviors can elicit an array of negative feelings from the caregiver. The existence of negative feelings by the nurse or therapist must be acknowledged but must not be allowed to interfere with the therapeutic process.*

Table 31–3 | CARE PLAN FOR THE PATIENT WITH BORDERLINE PERSONALITY DISORDER

NURSING DIAGNOSIS: MALADAPTIVE GRIEVING
RELATED TO: Maternal deprivation during rapprochement phase of development (internalized as a loss, with fixation in anger stage of grieving process); possible childhood physical or sexual abuse
EVIDENCED BY: Depressed mood, acting-out behaviors

OUTCOME CRITERIA	NURSING INTERVENTIONS	RATIONALE
Short-Term Goal ■ Within 5 days, the patient discusses with nurse or therapist maladaptive patterns of expressing anger. **Long-Term Goal** ■ By time of discharge from treatment, the patient is able to identify the true source of angry feelings, accept ownership of these feelings, and express them in a socially acceptable manner, in an effort to satisfactorily progress through the grieving process.	1. Convey an accepting attitude—one that creates a nonthreatening environment for the patient to express feelings. Be honest and keep all promises. 2. Identify the function that anger, frustration, and rage serve for the patient. Allow them to express these feelings within reason. 3. Encourage the patient to discharge pent-up anger through participation in large motor activities (e.g., brisk walks, jogging, physical exercises, volleyball, exercise bike). 4. Explore with the patient the true source of the anger. This is a painful therapy that often leads to regression as the patient confronts feelings of early abandonment or issues of abuse. 5. As anger is displaced onto the nurse or therapist, caution must be taken to guard against the negative effects of countertransference. These patients may elicit negative feelings in the therapist. 6. Explain the behaviors associated with the normal grieving process. Help the patient recognize their position in this process. 7. Help the patient understand appropriate ways to express anger. Give positive reinforcement for behaviors used to express anger appropriately. Act as a role model. It is important to let the patient know when they have done something that has generated angry feelings in you. 8. Set limits on acting-out behaviors and explain consequences of violation of those limits. Be supportive, yet consistent and firm, in caring for this patient.	1. An accepting attitude conveys to the patient that you believe they are a worthwhile person. Trust is enhanced. 2. Verbalization of feelings in a nonthreatening environment may help the patient come to terms with unresolved issues. 3. Physical exercise provides a safe and effective method for discharging pent-up tension. 4. Reconciliation of the feelings associated with this stage is necessary before progression through the grieving process can continue. 5. The existence of negative feelings by the nurse or therapist must be acknowledged, but they must not be allowed to interfere with the therapeutic process. 6. Knowledge of the acceptability of the feelings associated with normal grieving may help to relieve some of the guilt that these responses generate. 7. Positive reinforcement enhances self-esteem and encourages repetition of desirable behaviors. Role-modeling expression of anger in an appropriate manner is a powerful learning tool. 8. These patients lack sufficient self-control to limit maladaptive behaviors, so assistance is required. Without consistency on the part of all staff members working with this patient, a positive outcome will not be achieved.

■ Explain the behaviors associated with the normal grieving process. Help the patient recognize their position in this process. *Knowledge of the acceptability of the feelings associated with normal grieving may help to relieve some of the guilt that these responses generate.*

■ Help the patient understand appropriate ways of expressing anger. Give positive reinforcement for behaviors used to express anger appropriately. Act as a role model. It is appropriate to let the patient know when they have done something that has generated angry feelings in you. *Role-modeling ways to express anger in an appropriate manner is a powerful learning tool.*

■ Clearly identify expected behaviors within the milieu and set limits on behaviors that are in violation of stated expectations with clearly stated consequences. For example, the nurse states clearly to the patient on admission that physical contact among patients is not permitted. When the patient is noticed hugging another patient, the nurse clarifies the limit, indicates that the behavior is not acceptable, and communicates that if the behavior continues, the patient will not be permitted to continue participating in the current activity. Be supportive, yet consistent and firm, in caring for this patient. *The patient lacks sufficient self-control to limit maladaptive behaviors, so assistance is required. Without consistency on the part of all staff members working with this patient, a positive outcome will not be achieved.*

Impaired Social Interaction

Impaired social interaction is defined as "insufficient or excessive quantity or ineffective quality of social exchange" (Herdman et al., 2021, p. 384).

Patient Goals

Outcome criteria include short- and long-term goals. Timelines are individually determined.

Short-term goal

■ Within 5 days, the patient will discuss with the nurse or therapist behaviors that impede the development of satisfactory interpersonal relationships.

Long-term goal

■ By the time of discharge from treatment, the patient will interact appropriately with others in the therapy setting in both social and therapeutic activities (evidencing discontinuation of splitting and clinging and distancing behaviors).

Interventions

■ Encourage the patient to examine these behaviors and associated feelings (to recognize that they are occurring). They may be unaware of splitting or

of clinging and distancing patterns of interaction with others. Recognition must take place before change can occur. *For example, when a patient begins to recognize that they feel less anxious when engaging in disruptive behaviors, a foundation is laid for exploring healthier strategies for anxiety reduction.*

■ Help the patient understand that you will be available, without reinforcing dependent behaviors. *Knowledge of your availability may provide needed security.*

■ Rotate staff members who work with the patient to avoid the development of dependence on particular individuals. The patient must learn to relate to more than one staff member to decrease the use of splitting and diminish fears of abandonment. *Communication and consistency among the staff team members in adherence to the established plan of care are essential to minimize opportunities for the patient to manipulate or split staff members.*

■ Explore feelings that relate to fears of abandonment and engulfment. Help the patient understand that clinging and distancing behaviors are engendered by these fears. *Exploration of feelings with a trusted individual may help the patient come to terms with unresolved issues.*

■ Help the patient understand how these behaviors interfere with satisfactory relationships. *They may be unaware of how others perceive these behaviors and why they are not acceptable.*

■ Help the patient work toward achievement of object constancy. Be available without promoting dependency. Give positive reinforcement for independent behaviors. *The patient must resolve fears of abandonment to establish satisfactory intimate relationships.*

■ Provide education, support, and referral resources for family members and significant others who may also experience anger and frustration at failed attempts to navigate interpersonal relationships with the patient. *Family members and significant others often experience guilt and frustration in attempts to communicate and support their loved ones with BPD, particularly when the patient uses manipulation, lying, or splitting behaviors. Reinforcing that they are not responsible for the patient's manipulative behaviors and providing tools for therapeutic communication support the family and the patient's recovery process.*

CLINICAL PEARL Recognize when the patient is playing one staff member against another. Remember that splitting is the primary defense mechanism of individuals with BPD, and the impressions they have of others as either "all good" or "all bad" are a manifestation of this defense. Do not engage the patient in discussions that are attempts to degrade other staff members. Suggest instead that the patient discuss problems directly with the staff person involved.

Concept Care Mapping

The concept map care plan is a diagrammatic teaching and learning strategy that allows visualization of interrelationships between medical diagnoses, nursing diagnoses, assessment data, and treatments (see Chapter 8, "The Nursing Process in Psychiatric-Mental Health Nursing"). An example

of a concept map care plan for a patient with BPD is presented in Figure 31–1.

Evaluation

Reassessment is conducted to determine whether the nursing actions have been successful in achieving the objectives of care. Evaluation of the nursing

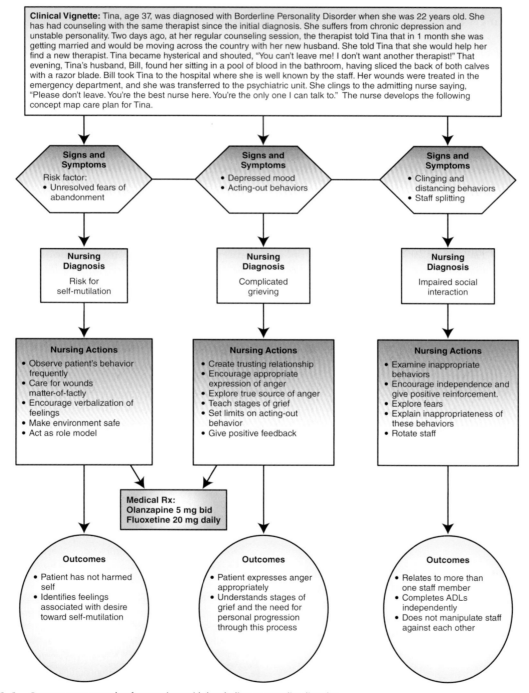

Clinical Vignette: Tina, age 37, was diagnosed with Borderline Personality Disorder when she was 22 years old. She has had counseling with the same therapist since the initial diagnosis. She suffers from chronic depression and unstable personality. Two days ago, at her regular counseling session, the therapist told Tina that in 1 month she was getting married and would be moving across the country with her new husband. She told Tina that she would help her find a new therapist. Tina became hysterical and shouted, "You can't leave me! I don't want another therapist!" That evening, Tina's husband, Bill, found her sitting in a pool of blood in the bathroom, having sliced the back of both calves with a razor blade. Bill took Tina to the hospital where she is well known by the staff. Her wounds were treated in the emergency department, and she was transferred to the psychiatric unit. She clings to the admitting nurse saying, "Please don't leave. You're the best nurse here. You're the only one I can talk to." The nurse develops the following concept map care plan for Tina.

Signs and Symptoms
Risk factor:
• Unresolved fears of abandonment

Signs and Symptoms
• Depressed mood
• Acting-out behaviors

Signs and Symptoms
• Clinging and distancing behaviors
• Staff splitting

Nursing Diagnosis
Risk for self-mutilation

Nursing Diagnosis
Complicated grieving

Nursing Diagnosis
Impaired social interaction

Nursing Actions
• Observe patient's behavior frequently
• Care for wounds matter-of-factly
• Encourage verbalization of feelings
• Make environment safe
• Act as role model

Nursing Actions
• Create trusting relationship
• Encourage appropriate expression of anger
• Explore true source of anger
• Teach stages of grief
• Set limits on acting-out behavior
• Give positive feedback

Nursing Actions
• Examine inappropriate behaviors
• Encourage independence and give positive reinforcement.
• Explore fears
• Explain inappropriateness of these behaviors
• Rotate staff

Medical Rx:
Olanzapine 5 mg bid
Fluoxetine 20 mg daily

Outcomes
• Patient has not harmed self
• Identifies feelings associated with desire toward self-mutilation

Outcomes
• Patient expresses anger appropriately
• Understands stages of grief and the need for personal progression through this process

Outcomes
• Relates to more than one staff member
• Completes ADLs independently
• Does not manipulate staff against each other

FIGURE 31–1   Concept map care plan for a patient with borderline personality disorder.

actions for the patient with BPD may be facilitated by gathering information using the following types of questions:

Has the patient:

- Been able to seek out staff when feeling the desire for self-harm?
- Avoided self-harm?
- Correlated times of desire for self-harm to times of elevation in level of anxiety?
- Discussed feelings with staff (particularly feelings of depression and anger)?
- Identified the true sources of their anger?
- Verbalized understanding of the basis for their anger?
- Expressed anger appropriately?
- Demonstrated ability to function independently?
- Related to more than one staff member?
- Verbalized the knowledge that the staff members will return and are not abandoning them when leaving for the day?
- Separated from the staff in an appropriate manner?
- Demonstrated ability to delay gratification and refrain from manipulating others in order to fulfill own desires?
- Identified resources within the community from whom they may seek assistance in times of extreme stress?

Antisocial Personality Disorder (Background Assessment Data)

In the *DSM-I*, antisocial behavior was categorized as a "sociopathic or psychopathic" reaction that could be symptomatic of any of several underlying personality disorders. The *DSM-II* represented it as a separate personality type, a distinction that has been retained in subsequent editions. The *DSM-5-TR* diagnostic criteria for antisocial personality disorder are presented in Box 31–3.

Individuals with antisocial personality disorder are seldom seen in most clinical settings, and when they are, it is commonly a way to avoid legal consequences. Sometimes they are admitted to the health-care system by court order for psychological evaluation. Most frequently, however, these individuals are encountered in prisons, jails, and rehabilitation services.

Although the *DSM-5-TR* continues to identify antisocial personality disorder as synonymous with psychopathy, the terms can be confusing and although there are overlapping symptoms there are also distinctions between the two conditions. Abdalla-Filho and Völlm (2020) clarified that only one-third of individuals with antisocial personality disorder meet criteria for psychopathy. Antisocial personality disorder as a distinct entity is characterized by *behaviors* that are reactive to perceived threats, control, and a negative affect; psychopathy is described as *personality traits* that include low fear, low empathy, domination, callous cruelty, and emotional insensitivity. Those with either diagnosis may be considered prone to violence, but with different etiologies and potentially different responses in treatment. For the purpose of this text, they are discussed together as antisocial personality disorder.

Clinical Picture

Antisocial personality disorder is a pattern of socially irresponsible, exploitative, and guiltless behavior

---

BOX 31–3 Diagnostic Criteria for Antisocial Personality Disorder

A. A pervasive pattern of disregard for and violation of the rights of others occurring since age 15 years, as indicated by three (or more) of the following:
　1. Failure to conform to social norms with respect to lawful behaviors as indicated by repeatedly performing acts that are grounds for arrest
　2. Deceitfulness, as indicated by repeated lying, use of aliases, or conning others for personal profit or pleasure
　3. Impulsivity or failure to plan ahead
　4. Irritability and aggressiveness, as indicated by repeated physical fights or assaults
　5. Reckless disregard for safety of self or others
　6. Consistent irresponsibility, as indicated by repeated failure to sustain consistent work behavior or honor financial obligations
　7. Lack of remorse, as indicated by being indifferent to or rationalizing having hurt, mistreated, or stolen from another
B. Individual is at least 18 years.
C. There is evidence of conduct disorder with onset before age 15 years.
D. The occurrence of antisocial behavior is not exclusively during the course of schizophrenia or bipolar disorder.

that reflects a general disregard for the rights of others. Individuals with antisocial personality disorder exploit and manipulate others for personal gain and are unconcerned with obeying the law. They have difficulty sustaining consistent employment and developing stable relationships. They appear cold and callous, often intimidating others with their brusque and belligerent manner. They tend to be argumentative and, at times, cruel and malicious. They lack warmth and compassion and are often suspicious of these qualities in others.

Individuals with antisocial personality have a very low tolerance for frustration, act impulsively, and are unable to delay gratification. They are restless and easily bored, often taking chances and seeking thrills as if they were immune to danger. Their pattern of impulsivity may be manifested in failure to plan ahead culminating in sudden job, residence, or relationship changes (APA, 2022).

When things go their way, individuals with this disorder act cheerful, even gracious and charming. But because of their low tolerance for frustration, this pleasant exterior can change very quickly. When momentary desires are challenged, they are likely to become furious and vindictive. Easily provoked to attack, their first inclination is to demean and dominate. They believe that "good guys finish last," and they show contempt for the weak and underprivileged. They exploit others to fulfill their own desires, showing no trace of shame or guilt for their behavior. Individuals with antisocial personalities see themselves as victims, using projection, devaluing, and denial as primary ego defense mechanisms. They do not accept responsibility for the consequences of their behavior. Instead, the perception of victimization by others justifies their malicious behavior, lest they be the recipient of unjust persecution and hostility from others. Physical attacks or other acts of aggression are not uncommon.

Satisfying interpersonal relationships are not possible because individuals with antisocial personality disorder have learned to trust only themselves. They have a philosophy that "it's everyone for themselves" and that one should stop at nothing to avoid being manipulated by others. They may disregard their safety and that of others through reckless sexual activity, substance use, reckless driving, or child neglect (APA, 2022).

One of the most distinctive characteristics of individuals with antisocial personality is their tendency to ignore conventional authority and rules. They act as if established social norms and guidelines for self-discipline and cooperative behavior do not apply to them. They are flagrant in their disrespect for the law and the rights of others.

Predisposing Factors to Antisocial Personality Disorder

Biological Influences

Antisocial personality is more common among first-degree biological relatives of those with the disorder than among the general population. Twin and adoptive studies have implicated the role of genetics in antisocial personality disorder as well as environmental influences, and the fact that both biological and adoptive children of parents with antisocial personality disorder are at greater risk for this personality disorder suggests that it has both genetic and environmental influences (Boland & Verduin, 2022). Research has linked *MAO-A* gene variants to antisocial personality disorders and BPD, which may be moderated after exposure to violence such as child maltreatment, physical abuse, or sexual abuse (Kolla & Vinette, 2017). Moderation of this gene is believed to be associated with the eventual development of differential features of antisocial personality and BPD, although the authors note that study results have been mixed and more research is needed. Nonetheless, it lends support to the idea that a complex interaction of genetics and environment is involved in the development of antisocial personality disorder and underscores the significance of childhood trauma.

Characteristics associated with temperament in the newborn may be significant in the predisposition to antisocial personality disorder. Parents who bring children with behavior disorders to clinics often report that the child has displayed temper tantrums from infancy and became furious when awaiting a bottle or a diaper change. As these children mature, they commonly develop a bullying attitude toward other children. Parents report that they are undaunted by punishment and generally quite unmanageable.

The likelihood of developing antisocial personality disorder is increased if the individual had attention deficit-hyperactivity disorder and conduct disorder as a child (APA, 2022). Brain imaging studies have identified decreases in prefrontal cortex gray matter volume, which regulates cognitive control and inhibition, decreased activity in the amygdala, which is responsible for modulating fearful or threatening stimuli, and lower right thalamic volume (associated with impaired control inhibition) (Johanson et al., 2020). Johanson and associates also noted that variations in imaging findings, compared with individuals with psychopathy, support that these two conditions might stem from dissimilar biological processes.

Other studies have implicated dysregulation of dopamine and serotonin neurotransmitters (Boland & Verduin, 2022). Overactivity in dopamine reward circuitry has been hypothesized to be linked to antisocial personality disorder as well as commonly comorbid substance use disorders, whereas low levels of serotonin have been associated with impulsiveness.

Family Dynamics

Antisocial personality disorder frequently arises from a chaotic home environment. Parental deprivation during the first 5 years of life appears to be a critical predisposing factor in the development of antisocial personality disorder. Separation due to parental delinquency appears to be more highly correlated with the disorder than is parental loss from other causes.

Studies have shown that antisocial personality disorder in adulthood is highly associated with physical abuse and neglect, teasing, and lack of parental bonding in childhood (Afifi et al., 2019; Delisi et al., 2019). Severe physical abuse in childhood is particularly correlated to aggression and violent offending. The abuse also contributes to the development of antisocial behavior in that it provides a model for behavior and may result in injury to the child's central nervous system, thereby impairing the child's ability to function appropriately. Although a diagnosis of antisocial personality disorder is only made when the individual is at least 18 years old, these behavioral patterns first appear in childhood and adolescence. When they are identified in children and adolescents, the diagnosis is *conduct disorder*, and the common symptoms are bullying, fighting, physical cruelty to animals, destruction of property and theft, and others (APA, 2022). Whether better identification and early intervention might prevent more dangerous behavior in adulthood is yet to be determined through ongoing research.

Diagnosis and Outcome Identification

Nursing diagnoses are formulated from the data gathered during the assessment phase and with background knowledge regarding predisposing factors to the disorder. Table 31–4 presents a list of patient behaviors and the NANDA-I nursing diagnoses that correspond to those behaviors, which may be used in planning care for patients with antisocial personality disorder.

Outcome Criteria

The following criteria may be used for measurement of outcomes in the care of the patient with antisocial personality disorder.

The patient:

- Discusses angry feelings with staff and in group sessions
- Has not harmed self or others
- Can rechannel hostility into socially acceptable behaviors
- Follows rules and regulations of the therapy environment

TABLE 31–4 Assigning Nursing Diagnoses to Behaviors Commonly Associated With Antisocial Personality Disorder

BEHAVIOR	NURSING DIAGNOSES
Risk factors: Body language (e.g., rigid posture, clenching of fists and jaw, hyperactivity, pacing, breathlessness, threatening stances); cruelty to animals; rage reactions; history of childhood abuse; history of violence against others; impulsivity; substance abuse; negative role-modeling; inability to tolerate frustration	Risk for other-directed violence
Disregard for societal norms and laws; absence of guilty feelings; inability to delay gratification; denial of obvious problems; grandiosity; hostile laughter; projection of blame and responsibility; ridicule of others; superior attitude toward others	Defensive coping
Manipulation of others to fulfill own desires; inability to form close, personal relationships; frequent lack of success in life events; passive-aggressiveness; overt aggressiveness (hiding feelings of low self-esteem)	Chronic low self-esteem
Inability to form a satisfactory, enduring, intimate relationship with another; dysfunctional interaction with others; use of unsuccessful social interaction behaviors	Impaired social interaction
Demonstration of inability to take responsibility for meeting basic health practices; history of lack of health-seeking behavior; demonstrated lack of knowledge regarding basic health practices; lack of expressed interest in improving health behaviors	Ineffective health maintenance

■ Can verbalize which of their behaviors are not acceptable

■ Shows regard for the rights of others by delaying gratification of own desires when appropriate

■ Does not manipulate others in an attempt to increase feelings of self-worth

■ Verbalizes understanding of knowledge required to maintain basic health needs

Planning and Implementation

The following section presents a group of selected nursing diagnoses common to patients with antisocial personality disorder, with short- and long-term goals and nursing interventions for each. Rationales for nursing interventions are italicized.

Risk for Other-Directed Violence

Risk for other-directed violence is defined as "susceptible to behaviors in which an individual demonstrates that he or she can be physically, emotionally, and/or sexually harmful to others" (Herdman et al., 2021, p. 523).

Patient Goals

Outcome criteria include short- and long-term goals. Timelines are individually determined.

Short-term goals

■ Within 3 days, the patient will discuss angry feelings and situations that precipitate hostility.

■ The patient will not harm others.

Long-term goal

■ The patient will not harm others.

Interventions

■ Convey an accepting attitude toward the patient. Work on development of trust. Be honest, keep all promises, and convey the message to the patient that it is not *them* but the *behavior* that is unacceptable. *An attitude of acceptance promotes feelings of self-worth. Trust is the basis of a therapeutic relationship. Be alert, however, to the tendency of this patient to manipulate others. Do not misconstrue charm or compliments as indicative of mutual trust. Maintaining clear, professional boundaries is essential.*

■ Maintain a low level of stimuli in the patient's environment (low lighting, few people, simple decor, low noise level). *A stimulating environment may increase agitation and promote aggressive behavior.*

■ Observe the patient's behavior frequently through routine activities and interactions; avoid appearing watchful and suspicious. *Close observation is required so that intervention can occur if needed to ensure the patient's (and others') safety.*

■ Remove dangerous objects from the patient's environment so that they may not purposefully or inadvertently use them to inflict harm to self or others. *Patient safety is a priority.*

■ Help the patient identify the true object of their hostility (e.g., "You seem to be upset with..."). *Because of weak ego development, the patient may misuse the defense mechanism of displacement. Helping them recognize this in a nonthreatening manner may help reveal unresolved issues so that they may be confronted.*

■ Encourage the patient to gradually verbalize hostile feelings. *Verbalization of feelings in a nonthreatening environment may help the patient come to terms with unresolved issues.*

■ Explore with the patient alternative ways of handling frustration (e.g., large motor skills that channel hostile energy into socially acceptable behavior). *Physically demanding activities help to relieve pent-up tension.*

■ The staff should maintain and convey a calm attitude toward the patient. *Anxiety is contagious and can be transferred from staff to patient. A calm attitude provides the patient with a feeling of safety and security.*

■ Administer sedative medications as ordered by the physician or obtain an order if necessary. Monitor the patient for effectiveness of the medication as well as for appearance of adverse side effects. Antianxiety agents (e.g., lorazepam, chlordiazepoxide, oxazepam) produce a calming effect and may help to allay hostile behaviors. *(Note: Medications are not often prescribed for patients with antisocial personality disorder because of these individuals' strong susceptibility to substance use disorders.)*

■ Ensure that sufficient staff is available to control the patient if necessary due to imminent threats of violence. *This promotes safety for the patient, staff, and others.*

■ If the patient is not calmed by "talking down" or by medication, use of mechanical restraints may be necessary. *The "least restrictive alternative" must be applied when planning interventions for a violent patient. Restraints should be used only as a last resort, after all other interventions have been unsuccessful, and when the patient is clearly at risk of harm to self or others.*

■ If restraint is deemed necessary, ensure that sufficient staff is available to assist. Follow protocol established by the institution. *This ensures patient and staff safety.* As agitation decreases, assess the patient's readiness for restraint removal or reduction. Remove one restraint at a time while assessing the patient's response. *This minimizes the risk of injury to patient and staff.*

Defensive Coping

Defensive coping is defined as "repeated projection of falsely positive self-evaluation based on a self-protective pattern that defends against underlying perceived threats to positive self-regard" (Herdman et al., 2021, p. 407).

Patient Goals

Outcome criteria include short- and long-term goals. Timelines are individually determined.

Short-term goals

■ Within 24 hours after admission, the patient will verbalize understanding of treatment setting rules and regulations and the consequences for violation.
■ The patient will verbalize personal responsibility for difficulties experienced in interpersonal relationships within (time period reasonable for patient).

Long-term goals

■ By the time of discharge from treatment, the patient will be able to cope more adaptively by delaying gratification of their desires and following rules and regulations of the treatment setting.
■ By the time of discharge from treatment, the patient will demonstrate ability to interact with others without becoming defensive, rationalizing behaviors, or expressing grandiose ideas.

Interventions

■ From the time of admission, the patient should be made aware of which behaviors are acceptable and which are not. Explain consequences of violation of the limits. A consequence must involve something of value to the patient. All staff must be consistent in enforcing these limits. Consequences should be administered in a matter-of-fact manner immediately after the infraction. *Because the patient cannot (or will not) self-impose limits on maladaptive behaviors, these behaviors must be delineated and enforced by staff. Undesirable consequences may help to decrease repetition of these behaviors.*
■ The ideal goal would be for this patient to eventually internalize societal norms, beginning with a step-by-step, "either/or" approach on the unit (*either* you do [don't do] this, *or* this will occur). *Explanations must be concise, concrete, and clear, with little or no capacity for misinterpretation.*

> **CLINICAL PEARL** Do not attempt to coax or convince the patient to do the "right thing." Do not use the words "You should (or shouldn't)…"; instead, use the words "You will be expected to…."

■ Provide positive feedback or reward for acceptable behaviors. *Positive reinforcement enhances self-esteem and encourages repetition of desirable behaviors.*

■ To assist the patient in delaying gratification, increase the length of time required for acceptable behavior to achieve the reward. For example, 2 hours of acceptable behavior may be exchanged for a phone call; 4 hours of acceptable behavior for 2 hours of television; 1 day of acceptable behavior for a recreational therapy bowling activity; 5 days of acceptable behavior for a weekend pass.
■ A therapeutic milieu provides the appropriate environment for the patient with antisocial personality. *The democratic approach, with specific rules and regulations, community meetings, and group therapy sessions, emulates the type of societal situation in which the patient must learn to live. Feedback from peers is often more effective than confrontation from an authority figure. The patient learns to follow the rules of the group as a positive step in the progression toward internalizing the rules of society.*
■ Help the patient gain insight into their behavior. Often, these individuals deny that their behavior is inappropriate. For example, rationalizing may be reflected in statements such as, "The owner of this store has so much money, he'll never miss the little bit I take. He has everything, and I have nothing. It's not fair! I deserve to have some of what he has." *The patient must come to understand that certain behaviors will not be tolerated within society and that severe consequences are imposed on those individuals who refuse to comply.* The patient must *want* to change behavior before they can be helped. One of the difficulties posed in interventions for personality disorders is that often the behaviors are ego-syntonic; in other words, the patient may not perceive these behaviors as requiring change.
■ Talk about past behaviors with the patient. Discuss which are acceptable by societal norms and which are not. Help the patient identify ways in which they have exploited others and the benefits versus consequences of previous behavior. Explore the patient's insight into feelings associated with their behavior. *This attempts to enlighten the patient to the sensitivity of others by promoting self-awareness to help the patient gain insight into their behavior.*
■ Throughout the relationship with the patient, maintain an attitude of "It is not *you*, but *your* behavior, that is unacceptable." *An attitude of acceptance promotes feelings of dignity and self-worth.*

Concept Care Mapping

The concept map care plan care (see Chapter 8, "The Nursing Process in Psychiatric-Mental Health Nursing") is a diagrammatic teaching and learning strategy that allows visualization of interrelationships between medical diagnoses, nursing diagnoses, assessment data, and treatments. An example of a concept map care plan for a patient with antisocial personality disorder is presented in Figure 31–2.

Evaluation

Reassessment is conducted to determine whether the nursing actions have been successful in achieving the objectives of care. Evaluation of the nursing actions

for the patient with antisocial personality disorder may be facilitated by gathering information using the following types of questions:

Has the patient:

■ Recognized when anger is getting out of control?
■ Sought out staff instead of expressing anger in an inappropriate manner?

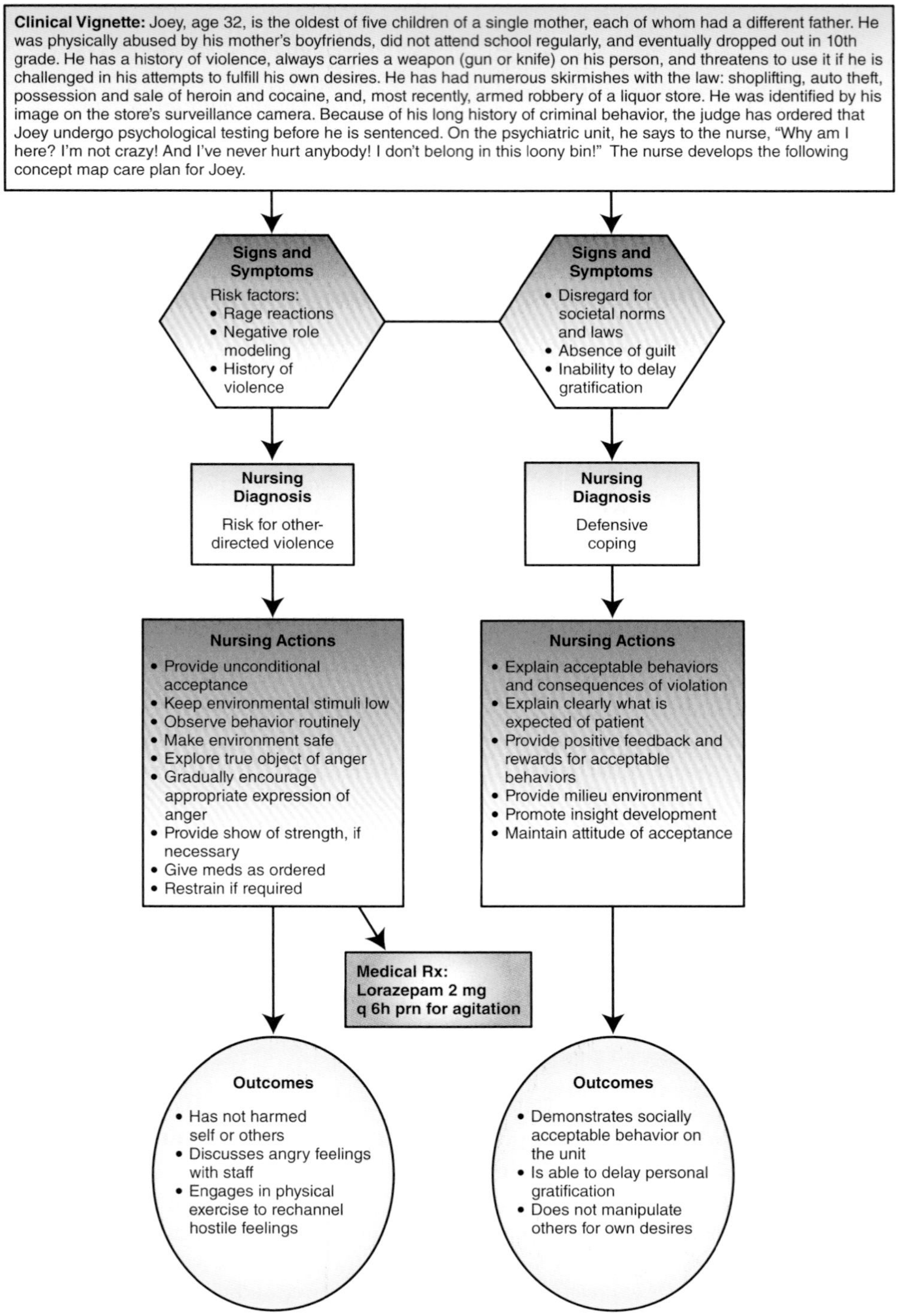

Clinical Vignette: Joey, age 32, is the oldest of five children of a single mother, each of whom had a different father. He was physically abused by his mother's boyfriends, did not attend school regularly, and eventually dropped out in 10th grade. He has a history of violence, always carries a weapon (gun or knife) on his person, and threatens to use it if he is challenged in his attempts to fulfill his own desires. He has had numerous skirmishes with the law: shoplifting, auto theft, possession and sale of heroin and cocaine, and, most recently, armed robbery of a liquor store. He was identified by his image on the store's surveillance camera. Because of his long history of criminal behavior, the judge has ordered that Joey undergo psychological testing before he is sentenced. On the psychiatric unit, he says to the nurse, "Why am I here? I'm not crazy! And I've never hurt anybody! I don't belong in this loony bin!" The nurse develops the following concept map care plan for Joey.

Signs and Symptoms

Risk factors:
• Rage reactions
• Negative role modeling
• History of violence

Signs and Symptoms

• Disregard for societal norms and laws
• Absence of guilt
• Inability to delay gratification

Nursing Diagnosis

Risk for other-directed violence

Nursing Diagnosis

Defensive coping

Nursing Actions

• Provide unconditional acceptance
• Keep environmental stimuli low
• Observe behavior routinely
• Make environment safe
• Explore true object of anger
• Gradually encourage appropriate expression of anger
• Provide show of strength, if necessary
• Give meds as ordered
• Restrain if required

Nursing Actions

• Explain acceptable behaviors and consequences of violation
• Explain clearly what is expected of patient
• Provide positive feedback and rewards for acceptable behaviors
• Provide milieu environment
• Promote insight development
• Maintain attitude of acceptance

Medical Rx:
Lorazepam 2 mg
q 6h prn for agitation

Outcomes

• Has not harmed self or others
• Discusses angry feelings with staff
• Engages in physical exercise to rechannel hostile feelings

Outcomes

• Demonstrates socially acceptable behavior on the unit
• Is able to delay personal gratification
• Does not manipulate others for own desires

FIGURE 31–2 Concept map care plan for a patient with antisocial personality disorder.

■ Used other sources for rechanneling anger (e.g., physical activities)?

■ Expressed anger without physical aggression or harm to others?

■ Followed the rules and regulations of the therapeutic milieu with little or no reminding?

■ Verbalized which behaviors are appropriate and which are not?

■ Expressed a desire to change?

■ Demonstrated ability to delay gratification of own desires in deference to those of others when appropriate?

■ Refrained from manipulating others to fulfill own desires?

■ Fulfilled activities of daily living willingly and independently?

■ Verbalized methods of achieving and maintaining optimal wellness?

■ Demonstrated knowledge of community resources from which they can seek assistance with daily living and health-care needs when required?

Treatment Modalities

Treatment of individuals with personality disorders is complex. Personality characteristics are learned very early in life and may be genetically influenced. Many of the symptoms of a personality disorder are viewed by the individual as ego-syntonic, so there may be little motivation to seek treatment or to explore change. It is not surprising that these enduring patterns of behavior may take years to change, if change does indeed occur. However, we now understand the personality as a dynamic, adaptive system and, as such, may be modifiable.

Zimmerman (2017) stresses that psychological screening is imperative for appropriate treatment. In particular, BPD is a comorbid condition in 40% of hospitalized psychiatric patients, but it often goes undetected. Although extended inpatient hospitalization for treatment of personality disorders has historically been believed to be associated with adverse events and deterioration, evidence supports that longer-term inpatient hospitalizations of 40 days or more resulted in significant improvement for patients with BPD (Fowler et al., 2018; Oldham, 2019). Such treatment programs, however, are in short supply. The main treatment modalities for personality disorders are psychosocial and pharmacological, although most of the available evidence comes from studies of borderline and antisocial personality disorders.

Comorbid conditions are common in most personality disorders, and there is evidence that treating these conditions may have positive outcomes.

There is general agreement that all treatment modalities for personality disorders require intensive long-term plans of care. Selection of intervention is generally based on the area of greatest dysfunction, such as cognition, affect, behavior, or interpersonal relations. Following is a brief description of various types of therapies and the disorders to which they are customarily suited.

Individual Psychotherapy

Depending on the therapeutic goals, psychotherapy with personality disorders may be time-limited interpersonal psychotherapy or may involve long-term psychoanalytic therapy. Interpersonal psychotherapy may be particularly appropriate because personality disorders largely reflect problems in interpersonal relationship skills.

Long-term psychotherapy attempts to understand and modify the maladjusted behaviors, cognition, and affects of clients with personality disorders that dominate their personal lives and relationships.

Milieu or Group Therapy

This treatment is especially appropriate for individuals with antisocial personality disorder, who respond more adaptively to support and feedback from peers. In milieu or group therapy, feedback from peers is more effective than one-to-one interaction with a therapist.

Group therapy—particularly homogenous supportive groups that emphasize the development of social skills—may also be helpful in overcoming social anxiety and developing interpersonal trust and rapport in clients with avoidant personality disorder. Saeed and Kallis (2022) cited evidence that supports combined treatment programs (Antonsen et al., 2016), which include short-term day-hospital treatment followed by outpatient group therapy combined with individual psychotherapy as superior to individual psychotherapy alone, particularly for reduction in symptom distress and self-control and identity integration.

Cognitive Behavior Therapy

Behavioral strategies offer reinforcement for positive change. Social skills training and assertiveness training teach alternative ways to deal with frustration. Cognitive strategies help the client recognize and correct distorted and irrational thinking patterns. Cognitive behavior therapy (CBT) is generally supported as an evidence-based treatment for personality disorders. Davidson and associates (2009) found that the addition of CBT to the usual treatment for clients with antisocial personality disorders afforded a reduction in both verbal and physical aggression. However, a more recent systematic review of psychological interventions for antisocial personality disorder concluded that there are none that demonstrate compelling evidence of behavior change in this population (Gibbon et al., 2020). There is also limited evidence that CBT is beneficial for clients with schizotypal personality disorder (Bateman et al., 2015).

Dialectical Behavior Therapy

Dialectical behavior therapy (DBT) is a type of psychotherapy originally developed by Marsha Linehan, specifically as a treatment for the chronic self-injurious and parasuicidal behavior of clients with BPD. Rooted in a belief that the primary problem for this client is emotional dysregulation (a kind of emotional reactivity to perceived threats), DBT has become a well-established treatment for clients with BPD. It is a complex, eclectic treatment that combines the concepts of cognitive, behavioral, and interpersonal therapies with Eastern mindfulness practices. The four primary modes of treatment in DBT are as follows:

1. **Group skills training:** In these groups, clients are taught skills relevant to the problems experienced by people with BPD, such as core mindfulness skills, interpersonal effectiveness skills, emotion modulation skills, and distress tolerance skills.
2. **Individual psychotherapy:** Weekly sessions address dysfunctional behavioral patterns, personal motivation, and skills strengthening.
3. **Telephone contact:** The therapist is available to the client by telephone, according to limits set by the therapist, usually for 24 hours a day. The purpose is to provide appropriate support, to counter abandonment fears, and to reduce episodes of self-harming behavior.
4. **Therapist consultation/team meeting:** Therapists meet regularly to review their work with their clients. These meetings are focused specifically on providing support for each other, keeping the therapists motivated, and providing effective treatment to their clients.

DBT has been well studied since the 1990s, and evidence supports the benefits of this treatment for clients with BPD (May et al., 2016). It has demonstrated benefits in decreasing suicidal behaviors, reducing the number of hospitalizations, and increasing adherence to the treatment plan.

This method of treatment is now being used with other disorders, including substance use disorders, eating disorders, schizophrenia, and post-traumatic stress disorder (PTSD) (Boland & Verduin, 2022). Bateman and associates (2015) cautioned, however, that of the many interventions specialized for the treatment of personality disorders, improvement is more often evidenced by symptom reduction rather than significant improvements in social functioning.

Psychoanalytic Therapies

Two psychoanalytically oriented approaches that have demonstrated benefit in the treatment of BPD are mentalization-based treatment and transference therapy. Mentalization-based treatment combines aspects of CBT, psychoanalysis, attachment theory, and social cognition research to assist clients in improving their ability to reflect on and understand internal states (their own and others) and how these states affect behavior. The goal is to teach clients to use mentalization when they are experiencing stressful situations and ultimately improve their ability to relate to others (Yasgur, 2017). A follow-up study demonstrated that this treatment resulted in significantly less incidents of self-harm, suicide attempts, and inpatient hospitalizations over an 8-year period compared with structured clinical management (Bateman et al., 2021). The authors also found that this treatment group spent fewer months receiving psychotropic medications. Transference therapy seeks to use the transference that occurs in a client-therapist relationship to help the client improve self-perception and relationship skills. Fischer-Kern and associates (2015) found that there was only significant improvement in reflective functioning (mentalization) as an outcome of this treatment approach.

Biological Interventions

Psychopharmacology may be helpful in some instances. Although these drugs have no effect in the direct treatment of the disorder itself, some symptomatic relief can be achieved.

For the treatment of BPD, symptom-targeted pharmacotherapy has been identified as an important adjunct. Antipsychotic medications show benefit in treating cognitive-perceptual symptoms, selective serotonin reuptake inhibitors show some benefit in treating emotional dysregulation, and although clinical treatment guidelines recommend use of mood stabilizers for BPD, there is little evidence of effectiveness and no U.S. Food and Drug Administration (FDA)-approved medications for this purpose (Saeed & Kallis, 2022).

Lithium may be of benefit to the patient with narcissistic personality disorder who has mood swings (Boland & Verduin, 2022). For antisocial personality disorder, pharmacotherapy is generally not recommended unless it is being used to treat a comorbid condition, although anticonvulsants may be of benefit to treat aggressive behavior, especially in the presence of abnormal electroencephalogram (EEG) waveforms (Boland & Verduin, 2022). As mentioned previously, some current research (Domes et al., 2019) identified the benefits of adjunctive oxytocin therapy in the treatment of women with BPD.

Caution must be used when prescribing medications outside the structured setting because of the high risk for substance use disorders in this population. In addition, benzodiazepines should be avoided, particularly in patients with BPD, because of the increased risk for disinhibition, which may increase acting out and self-harm behaviors (Black, 2021).

Transcranial direct current stimulation (tDCS), in one study, demonstrated benefits in the treatment of patients with BPD, particularly in reducing symptoms of impulsivity, aggression, and craving (Lisoni et al., 2020). In another study tDCS was found to improve executive function, emotional regulation, and emotional processing (Molavi et al., 2020). However, in both studies the sample sizes were small, there were no functional neuroimaging studies to support biological changes, and there were no follow-up studies (Saeed & Kallis, 2022); more research is needed.

CLINICAL JUDGMENT IN ACTION: CASE STUDY AND SAMPLE CARE PLAN

NURSING HISTORY AND ASSESSMENT

Recognizing cues: The nurse must demonstrate ability to recognize what information is most important to making an assessment (National Council of State Boards of Nursing [NCSBN], 2021). This information is italicized in the following.

Anthony, age 34, has been admitted to the psychiatric unit with a ***diagnosis of antisocial personality disorder.*** He was recently ***arrested and convicted for armed robbery*** of a convenience store and ***attempted murder of the store clerk.*** Due to the actions of the store clerk, who quickly alerted police, and to the store surveillance camera, Anthony was identified and apprehended within hours of the crime. The judge has ordered physical, neurological, and psychiatric evaluations before sentencing Anthony.

Anthony was ***physically and psychologically abused as a child by his alcoholic father.*** He was ***suspended from high school because of failing grades and habitual truancy.*** He has a ***long history of arrests,*** beginning with shoplifting at age 7, progressing in adolescence to burglary, auto theft, and sexual assault, and finally to armed robbery and attempted murder. He ***was on probation when he committed his latest crime.***

On the psychiatric unit, Anthony is ***loud, belligerent, and uncooperative.*** When Julie, his admitting nurse, arrives to work the evening shift on Anthony's second hospital day, he says to her, ***"I'm so glad you are finally here. You are the best nurse on the unit. I can't talk to anyone but you. These people are nothing but a bunch of loonies around here—and that includes staff as well as patients! Maybe you and I could walk down to the coffee shop together later. Are you married? I'd sure like to get to know you better after I get out of this nuthouse!"***

Analyzing cues: The nurse must be able to interpret the information (NCSBN, 2021).

The nurse interprets Anthony's long history of arrests, lack of remorse for his actions, and history of trauma as consistent with the diagnosis of antisocial personality disorder. His recent behavior is interpreted as posing safety risks for violence toward others. Anthony's communication with the nurse is interpreted as outside the boundaries of a professional nurse–patient relationship and suggests attempts to manipulate the nurse by showing special interest in the nurse on a personal level.

Prioritize hypotheses: The nurse must be able to identify the client's most important needs (NCSBN, 2021).

Recognizing that patient safety and safety of others is always a priority, the nurse identifies the risk of violence toward others as the primary concern. Inferring that Anthony's history of trauma is influential in his current maladaptive behaviors, the nurse also prioritizes a focus on coping skills.

NURSING DIAGNOSES AND OUTCOME IDENTIFICATION

Generate solutions: The nurse must be able to connect their prioritized understanding of client needs to a course of action or plan of care (NCSBN, 2021).

From the assessment data, the nurse develops the following nursing diagnoses for Anthony:

1. Risk for other-directed violence related to history of violence against others and history of childhood abuse.
   a. Short-term goals:
      - The patient will discuss angry feelings and situations that precipitate hostility.
      - The patient will not harm others.
   b. Long-term goal:
      - The patient will not harm others.
2. Defensive coping related to low self-esteem, dysfunctional nuclear family, underdeveloped ego and superego, evidenced by absence of guilt feelings, disregard for societal laws and norms, inability to delay gratification, superior attitude toward others, denial of problems, and projection of blame and responsibility.
   a. Short-term goal:
      - The patient will verbalize understanding of unit rules and regulations and consequences for violation of them.

Continued

CLINICAL JUDGMENT IN ACTION: CASE STUDY AND SAMPLE CARE PLAN—cont'd

b. Long-term goals:
- The patient will be able to delay gratification and follow rules and regulations of the unit.
- The patient will verbalize personal responsibility for own actions and behaviors.

PLANNING AND IMPLEMENTATION

Take Action: The nurse must be able to identify what actions need to be taken and how they will be implemented (NCSBN, 2021).

RISK FOR OTHER-DIRECTED VIOLENCE

The following nursing interventions have been identified for Anthony.

1. Develop a trusting relationship with Anthony by conveying an accepting attitude. Ensure that he understands it is not him but his behavior that is unacceptable.
2. Try to keep excess stimuli out of the environment. Speak to Anthony in a calm, quiet voice.
3. Observe Anthony's behavior regularly through routine activity so that he does not become suspicious and angry about being watched. If hostile and aggressive behaviors are observed, intervention may prevent harm to Anthony, staff members, and/or other patients.
4. Assess Anthony's trauma history at his comfort level and encourage him to talk about his anger and hostile feelings. Help him understand where these feelings originate and identify the true target of the hostility.
5. Help him develop adaptive ways of dealing with frustration, such as exercise and other physical activities.
6. Administer sedative medication as ordered by the physician.
7. If Anthony should become out of control and mechanical restraints become necessary, ensure that sufficient staff is available to intervene. Do not use restraints as a punishment, but only as a last resort, protective measure for Anthony and the other patients.

DEFENSIVE COPING

The following nursing interventions have been identified for Anthony.

1. Explain to Anthony which of his behaviors are acceptable on the unit and which are not. Simply state that unacceptable behaviors will not be tolerated.

2. Determine appropriate consequences for violation of these limits (e.g., no TV or movies; no phone calls; time-out room). Ensure that all staff members follow through with these consequences.
3. Do not be taken in by Anthony's attempts to flatter or "charm" staff members. Compliments from Anthony are another form of manipulative behavior. Explain to Anthony that you will not accept these types of comments from him, and if they continue, impose consequences.
4. Encourage Anthony to talk about his past misdeeds. Try to help him understand how he would feel if someone treated him in the manner that he has treated others.

EVALUATION

Evaluate outcomes: The nurse must be able to evaluate actions taken and determine whether they have had a positive, neutral, or negative effect (NCSBN, 2021).

The outcome criteria for Anthony have only partially been met. Personality characteristics such as those of Anthony's are deep-rooted and enduring. He does not present any evidence of intent to change his behavior and feels that many of his actions are justified because he has to "do what [he thinks] needs to be done." The nurse evaluates that he is likely to continue to endure legal consequences and prison sentences until he develops insight and willingness to engage in behavior change. During his time on the psychiatric unit, harm to self and others has been avoided. He has discussed his anger and hostile feelings with Julie and other staff members. He continues to become belligerent when told that he cannot smoke on the unit and must wait for someone to escort him to the smoking area. He yells at the other patients and calls them "nut cases." He refuses to take responsibility for his actions and blames negative behavioral outcomes on others. He has begun a regular exercise program in the fitness room and receives positive feedback from the staff for this attempt to integrate healthier coping strategies.

Summary and Key Points

- People with personality disorders may present with some of the most challenging symptoms healthcare workers are likely to encounter.
- Personality characteristics are formed very early in life and are difficult to change. In fact, some clinicians believe the therapeutic approach is not

to try to change the characteristics but rather to decrease the inflexibility of the maladaptive traits and reduce their interference with everyday functioning and meaningful relationships.

- The concept of a personality disorder has been present throughout the history of medicine. There have been controversies over the best way to classify these disorders.

■ The *DSM-5-TR* identifies 10 individual personality disorders: antisocial, avoidant, borderline, histrionic, dependent, narcissistic, obsessive-compulsive, paranoid, schizoid, and schizotypal.

■ Nursing care of the patient with a personality disorder is accomplished using the steps of the nursing process.

■ Other treatment modalities include interpersonal psychotherapy, psychoanalytical psychotherapy (including mentalization-based treatment and transference therapy), milieu or group therapy, cognitive behavior therapy, dialectical behavior therapy, psychopharmacology, and transcranial direct current stimulation.

■ Individuals with BPD may enter the health-care system because of their instability and frequent attempts at self-destructive behavior.

■ The individual with antisocial personality disorder may become part of the health-care system to avoid legal consequences or because of a court order for psychological evaluation.

■ Nurses who work in all types of clinical settings should be familiar with the characteristics associated with personality disorders.

■ Nurses working in psychiatry must be knowledgeable about appropriate interventions, have good therapeutic communication skills, and have a clear sense of professional boundaries to meet the complex needs of patients with personality disorders.

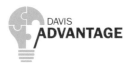 DAVIS ADVANTAGE | Go to **Davis Advantage** to complete your learning: strengthen understanding, apply your knowledge, and prepare for the Next Gen NCLEX®.

Review Questions

1. A client diagnosed with borderline personality disorder manipulates the staff in an effort to fulfill their own desires. All of the following may be examples of manipulative behaviors in the borderline patient *except:*
   a. Refusal to stay in a room alone, stating, "It's so lonely."
   b. Asking the nurse for cigarettes after 30 minutes, knowing the assigned nurse has explained they must wait 1 hour.
   c. Stating to the nurse, "I really like having you for my nurse. You're the best one around here."
   d. Cutting arms with razor blade after discussing dismissal plans with physician.

2. A client on the psychiatric unit has a diagnosis of antisocial personality disorder. Which of the following characteristics is consistent with this diagnosis?
   a. Lack of guilt for wrongdoing
   b. Insight into their own behavior
   c. Ability to learn from past experiences
   d. Compliance with authority

3. A nurse on the psychiatric unit documents that the client was attempting to use "splitting" behaviors with staff. This should be interpreted to mean that the client is exhibiting what behavior?
   a. Trying to keep staff away from other patients
   b. Characterizing staff members as either all good or all bad
   c. Having brief psychotic episodes
   d. Manifesting two or more distinct subpersonalities when communicating with staff

4. According to researchers, which of the following is a common theme in the health history of the client with borderline personality disorder?
   a. Autism
   b. Attention deficit-hyperactivity disorder
   c. Positive and fulfilling interpersonal relationships
   d. Early childhood trauma

5. Which of the following behavioral patterns is characteristic of individuals with narcissistic personality disorder?
   a. Overly self-centered and exploitative of others
   b. Suspicious and mistrustful of others
   c. Rule conscious and disapproving of change
   d. Anxious and socially isolated

6. Which of the following behavioral patterns is characteristic of individuals with schizoid personality disorder?
   a. Belittling themselves and their abilities
   b. A lifelong pattern of social withdrawal
   c. Suspicious and mistrustful of others
   d. Overreacting inappropriately to minor stimuli

Clinical Judgment Questions

7. A client with a diagnosis of borderline personality disorder exhibits alternating clinging and distancing behaviors with the nurse who has been assigned to their care. Which is the most appropriate nursing intervention for the client with this type of behavior?
   a. Encourage the client to establish trust in one staff person with whom all therapeutic interaction should take place.
   b. Secure a verbal contract from the client to discontinue these behaviors.
   c. Withdraw attention if these behaviors continue.
   d. Rotate staff members who work with the client so that the client will learn to relate to more than one person.

8. A client diagnosed with antisocial personality disorder approaches the nurse and says, "You're so cute, are you married?" Which of these is the most appropriate response by the nurse?
   a. "I'm married, but that's none of your business."
   b. "Let's talk about your love life instead."
   c. "Thank you so much for the compliment but I'm married."
   d. "Our relationship is strictly professional. It is not appropriate for us to have that kind of discussion."

9. A client with borderline personality disorder reports to the nurse that she is having abdominal pain and is requesting pain medication. Which action by the nurse is a priority?
   a. Explore alternative pain management strategies
   b. Confront the client about their manipulation to try to get drugs
   c. Assess the client's pain in more detail
   d. Set limits on the client's attempts to cling to the nurse

10. A male client with antisocial personality disorder was found on the bed in a female patient's room. When instructed to leave the room, the client states, "I'm sick of you telling me what I can or can't do. If I want to carry on a relationship with one of these ladies, it's my right. I'll do exactly as I please!" Which of these actions by the nurse is a priority at this point?
    a. Reassure the client that he will have plenty of opportunities with women after he is discharged.
    b. Reinforce the rules of the treatment program that all clients are expected to follow.
    c. Escort the client to seclusion.
    d. Establish a trusting relationship by telling the client that you will make an exception just this once.

IMPLICATIONS OF RESEARCH FOR EVIDENCE-BASED PRACTICE

Yen, S., Peters, J. R., Nishar, S., Grilo, C. M., Sanislow, C. A., Shea, M. T., Zanarini, M. C., McGlashan, T. H., Morey, L. C., & Skodol, A. E. (2020). Association of borderline personality disorder criteria with suicide attempts: Findings from the collaborative longitudinal study of personality disorders over 10 years of follow-up. *JAMA Psychiatry, 78*(2), 187–194. https//doi.org/10.1001/jamapsychiatry.2020.3598

DESCRIPTION OF THE STUDY: This longitudinal follow-up study of treatment-seeking individuals (n = 701) with personality disorders sought to identify factors associated with risk for suicide behavior, including suicide attempts. The intent was to identify those risk factors that could inform interventions. Participants were assessed annually using semistructured diagnostic interviews and a variety of self-report measures for up to 10 years.

RESULTS OF THE STUDY: Of all disorders, BPD emerged as the most robust factor associated with prospectively

observed suicide attempt(s) (odds ratio, even after controlling for significant demographic [sex, employment, and education] and clinical [childhood sexual abuse, alcohol use disorder, substance use disorder, and post-traumatic stress disorder] factors). Among BPD criteria, identity disturbance (inconsistency in beliefs, values, and actions), chronic feelings of emptiness, and frantic efforts to avoid abandonment emerged as significant independent factors associated with suicide attempt(s) over follow-up.

IMPLICATIONS FOR NURSING PRACTICE: BPD has long been identified as a disorder associated with frequent suicidal behavior. Understanding the features that may increase risk for these behaviors can guide the nurse's assessment and interventions directed toward suicide prevention.

TEST YOUR CLINICAL REASONING AND CLINICAL JUDGMENT SKILLS

Dana, age 32, was diagnosed with borderline personality disorder when she was 26 years old. Her husband took her to the emergency department when he walked into the bathroom and found her cutting her legs with a razor blade. At that time, assessment revealed that Dana had a long history of self-mutilation, which she had carefully hidden from her husband and others. Dana began long-term psychoanalytical psychotherapy on an outpatient basis. Therapy revealed that Dana had been physically and sexually abused as a child by both her mother and her father, both now deceased. She admitted to having chronic depression, and her husband related episodes of rage reactions. Dana has been hospitalized on the psychiatric unit for a week because of suicidal ideations. After a reassessment for suicide risk, it is determined that she is ready to be discharged and is scheduled to attend an outpatient therapy session later in the day. She has just returned to the inpatient unit and says to her nurse, "You are so much more helpful than those outpatient therapists. I just took 20 Desyrel while I was sitting in my car in the parking lot and I probably need to be readmitted."

Answer the following questions related to Dana:

1. The nurse is well acquainted with Dana and believes this is a manipulative gesture. How should the nurse handle this situation?
2. What is the priority nursing diagnosis for Dana?
3. Dana likes to "split" the staff into "good guys" and "bad guys." What is the most important intervention for splitting by a person with borderline personality disorder?

Communication Exercises

1. Nathan, age 37, has been admitted to the hospital for a psychiatric evaluation after being arrested for armed robbery of a convenience store. He has a history of encounters with law enforcement since early adolescence. He has been diagnosed with antisocial personality disorder. Nathan says to the nurse, "Hey pretty lady! Where have you been all my life?"

   How would the nurse respond appropriately to this statement by Nathan?
2. "I really got a bum rap! I had no intentions of hurting anyone. The gun only had one bullet in it! I just wanted to scare that clerk into giving me a few bucks! Just my bad luck an off-duty cop had to walk in about that time."

   How would the nurse respond appropriately to this statement by Nathan?
3. "You're really cute. Are you married? I'm pretty sure my lawyer can get me out of this rap, and I'll be a free man! Why don't you give me your phone number and I'll call you sometime. We could go out and have some fun!"

   How would the nurse respond appropriately to this statement by Nathan?

MOVIE CONNECTIONS

Taxi Driver (schizoid personality) • *One Flew Over the Cuckoo's Nest* (antisocial) • *The Boston Strangler* (antisocial) • *Just Cause* (antisocial) • *The Dream Team* (antisocial) • *Goodfellas* (antisocial) • *Fatal Attraction* (BPD) • *Play Misty for Me* (BPD) • *Girl, Interrupted* (BPD) • *Gone With the Wind* (histrionic) • *Wall Street* (narcissistic) • *The Odd Couple* (obsessive-compulsive) • *Welcome to Me* (BPD)

References

Abdalla-Filho, E. & Völlm, B. (2020). Does every psychopath have an antisocial personality disorder? *Brazilian Journal of Psychiatry, 42*(3), 241–242. doi:10.1590/1516-4446-2019-0762

Afifi, T. O., Fortier, J., Sareen, J., & Taillieu, T. (2019). Associations of harsh physical punishment and child maltreatment in childhood with antisocial behaviors in adulthood. *JAMA Network Open, 2*(1), e187374. doi:10.1001/jamanetworkopen.2018.7374

American Psychiatric Association (APA). (2022). *Diagnostic and statistical manual of mental disorders, fifth edition, text revision (DSM-5-TR).* American Psychiatric Association.

Antonsen, B. T., Kvarstein, E. H., Urnes, Ø., Hummelen, B., Karterud, S., & Wilberg, T. (2017). Favourable outcome of long-term combined psychotherapy for patients with borderline personality disorder: Six-year follow-up of a randomized study. *Psychotherapy Research, (1),* 51–63. doi:10.1080/10503307.2015.1072283

Bateman, A., Constantinou, M. P., Fonagy, P., & Holzer, S. (2021). Eight-year prospective follow-up of mentalization-based treatment versus structured clinical management for people with borderline personality disorder. *Personality Disorders: Theory, Research, and Treatment, 12*(4), 291–299. https://doi.org/10.1037/per0000422

Bateman, A. W., Gunderson, J., & Mulder, R. (2015). Treatment of personality disorder. *Lancet, 385,* 735–743. doi:10.1016/S0140-6736(14)61394-5

Bierzynska, M., Sobczak, P. A., Kozak, A., Bielecki, M., Strelau, J., & Kossut, M. M. (2019). No risk, no differences. Neural correlates of temperamental traits revealed using naturalistic fMRI method. *Frontiers in Psychology, 6*(10), 1757. doi:10.3389/fpsyg.2019.01757

Black, D. (2021). A clinical approach to pharmacotherapy for personality disorders. *Current Psychiatry, 20*(4), 27–32.

Boland, R., & Verduin, M. L. (2022). *Kaplan & Sadock's synopsis of psychiatry* (P. Ruiz, Ed.). (12th ed.). Wolters Kluwer.

Bozzatello, P., Rocca, P., Baldassarri, L., Bosia, M., & Bellino, S. (2021). The role of trauma in early onset borderline personality disorder: A biopsychosocial perspective. *Frontiers in Psychiatry 12,* 721361. doi:10.3389/fpsyt.2021.721361

Cattane, N., Rossi, R., Lanfredi, M., Cattaneo, A. (2017). Borderline personality disorder and childhood trauma: Exploring the affected biological systems and mechanisms. *BMC Psychiatry 17,* 221. https://doi.org/10.1186/s12888-017-1383-2

Cloninger, C. R., & Svrakic, D. M. (2017). Personality disorders. In Sadock, B.J., Sadock, V. A., & Ruiz, P. (Eds.), *Comprehensive textbook of psychiatry* (10th ed., pp. 2126–2176). Wolters Kluwer.

Davidson, K. M., Tyrer, P., Tata, P., Cook, D., Gumely, A., Ford, I., Walker, A., Bezlyak, V., Sievewright, H., Robertson, H., & Crawford, M. J. (2009). Cognitive behaviour therapy for violent men with antisocial personality disorder in the community: An exploratory randomized controlled trial. *Psychological Medicine, 39*(4), 569–577. doi:10.1017/S00332910708004066

DeLisi, M., Drury, A. J., & Elbert, M. J. (2019). The etiology of antisocial personality disorder: The differential roles of adverse childhood experiences and childhood psychopathology. *Comprehensive Psychiatry, 92,* 1–6. https://doi.org/10.1016/j.comppsych.2019.04.001

Ditrich, I., Philipsen, A., & Matthies, S. (2021). Borderline personality disorder (BPD) and attention deficit hyperactivity disorder (ADHD) revisited—A review-update on common grounds and subtle distinctions. *Borderline Personality Disorder and Emotional Dysregulation 8*(22). https://doi.org/10.1186/s40479-021-00162-w

Domes, G., Ower, N., von Dawans, B., Spengler, F. B., Dziobek, I., Bohus, M., Matthies, S., Philipsen, A., & Heinrichs, M. (2019). Effects of intranasal oxytocin administration on empathy and approach motivation in women with borderline personality disorder: A randomized controlled trial. *Translational Psychiatry 9,* 328 (2019). https://doi.org/10.1038/s41398-019-0658-4

Fischer-Kern, M., Doering, S., Taubner, S., Hörz, S., Zimmermann, J., Rentrop, M., Schuster, P., Buchheim, P., & Buchheim, A. (2015). Transference-focused psychotherapy for borderline personality disorder: Change in reflective function. *British Journal of Psychiatry. 207*(2):173–174. doi:10.1192/bjp.bp.113.143842

Fowler, J. C., Clapp, J. D., Madan, A., Allen, J. G., Frueh, C., Fonagy, P., & Oldham, J. M. (2018). A naturalistic longitudinal study of extended inpatient treatment for adults with borderline personality disorder: An examination of treatment response, remission and deterioration. *Journal of Affective Disorders, 235,* 323–331. doi:https://doi.org/10.1016/j.jad.2017.12.054

Gibbon, S., Khalifa, N. R., Cheung, N. H., Völlm, B. A., McCarthy, L. (2020). Psychological interventions for antisocial personality disorder. *Cochrane Database of Systematic Reviews. 9*(9), CD007668. doi:10.1002/14651858.CD007668.pub3

Gregory, C., & Soriano, K. (2022). *Tell me all I need to know about narcissistic personality disorder.* https://www.psycom.net/personality-disorders/narcissistic/

Herdman, T. H., Kamitsuru, S., & Lopes, C. T. (Eds.). (2021). *NANDA-I, Inc. nursing diagnoses: Definitions and classification, 2021–2023.* Thieme.

Johanson, M., Vaurio, O., Tiihonen, J., & Lähteenvuo, M. (2020). A systematic literature review of neuroimaging of psychopathic traits. *Frontiers in Psychiatry 10,* 1027. doi:10.3389/fpsyt.2019.01027

Junewicz, A., & Billick, S. B. (2021). Preempting the development of antisocial behavior and psychopathic traits. *The Journal of the American Academy of Psychiatry and the Law, 49*(1), 66–76. doi:10.29158/JAAPL.200060-20

Kolla, N. J., & Vinette, S. A. (2017). Monoamine oxidase a in antisocial personality disorder and borderline personality disorder. *Current Behavioral Neuroscience Reports, 4*(1), 41–48. doi:10.1007/s40473-017-0102-0

Lisoni, J., Miotto, P., Barlati, S., Calza, S., Crescini, A., Deste, G., Sacchetti, E., & Vita, A. (2020). Change in core symptoms of borderline personality disorder by tDCS: A pilot study. *Psychiatry Research, 291,* 113261. doi:10.1016/j.psychres.2020.113261

May, J. M., Richardi, T. M., & Barth, K. S. (2016). Dialectical behavior therapy as treatment for borderline personality disorder. *Mental Health Clinics, 6*(2), 62–67. doi:10.9740/mhc.2016.03.62

Mayo Clinic. (2022). *Narcissistic personality disorder.* https://www.mayoclinic.org/diseases-conditions/narcissistic-personality-disorder/symptoms-causes/syc-20366662

McNee, L., Donogue, C., & Coppola, A. M. (2014). A team approach to borderline personality disorder. *Mental Health Practice, 17*(10), 33–35. doi:http://dx.doi.org/10.7748/mhp.17.10.33.e887

Molavi, P., Aziziaram, S., Basharpoor, S., Atadokht, A., Nitsche, M. A., & Salehinejad, M. A. (2020). Repeated transcranial direct current stimulation of dorsolateral-prefrontal cortex improves executive functions, cognitive reappraisal emotion regulation, and control over emotional processing in borderline personality disorder: A randomized, sham-controlled, parallel-group study. *Journal of Affective Disorders, 274*, 93–102. doi:10.1016/j.jad.2020.05.007

National Council of State Boards of Nursing (NCSBN). (2021). *Next generation NCLEX®: Comparison between case studies and stand-alone items.* https://www.ncsbn.org/public-files/NGN_Fall21_English_Final.pdf

Oldham, J. (2019). Inpatient treatment for patients with borderline personality disorder. *Journal of Psychiatric Practice, 25*(3), 177–178.

Paris, J. (2019). Suicidality in borderline personality disorder. *Medicina (Kaunas), 55*(6), 223. doi:10.3390/medicina55060223

Richmond, J. R., Tull, M. T., & Gratz, K. L. (2020). The roles of emotion regulation difficulties and impulsivity in the associations between borderline personality disorder symptoms and frequency of nonprescription sedative use and prescription sedative/opioid misuse. *Journal of Contextual and Behavioral Sciences, 16*, 62–70. doi:10.1016/j.jcbs.2020.03.002.

Rodriguez, T. (2017). *Bipolar disorder, borderline personality disorder may represent the same disorder.* http://www.psychiatryadvisor.com/bipolar-disorder/bipolar-disordersame-as-borderline-personality-disorder/article/712397

Saeed, S. A., & Kallis, A. C. (2021). Borderline personality disorder: 6 studies of biological interventions. *Current Psychiatry, 20*(11), 27–36.

Yasgur, B. S. (2017). Borderline personality disorder: Not just an adult condition. *Psychiatric Advisor.* http://www.psychiatryadvisor.com/childadolescent-psychiatry/borderlinepersonality-adult-adolescent/article/708450/2/

Yen, S., Peters, J. R., Nishar, S., Grilo, C. M., Sanislow, C. A., Shea, M. T., Zanarini, M. C., McGlashan, T. H., Morey, L. C., & Skodol, A. E. (2020). Association of borderline personality disorder criteria with suicide attempts: Findings from the collaborative longitudinal study of personality disorders over 10 years of follow-up. *JAMA Psychiatry, 78*(2), 187–194. https//doi.org/10.1001/jamapsychiatry.2020.3598

Zimmerman, M. (2017). Improving the recognition of borderline personality disorder. *Current Psychiatry, 16*(10), 13–19.

Zimmerman, M. (2019). Borderpolar: Patients with borderline personality disorder and bipolar disorder. *Psychiatric Times, 36*(12). https://www.psychiatrictimes.com/view/borderpolar-patients-borderline-personality-disorder-and-bipolar-disorder

Zwir, I., Arnedo, J., Del-Val, C., Pulkki-Råback, L., Konte, B., Yang, S. S., Romero-Zaliz, R., Hintsanen, M., Cloninger, K. M., Garcia, D., Svrakic, D., Rozsa, S., Martinez, M., Lyytikäinen, L., Giegling, I., Kähönen, M., Hernandez-Cuervo, H., Seppälä, I., Raitoharju, E., ... Cloninger, C. R. (2020). Uncovering the complex genetics of human character. *Molecular Psychiatry 25*, 2295–2312 (2020). https://doi.org/10.1038/s41380-018-0263-6

Classical References

Erikson, E. (1963). *Childhood and society* (2nd ed.). WW Norton.

Mahler, M., Pine, F., & Bergman, A. (1975). *The psychological birth of the human infant.* Basic Books.

Sullivan, H. S. (1953). *The interpersonal theory of psychiatry.* WW Norton.

UNIT 5

Psychiatric-Mental Health Nursing of Special Populations

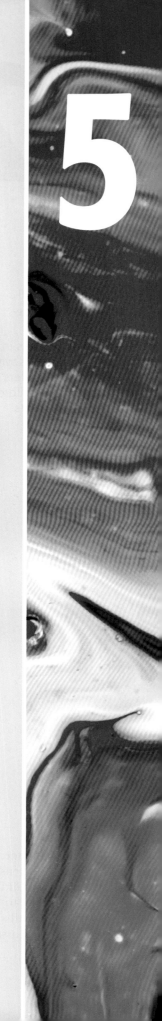

32 Children and Adolescents

CORE CONCEPTS

Growth and
Development

Health Promotion

Stress and Coping

Professionalism:
Nursing process in the
care of patients with
selected disorders
occurring in children
and adolescents

KEY TERMS

aggression
attention deficit-hyperactivity disorder (ADHD)
autism spectrum disorder (ASD)
clinging
conduct disorder
echolalia
hyperactivity
impulsivity

intellectual developmental disorder
(intellectual disability)
negativism
oppositional defiant disorder (ODD)
palilalia
separation anxiety disorder
temperament
Tourette's disorder

OBJECTIVES
After reading this chapter, the student will be able to:

1. Identify psychiatric disorders that
commonly have their onset in infancy,
childhood, or adolescence.
2. Discuss predisposing factors implicated in
the etiology of intellectual developmental
disorder, autism spectrum disorder, attention
deficit-hyperactivity disorder, conduct disorder, oppositional defiant disorder, Tourette's
disorder, and separation anxiety disorder.
3. Identify symptomatology and use the
information in the assessment of patients
with the aforementioned disorders.

4. Identify nursing diagnoses common to
patients with these disorders and select
appropriate nursing interventions for each.
5. Discuss relevant criteria for evaluating
nursing care of patients with selected
infant, childhood, and adolescent psychiatric disorders.
6. Describe treatment modalities relevant to
selected disorders of infancy, childhood,
and adolescence.

This chapter examines various disorders in which
symptoms usually first become evident during
infancy, childhood, or adolescence. However, it is
important to note that some of the disorders discussed in this chapter may appear later in life, and
symptoms associated with other disorders, such as

major depressive disorder or bipolar disorder, may
appear in childhood or adolescence.

All nurses working with children or adolescents
should be knowledgeable about "normal" stages of
growth and development. Online Chapter 38, "Theoretical Models of Personality Development," discusses

this topic, and Chapter 31, "Personality Disorders," includes a summary of personality development theories. The developmental process is fraught with challenges. Behavioral responses are individual and idiosyncratic. They are, indeed, *human* responses.

Whether or not a child's behavior indicates emotional problems is often difficult to determine. Guidelines for making such a determination should consider the appropriateness of the behavior according to age and cultural norms and whether the behavior interferes with adaptive functioning. This chapter focuses on the nursing process in the care of patients with intellectual developmental disorder, autism spectrum disorder (ASD), attention deficit-hyperactivity disorder (ADHD), conduct disorder, oppositional defiant disorder (ODD), Tourette's disorder, and separation anxiety disorder. Additional treatment modalities are included.

Neurodevelopmental Disorders

Intellectual Developmental Disorder

The *Diagnostic and Statistical Manual of Mental Disorders, Fifth Edition, Text Revision (DSM-5-TR)* defines **intellectual developmental disorder** (equivalent to *intellectual disability*) as a "disorder with onset during the developmental period that includes both intellectual and adaptive functioning deficits in conceptual, social, and practical domains" (American Psychiatric Association [APA], 2022, p. 37). The prevalence in the general population is about 10 per 1,000 (APA, 2022). The level of severity (mild, moderate, severe, or profound) is based on adaptive functioning within the three domains. General intellectual functioning (cognitive and learning function) is measured by both clinical assessment and an individual's performance on intelligence quotient (IQ) tests. Adaptive functioning refers to the person's ability to adapt to the requirements of daily living (such as communication, social, and independent functioning) and the expectations of the individual's age and cultural group (APA, 2022).

Predisposing Factors

The etiology of intellectual developmental disorder may be primarily biological, primarily psychosocial, a combination of both, and in some instances unknown. Regardless of etiology, the common factors are significant impairments in intellectual functions and social adaptation.

Genetic Factors

Genetic factors are implicated as the cause of intellectual developmental disorder in approximately 5% of cases. These factors include inborn errors of metabolism, such as Tay-Sachs disease; phenylketonuria; and hyperglycinemia (abnormally high levels of glycine). Also included are chromosomal disorders, such as Down's syndrome and Klinefelter's syndrome, and single-gene abnormalities, such as fragile X syndrome, tuberous sclerosis, and neurofibromatosis.

Disruptions in Embryonic Development

Conditions that result in early alterations in embryonic development account for approximately 30% of intellectual developmental disorder cases. Damage may occur in response to toxicity associated with maternal ingestion of alcohol or other drugs. For example, fetal alcohol syndrome (one of the fetal alcohol spectrum disorders) has been identified as one of the leading preventable causes of intellectual developmental disorder. Maternal illnesses and infections during pregnancy (e.g., rubella, cytomegalovirus) and complications of pregnancy (e.g., toxemia, uncontrolled diabetes) also can result in congenital intellectual developmental disorder (Boland & Verduin, 2022).

Pregnancy and Perinatal Factors

Approximately 10% of cases of intellectual developmental disorder are the result of circumstances that occur during pregnancy (e.g., fetal malnutrition, viral and other infections, and prematurity) or during the birth process. Examples of the latter include trauma to the head incurred during the process of birth, placenta previa or premature separation of the placenta, and prolapse of the umbilical cord.

General Medical Conditions Acquired in Infancy or Childhood

General medical conditions acquired during infancy or childhood account for approximately 5% of cases of intellectual developmental disorder. They include infections, such as meningitis and encephalitis; poisonings, such as from insecticides, medications, and lead; and physical trauma, such as head injuries, asphyxiation, and hyperpyrexia. Universal use of the measles vaccine had virtually eliminated measles encephalitis but recent refusal to vaccinate by some individuals and communities has increased this risk (Boland & Verduin, 2022).

Sociocultural Factors and Other Mental Disorders

Between 15% and 20% of cases of intellectual developmental disorder may be attributed to deprivation of nurturance and social stimulation and to impoverished environments associated with poor prenatal and perinatal care and inadequate nutrition. In approximately 30% of cases, ASD and intellectual developmental disorder are comorbid, and research suggests that there are phenotypic and genetic overlaps between the two disorders (Bhatia, 2022).

Recognition of the cause and time of inception provides information regarding what to expect in terms of behavior and potential. However, each child is different, and consideration must be given on an individual basis.

Application of the Nursing Process to Intellectual Developmental Disorder

Background Assessment Data (Symptomatology)

The degree of severity of intellectual developmental disorder may be measured by the individual's IQ level, but as the APA notes in the *DSM-5-TR* (2022) "neuropsychological testing as well as cross-battery intellectual assessment (using multiple IQ or other cognitive tests to create a profile) are more useful for understanding intellectual abilities than a single IQ score" (p. 38). Four levels have been delineated: mild, moderate, severe, and profound. The various behavioral manifestations and abilities associated with each of these levels of severity are outlined in Table 32–1.

Nurses should assess and focus on each child's strengths and individual abilities. Knowledge regarding a child's level of independence in the performance of self-care activities is essential to the development of an adequate plan for nursing care.

Nursing Diagnosis

Selection of appropriate nursing diagnoses for the patient with intellectual developmental disorder depends largely on the degree of severity of the condition and the patient's capabilities. Possible nursing diagnoses include the following:

■ Risk for injury related to altered physical mobility or aggressive behavior
■ Self-care deficit related to altered physical mobility or lack of maturity
■ Impaired verbal communication related to developmental alteration

TABLE 32–1	Developmental Characteristics of Intellectual Developmental Disorder by Degree of Severity			
LEVEL	**ABILITY TO PERFORM SELF-CARE ACTIVITIES**	**COGNITIVE/EDUCATIONAL CAPABILITIES**	**SOCIAL/COMMUNICATION CAPABILITIES**	**PSYCHOMOTOR CAPABILITIES**
Mild	May need some support with complex activities of daily living. As an adult is generally capable of independent living with assistance during times of stress.	Capable of academic skills to sixth-grade level. As an adult, can achieve vocational skills for minimum self-support.	Capable of developing social skills. Social judgment is immature for age and may increase risk of being manipulated. Communication and language is more concrete or immature than expected for age.	Psychomotor skills usually not affected, although may have some slight problems with coordination.
Moderate	Can perform some activities independently. Requires supervision.	Unlikely to achieve academic skill beyond second-grade level. As adult may be able to contribute to own support in a sheltered workshop.	May experience some limitation in speech communication. Difficulty adhering to social convention may interfere with peer relationships.	Motor development is fair. Vocational capabilities may be limited to unskilled gross motor activities.
Severe	Requires support for all activities of daily living. Requires complete supervision.	Unable to benefit from vocational training. Attainment of conceptual skills is limited. Profits from systematic habit training.	Minimal verbal skills. Wants and needs often communicated by acting-out behaviors.	Poor motor development. Able to perform only simple tasks under close supervision.
Profound	No capacity for independent functioning. Requires constant aid and supervision.	Unable to profit from academic or vocational training. May respond to minimal training in self-help if presented in the close context of a one-to-one relationship.	Little, if any, speech development. Needs are typically expressed nonverbally. May respond to relationship with close, well-known others and initiate social interaction through gestures and emotions.	Lack of ability for both fine and gross motor movements. Requires constant supervision and care. May be associated with other physical disorders.

Adapted from American Psychiatric Association. (2022). *Diagnostic and statistical manual of mental disorders, fifth edition, text revision (DSM-5-TR)*. American Psychiatric Association; and Boland, R., & Verduin, M. L. (2022). *Kaplan & Sadock's synopsis of psychiatry* (P. Ruiz, Ed.). (12th ed.). Wolters Kluwer.

■ Impaired social interaction related to speech deficiencies or difficulty adhering to conventional social behavior
■ Delayed growth and development related to isolation from significant others, inadequate environmental stimulation, genetic factors
■ Anxiety (moderate to severe) related to hospitalization and absence of familiar surroundings
■ Defensive coping related to feelings of powerlessness and threat to self-esteem
■ Ineffective coping related to inadequate coping skills secondary to developmental delay

Outcome Identification

Outcome criteria include short- and long-term goals. Timelines are individually determined. The following criteria may be used for measurement of outcomes in the care of the patient with intellectual developmental disorder.

The patient:

■ Has experienced no physical harm
■ Has had self-care needs fulfilled
■ Interacts with others in a socially appropriate manner
■ Has maintained anxiety at a manageable level
■ Is able to accept direction without becoming defensive
■ Demonstrates adaptive coping skills in response to stressful situations

Planning and Implementation

Table 32–2 provides a plan of care for the child with intellectual developmental disorder using selected nursing diagnoses, outcome criteria, and appropriate nursing interventions and rationales.

Although this plan of care is directed toward the individual patient, it is essential that family members or primary caregivers participate in the ongoing

Table 32–2 | CARE PLAN FOR THE CHILD WITH INTELLECTUAL DEVELOPMENTAL DISORDER (INTELLECTUAL DISABILITY)

NURSING DIAGNOSIS: RISK FOR INJURY

RELATED TO: Altered physical mobility or aggressive behavior

OUTCOME CRITERIA	NURSING INTERVENTIONS	RATIONALE
Short- and long-term goal ■ Patient does not experience injury.	1. Create a safe environment for the patient. 2. Ensure that small items are removed from area where the patient will be ambulating and that sharp items are out of reach. 3. Store items that the patient uses frequently within easy reach. 4. Pad side rails and headboard of the patient with history of seizures. 5. Prevent physical aggression and acting-out behaviors by learning to recognize signs that the patient is becoming agitated.	1–5. Patient safety is a nursing priority.

NURSING DIAGNOSIS: SELF-CARE DEFICIT

RELATED TO: Altered physical mobility or lack of maturity

OUTCOME CRITERIA	NURSING INTERVENTIONS	RATIONALE
Short-term goal ■ Patient is able to participate in aspects of self-care. Long-term goal ■ Patient has all self-care needs met.	1. Identify aspects of self-care that may be within the patient's capabilities. Work on one aspect of self-care at a time. Provide simple, concrete explanations. Offer positive feedback for efforts.	1. Positive reinforcement enhances self-esteem and encourages repetition of desirable behaviors.

Continued

Table 32–2 | CARE PLAN FOR THE CHILD WITH INTELLECTUAL DEVELOPMENTAL DISORDER (INTELLECTUAL DISABILITY)—cont'd

OUTCOME CRITERIA	NURSING INTERVENTIONS	RATIONALE
	2. When one aspect of self-care has been mastered to the best of the patient's ability, move on to another. Encourage independence but intervene when the patient is unable to perform.	2. Patient comfort and safety are nursing priorities.

NURSING DIAGNOSIS: IMPAIRED VERBAL COMMUNICATION
RELATED TO: Developmental alteration

OUTCOME CRITERIA	NURSING INTERVENTIONS	RATIONALE
Short-term goal ■ Patient will establish trust with caregiver and a means of communication of needs.	1. Maintain consistency of staff assignment over time.	1. Consistency of staff assignments facilitates trust and the ability to understand the patient's actions and communications.
Long-term goal ■ Patient's needs are being met through established means of communication. ■ If patient cannot speak or communicate by other means, needs are met by caregiver's anticipation of patient's needs.	2. Anticipate and fulfill the patient's needs until satisfactory communication patterns are established. Learn (from family, if possible) special words the patient uses that are different from the norm. Identify nonverbal gestures or signals that patient may use to convey needs if verbal communication is absent. Practice these communications skills repeatedly.	2. Some children with intellectual developmental disorder, particularly at a severe level, can learn only by systematic habit training.

NURSING DIAGNOSIS: IMPAIRED SOCIAL INTERACTION
RELATED TO: Speech deficiencies or difficulty adhering to conventional social behavior

OUTCOME CRITERIA	NURSING INTERVENTIONS	RATIONALE
Short-term goal ■ Patient attempts to interact with others in the presence of trusted caregiver. Long-term goal ■ Patient is able to interact with others using behaviors that are socially acceptable and appropriate to developmental level.	1. Remain with the patient during initial interactions with others on the unit. 2. Explain to other patients the meaning behind some of this patient's nonverbal gestures and signals. Use simple language to explain to the patient which behaviors are acceptable and which are not. Establish a procedure for behavior modification with rewards for appropriate behaviors and aversive reinforcement for inappropriate behaviors.	1. Presence of a trusted individual provides a feeling of security. 2. Positive, negative, and aversive reinforcements can contribute to desired changes in behavior. These privileges and penalties are individually determined as staff learns the patient's likes and dislikes.

care of the child with intellectual developmental disorder. They need information regarding the scope of the condition, realistic expectations and the child's potential, methods for modifying behavior as required, and community resources from which they may seek assistance and support.

Evaluation

Evaluation of care given to the patient with intellectual developmental disorder should reflect positive behavioral changes. Evaluation is accomplished by determining whether the goals of care (as identified previously) have been met through implementation of the nursing actions selected. The nurse reassesses the plan and makes changes as required. Reassessment data may include information gathered by asking the following questions:

Has the patient:

- Remained free from injury?
- Had self-care needs fulfilled? Been able to fulfill some of these needs independently?
- Been able to communicate needs and desires so that they can be understood?
- Learned to interact appropriately with others?
- Accepted constructive feedback and discontinued the inappropriate behavior when regressive behaviors surface?
- Maintained anxiety at a manageable level?
- Learned new coping skills through behavior modification? Demonstrated evidence of increased self-esteem because of the accomplishment of these new skills and adaptive behaviors?

Have primary caregivers:

- Demonstrated understanding of realistic expectations for the child's behavior and methods for attempting to modify unacceptable behaviors?
- Demonstrated awareness of various resources from which they can seek assistance and support within the community?

CORE CONCEPT

Autism Spectrum Disorder

Autism spectrum disorder (ASD) is defined as a heterogenous group of neurodevelopmental syndromes characterized by a wide range of communication impairments and restricted, repetitive behaviors (Boland & Verduin, 2022).

Autism Spectrum Disorder
Clinical Findings

In the older edition of the *DSM* (4th ed., text revision; APA, 2000), the category of ASD encompassed a broad spectrum of associated diagnoses that included autistic disorder, Rett's disorder, childhood disintegrative disorder, pervasive developmental disorder not otherwise specified, and Asperger's disorder. The *DSM-5-TR* groups these disorders into a single diagnostic category—ASD. The diagnosis is adapted to each individual by clinical specifiers (e.g., level of required support, presence or absence of language impairment, and presence or absence of intellectual impairment) and associated features (e.g., known genetic or other medical conditions or environmental factors, or associated with a neurodevelopmental, mental, or behavior problem) (APA, 2022). ASD includes a wide range of symptoms and levels of severity that affect thinking, feeling, communication, and social relationships. Behavior is often limited and repetitive, but each child is likely to have a unique pattern of behavior and level of severity from low to high functioning (Mayo Clinic, 2022a).

Epidemiology and Course

The Autism and Developmental Disabilities Monitoring (ADDM) Network estimates that 1 in 44 8-year-old children in the United States is identified with ASD; the disorder occurs about four times more often in boys than in girls and about one-third (35.2 %) of the children had intellectual disability (Centers for Disease Control and Prevention [CDC], 2022). Onset of the disorder occurs in early childhood, and in most cases it runs a chronic course, with symptoms persisting into adulthood. Evidence supports an overrepresentation (3.03 to 6.36 times greater) of autism among transgender and gender-diverse individuals (Warrier et al., 2020). The researchers note that transgender and gender-diverse individuals also had elevated rates of ADHD, bipolar disorder, depression, obsessive-compulsive disorder (OCD), learning disorders, and schizophrenia compared with cisgender individuals. Genetic evidence suggests a "shared underlying liability for many co-occurring neurodevelopmental and psychiatric conditions" (p. 7).

Predisposing Factors
Neurological Implications

Imaging studies have revealed several alterations in major brain structures of individuals with ASD: widespread white matter anomalies; overgrowth of the uncinated fasciculus (which is a region associated with socioemotional processing); and lower connectivity between voice-specific left hemisphere posterior superior temporal sulcus and the orbitofrontal cortex, the amygdala, and areas associated with reward circuitry (Bhatia, 2022). Boland and Verduin (2022) identified that there are patterns of change in total brain volume over time, lending support for the hypothesis that there are critical periods in the brain's plasticity that, when disrupted, may contribute to the development of ASD. These findings related to brain plasticity also support that early recognition and intervention can be meaningful in improving functional abilities over time. Volkmar and associates (2017) reported that the Infant Brain Imaging Study, a national study of developmental changes in at-risk infants, has consistently demonstrated abnormal organizational properties in white matter within the first year of life that increase over time. In one study it was found that nonlinear electroencephalogram (EEG) measurements in infants predicted with high accuracy a later diagnosis of ASD (Bosl et al., 2018). All of this research holds the promise that early recognition and intervention may provide avenues for better treatment options or prevention.

Genetics

Family and twin studies support that genetic factors play a significant role in the etiology of ASD; about 15% of ASD cases are related to a known genetic mutation, but, in most cases, its expression is related to multiple genes (Boland & Verduin, 2022). Genetic studies have identified genes that confer risk for both autism and schizophrenia, suggesting that these conditions are related (Gilman et al., 2012), but the same genetic variations also appear to confer risk for some other neurodevelopmental disorders as well (Volkmar et al., 2017). Kranjac (2016) reported that rare genetic variants such as copy number variations increase the risk for autism by 20% to 60%. DNA studies have implicated areas on several chromosomes containing genes that may contribute to the development of ASD. Genetic studies have also identified disruptions in serotonin (5-HT), and because 5-HT is important in brain development, it is postulated that changes in 5-HT may be associated with enlargement in the brain (Boland & Verduin, 2022).

Prenatal and Perinatal Influences

Some of the prenatal risk factors that have been associated with development of ASD include advanced parental age, fetal exposure to valproate, gestational diabetes, and maternal gestational bleeding (APA, 2022; Boland & Verduin, 2022). Perinatal influences include low birth weight, obstetrical complications (particularly those associated with neonatal hypoxia), hyperbilirubinemia, congenital malformation, and ABO or Rh factor incompatibilities (Boland & Verduin, 2022). Exposure to environmental toxins, including air pollution and pesticides, showed the strongest links to ASD when it occurred during preconception, gestation, and early childhood stages (Rossignol & Frye, 2016). Volkmar and associates (2017) noted that "despite multiple focused investigations, there is no evidence that vaccinations play a role in the environmental liability for ASD" (p. 3576).

Application of the Nursing Process to Autism Spectrum Disorder

Background Assessment Data (Symptomatology)

The symptomatology presented here is common among children with ASD, but it is important to understand these disorders occur along a spectrum with varying levels of functionality. Some individuals who meet criteria for ASD may be highly functional and highly intelligent despite communication impairments and repetitive or restrictive behaviors. The dramatic increase in the prevalence of ASD has led to research focused on differential and common features along the continuum as well as on etiological factors. This information is important in creating an accurate plan of care for the patient. Because ASD is a *spectrum* disorder, the symptomatology described here should be understood on a continuum ranging from mild to severe.

Impairment in Social Interaction Children with ASD have difficulty forming interpersonal relationships with others. They show little interest in people and often do not respond to others' attempts at interaction. As infants, they may have an aversion to affection and physical contact. As toddlers, the attachment to a significant adult may be either absent or manifested as exaggerated adherence behaviors. In childhood, a lack of spontaneity is manifested in less cooperative play, less imaginative play, and fewer friendships. Those children with minimal handicaps may progress to the point of recognizing other children as part of their environment, but they struggle, nonetheless, in interpersonal relationships. Social interaction is further impaired by deficits in ability to accurately process others' feelings or affect. Higher-functioning children may recognize their difficulty with social skills even though they may desire friendship. In one study (Strunz et al., 2015), researchers noted that as these relational struggles unfold into adulthood, it is difficult at times to distinguish ASD from personality disorders because there are disruptions in interpersonal relationships within both groups. They found that the differential features in ASD were less extroversion, less openness to experience, increased inhibition, and increased compulsivity than among those with personality disorders.

Impairment in Communication and Imaginative Activity Both verbal and nonverbal skills are affected. In more severe ASD, language may be totally absent or characterized by immature structure or idiosyncratic utterances whose meaning is clear only to those who are familiar with the child's past experiences. Nonverbal communication, such as facial expression or gestures, may be absent or socially inappropriate. Sometimes children with ASD are misdiagnosed as being hearing-impaired as a result of their lack of response to sounds, whereas other children may overreact to sound or other stimuli. In some cases, children with ASD demonstrate special abilities, such as fluent reading skills while still in preschool (Boland & Verduin, 2022). The pattern of play is often restricted and repetitive.

Restricted Activities and Interests Even minor changes in the environment are often met with resistance or sometimes with agitated irritability. Attachment to or extreme fascination with objects that move or spin (e.g., fans) is common. Stereotyped body movements (hand-clapping, rocking, whole-body swaying) and verbalizations (repetition of words or phrases) are typical. Diet abnormalities may include eating only a few specific foods or consuming an excessive amount of fluids. Self-injurious behaviors, such as head banging or biting the hands or arms, may be evident. Harrop and associates (2014) compared children with ASD to children without this disorder and found that all children demonstrated some repetitive behaviors as part of their development of skill mastery, but children with ASD displayed a wider range of repetitive behaviors in many different circumstances.

The *DSM-5-TR* diagnostic criteria for ASD are presented in Box 32–1. The criteria specify a range of behaviors, with varying levels of severity, thus addressing the spectrum of symptomatology associated with this diagnosis.

Nursing Diagnosis

Based on data collected during the nursing assessment, possible nursing diagnoses for the patient with ASD include the following:

- Risk for self-mutilation or self-injury related to neurological, cognitive, or social deficits
- Impaired social interaction related to inability to trust; neurological alterations, evidenced by lack of responsiveness to, or interest in, people
- Impaired verbal communication related to withdrawal into the self; neurological alterations, evidenced by inability or unwillingness to speak; lack of nonverbal expression
- Disturbed personal identity related to neurological alterations; delayed developmental stage, evidenced by difficulty separating own physiological and emotional needs and personal boundaries from those of others

Outcome Identification

Outcome criteria include short- and long-term goals. Timelines are individually determined. The following criteria may be used for measurement of outcomes in the care of the patient with ASD.

The patient:

- Exhibits no evidence of self-harm
- Interacts appropriately with at least one staff member
- Demonstrates trust in at least one staff member
- Is able to communicate so that they can be understood by at least one staff member
- Demonstrates behaviors that indicate they have begun the separation/individuation process

Planning and Implementation

Table 32–3 provides a plan of care for the child with ASD, including selected nursing diagnoses, outcome criteria, and appropriate nursing interventions and rationales.

Evaluation

Evaluation of care for the child with ASD reflects whether the nursing actions have been effective in achieving the established goals. The nursing process calls for reassessment of the plan. Questions for gathering reassessment data may include the following:

Has the child:

- Been able to establish trust with at least *one* caregiver?
- Remained free from mutilative behaviors or other forms of self-harm?
- Attempted to interact with others? Received positive reinforcement for these efforts?
- Improved in ability to indicate that attention is being paid?
- Established a means of communicating their needs and desires to others? Had all self-care needs met?
- Demonstrated an awareness of self as separate from others?
- Accept touch from others and been appropriate in touching others?

Psychopharmacological Intervention for ASD

Behavioral interventions are first-line treatments for core symptoms of ASD. Pharmacological interventions are directed toward relief of associated symptoms, such as aggression, hyperactivity, self-harm, impulsivity, and temper tantrums. There are no medications that treat the core symptoms of ASD. The U.S. Food and Drug Administration (FDA) has approved two medications for the treatment of irritability associated with ASD: risperidone (Risperdal) in children and adolescents 5 to 16 years, and aripiprazole (Abilify) in children and adolescents 6 to 17 years. When administering risperidone, caution must be maintained concerning less common but more serious side effects, including neuroleptic malignant syndrome, tardive dyskinesia, hyperglycemia, and diabetes. A review and meta-analysis (Fallah et al., 2019) concluded that risperidone was

BOX 32-1 Diagnostic Criteria for Autism Spectrum Disorder

A. Persistent deficits in social communication and social interaction across multiple contexts, as manifested by the following, currently or by history (examples are illustrative, not exhaustive):
   1. Deficits in social-emotional reciprocity, ranging, for example, from abnormal social approach and failure of normal back-and-forth conversation; to reduced sharing of interests, emotions, or affect; to failure to initiate or respond to social interactions.
   2. Deficits in nonverbal communicative behaviors used for social interaction, ranging, for example, from poorly integrated verbal and nonverbal communication; to abnormalities in eye contact and body language or deficits in understanding and use of gestures; to a total lack of facial expressions and nonverbal communication.
   3. Deficits in developing, maintaining, and understanding relationships, ranging, for example, from difficulties adjusting behavior to suit various social contexts; to difficulties in sharing imaginative play or in making friends; to absence of interest in peers.
B. Restricted, repetitive patterns of behavior, interests, or activities, as manifested by at least two of the following, currently or by history (examples are illustrative, not exhaustive):
   1. Stereotyped or repetitive motor movements, use of objects, or speech (e.g., simple motor stereotypies, lining up toys or flipping objects, echolalia, idiosyncratic phrases).
   2. Insistence on sameness, inflexible adherence to routines, or ritualized patterns of verbal or nonverbal behavior (e.g., extreme distress at small changes, difficulties with transitions, rigid thinking patterns, greeting rituals, need to take same route or eat same food every day).
   3. Highly restricted, fixated interests that are abnormal in intensity or focus (e.g., strong attachment to or preoccupation with unusual objects, excessively circumscribed or perseverative interests).
   4. Hyper- or hyporeactivity to sensory input or unusual interest in sensory aspects of environment (e.g., apparent indifference to pain/temperature, adverse response to specific sounds or textures, excessive smelling or touching of objects, visual fascination with lights or movement).

C. Symptoms must be present in the early developmental period (but may not become fully manifest until social demands exceed limited capacities, or may be masked by learned strategies in later life).
D. Symptoms cause clinically significant impairment in social, occupational, or other important areas of current functioning.
E. These disturbances are not better explained by intellectual developmental disorder (intellectual disability) or global developmental delay. Intellectual developmental disorder and autism spectrum disorder frequently co-occur; to make comorbid diagnoses of autism spectrum disorder and intellectual developmental disorder, social communication should be below that expected for general developmental level.

Note: Individuals with a well-established DSM-IV diagnosis of autistic disorder, Asperger's disorder, or pervasive developmental disorder not otherwise specified should be given the diagnosis of autism spectrum disorder. Individuals who have marked deficits in social communication, but whose symptoms do not otherwise meet criteria for autism spectrum disorder, should be evaluated for social (pragmatic) communication disorder.

Specify current severity based on social communication impairments and restricted, repetitive patterns of behavior:

Requiring very substantial support
Requiring substantial support
Requiring support

   Specify if:

With or without accompanying intellectual impairment
With or without accompanying language impairment

   Specify if:

Associated with a known genetic or other medical condition or environmental factor
Associated with a neurodevelopmental, mental, or behavioral problem

   Specify if:

With catatonia

Reprinted with permission from the *Diagnostic and Statistical Manual of Mental Disorders, Fifth Edition, Text Revision.* (Copyright 2022). American Psychiatric Association.

more effective than aripiprazole, lurasidone, or placebo in reducing irritability symptoms.

In clinical studies with aripiprazole, the most frequently reported adverse events included sedation, fatigue, weight gain, vomiting, somnolence, and tremor. The most common reasons for discontinuation of aripiprazole were sedation, drooling, tremor, vomiting, and extrapyramidal disorder.

Recent studies and meta-analyses as cited by Kothadia and associates (2021) have identified several other medications for the treatment of ASD-associated symptoms: donepezil and a choline supplement improved receptive language skills in children age 5 to 10 years (Gabis et al., 2019); bumetanide improved social communication, interaction, and restricted interests in children with moderate

Table 32–3 | CARE PLAN FOR THE CHILD WITH AUTISM SPECTRUM DISORDER

NURSING DIAGNOSIS: RISK FOR SELF-MUTILATION

RELATED TO: Neurological alterations; history of self-mutilative behaviors; hysterical reactions to changes in the environment

OUTCOME CRITERIA	NURSING INTERVENTIONS	RATIONALE
Short-term goal ■ Patient demonstrates alternative behavior (e.g., initiating interaction between self and nurse) in response to anxiety within specified time. (Length of time required for this objective will depend on severity and chronicity of the disorder.) **Long-term goal** ■ Patient does not harm self.	1. Work with the child on a one-to-one basis. 2. Try to determine whether the self-mutilative behavior occurs in response to increasing anxiety, and if so, to what the anxiety may be attributed. 3. Try to intervene with diversion or replacement activities and offer self to the child as anxiety level starts to rise. 4. Protect the child when self-mutilative behaviors occur. Devices such as a helmet, padded hand mitts, or arm covers may provide protection when the risk for self-harm exists.	1. One-to-one interaction facilitates trust. 2. Mutilative behaviors may be averted if the cause can be determined and alleviated. 3. Diversion and replacement activities may provide needed feelings of security and substitute for self-mutilative behaviors. 4. Patient safety is a priority nursing intervention.

NURSING DIAGNOSIS: IMPAIRED SOCIAL INTERACTION

RELATED TO: Inability to trust; neurological alterations

EVIDENCED BY: Lack of responsiveness to, or interest in, people

OUTCOME CRITERIA	NURSING INTERVENTIONS	RATIONALE
Short-term goal ■ Patient will demonstrate trust in one caregiver (as evidenced by facial responsiveness and eye contract) within a specified time (depending on severity and chronicity of disorder). **Long-term goal** ■ Patient will initiate social interactions (physical, verbal, nonverbal) with a caregiver by the time of discharge from treatment.	1. Assign a limited number of caregivers to the child. Ensure that warmth, acceptance, and availability are conveyed. 2. Provide the child with familiar objects, such as familiar toys or a blanket. Support the child's attempts to interact with others. 3. Give positive reinforcement for eye contact with something acceptable to the child (e.g., food, familiar object). Gradually replace with social reinforcement (e.g., touch, smiling, hugging).	1. Warmth, acceptance, and availability, along with consistency of assignment, enhance the establishment and maintenance of a trusting relationship. 2. Familiar objects and the presence of a trusted individual provide security during times of distress. 3. Being able to establish eye contact is essential to the child's ability to form satisfactory interpersonal relationships.

Continued

Table 32–3 | CARE PLAN FOR THE CHILD WITH AUTISM SPECTRUM DISORDER—cont'd

NURSING DIAGNOSIS: IMPAIRED VERBAL COMMUNICATION

RELATED TO: Withdrawal into the self; neurological alterations

EVIDENCED BY: Inability or unwillingness to speak; lack of nonverbal expression

OUTCOME CRITERIA	NURSING INTERVENTIONS	RATIONALE
Short-term goal ■ Patient establishes trust with one caregiver (as evidenced by facial responsiveness and eye contact) by a specified time (depending on severity and chronicity of disorder). **Long-term goal** ■ Patient establishes a means of communicating needs and desires to others.	1. Maintain consistency in assignment of caregivers. 2. Anticipate and fulfill the child's needs until communication can be established. 3. Seek clarification and validation. 4. Give positive reinforcement when eye contact is used to convey nonverbal expressions.	1. Consistency facilitates trust and enhances the caregiver's ability to understand the child's attempts to communicate. 2. Anticipating needs helps to minimize frustration while the child is learning communication skills. 3. Validation ensures that the intended message has been conveyed. 4. Positive reinforcement increases self-esteem and encourages repetition.

NURSING DIAGNOSIS: DISTURBED PERSONAL IDENTITY

RELATED TO: Neurological alterations; delayed developmental stage

EVIDENCED BY: Difficulty separating own physiological and emotional needs and personal boundaries from those of others

OUTCOME CRITERIA	NURSING INTERVENTIONS	RATIONALE
Short-term goal ■ Patient names own body parts as separate and individual from those of others. **Long-term goal** ■ Patient develops ego identity (evidenced by ability to recognize physical and emotional self as separate from others) by time of discharge from treatment.	1. Assist the child to recognize separateness during self-care activities, such as dressing and feeding. 2. Assist the child in learning to name own body parts. This can be facilitated by the use of mirrors, drawings, and pictures of the child. Encourage appropriate touching of, and being touched by, others.	1. Recognition of body parts during dressing and feeding increases the child's awareness of self as separate from others. 2. All of these activities may help increase the child's awareness of self as separate from others.

to severe ASD (James et al., 2019); and vitamin D with omega-3 long chain polyunsaturated fatty acids reduced associated irritability and hyperactivity (Mazahery et al., 2019).

Nonpharmacological Treatments for ASD

Conventional nonpharmacological treatments include behavior and communication therapies, education therapies, and family therapies (Mayo Clinic, 2022a). These programs may focus on reducing problem behaviors or teaching social and communication skills.

Applied behavior analysis (ABA) is referred to as the gold standard behavioral treatment for ASD; it involves tailoring a reward-based motivation program specific to each child's needs (Raypole, 2021).

Pivotal response treatment, which is based on ABA principles, is another evidence-based approach that uses play therapy to prompt development in the pivotal areas of motivation, self-regulation, initiation of social interactions, and the ability to respond to multiple cues (Lei & Ventola, 2017). Family therapies involve engaging family members in learning how to interact with their children to promote social interaction skills and manage problem behaviors. Education programs are typically highly structured to facilitate learning and meet the individual needs of the child. Speech therapy, occupational therapy, and physical therapy may also be beneficial. Adjunctive treatments may include art, music, or sensory-based therapies aimed at reducing the child's sensitivity to touch or sound, but while these approaches may support evidence-based treatment approaches, more research is needed to support their efficacy alone (DeBoth & Reynolds, 2017).

CORE CONCEPT
Hyperactivity
Excessive psychomotor activity that may be purposeful or aimless, accompanied by physical movements and verbal utterances that are usually more rapid than normal is termed **hyperactivity**. Inattention and distractibility are common with hyperactive behavior.

Attention Deficit-Hyperactivity Disorder
Clinical Findings, Epidemiology, and Course

The essential behavior pattern of a child with **attentive deficit-hyperactivity disorder (ADHD)** is one of inattention or hyperactivity/impulsivity or both. The most frequently cited characteristics (in order of frequency) are hyperactivity, attention deficit, impulsivity, memory and thinking deficits, specific learning disabilities, and speech and hearing deficits (Boland & Verduin, 2022). Children with this disorder are highly distractible and unable to contain stimuli. Motor activity is excessive, and movements are random and impulsive. Onset of the disorder is difficult to diagnose in children younger than age 4 years because characteristic behavior at that age is much more variable than that of older children. Frequently, the disorder is not recognized until the child enters school. It is more common in boys (11.7%) than girls (5.7%), and the overall prevalence among school-age children is 8.8% (CDC, 2021). It is estimated that in 50% to 70% of the cases, ADHD persists into young adulthood and beyond, and unlike other psychiatric disorders that are typically episodic, the adult with ADHD has symptoms that are chronic and unrelenting (McGough, 2017). Some symptoms may change as a child progresses into adolescence. For example, adolescents are more likely than children to have affective symptoms such as depression, whereas hyperactivity may decline in intensity (Jain, 2022). Without prompt diagnosis and treatment, the child with ADHD is at higher risk for substance abuse and negative consequences associated with risky behavior; the adult is at higher risk for restlessness and functional impairment, occupation difficulties, and disorganization. See "Real People, Real Stories" to learn more about Myrle's experience as an adult living with ADHD.

In making the diagnosis of ADHD, the *DSM-5-TR* criteria are further specified according to current clinical presentation. These subtypes include a combined presentation (meeting the criteria for both inattention and hyperactivity/impulsivity), a predominantly inattentive presentation, and a predominantly hyperactive/impulsive presentation.

CORE CONCEPT
Impulsivity
The definition of **impulsivity** is the trait of acting without reflection and without thought to the consequences of the behavior; an abrupt inclination to act (and the inability to resist acting) on certain behavioral urges.

Predisposing Factors
Biological Influences

Genetics: Several studies have revealed supportive evidence of genetic influences in the etiology of ADHD. Twin and family studies showed that the heritability for ADHD exceeds 75% (McGough, 2017). Adoption studies reveal that biological parents of children with ADHD more often display psychopathology than do the adoptive parents.

Studies of genetic evidence for ADHD have found genetic variants and mutations such as copy number variants on a specific region of chromosome 16 and copy number variants overlap with chromosomal regions previously linked to ASD and schizophrenia (Acosta et al., 2016; Kushima, 2018). Most molecular research has implicated genes that influence the metabolism or action of dopamine (Boland & Verduin, 2022).

Biochemical Theory: Hypotheses about the effect of neurotransmitters have been based on the benefits associated with taking stimulant medications, which are thought to increase the availability of dopamine. Several studies, using single-photon emission computed tomography (SPECT), have now demonstrated increased dopamine transporter-binding densities in the striatal regions (McGough, 2017) (Fig. 32–1). Not surprisingly, researchers have also found a significant risk of new-onset psychosis in ADHD patients taking amphetamines, almost double the risk than for those taking methylphenidate (Griffin & Harari, 2019).

Anatomical Changes: Brain imaging studies show decreased volume and activity in the prefrontal cortex, anterior cingulate cortex, globus pallidus,

Real People, Real Stories: Attention Deficit/Hyperactivity Disorder

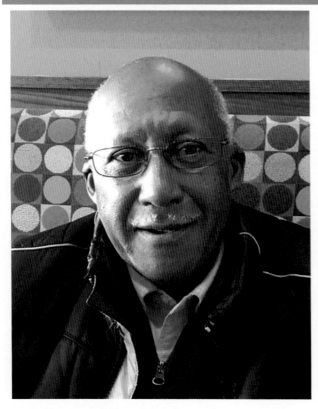

Karyn: When did you first become aware that you had ADHD?

Myrle: I had symptoms as a child, but I didn't get diagnosed or treated until I was 50 years old. They put me on Ritalin first and then on Ritalin-XR. When I first started to take it, I got very high and very talkative, then after a little while I could focus better and then it wears off.

Karyn: What symptoms do you remember having as a child?

Myrle: I guess I thought of myself as selfish. I was easily distracted and I couldn't handle noise, like the noise at a basketball game was unmanageable and agitating. I was the youngest child but even so, I wanted my way right now. No one else had anything important to say. Later I realized it wasn't that I was so smart but that everyone else seemed to go too slow.

Karyn: How did you get along in school?

Myrle: I didn't have any trouble. I went to school in the country and the classrooms were very small and very quiet so that helped me. When I graduated from high school I went into the military and that was when I really realized I had a problem. I got into fights a lot because the noise and the talking and all the activity really agitated me.

Karyn: Impulsivity is a common symptom in ADHD. Did you experience that?

Myrle: I don't think so. I was pretty forward, outgoing, and I liked to take the lead, but I had trouble paying attention. I did become hypersexual as I got older and as an adult, I started smoking pot because it improved my sexual performance, and I started drinking alcohol because it helped me sleep. Then those became problems, too. I always wanted to be a lawyer so I went to law school after I got out of the military, but I was on probation because I got involved in too many things and couldn't focus on my studies. I eventually did graduate with a PhD but then I took the bar exam four times and couldn't pass it; sometimes I would get sick and couldn't study; even after I got accommodations when I had less noise and twice the time, I would second guess myself and change my answers. I had a lot of anxiety. Then I got fired from a job I had at the sewer department and since I had admitted to lying, I was unable to take the bar exam for another five years. I never was able to pass.

I got a job at the Department of Education as a disabilities' investigator, and I was good at handling these cases. I had cases of people with attention deficit disorder that were being discriminated against. I was very detailed, but it took me a lot longer to get things done. I collected a lot of information, but I was unable to shorten the process compared to my coworkers. It was there that I had the epiphany that I had a lot of the same symptoms that my clients were describing. In general, I've always had a lot of trouble separating myself from the noise and other distractions.

Karyn: How would you describe your ability to function now that you are being treated with medication?

Myrle: Well, just like I'm doing now, I can go on and on talking about nothing. (There were several subject changes and refocusing; at times Myrle had difficulty refocusing, stating that he just had to finish one more point.)

Myrle: I'm still very disorganized and sometimes have trouble with attention. The meds help somewhat but I still can't stop talking. My current medical record says I also have OCD, hoarding disorder, and depression. I see a psychiatrist for medications, but I still have symptoms. I never feel very confident, and I can't seem to get all my ducks in a row. The medication helps me not get quite so agitated as I used to. So I am able to conduct my current role as a minister and I am better able to listen.

Karyn: Yes, I heard you preach, and it sounded like a very focused message.

Myrle: Well, I do better with structured time limits, and I let the Spirit take over when I preach. I know this is what I was called to do, and I serve a congregation that has a lot of disabilities, so I understand their needs because of my own experiences.

Real People, Real Stories: Attention Deficit/Hyperactivity Disorder–cont'd

Karyn: What is the most important thing that nurses need to know about an adult with ADHD?

Myrle: They need to understand the impact my attention deficit symptoms have on getting my health-care needs met.

I was admitted to a medical unit and was told I needed to stay in a situation that was literally driving me crazy. I was in a room with three patients, nurses were talking outside the door, buzzers and alarms were beeping and they weren't being shut off. The more I asked for help, the more I felt like they weren't listening and then I started to think they were retaliating or doing it deliberately . . . or maybe I was getting a little paranoid as I was becoming more agitated.

It's really important that nurses listen to me when I'm telling them I can't tolerate the noise and try to reduce the noise as much as possible. I ask for a private room if that's possible. Sometimes I might get pegged as a problem patient because I do get agitated, but a lower stimulation environment could prevent that.

---

caudate, thalamus, and cerebellum (Boland & Verduin, 2022). Several alterations occur in neural connectivity with evidence of decreased activation in frontoparietal areas and overactivation in visual, dorsal attention, and default networks (McGough, 2017). A study by Humphreys and associates (2018) found a correlation between brain volume changes, elevated ADHD symptoms, and the number of childhood stressors. This finding underscores the interaction between genetics and environmental influences and reinforces the need for trauma-informed care.

Environmental Influences

In a systematic review Kim et al. (2020) identified five environmental influences that were most convincing (in evidence-based literature) of their association with development of ADHD: prepregnancy obesity, childhood eczema, hypertensive disorders, preeclampsia, and maternal acetaminophen exposure during pregnancy. Four influences were identified as "highly suggestive" of an association with development of ADHD: maternal smoking during pregnancy, childhood asthma, prepregnancy overweight, and lower levels of serum vitamin D. Several other risk factors evidenced in some studies included perinatal hypoxic conditions, breech or transverse presentation, and preterm birth. Kim and associates (2020) also found that in children with ADHD three biomarkers were apparent: the biomarker most supported in studies was low levels of vitamin D followed by high blood lead levels and low magnesium levels.

Psychosocial Influences

Disorganized or chaotic environments or disruption in family equilibrium may contribute to ADHD in some individuals. Psychosocial risk factors include nonintact or single-parent families, young maternal age at birth of the target child, paternal history of antisocial behavior, maternal depression, and lower socioeconomic class (ADHD Institute, 2021).

Application of the Nursing Process to ADHD

Background Assessment Data (Symptomatology)

A major portion of the hyperactive child's problems relate to difficulties in performing age-appropriate tasks. Hyperactive children are highly distractible and have extremely limited attention spans. They often shift from one uncompleted activity to another. Impulsivity, or deficit in inhibitory control, is also common.

Children with ADHD have difficulty forming satisfactory interpersonal relationships, often demonstrating behaviors that interfere with acceptable social interaction. They tend to be disruptive and intrusive in group endeavors. They have difficulty complying with social norms. Some children with ADHD are very aggressive or oppositional, whereas others exhibit more regressive and immature behaviors. Low frustration tolerance and outbursts of temper are common.

Children with ADHD who manifest with hyperactivity symptoms have boundless energy, exhibiting excessive levels of activity, restlessness, and fidgeting. They have been described as "perpetual motion machines," continuously running, jumping, wiggling, or squirming. They experience a greater than average number of accidents, from minor mishaps to more serious incidents that may lead to physical injury or the destruction of property. The *DSM-5-TR* diagnostic criteria for ADHD are presented in Box 32–2.

Comorbidity Several comorbidities are common in children with ADHD, but the most common are ODD, anxiety, and depression (Jain, 2022). The APA (2022) reported that in children with ADHD who have both symptoms of inattention and hyperactivity/impulsivity, ODD co-occurs about 50% of the time. They further identify that most children and adolescents with disruptive mood dysregulation disorder also meet criteria for ADHD. Other comorbidities

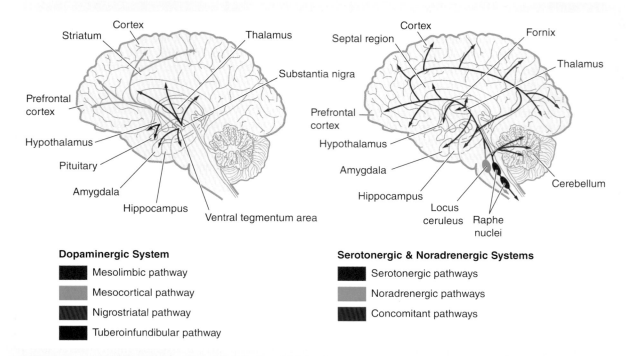

FIGURE 32–1   Neurobiology of attention deficit-hyperactivity disorder.

NEUROTRANSMITTERS

The major neurotransmitters implicated in the pathophysiology of ADHD are dopamine, norepinephrine, and possibly serotonin. Dopamine and norepinephrine appear to be depleted in ADHD. Serotonin in ADHD has been studied less extensively, but recent evidence suggests that it also is reduced in children with ADHD.

NEUROTRANSMITTER FUNCTIONS

- Norepinephrine is thought to play a role in the ability to perform executive functions, such as analysis and reasoning, and in the cognitive alertness essential for processing stimuli and sustaining attention and thought.
- Dopamine is thought to play a role in sensory filtering, memory, concentration, controlling emotions, locomotor activity, and reasoning.
- Deficits in norepinephrine and dopamine have both been implicated in the inattention, impulsiveness, and hyperactivity associated with ADHD.
- Serotonin appears to play a role in ADHD, although possibly a less significant role than norepinephrine and dopamine. It has been suggested that alterations in serotonin may be related to the disinhibition and impulsivity observed in children with ADHD. It may play a role in mood disorders, particularly depression, which is a common comorbid disorder associated with ADHD.

FUNCTIONAL AREAS OF THE BRAIN AFFECTED

- **Prefrontal cortex:** Associated with maintaining attention, organization, and executive function. Also serves to modulate behavior inhibition, with serotonin as the predominant central inhibiting neurotransmitter for this function.
- **Basal ganglia (particularly the caudate nucleus and globus pallidus):** Involved in the regulation of high-level movements. In association with its connecting circuits to the prefrontal cortex, may also be important in cognition. Interruptions in these circuits may result in inattention or impulsivity.
- **Hippocampus:** Plays an important role in learning and memory.
- **Limbic system** (composed of the amygdala, hippocampus, mammillary body, hypothalamus, thalamus, fornix, cingulate gyrus, and septum pellucidum): Regulation of emotions. A neurotransmitter deficiency in this area may result in restlessness, inattention, or emotional volatility.
- **Reticular activating system** (composed of the reticular formation [located in the brainstem] and its connections): It is the major relay system among the many pathways that enter and leave the brain. It is thought to be the center of arousal and motivation and is crucial for maintaining a state of consciousness.

MEDICATIONS FOR ADHD

Central Nervous System (CNS) Stimulants

• Amphetamines (dextroamphetamine, lisdexamfetamine, methamphetamine, and mixtures): Cause the release of norepinephrine from central noradrenergic neurons. At higher doses, dopamine may be released in the mesolimbic system.

• Methylphenidate and dexmethylphenidate: Block the reuptake of norepinephrine and dopamine into the presynaptic neuron and increase the release of these monoamines into the extraneuronal space.

Side effects of CNS stimulants include restlessness, insomnia, headache, palpitations, weight loss, suppression of growth in children (with long-term use), increased blood pressure, abdominal pain, anxiety, tolerance, and physical and psychological dependence.

Others

• Atomoxetine: Selectively inhibits the reuptake of norepinephrine by blocking the presynaptic transporter.

Side effects include headache, upper abdominal pain, nausea and vomiting, anorexia, cough, dry mouth, constipation, increase in heart rate and blood pressure, and fatigue.

• Bupropion: Inhibits the reuptake of norepinephrine and dopamine into presynaptic neurons.

Side effects include headache, dizziness, insomnia or sedation, tachycardia, increased blood pressure, dry mouth, nausea and vomiting, weight gain or loss, and seizures (dose dependent).

• Viloxazine (Qelbree): Inhibits the reuptake of serotonin and norepinephrine (SNRI)

• Alpha agonists (clonidine, guanfacine): Stimulate central alpha-adrenoreceptors in the brain, resulting in reduced sympathetic outflow from the CNS.

Side effects include palpitations, bradycardia, constipation, dry mouth, and sedation.

BOX 32–2 Diagnostic Criteria for Attention Deficit-Hyperactivity Disorder

A. A persistent pattern of inattention and/or hyperactivity-impulsivity that interferes with functioning or development, as characterized by (1) and/or (2):

1. **Inattention:** Six (or more) of the following symptoms have persisted for at least 6 months to a degree that is inconsistent with developmental level and that negatively effects directly on social and academic/occupational activities. **Note:** The symptoms are not solely a manifestation of oppositional behavior, defiance, hostility, or failure to understand tasks or instructions. For older adolescents and adults (age 17 and older), at least five symptoms are required.

    a. Often fails to give close attention to details or makes careless mistakes in schoolwork, at work, or during other activities (e.g., overlooks or misses details, work is inaccurate).

    b. Often has difficulty sustaining attention in tasks or play activities (e.g., has difficulty remaining focused during lectures, conversations, or reading lengthy reading).

    c. Often does not seem to listen when spoken to directly (e.g., mind seems elsewhere, even in the absence of any obvious distraction).

    d. Often does not follow through on instructions and fails to finish schoolwork, chores, or duties in the workplace (e.g., starts tasks but quickly loses focus and is easily sidetracked).

    e. Often has difficulty organizing tasks and activities (e.g., difficulty managing sequential tasks; difficulty keeping materials and belongings in order; messy, disorganized, work; has poor time management; fails to meet deadlines).

    f. Often avoids, dislikes, or is reluctant to engage in tasks that require sustained mental effort (e.g., schoolwork or homework; for older adolescents and adults, preparing reports, completing forms, reviewing lengthy papers).

    g. Often loses things necessary for tasks or activities (e.g., school materials, pencils, books, tools, wallets, keys, paperwork, eyeglasses, or mobile telephones).

    h. Is often easily distracted by extraneous stimuli (for older adolescents and adults, may include unrelated thoughts).

    i. Is often forgetful in daily activities (e.g., chores, running errands; for older adolescents and adults, returning calls, paying bills, keeping appointments).

2. **Hyperactivity and Impulsivity:** Six (or more) of the following symptoms have persisted for at least 6 months to a degree that is inconsistent with developmental level and that negatively effects directly on social and academic/occupational activities. **Note:** The symptoms are not solely a manifestation of oppositional behavior, defiance, hostility, or a failure

Continued

BOX 32–2 Diagnostic Criteria for Attention Deficit-Hyperactivity Disorder—cont'd

to understand tasks or instructions. For older adolescents and adults (age 17 and older), at least five symptoms are required.

   a. Often fidgets with or taps hands or feet or squirms in seat.

   b. Often leaves seat in situations when remaining seated is expected (e.g., leaves his or her place in the classroom, in the office or other workplace, or in other situations that require remaining in place).

   c. Often runs about or climbs in situations where it is inappropriate. (**Note:** In adolescents or adults, may be limited to feeling restless.)

   d. Often unable to play or engage in leisure activities quietly.

   e. Is often "on the go," acting as if "driven by a motor" (e.g., is unable to be or uncomfortable being still for extended time, as in restaurants, meetings; may be experienced by others as being restless and difficult to keep up with).

   f. Often talks excessively.

   g. Often blurts out an answer before a question has been completed (e.g., completes people's sentences, cannot wait for turn in conversation).

   h. Often has difficulty waiting his or her turn (e.g., while waiting in line).

   i. Often interrupts or intrudes on others (e.g., butts into conversations, games, or activities; may start using other people's things without asking or receiving permission; for adolescents or adults, may intrude into or take over what others are doing).

B. Several inattentive or hyperactive-impulsive symptoms were present before age 12 years.

C. Several inattentive or hyperactive-impulsive symptoms are present in two or more settings (e.g., at home, school or work, with friends or relatives, in other activities).

D. There is clear evidence that the symptoms interfere with or reduce the quality of social, academic, or occupational functioning.

E. The symptoms do not occur exclusively during the course of schizophrenia or another psychotic disorder and are not better explained by another mental disorder (e.g., mood disorder, anxiety disorder, dissociative disorder, personality disorder, substance intoxication or withdrawal).

Specify whether:

1. **Combined presentation:** If both Criterion A1 (inattention) and Criterion A2 (hyperactivity-impulsivity) are met for the past 6 months.

2. **Predominantly inattentive presentation:** If Criterion A1 (inattention) is met but Criterion A2 (hyperactivity-impulsivity) is not met for the past 6 months.

3. **Predominantly hyperactive/impulsive presentation:** If Criterion A2 (hyperactivity-impulsivity) is met and Criterion A1 (inattention) is not met for the past 6 months.

Specify if:

In partial remission: When full criteria were previously met, fewer than the full criteria have been met for the past 6 months, and the symptoms still result in impairment in social, academic, or occupational functioning.
Specify current severity:

Mild: Few, if any, symptoms in excess of those required to make the diagnosis are present, and symptoms result in no more than minor impairments in social or occupational functioning.

Moderate: Symptoms or functional impairment between "mild" and "severe" are present.

Severe: Many symptoms in excess of those required to make the diagnosis, or several symptoms that are particularly severe, are present, or the symptoms result in marked impairment in social or occupational functioning.

include conduct disorder, specific learning disorder, and intermittent explosive disorder. Boland and Verduin (2022) identified that although bipolar mania and ADHD share many core features, such as distractibility, excessive talking, and hyperactivity, children with bipolar I disorder exhibit symptoms that wax and wane, whereas children with ADHD have more persistent, continuous symptoms. They note that bipolar disorder and ADHD can coexist and that when certain features of ADHD occur, they appear to predict future mania. In a systematic review and meta-analysis, Schiweck and associates (2022) found that 7.95% of those with ADHD were also diagnosed with bipolar disorder and 17.1% of those diagnosed with bipolar disorder also had ADHD. They also found that the age of onset for bipolar disorder was earlier among those with comorbid ADHD.

Nursing Diagnosis

Based on the data collected during the nursing assessment, possible nursing diagnoses for the child with ADHD include the following:

■ Risk for injury related to impulsive and accident-prone behavior and the inability to perceive self-harm

■ Impaired social interaction related to intrusive and immature behavior
■ Low self-esteem related to dysfunctional family system and negative feedback
■ Ineffective health self-management of task expectations related to low frustration tolerance and short attention span

Outcome Identification

Outcome criteria include short- and long-term goals. Timelines are individually determined. The following criteria may be used for measurement of outcomes in the care of the child with ADHD.

The patient:

■ Experiences no physical harm
■ Interacts with others appropriately
■ Verbalizes positive aspects about self
■ Demonstrates fewer demanding behaviors
■ Cooperates with staff to complete assigned tasks

Planning and Implementation

Table 32–4 provides a plan of care for the child with ADHD using nursing diagnoses common to the disorder, outcome criteria, and appropriate nursing interventions and rationales.

Table 32–4 | CARE PLAN FOR THE CHILD WITH ATTENTION-DEFICIT/HYPERACTIVITY DISORDER

NURSING DIAGNOSIS: RISK FOR INJURY

RELATED TO: Impulsive and accident-prone behavior and the inability to perceive self-harm

OUTCOME CRITERIA	NURSING INTERVENTIONS	RATIONALE
Short- and long-term goal ■ Patient remains free of injury.	1. Ensure that the patient has a safe environment. Remove objects from immediate area on which the patient could injure self as a result of random, hyperactive movements.	1. Objects that are appropriate to the normal living situation can be hazardous to a child whose motor activities are out of control.
	2. Identify deliberate behaviors that put the child at risk for injury. Institute consequences for repetition of this behavior.	2. Behavior can be modified with aversive reinforcement.
	3. If there is risk of injury associated with specific therapeutic activities, provide adequate supervision and assistance, or limit the patient's participation if adequate supervision is not possible.	3. Patient safety is a nursing priority.

NURSING DIAGNOSIS: IMPAIRED SOCIAL INTERACTION

RELATED TO: Intrusive and immature behavior

OUTCOME CRITERIA	NURSING INTERVENTIONS	RATIONALE
Short-term goal ■ Patient interacts in age-appropriate manner with nurse in one-to-one relationship within 1 week. ■ Patient observes limits set on intrusive behavior and demonstrates ability to interact appropriately with others.	1. Develop a trusting relationship with the child. Convey acceptance of the child separate from the unacceptable behavior. 2. Discuss with the patient those behaviors that are and are not acceptable. Describe in a matter-of-fact manner the consequences of unacceptable behavior. Follow through.	1. Unconditional acceptance increases feelings of self-worth. 2. Aversive reinforcement can alter undesirable behaviors.

Continued

Table 32–4 | CARE PLAN FOR THE CHILD WITH ATTENTION-DEFICIT/HYPERACTIVITY DISORDER—cont'd

	3. Provide group situations for the patient.	3. Appropriate social behavior is often learned from the positive and negative feedback of peers.

NURSING DIAGNOSIS: LOW SELF-ESTEEM

RELATED TO: Dysfunctional family system and negative feedback

OUTCOME CRITERIA	NURSING INTERVENTIONS	RATIONALE
Short-term goal ■ Patient independently directs own care and activities of daily living within 1 week. Long-term goal ■ Patient demonstrates increased feelings of self-worth by verbalizing positive statements about self and exhibiting fewer demanding behaviors.	1. Ensure that goals are realistic. 2. Plan activities that provide opportunities for success. 3. Convey unconditional acceptance and positive regard. 4. Offer recognition of successful endeavors and positive reinforcement for attempts made. Give immediate positive feedback for acceptable behavior.	1. Unrealistic goals set the patient up for failure, which diminishes self-esteem. 2. Success enhances self-esteem. 3. Affirmation of the patient as a worthwhile human being may increase self-esteem. 4. Positive reinforcement enhances self-esteem and may increase the desired behaviors.

NURSING DIAGNOSIS: INEFFECTIVE HEALTH SELF MANAGEMENT

RELATED TO: Low frustration tolerance and short attention span

OUTCOME CRITERIA	NURSING INTERVENTIONS	RATIONALE
Short-term goal ■ Patient participates in and cooperates during therapeutic activities. Long-term goal ■ Patient is able to complete assigned tasks independently or with a minimum of assistance.	1. Provide an environment for task efforts that is as free of distractions as possible. 2. Provide assistance on a one-to-one basis, beginning with simple, concrete instructions. 3. Ask the patient to repeat instructions to you. 4. Establish goals that allow the patient to complete a part of the task, rewarding each step-completion with a break for physical activity. 5. Gradually decrease the amount of assistance given while assuring the patient that assistance is still available if deemed necessary.	1. This patient is highly distractible and is unable to perform in the presence of even minimal stimulation. 2. This patient lacks the ability to assimilate information that is complicated or has abstract meaning. 3. Repetition of the instructions helps to determine the patient's level of comprehension. 4. Short-term goals are not so overwhelming to one with such a short attention span. The positive reinforcement (physical activity) increases self-esteem and provides an incentive for the patient to pursue the task to completion. 5. This process encourages the patient to perform independently while providing a feeling of security with the presence of a trusted individual.

Concept Care Mapping

The concept map care plan (see Chapter 8, "The Nursing Process in Psychiatric-Mental Health Nursing") is a diagrammatic teaching and learning strategy that allows visualization of interrelationships between medical diagnoses, nursing diagnoses, assessment data, and treatments. An example of a concept map care plan for a patient with ADHD is presented in Figure 32–2.

Evaluation

Evaluation of the care of a patient with ADHD involves examining patient behaviors after implementation of the nursing actions to determine whether the

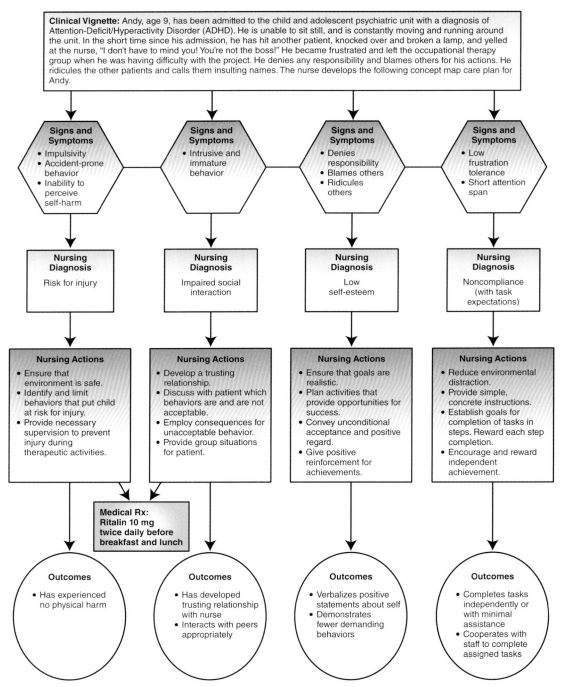

FIGURE 32–2 Concept map care plan for a patient with attention deficit-hyperactivity disorder.

treatment goals have been achieved. Collecting data by using the following types of questions may provide appropriate information for evaluation.

Has the child:

- Remained free from injury?
- Been able to establish a trusting relationship with the primary caregiver?
- Responded to limits set on unacceptable behaviors?
- Been able to interact appropriately with others?
- Been able to verbalize positive statements about self?
- Been able to complete tasks independently or with a minimum of assistance? Can they follow through after listening to simple instructions?
- Been able to apply self-control to decrease motor activity?

Psychopharmacological Intervention for ADHD

Indications

Pharmacological intervention, particularly central nervous system (CNS) stimulants, are considered the first line of treatment for ADHD (Boland & Verduin, 2022). For a list of agents used to treat ADHD, see Table 32–5. The mechanism of action is unclear, but because these drugs are believed to elevate dopamine and norepinephrine levels, it is hypothesized that their effectiveness is in response to neurotransmitter dysregulation. They have

generally mild side effects but are contraindicated in anyone with cardiac problems or risks for cardiac problems. As previously mentioned, there is an increased risk for new-onset psychosis with amphetamine stimulants, which release about four times as much dopamine as methylphenidate (Griffin & Harari, 2019).

One study (Van Den Ban et al., 2014) explored whether use of stimulants had an effect on reducing injuries and hospital admissions for children with ADHD. This topic is relevant because this population has a high incidence of injury and hospital admissions related to hyperactivity and impulsivity. About 60% of children with ADHD demonstrate suboptimal motor performance, which may also increase their risks for injury. The researchers found that children taking ADHD drugs (mostly stimulants) had a twofold higher risk of injury-related hospital admissions than among those not treated with ADHD drugs. They also found that children who were on ADHD drugs and psychotropic drugs such as antipsychotics and benzodiazepines had a fivefold increase in risk for injuries and hospital admissions compared with those who were on ADHD medication alone. The severity of ADHD in children on medication may, in part, account for these findings, but it is significant that while mediating other core symptoms of ADHD, medication may not reduce risks for injury. Amphetamines

TABLE 32–5 Medications for Attention Deficit-Hyperactivity Disorder

CHEMICAL CLASS	GENERIC (TRADE) NAME	DAILY DOSAGE RANGE (mg)	CONTROLLED CATEGORIES
CNS STIMULANTS			
Amphetamines	Dextroamphetamine sulfate (Dexedrine; Dextrostat)	2.5–40	CII
	Methamphetamine (Desoxyn)	5–25	CII
	Lisdexamfetamine (Vyvanse)	20–70	CII
Amphetamine mixtures	Dextroamphetamine/amphetamine (Adderall; Adderall XR)	2.5–40	CII
	Adzenys XR-ODT	6.3–18.8	CII
Miscellaneous	Methylphenidate (Ritalin; Ritalin-SR; Ritalin LA; Methylin; Methylin ER; Metadate ER; Metadate CD; Concerta; Daytrana)	10–60	CII
	Dexmethylphenidate (Focalin)	5–20	CII
	Serdexmethylphenidate and dexmethylphenidate (Azstarys)	39.2–52.3	CII
Alpha agonists	Clonidine (Catapres)	0.05–0.3	—
	Guanfacine (Tenex; Intuniv)	1–4	—
Miscellaneous	Atomoxetine (Strattera)	>70 kg: 40–100; ≤ 70 kg: 0.5–1.4 mg/kg (or 100 mg, whichever is less)	—
	Bupropion (Wellbutrin; Wellbutrin SR; Wellbutrin XL)	3 mg/kg (ADHD); 100–300 (depression)	—
	Viloxazine (Qelbree)	100–200 mg	—

have been a common substance of abuse and demonstrate a high risk for dependence, and similar concerns have been identified for individuals with ADHD. In addition, there are concerns that children with ADHD may be at risk for diversion of these medications; Jain (2022) reported that up to 23% of children on amphetamine stimulants identify having been approached to give, sell, or trade their medication to someone else.

In January of 2016 the FDA approved Adzenys XR-ODT, a flavored, chewable amphetamine mixture tablet for use in the treatment of ADHD in children. See Chapter 4, "Psychopharmacology," for a complete discussion of the medications used in the treatment of ADHD, including safety and education issues.

Other advances in the pharmacological treatment of ADHD, include a delayed-release stimulant (methylphenidate hydrochloride) given at bedtime so that it reaches effectiveness levels in the morning; FDA approval of a selective norepinephrine reuptake inhibitor (SNRI), viloxazine (Qelbree), as another nonstimulant option; and a combination CNS stimulant drug, serdexmethylphenidate and dexmethylphenidate (Azstarys), which is advanced as offering all-day relief in a single daily dose.

Nonpharmacological Treatment for ADHD

Recently the FDA (2020) approved a novel interactive video game, EndeavorRx, for the treatment of ADHD. Its developers identify that it directly targets neurological function and that studies support its effectiveness in improving attention (Tumolo, 2020). It requires a prescription and is currently advanced as a nondrug adjunctive treatment option.

A second FDA-approved device is the Monarch external Trigeminal Nerve Stimulation (eTNS) System. The device stimulates the trigeminal nerve through the skin on the forehead, activating a part of the brain thought to be involved in ADHD. As Greenhill (2022) noted, FDA approvals for devices only require evidence of safety (unlike medications, which also require evidence of efficacy). More research is needed to evaluate the therapeutic benefits of these treatments.

Tourette's Disorder
Clinical Findings, Epidemiology, and Course

Tourette's disorder is characterized by the presence of multiple motor tics and one or more vocal tics, which may appear simultaneously or at different periods during the illness (APA, 2022). The disturbance may cause distress or interfere with social, occupational, or other important areas of functioning. The age at onset of Tourette's disorder can be as early as 2 years, but the disorder occurs most commonly around age 6 to 7 years. Prevalence of the disorder is estimated between 3 and 9 per 1,000 in school-age children (APA, 2022). The lifetime prevalence is estimated to be about 1% (Boland & Verduin, 2022). It is two to four times more common in boys than in girls. Although the disorder can be lifelong, most people with this condition experience the worst tic symptoms in their early teens with gradual improvement thereafter (National Institutes of Health [NIH], 2021).

Predisposing Factors
Biological Factors

Genetics: Various genetic studies, including twin studies and adoption studies, support a genetic basis for this neurological disorder (Boland & Verduin, 2022). Recent studies suggest that the pattern of inheritance is complex, probably involving several genes influenced by environmental factors (NIH, 2021). In addition, genetic studies suggest that ADHD and OCD are genetically related to Tourette's disorder; both are common comorbidities of patients with Tourette's disorder (NIH, 2021).

Biochemical Factors: Abnormalities in levels of dopamine, choline, *N*-acetylaspartate, creatine, myoinositol, and norepinephrine have all been demonstrated in neuroimaging studies. The effectiveness of antipsychotic medication (particularly haloperidol and fluphenazine) in suppressing tics also supports neurotransmitter involvement in Tourette's disorder (Boland & Verduin, 2022). However, Boland and Verduin added that there is variability in response to antipsychotic medications, and sometimes Tourette's disorder has emerged in patients being treated with antipsychotics. Based on current evidence, although there appear to be several biochemical influences in this disorder, these are complex interactions and are not well understood.

Structural Factors: Abnormalities in the basal ganglia, frontal lobes, cortex, and circuits that connect these regions have also been implicated in the pathology of Tourette's disorder (NIH, 2021). Although many structural influences have been identified, the direct cause is not yet known. It is probably a complex interaction of genetics, biochemistry, and environmental influences.

Environmental Factors

Some studies have shown that environmental influences, such as maternal alcohol use during pregnancy, low birth weight, complications during childbirth, and infection, may be associated with the development of Tourette's disorder (Boland & Verduin, 2022; CDC,

2020). Further research is needed to confirm these influences.

Application of the Nursing Process to Tourette's Disorder

Background Assessment Data (Symptomatology)

The motor tics of Tourette's disorder may involve the head, torso, and upper and lower limbs. Initial symptoms may begin with a single motor tic, most commonly eye blinking, or with multiple symptoms. Tics tend to first occur in the face and neck and progress downward to the torso and lower limbs over time (Boland & Verduin, 2022). Simple motor tics include movements such as eye blinking, neck jerking, shoulder shrugging, and facial grimacing. The more complex motor tics include squatting, hopping, skipping, tapping, touching behaviors, grooming rituals, echopraxia (repetition or imitation of the movements of others), and retracing steps. Some tics involve self-harm, such as punching oneself in the face (NIH, 2021).

Vocal tics include various words or sounds such as squeaks, grunts, barks, sniffs, snorts, coughs, and, in rare instances, a complex vocal tic involving the uttering of obscenities. Vocal tics may include repeating certain words or phrases out of context, repeating one's own sounds or words **(palilalia),** or repeating what others say **(echolalia).**

The movements and vocalizations are experienced as compulsive and irresistible but can be suppressed for varying lengths of time. Many report a buildup of tension as they attempt to suppress tics to the point where they feel the tic must be expressed against their will. Tics are often worse during periods of stress or excitement and better during periods of calm, focused activity (NIH, 2021). In most cases, tics are diminished during sleep. Neurobehavioral disorders that are common in conjunction with Tourette's disorder (and may be more troublesome than the tics themselves) are inattention, hyperactivity, and impulsivity as are seen in ADHD and OCD, depression, and anxiety. Many children with Tourette's disorder also manifest difficulty with reading, writing, and arithmetic (NIH, 2021). The *DSM-5-TR* diagnostic criteria for Tourette's disorder require that both motor and vocal tics have been present at some time during the illness and are persistent for more than 1 year.

Nursing Diagnosis

Based on data collected during the nursing assessment, possible nursing diagnoses for the patient with Tourette's disorder include the following:

- Risk for self-directed or other-directed violence related to low tolerance for frustration
- Impaired social interaction related to impulsiveness and oppositional and aggressive behavior
- Low self-esteem related to embarrassment associated with tic behaviors

Outcome Identification

Outcome criteria include short- and long-term goals. Timelines are individually determined. The following criteria may be used for measurement of outcomes in the care of the patient with Tourette's disorder.

The patient:

- Has not harmed self or others
- Interacts with staff and peers in an appropriate manner
- Demonstrates self-control by managing tic behavior
- Follows rules without becoming defensive
- Verbalizes positive aspects about self

Planning and Implementation

Table 32–6 provides a plan of care for the child or adolescent with Tourette's disorder using selected nursing diagnoses, outcome criteria, and appropriate nursing interventions and rationales.

Evaluation

Evaluation of care for the child with Tourette's disorder reflects whether the nursing actions have been effective in achieving the established goals. The nursing process calls for reassessment of the plan. Questions for gathering reassessment data may include the following:

Has the patient:

- Refrained from causing harm to self or others during times of increased tension?
- Developed adaptive coping strategies for dealing with frustration to prevent resorting to self-destruction or aggression to others?
- Been able to interact appropriately with staff and peers?
- Been able to suppress tic behaviors when they choose to do so?
- Set a time for "release" of the suppressed tic behaviors?
- Verbalized positive aspects about self, particularly as they relate to their ability to manage the illness?
- Complied with treatment in a nondefensive manner?

Psychopharmacological Intervention for Tourette's Disorder

Systematic review of current evidence supports the efficacy of antipsychotic agents, both typical and atypical agents, and the use of alpha-2-adrenergic agonist agents (such as clonidine and guanfacine) in treating tics (Weisman et al., 2013). Medications are reserved for those with significant impairment and

Table 32–6 | CARE PLAN FOR THE CHILD OR ADOLESCENT WITH TOURETTE'S DISORDER

NURSING DIAGNOSIS: RISK FOR SELF-DIRECTED OR OTHER-DIRECTED VIOLENCE

RELATED TO: Low tolerance for frustration

OUTCOME CRITERIA	NURSING INTERVENTIONS	RATIONALE
Short-term goal ■ Patient seeks out staff or support person at any time if thoughts of harming self or others should occur. **Long-term goal** ■ Patient does not harm self or others.	1. Observe the patient's behavior frequently through routine activities and interactions. Become aware of behaviors that indicate a rise in agitation.	1. Stress commonly increases tic behaviors. Recognition of behaviors that precede the onset of aggression may provide the opportunity to intervene before violence occurs.
	2. Monitor for self-destructive behavior and impulses. A staff member may need to stay with the patient to prevent self-mutilation.	2. Patient safety is a nursing priority.
	3. Provide hand coverings and other restraints that prevent the patient from self-mutilative behaviors.	3. For the patient's protection, provide immediate external controls against self-aggressive behaviors.
	4. Redirect violent behavior with physical outlets for frustration.	4. Excess energy is released through physical activities, and a feeling of relaxation is induced.

NURSING DIAGNOSIS: IMPAIRED SOCIAL INTERACTION

RELATED TO: Impulsiveness; oppositional and aggressive behavior

OUTCOME CRITERIA	NURSING INTERVENTIONS	RATIONALE
Short-term goal ■ Patient develops a one-to-one relationship with a nurse or support person within 1 week. **Long-term goal** ■ Patient is able to interact with staff and peers using age-appropriate, acceptable behaviors.	1. Develop a trusting relationship with the patient. Convey acceptance of the person separate from the unacceptable behavior.	1. Unconditional acceptance increases feeling of self-worth.
	2. Discuss with the patient which behaviors are and are not acceptable. Describe in matter-of-fact manner the consequence of unacceptable behavior. Follow through.	2. Aversive reinforcement can alter or extinguish undesirable behaviors.
	3. Provide group situations for the patient.	3. Appropriate social behavior is often learned from the positive and negative feedback of peers.

Continued

Table 32–6 | CARE PLAN FOR THE CHILD OR ADOLESCENT WITH TOURETTE'S DISORDER–cont'd

NURSING DIAGNOSIS: LOW SELF-ESTEEM

RELATED TO: Embarrassment associated with tic behaviors

OUTCOME CRITERIA	NURSING INTERVENTIONS	RATIONALE
Short-term goal ■ Patient verbalizes positive aspects about self not associated with tic behaviors.	1. Convey unconditional acceptance and positive regard.	1. Communicating a perception of the patient as a worthwhile human being may increase self-esteem.
Long-term goal ■ Patient exhibits increased feeling of self-worth as evidenced by verbal expression of positive aspects about self, past accomplishments, and future prospects.	2. Set limits on manipulative behavior. Take caution not to reinforce manipulative behaviors by providing desired attention. Identify the consequences of manipulation. Administer consequences matter-of-factly when manipulation occurs.	2. Aversive consequences may work to decrease unacceptable behaviors.
	3. Help the patient understand that they use manipulation to try to increase self-esteem. Interventions should reflect other actions to accomplish this goal.	3. When the patient feels better about self, the need to manipulate others will diminish.
	4. If the patient chooses to suppress tics in the presence of others, provide a specified "tic time" during which they "vent" tics, feelings, and behaviors (alone or with staff).	4. Allows for release of tics and assists in sense of control and management of symptoms.
	5. Ensure that the patient has regular one-to-one time with nursing staff.	5. One-to-one time gives the nurse the opportunity to provide the patient with information about the illness and healthy ways to manage it. Exploring feelings about the illness helps the patient incorporate the illness into a healthy sense of self.

unresponsive to psychological therapies. Weisman and associates (2013) noted that alpha-2 agonists are more efficacious in treating tics among patients with ADHD. Other medications that have demonstrated potential benefits, but need more research, include tetrabenazine, topiramate, botulinum, and tetrahydrocannabinol. Pharmacotherapy is most effective when combined with psychosocial therapy, such as behavioral therapy, individual counseling or psychotherapy, or family therapy.

Antipsychotics

Haloperidol (Haldol), pimozide (Orap), and aripiprazole (Abilify) have been approved by the FDA for control of tics and vocal utterances associated with Tourette's disorder. Although antipsychotics have demonstrated efficacy in treating symptoms, they are often not the first-line choice of therapy (particularly first generation antipsychotics) because of their propensity for severe adverse effects such as extrapyramidal symptoms, neuroleptic malignant syndrome, tardive dyskinesia, and electrocardiographic changes. Haloperidol is not recommended for children younger than 3 years of age, and pimozide should not be administered to children younger than 12 years.

Although not presently approved by the FDA for use in Tourette's disorder, some clinicians prefer to prescribe other atypical antipsychotics, such as risperidone (Risperdal), olanzapine (Zyprexa), or ziprasidone (Geodon), because of their more favorable side-effect profiles. Boland and Verduin (2022) identified risperidone as the most well-studied atypical antipsychotic for the treatment of tics and reported that there is considerable evidence for its efficacy. These medications have a lower incidence of neurological side effects than the typical antipsychotics, although extrapyramidal symptoms have been observed with risperidone. Common side effects include weight gain, metabolic side effects, and hyperprolactinemia. Ziprasidone has been associated with an increased risk of QTc interval prolongation. Hyperglycemia has also been reported in some patients taking atypical antipsychotics.

Alpha-Adrenergic Agonists

Clonidine (Catapres) and guanfacine (Tenex, Intuniv) are alpha-adrenergic agonists that are approved for use as antihypertensive agents. The extended-release forms have been approved by the FDA for the treatment of ADHD. Atomoxetine, an SNRI, has also been used, but more research is needed to confirm safety and efficacy in treating children with Tourette's disorder (Boland & Verduin, 2022). These medications may be preferred for the treatment of Tourette's disorder symptoms because of their favorable side-effect profile and because they are often effective for comorbid symptoms of ADHD, anxiety and insomnia. Common side effects include dry mouth, sedation, headaches, fatigue, and dizziness or postural hypotension. Guanfacine is longer lasting and less sedating than clonidine; however, its efficacy in reducing tics is controversial (Boland & Verduin, 2022). Alpha-adrenergic agonists should not be prescribed for children and adolescents with preexisting cardiac or vascular disease and they should not be discontinued abruptly; doing this could result in symptoms of nervousness, agitation, tremor, and a rapid rise in blood pressure.

Nonpharmacological Treatments for Tourette's Disorder

Nonpharmacological treatment options for patients with Tourette's disorder include comprehensive behavioral intervention for tics (CBIT), speech therapies, and deep brain stimulation. CBIT is an evidence-based treatment to reduce the severity of tics. The intervention teaches individuals how to recognize and manage environmental factors that trigger or worsen tics. Studies in both children and adults have demonstrated sustained improvement at least 6 months after the intervention (Tourette's Association of America, n.d.) and habit reversal

training is currently the first-line behavioral treatment for tic disorders (Boland & Verduin, 2022). Individuals with Tourette's syndrome who also have other co-occurring conditions such as social language impairments, learning disabilities, or other communication disorders may benefit from speech therapies. Deep brain stimulation is an experimental surgical treatment that involves connecting electrodes to brain centers and implanting a pulse generator to stimulate areas of the brain associated with communication. It is yet to be determined which center or centers of the brain are the best targets for neuromodulation, but it has demonstrated success in some patients. Researchers (Xu et al., 2020) reported that the treatments do not eliminate tics but significantly reduce (53%) their intensity. This treatment is reserved for cases where all other treatments have been tried and found ineffective.

Disruptive Behavior Disorders

Oppositional Defiant Disorder
Clinical Findings, Epidemiology, and Course

Oppositional defiant disorder (ODD) is characterized by a frequent and persistent pattern of angry mood and defiant behavior that occurs more frequently than is usually observed in individuals of comparable age and developmental level and interferes with social, educational, occupational, or other important areas of functioning (APA, 2022). The behavior must be distinct, pervasive, and more disruptive than the sometimes negativistic and oppositional behavior that is typical in children and adolescents. The disorder typically begins by 8 years of age and usually no later than early adolescence. Prevalence estimates range from 1% to 11%, and common comorbid disorders include ADHD, anxiety, major depressive disorder, conduct disorder, and substance use disorders (APA, 2022). It is more prevalent in boys than in girls before puberty, but the rates are more closely equal after puberty. The *DSM-5-TR* identifies that ODD often precedes conduct disorder, especially in children with onset of conduct disorder before age 10 years (APA, 2022).

Predisposing Factors
Biological Influences

What role, if any, that genetics, temperament, or biochemical alterations play in the etiology of ODD is still unclear. Some studies have identified genetic influences in the establishment of a child's temperament, but there is no clear evidence of this connection in ODD. However, having a temperament in which the child has difficulty regulating emotions and has low frustration tolerance is an identified risk factor for ODD (Mayo Clinic, 2022b).

Family Influences

Opposition during various developmental stages is both normal and healthy. Children first exhibit oppositional behaviors at around age 10 or 11 months, again as toddlers between ages 18 and 36 months, and finally during adolescence. Pathology is considered only when the developmental phase is prolonged or when there is overreaction in the child's environment to their behavior.

Some children exhibit these behaviors in a more intense form than others. Boland and Verduin (2022) reported, "Epidemiological studies of negativistic traits in nonclinical populations found such behavior in 16% to 22% of school-age children" (p. 189).

Some parents interpret an average or increased level of developmental oppositional behavior as hostility and a deliberate effort on the part of the child to be in control. If power and control are issues for parents or if they exercise authority for their own needs, a power struggle can be established between the parents and the child that sets the stage for the development of ODD. Lubit (2022) suggested the following pattern of family dynamics:

- There is the combination of a child with a temperament that includes poor emotion regulation, high levels of emotional reactivity, and poor frustration tolerance in an environment of harsh or neglectful and highly authoritarian parenting.
- The child sees the parent as overly domineering and the parents see the child as unreasonable and disrespectful.
- Both children and parents become angry and increasingly rigid in their stances.

Lubit (2022) stated:

These patterns develop when parents inadvertently reinforce disruptive and deviant behaviors in a child by giving those behaviors a significant amount of negative attention. At the same time, the parents, who are often exhausted by the struggle to obtain compliance with simple requests, usually fail to provide positive attention; often, the parents have infrequent positive interactions with their children. The pattern of negative interactions evolves quickly as the result of repeated, ineffective, emotionally expressed commands and comments; ineffective harsh punishments; and insufficient attention and modeling of appropriate behaviors.

A childhood history of trauma can be influential in the appearance of oppositional defiant behaviors, so it is essential to assess the child for a history of abuse, neglect, or other traumas.

Application of the Nursing Process to ODD

Background Assessment Data (Symptomatology)

ODD is characterized by passive-aggressive behaviors such as stubbornness, procrastination, disobedience, carelessness, **negativism** (an attitude of persistent resistance and contradictory behavior toward others), testing of limits, resistance to directions, deliberately ignoring the communication of others, and unwillingness to compromise. Other symptoms that may be evident are running away, school avoidance, school underachievement, temper tantrums, fighting, and argumentativeness.

Initially, the oppositional attitude is directed toward the parents, but in time, relationships with peers and teachers become affected. These impairments in social interaction often lead to depression, anxiety, and additional problematic behavior (Lubit, 2022).

Usually, these children do not see themselves as being oppositional but believe the problem is caused by the unreasonable demands of others. They are often friendless, perceiving human relationships as negative and unsatisfactory. School performance is usually poor because of their refusal to participate and their resistance to external demands.

The *DSM-5-TR* diagnostic criteria for ODD are presented in Box 32–3.

Nursing Diagnosis

Based on the data collected during the nursing assessment, possible nursing diagnoses for the patient with ODD include the following:

- Defensive coping related to retarded ego development, low self-esteem, unsatisfactory parent/child relationship, denial of problems, underlying hostility
- Low self-esteem related to lack of positive feedback, retarded ego development
- Impaired social interaction related to negative temperament, underlying hostility, manipulation of others

Outcome Identification

Outcome criteria include short- and long-term goals. Timelines are individually determined. The following criteria may be used for measurement of outcomes in the care of the patient with ODD.

The patient:

- Participates in therapies without negativism
- Accepts responsibility for their part in the problem
- Takes direction from staff without becoming defensive
- Does not manipulate other people
- Verbalizes positive aspects about self
- Interacts with others in an appropriate manner

BOX 32–3 Diagnostic Criteria for Oppositional Defiant Disorder

A. A pattern of angry/irritable mood, argumentative/defiant behavior, or vindictiveness lasting at least 6 months as evidenced by at least four symptoms from any of the following categories and exhibited during interaction with at least one individual that is not a sibling.

ANGRY/IRRITABLE MOOD
1. Often loses temper.
2. Is often touchy or easily annoyed.
3. Is often angry and resentful.

ARGUMENTATIVE/DEFIANT BEHAVIOR
4. Often argues with authority figures or, for children and adolescents, with adults.
5. Often actively defies or refuses to comply with requests from authority figures or with rules.
6. Often deliberately annoys others.
7. Often blames others for his or her mistakes or misbehavior.

VINDICTIVENESS
8. Has been spiteful or vindictive at least twice within the past 6 months.

Note: The persistence and frequency of these behaviors should be used to distinguish a behavior that is within normal limits from a behavior that is symptomatic. For children younger than 5 years, the behavior should occur on most days for a period of at least 6 months unless otherwise noted (Criterion A8). For individuals 5 years or older, the behavior should occur at least once per week for at least 6 months, unless otherwise noted (Criterion A8). Although these frequency criteria provide guidance on a minimal level of frequency to define symptoms, other factors should also be considered, such as whether the frequency and intensity of the behaviors are outside a range that is normative for the individual's developmental level, gender, and culture.

B. The disturbance in behavior is associated with distress in the individual or others in his or her immediate social context (e.g., family, peer group, work colleagues), or it effects negatively on social, educational, occupational, or other important areas of functioning.
C. The behaviors do not occur exclusively during the course of a psychotic, substance use, depressive, or bipolar disorder. Also, the criteria are not met for disruptive mood dysregulation disorder.

Specify current severity:

Mild: Symptoms are confined to only one setting (e.g., at home, at school, at work, with peers).

Moderate: Some symptoms are present in at least two settings.

Severe: Some symptoms are present in three or more settings.

Reprinted with permission from the *Diagnostic and Statistical Manual of Mental Disorders, Fifth Edition, Text Revision* (Copyright 2022). American Psychiatric Association.

Planning and Implementation

Table 32–7 provides a plan of care for the child with ODD using nursing diagnoses common to the disorder, outcome criteria, and appropriate nursing interventions and rationales.

Evaluation

The evaluation step of the nursing process calls for reassessment of the plan of care to determine whether the nursing actions have been effective in achieving the goals of therapy. The following questions can be used with the child or adolescent with ODD to gather information for the evaluation.

Is the patient:

■ Cooperating with the schedule of therapeutic activities? Is level of participation adequate?
■ Manifesting a less negative attitude toward therapy?
■ Accepting responsibility for problem behavior?
■ Verbalizing the unacceptability of their passive-aggressive behavior?
■ Able to identify which behaviors are unacceptable and substitute more adaptive behaviors?
■ Able to interact with staff and peers without defending behavior in an angry manner?
■ Able to verbalize positive statements about self?
■ Manifesting fewer manipulative behaviors?
■ Able to make compromises with others when issues of control emerge?
■ Expressing anger and hostility appropriately and verbalizing ways of releasing anger adaptively?
■ Able to verbalize true feelings instead of allowing them to emerge through use of passive-aggressive behaviors?

Conduct Disorder

Clinical Findings, Epidemiology, and Course

With **conduct disorder,** there is a repetitive and persistent pattern of behavior in which the basic rights of others or major age-appropriate societal norms or rules are violated (APA, 2022). This feature distinguishes it from ODD. Physical **aggression** (behavior that is intended to be harmful toward others) is common, and peer relationships are disturbed. Conduct disorder is one of the most frequent reasons that children and adolescents are referred for psychiatric

Table 32–7 | CARE PLAN FOR THE CHILD/ADOLESCENT WITH OPPOSITIONAL DEFIANT DISORDER

NURSING DIAGNOSIS: DEFENSIVE COPING

RELATED TO: Negative temperament; denial of problems; underlying hostility, low self-esteem, conflict in relationship with parents

OUTCOME CRITERIA	NURSING INTERVENTIONS	RATIONALE
Short-term goals ■ Patient participates in and cooperates during therapeutic activities. ■ Patient verbalizes personal responsibility for difficulties experienced in interpersonal relationships within a time period reasonable for the patient. **Long-term goals** ■ Patient completes assigned tasks willingly and independently or with a minimum of assistance. ■ Patient accepts responsibility for own behaviors and interacts with others without becoming defensive.	1. Set forth a structured plan of therapeutic activities. Start with minimum expectations and increase as the patient begins to manifest evidence of adherence. 2. Establish a system of rewards for follow through with therapy and consequences for negative behavior. Ensure that the rewards and consequences are concepts of value to the patient. 3. Convey acceptance of the patient separate from the undesirable behaviors being exhibited. ("It is not *you* but your *behavior* that is unacceptable.") 4. Help the patient recognize that feelings of inadequacy provoke defensive behaviors, such as blaming others for problems, and the need to "get even." 5. Provide immediate, nonthreatening feedback for passive-aggressive behavior. 6. Help identify situations that provoke defensiveness and practice through role-play more appropriate responses. 7. Provide immediate positive feedback for acceptable behaviors.	1. Structure provides security, and one or two activities may not seem as overwhelming as the whole schedule of activities presented at one time. 2. Positive, negative, and aversive reinforcements can contribute to desired changes in behavior. 3. Unconditional acceptance enhances self-worth and may contribute to a decrease in the need for passive-aggression toward others. 4. Recognition of the problem is the first step toward initiating change. 5. Because the patient denies responsibility for problems, they are denying the inappropriateness of behavior. 6. Role-playing provides confidence to deal with difficult situations when they actually occur. 7. Positive feedback encourages repetition, and immediacy is significant for these children who respond to immediate gratification.

NURSING DIAGNOSIS: LOW SELF-ESTEEM

RELATED TO: Lack of positive feedback; retarded ego development

OUTCOME CRITERIA	NURSING INTERVENTIONS	RATIONALE
Short-term goal ■ Patient participates in own self-care and discusses with nurse aspects of self about which they feel good.	1. Ensure that goals are realistic.	1. Unrealistic goals set the patient up for failure, which diminishes self-esteem.

Table 32–7 | CARE PLAN FOR THE CHILD/ADOLESCENT WITH OPPOSITIONAL DEFIANT DISORDER—cont'd

OUTCOME CRITERIA	NURSING INTERVENTIONS	RATIONALE
Long-term goal ■ Patient demonstrates increased feelings of self-worth by verbalizing positive statements about self and exhibiting fewer manipulative behaviors.	2. Plan activities that provide opportunities for success. 3. Convey unconditional acceptance and positive regard. 4. Set limits on manipulative behavior. Take caution not to reinforce manipulative behaviors by providing desired attention. Identify the consequences of manipulation. Administer consequences matter-of-factly when manipulation occurs. 5. Help the patient understand that they use this behavior to try to increase own self-esteem. Interventions should reflect other actions to accomplish this goal.	2. Success enhances self-esteem. 3. Affirmation of the patient as a worthwhile human being may increase self-esteem. 4. Aversive reinforcement may work to decrease unacceptable behaviors. 5. When the patient feels better about self, the need to manipulate others will diminish.

NURSING DIAGNOSIS: IMPAIRED SOCIAL INTERACTION

RELATED TO: Negative temperament; underlying hostility; manipulation of others

OUTCOME CRITERIA	NURSING INTERVENTIONS	RATIONALE
Short-term goal ■ Patient interacts in age-appropriate manner with nurse in one-to-one relationship within 1 week. **Long-term goal** ■ Patient is able to interact with staff and peers using age-appropriate, acceptable behaviors.	1. Develop a trusting relationship with the patient. Convey acceptance of the person separate from the unacceptable behavior. 2. Explain to the patient about passive-aggressive behavior. Explain how these behaviors are perceived by others. Describe which behaviors are not acceptable and role-play more adaptive responses. Give positive feedback for acceptable behaviors. 3. Provide peer group situations for the patient.	1. Unconditional acceptance increases feelings of self-worth and may serve to diminish feelings of rejection that have accumulated over a long period. 2. Role-playing is a way to practice behaviors that do not come readily to the patient, making it easier when the situation actually occurs. Positive feedback enhances repetition of desirable behaviors. 3. Appropriate social behavior is often learned from the positive and negative feedback of peers. Groups also provide an atmosphere for using the behaviors rehearsed in role-play.

intervention (Boland & Verduin, 2022). Prevalence estimates range from 2% to more than 10%, rises from childhood to adolescence, and is more common in males than females (APA, 2022). There is a higher male predominance among those with the childhood-onset subtype. Several comorbidities are common with conduct disorder, including ADHD, mood disorders, learning disorders, and substance use disorders. The symptoms of ODD are generally considered less severe than those of conduct disorder. However, ODD may progress to conduct disorder, and both ODD and conduct disorder confer greater risk for antisocial personality disorder in adulthood (Connor, 2017). When the disorder begins in childhood, there is more likely to be a history of ODD and a greater likelihood of antisocial personality disorder in adulthood than if the disorder is diagnosed in adolescence.

CORE CONCEPT

Temperament

Personality characteristics that define an individual's mood and behavioral tendencies are termed **temperament**. The sum of physical, emotional, and intellectual components that affect or determine a person's actions and reactions.

Predisposing Factors

Biological Influences

Genetics: Family, twin, and adoptive studies have revealed a significantly higher number of individuals with conduct disorder among those who have family members with the disorder. Although genetic factors appear to be involved in the etiology of conduct disorder, little is yet known about the actual mechanisms involved in genetic transmission. A potential role for X-linked monoamine oxidase, a gene in the etiology of antisocial behavior, suggests the need for more research into its potential role in conduct disorder (Boland & Verduin, 2022).

There is some evidence, however, of the distinction between behaviors that appear to be genetic versus environmental risk factors. In a large study of male twins (N = 2,769), researchers attempted to determine the structure of genetic and environmental influences in conduct disorder. They found the familial risk to conduct disorder is composed of two discrete dimensions of genetic risk, rule-breaking (such as truancy) and overt aggression (harming other people), and one dimension of shared environmental risk, reflecting covert delinquency (such as stealing and hurting animals) (Kendler et al., 2013). Studies such as these support a complex dynamic of both genetic and environmental factors in the development of conduct disorder.

Temperament: The term *temperament* refers to personality traits that become evident very early in life and may be present at birth. Children who show signs of an irritable temperament, poor compliance, inattentiveness, and impulsivity as early as age 2 may show signs of conduct disorder at later ages (Bernstein, 2022). Bernstein added that children with severe temperamental disturbances, including poor attachment, may develop ODD and conduct disorder despite adequate parental intervention. More commonly, however, these children come from unstable families, with frequent changes in residence and economic stress. Evidence suggests a genetic influence in temperament and an association between temperament and behavioral problems later in life.

Neurobiological Factors: Boland and Verduin (2022) identified three neurobiological findings relevant to conduct disorders. First, neuroimaging studies identify decreased gray matter in limbic structures, bilateral insula (an area of the cortex that plays a role connecting emotional responses to pain), and the left amygdala. Second, studies have found high plasma concentration of serotonin and low levels in cerebrospinal fluid, both of which are correlated with aggression and violence. The third finding is that aggressive children had "significantly greater relative right frontal brain activity at rest than healthy controls" (p. 194). Bernstein (2022) added that decreased dopamine response to reward and increased risk-taking behaviors related to several disrupted structures within the frontal cortex worsen over time due to activation of brain stress systems and increases in corticotropin-releasing factor.

Psychosocial Influences

Poor academic performance and social maladaptation often lead to affiliations with a deviant peer group. "Considerable research indicates that the deviant peer group provides training in criminal and delinquent behavior including substance abuse" (Bernstein, 2022). In addition to evidence that engaging in risk-taking behaviors can yield reinforcement on a social level (acceptance within a peer group), Bernstein noted that "studies of neural processing show that risk-taking may be associated with reward-related brain activation."

Family Influences

The following factors related to family dynamics have been implicated as contributors in the predisposition to conduct disorder and typically combine to create a pattern of chaotic disruption in family life (Bernstein, 2022; Boland & Verduin, 2022; Mayo Clinic, 2022b):

- Parental rejection, neglect, or severe physical and verbal aggression
- Inconsistent or harsh, punitive discipline
- Parental psychopathology, antisocial personality disorder, or substance use disorders
- Lack of parental supervision
- Frequent changes in residence
- Economic stressors
- Marital conflict and divorce (particularly with persistent hostility)

Application of the Nursing Process to Conduct Disorder

Background Assessment Data (Symptomatology)

The classic characteristic of conduct disorder is the use of physical aggression to violate the rights of others. The behavior pattern manifests itself in virtually all areas of the child's life (home, school, with peers, and in the community). Stealing, lying, and truancy are common problems. The child lacks feelings of guilt or remorse.

The use of tobacco, liquor, or nonprescribed drugs, as well as the participation in sexual activities, occurs earlier than at the expected age for the peer group. Projection is a common defense mechanism.

Low self-esteem is manifested by a "tough guy" image. Characteristics include poor frustration tolerance, irritability, and frequent temper outbursts. Symptoms of anxiety and depression are not uncommon.

Level of academic achievement may be low in relation to age and IQ. Manifestations associated with ADHD (e.g., attention difficulties, impulsiveness, and hyperactivity) are common in children with conduct disorder.

The *DSM-5-TR* diagnostic criteria for conduct disorder are presented in Box 32–4.

Nursing Diagnosis

Based on the data collected during the nursing assessment, possible nursing diagnoses for the patient with conduct disorder include the following:

- Risk for other-directed violence related to characteristics of temperament, peer rejection, negative parental role models, dysfunctional family dynamics
- Impaired social interaction related to negative parental role models, impaired peer relations leading to inappropriate social behaviors
- Defensive coping related to low self-esteem and dysfunctional family system
- Low self-esteem related to lack of positive feedback and unsatisfactory parent-child relationship

Outcome Identification

Outcome criteria include short- and long-term goals. Timelines are individually determined. The following criteria may be used for measurement of outcomes in the care of the patient with conduct disorder.

The patient:

- Has not harmed self or others
- Interacts with others in a socially appropriate manner
- Accepts direction without becoming defensive
- Demonstrates evidence of increased self-esteem by discontinuing exploitative and demanding behaviors toward others

Planning and Implementation

Table 32–8 provides a plan of care for the child with conduct disorder using nursing diagnoses common to the disorder, outcome criteria, and appropriate nursing interventions and rationales.

Evaluation

Following the planning and implementation of care, evaluation is made of the behavioral changes in the child with conduct disorder. This evaluation is accomplished by determining whether the goals of therapy have been achieved. Reassessment, the next step in the nursing process, may be initiated by gathering information using the following questions:

Has the patient:

- Been able to manage aggressive impulses?
- Been able to prevent harm to others or others' property?
- Been able to express anger in an appropriate manner?
- Developed more adaptive coping strategies to deal with anger and feelings of aggression?
- Demonstrated the ability to trust others and interact with staff and peers in an appropriate manner?
- Been able to accept responsibility for their own behavior? Is there less blaming of others?
- Been able to accept feedback from others without becoming defensive?
- Been able to verbalize positive statements about self?
- Been able to interact with others without engaging in manipulation?

Anxiety Disorders

Separation Anxiety Disorder
Clinical Findings, Epidemiology, and Course

Separation anxiety disorder is characterized by excessive fear or anxiety concerning separation from those to whom the individual is attached (APA, 2022). The

BOX 32–4 **Diagnostic Criteria for Conduct Disorder**

A. A repetitive and persistent pattern of behavior in which the basic rights of others or major age-appropriate societal norms or rules are violated, as manifested by the presence of at least 3 of the following 15 criteria in the past 12 months from any of the categories below, with at least one criterion present in the past 6 months:

AGGRESSION TO PEOPLE AND ANIMALS
1. Often bullies, threatens, or intimidates others.
2. Often initiates physical fights.
3. Has used a weapon that can cause serious physical harm to others (e.g., a bat, brick, broken bottle, knife, gun).
4. Has been physically cruel to people.
5. Has been physically cruel to animals.
6. Has stolen while confronting a victim (e.g., mugging, purse snatching, extortion, armed robbery).
7. Has forced someone into sexual activity.

DESTRUCTION OF PROPERTY
8. Has deliberately engaged in fire setting with the intention of causing serious damage.
9. Has deliberately destroyed others' property (other than by fire setting).

DECEITFULNESS OR THEFT
10. Has broken into someone else's house, building, or car.
11. Often lies to obtain goods or favors or to avoid obligations (i.e., "cons" others).
12. Has stolen items of nontrivial value without confronting a victim (e.g., shoplifting, but without breaking and entering; forgery).

SERIOUS VIOLATIONS OF RULES
13. Often stays out at night despite parental prohibitions, beginning before age 13 years.
14. Has run away from home overnight at least twice while living in parental or parental surrogate home, or once without returning for a lengthy period.
15. Is often truant from school, beginning before age 13 years.

B. The disturbance in behavior causes clinically significant impairment in social, academic, or occupational functioning.

C. If the individual is age 18 years or older, criteria are not met for antisocial personality disorder.

Specify whether:

Childhood-Onset Type: Individuals show at least one symptom characteristic of conduct disorder before age 10 years.

Adolescent-Onset Type: Individuals show no symptom characteristic of conduct disorder before age 10 years.

Unspecified Onset: Criteria for a diagnosis of conduct disorder are met, but there is not enough information available to determine whether the onset of the first symptom was before or after age 10 years.

Specify if:

With limited prosocial emotions: To qualify for this specifier, an individual must have displayed at least two of the following characteristics persistently over at least 12 months and in multiple relationships and settings. These characteristics reflect the individual's typical pattern of interpersonal and emotional functioning over this period and not just occasional occurrences in some situations. Thus, to assess the criteria for the specifier, multiple information sources are necessary. In addition to the individual's self-report, it is necessary to consider reports by others who have known the individual for extended periods of time (e.g., parents, teachers, coworkers, extended family members, peers).

Lack of remorse or guilt: Does not feel bad or guilty when he or she does something wrong (exclude remorse when expressed only when caught and/or facing punishment). The individual shows a general lack of concern about the negative consequences of his or her actions. For example, the individual is not remorseful after hurting someone or does not care about the consequences of breaking rules.

Callous–lack of empathy: Disregards and is unconcerned about the feelings of others. The individual is described as cold and uncaring. The individual appears more concerned about the effects of his or her actions on himself or herself, rather than their effects on others, even when they result in substantial harm to others.

Unconcerned about performance: Does not show concern about poor/problematic performance at school, at work, or in other important activities. The individual does not put forth the effort necessary to perform well, even when expectations are clear, and typically blames others for his or her poor performance.

Shallow or deficient affect: Does not express feelings or show emotions to others, except in ways that seem shallow, insincere, or superficial (e.g., actions contradict the emotion displayed, can turn emotions "on" or "off" quickly) or when emotional expressions are used for gain (e.g., emotions displayed to manipulate or intimidate others).

Specify current severity:

Mild: Few if any conduct problems in excess of those required to make the diagnosis are present, and conduct problems cause relatively minor harm to others (e.g., lying, truancy, staying out after dark without permission, other rule breaking).

Moderate: The number of conduct problems and the effect on others are intermediate between those specified in "mild" and those in "severe" (e.g., stealing without confronting a victim, vandalism).

Severe: Many conduct problems in excess of those required to make the diagnosis are present, or conduct problems cause considerable harm to others (e.g., forced sex, physical cruelty, use of a weapon, stealing while confronting a victim, breaking and entering).

Table 32–8 | CARE PLAN FOR CHILD/ADOLESCENT WITH CONDUCT DISORDER

NURSING DIAGNOSIS: RISK FOR OTHER-DIRECTED VIOLENCE

RELATED TO: Characteristics of temperament, peer rejection, negative parental role models, dysfunctional family dynamics

OUTCOME CRITERIA	NURSING INTERVENTIONS	RATIONALE
Short-term goal ■ Patient discusses feelings of anger with nurse or therapist. **Long-term goal** ■ Patient does not harm others or others' property.	1. Observe the patient's behavior frequently through routine activities and interactions. Become aware of behaviors that indicate a rise in agitation.	1. Recognition of behaviors that precede the onset of aggression may provide the opportunity to intervene before violence occurs.
	2. Redirect violent behavior with physical outlets for suppressed anger and frustration.	2. Excess energy is released through physical activities, inducing a feeling of relaxation.
	3. Encourage the patient to express anger, and act as a role model for appropriate expression of anger. Explore the child's perceptions and feelings about contributing factors and triggers for anger and violent behavior.	3. Discussion of situations that create anger may lead to more effective ways of dealing with them.
	4. Ensure that a sufficient number of staff is available to indicate a show of strength if necessary.	4. This conveys evidence of control over the situation and provides physical security for staff and others.
	5. Administer tranquilizing medication, if ordered, or use mechanical restraints or isolation room only if situation cannot be controlled with less restrictive means.	5. It is the patient's right to expect the use of techniques that ensure safety of the patient and others by the least restrictive means.

NURSING DIAGNOSIS: IMPAIRED SOCIAL INTERACTION

RELATED TO: Negative parental role models; impaired peer relations leading to inappropriate social behavior

OUTCOME CRITERIA	NURSING INTERVENTIONS	RATIONALE
Short-term goal ■ Patient will interact in age-appropriate manner with nurse in one-to-one relationship within 1 week. **Long-term goal** ■ Patient is able to interact with staff and peers using age-appropriate, acceptable behaviors.	1. Develop a trusting relationship with the patient. Convey acceptance of the person separate from the unacceptable behavior.	1. Unconditional acceptance increases feelings of self-worth.
	2. Discuss with the patient which behaviors are and are not acceptable. Describe in a matter-of-fact manner the consequences of unacceptable behavior. Follow through.	2. Aversive reinforcement can alter undesirable behaviors.
	3. Provide group situations for the patient.	3. Appropriate social behavior is often learned from the positive and negative feedback of peers.

Continued

Table 32–8 | CARE PLAN FOR CHILD/ADOLESCENT WITH CONDUCT DISORDER—cont'd

NURSING DIAGNOSIS: DEFENSIVE COPING

RELATED TO: Low self-esteem and dysfunctional family system

OUTCOME CRITERIA	NURSING INTERVENTIONS	RATIONALE
Short-term goal ■ Patient verbalizes personal responsibility for difficulties experienced in interpersonal relationships within a time period reasonable for the patient. **Long-term goal** ■ Patient accepts responsibility for own behaviors and interacts with others without becoming defensive.	1. Explain to the patient the correlation between feelings of inadequacy and the need for acceptance from others and how these feelings provoke defensive behaviors, such as blaming others for own behaviors. 2. Provide immediate, matter-of-fact, nonthreatening feedback for unacceptable behaviors. 3. Help identify situations that provoke defensiveness, and practice through role-play more appropriate responses. 4. Provide immediate positive feedback for acceptable behaviors.	1. Recognition of the problem is the first step in the change process toward resolution. 2. The patient may not realize how these behaviors are being perceived by others. 3. Role-playing provides confidence to deal with difficult situations when they actually occur. 4. Positive feedback encourages repetition, and immediacy is significant for these children, who respond to immediate gratification.

NURSING DIAGNOSIS: LOW SELF-ESTEEM

RELATED TO: Lack of positive feedback and unsatisfactory parent/child relationship

OUTCOME CRITERIA	NURSING INTERVENTIONS	RATIONALE
Short-term goal ■ Patient participates in own self-care and discusses with nurse aspects of self about which they feel good. **Long-term goal** ■ Patient demonstrates increased feelings of self-worth by verbalizing positive statements about self and exhibiting fewer manipulative behaviors.	1. Ensure that goals are realistic. 2. Plan activities that provide opportunities for success. 3. Convey unconditional acceptance and positive regard. 4. Set limits on manipulative behavior. Take caution not to reinforce manipulative behaviors by providing desired attention. Identify the consequences of manipulation. Administer consequences matter-of-factly when manipulation occurs. 5. Help the patient understand that they use this behavior to try to increase own self-esteem. Interventions should reflect other actions to accomplish this goal.	1. Unrealistic goals set the patient up for failure, which diminishes self-esteem. 2. Success enhances self-esteem. 3. Communicating that the patient is a worthwhile human being helps to increase self-esteem. 4. Aversive consequences may work to decrease unacceptable behaviors. 5. When the patient feels better about self, the need to manipulate others will diminish.

anxiety is beyond that which would be expected for the individual's developmental level and interferes with social, academic, occupational, or other areas of functioning. Onset may occur at any time before age 18 years but is most commonly diagnosed around age 5 or 6, when the child goes to school. Diagnosis at this time may be related to the surfacing of symptoms when the child is faced with new stressors. Typically, school-teachers and counselors are the first to recognize anxiety and associated behavioral disturbances. Because there is also a high prevalence of separation anxiety disorders (43%) with onset after age 18, the *DSM-5-TR* removed the diagnostic criteria that specified this disorder as one that occurs only in children and adolescents. Prevalence estimates for the disorder average about 4%. Among clinical samples the disorder is equally common in boys and girls but in community samples the disorder is more frequent in girls (APA, 2022). It is more common in young children than in adolescents or adults (Boland & Verduin, 2022). Over 50% experience remission of symptoms within 10 years of onset, but there are several common comorbidities, including panic disorder, social anxiety disorders, specific phobias, depression, and bipolar disorders (Kimmel & Roy-Byrne, 2017).

Predisposing Factors

Biological Influences

Genetics: A greater number of children with relatives who manifest anxiety problems develop anxiety disorders than do children with no such family patterns. The results are significant enough to speculate that there is a hereditary influence in the development of separation anxiety disorder, but the mode of genetic transmission has not been determined. Boland and Verduin (2022) stated:

> Current consensus on the genetics of anxiety disorders suggests that what is inherited is a general predisposition toward anxiety, with resulting heightened levels of arousability, emotional reactivity, and increased negative affect, all of which increase the risk for the development of separation anxiety disorder [and other anxiety disorders]. (p. 201)

Temperament: It is well established that children differ in temperament starting at birth or shortly thereafter. Although the temperamental traits of behavioral inhibition, excessive shyness, and the tendency to withdraw from unfamiliar situations represent a genetic contribution to development of anxiety disorders later in life, "one third to two thirds of young children with behavioral inhibition do not develop anxiety disorders" (Boland & Verduin, p. 2022). So heritable temperament traits may influence the risk of anxiety disorders, but they are not predictive.

Environmental Influences

Stressful Life Events: Studies have shown a relationship between life events and the development of anxiety disorders. Significant change or loss often coincides with the development of the disorder (Boland & Verduin, 2022). Children of mothers who were stressed during pregnancy also appear to be at greater risk for developing separation anxiety disorder (Dryden-Edwards, 2022).

Family Influences

Various theories expound on the idea that anxiety disorders in children are related to an attachment issue with the mother. Three family influences that have demonstrated an increased risk for anxiety disorders in children include parental overprotection, insecure parent-child attachment, and maternal depression (Boland & Verduin, 2022).

Some parents may also transfer their fears and anxieties to their children through role-modeling. For example, a parent who becomes significantly fearful and apprehensive when confronted with unfamiliar circumstances, such as a job or residence change, teaches the child that this is an appropriate response.

Application of the Nursing Process to Separation Anxiety Disorder

Background Assessment Data (Symptomatology)

Onset of this disorder may occur as early as preschool age; it rarely begins as late as adolescence. In most cases, the child has difficulty separating from the mother. Occasionally, the separation reluctance is directed toward the father, siblings, or other significant individual to whom the child is attached. Anticipation of separation may result in tantrums, crying, screaming, complaints of physical problems, and **clinging** behaviors (overattachment and clinging to the primary caregiver accompanied by acute distress over the thought of or the actuality of separation).

Reluctance or refusal to attend school occurs in the majority of these children. Up to 80% of children with school refusal meet criteria for separation anxiety disorder (Dryden-Edwards, 2022). Younger children may "shadow" or follow the person from whom they are afraid to be separated. During middle childhood or adolescence, they may refuse to sleep away from home (e.g., at a friend's house or at camp). Interpersonal peer relationships are usually not a problem with these children. They are generally well liked by their peers and are reasonably socially skilled.

Worrying is common and relates to the possibility of harm to self or to the attachment figure. Younger children may even have nightmares to this effect. Specific phobias are not uncommon (e.g., fear of the dark, ghosts, animals). Depressed mood is frequently present and often precedes the onset of the anxiety symptoms, which commonly occur following a major stressor. The *DSM-5-TR* diagnostic criteria for separation anxiety disorder are presented in Box 32–5.

Nursing Diagnosis

Based on the data collected during the nursing assessment, possible nursing diagnoses for the patient with separation anxiety disorder include the following:

- Anxiety (severe) related to family history, temperament, overattachment to parent, negative role modeling
- Ineffective coping related to unresolved separation conflicts and inadequate coping skills evidenced by numerous somatic complaints
- Impaired social interaction related to reluctance to be away from attachment figure

Outcome Identification

Outcome criteria include short- and long-term goals. Timelines are individually determined. The following criteria may be used for measurement of outcomes in the care of the patient with separation anxiety disorder.

The patient:

- Is able to maintain anxiety at manageable level
- Demonstrates adaptive coping strategies for dealing with anxiety when separation from attachment figure is anticipated
- Interacts appropriately with others and spends time away from attachment figure to do so

Planning and Implementation

Table 32–9 provides a plan of care for the child or adolescent with separation anxiety, using nursing diagnoses common to this disorder, outcome criteria, and appropriate nursing interventions and rationales.

Evaluation

Evaluation of the child or adolescent with separation anxiety disorder requires reassessment of the behaviors for which the family sought treatment. Both the patient and the family members need to change their behavior. The following types of questions may provide assistance in gathering data required for evaluating whether the nursing interventions have been effective in achieving the goals of therapy.

BOX 32–5 Diagnostic Criteria for Separation Anxiety Disorder

A. Developmentally inappropriate and excessive fear or anxiety concerning separation from those to whom the individual is attached, as evidenced by at least three of the following:
   1. Recurrent excessive distress when anticipating or experiencing separation from home or major attachment figures.
   2. Persistent and excessive worry about losing major attachment figures or about possible harm to them, such as illness, injury, disasters, or death.
   3. Persistent and excessive worry about experiencing an untoward event (e.g., getting lost, being kidnapped, having an accident, becoming ill) that causes separation from a major attachment figure.
   4. Persistent reluctance or refusal to go out, away from home, to school, to work, or elsewhere because of fear of separation.
   5. Persistent and excessive fear of or reluctance about being alone or without major attachment figures at home or in other settings.
   6. Persistent reluctance or refusal to sleep away from home or to go to sleep without being near a major attachment figure.
   7. Repeated nightmares involving the theme of separation.
   8. Repeated complaints of physical symptoms (e.g., headaches, stomachaches, nausea, vomiting) when separation from major attachment figures occurs or is anticipated.

B. The fear, anxiety, or avoidance is persistent, lasting at least 4 weeks in children and adolescents and typically 6 months or more in adults.

C. The disturbance causes clinically significant distress or impairment in social, academic, occupational, or other important areas of functioning.

D. The disturbance is not better accounted for by another mental disorder, such as refusing to leave home because of excessive resistance to change in autism spectrum disorder, delusions or hallucinations concerning separation in psychotic disorders, refusal to go outside without a trusted companion in agoraphobia, worries about ill health or other harm befalling significant others in generalized anxiety disorder, or concerns about having an illness in illness anxiety disorder.

Table 32–9 | CARE PLAN FOR THE PATIENT WITH SEPARATION ANXIETY DISORDER

NURSING DIAGNOSIS: ANXIETY (SEVERE)

RELATED TO: Family history; temperament; overattachment to parent; negative role modeling

OUTCOME CRITERIA	NURSING INTERVENTIONS	RATIONALE
Short-term goal ■ Patient discusses fears of separation with trusted individual. Long-term goal ■ Patient maintains anxiety at no higher than moderate level in the face of events that formerly have precipitated panic.	1. Establish an atmosphere of calm, trust, and genuine positive regard.	1. Trust and unconditional acceptance are necessary for satisfactory nurse-patient relationship. Calmness is important because anxiety is easily transmitted from one person to another.
	2. Assure the patient of their safety and security.	2. Symptoms of panic anxiety are very frightening.
	3. Explore child's or adolescent's fears of separating from the parents. Explore with parents possible fears they may have of separation from child.	3. Some parents may have an underlying fear of separation from the child of which they are unaware and which they are unconsciously transferring to child.
	4. Help parents and child initiate realistic goals (e.g., child to stay with sitter for 2 hours with minimal anxiety; or child to stay at friend's house without parents until 9 p.m. without experiencing panic anxiety).	4. Parents may be so frustrated with child's clinging and demanding behaviors that assistance with problem-solving may be required.
	5. Give, and encourage parents to give, positive reinforcement for desired behaviors.	5. Positive reinforcement encourages repetition of desirable behaviors.

NURSING DIAGNOSIS: INEFFECTIVE COPING

RELATED TO: Unresolved separation conflicts and inadequate coping skills

EVIDENCED BY: Numerous somatic complaints

OUTCOME CRITERIA	NURSING INTERVENTIONS	RATIONALE
Short-term goal ■ Patient verbalizes correlation of somatic symptoms to fear of separation. Long-term goal ■ Patient demonstrates use of more adaptive coping strategies (rather than physical symptoms) in response to stressful situations.	1. Encourage the child or adolescent to discuss specific situations in life that produce the most distress and describe their response to these situations. Include parents in the discussion.	1. The patient and family may be unaware of the correlation between stressful situations and the exacerbation of physical symptoms.
	2. Help the child or adolescent who is perfectionistic to recognize that self-expectations may be unrealistic. Connect times of unmet self-expectations to the exacerbation of physical symptoms.	2. Recognition of maladaptive patterns is the first step in the change process.

Continued

Table 32–9 | CARE PLAN FOR THE PATIENT WITH SEPARATION ANXIETY DISORDER–cont'd

OUTCOME CRITERIA	NURSING INTERVENTIONS	RATIONALE
	3. Encourage parents and child to identify more adaptive coping strategies that the child could use in the face of anxiety that feels overwhelming. Practice through role-play.	3. Practice facilitates the use of the desired behavior when the individual is actually faced with the stressful situation.

NURSING DIAGNOSIS: IMPAIRED SOCIAL INTERACTION

RELATED TO: Reluctance to be away from attachment figure

OUTCOME CRITERIA	NURSING INTERVENTIONS	RATIONALE
Short-term goal ■ Patient spends time with staff or other support person, without presence of attachment figure, without excessive anxiety. Long-term goal ■ Patient is able to spend time with others (without presence of attachment figure) without excessive anxiety.	1. Develop a trusting relationship with the patient.	1. This is the first step in helping the patient learn to interact with others.
	2. Attend groups with the child and support efforts to interact with others. Give positive feedback.	2. Presence of a trusted individual provides security during times of distress. Positive feedback encourages repetition.
	3. Convey to the child the acceptability of their not participating in group in the beginning. Gradually encourage small contributions until the patient is able to participate more fully.	3. Small successes will gradually increase self-confidence and decrease self-consciousness, so that the patient will feel less anxious in the group situation.
	4. Help the patient set small personal goals (e.g., "Today I will speak to one person I don't know").	4. Simple, realistic goals provide opportunities for success that increase self-confidence and may encourage the patient to attempt more difficult objectives in the future.

Has the patient:

■ Been able to maintain anxiety at a manageable level (i.e., without temper tantrums, screaming, or clinging)?
■ Had fewer complaints of physical symptoms?
■ Demonstrated the ability to cope in more adaptive ways in the face of escalating anxiety?
■ (Parents) Identified more adaptive coping strategies?
■ Verbalized an intention to return to school?
■ Been able to sleep without nightmares?
■ Been able to interact with others away from the attachment figure?

General Therapeutic Approaches

Treatment for neurodevelopmental disorders, disruptive behavior disorders, and anxiety disorders poses many challenges and requires a comprehensive treatment plan that may include individual, group, and family therapies; family education; pharmacotherapy; and psychotherapeutic interventions specifically designed for the unique clinical issues presented in each disorder. The following general therapeutic approaches are described.

Behavior Therapy

Behavior therapy is based on the concepts of classical conditioning and operant conditioning and is a common and effective treatment with disruptive behavior disorders such as ADHD, ODD, and conduct disorder. With this approach, rewards are given for appropriate behaviors and withheld when behaviors are disruptive or otherwise inappropriate. The principle behind behavior therapy is that positive reinforcements encourage repetition of desirable behaviors and aversive reinforcements (punishments) discourage repetition of undesirable behaviors. Behavior modification techniques—the system of rewards and consequences—can be taught to parents to be used in the home environment. Consistency is an essential component. In the treatment setting, individualized behavior modification programs are designed for each client.

As mentioned previously, ABA is a type of behavior therapy that is considered the gold standard treatment for children with autism (although it is used to treat other conditions, too). It begins with a thorough consultation and assessment by an ABA-trained therapist and culminates in the development of a specific, individualized, behavioral treatment plan to teach social and communication skills and reduce problem behaviors such as tantrums or self-injury. ABA relies on caregiver training to ensure that parents and other caregivers are reinforcing the treatment plan outside of the formal therapy setting (Raypole, 2021).

Family Therapy

Therapy for children and adolescents must involve the entire family if treatment is to be successful. Parents should be involved in designing and implementing the treatment plan for the child and all other aspects of the treatment process.

The genogram can be used to identify problem areas between family members. It provides an overall picture of the family over several generations, including roles that various family members play and emotional distance between specific individuals. Areas for change can be easily identified.

The effect of family dynamics on disruptive behavior disorders has been identified. Family coping can become severely compromised by the chronic stress of dealing with a child with a behavior disorder. It is therefore imperative that the treatment plan for the identified client be instituted within the context of family-centered care.

Group Therapy

Group therapy provides children and adolescents with the opportunity to interact within an association of their peers. This experience can be both gratifying and overwhelming, depending on the child.

Group therapy provides several benefits. Appropriate social behavior often is learned from the positive and negative feedback of peers. Group members learn to tolerate and accept differences in others, discover that it is acceptable to disagree, offer and receive support from others, and practice these new skills in a safe environment. Group therapy is also a way to learn from the experiences of others.

Group therapy with children and adolescents can take several forms. Music therapy groups provide the opportunity to express feelings through music; some children may be unable to express themselves in any other way. Art and activity/craft therapy groups allow individual expression through artistic means.

Group play therapy is the treatment of choice for many children between 3 and 9 years, and evidence supports its effectiveness for many different childhood problems. The Association for Play Therapy (n.d.) defined play therapy as:

> "the systematic use of a theoretical model to establish an interpersonal process wherein trained play therapists use the therapeutic powers of play to help clients prevent or resolve psychosocial difficulties and achieve optimal growth and development."

Child play therapy is a way of being with the child that honors their unique developmental level and looks for ways of helping in the "language" of the child—play. Licensed mental health professionals therapeutically use play to help their clients better express themselves and resolve their problems.

Psychoeducational groups are very beneficial for adolescents. The only drawback to this type of group is that it works best when the group is closed-ended; that is, once the group has been formed, no one is allowed to join until the group has reached its preestablished closure. Members are allowed to propose topics for discussion. The leader serves as teacher much of the time and facilitates discussion of the proposed topic. Members may, from time to time, be presenters and serve as discussion leaders. Sometimes, psychoeducation groups evolve into traditional therapy discussion groups.

Cognitive behavior therapy (CBT) has demonstrated benefit in the treatment of tic disorders (Tourette's); separation anxiety disorder; and disruptive behavior disorders including ADHD, ODD, and OCD. It has also been identified as beneficial for higher functioning patients with ASD to treat secondary issues such as depression, anger, anxiety, and social skills deficits (Grossman, 2021).

Psychopharmacology

Several of the disorders presented in this chapter are treated with medications. The appropriate pharmacology was presented in the section in which the disorder was discussed. Medication should not be the sole method of treatment. Although medication can improve quality of life for families of children and adolescents with these disorders, research has indicated that medication alone is not as effective as a combination of medication and psychosocial therapy. It is important for families to understand that there is no way to "give him a pill and make him well." The importance of psychosocial therapies in the treatment process cannot be overstressed. Some clinicians will not prescribe medications for child and adolescent patients unless they also participate in concomitant psychotherapy sessions.

Summary and Key Points

- Intellectual developmental disorder (intellectual disability) is defined by the presence of deficits in general intellectual functioning and adaptive functioning.
- Four levels of intellectual developmental disorder—mild, moderate, severe, and profound—are associated with various behavioral manifestations and abilities.
- Autism spectrum disorder (ASD) includes a wide range of symptoms and levels of severity that affect thinking, feeling, communication, and social relationships. Behavior is often limited and repetitive, but each child is likely to have a unique pattern of behavior and level of severity from low to high functioning.
- It is generally accepted that ASD is caused by abnormalities in brain structures or functions. Genetic factors are also thought to play a significant role in ASD.
- Children with ADHD may exhibit symptoms of inattention, hyperactivity/impulsivity, or a combination of the two.

- Genetics plays a role in the etiology of ADHD. Neurotransmitters that have been implicated include dopamine, norepinephrine, and serotonin. Exposure to tobacco smoke, maternal smoking, and alcohol use during pregnancy have been linked to hyperactive behavior in offspring.
- Central nervous system stimulants, alpha-adrenergic agonists, atomoxetine, bupropion, and viloxazine are commonly used to treat ADHD.
- The essential feature of Tourette's disorder is the presence of multiple motor tics and one or more vocal tics.
- Common medications used with Tourette's disorder include antipsychotics such as haloperidol, pimozide, and others (off-label). Alpha-adrenergic agents clonidine and guanfacine are also approved by the FDA approved for treatment of this disorder.
- Deep brain stimulation has demonstrated success in reducing the intensity of tics for some patients. It is only used in patients that have failed to respond to other, less invasive treatments.
- Oppositional defiant disorder (ODD) is characterized by a pattern of negativistic, defiant, disobedient, and hostile behavior toward authority figures that occurs more frequently than is usually observed in individuals of comparable age and developmental level.
- Conduct disorder is characterized by a repetitive and persistent pattern of behavior in which the basic rights of others or major age-appropriate societal norms or rules are violated.
- The essential feature of separation anxiety disorder is excessive anxiety concerning separation from the home or from those to whom the person is attached.
- Children with separation anxiety disorder may have temperamental characteristics present at birth that predispose them to the disorder.
- General therapeutic approaches for child and adolescent psychiatric disorders include behavior therapy, family therapy, group therapies (including music, art, crafts, play, and psychoeducation groups), and psychopharmacology.

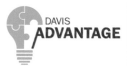

Go to **Davis Advantage** to complete your learning: strengthen understanding, apply your knowledge, and prepare for the Next Gen NCLEX®.

Review Questions

1. Which of the following groups is most commonly used for drug management of the child with ADHD?
   a. CNS depressants (e.g., diazepam [Valium])
   b. CNS stimulants (e.g., methylphenidate [Ritalin])
   c. Anticonvulsants (e.g., phenytoin [Dilantin])
   d. Major tranquilizers (e.g., haloperidol [Haldol])

2. The nursing history and assessment of an adolescent with conduct disorder might reveal all of the following behaviors *except:*
   a. Manipulation of others for fulfillment of own desires.
   b. Chronic violation of rules.
   c. Feelings of guilt associated with the exploitation of others.
   d. Inability to form close peer relationships.

3. Certain family dynamics often predispose adolescents to the development of conduct disorder. Which of the following patterns is thought to be a contributing factor?
   a. Parents who are overprotective
   b. Parents who have high expectations for their children
   c. Parents who consistently set limits on their children's behavior
   d. Parents who are alcohol dependent

4. Which of the following is *least* likely to predispose a child to Tourette's disorder?
   a. Absence of parental bonding
   b. Family history of the disorder
   c. Abnormalities of brain neurotransmitters
   d. Structural abnormalities of the brain

5. Which of the following medications is used to treat Tourette's disorder?
   a. Methylphenidate (Ritalin)
   b. Haloperidol (Haldol)
   c. Imipramine (Tofranil)
   d. Phenytoin (Dilantin)

Clinical Judgment Questions

6. The child with ADHD has a nursing diagnosis of impaired social interaction. Which of the following nursing interventions are appropriate for this child? (Select all that apply.)
   a. Socially isolate the child when interactions with others are inappropriate.
   b. Set limits with consequences on inappropriate behaviors.
   c. Provide rewards for appropriate behaviors.
   d. Provide group situations for the child.

7. To help the child with mild to moderate intellectual developmental disorder develop satisfying relationships with others, which of the following nursing interventions is most appropriate?
   a. Interpret the child's behavior for others.
   b. Set limits on behavior that is socially inappropriate.
   c. Allow the child to behave spontaneously because they have no concept of right or wrong.
   d. This child is not capable of forming social relationships.

8. The child with ASD often has difficulty with trust. With this in mind, which of the following nursing actions would be most appropriate?
   a. Encourage all staff to hold the child as often as possible, conveying trust through touch.
   b. Assign a different staff member each day so the child will learn that everyone can be trusted.
   c. Assign the same staff person as often as possible to promote feelings of security and trust.
   d. Avoid eye contact because it is extremely uncomfortable for the child and may even discourage trust.

9. Which of the following nursing diagnoses would be considered the priority in planning care for the child with severe ASD?
   a. Risk for self-mutilation evidenced by banging head against wall
   b. Impaired social interaction evidenced by unresponsiveness to people
   c. Impaired verbal communication evidenced by absence of verbal expression
   d. Disturbed personal identity evidenced by inability to differentiate self from others

10. A client with ODD has been admitted to a residential treatment setting and tells the nurse, "I don't want to be here and you're not in charge of me." Which intervention by the nurse is a priority?
   a. Instruct the client that they will have to follow the rules, or they will be put in seclusion.
   b. Provide information about the structured activities and behavioral expectations in the treatment program.
   c. Give positive feedback to the client for their assertive communication.
   d. Ask the patient whether they would rather go to jail.

IMPLICATIONS OF RESEARCH FOR EVIDENCE-BASED PRACTICE

Lavallee, K., Schuck, K., Blatter-Meunier, J., & Schneider, S. (2019). Transgenerational improvements following child anxiety treatment: An exploratory examination. *PLOS ONE, 14*(2), Article e0212667. https://doi.org/10.1371/journal.pone.021266

DESCRIPTION OF THE STUDY: This study was a secondary analysis of a randomized controlled trial to examine the transgenerational relationship between CBT for child separation anxiety disorder and the mental health of parents. One hundred and seven children ages 4 to 14 years with separation anxiety disorder received one of two CBT programs. Their parents (N = 189; 101 mothers and 88 fathers) were assessed at baseline and post-treatment for symptoms of separation anxiety, general anxiety, and depression. A comparison group of parents (N = 74; 42 mothers and 32 fathers) of 45 children without separation anxiety disorder, who did not receive any treatment, were also assessed.

RESULTS OF THE STUDY: Maternal symptoms of depression and separation anxiety improved in the child treatment group compared with mothers of healthy children. There was no significant improvement in parental pathology levels among fathers of children treated for separation anxiety disorder.

IMPLICATIONS FOR NURSING PRACTICE: This study has implications for nurses who work with children that have separation anxiety disorder. Providing care and intervention for a child always involves working with parents. This study expands the focus of treatment to understanding the benefits not just for the child but also for evaluating the anxiety and depression in parents as well. Although the authors acknowledge that more research is needed to better understand the mechanisms, nurses can educate parents about research findings such as these to promote confidence in the treatment process.

TEST YOUR CLINICAL REASONING AND CLINICAL JUDGMENT SKILLS

Jimmy, age 9, has been admitted to the child psychiatric unit with a diagnosis of attention deficit-hyperactivity disorder. He has been unmanageable at school and at home and has had several suspensions from school for continuous disruption of his class. He refuses to sit in his chair or do his work. He yells out in class, interrupts the teacher and the other students, and lately has become physically aggressive when he cannot have his way. Most recently, he was suspended after hitting his teacher when she asked him to return to his seat.

Jimmy's mother describes him as a restless and demanding baby who grew into a restless and demanding toddler. He has never gotten along well with his peers. Even as a small child, he would take his friends' toys away from them or bite them if they tried to hold their own with him. His 5-year-old sister is afraid of him and refuses to be alone with him.

During the nurse's intake assessment, Jimmy paced the room or rocked in his chair. He talked incessantly on a superficial level and jumped from topic to topic. He told the nurse that he did not know why he was there. He acknowledged that he had some problems at school but said that it was only because the other kids picked on him and the teacher did not like him. He said he got into trouble at home sometimes but that it was because his parents liked his little sister better than they liked him.

The physician has ordered methylphenidate 5 mg twice a day for Jimmy. His response to this order is, "I'm not going to take drugs. I'm not sick!"

Answer the following questions related to Jimmy:

1. What are the pertinent assessment data to be noted by the nurse?
2. What is the primary nursing diagnosis for Jimmy?
3. Aside from patient safety, to what problems would the nurse want to direct intervention with Jimmy?

MOVIE CONNECTIONS

Bill (intellectual disability) • *Bill, On His Own* (intellectual disability) • *Sling Blade* (intellectual disability) • *Forrest Gump* (intellectual disability) • *Rain Man* (autism spectrum disorder [ASD]) • *Mercury Rising* (ASD) • *Niagara, Niagara* (Tourette's disorder) • *Toughlove* (conduct disorder)

References

Acosta, M. T., Swanson, J., Stehli, A., Molina, B., Martinez, A. F., the MTA team, Arcos-Burgos, M., & Muenke, M. (2016). ADGRL3 (LPHN3) variants are associated with a refined phenotype of ADHD in the MTA study. *Molecular Genetics and Genomic Medicine, 4*(5), 540–547. doi:10.1002/mgg3.230

ADHD Institute. (2021). *Socioeconomic risk factors for ADHD.* https://adhd-institute.com/burden-of-adhd/aetiology/

American Psychiatric Association (APA). (2000). *Diagnostic and statistical manual of mental disorders* (4th ed., text rev.). American Psychiatric Publishing.

American Psychiatric Association (APA). (2022). *Diagnostic and statistical manual of mental disorders, fifth edition, text revision (DSM-5-TR).* American Psychiatric Association.

Association for Play Therapy. (n.d.). *Play therapy makes a difference.* www.a4pt.org/?page=PTMakesADifference

Bernstein, B. E. (2022). *Conduct disorder.* http://emedicine.medscape.com/article/918213-overview#a3

Bhatia, R. (2022). Autism spectrum disorder: Keys to early detection and accurate diagnosis. *Current Psychiatry, 21*(3), 10–20. doi:10.12788/cp.0146

Boland, R., & Verduin, M. L. (2022). *Kaplan & Sadock's synopsis of psychiatry* (P. Ruiz, Ed.). (12th ed.). Wolters Kluwer

Bosl, W. J., Tager-Flusberg, H., & Nelson, C. A. (2018). EEG analytics for early detection of autism spectrum disorder: A data-driven approach. *Scientific Reports, 8*(1), 6828. doi:10.1038/s41598-018-24318-x. PMID: 29717196; PMCID: PMC5931530

Centers for Disease Control and Prevention (CDC). (2020). *Tourette syndrome: Risk factors and causes.* www.cdc.gov/ncbddd/tourette/riskfactors.html

Centers for Disease Control and Prevention (CDC). (2021). *FastStats: Attention deficit hyperactivity disorder (ADHD).* www.cdc.gov/nchs/fastats/adhd.htm

Centers for Disease Control and Prevention (CDC). (2022). *Autism spectrum disorders. Autism and developmental disabilities monitoring network.* http://www.cdc.gov/ncbddd/autism/addm.html

Connor, D. (2017). Disruptive behavior disorders in children and adolescents. In Sadock, B. J., Sadock, V. A., & Ruiz, P. (Eds.), *Comprehensive textbook of psychiatry* (10th ed., pp. 3605–3621). Wolters Kluwer.

DeBoth, K. K., & Reynolds, S. (2017). A systematic review of sensory-based autism subtypes. *Research in Autism Spectrum Disorders, 36,* 44–56. https://doi.org/10.1016/j.rasd.2017.01.005

Dryden-Edwards, R. (2022). *Separation anxiety disorder.* www.medicinenet.com/separation_anxiety/page4.htm

Fallah, M. S., Shaikh, M. R., Neupane, B., Rusiecki, D., Bennett, T. A., & Beyene, J. (2019). Atypical antipsychotics for irritability in pediatric autism: A systematic review and network meta-analysis. *Journal of Child and Adolescent Psychopharmacology, 29*(3), 168–180. http://doi.org/10.1089/cap.2018.0115

Food and Drug Administration (FDA). (2020). *FDA permits marketing of first game-based digital therapeutic to improve attention function in children with ADHD.* https://www.fda.gov/news-events/press-announcements/fda-permits-marketing-first-game-based-digital-therapeutic-improve-attention-function-children-adhd

Gabis, L. V., Ben-Hur, R., Shefer, S., Jokel, A., & Shalom, D. B. (2019). Improvement of language in children with autism with combined donepezil and choline treatment. *Journal of Molecular Neuroscience, 69*(2), 224–234. https://doi.org/10.1007/s12031-019-01351-7

Gilman, S. R., Chang, J., Xu, B., Bawa, T. S., Gogos, J. A., Karayiorgou, M., & Vitkup, D. (2012). Diverse types of genetic variation converge on functional gene networks involved in schizophrenia. *Nature Neuroscience, 15*(12), 1723–1728. doi:10.1038/nn.3261

Greenhill, L. (2022). Advances in treatment for ADHD. *Psychiatric Times, 39*(1). https://www.psychiatrictimes.com/view/advances-in-treatments-for-adhd

Griffin, M., & Harari, E. (2019). Research sheds light on two types of treatment for ADHD. *Psychiatric Times, 36*(7). https://www.psychiatrictimes.com/adhd/research-sheds-light-two-types-treatment-adhd

Grossman, H. (2021). *CBT shows promise for anxious youth with autism spectrum disorders.* https://beckinstitute.org/blog/cbt-shows-promise-for-anxious-youth-with-autism-spectrum-disorders/

Harrop, C., McConachie, H., Emsly, R., Leadbitter, K., Green, J., & the PACT Consortium. (2014). Restricted and repetitive behaviors in autism spectrum disorders and typical development: Cross-sectional and longitudinal comparisons. *Journal of Autism and Developmental Disorders, 44*(5), 1207–1219. doi:10.1007/s10803-13-1986-5

Humphreys, K. L., Watts, E. L., Dennis, E. L., King, L. S., Thompson, P. M., & Gotlib, I. H. (2018). Stressful life events, ADHD symptoms, and brain structure in early adolescence. *Journal of Abnormal Child Psychology.* doi:10.1007/s10802-018-0443-5

Jain, R. (2022). Cases and concepts in ADHD: Could you manage these patients? [supplement]. *Current Psychiatry, 21*(1), 3–12.

James, B. J., Gales, M. A., & Gales, B. J. (2019). Bumetanide for autism spectrum disorder in children: A review of randomized controlled trials. *Annals of Pharmacotherapy, 53*(5), 537–544.

Kendler, K. S., Aggen, S. H., & Patrick, C. J. (2013). Familial influences on conduct disorder reflect 2 genetic factors and 1 shared environmental factor. *JAMA Psychiatry, 70*(1), 78–86. Doi:10.1001/jamapsychiatry.2013.267

Kim, J. H., Kim, J. Y., Lee, J., Jeong, G. H., Lee, E., Lee, S., Lee, K. H., Kronbichler, A., Stubbs, B., Solmi, M., Koyanagi, A., Hong, S. H., Dragioti, E., Jacob, L., Brunoni, A. R., Carvalho, A. F., Radua, J., Thompson, T., Smith, L., Oh, H.... Fusar-Poli P. (2020). Environmental risk factors, protective factors, and peripheral biomarkers for ADHD: An umbrella review. *Lancet Psychiatry, 7*(11), 955–970. doi:10.1016/S2215-0366(20)30312-6. PMID: 33069318

Kimmel, R. J., & Roy-Byrne, P. (2017). Clinical features of anxiety disorders. In Sadock, B. J., Sadock, V. A., & Ruiz, P. (Eds.), *Comprehensive textbook of psychiatry* (10th ed., pp. 1723–1730). Wolters Kluwer.

Kothadia, R. J., Krause, M., & Saeed, S. A. (2021). Pharmacologic management of autism spectrum disorder: A review of 7 studies. *Current Psychiatry, 20*(1), 33–38.

Kranjac, D. (2016). *In vitro modeling of early brain overgrowth in autism.* www.psychiatryadvisor.com/neurodevelopmental-disorder/modeling-early-brain-overgrowth-in-autism/article/508852/

Kushima, I., Aleksic, B., Nakatochi, M., Shimamura, T., Okada,T., Uno, Y., Morikawa, M., Ishizuka, K., Shiino, T., Kimura, H., Arioka, Y., Yoshimi, A., Takasaki, Y., Yu, Y., Nakamura, Y., Yamamoto, M., Iidaka, T., Iritani, S., Inada, T., Ogawa, N., Shishido, E., Torii, Y., Kawano, N., Omura, Y., Yoshikawa, T., Uchiyama, T., Yamamoto, T., Ikeda, M., Hashimoto, R., Yamamori, H., Yasuda, Y., Someya, T., Watanabe, Y., Egawa, J., Nunokawa, A., Itokawa, M.,...Ozaki, N. (2018). Comparative analyses of copy-number variation in autism spectrum disorder and schizophrenia reveal etiological overlap and biological insights. *Cell Reports 24*, 2838–2856. https://doi.org/10.1016/j.celrep.2018.08.022

Lavallee, K., Schuck, K., Blatter-Meunier, J., & Schneider, S. (2019). Transgenerational improvements following child anxiety treatment: An exploratory examination. *PLOS ONE, 14*(2), Article e0212667. https://doi.org/10.1371/journal.pone.021266

Lei, J., & Ventola, P. (2017). Pivotal response treatment for autism spectrum disorder: Current perspectives. *Neuropsychiatric Disease and Treatment, 13,* 1613–1626. https://doi.org/10.2147/NDT.S120710

Lubit, R. H. (2022). *Oppositional defiant disorder.* http://emedicine.medscape.com/article/918095-overview#a4

Mayo Clinic. (2022a). *Autism spectrum disorder.* https://www.mayoclinic.org/diseases-conditions/autism-spectrum-disorder/symptoms-causes/syc-20352928

Mayo Clinic. (2022b). *Oppositional defiant disorder.* www.mayoclinic.org/diseases-conditions/oppositional-defiant-disorder/basics/risk-factors/con-20024559

Mazahery, H., Conlon, C. A., Beck, K. L., Mugridge, O., Kruger, M. C., Stonehouse, W., Camargo, C. A. Jr., Meyer, B. J., Jones, B., & von Hurst, P. R. (2019). A randomised controlled trial of vitamin D and omega-3 long chain polyunsaturated fatty acids in the treatment of irritability and hyperactivity among children with autism spectrum disorder. *Journal of Steroid Biochemistry and Molecular Biology, 187,* 9–16. https://doi.org/10.1016/j.jsbmb.2018.10.017

McGough, J. J. (2017). Adult manifestations of attention-deficit hyperactivity disorder. In Sadock, B. J., Sadock, V. A., & Ruiz, P. (Eds.), *Comprehensive textbook of psychiatry* (10th ed., pp. 3598–3604). Wolters Kluwer.

National Institutes of Health (NIH). (2021). *Tourette's syndrome information page.* https://www.ninds.nih.gov/Disorders/All-Disorders/Tourette-Syndrome-Information-Page

Raypole, C. (2021). *Is applied behavioral analysis (ABA) right for your child?* https://www.healthline.com/health/aba-therapy

Rossignol, D. A., & Frye, R. E. (2016). *Environmental toxicants and autism spectrum disorder.* https://www.psychiatrictimes.com/view/environmental-toxicants-and-autism-spectrum-disorder

Schiweck, C., Arteaga-Henriquez, G., Aichholzer, M., Thanarajah, S. E., Vargas-Cáceres, S., Matura, S., Grimm, O., Haavik, J., Kittel-Schneider, S., Ramos-Quiroga, J. A., Faraone, S. V., Reif, A. (2021). Comorbidity of ADHD and adult bipolar disorder: A systematic review and meta-analysis. *Neuroscience and Biobehavioral Reviews, 124,* 100–123. doi:10.1016/j.neubiorev.2021.01.017

Strunz, S., Westphal, L., Ritter, K., Heuser, I., Dziobek, I., & Roepke, S. (2015). Personality pathology of adults with autism spectrum disorder without accompanying intellectual impairment in comparison to adults with personality disorders. *Journal of Autism and Developmental Disorders, 45,* 4026–4038. doi:10.1007/s10803-14-2183-x

Tourette's Association of America. (n.d.). *What is Tourette.* https://tourette.org/about-tourette/overview/what-is-tourette/

Tumolo, J. (2020). FDA clears video game as treatment for ADHD. *Psych Congress Network.* https://www.hmpgloballearningnetwork.com/site/pcn/article/fda-clears-video-game-treatment-adhd?key=FDA+clears+video+game+as+treatment+for+ADHD&elastic%5B0%5D=learning_network%3APsychiatry+%26+Behavioral+Health

Van Den Ban, E., Souverein, P., Meijer, W., Van Engeland, H., Swaab, H., Egber, T., & Heerdinle, E. (2014). Association between ADHD drug use and injuries among children and adolescents. *European Child and Adolescent Psychiatry, 23,* 95–102. doi:10.1007/s00787-013-0432-8

Volkmar, F. R., Klin, A., Schultz, R. T., & State, M. W. (2017). Autism spectrum and social communication disorder. In Sadock, B. J., Sadock, V. A., & Ruiz, P. (Eds.), *Comprehensive textbook of psychiatry* (10th ed., pp. 3571–3586). Wolters Kluwer.

Warrier, V., Greenberg, D. M., Weir, E., Buckingham, C., Smith, P., Lai, M. C., Allison, C., & Baron-Cohen, S. (2020). Elevated rates of autism, other neurodevelopmental and psychiatric diagnoses, and autistic traits in transgender and gender-diverse individuals. *Nature Communications, 11*(1), 1–12. https://doi.org/10.1038/s41467-020-17794-1

Weisman, H., Qureshi, I. A., Leckman, J. F., Scahill, L., & Bloch, M. H. (2013). Systematic review: Pharmacological treatment of tic disorders—efficacy of antipsychotic and alpha-2 adrenergic agonist agents. *Neuroscience and Biobehavioral Reviews, 37*(6), 1162–1171. doi:10.1016/j.neubiorev.2012.09.008

Xu, W., Zhang, C., Deeb, W., Patel, B., Wu, Y., Voon, V., Oku, M. S., & Sun, B. (2020). Deep brain stimulation for Tourette's syndrome. *Translational Neurodegeneration 9* (4). https://doi.org/10.1186/s40035-020-0183-7

The Aging Individual

CHAPTER OUTLINE

Objectives

How Old Is *Old*?

Epidemiology

Theories of Aging

The Normal Aging Process

Special Concerns of the Elderly Population

Application of the Nursing Process

Summary and Key Points

Review Questions

Clinical Judgment Questions

Implications of Research for Evidence-Based Practice

Test Your Clinical Reasoning and Clinical Judgment Skills

Movie Connections

CORE CONCEPTS

Health Promotion

Grief and Loss

Professionalism: Nursing process in the care of older adults

Clinical Judgment

KEY TERMS

attachment

bereavement overload

conscientiousness

disengagement theory

elder abuse

geriatrics

gerontology

geropsychiatry

long-term memory

Medicaid

Medicare

reminiscence therapy

short-term memory

transcendence

OBJECTIVES

After reading this chapter, the student will be able to:

1. Discuss societal perspectives on aging.
2. Describe an epidemiological profile of aging in the United States.
3. Explain the various theories of aging.
4. Describe biological, psychological, sociocultural, and sexual aspects of the normal aging process.
5. Discuss retirement as a special concern to the aging individual.
6. Explain personal and sociological perspectives of long-term care of the aging individual.
7. Describe the problem of elder abuse as it exists in today's society.
8. Discuss the implications of the increasing number of suicides among the elderly population.
9. Apply the steps of the nursing process to the care of aging individuals.

What is it like to grow old? It is not likely that many people in American culture would state that it is something they want to do. Most would agree, however, that it is "better than the alternative."

Supreme Court Justice Oliver Wendell Holmes, Jr., who retired at the age of 91, is quoted as saying, "Old is fifteen years older than I am." Obviously, being old is relative to the individual experiencing it and as the population of older adults continues to grow, our norms about aging will no doubt be reconceptualized. Growing old has not historically been desirable among the youth-oriented American culture. However, with 66 million baby boomers reaching their 65th birthdays by the year 2030, greater emphasis is being placed on the needs of an aging population. The disciplines of **gerontology** (the study of the aging process), **geriatrics** (the branch of clinical medicine specializing in problems of the older adult), and **geropsychiatry** (the branch of clinical medicine focused on psychiatric disorders in older adults) are expanding rapidly in response to this demand.

Growing old in a society that has been obsessed with youth may have a critical effect on the mental health of many people. This situation has serious implications for psychiatric nursing.

What is it like to grow old? More and more people will be able to answer this question as the 21st century progresses. Perhaps they will also be asking the question that Roberts (1991) asked: "How did I get here so fast?"

This chapter focuses on physical and psychological changes associated with the aging process, as well as special concerns of the older adult population, such as retirement, long-term care, elder abuse, and high suicide rates. The nursing process is presented as the vehicle for delivery of nursing care to older adults.

How Old Is *Old?*

The concept of "old" has changed drastically over the years. Our prehistoric ancestors probably had a life span of 40 years, with the average individual living around 18 years. As civilization developed, mortality rates remained high as a result of periodic famine and frequent malnutrition. An improvement in the standard of living was not truly evident until about the middle of the 17th century. Since that time, assured food supply, changes in food production, better housing conditions, and more progressive medical and sanitation facilities have contributed to population growth, declining mortality rates, and substantial increases in longevity.

In 1900 the average life expectancy in the United States was 47 years, and only 4% of the population was age 65 or older. According to the National Center for Health Statistics (NCHS) (2022) the current average life expectancy is 77 years (as of 2020). This represents a decrease of 1.8 years from the previous year (NCHS, 2022).

The U.S. Census Bureau has created a system for classification of older Americans:

- Older: 55 through 64 years
- Elderly: 65 through 74 years
- Aged: 75 through 84 years
- Very old: 85 years and older

Some gerontologists have elected to use a simpler classification system:

- Young old: 60 through 74 years
- Middle old: 75 through 84 years
- Old old: 85 years and older

So how old is *old?* Obviously, the term cannot be defined by a number. Myths and stereotypes of aging have long obscured our understanding of the aged and the process of aging. Ideas that all older individuals are sick, depressed, obsessed with death, senile, and incapable of change affect the way older adults are treated. They even shape the pattern of aging for people who believe them by becoming self-fulfilling prophecies—people start to believe they should behave in certain ways and therefore act according to those beliefs. Generalized assumptions can be demeaning and can interfere with the quality of life for older individuals.

Just as there are many differences in individual adaptation at earlier stages of development, so it is in the elderly population. Erikson (1963) has suggested that the mentally healthy older person possesses a sense of ego integrity and self-acceptance that will help in adapting to the ambiguities of the future with a sense of security and optimism.

The World Health Organization (WHO; 2017) reported that over 20% of adults over 60 have a mental or neurological disorder and that the keys to mental health in older adulthood are resources to meet their needs, including security and freedom, adequate housing, social support, programs to prevent elder abuse, availability of health and social programs for vulnerable populations such as those who live alone, and community development programs. The WHO also estimates that common mental disorders such as depression and anxiety have increased by 25% since the beginning of the COVID-19 pandemic, and mental health services, particularly for older adults, were most affected by the pandemic-related disruptions (WHO, 2022).

Everyone, particularly health-care workers, should see aging people as individuals, each with specific needs and abilities, rather than as a stereotypical group. Some individuals may seem "old" at 40, whereas others may not seem "old" at 70. Variables such as attitude, mental health, physical health, and degree of independence strongly influence how an individual perceives themselves. Surely, in the final analysis, whether one is considered "old" must be self-determined.

Epidemiology

The Population

In 1980 Americans age 65 years or older numbered 25.5 million. By 2017 these numbers had increased to 54.1 million and are expected to increase by 2060 to 94.7 million (Administration on Aging [AoA], 2021). The 85 and older population, which numbered 6.6 million in 2020, is expected to more than double by 2040. In 2019 there were 100,322 people age 100 years or older (more than triple the number since 1980).

Marital Status

In 2020, of individuals age 65 years and older, 70% of men and 48% of women were married and 30% of all women in this age-group were widowed (AoA, 2021). There were three times as many widows as widowers.

Living Arrangements

About 27% of older adults and 42% of women older than age 75 years live alone (AoA, 2021). Approximately 1.1 million grandparents age 60 years and older were responsible for the basic needs of one or more grandchildren younger than age 18 years living with them in 2019. This trend continues to grow and has significant implications for the changing complexion of older adult life. A relatively small number (1.2 million) of adults older than 65 years lived in nursing homes in 2019. This percentage increases dramatically with age, ranging from 1% for people age 65 to 74 years to 8% for people age 85 years and older (AoA, 2021). See Figure 33–1 for a distribution of living arrangements for people age 65 years and older.

Economic Status

About 8.9% of adults age 65 and older lived below the poverty level in 2019. When the U.S. Census Bureau figures adjusted for regional variations in the costs of housing, other benefits, and out-of-pocket expenses for needs such as medical care, the percentage of those living below the poverty level rose to 12.8%; medical out-of-pocket expenses were the major source of differences in these poverty measures (AoA, 2021).

Older women had a higher poverty rate than older men, and the highest poverty rates were among Hispanic women living alone (32.1%) and African

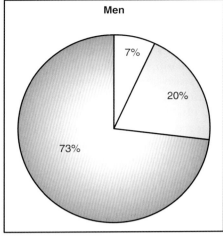

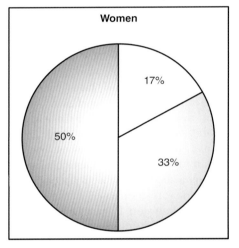

FIGURE 33–1 Living arrangements of noninstitutionalized persons age 65 and older. (Source: Administration on Aging (AoA). (2021). *2020 profile of older Americans.* https://acl.gov/sites/default/files/Profile%20of%20OA/2020ProfileOlderAmericans_RevisedFinal.pdf)

American women who live alone (31.7%). Of those age 75 years and older who were living in a house, 75% were homeowners, and 45% of householders spent one-third or more of their income on housing costs (36% for homeowners and 76% for renters) (AoA, 2021).

Poor people who have worked all their lives can expect to become poorer in old age, and others will become poor only after becoming old. However, there is a substantial number of affluent and middle-income older people.

Employment

With the passage of the Age Discrimination in Employment Act in 1967, forced retirement or age discrimination for employees over the age of 40 is now illegal, although there are some exceptions to protections under this law. It is well accepted that involvement in purposeful activity is vital to successful adaptation and perhaps even to survival at any age. Increasing numbers of adults older than age 65 years are remaining active in employment environments. In 2020 approximately 10.6 million Americans (19.4%) age 65 years and older were in the labor force (working or actively seeking work), and that number represents a steady increase for women from the year 2000 through 2019 (there was a decline in employment rates for older adult women in 2020, which is believed to be effected by the COVID-19 pandemic) (AoA, 2021). These data do not clarify whether this tendency to remain in the workforce during older adulthood is related to the desire to remain active and productive or is based on economic necessity.

Health Status

The number of days in which usual activities are restricted because of illness or injury increases with age. Most adults age 65 years and older have at least one chronic illness, and many have two to three. The most commonly occurring conditions (in order of prevalence) are hypertension, arthritis, heart disease, diabetes, cancer, and stroke (AoA, 2021).

Emotional and mental illnesses increase over the life span. Depression is particularly prevalent, and suicide is a serious problem among older adult Americans. The prevalence of major depression is estimated to be between 1% and 5% for the general population of older adults but may rise to as high as 13.5% for older adults requiring hospitalization or home health care (Centers for Disease Control and Prevention [CDC], 2021). The CDC adds that depression in this age-group is particularly underdiagnosed and undertreated by both health-care providers and older adults themselves, perhaps related to a misperception that this is a normal part of aging or a natural reaction to illnesses. Neurocognitive disorders (NCDs) increase dramatically in old age.

Theories of Aging

Several theories related to the aging process have been described. These theories are grouped into two broad categories: biological and psychosocial.

Biological Theories

Biological theories attempt to explain the physical process of aging, including molecular and cellular changes in the major organ systems and the body's ability to function adequately and resist disease. They also attempt to explain why people age differently and what factors affect longevity and the body's ability to resist disease.

Genetic Theory

According to one genetic theory, aging is an involuntarily inherited process that operates over time to alter cellular or tissue structures. This theory suggests that life span and longevity changes are predetermined. The theory is supported by the finding that there are similar life spans among identical twins and children of parents with a long life span (Rogers et al., 2020). A second genetic theory, involving epigenetics, identifies aging as a process of genetic mutations that essentially create errors in transmission of information, causing molecules to become dysfunctional. Epigenetics is the study of heritable changes in how genes are expressed and whether they are active or inactive. These changes can be influenced by factors such as aging, environment, or disease. Epigenetics research has confirmed fascinating findings that have implications for aging and illness. First, it was discovered that DNA methylation (the addition of a methyl group to a DNA base) is a mechanism responsible for gene regulation. Genome studies of aging cells and tissues have shown a variable "DNA methylation drift," which creates changes in aging stem cells that culminates in reduced stem cell plasticity, stem cell exhaustion, and focal defects that can promote chronic inflammation and increase in illness (Bell et al., 2019). Environmental influences such as smoking may also influence DNA methylation shift and contribute to aging. With ongoing research, we may discover what aging will look like for an individual and what their disease risks are. If epigenetic drift can be prevented, it may be possible to prevent diseases associated with aging.

Wear-and-Tear Theory

Proponents of this theory believe that the body wears out on a scheduled basis. Because animals have some ability to repair themselves, this theory does not seem to fit what we know about biological systems (Rogers et al., 2020). A related theory suggests that free radicals, the waste products of metabolism, accumulate and cause damage to important biological structures. Free radicals are molecules with unpaired electrons that exist normally in the body; they also are produced by ionizing radiation, ozone, and chemical toxins. According to this theory, these free radicals cause DNA damage, cross-linkage of collagen, and the accumulation of age pigments.

Environmental Theory

According to this theory, factors in the environment (e.g., industrial carcinogens, sunlight, trauma, and infection) bring about changes in the aging process.

Although these factors are known to accelerate aging, the effect of the environment is a secondary rather than a primary factor in aging. Science is only beginning to uncover the many environmental factors that affect aging.

Autoimmune Theory

The autoimmune theory describes an age-related decline in the immune system. As people age, their ability to defend against foreign organisms decreases, resulting in susceptibility to infection and diseases such as cancer. An increase in the body's autoimmune response occurs in which aging cells can no longer distinguish foreign cells and instead begin to attack the body's own tissues. This misdirected immune response leads to the development of autoimmune diseases, such as rheumatoid arthritis and allergies to food and environmental agents. This theory, however, is based on clinical rather than experimental evidence (Rogers et al., 2020).

Neuroendocrine Theory

The neuroendocrine theory was first developed in 1954 by Vladimir Dilman, MD, who subsequently worked with another physician, Ward Dean, to update this theory in the early 1990s. The theory suggests that as humans age, the hypothalamus' ability to regulate hormones decreases, and it becomes less responsive to hormonal effects. Consequently, hormone secretion and function also decline. Dilman (1954) identified several hypotheses about why this decrease in sensitivity occurs, including reduced neurotransmitter levels (serotonin in particular), decline in the secretion of pineal gland hormones, reduced glucose utilization and fat accumulation, development of neuronal lesions caused by chronically elevated cortisol levels secondary to stress, and accumulation of cholesterol in plasma membranes of neurons (Dean, 2021). Some researchers believe that therapeutic replacement of the hormones affected by the decline in hypothalamic activity may be a future treatment to counter the effects of aging, but more research is needed.

Psychosocial Theories

Psychosocial theories focus on social and psychological changes that accompany advancing age, as opposed to the biological implications of anatomic deterioration. Several theories have attempted to describe how attitudes and behavior in the early phases of life affect people's reactions during the late phase. This work is called the process of "successful aging."

Personality Theory

In a review of research on personality and aging that studied people between 60 and 80 years of age, Srivastava and Das (2013) identified support for the premise that personality traits are relatively stable but may change somewhat over the long term related to aging and possibly in response to intervention. The personality trait of conscientiousness, for example, when viewed over the course of a lifetime, was found to be relatively stable, but recent research found that conscientiousness can be changed with intervention even when study participants were unaware that conscientiousness was the target of the intervention (Hudson, 2021). As the population of older adults continues to grow, research has focused not only on what constitutes aging but more specifically what constitutes successful aging. Srivastava and Das (2013) stressed that personality is undeniably influential in successful aging (they note that the term "successful aging" is often used but is controversial to some). Rowe and Kahn (1997) provided the classic paradigm for successful aging, identifying three criteria that must be met: (a) absence of disease, disability, and risk factors; (b) maintaining physical and mental functioning; and (c) active engagement in life.

So what role do personality factors play in these aspects of successful aging? Several studies have focused on the personality trait of conscientiousness as most associated with health-promoting behaviors (Ormstad et al., 2020, Sun et al., 2022). Research also supports that the personality trait of conscientiousness is protective against dementia, and the facets of **conscientiousness** most protective against cognitive impairment are one's sense of personal responsibility, one's belief in one's ability to control their behavior, and one's sense of themselves as hard working (Aschenbrenner et al., 2020; Sutin et al., 2018; Yoneda et al., 2022). This research suggested that personality may indeed play a significant role in aging and age-related illness. The significance of these findings for intervention in and possible improvement of the aging process is still unknown. Future research may begin to reveal the intricate interaction between genetic and environmental influences such that personality traits may become alterable to promote healthier, more successful aging.

Developmental Task Theory

In contrast to the personality theories of aging, which discuss a largely stable process that continues into old age, developmental task theory holds that there are activities and challenges that one must accomplish at predictable, changing stages in life to achieve successful aging. Erikson (1963) described the primary task of old age as being able to see one's life as having been lived with integrity. In the absence of achieving the sense of having lived well, the older adult is at risk of becoming preoccupied with feelings of regret or despair. As noted previously, the life span was significantly shorter when Erikson's developmental tasks and stages were first identified. In the late 1990s, Erikson added the concept of **transcendence** as the stage that occurs after the stage of integrity versus despair (Erikson & Erikson, 1997). McCarthy and associates (2013) identified transcendence as a concept within the spiritual domain, and they cited McCarthy and Bockweg's (2012) definition:

> Transcendence [is] an inherent developmental process, resulting in a shift from a rational, materialistic view to a wider world view characterized by broadened personal boundaries, within interpersonal, intrapersonal, transpersonal, and temporal dimensions resulting in an increased sense of meaning in life, well-being, and life satisfaction (p. 180).

Research on transcendence suggests that transcendence and spirituality are significant contributors to successful aging (Kruse & Schmitt, 2019; McCarthy et al., 2013). McCarthy added that even in the face of chronic illness and functional limitations, individuals can age successfully depending on their ability to cope and adapt while maintaining a sense of connectedness and meaning in life (News Medical, 2014).

Disengagement Theory

Disengagement theory describes the process of withdrawal by older adults from societal roles and responsibilities. According to the theory, this withdrawal process is predictable, systematic, inevitable, and necessary for the proper functioning of a growing society. Older adults were believed to be happy when social contacts diminished and responsibilities were assumed by a younger generation, providing time for reflecting on life's accomplishments and coming to terms with unfulfilled expectations. For society, the benefit is an orderly transfer of power from old to young.

There have been many critics of this theory, and the postulates have been challenged. For many healthy and productive older individuals, the prospect of a slower pace and fewer responsibilities is undesirable.

Activity Theory

In direct opposition to the disengagement theory is the activity theory of aging, which holds that the way to age successfully is to stay active. Boland and Verduin (2022) reported that growing evidence supports the importance of remaining socially active for both physical and emotional well-being. Cultural expectations are influential, and as older Americans increasingly reap the benefits of physical and social activities, cultural expectations begin to shift. Many fitness classes, for example, are now finding a membership of people in their 80s and beyond.

Continuity Theory

This theory, also known as the *developmental theory*, is a follow-up to the disengagement and activity theories. It emphasizes the individual's previously established coping abilities and personal character traits as a basis for predicting how the person will adjust to the changes of aging. Basic lifestyle characteristics are likely to remain stable in old age, barring physical or other types of complications that necessitate change. A person who has enjoyed the company of others and an active social life will continue to enjoy this lifestyle into old age. One who has preferred solitude and a limited number of activities will probably find satisfaction in a continuation of this lifestyle.

Maintenance of internal continuity is motivated by the need for preservation of self-esteem, ego integrity, cognitive function, and social support. As individuals age, they maintain self-concept by reinterpreting current experiences so that old values can take on new meanings in keeping with present circumstances. Internal self-concepts and beliefs are not readily vulnerable to environmental change, and external continuity in skills, activities, roles, and relationship styles can remain remarkably stable into the 70s and beyond.

The Normal Aging Process

Biological Aspects of Aging

Individuals are unique in their physical and psychological aging processes, as influenced by their predisposition or resistance to illness; the effects of their external environment and behaviors; their exposure to trauma, infections, and past diseases; and the health and illness practices they have adopted during their life spans. As the individual ages, a quantitative loss of cells and changes in many of the enzymatic activities within cells result in diminished responsiveness to biological demands made on the body. Age-related changes occur at different rates for different individuals, although in fact, when growth stops, aging begins. This section presents a brief overview of the normal biological changes that occur with the aging process.

Integumentary System

One of the most dramatic changes that occurs in aging is the loss of elastin in the skin. This effect, along with changes in collagen, causes aged skin to wrinkle and sag. Excessive exposure to sunlight compounds these changes and increases the risk of skin cancer.

Fat redistribution results in a loss of the subcutaneous cushion of adipose tissue. Thus, older people lose "insulation," the skin appears thinner, and they are more sensitive to extremes of ambient temperature than younger people. A diminished supply of blood vessels to the skin results in a slower rate of healing.

Cardiovascular System

The age-related decline in the cardiovascular system is thought to be the major influence in decreased tolerance for exercise, loss of conditioning, and the overall decline in energy reserve. The aging heart is characterized by modest hypertrophy and loss of pacemaker cells, resulting in a decrease in maximal heart rate and diminished cardiac output. These changes result in a decrease in response to work demands and some diminishment of blood flow to the brain, kidneys, liver, and muscles. Heart rate also slows with age. If arteriosclerosis is present, cardiac function is further compromised.

Respiratory System

Thoracic expansion is diminished by an increase in fibrous tissue and loss of elastin. Pulmonary vital capacity decreases, and the amount of residual air increases. Scattered areas of fibrosis in the alveolar septa interfere with the exchange of oxygen and carbon dioxide. These changes are accelerated by the use of cigarettes or other inhaled substances. Cough and laryngeal reflexes are reduced, causing decreased ability to defend the airway. Decreased pulmonary blood flow and diffusion ability result in reduced efficiency in responding to sudden respiratory demands.

Musculoskeletal System

Skeletal aging involving the bones, muscles, ligaments, and tendons probably generates the most frequent limitations on activities of daily living for aging individuals. Loss of muscle mass is significant, although this occurs more slowly in men than in women. Demineralization of the bones occurs at a rate of about 1% per year throughout the life span in both men and women. However, bone loss increases to approximately 10% in women around menopause, making them particularly vulnerable to osteoporosis.

Individual muscle fibers become thinner and less elastic with age. Muscles become less flexible after disuse. Diminished storage of muscle glycogen results in loss of energy reserve for increased activity. These changes are accelerated by nutritional deficiencies and inactivity.

Gastrointestinal System

In the oral cavity, the teeth show a reduction in dentine production, shrinkage and fibrosis of root pulp, gingival retraction, and loss of bone density in the alveolar ridges. There is some loss of peristalsis in the stomach and intestines, and gastric acid production decreases. Levels of intrinsic factor may also decrease, resulting in vitamin B12 malabsorption in some aging individuals. A significant decrease in the absorptive surface area of the small intestine may be associated with some decline in nutrient absorption. Motility slows in the large intestine, and, combined with poor dietary habits, dehydration, lack of exercise, and some medications, may give rise to problems with constipation.

A modest decrease in the size and weight of the liver results in losses in enzyme activity required to deactivate certain medications by the liver, which can influence their metabolism and excretion. Along with the pharmacokinetics of the drug, these age-related changes must be considered when giving medications to older adults.

Endocrine System

A decreased level of thyroid hormones causes a lowered basal metabolic rate. Decreased amounts of adrenocorticotropic hormone may result in a less efficient stress response.

Impairments in glucose tolerance are more evident in older adults. Studies of glucose challenge test results in older individuals show that insulin levels are equivalent to or slightly higher than results from younger individuals, although peripheral insulin resistance appears to play a significant role in carbohydrate intolerance. The observed glucose clearance abnormalities and insulin resistance in older people may be related to many factors other than biological aging (e.g., obesity, family history of diabetes) and may be influenced substantially by diet or exercise.

Genitourinary System

Age-related declines in renal function occur because of steady attrition of nephrons and sclerosis within the glomeruli over time. Vascular changes affect blood flow to the kidneys, resulting in reduced glomerular filtration and tubular function. Older adults are prone to develop inappropriate antidiuretic hormone secretion, causing slight elevation in levels of blood urea nitrogen and creatinine. The overall decline in renal function has important implications for physicians who prescribe medications for older adults.

In men, enlargement of the prostate gland is common as aging occurs. Symptoms include urgency, difficulty urinating, nocturia, and inability to empty the bladder completely. In addition to changes that may occur as part of the normal aging process, obesity, lack of activity, and erectile dysfunction can also increase the risk (American Urological Association, 2022). Loss of muscle and sphincter control, as well as the use of some medications, may cause urinary incontinence in women. Not only is this problem a cause of social stigma, but it also increases the risk of urinary tract infection and local skin irritation if left untreated. Normal changes in the genitalia are discussed in the section "Sexual Aspects of Aging."

Immune System

Aging causes changes in both cell-mediated and antibody-mediated immune responses. The size of the thymus gland declines continuously beginning just after puberty, decreasing to about 15% of its original size by age 50. The consequences of these changes include an increased susceptibility to infections and a diminished inflammatory response that results in delayed healing. There is also evidence of an increase in various autoantibodies as a person ages, increasing the risk of autoimmune disorders such as rheumatoid arthritis (National Institutes of Health [NIH], 2022). Because of the overall decrease in the efficiency of the immune system, the proliferation of abnormal cells is facilitated in the elderly individual. Cancer is the best example of aberrant cells allowed to proliferate due to the ineffectiveness of the immune system.

Nervous System

Neuroimaging studies have found changes in brain structure and cognitive functions associated with aging, the most common of which are loss of gray matter volume and cortical thinning, a reduction in white matter integrity and volume, and abnormal functional connectivity (Wrigglesworth et al., 2021). The loss of cells in the cerebellum, the locus ceruleus, the substantia nigra, and olfactory bulbs may account for some of the characteristic signs of aging, including mild gait disturbances, sleep disruptions, and decreased smell and taste perception.

Neurochemical changes in the brain consistently associated with aging include reduction in N-acetyl-aspartate (NAA) concentration and increased myo-inositol (mI) concentration, both of which mirror neurometabolite changes often seen in Alzheimer's disease (AD) (Cleland et al., 2019). Evidence supports that schizophrenia and AD are both associated with accelerated brain aging (Wrigglesworth et al., 2021).

Sensory Systems

Vision

Visual acuity begins to decrease in midlife. Presbyopia (blurred near vision) is the standard sign of aging of the eye. It is caused by a loss of elasticity of the crystalline lens and results in compromised accommodation.

Cataract development is inevitable if the individual lives long enough for vision changes to occur. Cataracts occur when the lens of the eye becomes less resilient due to compression of fibers and increasingly opaque as proteins lump together, ultimately resulting in a loss of visual acuity.

The color in the iris may fade, and the pupil may become irregular in shape. A decrease in production of secretions by the lacrimal glands may cause dryness and result in increased irritation and infection. The pupil may become constricted, requiring an increase in the amount of light needed for reading.

Hearing

Hearing changes significantly with age. Gradually, sensitivity to changes in sound discrimination decreases because of damage to the hair cells of the cochlea. The most dramatic decline appears to be in the perception of high-frequency sounds.

Age-related hearing loss, called *presbycusis*, is common and affects more than one-half of all adults by age 75 years and nearly all those older than 90 years (Blevins, 2022). It occurs more frequently in men than in women, a fact that may be related to differences in levels of lifetime noise exposure. A genetic influence also predisposes older adults to age-related hearing loss.

Taste and Smell

Beyond 70 years of age, taste sensitivity begins to decline related to atrophy and loss of taste buds (Shock, 2020). Taste discrimination decreases, and bitter taste sensations predominate. Sensitivity to sweet and salty tastes is diminished.

The deterioration of the olfactory bulbs is accompanied by loss of smell acuity. The effect of aging on the sense of smell has not been precisely identified and is difficult to evaluate because so many environmental factors influence sensitivity to smell (Shock, 2020). However, some decreased sensitivity may be related to the loss of nerve endings in the nose and decreased mucus production.

Touch and Pain

Although the primary sensory changes related to aging are in hearing and vision, sensitivity to touch and pain may also decline or change because of decreased blood flow to nerve endings, in the spinal cord, or to the brain. These changes have critical implications for older adults in their potential inability to respond to sensory warnings to escape serious injury.

Psychological Aspects of Aging

Memory Functioning

Age-related memory deficiencies and slower response times have been reported extensively in the literature. Although **short-term memory** (ability to recall information that one has just received) seems to deteriorate with age, perhaps because of poorer sorting strategies, **long-term memory** (ability to recall remote information received from hours to decades ago) does not show similar changes. However, in nearly every instance, well-educated, mentally active people do not exhibit the same decline in memory functioning as their peers who lack similar opportunities to flex their minds. Nevertheless, with few exceptions, the time required for memory scanning is longer for both recent and remote recall among older people. This change can sometimes be attributed to social or health factors (e.g., stress, fatigue, illness), but it can also occur because of certain normal physical changes associated with aging (e.g., decreased blood flow to the brain).

Intellectual Functioning

There appears to be a high degree of regularity in intellectual functioning across the adult age span. Crystallized abilities, knowledge acquired in the course of education and life experiences, tend to remain stable or may even increase over the adult life span. Fluid abilities, those involved in solving novel problems, tend to decline gradually from youth to old age and are thought to be more associated with the integrity of brain function.

Learning Ability

The ability to learn is not diminished by age. However, studies have shown that some aspects of learning do change with age. The ordinary slowing of reaction time with age for nearly all tasks or the over-arousal of the central nervous system may account for lower performance levels on tests requiring rapid responses. Under conditions that allow for self-pacing by the participant, differences in accuracy of performance diminish. The ability to learn continues throughout life, although it is strongly influenced by interests, activity, motivation, health, and experience. Adjustments need to be made in teaching methodology and the time allowed for learning.

Adaptation to the Tasks of Aging

Loss and Grief

Individuals experience losses from the very beginning of life. By the time individuals reach their 60s and 70s, they have experienced numerous losses, and mourning has become a lifelong process. Unfortunately, with the aging process comes a convergence of losses, the timing of which makes it difficult for the aging individual to complete the grief process in response to one loss before another occurs. Because grief is cumulative, this can result in **bereavement overload,** which has been implicated in the predisposition to depression in the elderly.

Attachment to Others

Many studies have confirmed the importance of interpersonal relationships at all stages in the life cycle. Benefits include decreased sense of loneliness, increased life satisfaction, and support systems to facilitate coping with stressful changes and events.

This need for **attachment** (emotional bonds with others) is consistent with the activity theory of aging that correlates the importance of social integration with successful adaptation in later life. Evidence supports that in addition to the psychosocial benefits, social engagement is also correlated with physical and cognitive health in older adulthood (Luo et al., 2020; Myhre et al., 2017; Steppe et al., 2022).

Maintenance of Self-Identity

Maintaining a positive self-concept and identity is important in successful aging. Individuals who tend toward a rigid self-identity and a negative self-concept will no doubt struggle with any of the changes and adaptations faced in the aging process. For example, someone whose identity centers entirely around their job may struggle more with identity in retirement than someone whose identity includes job, family, travel, and hobbies. Researchers have found that maintaining a youthful age identity and positive perceptions and experiences related to aging had a self-enhancing function for self-esteem and identity (Chen et al., 2018). The authors compared citizens in the United States with those in the Netherlands and found that for the former, this self-enhancing function was stronger than for those from the latter. They concluded that factors influencing self-identity and self-concept in older age need to be considered within the cultural context.

Dealing With Death

Death anxiety is believed to be a universal phenomenon, and attitudes about death are influenced by cumulative life experiences. As the average life span has increased, there has been a resurgence of interest in research about death anxiety. Kübler-Ross's (1969) pioneering research on attitudes about death and the experience of dying paved the way for discussions of this issue. More recent research supports that death anxiety is lower among individuals who have dimensions of meaning in life, presence of meaning, search for meaning, and positive self-esteem (Zhang et al., 2019). Conversely significant death anxiety is associated with several psychiatric disorders including somatoform and illness anxiety, disorders, obsessive compulsive disorders, depression, and others (Menzies & Menzies, 2018). Assessment of individuals for death anxiety and intervention when it is identified may be beneficial in preventing longer-term consequences. In a systematic review (Grossman et al., 2018), researchers found that interventions focused on creating meaning in life were the most effective in reducing death anxiety. Menzies and Menzies (2018) reported the finding that cognitive behavior therapy (CBT) interventions were also effective in reducing death fears.

Psychiatric Disorders in Later Life

Cognitive disorders, depressive disorders, phobias, and alcohol use disorders are among the most common psychiatric illnesses in later life (Boland & Verduin, 2022). Many factors influence symptomatology, including medical conditions and medications. It should never be assumed that psychiatric symptoms are a usual part of aging. A thorough assessment is essential to distinguish the multiple factors that may be concurrently influencing symptomatology.

Neurocognitive Disorders

NCDs are common causes of psychopathology in older adults and are expected to increase over the next few decades as the population of older adults increases and research on early identification of NCDs improves. The Global Burden of Disease Dementia Forecasting Collaborators (2022) estimated that the incidence of dementia will triple by 2050. About one-half of these disorders are of the Alzheimer's type, characterized by an insidious onset and a gradually progressive course of cognitive impairment. No curative treatment is currently available. Symptomatic treatments, including pharmacological interventions, attention to the environment, and family support, can help to maximize the client's level of functioning. Current research identifies 12 modifiable risk factors for dementia: less education, hypertension, hearing impairment, smoking, midlife obesity, depression, physical inactivity, diabetes, social isolation, excessive alcohol consumption, head injury, and air pollution (Livingston et al., 2020).

Delirium

Delirium is one of the most common and critical forms of psychopathology in later life. Several factors have been identified that predispose elderly people to delirium, including structural brain disease, reduced capacity for homeostatic regulation, impaired vision and hearing, a high prevalence of chronic disease, reduced resistance to acute stress, and age-related changes in the pharmacokinetic and pharmacodynamics of drugs. Delirium needs to be recognized and the underlying condition treated as soon as possible. A high mortality rate is associated with this condition.

Depression

Depressive disorders are the most common affective illnesses occurring after the middle years. The increased incidence of depression among older adults is influenced by the variables of physical illness, functional disability, cognitive impairment, and loss of a spouse. Somatic symptoms such as changes in appetite and complaints of pain are common in older adults with depression but should always be assessed to rule out other illnesses. Symptomatology often mimics that of NCDs, a condition called *pseudodementia*. (See Chapter 22, "Neurocognitive Disorders," Table 22–1, for a comparison of the symptoms of NCDs and pseudodementia.)

Suicide is prevalent in older adults, with declining health and decreased economic status considered important influencing factors. Treatment of depression in the older adult may include psychotropic medications or electroconvulsive therapy. Because tricyclic antidepressants pose a risk for orthostatic hypotension and other anticholinergic effects, and selective serotonin reuptake inhibitors (SSRIs) pose a higher risk for hyponatremia in the elderly, the risks and benefits of medication use should be carefully reviewed. Depression in the presence of coronary artery disease is associated with significant increases in risk for poorer outcomes and death, underscoring the importance of screening and treatment for depression in older adults (May et al., 2017).

Schizophrenia

Schizophrenia typically begins in young adulthood. In most instances, individuals who manifest psychotic disorders early in life show a decline in psychopathology as they age. Late-onset schizophrenia (after age 60) is rare, and when it does occur, it is more common in women and often characterized by paranoid delusions or hallucinations. Antipsychotic agents may be beneficial but should be used judiciously and at lower than usual doses (Boland & Verduin, 2022).

Anxiety Disorders

Anxiety disorders are common in older adults. Most anxiety disorders begin in early to middle adulthood, but some appear for the first time after age 60. Because the autonomic nervous system is more fragile in older persons, the response to a major stressor is often quite intense. The presence of physical disability frequently compounds the situation, resulting in a more severe post-traumatic stress response than is commonly observed in younger persons. In older adults, symptoms of anxiety and depression often accompany each other, making it difficult to determine which disorder is dominant.

Anxiety disorders, like depression, are also associated with cardiac disease in older adults and to adverse cardiovascular outcomes (Celano et al., 2016; Karlsen et al., 2021). There may be physiological (inflammation, autonomic and endothelial dysfunction, platelet aggregation) as well as behavioral mechanisms involved in the link between anxiety and cardiovascular disease, but careful identification and treatment of both are essential.

Substance Use Disorders

It is believed that the incidence of substance misuse and addiction in older adults may have been underdiagnosed, but nationwide attention to the epidemic use and misuse of opioid pain medication has shed light on this problem in the older adult population. Older adults often combine prescription and over-the-counter (OTC) medications and may have more difficulty tolerating some drugs, particularly some long-acting drugs, sedative-hypnotics, and benzodiazepines. For these reasons (and others), older adults are an at-risk population for substance use disorders and should be screened for prescription, OTC, and other substance use to conduct a thorough assessment and identify potential health risks. Benzodiazepines used concomitantly with opiate medication has been identified as a potentially fatal combination of drugs, and prescriptions for benzodiazepines among older adults have been rising over the past 15 years (Neft et al., 2019).

Older adults with alcohol dependence often have a long-standing history, and consequently many have Wernicke's encephalopathy or Korsakoff syndrome. "The sudden onset of delirium in older adults hospitalized for a medical illness is most often caused by alcohol withdrawal" (Boland & Verduin, 2022, p. 807), so careful evaluation for alcohol use history is important in assessment of this population.

Sleep Disorders

Sleep disorders are very common in older adults. Boland and Verduin (2022) identified that advanced age is the single most important factor related to the increased prevalence of sleep disorders. Contributing factors may include medical conditions, medications, age-related changes in circadian rhythms, sleep apnea, and restless legs syndrome. Sedative-hypnotics, along with nonpharmacological approaches, are often used as sleep aids for the elderly. Changes in aging associated with metabolism and elimination must be considered when maintenance medications are administered for chronic insomnia in the aging individual.

Sociocultural Aspects of Aging

Old age brings many important socially induced changes, some of which have the potential for negative effects on both the physical and mental well-being of older persons. In American society, *old age* is defined arbitrarily as 65 years or older because that is the age when most people have been able to retire with full Social Security and other pension benefits. Recent legislation has increased the age beyond 65 years for full Social Security benefits. Currently, the age increases yearly (based on year of birth) until 2027, when the age for full benefits will be 67 for all individuals.

Older adults in virtually all cultures share some basic needs and interests. There is little doubt that most individuals choose to live the most satisfying life possible for as long as possible. They want protection from hazards and release from the weariness of everyday tasks. They want to be treated with the respect and dignity that individuals who have reached this pinnacle in life deserve, and they want to die with the same respect and dignity.

Historically, the aged have had a special status in society. Even today, in some cultures, the aged are the most powerful, the most engaged, and the most respected members of society. This elevated status has not been the case in modern industrial societies, although trends in the status of the aged differ widely among industrialized countries. For example, the status and integration of the aged in Japan have remained relatively high compared with other industrialized nations, such as the United States.

Many negative stereotypes influence the perspective on aging in the United States. Views of older adults as always tired or sick, slow and forgetful, isolated and lonely, unproductive, and angry determine the way younger individuals relate to this population. Increasing disregard for the elderly has resulted in a type of segregation as aging individuals voluntarily seek out or are involuntarily placed in special residences for the aged.

Retirement apartment complexes, assisted living centers, and even entire retirement communities intended solely for individuals over age 50 are becoming increasingly common. Geographic distribution of older populations varies significantly in different states. In 2019 the highest percentage of those aged 65 or older were living in Maine, Florida, West Virginia, and Vermont (AoA, 2021). Older adults may be migrating to these areas in an effort to achieve integration with others in their age-group. As the older adult population continues to increase and assert their voice, their status, benefits, and privileges within society may improve.

Sexual Aspects of Aging

Sexuality and the sexual needs of older adults are frequently misunderstood, condemned, stereotyped, ridiculed, repressed, and ignored. Americans have grown up in a society that has liberated sexual expression for all other age-groups but still retains certain rigid standards regarding sexual expression by the elderly. Negative stereotyped notions concerning sexual interest and activity among the elderly are common. Some of these include ideas that older people have no sexual interests or desires, that they are sexually undesirable, or that they are too fragile or too ill to engage in sexual activity.

These cultural stereotypes undoubtedly play a large part in the misperception many people hold regarding the sexuality of the aged, and they may be reinforced by the common tendency of the young to deny the inevitability of aging. With reasonably good health and an interesting and interested partner, there is no inherent reason why individuals should not enjoy an active sexual life well into late adulthood.

Physical Changes Associated With Sexuality

Many of the changes in sexuality that occur in later years are related to the physical changes that take place at that time of life.

Changes in Women

Menopause may begin anytime during the 40s or early 50s. During this time, there is a gradual decline in ovarian function and the subsequent production of estrogen, which results in several changes. The walls of the vagina become thin and inelastic, the vagina itself shrinks in both width and length, and the amount of vaginal lubrication noticeably decreases. Orgastic uterine contractions may become spastic. All of these changes can result in painful penetration, vaginal burning, pelvic aching, or irritation on urination. In some women, the discomfort may be severe enough to result in avoidance of intercourse. Paradoxically, these symptoms are more likely to occur with infrequent intercourse (once a month or less). Regular and more frequent sexual activity results in a greater sexual satisfaction (Smith et al., 2019; Velten & Margraf, 2017). Other symptoms associated with menopause in some women include hot flashes, night sweats, sleeplessness, irritability, mood swings, migraine headaches, urinary incontinence, and weight gain.

Changes in Men

Testosterone production declines gradually over the years, beginning between ages 40 and 60. A major change resulting from this hormone reduction is that erections occur more slowly and require more direct genital stimulation to achieve. There may also be a modest decrease in the firmness of the erection in men older than age 60. The refractory period lengthens with age, increasing the amount of time after orgasm before the man may achieve another erection. The volume of ejaculate gradually decreases, and the force of ejaculation lessens. The testes become somewhat smaller, but most men continue to produce viable sperm well into old age. Prolonged control over ejaculation in middle-aged and elderly men may bring increased sexual satisfaction for both partners. Adverse effects of some medications and circulatory problems may increase risks for erectile dysfunction in older adult men. Vasodilator medications such as sildenafil (Viagra) and tadalafil (Cialis) are treatment options.

Sexual Behavior in Older Adults

Although sexual interest and behavior do appear to decline somewhat with age, studies show that significant numbers of older men and women have active and satisfying sex lives well into their 80s. According to a University of Michigan national poll (2018) on sexual behavior and health among adults ages 65 to 80, 40% identified being sexually active. Some statistics from the survey are summarized in Table 33–1. A large, longitudinal study ($n = 6021$) on sexual health and well-being in older adults within the United Kingdom (Lee et al., 2016) also included the age-group of 80 to >90 years and found that roughly 14% of women and 37% of men reported being sexually active. The information from these surveys clearly indicates that sexual activity can and does continue well past the 70s for healthy, active individuals who have regular opportunities for sexual expression.

Special Concerns of the Elderly Population

Retirement

It is estimated that about 29% of Americans reenter the workforce after retirement, even though current estimates suggest that there will still be dramatic

TABLE 33–1 Sexuality at Midlife and Beyond

	Sex is an important part of a romantic relationship at any age (n = 989) Percentage that agreed or strongly agreed	Sex is important to my overall quality of life (n = 979) Percentage that agreed or strongly agreed	How would you describe your interest in sex? (n = 979) Percentage that were extremely or strongly interested	How satisfied are you with your sex life? (n = 956) Percentage that were extremely or very satisfied
ALL RESPONDENTS				
	76%	54%	30%	37%
AGE				
65–70	78%	57%	34%	38%
71–75	72%	52%	28%	37%
76–80	77%	50%	19%	36%
GENDER				
Male	84%	70%	50%	31%
Female	69%	40%	12%	43%
RELATIONSHIP STATUS				
Married/Partnered/In a relationship	76%	61%	34%	40%
Not in a relationship	75%	36%	19%	30%
PHYSICAL HEALTH				
Excellent/Very good/Good	77%	56%	32%	40%
Fair/Poor	71%	49%	21%	28%
SEXUALLY ACTIVE				
Yes	92%	83%	52%	49%
No	66%	35%	16%	29%

Solway, E., Clark, S., Singer, D., Kirch, M., Malani, P. Let's Talk about Sex. *University of Michigan National Poll on Healthy Aging.* May 2018. Available at: http://hdl.handle.net/2027.42/143212 With permission.

shortages in the number of needed employees (Sullivan & Ariss, 2018). In the field of nursing, for example, the American Association of Colleges of Nursing (AACN, 2020) predicted that, as more nurses retire, there will be an annual shortage of 175,900 nurses through 2029. Sullivan and Ariss (2018) proposed that anticipated shortages, a larger number of retirees, and longer life spans require the development of a new paradigm for examining the role of older adults in the workforce. The authors also cited reasons for older adults not wanting to return to the workforce included ageism, unsupportive work climates, lack of flexibility in the availability of part-time positions, and their own inability to effectively search for employment. Retirement has both social and economic implications for elderly individuals.

The role is fraught with ambiguity and requires many adaptations on the part of those involved.

Social Implications

Retirement is often anticipated as an achievement, in principle, but is met with many mixed feelings when it actually occurs. Our society places a great deal of importance on productivity, making as much money as possible, and doing it at as young an age as possible. These types of values contribute to the ambiguity associated with retirement. Although leisure has been acknowledged as a legitimate reward for workers, leisure during retirement historically has lacked the same social value. Adjustment to this life cycle event becomes more difficult in the face of societal values that are in direct conflict with the new lifestyle.

American society often identifies an individual by their occupation. Almost everyone has either asked or been asked at some point in time, "What do you do?" or "Where do you work?" Occupation determines status, and retirement represents a significant change in status. The basic ambiguity of retirement occurs in an individual's or society's definition of this change. Is it undertaken voluntarily or involuntarily? Is it desirable or undesirable? Is one's status made better or worse by the change? With the population of older adults growing, retirement versus remaining in the workforce will continue to be an important issue for this age-group. Clearly, retirement is a major life event that requires planning and realistic expectations of life changes.

Economic Implications

Because retirement is generally associated with a 20% to 40% reduction in personal income, the standard of living after retirement may be adversely affected. Most older adults derive postretirement income from a combination of Social Security benefits, public and private pensions, and income from savings or investments.

The Social Security Act of 1935 promised assistance with financial security for the elderly. Since then, the original legislation has been modified, yet the basic philosophy remains intact. Its effectiveness, however, is now in question. Faced with deficits, the program is forced to pay benefits to the currently retired from both the reserve funds and monies being collected at present. There is genuine concern about future generations when there may be no reserve funds from which to draw. Because many of the programs that benefit older adults depend on contributions from the younger population, the growing ratio of older Americans to younger people may affect society's ability to supply the goods and services necessary to meet this expanding demand.

Medicare and **Medicaid** were established by the government to provide medical care benefits for elderly and indigent Americans. The Medicaid program is jointly funded by state and federal governments, and coverage varies significantly from state to state. Medicare covers only a percentage of health-care costs; therefore, to reduce risk related to out-of-pocket expenditures, many older adults purchase private "medigap" policies designed to cover charges in excess of those approved by Medicare.

The magnitude of retirement earnings depends almost entirely on preretirement income. The poor will remain poor and the wealthy are unlikely to lower their status during retirement; however, for many in the middle classes, the relatively fixed income sources may be inadequate, possibly forcing them to face financial hardship for the first time in their lives.

Long-Term Care

Long-term care facilities are defined by the level of care they provide. They may be skilled nursing facilities, intermediate care facilities, or a combination of the two. Some institutions provide convalescent care for individuals recovering from acute illness or injury, some provide long-term care for individuals with chronic illness or disabilities, and still others provide both types of assistance.

Most elderly individuals prefer to remain in their own homes or in the homes of family members for as long as it is possible without deterioration of family or social patterns. Many elderly individuals are placed in institutions as a last resort only after heroic efforts have been made to keep them in their own or a relative's home. The increasing emphasis on home health care has extended the period of independence for aging individuals.

As mentioned previously, a relatively small number of older adults reside in long-term care facilities in the United States, but the number rises rapidly from 1% (in those age 65 to 74 years) to 8% in those age 85 years and older (AoA, 2021). A profile of the "typical" elderly nursing home resident is about 80 years of age, white, female, and widowed, with multiple chronic health conditions.

Risk Factors for Institutionalization

In determining who in our society will need long-term care, several factors have been identified that appear to place people at risk. Factors that influence the need for long-term care include prevalence of chronic health conditions and disabilities, level of ability to independently provide self-care, presence of mental disorders (particularly NCDs), financial hardships that prohibit exploring other options (such as senior living settings), and lack of a spouse or other support network to provide care or assistance.

Attitudinal Factors

Many people dread the thought of even visiting a nursing home, let alone moving to one or placing a relative in one. Negative perceptions exist of nursing homes as "places to go to die." The media picture and subsequent reputation of nursing homes have not been positive. Stories of substandard care and patient abuse have scarred the industry, making it difficult for those facilities that are clean, are well managed, and provide innovative, quality care to their residents to rise above the stigma.

State and national licensing boards perform periodic inspections to ensure that standards set forth by the federal government are met. These standards address the quality of patient care as well as adequacy of the nursing home facility. Yet many elderly individuals and their families still perceive nursing homes as a place to go to die, and the fact that many of these institutions are poorly equipped, understaffed, and disorganized keeps this societal perception alive. There are, however, many excellent nursing homes that strive to go beyond the minimum federal regulations for Medicaid and Medicare reimbursement. In addition to medical, nursing, rehabilitation, and dental services, social and recreational services are provided to increase the quality of life for those living in nursing homes. These activities include playing cards, bingo, and other games; parties; church activities; books; television; movies; and arts, crafts, and other classes. Some nursing homes provide occupational and professional counseling. These facilities strive to enhance opportunities for improving quality of life and for becoming "places to live" rather than "places to die."

Elder Abuse

Elder abuse is defined as the psychological, physical, or financial abuse, or intentional or unintentional neglect, of an older adult. Elder abuse occurs within families and inside of institutions such as nursing homes and long-term care facilities. Psychological abuse includes yelling, insulting, harsh commands, threats, silence, and social isolation. Physical abuse is described as striking, shoving, beating, or restraint. Financial abuse refers to misuse or theft of finances, property, or material possessions. Neglect implies the failure to fulfill the physical needs of an individual who cannot do so independently. Unintentional neglect is inadvertent, whereas intentional neglect is deliberate. In addition, older individuals may be the victims of sexual abuse, which is sexual activity between two persons that occurs without the consent of one of the persons involved. Types of elder abuse are summarized in Box 33–1.

Statistics regarding the prevalence of elder abuse are difficult to determine. It is estimated that 1 in 10 older adults in the United States is a victim of abuse (National Council on Aging [NCoA], 2021). However, one study found that only 1 in 24 cases of violence in older adults were reported to authorities (NCoA, 2021). The abuser is often a relative who lives with the elderly person and may be the assigned caregiver. Factors that may contribute to risks for caregiver elder abuse include economic stress, substance use disorders, difficulty coping with the caregiver role, and history of violent behavior. Identified risk factors for victims of abuse may include social isolation, being mentally or physically impaired, being unable to meet daily self-care needs, and having care needs that exceed the caretaker's ability (National Center on Elder Abuse [NCEA], n.d.).

Victims often minimize the abuse or deny that it has occurred. The older adult victim may be unwilling to disclose information because of fear of retaliation, embarrassment about the existence of abuse

---

BOX 33–1 Examples of Elder Abuse

PHYSICAL ABUSE
Striking, hitting, beating
Shoving
Bruising
Cutting
Restraining

PSYCHOLOGICAL ABUSE
Yelling
Insulting, name-calling
Harsh commands
Threats
Ignoring, silence, social isolation
Withholding of affection

NEGLECT (INTENTIONAL OR UNINTENTIONAL)
Withholding food and water
Inadequate heating

Unclean clothes and bedding
Lack of needed medication
Lack of eyeglasses, hearing aids, false teeth

FINANCIAL ABUSE OR EXPLOITATION
Misuse of the elderly person's income by the caregiver
Forcing the elderly person to sign over financial affairs to another person against his or her will or without sufficient knowledge about the transaction

SEXUAL ABUSE
Sexual molestation; rape
Any type of sexual activity against the elderly person's will

in the family, protectiveness toward a family member, or unwillingness to institute legal action. Adding to this unwillingness to report is that infirm elders are often isolated, so their mistreatment is less likely to be noticed by those who might be alert to symptoms of abuse. For these reasons, the detection of abuse in the elderly is difficult at best.

Identifying Elder Abuse

Because so many elderly individuals are reluctant to report personal abuse, health-care workers must be able to detect signs of mistreatment when they are in a position to do so. Box 33–1 lists the *types* of elder abuse. The following *manifestations* of various types of elder abuse have been identified:

- **Psychological and verbal abuse:** The elder adult may appear depressed, withdrawn, more confused, or agitated.
- **Physical abuse:** The victim has unexplained bruises, welts, lacerations, burns, punctures, evidence of hair-pulling, skeletal dislocations and fractures, or broken glasses.
- **Neglect:** The victim may present with unexplained weight loss, poor hygiene, inappropriate dress, consistent fatigue or listlessness, unattended physical problems or medical needs, or abandonment.
- **Sexual abuse:** The elderly person may present with pain or itching in the genital area; bruising or bleeding in external genitalia, vaginal, or anal areas; unexplained sexually transmitted disease; torn or ripped clothing.
- **Financial abuse:** There is evidence of disparity between assets and satisfactory living conditions, or the elderly person complains of a sudden lack of sufficient funds for daily living expenses.

Health-care workers often feel intimidated when confronted with cases of elder abuse. In these instances, referral to an individual experienced in the management of victims of such abuse may be the most effective approach to evaluation and intervention. Health-care workers are responsible for reporting suspicion of elder abuse. An investigation is then conducted by regulatory agencies, whose job it is to determine whether the suspicions are corroborated. Every effort must be made to ensure the client's safety, but it is important to remember that a competent elderly person has the right to choose their health-care options. As inappropriate as it may seem, some elderly individuals choose to return to an abusive situation. In this instance, they should be provided with names and phone numbers to call for assistance if needed. A follow-up visit by an adult protective services representative should be conducted.

Increased efforts need to be made to ensure that health-care providers have comprehensive training in the detection of and intervention in elder abuse. More research is needed to increase knowledge and understanding of the phenomenon of elder abuse and ultimately to develop more sophisticated strategies for prevention, intervention, and treatment.

Suicide

Men 65 years of age and older have the highest overall rate of suicide and older adults in general account for 18% of all suicides (NCoA, 2021). The suicide rate for white men over the age of 65 is five times higher than that of the general population (Boland & Verduin, 2022). Predisposing factors include loneliness, financial problems, physical illness, loss, and depression.

It has been suggested that social isolation and loneliness may be contributing factors to suicide among the elderly. Boland and Verduin (2022) identified that older suicide victims are more likely to be widowed, and the most common precipitants are physical illness and loss.

Many elderly individuals show symptoms associated with depression that are never recognized as such, particularly somatic symptoms. Any sign of helplessness or hopelessness should prompt screening for suicide risk using clear and often closed-ended questions to elicit a specific response such as the following:

- Have you thought of hurting yourself or taking your own life?
- Do you have a plan for hurting yourself?
- Have you ever acted on that plan?
- Have you ever attempted suicide?

Components of intervention with a suicidal older adult should include thorough assessment, demonstrations of genuine concern, interest, and caring; indications of empathy for their fears and concerns; and help in identifying, clarifying, and formulating a plan of action to manage the unresolved issue. Loneliness and social isolation are often compounding issues and should be addressed as part of collaborative suicide prevention plan.

Application of the Nursing Process

Assessment

Assessment of the older adult may follow the same framework used for all adults, but with consideration of the possible biological, psychological, sociocultural, and sexual changes that occur in the normal aging process described previously in this chapter. The practice of holistic nursing with older people is especially important. Older adults are likely to have multiple physical problems that contribute to problems in other areas of their lives. Obviously, these components cannot be addressed as separate entities. Nursing care with older adults is a multifaceted, challenging process because of the multiple changes occurring at this time in the life cycle and how each change affects every aspect of the individual.

Several considerations are unique to the assessment of older adults. Assessment of the older person's cognitive status is a primary responsibility. Knowledge about the presence and extent of disorientation or confusion will influence the way in which the nurse approaches care for this patient.

Information about sensory capabilities is also extremely important. Because hearing loss is common, the nurse should lower the pitch and loudness of their voice when addressing the older adult. Looking directly into the face of the older person when talking facilitates communication. Questions that require a declarative sentence in response should be asked; in this way, the nurse is able to assess the patient's ability to use words correctly. Visual acuity can be determined by assessing adaptation to the dark, color matching, and the perception of color contrast. Knowledge about these aspects of sensory functioning is essential in the development of an effective care plan.

The nurse should be familiar with the normal physical changes associated with the aging process. The following are examples of some of these changes:

■ Less effective response to changes in environmental temperature, resulting in hypothermia

■ Decreases in oxygen use and the amount of blood pumped by the heart, resulting in cerebral anoxia or hypoxia

■ Skeletal muscle wasting and weakness, resulting in difficulty in physical mobility

■ Limited cough and laryngeal reflexes, resulting in an increased risk of aspiration

■ Demineralization of bones, resulting in spontaneous fracturing

■ Decrease in gastrointestinal motility, resulting in constipation

■ Decrease in the ability to interpret painful stimuli, resulting in increased risk of injury

Common psychosocial changes associated with aging include the following:

■ Prolonged and exaggerated grief, resulting in depression

■ Physical changes, resulting in disturbed body image

■ Changes in status, resulting in loss of self-worth

This list is by no means exhaustive. The nurse should consider many other alterations in their assessment of the patient. Knowledge of the patient's functional capabilities is essential for determining the physiological, psychological, and sociological needs of the older adult. Age alone does not preclude the occurrence of all these changes. The aging process progresses at a wide range of variance, and each patient must be assessed as a unique individual.

Diagnosis and Outcome Identification

Virtually any nursing diagnosis may be applicable to the aging patient, depending on individual needs for assistance. Based on normal changes that occur in the older adult, the following nursing diagnoses may be considered.

Physiologically Related Diagnoses

■ Risk for trauma related to confusion, disorientation, muscular weakness, spontaneous fractures, and falls

■ Risk for frail elderly syndrome

■ Hypothermia related to loss of adipose tissue under the skin, evidenced by increased sensitivity to cold and body temperature below 98.6°F

■ Decreased cardiac output related to decreased myocardial efficiency secondary to age-related changes, evidenced by decreased tolerance for activity and decline in energy reserve

■ Ineffective breathing pattern related to an increase in fibrous tissue and loss of elasticity in lung tissue, evidenced by dyspnea and activity intolerance

■ Risk for aspiration related to diminished cough and laryngeal reflexes

■ Impaired physical mobility related to muscular wasting and weakness, evidenced by a need for assistance in ambulation

■ Imbalanced nutrition less than body requirements, related to inefficient absorption from the gastrointestinal tract, difficulty chewing and swallowing, anorexia, and difficulty in feeding self, evidenced by wasting syndrome, anemia, and weight loss

■ Constipation related to decreased motility; inadequate diet; insufficient activity or exercise, evidenced by decreased bowel sounds; hard, formed stools; or straining at stool

■ Stress urinary incontinence related to degenerative changes in pelvic muscles and structural supports associated with increased age, evidenced by reported or observed dribbling with increased abdominal pressure or urinary frequency

■ Urinary retention related to prostatic enlargement, evidenced by bladder distention, frequent voiding of small amounts, dribbling, or overflow incontinence

■ Disturbed sensory perception related to age-related alterations in sensory transmission, evidenced by

decreased visual acuity, hearing loss, diminished sensitivity to taste and smell, or increased touch threshold (this diagnosis has been retired by NAN-DA-I but retained in this text because of its appropriateness to the specific behaviors described)
■ Insomnia related to age-related cognitive decline, decrease in ability to sleep ("sleep decay"), or medications, evidenced by interrupted sleep, early awakening, or falling asleep during the day
■ Chronic pain related to degenerative changes in joints, evidenced by verbalization of pain or hesitation to use weight-bearing joints
■ Self-care deficit (specify) related to weakness, confusion, or disorientation, evidenced by an inability to feed self, maintain hygiene, dress or groom self, or use the toilet without assistance
■ Risk for impaired skin integrity related to alterations in nutritional state, circulation, sensation, or mobility

Psychosocially Related Diagnoses

■ Disturbed thought processes related to age-related changes that result in cerebral anoxia, evidenced by short-term memory loss, confusion, or disorientation.
■ Maladaptive grieving related to bereavement overload, evidenced by symptoms of depression
■ Risk for suicidal behavior related to depressed mood and feelings of low self-worth
■ Powerlessness related to a lifestyle of helplessness and dependency on others, evidenced by depressed mood, apathy, or verbal expressions of having no control or influence over life situation
■ Low self-esteem related to loss of preretirement status, evidenced by verbalization of negative feelings about self and life
■ Fear related to nursing home placement, evidenced by symptoms of severe anxiety and statements such as, "Nursing homes are places to go to die"
■ Disturbed body image related to age-related changes in skin, hair, and fat distribution, evidenced by verbalization of negative feelings about body
■ Ineffective sexuality pattern related to pain associated with vaginal dryness, evidenced by reported dissatisfaction with a decrease in frequency of sexual intercourse
■ Sexual dysfunction related to medications (e.g., antihypertensives) evidenced by erectile dysfunction
■ Social isolation related to total dependence on others, evidenced by expression of inadequacy in or absence of significant purpose in life
■ Risk for trauma (elder abuse) related to caregiver role strain

■ Caregiver role strain related to severity and duration of the care receiver's illness; lack of respite and recreation for the caregiver, evidenced by feelings of stress in relationship with care receiver; feelings of depression and anger; or family conflict around issues of providing care

Outcome Criteria

The following criteria may be used for the measurement of outcomes in the care of the older adult patient.

The patient:

■ Has not experienced injury
■ Maintains reality orientation consistent with cognitive level of functioning
■ Manages own self-care with assistance
■ Expresses positive feelings about self, past accomplishments, and hope for the future
■ Compensates adaptively for diminished sensory perception

Caregivers:

■ Can problem solve effectively regarding care of the older adult
■ Demonstrate adaptive coping strategies for dealing with stress of caregiver role
■ Openly express feelings
■ Express desire to join a support group of other caregivers

Planning and Implementation

In Table 33–2, selected nursing diagnoses are presented for the older adult patient. Outcome criteria are included, along with appropriate nursing interventions and rationale for each.

Reminiscence therapy is especially helpful with this population. This therapeutic intervention is highlighted in Box 33–2.

Evaluation

Reassessment is conducted to determine whether the nursing actions have been successful in achieving the objectives of care. Evaluation of nursing actions for the older adult patient may be facilitated by gathering information using the following types of questions:

Has the patient:

■ Avoided injury from falls, burns, or other means to which they are vulnerable because of age?
■ Maintained reality orientation at an optimum for their cognitive functioning?
■ Distinguished between reality-based and non–reality-based thinking?

Text continued on page 781

Table 33–2 | CARE PLAN FOR THE OLDER ADULT PATIENT

NURSING DIAGNOSIS: RISK FOR TRAUMA

RELATED TO: Confusion, disorientation, muscular weakness, spontaneous fractures, falls

OUTCOME CRITERIA	NURSING INTERVENTIONS	RATIONALE
Short-Term Goals: ■ Patient calls for assistance when ambulating or carrying out other activities. ■ Patient does not experience injury. Long-Term Goal: ■ Patient does not experience injury.	1. The following measures may be instituted: a. Arrange furniture and other items in the room to accommodate the patient's disabilities. b. Store frequently used items within easy access. c. Keep bed in unelevated position. Pad side rails and headboard if patient has history of seizures. Keep bed rails up when patient is in bed (if permitted by institutional policy). d. Assign room near nurses' station; observe frequently. e. Assist the patient with ambulation. f. Keep a dim light on at night. g. Frequently orient the patient to place, time, and situation.	1. To ensure patient safety.

NURSING DIAGNOSIS: DISTURBED THOUGHT PROCESSES

RELATED TO: Age-related changes that result in cerebral anoxia or other neurocognitive impairments

EVIDENCED BY: Short-term memory loss, confusion, or disorientation

OUTCOME CRITERIA	NURSING INTERVENTIONS	RATIONALE
Short-Term Goal: ■ Patient accepts explanations of inaccurate interpretations of the environment within (time to be determined based on patient condition). Long-Term Goal: ■ Patient interprets the environment accurately and maintains reality orientation to the best of their cognitive ability.	1. Frequently orient the patient to reality. Use clocks and calendars with large numbers that are easy to read. Notes and large, bold signs may be useful as reminders. Allow the patient to have personal belongings. 2. Keep explanations simple. Use face-to-face interaction. Speak slowly, and do not shout. 3. Discourage rumination on delusional thoughts. Talk about real events and real people.	1. To help maintain orientation and aid in memory and recognition. 2. To facilitate comprehension. Shouting may create discomfort and, in some instances, may provoke anger. 3. Rumination promotes disorientation. Reality orientation increases sense of self-worth and personal dignity.

Continued

Table 33–2 | CARE PLAN FOR THE OLDER ADULT PATIENT—cont'd

OUTCOME CRITERIA	NURSING INTERVENTIONS	RATIONALE
	4. Monitor for medication side effects.	4. Physiological changes in the older adult can alter the body's response to certain medications. Toxic effects may intensify altered thought processes.
	5. Conduct thorough physical assessment to rule out acute and reversible health problems.	5. Safety and early intervention for treatable health concerns that may be contributing to disturbed thought processes are a priority in caring for the older adult patient.

NURSING DIAGNOSIS: SELF-CARE DEFICIT (SPECIFY)

RELATED TO: Weakness, disorientation, confusion, or memory deficits

EVIDENCED BY: Inability to fulfill activities of daily living (ADLs)

OUTCOME CRITERIA	NURSING INTERVENTIONS	RATIONALE
Short-Term Goal: ■ Patient participates in ADLs with assistance from caregiver. Long-Term Goals: ■ Patient accomplishes ADLs to the best of their ability. ■ Unfulfilled needs are met by caregivers.	1. Provide a simple, structured environment: a. Identify self-care deficits and provide assistance as required. Promote independent actions as able. b. Allow plenty of time for the patient to perform tasks. c. Provide guidance and support for independent actions by talking the patient through the task one step at a time. d. Provide a structured schedule of activities that does not change from day to day. e. ADLs should follow home routine as closely as possible. f. Allow consistency in assignment of daily caregivers.	1. To minimize confusion.

NURSING DIAGNOSIS: CAREGIVER ROLE STRAIN

RELATED TO: Severity and duration of the care receiver's illness; lack of respite and recreation for the caregiver

EVIDENCED BY: Feelings of stress in relationship with care receiver; feelings of depression and anger; family conflict around issues of providing care

OUTCOME CRITERIA	NURSING INTERVENTIONS	RATIONALE
Short-Term Goal: ■ Caregivers verbalize understanding of ways to facilitate the caregiver role.	1. Assess prospective caregivers' ability to anticipate and fulfill the patient's unmet needs. Provide information to assist caregivers	1. Caregivers require relief from the pressures and strain of providing 24-hour care for their loved one. Studies have

Table 33–2 | CARE PLAN FOR THE OLDER ADULT PATIENT—cont'd

OUTCOME CRITERIA	NURSING INTERVENTIONS	RATIONALE
Long-Term Goal: ■ Caregivers achieve effective problem-solving skills and develop adaptive coping mechanisms to regain equilibrium.	with this responsibility. Ensure that caregivers are aware of available community support systems from which they can seek assistance when required. Examples include adult day-care centers, housekeeping and homemaker services, respite care services, or a local chapter of the Alzheimer's Association. This organization sponsors a nationwide 24-hour hotline to provide information and link families who need assistance with nearby chapters and affiliates: 800-272-3900.	shown that elder abuse may arise from caregiving situations in which the caregiver feels overwhelmed.
	2. Encourage caregivers to express feelings, particularly anger.	2. Release of these emotions can serve to prevent psychopathology, such as depression or psychophysiological disorders, from occurring.
	3. Encourage participation in support groups composed of members with similar life situations.	3. Hearing others who are experiencing the same problems discuss ways in which they have coped may help caregiver adopt adaptive strategies. Individuals with similar life experiences provide empathy and support for each other.

NURSING DIAGNOSIS: LOW SELF-ESTEEM

RELATED TO: Loss of preretirement status; early stages of cognitive decline

EVIDENCED BY: Verbalization of negative feelings about self and life

OUTCOME CRITERIA	NURSING INTERVENTIONS	RATIONALE
Short-Term Goal: ■ Patient verbalizes positive aspects of self and past accomplishments. **Long-Term Goal:** ■ Patient participates in group activities in which they can experience a feeling of enjoyment and accomplishment (to the best of their ability).	1. Encourage the patient to express honest feelings in relation to loss of prior status. Acknowledge pain of loss. Support the patient through process of grieving. Assess for depression and warning signs of risk for suicide.	1. The patient may be fixed in anger stage of grieving process, which is turned inward on the self, resulting in diminished self-esteem.

Continued

Table 33–2 | CARE PLAN FOR THE OLDER ADULT PATIENT—cont'd

OUTCOME CRITERIA	NURSING INTERVENTIONS	RATIONALE
	2. If lapses in memory are occurring, devise methods for assisting the patient with memory deficit. Examples: a. Name sign on door identifying the patient's room b. Identifying sign on outside of dining room door c. Identifying sign on outside of restroom door d. Large clock, with oversized numbers and hands, appropriately placed e. Large calendar, indicating 1 day at a time, with month, day, and year in bold print f. Printed, structured daily schedule, with one copy for the patient and one posted on unit wall g. "News board" on unit wall where current news of national and local interest may be posted	2. These aids may assist the patient to function more independently, thereby increasing self-esteem.
	3. Encourage the patient's attempts to communicate. If verbalizations are not understandable, express to the patient what you think they intended to say. It may be necessary to reorient the patient frequently.	3. The ability to communicate effectively with others may enhance self-esteem.
	4. Encourage reminiscence and discussion of life events (see Box 33–2). Sharing picture albums, if possible, is especially good. Also discuss present-day events.	4. Reminiscence and life review help the patient resume progression through the grief process associated with disappointing life events and increase self-esteem as successes are reviewed.
	5. Encourage participation in group activities. May need to accompany the patient at first until they feel secure that the group members will be accepting, regardless of limitations in verbal communication.	5. Positive feedback from group members increases self-esteem.

Table 33–2 | CARE PLAN FOR THE OLDER ADULT PATIENT—cont'd

OUTCOME CRITERIA	NURSING INTERVENTIONS	RATIONALE
	6. Encourage the patient to be as independent as possible in self-care activities. Provide written schedule of tasks to be performed. Intervene in areas where the patient requires assistance.	6. The ability to perform independently preserves self-esteem.

NURSING DIAGNOSIS: DISTURBED SENSORY PERCEPTION

RELATED TO: Age-related alterations in sensory transmission

EVIDENCED BY: Decreased visual acuity, hearing loss, diminished sensitivity to taste and smell, and increased touch threshold

OUTCOME CRITERIA	NURSING INTERVENTIONS*	RATIONALE

Short-Term Goal:
■ Patient does not experience injury due to diminished sensory perception.
Long-Term Goals:
■ Patient attains optimal level of sensory stimulation.
■ Patient does not experience injury due to diminished sensory perception.
	1. The following nursing strategies are indicated:
	  a. Provide meaningful sensory stimulation to all special senses through conversation, touch, music, or pleasant smells.
	  b. Encourage wearing of glasses, hearing aids, prostheses, and other adaptive devices.
	  c. Use bright, contrasting colors in the environment.
	  d. Provide large-print reading materials, such as books, clocks, calendars, and educational materials.
	  e. Maintain room lighting that distinguishes day from night and that is free of shadows and glare.
	  f. Teach the patient to scan the environment to locate objects.
	  g. Help the patient to locate food on plate using "clock" system and describe food if the patient is unable to visualize; assist with feeding as needed.
	  h. Arrange physical environment to maximize functional vision.
		1. To assist the patient with diminished sensory perception and because patient safety is a nursing priority.

Continued

Table 33–2 | CARE PLAN FOR THE OLDER ADULT PATIENT—cont'd

OUTCOME CRITERIA	NURSING INTERVENTIONS*	RATIONALE
	i. Place personal items and call light within the patient's field of vision.	
	j. Teach the patient to watch the person who is speaking.	
	k. Reinforce wearing of hearing aid; if the patient does not have an aid, may consider a communication device (e.g., amplifier).	
	l. Communicate clearly, distinctly, and slowly, using a low-pitched voice and facing the patient; avoid over-articulating.	
	m. Remove as much unnecessary background noise as possible.	
	n. Do not use slang or extraneous words.	
	o. As speaker, position self at eye level and no farther than 6 feet away.	
	p. Get the patient's attention before speaking.	
	q. Avoid speaking directly into the patient's ear.	
	r. If the patient does not understand what is being said, rephrase the statement rather than simply repeating it.	
	s. Help the patient select foods from the menu that will ensure discrimination between various tastes and smells.	
	t. Ensure that food has been properly cooled so that the patient with diminished pain threshold is not burned.	
	u. Ensure that bath or shower water is appropriate temperature.	
	v. Use backrubs and massage as therapeutic touch to stimulate sensory receptors.	

*The interventions for this nursing diagnosis were adapted from Rogers-Seidl, F. F. (1997). *Geriatric nursing care plans* (2nd ed.). Mosby.

BOX 33–2 Reminiscence Therapy With the Elderly

Studies have indicated that **reminiscence therapy**, defined as thinking about the past and reflecting on it, may promote better mental health in old age. Older individuals who spend time thinking about the past experience an increase in self-esteem and are less likely to suffer depression. Some psychologists believe that life review may help some people adjust to memories of an unhappy past. Others view reminiscence and life review as ways to bolster feelings of well-being, particularly in older people who can no longer remain active.

Reminiscence therapy can take place on a one-to-one basis or in a group setting. In reminiscence groups, older individuals share significant past events with peers. The nurse leader facilitates the discussion of topics that deal with specific life transitions, such as childhood, adolescence, marriage, childbearing, grandparenthood, and retirement. Members share both positive and negative aspects, including personal feelings, about these life cycle events.

Reminiscence on a one-to-one basis can provide a way for older adults to work through unresolved issues from the past. Painful issues may be too difficult to discuss in the group setting. As the individual reviews their life process, the nurse can validate feelings and help the older client come to terms with painful issues that may have been long suppressed. This process is necessary if the individual is to maintain (or attain) a sense of positive identity and self-esteem and ultimately achieve the goal of ego integrity as described by Erikson (1963).

A number of creative measures can be used to facilitate reminiscing with the older individual. Having the client keep a journal for sharing may be a way to stimulate discussion (as well as providing a permanent record of past events for significant others). Pets, music, and special foods have a way of provoking memories from the client's past. Showing the client photographs of family members and past significant events is an excellent way of guiding the older adult client to review life events.

Care must be taken in the reviewing of life events to assist clients to work through unresolved issues. Anxiety, guilt, depression, and despair may result if the individual is unable to work through the problems and accept them. Life review can work in a negative way if the individual maintains a negative or hopeless outlook. However, it can be a very positive experience for the person who can recognize past accomplishments and feel satisfied with their life, resulting in a sense of serenity and inner peace in the older adult.

■ Accomplished self-care activities independently to their optimum level of functioning?

■ Sought assistance for aspects of self-care that they are unable to perform independently?

■ Expressed positive feelings about themselves?

■ Reminisced about accomplishments that have occurred in their life?

■ Expressed some hope for the future?

■ Used eyeglasses or a hearing aid if needed to compensate for sensory deficits?

■ Consistently looks others in the face to facilitate hearing?

■ Used helpful aids, such as signs identifying various rooms, to help maintain orientation?

Have the caregivers:

■ Verbalized the means to provide a safe environment for the patient?

■ Verbalized strategies for reality orientation, if needed?

■ Worked through problems and made decisions regarding care of the older adult?

■ Included the older adult family member in the decision-making process, if appropriate?

■ Demonstrated adaptive coping strategies for dealing with the strain of long-term caregiving?

■ Been open and honest in expression of feelings?

■ Verbalized community resources to which they can go for assistance with their caregiving responsibilities?

■ Joined a support group?

Summary and Key Points

■ Care of the aging individual presents one of the greatest challenges for nursing.

■ The growing population of individuals age 65 and older suggests that the trend will progress well into the 21st century.

■ A growing number of older adults are living independently in residential communities designed specifically for them.

■ America is a youth-oriented society and, as such, older adults may be at risk for being stigmatized.

■ In some cultures, the elderly are revered and hold a special place of honor within the society, but in highly industrialized countries such as the United States, status declines with the decrease in productivity and participation in the mainstream of society.

■ Individuals experience many changes as they age. Physical changes occur in virtually every body system. Changes in liver function are relevant because they can influence how readily substances are metabolized and excreted. This is an important consideration when evaluating and managing medication use with the older adult.

■ Cognitively, there may be age-related, short-term memory deficits.

■ Intellectual functioning does not decline with age, but the length of time required for learning increases.

■ Aging individuals experience many losses, potentially leading to bereavement overload. They are vulnerable to depression and feelings of low self-worth.

■ The older adult population, especially white males 65 years and older, represents a disproportionately high percentage of individuals who die by suicide.

■ Neurocognitive disorders (dementias), depression, and anxiety are the most common psychiatric disorders in older adults. Sleep disorders are also very common.

■ The need for sexual expression among older adults is often misunderstood. Although many physical changes occur at this time of life that alter an individual's sexuality, if people have reasonably good health and a willing partner, sexual activity can continue well past the 70s for most people.

■ Retirement has both social and economic implications for elderly individuals. Society often equates an individual's status with an occupation, and loss of employment may result in the need for adjustment in the standard of living because retirement income may be reduced by 20% to 40% of preretirement earnings.

■ A relatively small number of older adults reside in long-term care facilities in the United States, but the number rises rapidly from 1% (in those ages 65 to 74 years) to 8% in those age 85 years and older (AoA, 2021).

■ The strain of the caregiver role has become a major dilemma in our society. Elder abuse is sometimes inflicted by caregivers for whom the role has become overwhelming and intolerable. There is an intense need to find assistance for these people, who must provide care for their loved ones on a 24-hour basis. Home health care, respite care, support groups, and financial assistance are needed to ease the burden of this role strain.

■ Caring for older adults requires a special kind of inner strength and compassion. The poem that follows conveys a vital message for nurses.

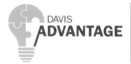 Go to **Davis Advantage** to complete your learning: strengthen understanding, apply your knowledge, and prepare for the Next Gen NCLEX®.

What Do You See, Nurse?

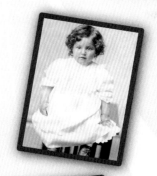

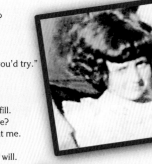

What do you see, nurse, what do you see?
 What are you thinking when you look at me?
A crabbed old woman, not very wise.
 Uncertain of habit, with faraway eyes.
Who dribbles her food and makes no reply
 When you say in a loud voice, "I do wish you'd try."
Who seems not to notice the things that you do
 And forever is losing a stocking or shoe.
Who unresisting or not, lets you do as you will
 With bathing and feeding, the long day to fill.
Is that what you're thinking, is that what you see?
 Then open your eyes, you're not looking at me.
I'll tell you who I am as I sit there so still.
 As I move at your bidding, as I eat at your will.
I'm a small child of ten with a father and a mother,
 Brothers and sisters who love one another.

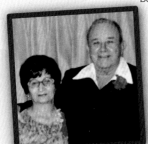

A young girl at sixteen with wings on her feet
 Dreaming that soon now a lover she'll meet.
A bride soon at twenty—my heart gives a leap
 Remembering the vows that I promised to keep.
At twenty-five, now, I have young of my own
 Who need me to build a secure happy home.
A woman of thirty, my young now grow fast
 Bound to each other with ties that should last.

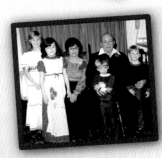

At forty my young will now soon be gone,
 But my man stays beside me to see I don't mourn.
At fifty once more babies play round my knee.
 Again we know children, my loved one and me.

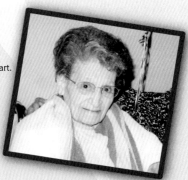

Dark days are upon me, my husband is dead.
 I look at the future, I shudder with dread.
For my young are all busy rearing young of their own.
 And I think of the years and the love I have known.

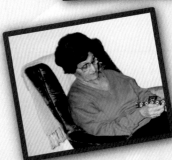

I'm an old woman now and nature is cruel.
 Tis her jest to make old age look like a fool.
The body it crumbles, grace and vigor depart.
 There is now just a stone where I once had a heart.
But inside this old carcass a young girl still dwells.
 And now and again my battered heart swells.

I remember the joys, I remember the pain.
 And I'm loving and living life all over again.
I think of the years all too few—gone so fast.
 And accept the stark fact that nothing can last.
So open your eyes, nurse, open and see.
 Not a crabbed old woman—look closer—SEE ME.

Author Unknown

Review Questions

1. During the admission assessment for a 72-year-old client the nurse notices an open sore on the client's arm. When questioned, the client says "I scraped it on the fence 2 weeks ago. It's smaller than it was." Which of the following is the best interpretation of this finding?
   a. Lower testosterone levels in older adults result in injury-prone skin.
   b. Confusion is common in the elderly, so the client probably doesn't remember how long ago the injury occurred.
   c. A diminished inflammatory response in older adults increases healing time.
   d. The supply of blood vessels to the skin increases with age and delays healing time.

2. What is the most appropriate way to communicate with an older person who is hard of hearing in their right ear?
   a. Speak loudly into their left ear.
   b. Speak to them from a position on their left side.
   c. Speak face-to-face in a high-pitched voice.
   d. Speak face-to-face in a low-pitched voice.

3. Which of the following factors are most associated with mental health in older adults?
   a. Pureed foods and warm beverages
   b. Physical activity and socialization
   c. Moderate alcohol and lower calorie intake
   d. Living alone and adhering to antidepressant medications

4. In a group for physical exercise, a 79-year-old client with major depression becomes tired and slightly short of breath. This symptom is most likely due to which of the following causes?
   a. Age-related changes in the cardiovascular system
   b. Anxiety
   c. The effects of pathological depression
   d. Medication the physician has prescribed for depression

5. The developmental task of transcendence suggests that mental health in older adulthood is contingent upon:
   a. Being able to ignore the stigmas associated with being elderly.
   b. Developing the ability to be alone.
   c. Transcending physical limitations imposed by age-related changes in the body.
   d. Having a sense of meaning in life and a sense of satisfaction.

Clinical Judgment Questions

6. A client, age 79, is admitted to the psychiatric unit for depression. He has lost weight and become socially isolated. His wife died 5 years ago, and his son tells the nurse, "He did very well when Mom died. He didn't even cry." Which would be the priority nursing diagnosis for Mr. B.?
   a. Maladaptive grieving
   b. Imbalanced nutrition: less than body requirements
   c. Social isolation
   d. Risk for injury

7. For the client identified in question #6, which would be the priority nursing intervention?
   a. Take blood pressure once each shift.
   b. Ensure that the client attends group activities.
   c. Encourage the client to eat all the food on his food tray.
   d. Encourage the client to talk about his wife's death.

8. A 75-year-old male client, who is taking an SSRI for depression, reports to the nurse that he recently began having erectile dysfunction. Which of these is the most appropriate action by the nurse?
   a. Set clear boundaries that this is not an appropriate topic to discuss with the nurse.
   b. Instruct the client that this is a potential side effect of his medication and ask if he would prefer to explore other treatment options.
   c. Educate the client that this is a normal age-related change and cannot be treated.
   d. Reinforce that this is a common symptom of depression and should subside after 4 to 6 weeks of antidepressant treatment.

9. An 80-year-old client says to the nurse, "I'm all alone now. My spouse is gone. My best friend is gone. My daughter is busy with her work and family. I might as well just go, too." Which is the best response by the nurse?
   a. "Are you having thoughts of wanting to hurt yourself or take your own life?"
   b. "You have lots to live for, but we need to talk to your daughter about her priorities."
   c. "It's hard getting old."
   d. "Tell me about your family."

10. An older adult client with depression says to the nurse, "I don't want to go to that crafts class. I'm too old to learn anything." Which of these is the most appropriate action by the nurse at this point?
    a. Tell the client that groups are mandatory and escort them by the hand.
    b. Pat the client on the shoulder and empathize about how annoying it is to get old.
    c. Educate the client that people don't typically lose the ability to learn as they age and encourage them to express their thoughts and feelings associated with aging.
    d. Assess the client for suicide risks and warning signs.

IMPLICATIONS OF RESEARCH FOR EVIDENCE-BASED PRACTICE

Estebsari, F., Dastoorpoor, M., Khalifehkandi, Z. R., Nouri, A., Mostafaei, D., Hosseini, M., Esmaeili, R., & Aghababaeian, H. (2020). The concept of successful aging: A review article. *Current Aging Science, 13*(1), 4–10. https://doi.org/10.2 174/1874609812666191023130117

DESCRIPTION OF THE STUDY: The authors sought to review the literature on successful aging to better explain this phenomenon. Twenty-seven articles met the quality criteria for inclusion in this review.

RESULTS OF THE STUDY: Definitions of successful aging covered a range of criteria depending on the article. The authors concluded that "successful aging" does not follow a universal standard and the concept depends on the cultural context of the community. The most common factors influencing successful aging were physical activity level, social interactions, and attitudes of the individual.

IMPLICATIONS FOR NURSING PRACTICE: The authors note that older adults need information, support, and encouragement to be empowered for successful aging. Nurses can play a key role in providing education about these principles. Discussing with older adults the importance of physical activity and social connection and assisting them to explore their personal attitudes about aging provides a framework for offering support and resources to promote successful aging.

TEST YOUR CLINICAL REASONING AND CLINICAL JUDGMENT SKILLS

Mrs. M., age 76, is seeing her primary physician for her regular 6-month physical examination. Mrs. M.'s husband died 2 years ago, at which time she sold her home in Kansas and came to live in California with her only child, a daughter. The daughter is married and has three children (one in college and two teenagers at home). The daughter reports that her mother is becoming increasingly withdrawn, stays in her room, and eats very little. She has lost 13 pounds since her last 6-month visit. The primary physician refers Mrs. M. to a psychiatrist, who hospitalizes her for evaluation. He diagnoses Mrs. M. with major depressive disorder.

Mrs. M. tells the nurse, "I didn't want to leave my home, but my daughter insisted. I would have been all right. I miss my friends and my church. Back home I drove my car everywhere. But there's too much traffic out here. They sold my car, and I have to depend on my daughter or grandkids to take me places. I hate being so dependent! I miss my husband so much. I just sit and think about him and our past life all the time. I don't have any interest in meeting new people. I want to go home!"

Mrs. M. admits to having some thoughts of dying, although she denies feeling suicidal. She denies having a plan or means for taking her life. "I really don't want to die, but I just can't see much reason for living. My daughter and her family are so busy with their own lives. They don't need me—or even have time for me!"

Answer the following questions about Mrs. M.:

1. What would be the *primary* nursing diagnosis for Mrs. M.?
2. Formulate a short-term goal for Mrs. M.
3. From the assessment data, identify the major problem that may be a long-term focus of care for Mrs. M.

 MOVIE CONNECTIONS

The Hiding Place (loss and grief, transcendence) • *On Golden Pond* (dementia) • *To Dance With the White Dog* (loss and grief) • *5 Flights Up* (aging, resilience) • *Still Alice* (Alzheimer's disease) • *The Second Best Exotic Marigold Hotel* (aging, resilience) • *A Man Called Ove* (depression, suicidal behavior) • *The Truth* (aging) • *Tea With the Dames* (reminiscence)

References

Administration on Aging (AoA). (2021). *2020 profile of older Americans.* https://acl.gov/sites/default/files/Profile%20 of%20OA/2020ProfileOlderAmericans_RevisedFinal.pdf

American Association of Colleges of Nursing (AACN). (2020). *The future of the nursing workforce in the United States: Data, trends and implications.* http://www.aacnnursing.org/News-Information/Nursing-Shortage-Resources

American Urological Association. (2022). *How to keep your prostate happy.* https://www.urologyhealth.org/healthy-living/care-blog/how-to-keep-your-prostate-happy

Aschenbrenner, A. J., Petros, J., McDade, E., Wang, G., Balota, D. A., Benzinger, T. L. S., Cruchaga, C., Goate, A., Xiong, C.,

Perrin, R., Fagan, A.M., Graff-Radford, N., Ghetti, B., Levin, J., Weidinger, E., Schofield, P., Gräber, S., Lee, J. H., Chhatwal, J. P.,...Hassenstab, J. for the Dominantly Inherited Alzheimer Network. (2020). Relationships between big-five personality factors and Alzheimer's disease pathology in autosomal dominant Alzheimer's disease. *Alzheimer's and Dementia Diagnosis, Assessment & Disease Monitoring, 12*(1), e12038. https://doi.org/10.1002/dad2.12038

Bell, C. G., Lowe, R., Adams, P. D., Baccarelli, A. A., Beck, S., Bell, J. T., Christensen, B. C., Gladyshev, V. N., Heijmans, B. T., Horvath, S., Ideker, T, Issa, J. J., Kelsey, K. T., Marioni, R. E., Reik, W., Relton, C. L., Schalkwyk, L. C., Teschendorff, A. E., Wagner, W., ... Rakyan, V. K. (2019). DNA methylation aging clocks: challenges and recommendations. *Genome Biology 20,* 249. https://doi.org/10.1186/s13059-019-1824-y

Blevins, N. H. (2022). *Presbycusis.* http://www.uptodate.com/contents/presbycusis

Boland, R., & Verduin, M. L. (Eds.). (2022). *Kaplan & Sadock's synopsis of psychiatry* (12th ed.). Wolters Kluwer.

Celano, C. M., Daunis, D. J., Lokko, H. N., Campbell, K. A., & Huffman, J. C. (2016). Anxiety disorders and cardiovascular disease. *Current Psychiatry Reports, 18*(11), 101. https://doi.org/10.1007/s11920-016-0739-5

Centers for Disease Control and Prevention. (2021). *Depression is not a normal part of growing older.* www.cdc.gov/aging/mentalhealth/depression.htm

Chen, J., Zheng, K., Xia, W., Wang, Q., Liao, Z., & Zheng, Y. (2018). Does inside equal outside? Relations between older adults' implicit and explicit aging attitudes and self-esteem. *Frontiers in Psychology, 9,* 2313. doi:10.3389/fpsyg.2018.02313

Cleland, C., Pipingas, A., Sholey, A., & White, D. (2019). Neurochemical changes in the aging brain: A systematic review. *Neuroscience & Biobehavioral Reviews, 98,* 306–316. https://doi.org/10.1016/j.neubiorev.2019.01.003

Dean, W. (2021). *Neuroendocrine theory of aging: Chapter 1.* https://warddeanmd.com/articles/neuroendocrine-theory-of-aging-chapter-1/

Estebsari, F., Dastoorpoor, M., Khalifehkandi, Z. R., Nouri, A., Mostafaei, D., Hosseini, M., Esmaeili, R., & Aghababaeian, H. (2020). The concept of successful aging: A review article. *Current Aging Science, 13*(1), 4–10. https://doi.org/10.2174/1874609812666191023130117

Global Burden of Disease (GBD) 2019 Dementia Forecasting Collaborators. (2022). Estimation of the global prevalence of dementia in 2019 and forecasted prevalence in 2050: an analysis for the Global Burden of Disease Study 2019. *Lancet Public Health, 7,* e105–125. https://doi.org/10.1016/S2468-2667(21)00249-8

Grossman, C. H., Brooker, J., Michael, N., & Kissane, D. (2018). Death anxiety interventions in patients with advanced cancer: A systematic review. *Palliative Medicine, 32,* 172–184.

Hudson, N. W. (2021). Does successfully changing personality traits via intervention require that participants be autonomously motivated to change? *Journal of Research in Personality, 95,* 104160. https://doi.org/10.1016/j.jrp.2021.104160

Karlsen, H. R., Matejschek, F., Saksvik-Lehouillier, I., & Langvik, E. (2021) Anxiety as a risk factor for cardiovascular disease independent of depression: A narrative review of current status and conflicting findings. *Health Psychology Open.* doi:10.1177/2055102920987462

Kruse, A., & Schmitt, E. (2019). Spirituality and transcendence. In R. Fernández-Ballesteros, A. Benetos, & J. Robine (Eds.), *The Cambridge handbook of successful aging* (Cambridge Handbooks in Psychology, pp. 426–454). Cambridge University Press. doi:10.1017/9781316677018.025

Lee, D. M., Nazroo, J., O'Connor, D. B., Blake, M., & Pendleton, N. (2016). Sexual health and well-being among older men and women in England: Findings from the English longitudinal study of ageing. *Archives of Sexual Behavior, 45*(1), 133–144. https://doi.org/10.1007/s10508-014-0465-1

Livingston, G., Huntley, J., Sommerlad, A., Ames, D., Ballard, C., Banerjee, S., Brayne, C., Burns, A., Cohen-Mansfield, J., Cooper, C., Costafreda, S. G., Dias, A., Fox, N., Gitlin, L. N., Howard, R., Kales, H. C., Kivimäki, M., Larson, E. B., Ogunniyi, A.,... Mukadam N. (2020). Dementia prevention, intervention, and care: 2020 report of the Lancet Commission. *Lancet, 396*(10248), 413–446. doi:10.1016/S0140-6736(20)30367-6

Luo, M., Ding, D., Bauman, A., Negin, J., & Phongsavan, P. (2020). Social engagement pattern, health behaviors and subjective well-being of older adults: An international perspective using WHO-SAGE survey data. *BMC Public Health 20,* 99. https://doi.org/10.1186/s12889-019-7841-7

May, H. T., Horne, B. D., Knight, S., Knowlton, K. U., Bair, T. L., Lappé, D. L., Le, V. T., & Muhlestein, J. B. (2017). The association of depression at any time to the risk of death following coronary artery disease diagnosis. *European Heart Journal— Quality of Care and Clinical Outcomes, 3*(4), 296–302, https://doi.org/10.1093/ehjqcco/qcx017

McCarthy, V. L., & Bockweg, M. (2012). The role of transcendence in a holistic view of successful aging: A concept analysis and model of transcendence in maturation and aging. *Journal of Holistic Nursing, 31*(2), 84–92. doi:10.1177/0898010112463492

McCarthy, V. L., Ling, J., & Carini, R. M. (2013). The role of self-transcendence: A missing variable in the pursuit of successful aging? *Research in Gerontological Nursing, 6*(3), 178–186. doi:10.3928/19404921-20130508-01

Menzies, R. E., & Menzies, R. G. (2018). Death anxiety. The worm at the core of mental health. *InPsych, 40*(6). https://psychology.org.au/for-members/publications/inpsych/2018/december-issue-6/death-anxiety-the-worm-at-the-core-of-mental-heal

Myhre, J. W., Mehl, M. R., & Glisky, E. L. (2017). Cognitive benefits of online social networking for healthy older adults. *The Journals of Gerontology: Series B, 72*(5), 752–760. https://doi.org/10.1093/geronb/gbw025

National Center for Health Statistics (NCHS). (2022). *Life expectancy.* https://www.cdc.gov/nchs/fastats/life-expectancy.htm

National Center on Elder Abuse (NCEA). (n.d.). *Research statistics and data.* https://ncea.acl.gov/What-We-Do/Research/Statistics-and-Data.aspx#prevalence

National Council on Aging (NCoA). (2021). Get the facts on elder abuse. https://www.ncoa.org/article/get-the-facts-on-elder-abuse

National Institutes of Health (NIH). (2022). *Aging changes in immunity.* https://www.nlm.nih.gov/medlineplus/ency/article/004008.htm

Neft, M. W., Oerther, S., Halloway, S., Hanneman, S. K., & Mitchell, A. M. (2019). Benzodiazepine and antipsychotic medication use in older adults. *Nursing Open, 7*(1), 4–6 https://doi.org/10.1002/nop2.425

News Medical. (2014). *Transcendence is the best predictor of positive aging, shows study.* https://www.news-medical.net/news/20140521/Transcendence-is-the-best-predictor-of-positive-aging-shows-study.aspx

Ormstad, H., Eilertsen, G., Heir, T., & Sandvik, L. (2020). Personality traits and the risk of becoming lonely in old age: A 5-year follow-up study. *Health and Quality of Life Outcomes 18,* 47. https://doi.org/10.1186/s12955-020-01303-5

Rogers, K., Simic, P., & Guarente, L. P. (2020). *Aging: Life process.* www.britannica.com/science/aging-life-process

Shock, N. W. (2020). *Human aging: Physiology and sociology.* www.britannica.com/science/human-aging

Smith, L., Yang, L., Veronese, N., Soysal, P., Stubbs, B., & Jackson, S. E. (2019). Sexual activity is associated with greater enjoyment of life in older adults. *Sexual Medicine, 7*(1), 11–18. doi:10.1016/j.esxm.2018.11.001

Srivastava, S., & Das, R. C. (2013). Personality pathways of successful ageing. *Industrial Psychiatry Journal, 22*(1), 1–3. doi:10.4103/0972-6748.123584

Steppe, J., Ramos, M. D., & Falvai, R. (2022). The role of social engagement in older adults' health. *Research in Gerontological Nursing, 15*(3). https://doi.org/10.3928/19404921-20220324-01

Sullivan, S., & Ariss, A. A. (2018). Employment after retirement: A review and framework for future research. *Journal of Management, 45*(1), 262–284. https://doi.org/10.1177/0149206318810411

Sun, X., Tang, S., Miyawaki, C. E., Li, Y., Hou, T., & Liu, M. (2022). Longitudinal association between personality traits and homebound status in older adults: Results from the National Health and Aging Trends Study. *BMC Geriatrics 22*(9). https://doi.org/10.1186/s12877-022-02771-8

Sutin, A. R., Stephan, Y., & Terracciano, A. (2018). Facets of conscientiousness and risk of dementia. *Psychological Medicine, 48,* 974–982. https://doi.org/10.1017/S0033291717002306

University of Michigan. (2018). *National poll on healthy aging.* https://deepblue.lib.umich.edu/bitstream/handle/2027.42/143212/NPHA-Sexual-Health-Report_050118_final.pdf?sequence=1&isAllowed=y

Velten, J., & Margraf, J. (2017). Satisfaction guaranteed? How individual, partner, and relationship factors impact sexual satisfaction within partnerships. *PLoS One, 12*(2), e0172855. doi:10.1371/journal.pone.0172855

World Health Organization (WHO). (2017). *Mental health of older adults.* https://www.who.int/en/news-room/fact-sheets/detail/mental-health-of-older-adults

World Health Organization (WHO). (2022). *WHO Director-General's opening remarks at mental health side event, Commonwealth Heads of Government Meeting, Rwanda—22 June 2022.* https://www.who.int/director-general/speeches/detail/who-director-general-s-opening-remarks-at-mental-health-side-event—commonwealth-heads-of-government-meeting—rwanda—22-june-2022

Wrigglesworth, J., Ward, P., Harding, I. H., Nilaweera, D., Wu, Z., Woods, R. L., & Ryan, J. (2021). Factors associated with brain ageing - a systematic review. *BMC Neurology 21,* 312. https://doi.org/10.1186/s12883-021-02331-4

Yoneda, T., Graham, E., Lozinski, T., Bennett, D. A., Mroczek, D., Piccinin, A. M., Hofer, S. M., & Muniz-Terrera, G. (2022). Personality traits, cognitive states, and mortality in older adulthood. *Journal of Personality and Social Psychology.* doi:10.1037/pspp0000418

Zhang, J., Peng, J., Gao, P., Huang, H., Cao, Y., Zheng, L., & Miao, D. (2019). Relationship between meaning in life and death anxiety in the elderly: self-esteem as a mediator. *BMC Geriatrics, 19,* 308. https://doi.org/10.1186/s12877-019-1316-7

Classical References

Dilman, V. (1954). Data regarding the origin of climacteric and the role of age-associated "perestroika" in the elevation of blood pressure, blood cholesterol levels, and body weight (Master's thesis, Leningrad).

Erikson, E. H. (1963). *Childhood and society* (2nd ed.). WW Norton.

Erikson, E. H., & Erikson, J. M. (1997). *The life cycle completed: Extended version with new chapters on the ninth stage of development.* WW Norton.

Kübler-Ross, E. (1969). *On death and dying.* Macmillan.

Roberts, C. M. (1991). *How did I get here so fast?* Warner Books.

Rogers-Seidl, F. F. (1997). *Geriatric nursing care plans* (2nd ed.). Mosby.

Rowe, J. W., & Kahn, R. L. (1997). Successful aging. *Gerontology, 37*(4), 433–440. doi:10.1093/geront/37.4.433

34 Survivors of Abuse or Neglect

CORE CONCEPTS

Stress and Coping

Safety

Professionalism:
Nursing process in
the care of survivors
of abuse or neglect

Clinical Judgment

KEY TERMS

abuse	emotional neglect	retraumatization
acquaintance rape	expressed response pattern	safe houses or shelters
adverse childhood experiences (ACEs)	forensic nursing	sexual assault
	incest	sexual exploitation of a child
child abuse	intimate partner violence (IPV)	sexual violence
child sexual abuse		silent rape reaction
compounded rape reaction	marital rape	stalking
controlled response pattern	physical neglect	statutory rape
cycle of battering	physical violence	trauma-informed care
date rape	psychological aggression	
emotional abuse	rape trauma syndrome	

OBJECTIVES
After reading this chapter, the student will be able to:

1. Describe the epidemiology of intimate partner violence, child abuse, and sexual assault.
2. Discuss characteristics of victims and victimizers.
3. Identify predisposing factors to abusive behaviors.
4. Describe physical and psychological effects on the survivors of intimate partner violence, child abuse, and sexual assault.
5. Identify nursing diagnoses, goals of care, and appropriate nursing interventions for care of survivors of intimate partner violence, child abuse, and sexual assault.
6. Evaluate nursing care of survivors of intimate partner violence, child abuse, and sexual assault.
7. Define the terms *forensic* and *forensic nursing*
8. Discuss modalities relevant to the treatment of survivors of abuse.

CORE CONCEPT
Abuse
The maltreatment of one person by another.

Abuse (the maltreatment of one person by another) is a significant and frightening public health problem that can take many forms including physical violence, sexual violence, stalking, human trafficking, psychological aggression, and bullying.

Epidemiology

The Centers for Disease Control and Prevention (CDC, 2021c) identified that 1 in 5 women and 1 in 7 men report having experienced severe physical **intimate partner violence (IPV)** in their lifetime. In addition, 1 in 5 women and 1 in 12 men have experienced contact sexual violence from an intimate partner. United States crime reports found that 1 in 5 homicide victims were killed by an intimate partner and over 50% of all female homicide victims are killed by a current or former male intimate partner (CDC, 2021c). These forms of violence most often occur before the age of 25 for both men and women. Commonly experienced IPV-related issues, reported by both women and men, included concern for safety, being fearful, injury, post-traumatic stress disorder (PTSD) symptoms, and needing help from law enforcement.

Child abuse includes physical or sexual abuse, psychological maltreatment, and neglect. It is well documented that **adverse childhood experiences (ACEs)**, which includes trauma associated with abuse and neglect, can have a major impact on health and well-being throughout one's life. ACE studies have found that as the number of ACE events increases, so do risks for heart disease, asthma, diabetes, cancer, depression, anxiety, PTSD, disability, unemployment, sexually transmitted infections, and other health problems (CDC, 2021a). The effect of trauma on physical, mental, emotional, and spiritual health is one of the primary reasons that nurses must assess for history of trauma and provide trauma-informed care.

Data from the U.S. Department of Health and Human Services (2022) identified that, based on data from 2020, 76.1% of abused children are neglected, 16.5% are physically abused, 9.4% are sexually abused, and 0.2% are sex trafficked. Nationally, in 2020 an estimated 1,750 children died of abuse or neglect.

Sex trafficking is another form of child abuse that is a significant public health concern. Federal law defines sex trafficking as

"the recruitment, harboring, transportation, provision, obtaining, patronizing, or soliciting of a person for the purpose of a commercial sex act, in which the commercial sex act is induced by force, fraud, or coercion, or in which the person induced to perform such act has not attained 18 years of age" (U.S. Department of Health and Human Services, n.d.)

Prevalence statistics are difficult to compile, but the sex trafficking of children has been reported in all 50 U.S. states, and traffickers have been known to prey on children as young as 9 years of age.

Elder abuse and neglect are also significant problems. The CDC (2021b) estimated that 1 in 10 people age 60 and older and living at home is a victim of physical or sexual abuse, neglect (the most common form of elder abuse), abandonment, and/or financial exploitation. *Institutional abuse* refers to elder adults who live in residential facilities and are victimized by any of the previously mentioned forms of abuse. There is general agreement that these statistics underestimate the scope of the problem. Despite mandatory reporting laws in most states and the recent trend toward more reporting of abuse, adult protective services vary markedly among states. One study estimated that for every case that these agencies know about, 24 have not been reported (National Center on Elder Abuse [NCEA], n.d.).

Abuse affects all populations equally. It occurs among all races, religions, economic classes, ages, and educational backgrounds. Many abusers were themselves victims of abuse as children.

Family violence is not a new problem; in fact, it is probably as old as humankind and has been documented as far back as biblical times. Child abuse became a mandatory reportable occurrence in the United States in 1968. Responsibility for the protection of older individuals from abuse rests primarily with the states. In 1987 Congress passed amendments to the Older Americans Act of 1965 that provide for state Area Agencies on Aging to assess the need for elder abuse prevention services. These laws have made it possible for individuals who once felt powerless to stop the abuse against them to come forward and seek advice, support, and protection.

This chapter discusses IPV, child abuse (including neglect), and sexual violence. Elder abuse is discussed in more detail in Chapter 33, "The Aging Individual." Factors that predispose individuals to commit acts of abuse against others, as well as the physical and psychological effects on the survivors, are examined. Forensic nursing, a field of nursing that specializes in the care of patients who are or have been victims of violence, is discussed. Nursing of individuals who have experienced abusive behavior from others is presented within the context of the nursing process, and various treatment modalities are described.

Predisposing Factors

What predisposes individuals to be abusive? Although no one knows for sure, several theories have been proposed. As researchers have sought to better understand aggression and violence, two distinct forms of aggression have been identified: reactive aggression (*hot-blooded aggression*), which is associated with impulsivity in response to provocation, and proactive aggression (*cold-blooded aggression*), which is goal-directed, instrumental, and intentional aggression that is associated with antisocial behavior (Boccadoro et al., 2021). Most research is associated with reactive aggression. The following sections briefly discuss the current evidence associated with the biological, psychological, and sociocultural influences of aggression and abusive behavior.

Biological Theories
Neurophysiological Influences

Research demonstrates consistently that the volume of the lower amygdala plays a role in aggression (Cupaioli et al., 2021). The amygdala, which is responsible for impulse control and affective processing, appears to be less modulated in people with aggression, and responses to fear are reduced. The limbic prefrontal cortex also has a primary role in aggression; smaller volumes of left-sided gray matter and greater right-sided volume have been noted in people with aggressive traits. Evidence has also demonstrated that reduced connectivity between the amygdala and the prefrontal cortex is associated with increased aggression. The striatum, an area of the brain that plays a critical role in the selection and inhibition of affective, cognitive, and motor responses, has been identified as dysfunctional in aggressive individuals. In addition, gene-gene, gene-environment interactions, and variations in proteins regulating the synthesis, degradation, and transport of serotonin and dopamine as well as their signal transduction have been found to be associated with behavioral variability observed in aggression (Boccadoro et al., 2021). Boccadoro and associates (2021) also noted that a major difference between reactive aggression and proactive aggression is that in the former there is a high state of physiological arousal and in the latter there is low physiological arousal.

Biochemical Influences

Biochemical influences in aggression are numerous. It is likely that these are complex interactions between several hormones, neurotransmitters, and the environment. Studies have associated increased dopamine release with aggression, and low levels of striatal serotonin have been associated with increases in impulsivity and aggression (Boccadoro et al., 2021). The role of testosterone, which has been classically associated with aggression, may actually be better understood as a complex interaction with other hormones such as serotonin and cortisol. Finally, gamma-aminobutyric acid (GABA) and more than 20 peptide hormones have been implicated in various aspects of aggression. Research is ongoing to explore the mechanisms of these biochemicals and their interactions in the brain, as well as the role of environmental factors. An explanation of selected biochemical influences on violent behavior is presented in Figure 34–1.

Genetic Influences

A study by Zhang-James and colleagues (2019) identified that at least 40 genes are associated with aggression, suggesting that the genetics underlying aggression are quite complex. It has also been demonstrated that stressful life events can influence some gene variants in the development of aggressive tendencies. The heritability of aggression is estimated at around 50%. Zhang-James and associates (2019) added to their findings that aggression in attention deficit-hyperactivity disorder (ADHD) and in adults with major depression share common DNA variants, and the lack of genetic correlations of either dataset with schizophrenia, bipolar disorder, autism, or PTSD suggests that for these disorders, aggression may arise from different causal factors. They conclude that future studies are needed to fully address the genetic bases of the comorbidity between aggression and psychiatric disorders.

Disorders of the Brain

Organic brain syndromes associated with various cerebral disorders have been implicated in the predisposition to aggressive and violent behavior. Brain tumors, particularly in the areas of the limbic system and the temporal lobes; trauma to the brain, resulting in cerebral changes; and diseases, such as encephalitis (or medications that may affect this syndrome) and epilepsy, particularly temporal lobe epilepsy, have all been implicated.

Psychological Theories
Psychodynamic Theory

The psychodynamic theorists imply that unmet needs for satisfaction and security result in an underdeveloped ego and a weak superego. It is thought that when frustration occurs, aggression and violence supply this individual with a dose of power and prestige that boosts self-image and validates a significance to their life that is lacking. The immature ego cannot prevent dominant id

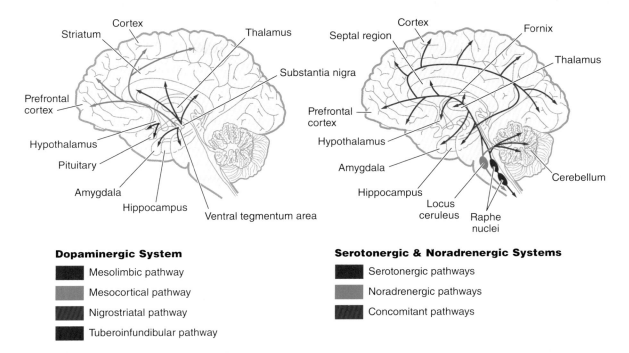

FIGURE 34-1   Neurobiology of violence.

NEUROTRANSMITTERS

Neurotransmitters that have been implicated in the etiology of aggression and violence include decreases in striatal serotonin and increases in norepinephrine and dopamine.

ASSOCIATED AREAS OF THE BRAIN

- Limbic structures: Emotional alterations
- Prefrontal and frontal cortices: Modulation of social judgment
- Amygdala: Anxiety, rage, fear
- Hypothalamus: Stimulates sympathetic nervous system in fight-or-flight response
- Hippocampus: Learning and memory

MEDICATIONS USED TO MODULATE AGGRESSION

1. Selective serotonin reuptake inhibitors (SSRIs) may reduce or increase irritability and aggression depending on the brain region measured and specific receptors where it acts. Catecholamines, gamma-aminobutyric acid (GABA), and glutamate modulate those effects.
2. Carbamazepine (Tegretol), phenytoin (Dilantin), and divalproex sodium (Depakote) have yielded positive results. Lithium has also been used effectively in violent individuals (Schatzberg et al., 2019).
3. Antiadrenergic agents such as beta blockers (e.g., propranolol) have been shown to reduce aggression in some individuals, presumably by dampening excessive noradrenergic activity (Schatzberg et al., 2019).
4. In their ability to modulate excessive dopaminergic activity, antipsychotics—both typical and atypical—have been helpful in the control of aggression and violence, particularly in individuals with comorbid psychosis.

behaviors from occurring, and the weak superego is unable to produce feelings of guilt.

Learning Theory

Children learn to behave by imitating their role models, usually their parents. Models are more likely to be imitated when they are perceived as prestigious or influential or when the behavior is followed by positive reinforcement. Children may have an idealistic perception of their parents during the very early developmental stages, but as they mature, they often begin to imitate the behavior patterns of their teachers, friends, and others. Individuals who were abused during childhood or who witnessed IPV as children are more likely to manifest reactive aggression as adults (Huecker et al., 2022).

Adults and children alike model many behaviors after individuals they observe on television and in movies. Unfortunately, modeling can result in maladaptive as well as adaptive behavior, particularly when children view heroes triumphing over villains by using violence. It is also possible that individuals who have a biological predisposition toward aggressive behavior may be more susceptible to negative role modeling.

Sociocultural Theories

Societal Influences

Although they agree that biological and psychological aspects are influential, social scientists believe that aggressive behavior is primarily a product of one's culture and social structure. Historically, American society has accepted some forms of aggression and violence as the means to solve problems (e.g., engaging in war, physical disciplining of children). However, there is widespread general acceptance that aggression or violence in certain situations is wrong (e.g., child abuse). The concept of relative deprivation has been shown to have a profound effect on collective violence within a society. Poverty, prolonged unemployment, family breakdown, emotional distress, lack of access to resources, and exposure to violence in the community and family have all been linked to increases in aggression (American Psychological Association [APA], 2022).

Application of the Nursing Process

Background Assessment Data

Data related to IPV, child abuse and neglect, and sexual assault are presented in this section. Characteristics of both victim and abuser are addressed. This information may be used as background knowledge in designing plans of care for these patients.

Intimate Partner Violence

> ## CORE CONCEPT
> **Battering**
> A pattern of coercive control founded on and supported by physical or sexual violence or threat of violence toward an intimate partner.

Various terms are used to describe the pattern of violence between intimate partners, including intimate partner violence, domestic violence, and battering. Tracy (2022) added to the definition of *battering* as follows:

> Battering is also known by the term "domestic violence" and refers to acts of violence between two parties in an intimate relationship. Battering

happens in heterosexual and homosexual relationships and either a male or a female can be the batterer or victim. Battering may occur in a marriage or in any other form of relationship.

The CDC (2021c) defined *intimate partner violence* as follows:

> Intimate partner violence (IPV) is abuse or aggression that occurs in a romantic relationship. "Intimate partner" refers to both current and former spouses and dating partners. IPV can vary in how often it happens and how severe it is. It can range from one episode of violence that could have lasting impact to chronic and severe episodes over multiple years. IPV can include any of the following types of behavior:

Physical violence is when a person hurts or tries to hurt a partner by hitting, kicking, or using another type of physical force.

Sexual violence is forcing or attempting to force a partner to take part in a sex act, sexual touching, or a nonphysical sexual event (e.g., sexting) when the partner does not or cannot consent.

Stalking is a pattern of repeated, unwanted attention and contact by a partner that causes fear or concern for one's own safety or the safety of someone close to the victim.

Psychological aggression is the use of verbal and nonverbal communication with the intent to harm another person mentally or emotionally and/or to exert control over another person.

The U.S. Department of Justice (n.d) defined *intimate partner violence* as follows:

> Domestic violence is a pattern of abusive behavior in any relationship that is used by one partner to gain or maintain power and control over another intimate partner. Domestic violence can be physical, sexual, emotional, economic, psychological, or technological actions or threats of actions or other patterns of coercive behavior that influence another person within an intimate partner relationship. This includes any behaviors that intimidate, manipulate, humiliate, isolate, frighten, terrorize, coerce, threaten, blame, hurt, injure, or wound someone.

According to the National Intimate Partner and Sexual Violence Survey (NISVS) (D'Inverno et al., 2019), an estimated 47% of men and women will be victims of psychological aggression in their lifetime; 32% of women will be victims of physical violence; 16% of women and 7% of men will be victims of contact sexual violence; and 9% of all homicides are committed by an intimate partner. Many of the victimizations are not reported to the police, and the main reason given for not reporting is that it is "considered a personal matter."

Profile of the Victim

For the purposes of this chapter, women are identified as the victim (and men as the victimizer) because the largest percentage of victims are women, and most of the available data speaks specifically about female victims. It should be noted that men may also be victims and victimized in similar ways. Likewise, female perpetrators of IPV may share many of the characteristics that are commonly identified as the profile of male victimizers.

Battered women represent all age, racial, religious, cultural, educational, and socioeconomic groups. They may be married or single, housewives or business executives. Many who are battered have low self-esteem, commonly adhere to feminine sex-role stereotypes, and often accept the blame for the batterer's actions. Feelings of guilt, anger, fear, and shame are common. They may be isolated from family and support systems.

Some women in violent relationships grew up in abusive homes and may have left those homes, sometimes to get married, at a very young age to escape the abuse. The battered woman views her relationship as male dominant, and as the battering continues, her ability to see the options available and make decisions concerning her life (and possibly those of her children) decreases. The phenomenon of *learned helplessness* may be applied to the woman's progressive inability to act on her own behalf. Learned helplessness occurs when an individual realizes that regardless of their behavior, the outcome is unpredictable and usually undesirable.

Profile of the Victimizer

Men who batter usually are characterized as persons with low self-esteem. Pathologically jealous, they present a "dual personality," one to the partner and one to the rest of the world. They are often under a great deal of stress with which they have a limited ability to cope. The typical abuser is very possessive and perceives his spouse as a possession. He becomes threatened when she shows any sign of independence or attempts to share herself and her time with others. Small children are often ignored by the abuser; however, they may also become the targets of abuse as they grow older, particularly if they attempt to protect their mother from abuse. The abuser also may use threats of taking the children away as a tactic of emotional abuse.

The perpetrator of abuse typically wages a continuous campaign of degradation against his partner. He insults and humiliates her and everything she does at every opportunity. He strives to keep her isolated from others and totally dependent on him. He demands to know where she is at every moment, and when she tells him, he challenges her honesty. He achieves power and control through intimidation.

The Cycle of Battering

In her classic studies of battered women and their relationships, Walker (1979) identified a **cycle of battering** as predictable behaviors that are repeated over time. The behaviors can be divided into three distinct phases that vary in time and intensity, both within the same relationship and among different couples. Figure 34–2 depicts a graphic representation of the cycle of battering.

Phase I. The Tension-Building Phase During this phase, the woman senses that the man's tolerance for frustration is declining. He becomes angry with little provocation, but after lashing out at her may be quick to apologize. The woman may become very nurturing and compliant, anticipating his every whim to prevent his anger from escalating. She may just try to stay out of his way.

Minor battering incidents may occur during this phase, and in a desperate effort to avoid more serious confrontations, the woman accepts the abuse as legitimately directed toward her. She denies her anger and rationalizes his behavior (e.g., "I need to do better," "He's under so much stress at work," "It's the alcohol. If only he didn't drink"). She assumes the guilt for the abuse, even reasoning that perhaps she *did* deserve the abuse, just as her aggressor suggests.

The minor battering incidents continue, and the tension mounts as the woman waits for the impending explosion. The abuser begins to fear that his partner will leave him. His jealousy and possessiveness increase, and he uses threats and

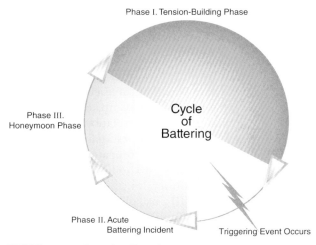

FIGURE 34–2 The cycle of battering.

brutality to keep her in his captivity. Battering incidents become more intense, after which the woman becomes less and less psychologically capable of restoring equilibrium. She withdraws from him, which he misinterprets as rejection, further escalating his anger toward her. Phase I may last from a few weeks to many months or even years.

Phase II. The Acute Battering Incident This phase is the most violent and the shortest, usually lasting up to 24 hours. It most often begins with the batterer justifying his behavior to himself. By the end of the incident, however, he cannot understand what has happened, only that in his rage, he has lost control over his behavior.

This incident may begin with the batterer wanting to "just teach her a lesson." In some instances, the woman may intentionally provoke the behavior. Having come to a point in phase I in which the tension is unbearable, long-term battered women know that once the acute phase is behind them, things will be better.

During phase II, women feel their only option is to find a safe place to hide from the batterer. Many women can describe the violence in great detail, almost as if dissociation from their bodies had occurred. The batterer generally minimizes the severity of the abuse. Help is usually sought only in the event of severe injury or if the woman fears for her life or the lives of her children.

Phase III. Calm, Loving, Respite ("Honeymoon") Phase In this phase, the batterer becomes extremely loving, kind, and contrite. He promises that the abuse will never recur and begs her forgiveness. He is afraid she will leave him and uses every bit of charm he can muster to ensure this does not happen. He believes he can now control his behavior, and because he has "taught her a lesson," he believes she will not "act up" again. He plays on her feelings of guilt, and she desperately wants to believe him. She wants to believe that he *can* change and that she will no longer have to suffer abuse. During this phase, the woman relives her original dream of ideal love and chooses to believe that *this* is what her partner is *really* like.

This loving phase becomes the focus of the woman's perception of the relationship. She bases her reason for remaining in the relationship on this "magical" ideal phase and hopes against hope that the previous phases will not be repeated. This hope is evident even in those women who have lived through a number of horrendous cycles.

Although phase III usually lasts somewhere between the lengths of time associated with phases I and II, it can be so short as to almost pass undetected. In most instances, the cycle soon begins again with renewed tensions and minor battering incidents. In an effort to "steal" a few precious moments of the phase III kind of love, the battered woman becomes a collaborator in her own abusive lifestyle. Victim and batterer become locked together in an intense, symbiotic relationship.

Why Do They Stay?

Probably the most common response that battered women give for staying is that they fear for their lives and the lives of their children. As the battering progresses, the man gains power and control through intimidation and fear, with threats such as, "I'll kill you and the kids if you try to leave." Challenged by these threats and compounded by her low self-esteem and sense of powerlessness, the woman sees no way out. In fact, she may try to leave, only to return when confronted by her partner and the psychological power he holds over her.

Victims have been known to stay in an abusive relationship for many reasons, some of which include the following:

■ **Fear of retaliation:** A woman may have been threatened with murder of herself and her children. Other perpetrator tactics include sleep deprivation, blackmail, and murdering pets. In the lesbian, gay, bisexual, and transgender community, fear of being outed is sometimes used to manipulate the victim.

■ **Fear of losing custody of children:** Women are sometimes threatened by the spouse or partner that they will take away the children. There may have been attempts to convince the woman that she is an unfit mother.

■ **Physical or financial dependence:** Victims may fear they are unable to care for themselves without the victimizer. Victims with disabilities may also be physically dependent on the victimizer for caregiving and physical support.

■ **Lack of a support network:** The victim may be under pressure from family members to stay in the marriage and try to work things out. In addition, the victimizer may have isolated the victim from family and friends.

■ **Fears about what others will think:** Cultural or religious convictions against divorce may dictate trying to save the marriage at all costs. The dual personality exhibited by perpetrators of abuse may lead the victim to think no one will believe them.

■ **Hopefulness:** The victim remembers good times and love in the relationship and has hope that her partner will change his behavior and they can have good times again.

■ **Lack of attention to the danger:** Low self-esteem may contribute to victim's belief that they are responsible for being abused and if they just change their behavior the abuse will stop. The honeymoon phase of the battering cycle provides reinforcement for the belief that it won't happen again. The dissociation that accompanies PTSD may contribute to the victim's numbness or lack of awareness of the reality of the situation. Or, as Leslie Morgan Steiner poignantly stated in a TED talk (cited by Dockterman, 2014):

Why did I stay? I didn't know he was abusing me. Even though he held those loaded guns to my head, pushed me down stairs, threatened to kill our dog, pulled the key out of the car ignition as I drove down the highway, poured coffee grinds on my head as I dressed for a job interview, I never once thought of myself as a battered wife. Instead I was a very strong woman in love with a deeply troubled man, and I was the only person on earth who could help [him] face his demons.

It is important to recognize that "75% of domestic violence–related homicides occur upon separation and there is a 75% increase of violence for at least 2 years" after the victim leaves an abusive relationship (Center for Relationship Abuse Awareness, 2022). Clients should be empowered to make that decision, informed of potential risks, and provided with resources and referrals to maximize their safety if they choose to leave, but the decision must be theirs to make.

Child Abuse

Erik Erikson (1963) stated, "The worst sin is the mutilation of a child's spirit." Children are vulnerable and relatively powerless, and the effects of maltreatment are infinitely deep and long-lasting. Federal law, through the Child Abuse Prevention and Treatment Act (CAPTA), identifies a minimum set of acts or behaviors that characterize child abuse or neglect. These include "any recent act or failure to act on the part of a parent or caretaker which results in death, serious physical or emotional harm, sexual abuse or exploitation, or an act or failure to act which presents an imminent risk of serious harm." In addition, "a child shall be considered a victim of 'child abuse and neglect' and of 'sexual abuse' if the child is identified, by a State or local agency employee of the State or locality involved, as being a victim of sex trafficking or a victim of severe forms of trafficking in persons" (Child Welfare Information Gateway [CWIG], 2019b). States may use these definitions as foundations on which to establish state legislation.

Physical Abuse

Physical abuse is "a nonaccidental physical injury to a child caused by a parent, caregiver, or other person responsible for a child and can include punching, beating, kicking, biting, shaking, throwing, stabbing, choking, hitting (with a hand, stick, strap, or other object), burning, or otherwise causing physical harm. Physical discipline, such as spanking or paddling, is not considered abuse as long as it is reasonable and causes no bodily injury to the child. Injuries from physical abuse could range from minor bruises to severe fractures or death" (CWIG, 2019b). Maltreatment is considered whether or not the caretaker intended to cause harm or even if the injury resulted from overzealous discipline or physical punishment. The most obvious way to detect this type of abuse is by outward physical signs. However, behavioral indicators also may be evident.

Signs of Physical Abuse Indicators of physical abuse may include any of the following (CWIG, 2019b). The child:

- Has unexplained burns, bites, bruises, broken bones, or black eyes
- Has fading bruises or other marks noticeable after an absence from school
- Seems frightened of the parents and protests or cries when it is time to go home
- Shrinks at the approach of adults
- Reports injury by a parent or another adult caregiver
- Abuses animals or pets

Physical abuse may be suspected when the parent or other adult caregiver (CWIG, 2019b):

- Offers conflicting, unconvincing, or no explanation for the child's injury
- Describes the child as "evil" or in some other very negative way
- Uses harsh physical discipline with the child
- Has a history of abuse as a child
- Has a history of abusing animals or pets

Emotional Abuse

Emotional abuse involves a pattern of behavior on the part of the parent or caretaker that results in serious impairment of the child's social, emotional, or intellectual functioning. Examples of emotional injury include belittling or rejecting the child, ignoring the child, blaming the child for things over which they have no control, isolating the child from normal social experiences, and using harsh and inconsistent discipline. Behavioral indicators of emotional maltreatment in the child may include the following (CWIG, 2019b):

- Extremes in behavior, such as overly compliant or demanding behavior, extreme passivity, or aggression
- Inappropriately adult (e.g., parenting other children) or inappropriately infantile (e.g., frequently rocking or head-banging) behavior

- Delays in physical or emotional development
- Shows signs of depression or suicidal thoughts (or attempts)
- Reports an inability to develop emotional bonds with others

Emotional abuse may be suspected when the parent or other adult caregiver (CWIG, 2019b):

- Constantly blames, belittles, or berates the child
- Is unconcerned about the child and refuses to consider offers of help for the child's problems
- Overtly rejects the child

Physical and Emotional Neglect

> ## CORE CONCEPT
> **Neglect**
> **Physical neglect** of a child includes refusal of or delay in seeking health care, abandonment, expulsion from the home or refusal to allow a runaway to return home, and inadequate supervision.
> **Emotional neglect** refers to a chronic failure by the parent or caretaker to provide the child with the hope, love, and support necessary for the development of a sound, healthy personality.

Indicators of Neglect The possibility of neglect may be considered when the child (CWIG, 2019b):

- Is frequently absent from school
- Begs or steals food or money
- Lacks needed medical or dental care, immunizations, or glasses
- Is consistently dirty and has severe body odor
- Lacks sufficient clothing for the weather
- Abuses alcohol or other drugs
- States that there is no one at home to provide care

The possibility of neglect may be considered when the parent or other adult caregiver (CWIG, 2019b):

- Appears to be indifferent to the child
- Seems apathetic or depressed
- Behaves irrationally or in a bizarre manner
- Is abusing alcohol or other drugs

Sexual Abuse of a Child

Various definitions of child sexual abuse are available in the literature. CAPTA defines *sexual abuse* as:

> Employment, use, persuasion, inducement, enticement, or coercion of any child to engage in, or assist any other person to engage in, any sexually explicit conduct or simulation of such conduct for the purpose of producing any visual depiction of such conduct; or the rape, and in cases of caretaker or interfamilial relationships, statutory rape, molestation, prostitution, or other form of sexual exploitation of children, or incest with children. (CWIG, 2019b)

Included in the definition is **sexual exploitation of a child,** in which a child is induced or coerced into engaging in sexually explicit conduct for the purpose of promoting any performance, and **child sexual abuse**, in which a child is being used for the sexual pleasure of an adult (parent or caretaker) or any other person.

Indicators of Sexual Abuse Child abuse may be considered a possibility when the child (CWIG, 2019b):

- Has difficulty walking or sitting
- Suddenly refuses to go to school
- Reports nightmares or bedwetting
- Experiences a sudden change in appetite
- Demonstrates bizarre, sophisticated, or unusual sexual knowledge or behavior
- Becomes pregnant or contracts a sexually transmitted disease, particularly if younger than age 14
- Runs away
- Reports sexual abuse by a parent or another adult caregiver
- Attaches very quickly to strangers or new adults in their environment

Sexual abuse may be considered a possibility when the parent or other adult caregiver (CWIG, 2019b; Rape, Abuse and Incest National Network [RAINN], 2022c):

- Is unduly protective of the child or severely limits the child's contact with other children, especially of the opposite sex
- Is secretive and isolated
- Does not respect boundaries or listen when someone tells them "no"
- Engages in touching that a child or child's parents/guardians have indicated is unwanted
- Tries to be a child's friend rather than filling an adult role in the child's life
- Does not seem to have age-appropriate relationships
- Makes up excuses to be alone with the child
- Expresses unusual interest in child's sexual development, such as commenting on sexual characteristics or sexualizing normal behaviors
- Gives gifts to a child without occasion or reason

Characteristics of the Abuser

A number of factors have been associated with adults who abuse or neglect their children. Parents who abuse their children were often victims of abuse in their own early lives and have impaired attachment with their child. Substance use disorders also increase the risk for child abuse and neglect.

Additional characteristics that may be associated with abusive parents include the following:

■ Repetitive shaming, blaming, or teasing in humiliating ways

■ Withholding care or demanding that a child earn the ability to have their basic needs met

■ Lacking adaptive coping strategies; angers easily; has difficulty trusting others

■ Expecting the child to be perfect or showing favoritism to siblings; exclusion or neglect

■ Overt or veiled threats of physical injury

Fingarson and associates (2019) found that the risks of child abuse were very high when the caregiver present was a nonbiological male, such as a mother's boyfriend. In addition, parents of children with disabilities or behavior problems who are ill-equipped to care for a child with complex needs may also pose a greater threat for child abuse. Maclean and associates (2017) found that 1 in 3 substantiated claims of maltreatment were among children with disabilities, particularly those with intellectual developmental disorders, mental/behavioral problems, and conduct disorder.

CORE CONCEPT

Incest

Incest is defined as the occurrence of sexual contacts or interaction between, or sexual exploitation of, close relatives, or between participants who are related to each other by a kinship bond that is regarded as a prohibition to sexual relations (e.g., caretakers, stepparents, stepsiblings).

The Incestuous Relationship

A great deal of attention has been given to the study of father-daughter incest but, by definition, incest could include sexual relations between any close relatives, including step or adoptive relatives. In fact, sibling sexual abuse is identified as the most common form of sexual abuse within families, but father-daughter incest is more often reported (Willacy, 2022).

In cases of father-daughter incest, there is usually an impaired sexual relationship between the parents. Communication between the parents is typically ineffective and the perpetrator is domineering, impulsive, and physically abusive. The other parent, most often the mother, is passive and submissive even though she may suspect that incest is occurring. At times, this passive response is born from fear of the perpetrator or denial that the child is being harmed. Families in which a single mother invites another man to live in the home triples the risk for incest

by the boyfriend or stepparent, and abuse by stepfathers is up to five times higher than that by biological fathers (Willacy, 2022).

The child victim may experience a variety of physical ailments connected to this abuse in addition to the conflicting emotions of fear, anger, and helplessness at odds with the desire for a loving relationship with the perpetrator. Often psychological symptoms are the most apparent signs of this child's conflict, including self-harming behaviors, school-related problems, withdrawal or aggression, nightmares, depression, eating disorders, PTSD, and overt sexual behavior with peers.

The incest is typically ongoing and, although the oldest daughter in a family is most vulnerable to becoming a participant in father-daughter incest, some fathers form sequential relationships with several daughters. If incest has been reported with one daughter, it should be suspected with all the daughters.

The Adult Survivor of Incest and Childhood Sexual Abuse

Several common characteristics have been identified in adults who have experienced childhood incest. Basic to these characteristics is a fundamental lack of trust resulting from an unsatisfactory parent-child relationship, which contributes to low self-esteem and a poor sense of identity. Children of incest often feel trapped, for they have been admonished not to talk about the experience and may even fear for their lives if they are exposed. If they do muster the courage to report the incest, often to the mother, they sometimes are not believed. This is confusing to the child, who is left with a sense of self-doubt and the inability to trust their own feelings. The child develops feelings of guilt with the realization over the years that the parents are using them in an attempt to solve their own problems.

Adult survivors of incest who come forward with their stories usually are estranged from nuclear family members, blamed for disclosing the "family secret," and often accused of overreacting to the incest. Frequently, the estrangement becomes permanent when family members continue to deny the behavior and the individual is accused of lying. In recent years, a number of celebrities have come forward with stories of their childhood sexual abuse. Some have chosen to make the disclosure only after the death of their parents. The revelation of these past activities can be one way of contributing to the healing process for survivors.

Many studies support that there are a multitude of long-term physical and mental consequences for the adult survivor of childhood maltreatment including brain damage, heart attack, diabetes, arthritis, high blood pressure, migraines, cancer, stroke, bowel disease, lung diseases, and chronic fatigue syndrome (CWIG, 2019a).

The conflicts associated with pain (either physical or emotional) and sexual pleasure experienced by children who are sexually abused are often repeated in adult relationships. Betrayal of trust and violations of personal boundaries in childhood contribute to trust issues and interpersonal difficulties in adulthood that increase the risk for revictimization (Papalia et al., 2021). Women who were abused as children often enter into relationships with men who abuse them physically, sexually, or emotionally. In addition, studies have shown that childhood sexual abuse victims are at greater risk for psychopathology, risky behaviors, physical illness, education and employment challenges, and crime and violence (Papalia et al., 2020). Langevin and associates (2021) added that child maltreatment demonstrates intergenerational continuity, and although many parents break these

cycles, mental illness, exposure to multiple forms of childhood adversity, lack of social support, disadvantage, and an environment of community violence increase the risks of childhood victims becoming adult perpetrators of child maltreatment.

Sexual Violence

Sexual violence is often equated with rape, but that is only one type of sexual assault. It is important for nurses and other health-care providers to be aware that sexual violence is any sexual activity when consent is not obtained or freely given and it can occur in person, online, or through technology, such as posting or sharing sexual pictures of someone without their consent, or nonconsensual sexting (CDC, 2022). All of these experiences can result in trauma, and assessment for a history of these events is foundational to providing trauma-informed care. Read about Diana's experiences in this chapter's "Real People, Real Stories" feature.

Real People, Real Stories: Diana's Journey

This individual wished to remain anonymous. Diana is not her real name. Her story is a poignant lesson in the various ways that one can be victimized, the long-term effect of such experiences on one's sense of self-esteem and personal safety, and the importance of nurses' understanding of trauma-informed care.

Karyn: I appreciate your willingness to talk about your experiences. If at any time you become uncomfortable discussing these events, we don't need to continue. All right?

Diana: I've had a lot of therapy, and I feel like it's important to tell and keep on telling so that, hopefully, something good will come out of it. When I was 6 years old, I had a crush on my best friend's brother. He was 12 years old, and when he started giving me attention, I thought he liked me; until he took me into a room, took my clothes off, and was touching me. He wanted me to take his clothes off, and I said no. I told my mom, and she intervened with his parents, but when a second incident occurred, my mother stopped me from going to my friend's house. I felt a lot of shame and embarrassment, but I never really talked about my feelings. For a long time, I carried around the belief that it was somehow my fault because I had a crush on him. I found out later that there were several other children who he molested and that his mom had implied they were "making it up."

When I was around 8 years old, I was in a toy store and a man came up from behind me and rubbed my rear end under my dress. I ran to get my father, but the perpetrator ran out of the store, and my parents decided not to call the police. They felt like I'd been scared enough. As an adult, I can understand that. But

as a child, I felt like someone did a bad thing to me, and I wished that someone had defended me. As a middle schooler, one of the neighborhood girls wanted to play Truth or Dare. I think she did this with a lot of girls. The dare was to take off my clothes after which she put her hands on me. I said no but felt paralyzed with fear when she touched me anyway. She was a year older, and again, I remember feeling powerless and thinking I didn't know what to do.

In another incident in middle school, one of the boys jumped out in front of me in the school hallway and grabbed my breasts. A teacher saw him do it and was going to send him to the principal's office, but the boy looked scared and I somehow thought it must be my job to protect him … or maybe I was trying to act like it was no big deal, so I told the teacher to just let him go. I didn't want to get the boy in trouble, and I was so embarrassed and humiliated, I just wanted it to go away. Part of me wishes the teacher hadn't listened to me, though. I don't think that boy had any idea how much he hurt me and how awful it was.

Karyn: I think that may be a common reaction by girls or women; even though someone has offended against us, we don't want to hurt them in return. And it minimizes the fact that *we* have been hurt.

Diana: Yes, and my parents were knee-deep in the Catholic training that if someone hurts you, you should just walk away or turn the other cheek. That influenced my own thinking, that you don't defend yourself—you should just walk away and avoid conflict. But that's a misunderstanding of the "turn the other cheek" teaching, which is really about showing forgiveness when

Real People, Real Stories: Diana's Journey—cont'd

people demonstrate remorse. It doesn't mean letting people hurt you without consequences. Around this time, I started putting on a lot of weight. I've always felt it was, in part, a reaction meant to keep people at a distance, so they couldn't hurt me.

Karyn: I've heard other people share a similar coping or defense mechanism; doing something simply to keep people away. Was that effective?

Diana: It only added to my self-esteem issues. I struggled with the question of why these things were happening to me. I felt like *I* must be doing *something* wrong. As a teenager, I struggled with anxiety and depression, and I was sent to a psychiatrist, but it wasn't helpful. Then when I moved to New York City for college, there were a couple of incidents on the subway. One was a frail-looking elderly man who stuck his hand between my legs, and when I turned around to confront him, he was laughing at me. I felt very powerless. I thought about kicking him, but, again, I didn't want to injure this shriveled-up old man, and I also didn't know if he had a knife, a gun. ... So there's the fear, the powerlessness, and the anger that someone was touching me and *laughing* at me, and I could do nothing. I wondered if I was sending out some vibe—i.e., it must be my fault. My friend told me I needed to learn how to put on an angry face and carry an umbrella to better defend myself. I knew I had anxiety and self-esteem issues, and that's when I decided I needed therapy.

Karyn: That took a lot of courage to identify what you needed to do to take some control back. What has been most helpful about that process?

Diana: I explored the underpinnings of my self-esteem issues and identified coping skills, but nonetheless, as an adult many things can trigger the feelings of vulnerability, anxiety, and low self-esteem: news stories about rape or abuse, or times when women or children are demeaned in the media, especially from people manipulating their power or authority. That brings up a lot of "stuff" for me. When my counselor challenged me to identify what was in the way of being able to set all this stuff aside—that's when I had the insight that I just wanted to know something good could come out of all this pain.

Karyn: One of the things you've told me is that you've been able to teach your daughters how to respond in such situations.

Diana: Yes, that was important and felt like a victory. I'm better able to identify potentially harmful situations. I've taught them to listen to that inner voice, where you get that "bad feeling" you can get that warns you when you're in a situation that may require defending or protecting yourself, and I taught my daughters how to be prepared. I've told them that if someone tries to touch them, it's okay to fight back. It's okay to tell me, school officials, tell *anyone,* and to keep telling until someone believes them and responds. I want them to

know that it's safe to talk to me about their feelings and that they are not powerless.

Karyn: I think that's an important message for health-care professionals as well: to listen, to not brush off someone's experiences but rather to explore the events, thoughts, and feelings and identify coping strategies.

Diana: Yes, I think sometimes adults who thought it was less traumatizing for me to walk away or try to forget about it thought they were helping, but that's not the answer. Even now, after all these years, I wasn't sure if you would think my story was important enough to tell, I mean, to some people, it might not seem so bad. I wasn't raped, it wasn't a family member—but it still left me feeling awful.

Karyn: I think your story is very important to tell. You are taking the opportunity to teach others that victimization can occur in a variety of ways, that it can have long-term effects on self-esteem, and that it is important to find ways to regain a sense of control and self-worth. I really appreciate your sharing this. What do you think are the most important things that nurses need to know about your and others' experience with victimization and trauma?

Diana: First of all, that 40 years later, those incidents still affect me. I saw a picture of the boy who molested me on a friend's Facebook page, and I felt sick and afraid all over again. And I beat myself up for still letting it get to me. Nurses need to know that even events that happened years ago can influence one's emotional responses in the present.

Second, the idea of "getting closure," even so many years later, is a misnomer. Certain things can trigger those memories and anxieties, and when they come back, all you can do is drag them out and talk about them again and again and again. It's another version of "you tell and you tell and you don't stop telling" until you remember that you survived it, that it wasn't your fault, and that you don't need to feel ashamed or embarrassed or humiliated (even if part of you still does).

Third, I want nurses to know that they are the front lines, and no matter what clinical area they practice in, a history of sexual trauma or abuse can affect how their patients experience and receive health care. I had a lot of trouble as an adult fertility patient, having to dress and undress so many times and deal with so many invasive procedures. It was important to tell my health-care providers why my heart was pounding, why I seemed so nervous, why I hated mammographies and regular GYN examinations a little bit more than the average woman. ... That, as always, a nurse's ability to care and offer compassion can make the biggest difference, and it all begins with trust and helping your patient to "tell." And I wanted to say thank you for the times those nurses held my hand, and squeezed tight, and told me that I would be okay.

CORE CONCEPT

Rape

The expression of power and dominance by means of sexual violence, most commonly by men over women, although men may also be rape victims.

Sexual assault is any type of sexual act in which an individual is threatened, coerced, or forced to submit to against their will. Rape, a type of sexual assault, occurs over a broad spectrum of experiences ranging from the surprise attack by a stranger to insistence on sexual intercourse by an acquaintance or spouse. Regardless of the defining source, one common theme always emerges: rape is an act of aggression, not one of passion.

Acquaintance rape (called **date rape** if the encounter occurs during a social engagement agreed to by the victim) is a term applied to situations in which the rapist is acquainted with the victim. They may be out on a first date, have been dating for a number of months, or merely be acquaintances or schoolmates. College campuses are the location for a staggering number of these types of rapes, a great many of which go unreported. An increasing number of colleges and universities are establishing programs for rape prevention and counseling for survivors of rape.

Marital rape, which has been recognized only in recent years as a legal category, is sexual assault committed against one's spouse. Historically, with societal acceptance of the concept of women as marital property, the legal definition of rape held an exemption within the marriage relationship. In 1993 marital rape became a crime in all 50 states, under at least one section of the sexual offenses code. In many states, there are no exemptions granted to husbands, but in a significant number of states, there are still some exemptions providing immunity to husbands from being prosecuted for rape. For example, some state laws related to spousal rape either explicitly require the use of force or provide immunity if one spouse is incapacitated, effectively providing immunity if the spouse was drugged, unconscious, or otherwise unable to give consent. In all states where husbands can be prosecuted, the criteria for proving marital rape are very stringent.

Statutory rape is unlawful intercourse between a person who is over the age of consent and a person who is under the age of consent. In the United States, legal age of consent varies from state to state, ranging from age 16 to 18 (LaMance, 2022). An adult who has intercourse with a person who is under the age of consent can be arrested for statutory rape, even if the interaction occurred between consenting individuals.

Profile of the Victimizer

It is difficult to profile a rapist because rapists comprise a heterogenous group and are not distinguished by looks or intelligence.

The majority of rapes are premeditated, and some behavioral characteristics that have been identified as associated with premeditation include the perpetrator seeking out a victim who appears to be vulnerable (capable of being overpowered or in an opportunistic position such as being alone or isolated from others); alcohol and drugs such as Rohypnol (flunitrazepam) may serve the purpose of increasing victim vulnerability. The perpetrator may also violate or ignore others' rights in a way that gives them information about whether a potential victim is passive or tolerant of those behaviors. But again, although these behaviors might be observed more commonly, they do not clearly define the complete profile of these perpetrators. Feminist theories suggest that rape is most common in societies that encourage aggressiveness in males, that have distinct gender roles, and in which men regard women's roles as inferior. Male aggressiveness as a cultural norm, however, does not explain why some men become perpetrators of criminal aggression and violence whereas others do not.

In 80% of rape and sexual assault cases, the offender was known to the victim, and many of the perpetrators have criminal histories (RAINN, 2022a). Although such statistics help describe aspects of the problem, understanding the essence of the perpetrator of aggression and violence is the subject of ongoing research.

The Victim

Rape can occur at any age; however, the most recent statistics suggest that the highest-risk age-group is females aged 12 to 34 (59%) and 90% of adult rape victims are females (RAINN, 2022b). Rapes are less likely to be reported than other violent crimes. Most sexual assault victims are single women, and the attack frequently occurs in or close to the victim's own neighborhood.

Although women are at highest risk for rape perpetrated by males, males may also be victimized by women or other men. Some groups that have been identified at higher risk (than the general population) for sexual violence victimization include male college students, TGQN (transgender, genderqueer, and nonconforming) college students, prisoners, military members, and American Indians (RAINN, 2022b).

Rape survivors who present themselves for care shortly after the crime has occurred likely are experiencing an overwhelming sense of violation and helplessness that began with the powerlessness and intimidation experienced during the rape. Burgess and Holmström (1974), who classically defined what has been described as **rape trauma syndrome,** identified two emotional patterns of response that may occur within hours after a rape and with which health-care workers may be confronted in the emergency department or rape crisis center. In the **expressed response pattern,** the survivor expresses feelings of fear, anger, and anxiety through such behaviors as crying, sobbing, restlessness, and tension. In the **controlled response pattern,** the feelings are masked or hidden, and a calm, composed, or subdued affect is seen.

Physical manifestations may occur days or weeks after the attack. Physical symptoms include bruises, cuts and abrasions, sleep difficulties, headaches, nausea and vomiting, vaginal discharge, burning on urination, and rectal pain and bleeding. Psychological manifestations are variable and may include numbness or rage, embarrassment, self-blame, desire for revenge, fear of another attack, and fear of death. Various long-term effects include increased restlessness, dreams and nightmares, and phobias (particularly those having to do with sexual interaction). Some women report that it takes years to get over the experience; they describe a sense of vulnerability and a loss of control over their own lives during this period. They feel defiled and unable to wash themselves clean, and some women are unable to remain living alone in their home or apartment. Trauma-informed care may be influential in reducing some long-term complications.

Some survivors develop a **compounded rape reaction,** in which additional symptoms such as depression and suicide, substance misuse, and even psychotic behaviors may be noted (Burgess & Holmström, 1974). Another variation has been called the **silent rape reaction,** in which the survivor tells no one about the assault. Anxiety is suppressed and the emotional burden may become overwhelming. The unresolved sexual trauma may not be revealed until the woman is forced to face another sexual crisis in her life that reactivates the previously unresolved feelings.

Diagnosis and Outcome Identification

Nursing diagnoses are formulated from the data gathered during the assessment phase and with background knowledge regarding predisposing factors to the situation. Some common nursing diagnoses for survivors of abuse include the following:

■ Rape trauma syndrome related to sexual assault evidenced by verbalizations of the attack; bruises and lacerations over areas of body; severe anxiety

■ Powerlessness related to the cycle of battering evidenced by verbalizations of abuse; bruises and lacerations over areas of body; fear for her safety and that of her children; verbalizations of no way to get out of the relationship

■ Risk for delayed child development related to an abusive family situation

Outcome Criteria

The following criteria may be used to measure outcomes in the care of abuse survivors:

The patient who has been sexually assaulted:

■ Is no longer experiencing panic anxiety
■ Demonstrates a degree of trust in the primary nurse
■ Has received immediate attention to physical injuries
■ Has initiated behaviors consistent with the grief response

The patient who has been physically battered:

■ Has received immediate attention to physical injuries
■ Verbalizes assurance of their immediate safety
■ Discusses life situation with primary nurse
■ Can verbalize choices from which they may receive assistance

The child who has been abused:

■ Has received immediate attention to physical injuries
■ Demonstrates trust in primary nurse by discussing abuse through the use of play therapy
■ Is demonstrating a decrease in regressive behaviors

Planning and Implementation

Table 34–1 provides a plan of care for the patient who is a survivor of abuse. Nursing diagnoses are presented, along with outcome criteria, appropriate nursing interventions, and rationales for each.

Evaluation

Evaluation of nursing actions to assist survivors of abuse must be considered on both a short- and a long-term basis. Short-term evaluation may be facilitated by gathering information using the following types of questions:

■ Has the individual been reassured of their safety?
■ Is this evidenced by a decrease in panic anxiety?
■ Has trauma-informed care been incorporated in assessment and provision of care?
■ Have wounds been properly cared for and provision made for follow-up care?
■ Have emotional needs been attended to?
■ Has trust been established with at least one person to whom the patient feels comfortable relating the abusive incident?

Table 34-1 | CARE PLAN FOR SURVIVORS OF ABUSE

NURSING DIAGNOSIS: RAPE TRAUMA SYNDROME
RELATED TO: Sexual assault
EVIDENCED BY: Verbalizations of the attack; bruises and lacerations over areas of body; severe anxiety

OUTCOME CRITERIA	NURSING INTERVENTIONS	RATIONALE
Short-Term Goal: ■ Patient's physical wounds heal without complication. Long-Term Goal: ■ Patient begins a healthy grief resolution, initiating the process of physical and psychological healing (time to be individually determined).	1. It is important to communicate the following to the individual who has been sexually assaulted: ■ "You are safe here." ■ "I'm sorry that it happened." ■ "I'm glad you survived." ■ "It's not your fault. No one deserves to be treated this way." ■ "You did the best that you could."	1. The victim of rape or sexual assault is often frightened and must be reassured of their safety. The patient may also be overwhelmed with self-doubt and self-blame, and these statements instill trust and validate self-worth.
	2. Explain every assessment procedure that will be conducted and why it is being conducted. Ensure that data collection is conducted in a caring, nonjudgmental manner. Engage the services of a sexual assault nurse examiner, where available, to facilitate evidence collection and patient advocacy.	2. This may serve to decrease fear and anxiety and increase trust.
	3. Ensure that the patient has adequate privacy for all immediate postcrisis interventions. Try to have as few people as possible providing the immediate care or collecting immediate evidence.	3. The post-trauma patient typically feels extremely vulnerable. Additional people in the environment increase this feeling of vulnerability and serve to escalate anxiety.
	4. Encourage the patient to give an account of the assault. Listen, but do not probe.	4. Nonjudgmental listening provides an avenue for catharsis that the patient needs to begin healing. A detailed account may be required for legal follow-up, and a caring nurse, as a patient advocate, may help to lessen the trauma of evidence collection.
	5. Discuss whom to call for support or assistance. Provide information about referrals for aftercare.	5. Because of severe anxiety and fear, the patient may need assistance from others during the immediate postcrisis period. Provide referral information in writing for later reference (e.g., psychotherapist, mental health clinic, community advocacy group).

Table 34–1 | CARE PLAN FOR SURVIVORS OF ABUSE –cont'd

NURSING DIAGNOSIS: POWERLESSNESS

RELATED TO: Cycle of battering

EVIDENCED BY: Verbalizations of abuse; bruises and lacerations over areas of body; fear for own safety and that of children; verbalizations of no way to get out of the relationship

OUTCOME CRITERIA	NURSING INTERVENTIONS	RATIONALE
Short-Term Goal: ■ Patient will recognize and verbalize choices available, thereby perceiving some control over life situation. **Long-Term Goal:** ■ Patient will exhibit control over life situation by making decisions about what to do regarding living with cycle of abuse.	1. In collaboration with physician, ensure that all physical wounds, fractures, and burns receive immediate attention. Take photographs if the patient permits.	1. Patient safety is a nursing priority. Photographs may be called as evidence if charges are filed.
	2. Take the patient to a private area to do the interview.	2. If the patient is accompanied by the person who did the battering, they are not likely to be truthful about the injuries.
	3. If the patient has come alone or with children, reassure them of their safety. Encourage discussion of the battering incident. Ask questions about whether this has happened before, whether the abuser takes drugs, whether the victim has a safe place to go, and whether they are interested in pressing charges.	3. Some victims attempt to keep secret how their injuries occurred to protect the partner or because they are fearful that the partner will kill them if they tell.
	4. Ensure that "rescue" efforts are not attempted by the nurse. Offer support but remember that the final decision must be made by patient.	4. Making their own decision gives the patient a sense of control over their life situation. Imposing judgments and giving advice are nontherapeutic.
	5. Stress to the patient the importance of safety. Provide information about available resources. These may include crisis hotlines, community groups for victims of abuse, shelters, counseling services, and information regarding the victim's rights in the civil and criminal justice system. Respect the patient's decision about whether to stay or leave the home or marriage.	5. Knowledge of available choices decreases the individual's sense of powerlessness. Respecting the patient's decision empowers critical thinking and decision making.

Continued

Table 34–1 | CARE PLAN FOR SURVIVORS OF ABUSE –cont'd

NURSING DIAGNOSIS: RISK FOR DELAYED CHILD DEVELOPMENT
RELATED TO: Child abuse

OUTCOME CRITERIA	NURSING INTERVENTIONS	RATIONALE
Short-Term Goal: ■ Patient develops trusting relationship with nurse and reports how evident injuries were sustained. **Long-Term Goal:** ■ Patient demonstrates behaviors consistent with age-appropriate growth and development.	1. Perform complete physical assessment of the child. Take particular note of bruises (in various stages of healing), lacerations, and patient complaints of pain in specific areas. Do not overlook or discount the possibility of sexual abuse. Assess for nonverbal signs of abuse: aggressive conduct, excessive fears, extreme hyperactivity, apathy, withdrawal, age-inappropriate behaviors.	1. An accurate and thorough physical assessment is required to provide appropriate care for the patient.
	2. Conduct an in-depth interview with the parent or adult who accompanies the child. Consider: If the injury is being reported as an accident, is the explanation reasonable? Is the injury consistent with the explanation? Is the injury consistent with the child's developmental capabilities?	2. Fear of imprisonment or loss of child custody may place the abusive parent on the defensive. Discrepancies may be evident in the description of the incident and lying to cover up involvement is a common defense that may be detectable in an in-depth interview.
	3. Use games or play therapy to gain child's trust. Use these techniques to assist in describing their side of the story.	3. Establishing a trusting relationship with an abused child is extremely difficult. They may not want to be touched. These types of play activities can provide a nonthreatening environment that may enhance the child's attempt to discuss these painful issues.

■ Have available support systems been identified and notified?
■ Have options for immediate circumstances been presented?

Long-term evaluation may be conducted by health-care workers who have contact with the individual long after the immediate crisis has passed and may include the following types of questions:

■ Is the individual able to conduct activities of daily living satisfactorily?
■ Have physical wounds healed properly?
■ Is the patient appropriately progressing through the phases of grieving?

■ Is the patient free of sleep disturbances (nightmares, insomnia), psychosomatic symptoms (headaches, stomach pains, nausea/vomiting), regressive behaviors (enuresis, thumb sucking, phobias), and psychosexual disturbances?
■ Is the individual free from problems with interpersonal relationships?
■ Has the individual (in an abusive relationship) considered the alternatives for change in their personal life?
■ Has a decision been made relative to the choices available?
■ Is the individual satisfied with the decision that has been made?

Forensic Nursing

Forensic nursing is a specialized nursing role in which nurses apply their skills to the care, evaluation, and advocacy for victims of crime in a variety of settings, including primary care facilities, hospitals, and correctional institutions. Catalano (2020) offered the following definition:

> Forensic nursing forms an alliance between nursing, law enforcement, and the forensic sciences. The term forensic means anything belonging to or pertaining to the law. . . . Forensic nurses provide a continuum of care to victims and their families, beginning in the emergency department [ED] or at the crime scene and leading to participation in the criminal investigation and the courts of law. (p. 700)

The International Association of Forensic Nurses (IAFN) (2022c) states:

> A forensic nurse is a Registered or Advanced Practice nurse who has received specific education and training. Forensic nurses provide specialized care for patients who are experiencing acute and long-term health consequences associated with victimization or violence, and/or have unmet evidentiary needs relative to having been victimized or accused of victimization. In addition, forensic nurses provide consultation and testimony for civil and criminal proceedings relative to nursing practice, care given, and opinions rendered regarding findings. Forensic nursing care is not separate and distinct from other forms of medical care, but rather integrated into the overall care needs of individual patients.

The sexual assault nurse examiner (SANE) is a clinical forensic registered nurse who has received specialized training to care for the sexual assault victim. Responsibilities include interviewing the victim, completing the physical examination, collecting specimens for forensic evidence, and documenting findings. The SANE also provides emotional support for victims and family members. The goal is to provide competent evidence collection and compassionate care that reduces psychological trauma. When the case goes to court, the SANE testifies as an expert legal witness regarding how the evidence was collected and the physical and psychological condition of the patient. Forensic mental health nurses may also be called upon to assess convicted perpetrators for physical fitness, criminal responsibility, disposition, and early release or to provide treatment for convicted offenders.

Preservation of Evidence

Crime-related evidence is essential to criminal investigation and must be protected in a manner consistent with the investigation. Brown (2013) identified common types of evidence as clothing, bullets, gunshot powder on the skin, bloodstains, hairs, fibers, grass, and any other debris found on the individual such as fragments of glass, paint, and wood. Often, this type of evidence is destroyed in the clinical setting when health-care personnel are unaware of its potential value in an investigation. This type of evidence must be saved and documented in all medical or accident cases that have legal implications.

Investigation of Wound Characteristics

When patients present in the emergency department with wounds from undiagnosed trauma, the clinical forensic nurse specialist documents the injuries. Failure to do so may interfere with the administration of justice should legal implications later arise. Nurses managing the care of a victim in the emergency department must be able to make assessments about the type of wound, the weapons involved, and an estimated length of time between the injury and presentation for treatment.

One type of wound that may go unnoticed is nonfatal strangulation. The IAFN (2022b) notes that 40% to 80% of women who report IPV and/or sexual violence have experienced one or more events of strangulation, and fatalities have occurred in victims who demonstrate no visible external injuries. Serious internal injuries, including fractured trachea, carotid aneurysm, cerebral artery infarct, and death, may occur days or weeks after the event. Child victims of strangulation are at increased risk for spinal cord injuries.

The IAFN (2022b) recommends universal screening for strangulation events using a collaborative, trauma-informed care approach, including protocols for medical/radiological evaluation, danger assessment, and safety plan development. They note that strangulation events are a strong predictor of future violence and risk for homicide. Brown (2019) stressed that direct inquiry about whether an attempt to strangle has occurred (in any assault victim) is essential because physical signs may be absent at the time of presentation, and victims may not be forthcoming with this information unless directly questioned. The IAFN (2022a) publishes a Nonfatal Strangulation Documentation Toolkit that details examples of direct questions and important aspects of documentation.

Treatment Modalities

Trauma-Informed Care

Trauma-informed care is foundational to all treatment modalities for survivors of abuse and neglect. At the outset, this requires awareness that trauma can have long-lasting physical, mental, emotional, and spiritual consequences. It will influence the ability to establish a trusting relationship and to collect accurate assessment data.

An individual's response to trauma is rooted in the fight-or-flight mechanism (the autonomic nervous system) that is designed to protect survival. When activated, however, this response disrupts the normal functions of body systems, including the brain. Notably, memories become fragmented and sensory experiences become intensified. When someone has also had previous traumas, the fight-or-flight response is easily reactivated. Thus, when a patient is interviewed immediately after a traumatic event, the patient may have extreme difficulty recalling events in sequence. In this situation, the nurse must recognize that collecting information will take time, and information may be shared in seemingly disconnected parts.

Sensory experiences may be so intensified that any loud noise, smell, visual experience, or touch can retrigger intense fear. Assuring the patient of their safety and working to establish trust, empathy, and compassionate care is not only good patient care in general, but for the trauma victim, it reduces the likelihood of retriggering fear, the fight-or-flight response, and its effects on the body and brain; a process called **retraumatization.** Health-care provider behaviors that may increase the risk for retraumatization include any behavior that violates the patient's trust, care that is imposed rather than collaborative, and punitive or shame-based approaches. Box 34–1 outlines four basic principles of trauma-informed care.

Crisis Intervention

The focus of the initial interview and follow-up with the patient who has been sexually assaulted is on the rape incident alone. Problems not associated with the rape are not dealt with at this time. The goal of crisis intervention is to help survivors return to their previous lifestyle as quickly as possible.

The patient should be involved in the intervention from the beginning. This promotes a sense of competency, control, and decision making. Because an overwhelming sense of powerlessness accompanies the rape experience, active involvement by the survivor is both a validation of personal worth and the beginning of the recovery process. Crisis intervention is time-limited, usually 6 to 8 weeks. If problems resurface beyond this time, the individual is referred for assistance from other agencies (e.g., long-term psychotherapy from a psychiatrist or mental health clinic).

During the crisis period, attention is given to coping strategies for dealing with the symptoms common to the post-trauma patient. Initially, the individual undergoes a period of disorganization during which there is difficulty making decisions,

BOX 34–1 Trauma-Informed Care: The Four R's	
FOUR DOMAINS OF TRAUMA-INFORMED APPROACHES	**DEFINITIONS AND ACTIVITIES**
REALIZE	**R**ealizes the widespread effect of trauma. Screens for trauma history. Understands potential paths for recovery.
RECOGNIZE	**R**ecognizes the signs and symptoms of trauma in clients, families, staff, and others involved with the system.
RESPOND	**R**esponds by fully integrating knowledge about trauma into policies, procedures, and practices.
RESIST	**R**esists retraumatization. Behaviors include trustworthiness, transparency, assuring client safety, collaboration, and empowerment.

Adapted from Substance Abuse and Mental Health Services Administration. (2014). *SAMHSA's concept of trauma and guidance for a trauma-informed approach.* HHS Publication No. (SMA) 14-4884. Substance Abuse and Mental Health Services Administration

extreme or irrational fears, and general mistrust. Observable manifestations may range from stark hysteria to expression of anger and rage to silence and withdrawal. Guilt and feelings of responsibility for the rape, as well as numerous physical manifestations, are common. The crisis counselor attempts to help the individual draw on previous successful coping strategies to regain control over their life.

If the client is a victim of IPV, the counselor ensures that various resources and options are discussed with the individual so that the victim may make a personal decision about moving forward. Discussing strategies for minimizing the dangers of leaving (sometimes called an escape plan) may be helpful if the client is considering leaving the relationship. Support groups provide a valuable forum for reducing isolation and learning new strategies for coping with the aftermath of physical or sexual abuse. Particularly for the survivor of rape, the peer support group provides a therapeutic forum for reducing the sense of isolation they may feel in the aftermath of predictable social and interpersonal responses to their experience.

The Safe House or Shelter

Most major cities in the United States now have **safe houses or shelters** where victims can reside temporarily in an environment that ensures physical protection for them and their children and resources for emotional healing. Safe houses have historically catered exclusively to the needs of female victims, but recently more safe houses for male victims of IPV are surfacing in the United States and in other countries. Shelters typically provide a variety of services, and the residents receive emotional support from staff and one another. Most shelters provide individual and group counseling; help with bureaucratic institutions such as the police, legal representation, and social services; childcare and children's programming; and aid for making future plans, such as employment counseling and linkages with housing authorities. Lengths of stay vary greatly depending on several factors, such as availability of outside support systems, financial resources, and personal resources.

Family-Based Interventions

The focus of therapy with families who experience violence is to help them develop democratic (respectful, interactive) ways of solving problems. The hope is that these interventions will reduce physical violence, but study results are mixed. The variables that influence violence within families are multifaceted, including the presence or absence of substance use disorders, support networks, and consensus about the need for change.

In a systematic review and meta-analysis (Vlahovicova et al., 2017), researchers concluded that there is evidence to support the benefits of social learning theory-based behavioral parenting programs to prevent recurrence of child abuse. The authors caution, though, that the effects were modest (an 11% lower recidivism to child protective services among families who received the training) and very few of the studies included follow-up beyond 6 months. A more recent systematic review focused on IPV (Ryan & Roman, 2019) concluded that family-centered IPV interventions yielded long-term positive results in improving parent-child interaction, including reductions in IPV, trauma symptoms of mothers, and problematic child behaviors. These authors cited follow-up studies that occurred up to 1 year postintervention.

Summary and Key Points

- Abuse is the maltreatment of one person by another.
- Intimate partner violence, child abuse, and sexual assault are widespread, and all populations are equally affected.
- Various factors have been theorized as influential in the predisposition to violent behavior. Physiological and biochemical influences within the brain have been suggested, as has the possibility of genetic influences.
- Organic brain syndromes associated with various cerebral disorders and traumatic brain injury have been implicated in the predisposition to aggressive and violent behavior.
- Psychoanalytical theorists relate the predisposition to violent behavior to underdeveloped ego and a weak superego.
- Learning theorists suggest that children imitate the abusive behavior of their parents. This theory has been substantiated by studies that show that individuals who were abused as children or whose parents disciplined them with physical punishment are more likely to be abusive as adults. Societal influences, such as acceptance of violence as a means of solving problems, have also been implicated.
- Although intimate partner violence is more frequently perpetrated by men against women, men may also be victims of domestic violence.
- Victims who are battered often blame themselves for their situations. They may have been reared in abusive families and thus expect this type of behavior.
- Battered women commonly see no way out of their present situation and may be encouraged by their social support network to remain in the abusive relationship.
- Child abuse includes physical and emotional abuse, physical and emotional neglect, and sexual abuse of a child.
- A child may experience many years of abuse without reporting it because of fear of retaliation by the abuser.
- Some children report incest experiences to their mothers, only to be rebuffed and told to remain secretive about the abuse.
- Research has identified a strong link between adverse childhood experiences (including abuse and neglect) and physical, psychosocial, and mental illness in adulthood.
- Sexual assault is identified as an act of aggression, not passion.
- A history of abuse and neglect in childhood increase one's risk of perpetrating abuse and neglect upon others in adulthood.
- Rape is a traumatic experience, and many women experience flashbacks, nightmares, rage, physical symptoms, depression, and thoughts of suicide for many years after the occurrence.
- Trauma-informed care is foundational to all interventions and treatment modalities for the patient who is a survivor of abuse or neglect.
- Nursing behaviors that are untrustworthy, noncollaborative, punitive, or shame-based or that

minimize or ignore trauma-associated fears and concerns can be retraumatizing to victims of abuse and neglect.

■ Forensic nursing is a specialized field of practice that seeks to provide care with attention to the needs of the victim as well as issues related to criminal proceedings.

■ Treatment modalities for survivors of abuse include crisis intervention with the sexual assault victim, safe shelters, psychological interventions focused on trauma recovery, and family-centered interventions.

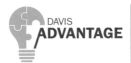 DAVIS **ADVANTAGE** | Go to **Davis Advantage** to complete your learning: strengthen understanding, apply your knowledge, and prepare for the Next Gen NCLEX®.

Review Questions

1. Trauma-informed care is foundational to all interventions with a victim of violence for which of the following reasons?
   a. It is a legal requirement in all 50 states.
   b. Trauma victims are unaware they have been traumatized until they are so informed.
   c. Victims of violence are at high risk for retraumatization.
   d. The client has a right to know what will happen to the perpetrator.

2. A sexual assault nurse examiner's primary role when intervening with a victim of violence is to:
   a. Conduct a sexual assault examination and preserve evidence
   b. Conduct a mini mental status examination
   c. Refer the client to a police officer
   d. Determine whether the client is lying about the events

3. A child, age 5, is sent to the school nurse's office with an upset stomach. She has vomited and soiled her blouse. When the nurse removes her blouse, she notices that the child has numerous bruises on her arms and torso in various stages of healing. She also notices some small scars, and her abdomen protrudes on her small, thin frame. From the objective physical assessment, the nurse should screen further for:
   a. Physical and sexual abuse.
   b. Physical abuse and neglect.
   c. Emotional neglect.
   d. Sexual and emotional abuse.

4. A school nurse notices bruises and scars on a child's body, but the child refuses to say how she received them. Which of the following is an evidence-based approach for further assessment by the nurse?
   a. Have her evaluated by the school psychologist.
   b. Tell her she may select a "treat" from the treat box (e.g., sucker, balloon, junk jewelry) if she answers the nurse's questions.
   c. Explain to her that if she answers the questions, she may stay in the nurse's office and not have to go back to class.
   d. Use a "family" of dolls to role-play the child's family with her.

5. The nurse is providing education to a support group for survivors of rape. Which of the following items is evidence-based information to include in this teaching?
   a. Rapists typically drink alcohol and are not in control of their actions.
   b. Rape is usually an event that occurs between two people who are sexually frustrated.
   c. Men who are born into poverty are predisposed to becoming rapists after puberty.
   d. Rape is an expression of power and dominance by means of sexual aggression and violence.

Clinical Judgment Questions

6. A client arrives at the emergency department and tells the nurse her husband inflicted the cuts to her face that required sutures. She says, "I didn't want to come. I'm really okay. He only does this when he has too much to drink. I just shouldn't have yelled at him." The best response by the nurse is:
   a. "How often does he drink too much?"
   b. "It is not your fault. You did the right thing by coming here."
   c. "How many times has he done this to you?"
   d. "He is not a good husband. You have to leave him before he kills you."

7. A woman who has a long history of being battered by her husband is staying at the woman's shelter. She has received emotional support from staff and peers and has been made aware of the alternatives open to her. Nevertheless, she decides to return to her home and marriage. The best response by the nurse to the woman's decision is:
   a. "I just can't believe you have decided to go back to that horrible man."
   b. "I'm just afraid he will kill you or the children when you go back."
   c. "What makes you think things have changed with him?"
   d. "I hope you have made the right decision. Call this number if you need help."

8. A school nurse notices bruises and scars on a child's body. The nurse suspects that the child is being physically abused. Which action by the nurse is a priority at this point?
   a. As a health-care worker, report the suspicion to child protective services.
   b. Check the child again in a week and see if there are any new bruises.
   c. Meet with the child's parents and ask them how she got the bruises.
   d. Initiate paperwork to have the child placed in foster care.

9. A college-age client is brought to the emergency department by her roommate after she confided that she was raped by her date who invited her to a frat party. The client says to the nurse, "It's all my fault. I shouldn't have gone to a party where I knew there was going to be alcohol." Which of these is the best response by the nurse?
   a. "Yes, you're right. You put yourself in a very vulnerable position when you allowed him to get you drunk."
   b. "You are not to blame for his behavior. You obviously made some right decisions, because you survived the attack."
   c. "There's no sense looking back now. Just look forward, and make sure you don't put yourself in the same situation again."
   d. "You'll just have to see that he is arrested so he won't do this to anyone else."

10. A young man who has just undergone a sexual assault is brought into the emergency department by a friend. What is the *priority* nursing intervention?
   a. Help him to bathe and clean himself up.
   b. Provide physical and emotional support during evidence collection.
   c. Provide him with a written list of community resources for survivors of rape.
   d. Discuss the importance of a follow-up visit to evaluate for sexually transmitted diseases.

IMPLICATIONS OF RESEARCH FOR EVIDENCE-BASED PRACTICE

Tso W. W., Chan K. L., Lee T. M., Rao N., Lee S. L., Jiang F., Chan S. H., Wong W. H., Wong R. S., Tung K. T., Yam J. C., Liu A. P., Chua G. T., Rosa Duque J. S., Lam A. L., Yip K. M., Leung L. K., Wang Y., Sun J., Wang G., Chan G. C., Wong I. C., & Ip P. (2022). Mental health & maltreatment risk of children with special educational needs during COVID-19. *Child Abuse & Neglect*, 105457.

DESCRIPTION OF THE STUDY: The authors sought to identify the effect of the COVID pandemic on the mental health of children with special education needs and their risk for child maltreatment. The study comprised 417 children with special education needs and 25,467 children with typical development who completed an online survey to explore and compare emotional/behavioral difficulties, quality of life, and parental stress during the pandemic.

RESULTS OF THE STUDY: Children in the special education needs group had significantly poorer quality of life; 23.5% of these children had at least one episode of severe physical assault and 1.9% experienced very severe physical assault during COVID-19. In general, rates of physical assault increased significantly and children with mental disorders had increased risk of severe physical assault compared with those without mental disorders

IMPLICATIONS FOR NURSING PRACTICE: The COVID-19 pandemic added a burden of stress to individuals and systems that has been unprecedented in our lifetime. Understanding the effect and concerns among vulnerable populations, such as children at risk for maltreatment, informs nurses on issues that need preventive attention in the event of a similar global crisis.

TEST YOUR CLINICAL REASONING AND CLINICAL JUDGMENT SKILLS

Sandy is a psychiatric registered nurse who works at a safe house for battered women. Lisa has just been admitted with her two small children after she was treated in the emergency department. She was beaten severely by her husband while he was intoxicated last night. She escaped with her children after he passed out in their bedroom.

In her initial assessment, Sandy learns from Lisa that she has been battered by her husband for 5 years, beginning shortly after their marriage. She explained that she "knew he drank quite a lot before we were married but thought he would stop after we had kids." Instead, the drinking has increased. Sometimes he does not even get home from work until midnight, after stopping to drink at the bar with his buddies.

Lately, he has begun to express jealousy and a lack of trust in Lisa, accusing her of numerous infidelities and indiscretions, none of which are true. Lisa says, "If only he wasn't under so much stress on his job, then maybe he wouldn't drink so much. Maybe if I tried harder to make everything perfect for him at home—I don't know. What do you think I should do to keep him from acting this way?"

Answer the following questions related to Lisa:

1. What is an appropriate response to Lisa's question?
2. Identify the priority psychosocial nursing diagnosis for Lisa.
3. What must the nurse do to ensure that Lisa learns from this experience?

Communication Exercises

1. Sarah is being treated in the emergency department for wounds inflicted by her husband. She says to the nurse, "He's really not a bad person. He's just under so much stress right now. His company is laying people off, and he thinks he will be next. He drinks a lot when he comes home from work. I just need to make things easier for him at home. I shouldn't have asked him to mow the lawn."

   How would the nurse respond appropriately to this statement by Sarah?

2. "I don't know what to do. I'm afraid he will hurt the kids."

   How would the nurse respond appropriately to this statement by Sarah?

3. "I don't want to press charges. I just want to go home!"

   How would the nurse respond appropriately to this statement by Sarah?

MOVIE CONNECTIONS

The Burning Bed (IPV) • *Life With Billy* (IPV) • *Two Story House* (child abuse) • *The Prince of Tides* (IPV) • *Radio Flyer* (child abuse) • *Flowers in the Attic* (child abuse) • *A Case of Rape* (sexual assault) • *The Accused* (sexual assault) • *Spotlight* (child molestation) • *What's Love Got to Do With It* (IPV)

References

American Psychological Association (APA). (2022). *Violence and socioeconomic status.* http://www.apa.org/pi/ses/resources/publications/violence.aspx

Boccadoro, S., Wagels, L., Henn, A. T., Hüpen, P., Graben, L., Raine, A., & Neuner, I. (2021). Proactive vs. reactive aggression within two modified versions of the Taylor aggression paradigm. *Frontiers in Behavioral Neuroscience, 15,* 749041. doi:10.3389/fnbeh.2021.749041

Brown, T. (2019). Strangulation victims: A forensic approach. *Medscape.* https://www.medscape.com/viewarticle/907317

Catalano, J. T. (2020). Developments in current nursing practice. In Catalano, J. T. (Ed.), *Nursing now! Today's issues, tomorrow's trends* (8th ed., pp. 700–716). F.A. Davis.

Center for Relationship Abuse Awareness. (2022). *Barriers to leaving an abusive relationship.* http://stoprelationshipabuse.org/educated/barriers-to-leaving-an-abusive-relationship/

Centers for Disease Control and Prevention (CDC). (2021a). *Adverse childhood experiences.* https://www.cdc.gov/violenceprevention/aces/index.html

Centers for Disease Control and Prevention (CDC). (2021b). *Fast facts: Preventing elder abuse.* https://www.cdc.gov/violenceprevention/elderabuse/fastfact.html

Centers for Disease Control and Prevention (CDC). (2021c). *Fast Facts: Preventing intimate partner violence.* https://www.cdc.gov/violenceprevention/intimatepartnerviolence/fastfact.html

Centers for Disease Control and Prevention (CDC). (2022). *Fast facts: Preventing sexual violence.* https://www.cdc.gov/violenceprevention/sexualviolence/fastfact.html

Child Welfare Information Gateway. (2019a). *Fact Sheet: Long-term consequences of child abuse and neglect.* https://www.childwelfare.gov/pubPDFs/long_term_consequences.pdf

Child Welfare Information Gateway. (2019b). *What is child abuse and neglect? Recognizing the signs and symptoms.* https://www.childwelfare.gov/pubs/factsheets/whatiscan

Cupaioli, F. A., Zucca, F. A., Caporale, C., Lesch, K. P., Passamonti, L., & Zecca, L. (2021). The neurobiology of human aggressive behavior: Neuroimaging, genetic, and neurochemical aspects. *Progress in Neuro-Psychopharmacology and Biological Psychiatry, 106,* 1–27. https://doi.org/10.1016/j.pnpbp.2020.110059

D'Inverno, A. S., Smith, S. G., Zhang, X., & Chen, J. (2019). The impact of intimate partner violence: A 2015 NISVS research-in brief. *National Center for Injury Prevention and Control, Centers for Disease Control and Prevention.* https://www.cdc.gov/violenceprevention/pdf/nisvs/nisvs-impactbrief-508.pdf

Dockterman, E. (2014). *Why women stay: The paradox of abusive relationships.* http://time.com/3309687/why-women-stay-in-abusive-relationships

Fingarson, A. K., Pierce, M. C., Lorenz, D. J., Kaczor, K., Bennett, B., Berger, R., Currie, M., Herr, S., Hickey, S., Magana, J., Makoroff, K., Williams, M., Young, A., & Zuckerbraun, N. (2019). Who's watching the children? Caregiver features associated with physical child abuse versus accidental injury. *Journal of Pediatrics, 212,* 180–187. doi:10.1016/j.jpeds.2019.05.040

Huecker, M. R., King, K. C., Jordan, G. A., & Smock, W. (2022). Domestic violence. *StatPearls.* https://www.ncbi.nlm.nih.gov/books/NBK499891/

International Association of Forensic Nurses. (2022a). *Nonfatal strangulation documentation toolkit.* https://www.forensicnurses.org/page/STAssessment

International Association of Forensic Nurses. (2022b). *The evaluation and treatment of non-fatal strangulation in the health care setting.* https://www.forensicnurses.org/wp-content/uploads/2022/08/2022-Strangulation-Position-Paper.pdf

International Association of Forensic Nurses. (2022c). *What is forensic nursing?* https://www.forensicnurses.org/page/WhatisFN

LaMance, K. (2022). *Statutory rape: The age of consent.* https://www.legalmatch.com/law-library/article/statutory-rape-the-age-of-consent.html

Langevin, R., Marshall, C., & Kingsland, E. (2021). Intergenerational cycles of maltreatment: A scoping review of psychosocial risk and protective factors. *Trauma Violence Abuse, 22*(4), 672–688. doi:10.1177/1524838019870917

Maclean, M. J., Sims, S., Bower, C., Leonard, H. M., Stanley, F. J., & O'Donnell, M. (2017). Maltreatment. *Pediatrics, 139*(4), e20161817

National Center on Elder Abuse. (n.d.). *Research statistics and data.* https://ncea.acl.gov/What-We-Do/Research/Statistics-and-Data.aspx

Papalia, N., Mann, E., & Ogloff, J. R. P. (2021). Child sexual abuse and risk of revictimization: impact of child demographics, sexual abuse characteristics, and psychiatric disorders. *Child Maltreatment, 26*(1), 74–86. doi:10.1177/1077559520932665

Rape, Abuse and Incest National Network (RAINN). (2022a). *Perpetrators of sexual violence: Statistics.* https://www.rainn.org/statistics/perpetrators-sexual-violence

Rape, Abuse and Incest National Network (RAINN) (2022b). *Victims of sexual violence: Statistics.* https://www.rainn.org/statistics/victims-sexual-violence

Rape, Abuse and Incest National Network (RAINN). (2022c). *Warning signs for young children.* https://www.rainn.org/articles/warning-signs-young-children

Ryan, J., & Roman, N. V. (2019). Family centered interventions for intimate partner violence: A systematic review. *Journal of Injury and Violence Prevention, 17*(1), 32–48.

Schatzberg, A. F., Cole, J. O., & DeBattista, C. (2019). *Manual of clinical psychopharmacology* (9th ed.). American Psychiatric Association Publishing.

Substance Abuse and Mental Health Services Administration. (2014). *SAMHSA's concept of trauma and guidance for a trauma-informed approach.* HHS Publication No. (SMA) 14-4884. Substance Abuse and Mental Health Services Administration.

Tracy, N. (2022). *What is battering?* www.healthyplace.com/abuse/domestic-violence/what-is-battering

Tso, W. W., Chan, K. L., Lee, T. M., Rao, N., Lee, S. L., Jiang, F., Chan, S. H., Wong, W. H., Wong, R. S., Tung, K. T., Yam, J. C., Liu, A. P., Chua, G. T., Rosa Duque, J. S., Lam, A. L., Yip, K. M., Leung, L. K., Wang, Y., Sun, J., Wang, G., Chan, G. C., Wong, I. C., & Ip, P. (2022). Mental health & maltreatment risk of children with special educational needs during COVID-19. *Child Abuse & Neglect,* 105457.

U.S. Department of Health and Human Services, Administration for Children and Families. (n.d). *Fact sheet: Human trafficking.* https://www.acf.hhs.gov/otip/fact-sheet/resource/fshumantrafficking

U.S. Department of Health & Human Services, Administration for Children and Families, Administration on Children, Youth and Families, Children's Bureau. (2022). *Child maltreatment 2020.* https://www.acf.hhs.gov/cb/data-research/child-maltreatment

U.S. Department of Justice. (n.d.). *Domestic violence*. https://www.justice.gov/ovw/domestic-violence

Vlahovicova, K., Melendez-Torres, G. J., Leijten, P., Knerr, W., & Gardner, F. (2017). Parenting programs for the prevention of child physical abuse recurrence: A systematic review and meta-analysis. *Clinical Child and Family Psychology Review, 20*(3), 35–365. https://doi.org/10.1007/s10567-017-0232-7

Willacy, H. (2022). *Incest: Family sexual abuse*. https://patient.info/doctor/incest

Zhang-James, Y., Fernàndez-Castillo, N., Hess, J. L., Malki, K., Glatt, S. J., Cormand, B., & Faraone, S. V. (2019). An integrated analysis of genes and functional pathways for aggression in human and rodent models. *Molecular Psychiatry, 24*(11), 1655–1667. https://doi.org/10.1038/s41380-018-0068-7

Classical References

Burgess, A. W., & Holmström, L. L. (1974). Rape trauma syndrome. *American Journal of Psychiatry, 131*(9), 981–986. doi:10.1176/appi.ajp.131.9.981

Erikson, E. H. (1963). *Childhood and society* (2nd ed.). WW Norton.

Walker, L. E. (1979). *The battered woman*. Harper & Row.

Community Mental 35
Health Nursing

CORE CONCEPTS

Health Promotion:
Primary, secondary,
and tertiary
prevention

Population Health:
Homelessness and
mental illness

Health Policy

Professionalism:
Nursing process in
the care of patients in
the community

KEY TERMS

case management

case manager

deinstitutionalization

diagnosis-related groups (DRGs)

mobile outreach units

prospective payment

serious mental illness (SMI)

shelters

storefront clinics

OBJECTIVES
After reading this chapter, the student will be able to:

1. Discuss the changes in mental health-care delivery.
2. Define the concepts of care associated with the public health model.
3. Discuss primary prevention of mental illness within the community.
4. Identify populations at risk for mental illness within the community.
5. Discuss nursing intervention in primary prevention of mental illness within the community.
6. Discuss secondary prevention of mental illness within the community.
7. Describe treatment alternatives related to secondary prevention within the community.

8. Discuss tertiary prevention of mental illness within the community as it relates to the seriously mentally ill and homeless mentally ill.
9. Recognize the history and epidemiology associated with caring for the seriously mentally ill and homeless mentally ill within the community.
10. Identify treatment alternatives for care of the seriously mentally ill and homeless mentally ill within the community.
11. Apply steps of the nursing process to care of the seriously mentally ill and homeless mentally ill within the community.

This chapter explores the concepts of primary and secondary prevention of mental illness within communities. Additional focus is placed on tertiary prevention of mental illness: treatment using community resources of individuals with serious and persistent mental illness, including homeless people with mental illness. Emphasis is given to the role of the psychiatric nurse in the various treatment alternatives within the community setting.

Historical Perspective

Before 1840 there was no known treatment for individuals with mental illness. Because mental illness was perceived as incurable, the only "reasonable" intervention was thought to be removing these individuals from the community to a place where they could not harm themselves or others.

In 1841 Dorothea Dix, a former schoolteacher, began a personal crusade on behalf of institutionalized individuals with mental illness. Her efforts resulted in the more humane treatment of these people and the establishment of several psychiatric hospitals across the country.

After the movement initiated by Dix, the number of hospitals for people with mental illness increased, although unfortunately not as rapidly as did the population with mental illness. Hospitals became overcrowded and understaffed, with conditions that fell far short of Dix's original intentions.

The community mental health movement had its impetus in the 1940s. With the establishment of the National Mental Health Act of 1946, the U.S. government awarded grants to the states to develop mental health programs outside of state hospitals. Outpatient clinics and psychiatric units in general hospitals were inaugurated. Then, in 1949, as an outgrowth of the National Mental Health Act, the National Institute of Mental Health (NIMH) was established. The U.S. government has charged this agency with the responsibility for mental health in the United States.

In 1955 the Joint Commission on Mental Health and Illness was established by Congress to identify the nation's mental health needs and make recommendations for improvement in psychiatric care. In 1961 the Joint Commission published the report *Action for Mental Health* in which recommendations were made for the treatment of people with mental illness, training for caregivers, and improvements in education and research on mental illness. With consideration given to these recommendations, Congress passed the Mental Retardation Facilities and Community Mental Health Centers Construction Act (often called the *Community Mental Health Centers Act*) of 1963. This act called for the construction of comprehensive community mental health centers, the cost of which would be shared by federal and state governments. The **deinstitutionalization** movement (the closing of state mental hospitals and discharging of individuals with mental illness) had begun.

Unfortunately, many state governments did not have the capability to match the federal funds required for the establishment of these mental health centers. Some communities found it difficult to follow the rigid requirements for services mandated by the legislation that provided the grant.

In 1980 the Community Mental Health Systems Act, which would have a major role in the renovation of mental health care, was established. Funding was authorized for community mental health centers, services to high-risk populations, and rape research and services. Approval was also granted for the appointment of an associate director for minority concerns at NIMH. However, before this plan could be enacted, the newly inaugurated administration set forth its intention to diminish federal involvement. Budget cuts reduced the number of mandated services, and federal funding for community mental health centers was terminated in 1984.

Meanwhile, the costs of care for hospitalized psychiatric patients continued to rise. The problem of the "revolving door" began to intensify. Individuals with serious and persistent mental illness had no place to go when their symptoms exacerbated except back to the hospital. Individuals without support systems remained in the hospital for extended periods because of the lack of appropriate community services. Hospital services were paid for by cost-based, retrospective reimbursement: Medicaid, Medicare, and private health insurance. Retrospective reimbursement encouraged hospital expenditure; the more services provided, the more payment received.

This system of health-care delivery was interrupted in 1983 with the advent of **prospective payment**—the Reagan administration's proposal for cost containment. It was directed at control of Medicare costs by designating preestablished amounts that would be reimbursed for specific diagnoses, or **diagnosis-related groups (DRGs)**. Since that time, prospective payment has also been integrated by the states (Medicaid) and by some private insurance companies, drastically affecting the amount of reimbursement for health-care services.

Mental health services have been influenced by prospective payment. General hospital services to psychiatric patients have been severely restricted. Patients who present with acute symptoms, such as acute psychosis, suicidal ideations or attempts, or manic exacerbations, constitute the largest segment of the psychiatric hospital census. People with less serious illnesses (e.g., moderate depression or adjustment disorders) may be hospitalized, but the length of stay has been shortened considerably by the reimbursement guidelines. People are being discharged from the hospital with a greater need for aftercare than in the past when hospital stays were longer.

A positive outgrowth of efforts to reduce costly hospital stays and restricted reimbursement has been the development of a broader continuum of outpatient treatment options than what has been available historically. In the past, individuals who needed psychiatric treatment saw an outpatient therapist or were hospitalized, but today there are partial hospitalization programs, intensive outpatient programs, aftercare programs, and a host of other community-based services available to individuals with mental health disorders.

For those with health insurance, inroads have been made to eliminate discrimination against those with mental illness and substance use disorders; the Paul Wellstone and Pete Domenici Mental Health Parity and Addictions Equity Act (2008) required that, for health insurance plans that provide mental health and substance use disorder benefits, the plan cannot provide less favorable benefits than those provided for medical/surgical issues. The Affordable Care Act (2010) also required some insurance plans to include mental health and substance use disorder benefits. In reality, however, many people with chronic mental illnesses are uninsured, undertreated, and homeless.

Deinstitutionalization continues to affect mental health care in the United States. Care for the client in the hospital has become cost-prohibitive, whereas care for the client in the community is considered cost-effective. However, the community mental health movement has also been criticized for being a continuation of an "overly narrow biomedical model" (Vanderplasschen et al., 2013, p. 1). Ironically, the prison populations of people who are homeless and mentally ill have risen dramatically during this same period, one of the problems that Dorothea Dix fought so adamantly against in the first place. The reality of the provision of health-care services today is often more of a political and funding issue than providers would care to admit. Decisions about how to treat are rarely made without consideration of cost and method of payment.

The recovery model (see Chapter 20, "The Recovery Model") promises the hope of integrating the support of community mental health services, peer support, and client empowerment to improve interventions and outcomes as we look to the future. We must serve the consumer by working collaboratively to provide essential services for health promotion and early intervention and to promote improvement in the quality of life for this population.

The Public Health Model

The premise of the model of public health is based largely on the concepts set forth by Gerald Caplan (1964) during the initial community mental health movement. They include primary prevention, secondary prevention, and tertiary prevention. These concepts have expanded beyond mental health treatment and are now widely accepted as guiding principles in clinical and community settings over a wide range of medical and nursing specialties.

CORE CONCEPT
Primary Prevention
Services aimed at reducing the incidence of mental disorders within the population.

Primary prevention targets both individuals and the environment. The emphasis is twofold:

1. Assisting individuals to increase their ability to cope effectively with stress
2. Targeting and diminishing harmful forces (stressors) within the environment

Nursing in primary prevention is focused on the targeting of groups at risk and the provision of educational programs. Examples include the following:

■ Teaching parenting skills and child development to prospective new parents
■ Teaching physical and psychosocial effects of alcohol and drugs to elementary school students
■ Teaching techniques of stress management to anyone who desires to learn
■ Teaching groups of individuals ways to cope with the changes associated with various maturational stages
■ Teaching concepts of mental health to various groups within the community
■ Providing education and support to unemployed or homeless individuals
■ Providing education and support to other individuals in various transitional periods (e.g., widows and widowers, new retirees, and women entering the workforce in middle life)

These are only a few examples of the types of services nurses provide in primary prevention. Such services can be offered in a variety of convenient public settings (e.g., churches, schools, colleges, community centers, YMCAs and YWCAs, workplaces of employee organizations, meetings of women's groups, or civic or social organizations such as parent–teacher associations, health fairs, and community shelters).

CORE CONCEPT
Secondary Prevention
Interventions aimed at minimizing early symptoms of psychiatric illness and directed toward reducing the prevalence and duration of the illness.

Secondary prevention is accomplished through early identification of problems and prompt initiation of effective treatment. Nursing in secondary prevention focuses on recognition of symptoms and provision of or referral for treatment. Examples include the following:

■ Ongoing assessment of individuals at high risk for illness exacerbation (e.g., during home visits, day care, community health centers, or in any setting where screening of high-risk individuals might occur).
■ Provision of care for individuals in whom illness symptoms have been assessed (e.g., individual or group counseling, medication administration, education and support during periods of increased stress [crisis intervention], staffing rape crisis centers, suicide hotlines, homeless shelters, shelters for abused persons, or mobile mental health units).
■ Referral for treatment of individuals in whom symptoms have been assessed. Referrals may come from support groups, community mental health centers, emergency services, psychiatrists or psychologists, and day or partial hospitalization programs. Inpatient therapy on a psychiatric unit of a general hospital or in a private psychiatric hospital may be necessary. Psychopharmacology and various adjunct therapies may be initiated as part of the treatment.
■ Providing education about the potential long-term health consequences associated with adverse childhood experiences and the importance of trauma recovery services.

Secondary prevention is addressed extensively in Unit 4, "Nursing Care of Patients with Alterations in Psychosocial Adaptation," of this text. Nursing assessment, diagnosis and outcome identification, planning and implementation, and evaluation are discussed for many of the mental illnesses identified in the *Diagnostic and Statistical Manual of Mental Disorders, Fifth Edition, Text Revision (DSM-5-TR)* (American Psychiatric Association [APA], 2022). These concepts may be applied in any setting where nursing is practiced.

CORE CONCEPT
Tertiary Prevention
Services directed at reducing the residual defects associated with serious and persistent mental illness.

Tertiary prevention is accomplished in two ways:

1. Preventing complications of the illness
2. Promoting rehabilitation directed toward the achievement of each individual's maximal level of functioning

Historically, individuals with serious and persistent mental illness often experienced long hospitalizations that resulted in a loss of social skills and increased dependency. With deinstitutionalization, many of these individuals may never have experienced hospitalization, but they still may not possess adequate support and skills to live productive lives within the community.

Nursing in tertiary prevention focuses on helping clients learn or relearn socially appropriate behaviors so that they may achieve a satisfying role within the community. Examples include the following:

■ Consideration of the rehabilitation process at the time of initial diagnosis and treatment planning
■ Teaching the client daily living skills and encouraging independence to their maximal ability
■ Referring clients for various aftercare services (e.g., support groups, day treatment programs, partial hospitalization programs, psychosocial rehabilitation programs, group homes, or other transitional housing)
■ Monitoring effectiveness of aftercare services (e.g., through home health visits or follow-up appointments in community mental health centers)
■ Making referrals for support services when required (e.g., some communities have programs linking individuals with serious mental disorders to volunteers who develop friendships with the individuals and may assist with household chores, shopping, and other activities of daily living with which the individual is having difficulty, in addition to participating in social activities with the individual)
■ Providing trauma-informed care, and when health consequences are associated with a history of trauma, referrals are made to specialized trauma recovery treatment programs

Nursing care at the tertiary level of prevention can be administered on an individual or group basis and in a variety of settings, such as inpatient hospitalization, day or partial hospitalization, group home or halfway houses, shelters, home health care, nursing homes, and community mental health centers.

The Community as Client

Primary Prevention

CORE CONCEPT
Community
A group, population, or cluster of people with at least one common characteristic, such as geographical location, occupation, ethnicity, or health concern.

Primary prevention within communities encompasses the twofold emphasis defined earlier in this chapter:

1. Identifying stressful life events that precipitate crises and targeting the relevant populations at high risk
2. Intervening with these high-risk populations to prevent or minimize harmful consequences

Populations at Risk

One way to view populations at risk is to focus on the types of crises that individuals typically experience in their lives. Two broad categories are maturational crises and situational crises.

Maturational Crises

Maturational crises are crucial experiences associated with various stages of growth and development. Erikson (1963) described eight stages of the life cycle during which individuals struggle with developmental "tasks." Crises can occur during any of these stages, although several developmental periods and life-cycle events have been recognized as having increased crisis potential: adolescence, marriage, parenthood, midlife, and retirement.

Adolescence

The task for adolescence according to Erikson (1963) is *identity versus role confusion*. This is the time in life when individuals ask questions such as "Who am I?" "Where am I going?" and "What is life all about?"

Adolescence is a transition into young adulthood. It can be a volatile time in families. Commonly, conflict arises over issues of control. Parents sometimes have difficulty relinquishing even a minimal amount of the control they have had throughout their child's infancy, toddlerhood, and school-aged years at this time when the adolescent is seeking increased independence. It may seem that the adolescent is 25 years old one day and 5 years old the next. An often-quoted definition of an adolescent, by an anonymous author, is: "A toddler with hormones and wheels."

At this time, adolescents are "trying out their wings," although they possess an essential need to know that the parents (or surrogate parents) are available if support is required. In fact, it is believed that the most frequent immediate precipitant to adolescent suicide is the loss, threat of loss, or abandonment by parents or closest peer relationship.

Adolescents have many issues to deal with and many choices to make. Some of these include issues that relate to self-esteem and body image (in a body that is undergoing rapid changes), peer relationships (with both genders), education and career selection, establishing a set of values and ideals,

sexuality and sexual experimentation (including issues of birth control and prevention of sexually transmitted infections), drug and alcohol use, and physical appearance.

Nursing interventions with adolescents at the primary level of prevention focus on providing support and accurate information to ease the transition they are undergoing. Educational programs can be presented in schools, churches, youth centers, or any location in which groups of teenagers gather. Types of programs may include the following:

- Alateen groups for adolescents with alcoholic parent(s)
- Other support groups for teenagers who need assistance to cope with stressful situations (e.g., children dealing with divorce of their parents, pregnant teenagers, teenagers coping with abortion, adolescents coping with the death of a parent)
- Educational programs that inform about and validate body changes and emotions about which there may be some concerns
- Educational programs that inform about positive self-esteem and resilience
- Educational programs that inform about sexuality, pregnancy, contraception, and sexually transmitted infections
- Educational programs that inform about the consequences of alcohol or other drug misuse

Marriage

Although there are many culturally accepted choices about the nature of relationships and living arrangements in lieu of marriage in today's society, crises may develop related to conflicting values between generations within a family and related to the many factors influencing those choices, including economic concerns.

Ideological changes that stress personal freedom, self-fulfillment, and individual choice have contributed to an increase in people delaying marriage to fulfill career aspirations or leaving marriages that do not fulfill their expectations (Casper & Coritz, 2018).

When young adults do decide to enter into marriage, a crisis may develop associated with unrealistic or uninformed expectations about this institution. It is well understood, too, that children raised in abusive, dysfunctional families are at higher risk for subconsciously choosing partners who perpetuate the negative experiences they were accustomed to while they were growing up. Both of these circumstances can increase the risk of crisis within a marriage.

Nursing interventions at the primary level of prevention with individuals in this stage of development involve education about what to expect from marriage and other committed relationships. Educating young adults about assertive communication skills, clarifying each person's expectations for the relationship, healthy boundaries, and, particularly, the risks associated with choosing a partner who perpetuates a cycle of violence are all important aspects of primary prevention. These interventions can be effective in individual or couples therapy and in support or educational groups of couples experiencing similar circumstances.

Parenthood

There is perhaps no developmental stage that creates an upheaval equal to that of the arrival of a child. Even when the child is desperately wanted and pleasurably anticipated, their arrival usually results in some degree of chaos within the family.

Because the family operates as a system, the addition of a new member influences all parts of the system as a whole. If it is a first child, the relationship between spouses is likely to be affected by the demands of caring for the infant on a 24-hour basis. If there are older children, they may resent the attention showered on the new arrival and show their resentment in a variety of creative ways.

The concept of having a child (particularly the first one) is often romanticized, with little or no consideration given to the realities and responsibilities that accompany this "bundle of joy." Many young parents are shocked to realize that such a tiny human can create so many changes in so many lives. It is unfortunate that although parenting is one of the most challenging positions an individual will hold in life, it is one for which new parents are often least prepared.

Nursing intervention at the primary level of prevention with those in the developmental stage of parenthood must begin long before the child is even born. How do we prepare individuals for parenthood? *Anticipatory guidance* is the term used to describe the interventions used to help new parents know what they might expect. Volumes have been written on the subject, but it is also important for expectant parents to have a support person or network with whom they can talk honestly and express feelings, excitement, and fears. Nurses can provide the following types of information to help ease the transition into parenthood (Spock & Needlman, 2018; Veltri et al., 2018):

- **Prepared childbirth classes:** These classes present what most couples can expect along with information about possible deviations from what is expected.
- **What to expect after the baby arrives:**
  - *Parent–infant bonding:* Expectant parents should know that it is common for parent–infant bonding not to occur immediately. The strong attachment will occur as parent and infant get to know each other.
  - *Changing communication patterns and relationship styles:* The couple should be encouraged to engage in open, honest communication with each other. Education should be offered about expected changes in communication patterns and the challenges of establishing communication with an infant, in addition to resources for referral if communication patterns are creating significant role strain. Frustrated attempts to adapt to these challenges can have consequences for the infant as well. In some cases, an infant's need may be neglected if the parents lack skills or resources to navigate communication challenges. As Veltri and colleagues note, "abusive head trauma, which includes shaken baby syndrome, is an extreme example of an inability to adapt to changed communication patterns with an infant" (Veltri et al., p. 367). Education should include strategies that family members may use to maintain motivation and morale and provide for comfort, rest, and self-care for each member.
  - *Clothing and equipment:* Expectant parents need to know what is required to care for a newborn child. Financing childbearing and child-rearing, arranging space for a child, and lifestyle should be considered.
  - *Feeding:* Advantages and disadvantages of breastfeeding and formula feeding should be presented. The couple should be supported in whatever method is chosen. Anticipatory guidance related to technique should be provided for one or both methods at the expectant parents' request.
  - *Other expectations:* It is important for expectant parents to receive anticipatory guidance about the infant's sleeping and crying patterns, bathing the infant, care of the circumcision and cord, toys that provide stimulation of the newborn's senses, aspects of providing a safe environment, and when to call the physician.
- **Stages of growth and development:** It is important for parents to understand what behaviors should be expected at what stage of development. It is also important to know that their child may not necessarily follow the age guidelines associated with these stages. However, a substantial deviation from these guidelines should be reported to the pediatrician.

Midlife

What is middle age? A colleague once remarked that upon turning 50 years of age, she stated, "'Now

I can say I am officially middle-aged' … until I began thinking about how few individuals I really knew who were 100!"

Midlife crises are not defined by a specific number. Various sources in the literature identify these conflicts as occurring anytime between the ages of 35 and 65.

What is a midlife crisis? It is very individual, but several patterns have been identified within three broad categories:

1. **An alteration in the perception of the self:** One's perception of self may change slowly, or a person may suddenly become aware of being "old" or "middle-aged." Other biological changes that occur naturally with the aging process may also affect the crises that occur at this time.

   - In women, a gradual decrease in estrogen production initiates menopause, which results in a variety of physical and emotional symptoms. Some physical symptoms include hot flashes, vaginal dryness, cessation of menstruation, loss of reproductive ability, night sweats, insomnia, headaches, and minor memory disturbances. Emotional symptoms include anxiety, depression, crying for no reason, and temper outbursts.

   - In men, lower testosterone levels may go unnoticed, but some men experience decreased energy, depressed mood, decline in sexual desire and activity, hot flashes, sweating, breast discomfort, and insomnia (Mayo Clinic, 2022). Alteration in sexual functioning is not uncommon.

2. **An alteration in the perception of others:** A change in relationship with adult children requires a sensitive shift in caring. Shajani and Snell (2019) identify several aspects of this change, including:

   - Navigating the new role between parent and adult child in place of the primary parent role
   - Renegotiating emotional and financial commitments
   - Adjusting to a multitude of exits from and entries into the family system

   These experiences are particularly difficult when parents' values conflict with the relationships and types of lifestyles their children choose. An alteration in perception of one's parents also begins to occur during this time. Having always looked to parents for support and comfort, the middle-aged individual may suddenly find that the roles are beginning to reverse. Aging parents may look to their children for assistance with decisions regarding their everyday lives and chores they have previously accomplished independently. When parents die, middle-aged individuals must come to terms with their own mortality. The process of recognition and resolution of one's own finitude begins in earnest at this time.

3. **An alteration in the perception of time:** Middle age has been defined as the end of youth and the beginning of old age. Individuals often experience a sense that time is running out: "I haven't done all I want to do or accomplished all I intended to accomplish!" Depression and a sense of loss may occur as individuals realize that some of the goals established in their youth may go unmet.

   - The term *empty nest syndrome* has been used to describe the adjustment period parents experience when the last child leaves home to establish an independent residence. The crisis is often more profound for the mother, who has devoted her life to nurturing her family. As the last child leaves, she may perceive her future as uncertain and meaningless.

   - Some women who have devoted their lives to rearing their children decide to develop personal interests and pursue personal goals once the children are grown. This occurs at a time when many husbands have begun to decrease what may have been a compulsive drive for occupational security during the earlier years of their lives. This disparity in common goals may create conflict and require numerous adaptations on the part of both spouses.

   - Finally, an alteration in one's perception of time may be related to the societal striving for eternal youth. The individual may try to delay the external changes that come with aging by the use of cosmetics, hormone creams, or even surgery. This yearning for youth may take the form of sexual promiscuity or extramarital affairs with much younger individuals to prove that one "still has what it takes." A negative view of oneself as an aging individual may lead to behaviors that are attempts to relive one's youth.

Nursing intervention at the primary level of prevention with those in the developmental stage of midlife involves providing accurate information regarding changes that occur during this time of life and support for adapting to these changes effectively. The community is an appropriate place for this education, as these experiences are shared by many of its members. These interventions might include the following:

- Nutrition classes to inform individuals in this age-group about the essentials of diet and exercise. Educational materials on how to avoid obesity and the importance of good nutrition can be included.

■ Assistance with ways to improve health (e.g., quit smoking, cease or reduce alcohol consumption, reduce fat intake).

■ Discussions of the importance of having regular physical examinations, including screening tests for breast and cervical cancer for women and prostate examinations for men.

■ Classes and support groups on menopause with information about what to expect.

■ Support and information related to physical changes occurring in the body during this time of life. Assist with the grief response that some individuals will experience in relation to loss of youth, the "empty nest syndrome," and change in the sense of identity.

■ Support and information related to the care of aging parents. Information and referral to community resources for respite and assistance *before* strain of the caregiver role threatens to disrupt the family system.

Retirement

Often anticipated as an achievement in principle, retirement may be met with ambivalence when it actually occurs. Our society places profound importance on productivity and earning as much money as possible at as young an age as possible. These types of values contribute to the ambivalence associated with retirement. Although leisure has been acknowledged as a legitimate reward for workers, leisure during retirement has never been accorded the same social value. Adjustment to this life-cycle event becomes more difficult in the face of societal values that are in direct conflict with the new lifestyle.

Termination of child-rearing activities can result in a loss of self-worth, and individuals who are unable to adapt satisfactorily may become depressed. It would appear that retirement is becoming, and will continue to become, more accepted by societal standards. With increasing numbers of individuals living longer, a growing number of aging persons will spend more time in retirement. Nursing intervention at the primary level of prevention with the developmental task of retirement involves providing information and support to individuals who have retired or are considering retirement. Support can be provided on a one-to-one basis to assist individuals in sorting out their feelings regarding retirement. Well-being in retirement is linked to factors such as stable health status, adequate income, the ability to pursue new goals or activities, extended social network of family and friends, and satisfaction with current living arrangements.

One trend that has been a hallmark of change for many older adults is the increasing numbers of grandparents who are caring for grandchildren and, in many cases, assuming primary responsibility for their care (Casper & Coritz, 2018). Nurses can promote primary prevention of crisis through education about resources for caregiving assistance and evidence-based information about this new role. In fact, evidence shows that despite the burdens associated with caregiving, many grandparents identify that this role revealed their inner strength and gave them a sense of accomplishment (White & Cartwright, 2018).

Support can also be provided in a group environment. Support groups of individuals undergoing the same types of experiences can be extremely helpful. Nurses can form and lead groups to assist retiring individuals through this critical period. These groups can also serve to provide information about available resources that offer assistance to individuals in or nearing retirement, such as information concerning Medicare, Social Security, and Medicaid; information related to organizations that specialize in hiring retirees; and information regarding ways to use newly acquired free time constructively.

Situational Crises

Situational crises are acute responses that occur as a result of an external stressor. The number and types of situational stressors are limitless. Some crises exist only in the perception of the individual. Types of situational crises that put individuals at risk for mental illness are discussed next.

Poverty

Many studies have identified poverty to be directly correlated with emotional illness. This may have to do with the direct consequences of poverty, such as inadequate and crowded living conditions, nutritional deficiencies, medical neglect, unemployment, or being homeless.

High Rate of Life-Change Events

Many studies have found that changes in life patterns when a large number of significant events occur close together tend to decrease a person's ability to manage stress, sometimes resulting in physical or emotional illness (McLeod, 2010). These include events such as death of a loved one, divorce, being fired from a job, a change in living conditions, a change in place of employment or residence, physical illness, or a change in body image caused by the loss of a body part or function.

Environmental Conditions

Environmental conditions can create situational crises. Tornados, floods, hurricanes, and earthquakes have wreaked devastation on thousands of individuals and families in recent years.

Trauma

Individuals who have encountered traumatic experiences must be considered at risk for physical, mental, emotional, and spiritual sequelae. These include those considered outside the range of typical human experience, such as physical or sexual abuse, rape, war, physical attack, torture, or natural or manmade disaster.

Nursing intervention at the primary level of prevention with individuals experiencing situational crises is aimed at how to manage specific situational crises (such as disaster planning) and offering support and assistance with problem-solving during the crisis period. Interventions for nursing of clients in crisis include the following:

- Use a reality-oriented approach. The focus of the problem is on the here and now.
- Remain with the individual who is experiencing panic anxiety.
- Establish a rapid working relationship by showing unconditional acceptance, active listening, and attending to immediate needs.
- Discourage lengthy explanations or rationalizations of the situation; promote an atmosphere for verbalization of true feelings.
- Set firm limits on aggressive, destructive behaviors. At high levels of anxiety, behavior is likely to be impulsive and regressive. Establish at the outset what is acceptable and what is not and maintain consistency.
- Clarify the problem the individual is facing. The nurse does this by describing their perception of the problem and comparing it with the individual's perception of the problem.
- Help the individual determine what they believe precipitated the crisis.
- Acknowledge feelings of anger, guilt, helplessness, and powerlessness, while taking care not to provide positive feedback for these feelings.
- Guide the individual through a problem-solving process by which they may move in the direction of positive life change:
  - Help the individual confront the source of the problem that is creating the crisis response.
  - Encourage the individual to discuss changes they would like to make. Jointly determine whether desired changes are realistic.
  - Encourage exploration of feelings about aspects that cannot be changed and explore alternative ways of coping more adaptively in these situations.
  - Discuss alternative strategies for creating change in situations that can realistically be changed.
  - Weigh the benefits and consequences of each alternative.
  - Assist the individual in selecting alternative coping strategies that will help alleviate future crises.
- Identify external support systems and new social networks from which the individual may seek assistance in times of stress.

Nursing at the level of primary prevention focuses largely on education of the consumer to prevent initiation or exacerbation of mental illness.

Secondary Prevention

Populations at Risk

Secondary prevention within communities relates to early detection of and prompt intervention with individuals experiencing mental illness symptoms. The same maturational and situational crises presented in the previous section on primary prevention are used to discuss intervention at the secondary level of prevention.

Maturational Crises

Adolescence

The need for intervention at the secondary level of prevention in adolescence occurs when disruptive and age-inappropriate behaviors become the norm and the family can no longer cope adaptively with the situation. All levels of dysfunction are considered—from dysfunctional family coping to the need for hospitalization of the adolescent.

Nursing intervention with the adolescent at this level may occur in the community setting at community mental health centers, physicians' offices, schools, public health departments, and crisis intervention centers. Nurses may work with families to problem-solve and improve coping and communication skills, or they may work on a one-to-one basis with the adolescent in an attempt to modify behavior patterns.

Adolescents may be hospitalized for a variety of problems, including (but not limited to) conduct disorders, adjustment disorders, eating disorders, substance-related disorders, depression, and anxiety disorders. Inpatient care is determined by the severity of the symptomatology. Nursing care of adolescents in the hospital setting focuses on identifying the problem and stabilizing a crisis situation. Once stability has been achieved, clients are commonly discharged to outpatient care. If an adolescent's home situation has been deemed unsatisfactory, the state may take custody, and the child is then discharged to a group or foster home.

Marriage

Problems that are not uncommon to the disruption of a marriage relationship include substance use disorders by one or both partners and disagreements on issues of sex, money, children, gender roles, and infidelity, among others.

Nursing intervention at the secondary level of prevention with individuals encountering marriage problems may include support groups for newly divorced individuals, referral to couples therapy, or referral to other specific treatment programs as needs are identified.

Divorce typically invokes a spectrum of troubling emotions including anger, mistrust, depression, and grief. Risks for clinical depression and suicide should always be a part of the assessment. Divorce also has an impact on the children involved. Group counseling with children who are manifesting behavioral or emotional problems associated with parental divorce is an important option for secondary prevention.

Parenthood

Intervention at the secondary level of prevention with parents may be required for many reasons, including the following:

■ Physical, emotional, or sexual abuse of a child
■ Physical or emotional neglect of a child
■ Birth of a child with special needs
■ Diagnosis of a terminal illness in a child
■ Death of a child

Nursing intervention at the secondary level of prevention includes recognition of the physical and behavioral signs that indicate possible abuse of a child. The child may be cared for in the emergency department or as an inpatient in the pediatric unit or child psychiatric unit of a general hospital.

Nursing intervention with parents may include teaching effective methods of disciplining children aside from physical punishment. Methods that emphasize the importance of positive reinforcement for acceptable behavior can be highly effective. Family members must be committed to the consistent use of this behavior modification technique for it to be successful.

Parents should also be informed about behavioral expectations at various levels of development. Knowledge of what to expect from children at these various stages may provide needed anticipatory guidance to deal with the crises commonly associated with each stage.

Referral to family therapy may help family members to resolve communication problems. Members are encouraged to express honest feelings in a manner that is nonthreatening to other family members. Active listening, assertiveness techniques, and respect for the rights of others are taught and encouraged. Barriers to effective communication are identified and resolved.

Referrals to agencies that promote effective parenting skills may be made (e.g., parent effectiveness training). Alternative agencies that may provide relief from the stress of parenting may also be considered (e.g., Mom's Day Out programs, sitter-sharing organizations, and day-care institutions). Support groups for abusive parents may also be helpful and assistance in locating or initiating such a group may be provided.

The nurse can assist parents who are grieving the loss of a child or the birth of a child with special needs by helping them express their feelings associated with the loss. Feelings such as shock, denial, anger, guilt, powerlessness, and hopelessness must be expressed for the parents to progress through the grief response.

Home health-care assistance can be provided for the family of a child with special needs by making referrals to other professionals, such as speech, physical, and occupational therapists; medical social workers; psychologists; and nutritionists. If the child with special needs is hospitalized, the home health nurse can provide specific information to hospital staff that may be helpful in providing continuity of care for the child and in the transition for the family.

Nursing intervention also includes providing assistance in the location of and referral to support groups that deal with the loss of a child or birth of a child with special needs. Some nurses may serve as leaders of these types of groups in the community.

Midlife

Nursing care at the secondary level of prevention during midlife becomes necessary when the individual is unable to integrate all the changes that are occurring during this period. An inability to accept the physical and biological changes, changes in relationships between themselves and their adult children and aging parents, and loss of the perception of youth may result in depression for which the individual may require help to resolve.

Retirement

Retirement can also result in depression for individuals who are unable to satisfactorily grieve for the loss of this aspect of their lives. This reaction is more likely to occur if the individuals have not planned for retirement or if they have derived most of their self-esteem from their employment.

Nursing intervention at the secondary level of prevention with depressed individuals takes place in both inpatient and outpatient settings. Severely depressed clients with suicidal ideations will need close observation in the hospital setting, whereas those with mild to moderate depression may be treated in the community. A plan of care for the patient with depression is found in Chapter 25, "Depressive Disorders." These concepts apply to the secondary level of prevention and may be used in all nursing care settings.

Situational Crises

Nursing care at the secondary level of prevention with clients undergoing situational crises occurs only if crisis intervention at the primary level has failed and the individual is unable to function socially or occupationally. Exacerbation of mental illness symptoms requires intervention at the secondary level of prevention. These disorders are addressed extensively in Unit 4, "Nursing Care of Patients With Alterations in Psychosocial Adaptation." Nursing assessment, diagnosis and outcome identification, planning, implementation, and evaluation are discussed for many of the mental illnesses identified in the *DSM-5-TR* (APA, 2022). These skills may be applied in any setting where nursing is practiced.

A case study of nursing care at the secondary level of prevention in a community setting is presented in Box 35–1.

Tertiary Prevention

Individuals With Serious and Persistent Mental Illness

Various terms such as *chronic mental illness, serious and persistent mental illness,* or **serious mental illness (SMI)**

BOX 35–1 Secondary Prevention Case Study: Parenthood

The identified patient was a petite, doll-like 4-year-old girl named Tanya. She was the older of two children. The other child was a boy named Joseph, age 2. The mother was 5 months pregnant with their third child. The family had been referred to the nurse after Tanya was placed in foster care after a report to child protective services by her nursery schoolteacher that the child had marks on her body suspicious of child abuse.

The parents, Paulo and Annette, were in their mid-20s. Paulo had lost his job at an aircraft plant 3 months ago and had been unable to find work since. Annette brought in a few dollars from cleaning houses for other people, but the family was struggling to survive.

Paulo and Annette were angry at having to see the nurse. After all, "parents have the right to discipline their children." The nurse did not focus on the *intent* of the behavior, but instead looked at factors in the family's life that could be viewed as stressors. This family had multiple stressors: poverty, the father's unemployment, the age and spacing of the children, the mother's chronic fatigue from work at home and in other people's homes, and finally, having a child removed from the home against the parents' wishes.

During therapy with this family, the nurse discussed the behaviors associated with various developmental levels. She also discussed possible deviations from these norms and when they should be reported to the physician. The nurse and the family discussed Tanya's behavior and how it compared with the norms.

The parents also discussed their own childhoods. They were able to relate some of the same types of behaviors that they observed in Tanya, but they both admitted that they came from families whose main method of discipline was physical punishment. Annette had been the oldest child in her large family and had been expected to "keep the younger ones in line." When she had not done so, she was punished with her father's belt. She expressed anger toward her father, although she had never been allowed to express it at the time.

Paulo's father had died when he was a small boy, and Paulo had been expected to be the "man of the family." From the time he was very young, he worked at odd jobs to bring money into the home. Consequently, he had little time for the usual activities of childhood and adolescence. He held much resentment toward the young men who "had everything and never had to work for it."

Paulo and Annette had high expectations for Tanya. In effect, they expected her to behave in a manner well beyond her developmental level. These expectations were based on the reflections of their own childhoods. They were uncomfortable with the spontaneity and playfulness of childhood because they had had little personal experience with these behaviors. When Tanya balked and expressed the verbal assertions common to early childhood, Paulo and Annette interpreted these behaviors as defiance toward them and retaliated with anger in the manner in which they had been parented.

With the parents, the nurse explored feelings and behaviors from their past so that they were able to understand the correlation to their current behaviors. They learned to negotiate ways to deal with Tanya's age-appropriate behaviors. In combined therapy with Tanya, they learned how to relate to her childishness and even how to enjoy playing with both of their children.

The parents ceased blaming each other for the family's problems. Annette had spent a good deal of her time deprecating Paulo for his lack of support of his family, and Paulo blamed Annette for being "unable to control her daughter." Communication patterns were clarified, and life in the family became more peaceful.

Without a need to "prove himself" to his wife, Paulo's efforts to find employment met with success because he no longer felt the need to turn down jobs that he believed his wife would perceive to be beneath his capabilities. Annette no longer works outside the home, and both she and Paulo participate in the parenting tasks. Tanya and her siblings continue to demonstrate age-appropriate developmental progression.

have been used to describe disorders that contribute to significant functional impairment. The term *chronic* has been replaced by the latter two descriptors because "chronic" may have a negative connotation, suggesting that recovery is not possible (Substance Abuse and Mental Health Services Administration [SAMHSA], 2016). In fact, those with SMI can respond to treatment, services, and recovery-oriented support (SAMHSA, 2016). Furthermore, not all SMIs are serious *and* persistent. The NIMH (2022) defines SMI as "a mental, behavioral, or emotional disorder resulting in serious functional impairment, which substantially interferes with or limits one or more major life activities." Those that are identified as "severe and persistent" are characterized by significant, ongoing, functional impairment and major disability. These disorders are identified by criteria listed in the *DSM-5-TR*. Diagnoses may include schizophrenia and related disorders, bipolar disorder, autism spectrum disorders, major depressive disorder, panic disorder, obsessive-compulsive disorder, post-traumatic stress disorder (PTSD), borderline personality disorder, and attention deficit-hyperactivity disorder.

Based on 2020 statistics, SMI affects about 5.6% of the population in the United States (NIMH, 2022). The actual number may be significantly higher because this research did not attempt to include the homeless; those in active military duty; or those who were in institutions such as correctional facilities, nursing homes, mental institutions, or long-term hospitals for the entire year.

History and Epidemiology

In 1955 more than half a million individuals resided in public mental hospitals, compared with fewer than 100,000 based on today's estimates. Deinstitutionalization of persons with SMI began in the 1960s as the national policy changed to one based on a strong belief in the individual's right to freedom. Other considerations included the deplorable conditions of some of the state asylums, introduction of psychotropic medications, and cost-effectiveness of caring for these individuals in the community setting.

Deinstitutionalization began to occur rapidly and without sufficient planning for the needs of these individuals as they reentered the community. Those who were fortunate to have support systems to provide assistance with living arrangements and sheltered employment experiences most often received the outpatient treatment they required. Those without adequate support, however, either managed to survive on a meager income or were forced into homelessness. Some ended up in nursing homes meant to provide care for individuals with physical disabilities.

Certain segments of our population with serious and persistent mental illness have been left untreated: the elderly, the working poor, the homeless, and those individuals previously covered by funds cut by various social reforms. These circumstances have promoted a greater number of crisis-oriented emergency department visits and hospital admissions for individuals with serious and persistent mental illness, in addition to frequent confrontations with law enforcement officials.

In 2002 President George W. Bush established the New Freedom Commission on Mental Health, charged with conducting a comprehensive study of the U.S. mental health service delivery system. They were to identify unmet needs and barriers to services and recommend steps for improvement in services and support for individuals with SMI. It is relevant to evaluate the current state of mental health services in comparison to problems that were identified over 20 years ago. In July 2003 the commission presented its final report to the president (President's New Freedom Commission on Mental Health, 2003). The commission identified the following five barriers:

1. **Fragmentation and gaps in care for children.** About 7% to 9% of all children (aged 9 to 17) have a serious emotional disturbance (SED). The commission found that services for children are even more fragmented than those for adults, with more uncoordinated funding and differing eligibility requirements. Only a small number of children with SED have access to school-based or school-linked mental health services. Children with SED who are identified for special education services have higher levels of absenteeism, higher drop-out rates, and lower levels of academic achievement than students with other disabilities.

2. **Fragmentation and gaps in care for adults with SMI.** The commission expressed concern that so many adults with SMI are homeless, dependent on alcohol or drugs, unemployed, and go without treatment. The commission identified public attitudes and the stigma associated with mental illness as major barriers to treatment. Stigma is often internalized by individuals with mental illness, leading to hopelessness, lower self-esteem, and isolation. Stigma deprives these individuals of the support they need to recover.

3. **High unemployment and disability for people with SMI.** Undiagnosed, untreated, and poorly treated mental disorders interrupt careers, leading many individuals into lives of disability, poverty, and long-term dependence. The commission found a 90% unemployment rate among adults

with SMI—the worst level of employment of any group of people with disabilities. Some surveys have shown that many individuals with SMI *want* to work and could do so with modest assistance. However, the largest "program" of assistance the United States has for people with mental illness is disability payments. Sadly, societal stigma is also reflected in employment discrimination against people with mental illness.

4. **Older adults with mental illnesses are not receiving care.** The commission reported that about 5% to 10% of older adults have major depression, yet most cases are not properly recognized and treated. The report stated:

Older people are reluctant to get care from specialists. They feel more comfortable going to their primary care physician. Still, they are often more sensitive to the stigma of mental illness, and do not readily bring up their sadness and despair. If they acknowledge problems, they are more likely than young people to describe physical symptoms. Primary care doctors may see their suffering as "natural" aging, or treat their reported physical distress instead of the underlying mental disorder. What is often missed is the deep impact of depression on older people's capacity to function in ways that are seemingly effortless for others.

5. **Mental health and suicide prevention are not yet national priorities.** The failure of the United States to prioritize mental health puts many lives at stake. Families struggle to maintain equilibrium, while communities strain (and often fail) to provide needed assistance for adults and children with mental illness. Over 30,000 lives are lost annually to suicide. About 90% of those who take their life have a mental disorder. Many individuals who die by suicide have not had care that would help them to affirm life in the months before their deaths.

Both the APA and the National Mental Health Association have since called on the U.S. Congress to pass parity legislation. As previously mentioned, in 2008 a federal law known as the Paul Wellstone and Pete Domenici Mental Health Parity and Addiction Equity Act was enacted that generally prevents group health plans and health insurance issuers that provide mental health or substance use disorder benefits from imposing less favorable limitations on those benefits than on medical/surgical benefits. In 2010 the Affordable Care Act amended this legislation to include individual insurance plans, and in 2014 a final regulation clarified and expanded the parity law (Centers for Medicare & Medicaid Services [CMS], n.d.). Many recent national initiatives since the commission's report have attempted to bridge the gaps,

particularly with efforts to address the national suicide rates and the opiate overdose epidemic. Clearly there is still much work to be done. The commission outlined the following goals and recommendations for mental health reform:

Goal 1. Americans will understand that mental health is essential to overall health.

Commission recommendations:

■ Advance and implement a national campaign to reduce the stigma of seeking care and a national strategy for suicide prevention.
■ Address mental health with the same urgency as physical health.

Goal 2. Mental health care will be consumer and family driven.

Commission recommendations:

■ Develop an individualized plan of care for every adult with a SMI and child with an SED.
■ Involve consumers and families fully in orienting the mental health system toward recovery.
■ Align relevant federal programs to improve access and accountability for mental health services.
■ Create a comprehensive state mental health plan.
■ Protect and enhance the rights of people with mental illness.

Goal 3. Disparities in mental health services will be eliminated.

Commission recommendations:

■ Improve access to quality care that is culturally competent.
■ Improve access to quality care in rural and geographically remote areas.

Goal 4. Early mental health screening, assessment, and referral to services will be common practice.

Commission recommendations:

■ Promote the mental health of young children.
■ Improve and expand school mental health programs.
■ Screen for co-occurring mental and substance use disorders and link with integrated treatment strategies.
■ Screen for mental disorders in primary health care across the life span and connect to treatment and supports.

Goal 5. Excellent mental health care will be delivered and research will be accelerated.

Commission recommendations:

■ Accelerate research to promote recovery and resilience, and ultimately to cure and prevent mental illnesses.

■ Advance evidence-based practices using dissemination and demonstration projects and create a public-private partnership to guide their implementation.

■ Improve and expand the workforce providing evidence-based mental health services and supports.

■ Develop the knowledge base in four understudied areas: mental health disparities, long-term effects of medications, trauma, and acute care.

Goal 6. Technology will be used to access mental health care and information.

Commission recommendations:

■ Use health technology and telehealth to improve access and coordination of mental health care, especially for Americans in remote areas or in underserved populations.

■ Develop and implement integrated electronic health records and personal health information systems.

The current state of mental health care delivery has changed and progressed on some of the goals established by the commission, but much more work is needed. The SAMHSA, in collaboration with several other federal agencies, is actively engaged in initiatives to address mental health issues for specific, underserved populations, suicide prevention, and other community and public health concerns. Suicide prevention has been identified as a national health priority, and the number of suicides continues to remain well above those identified by the commission in 2003. The surgeon general released a landmark report in 2016 identifying substance misuse as a national health priority in response to the rising death toll from opiate overdoses. In 2018 the National Institutes of Health launched the Helping End Addictions Long-term (HEAL) effort that includes 15 initiatives geared toward better treatment of opiate addiction and pain management. These initiatives are a response to the current national attention to mental health and addiction concerns, particularly those related to epidemic levels of suicide and opiate-related deaths. The SAMHSA strategic plan for 2019–2023 (2022b), again, identifies management of the opioid crisis and meeting the needs of those with SMI as top priorities. The solutions to the multitude of SMI and substance-use–related issues that affect individuals and communities are complex and will require ongoing individual, local, and nationwide efforts.

Many nurse leaders see this period of health-care reform as an opportunity for nurses to expand their roles and assume key positions in education, prevention, assessment, and referral. Nurses are, and will continue to be, in key positions to help individuals with serious and persistent mental illness remain as independent as possible, manage their illnesses within the community setting, and minimize the number of hospitalizations required.

Treatment Alternatives

In the current *Psychiatric Mental Health Nursing: Scope and Standards of Practice* (American Nurses Association et al., 2022), community-based care is identified as within the scope of practice for psychiatric–mental health registered nurses. It defines community-based care as "occurring in clinics, schools and colleges, homes, shelters, health maintenance organizations, crisis centers, senior centers, group homes, and businesses among others" and may include "developing and advocating for policies, promoting mental health literacy, serving as a consultant to a variety of entities, screening for risk, treating a variety of psychiatric presentations, and advocating for services across primary, secondary, and tertiary levels of prevention" (ANA et al., 2022, p. 44). Psychiatric nurses can and should play an active role in mental health care in the community.

Community Mental Health Centers

The goal of community mental health centers in caring for individuals with serious and persistent mental illness is to improve coping ability and prevent exacerbation of acute symptoms. A major obstacle in meeting this goal has been the lack of advocacy or sponsorship for clients who require services from a variety of sources. This gap has placed responsibility for health care on individuals with mental illness, who are often unable to cope with everyday life. Case management (discussed in Chapter 8, "The Nursing Process in Psychiatric-Mental Health Nursing") has become a recommended method of treatment for individuals with serious and persistent mental illness. The core elements of case management closely resemble the steps of the nursing process; thus nurses have a beneficial skill set for such roles. Giardino and De Jesus (2021) add that nurses (and social workers) are often seen as ideal for the role of case manager based on their clinical experience and training in communication and teamwork.

In its standards of practice, the Case Management Society of America (CMSA, 2020) defines **case management** as "a collaborative practice including patients, caregivers, nurses, social workers, physicians, payers, support staff, other practitioners and the community. The Case Management process facilitates communication and care coordination along a continuum through effective transitional care management" (p. 2).

Giardino and De Jesus (2021) identify six core elements that blend with the steps of the nursing process to form a framework for nursing case management:

1. **Patient identification and determination of eligibility:** This element involves identifying patients who are not currently receiving, but would benefit from, case management. Establishing rapport with patients through meaningful interpersonal connection is key to this process.

2. **Assessment:** During the assessment process, the nurse gathers pertinent information about a patient's ability to function, health care and social needs, and their access to resources in their family and community. Information may be obtained through physical examination, patient interviews, medical records, and reports from significant others.

3. **Planning:** A service care plan is devised with patient participation. The plan should include mutually agreed-on goals; specific actions directed toward goal achievement; and selection of essential resources and services through collaboration among health-care professionals, the patient, and the family or significant others.

4. **Implementation:** In this phase, the patient receives the needed services from the appropriate providers. In some instances, the nursing **case manager** is also a provider of care, whereas in others, they are only the coordinator of care. Nevertheless, coordination is an essential function to effective implementation. The case manager "partners with patients/families/caregivers/community-based organizations and the health care team to jointly communicate, problem solve and share accountability for optimal outcomes" and "respects and incorporates patients' goals of care and treatment preferences while respecting available resources" (CMSA, 2020). This collaborative effort involves the patient, physician, any other pertinent health-care providers, and family members or significant others concerned with the patient's care. The case manager ensures that all tests and treatments are conducted according to schedule and maintains close communication with all health-care providers to ensure that the individual's care is proceeding according to the plan.

5. **Monitoring:** The case manager monitors the effectiveness of the care plan by gathering pertinent information from various sources at regular intervals to determine the patient's response and progress (CMSA, 2020). If problems are identified, immediate adjustments are made.

6. **Transition and discharge:** The case manager evaluates the patient's responses to interventions and progress toward preestablished goals. Regular contact is maintained with the patient, family or significant others and direct service providers. Ongoing coordination of care continues until service gaps have been filled and outcomes have been achieved. If the expected outcomes are not achieved, the case manager reevaluates the plan to determine the reason and takes steps to intervene and modify the existing plan. Giardino and De Jesus (2021) state that "discharge represents the case management process component in which the patient's/client's case reaches the point of closure, goals are met, and the patient's needs warrant disengagement with the case management process."

A case study of nursing case management within a community mental health center is presented in Box 35–2.

Assertive Community Treatment (ACT)

The National Alliance on Mental Illness (NAMI, 2022) defines ACT as:

> a team-based treatment model that provides multidisciplinary, flexible treatment and support to people with mental illness 24/7. ACT is based around the idea that people receive better care when their mental health care providers work together. ACT team members help the person address every aspect of their life, whether it be medication, therapy, social support, employment or housing.

This approach includes members from psychiatry, social work, nursing, and addictions treatment and vocational rehabilitation. The ACT team provides these services 24 hours a day, 7 days a week, 365 days a year.

The ACT team provides treatment, rehabilitation, and support services to individuals with serious and persistent mental illness who are unable to receive treatment from a traditional model of case management. The team is usually able to provide most services with minimal referrals to other mental health programs or providers. Services are provided within community settings, such as a person's home, local restaurants, parks, nearby stores, or anywhere the individual requires assistance with living skills.

Partial Hospitalization Programs

Partial hospitalization programs (also called *day or evening treatment programs*) are designed to prevent institutionalization or to ease the transition from inpatient hospitalization to community living. Various types of treatment are offered. Many include therapeutic community (milieu) activities; individual, group, and family therapies; psychoeducation; alcohol and drug education; crisis intervention; therapeutic recreational activities; and occupational

BOX 35–2 Nursing Case Management in the Community Mental Health Center: A Case Study

William is a 63-year-old man with chronic schizophrenia who came into the community mental health center on the recommendation of a local church, where he sometimes attends their meal program. The nurse begins a comprehensive assessment and assures William that she wants to collaborate with him to identify how to best meet his needs. She assesses his basic physical health, management of daily living, family involvement, work history, involvement with any other social agencies, finances, medications, and other concerns identified by William.

She determines that William has not been taking antipsychotic medication for at least 3 months. Before that, he had been living in a house with several other individuals, most of whom were abusing substances. They were helping him access medications from a community medication program but were often taking or reselling most of his prescription. When the house was raided by police, William became homeless. He is currently disorganized in his thinking and actively hallucinating.

He expresses a desire to take medication but feels that finding a place to live is his most important priority. There is no family involvement, and William is unable to identify any support systems.

The nurse contacts the social worker for assistance with housing options and social resources such as food stamps and contacts the physician to schedule an appointment for medication evaluation.

The nurse recommends that William attend the partial hospitalization program offered at the community mental health center, and he agrees but says he does not have transportation. The local church has offered to help William in any way they can, so the nurse contacts them and asks about their availability to provide transportation.

The church informs her that they can provide transportation on Tuesdays and Thursdays.

During the assessment, William identified that sometimes the "people start fighting" in his mind, and when he starts to scream back, someone nearby always calls the police because they "don't get that I'm just trying to defend myself."

The nurse then engages a peer support specialist who introduces William to Alfonzo, a 65-year-old man with chronic schizophrenia who is willing to provide support to William regarding symptom management. Alfonzo is also willing to provide transportation to the partial hospitalization program on the days when the church resources are not available.

The nurse notices that William has some open sores on his feet. She cleans and bandages his feet, orders blood work to assess for infection, and accesses socks and footwear from the clothes bank offered through the Salvation Army.

She continues to meet regularly with William once a month on a day that he attends the partial hospitalization program and administers the fluphenazine (Prolixin) injection ordered by the physician. During her reassessment, William identifies that he has been "hanging out" with Alfonzo and states "he really understands me." He says that he still hears people fight sometimes in his head but is not as bothered by them. The social worker has facilitated group home placement, which is not available for another 3 months, but in the meantime the local homeless shelter has arranged for William to stay there. The local church has offered William a small stipend to help with stuffing envelopes, and when the nurse asks him how that job is going, William says, "They are nice people at the church, and they say I really help them, too."

---

therapy. Many programs offer medication administration and monitoring as part of their care. Some programs have established medication clinics for individuals on long-term psychopharmacological therapy. These clinics may include educational classes and support groups for individuals with similar conditions and treatments.

Partial hospitalization programs generally offer a comprehensive treatment plan formulated by an interdisciplinary team of psychiatrists, psychologists, nurses, occupational and recreational therapists, and social workers. Nurses play a leading role in the administration of partial hospitalization programs. They lead groups, provide crisis intervention, conduct individual counseling, act as role models, and make necessary referrals for specialized treatment. Use of the nursing process allows continuous evaluation of the program, and modifications can be made as necessary.

Partial hospitalization programs are an effective method of preventing hospitalization for many individuals with serious and persistent mental illness. They are a way of transitioning these individuals from the acute care setting back into the mainstream community. For some individuals who have been deinstitutionalized, they provide structure, support, opportunities for socialization, and an improvement in their overall quality of life.

Community Residential Facilities

Community residential facilities for people with serious and persistent mental illness are known by many names: group homes, halfway houses, foster homes, boarding homes, sheltered care facilities, transitional housing, independent living programs, social rehabilitation residences, and others. These facilities differ by the purpose for which they exist and the activities that they offer.

Some of these facilities provide food, shelter, housekeeping, and minimal supervision and assistance with activities of daily living. Others may also include a variety of therapies and serve as a transition between the hospital and independent living, such as individual and group counseling, medical care, job training or employment assistance, and leisure-time activities.

The concept of transitional housing for individuals with SMI is sound and has often been a successful means of therapeutic support and intervention for maintaining them within the community. However, without guidance and planning, the transition to the community can be problematic. These individuals may be ridiculed and rejected by the community or become targets of unscrupulous individuals who take advantage of their inability to care for themselves. These occurrences may increase maladaptive responses to the demands of community living and exacerbate the mental illness. Some facilities have live-in professionals who are available at all times, some have professional staff who are on call for intervention during crisis situations, and some are staffed by volunteers and individuals with little knowledge or background in understanding and treating persons with serious and persistent mental illness. A period of structured reorientation to the community in a supervised living situation monitored by professionals is more likely to result in a successful transition for the individual with serious and persistent mental illness.

Psychiatric Home Health Care

For the individual with SMI who no longer lives in a structured, supervised setting, home health care may help them maintain independent living. To receive home health care, individuals must validate their homebound status for the prospective payer (Medicare, Medicaid, most insurance companies, and the Department of Veterans Affairs [VA] benefits). An acute psychiatric diagnosis is not sufficient to qualify for the service. The client must show that they are unable to leave the home without considerable difficulty or the assistance of another person. The plan of treatment and subsequent charting must explain why the client's psychiatric disorder keeps them at home and justify the need for home services.

Homebound clients most often have a diagnosis of depressive disorder, neurocognitive disorder, anxiety disorder, bipolar disorder, or schizophrenia. Many older adult clients are homebound because of medical conditions that impair mobility and necessitate home care.

Nurses who provide psychiatric home care must have an in-depth knowledge of psychopathology, psychopharmacology, and how medical and physical problems can be influenced by psychiatric impairments. These nurses must be highly adept at performing biopsychosocial assessments. They must be sensitive to changes in behavior that signal that the client is decompensating psychiatrically or medically so that early intervention may be implemented.

Another important job of the psychiatric home health nurse is monitoring the client's adherence to the regimen of psychotropic medications. Some clients receiving injectable medications remain on home health care only until they can be placed on oral medications. Those clients receiving oral medications require close monitoring for adherence and assistance with the uncomfortable side effects of some of these drugs. Lack of adherence to the medication regimen is responsible for approximately two-thirds of psychiatric hospital readmissions. Home health nurses can assist clients with this problem by helping them see the relationship between control of their psychiatric symptoms and adherence to their medication regimen.

Client populations that benefit from psychiatric home health nursing include the following:

- **Older adults:** These individuals do not necessarily have a psychiatric diagnosis but may be experiencing emotional difficulties caused by medical, sociocultural, or developmental factors. Depressed mood and social isolation are common.
- **People with serious and persistent mental illness:** These individuals have a history of psychiatric illness and hospitalization. They require long-term medications and continual supportive care. Common diagnoses include recurrent major depressive disorder, schizophrenia, and bipolar disorder.
- **Individuals in acute crisis situations:** These individuals are in need of crisis intervention and/or short-term psychotherapy.

Psychiatric home nursing care is typically provided by nurses who have special training and/or experience beyond the standard curriculum required for a registered nurse. Preparation for psychiatric home health nursing, in addition to the registered nurse licensure, should include several years of psychiatric inpatient treatment experience. It is also recommended that the nurse have medical-surgical nursing experience because clients commonly have several physical comorbidities, and the holistic nursing perspective is beneficial for these complex patients. Additional training and experience in psychotherapy are viewed as helpful but are not required. Psychotherapy is not the primary focus of psychiatric home nursing care. In fact, most reimbursement sources do not pay for exclusively insight-oriented therapy.

Crisis intervention, client education, and hands-on care are common interventions in psychiatric home nursing care.

The psychiatric home health nurse provides comprehensive nursing care, incorporating interventions for physical and psychosocial problems into the treatment plan. The interventions are based on the client's mental and physical health status, cultural influences, and available resources. The nurse is accountable to the client at all times during the therapeutic relationship. Nursing interventions are carried out with appropriate knowledge and skill, and referrals are made when needs are outside the scope of nursing practice. Continued collaboration with other members of the health-care team (e.g., psychiatrist, social worker, psychologist, occupational therapist, and/or physical therapist) is essential for maintaining continuity of care.

A case study of psychiatric home health care and the nursing process is presented in Clinical Judgment in Action: Case Study and Sample Care Plan. A plan of care for Mrs. C. (the client in the case study) is presented in Table 35–1. Nursing diagnoses are presented, along with outcome criteria, appropriate nursing interventions, and rationale for each.

CLINICAL JUDGMENT IN ACTION: CASE STUDY AND SAMPLE CARE PLAN

NURSING HISTORY AND ASSESSMENT

Recognizing cues: The nurse must demonstrate ability to recognize what information is most important to making an assessment (National Council of State Boards of Nursing [NCSBN], 2021). This information is bold and italicized in the following:

Mrs. C., age 76, has been *living alone* in her small apartment for 6 months since the *death of her husband*, to whom she had been married for 51 years. Mrs. C. was an elementary school teacher for 40 years, retiring at age 65 with an adequate pension. She and her husband had *no children*. A *niece looks in on Mrs. C.* regularly. It was she who contacted Mrs. C.'s physician when she observed that Mrs. C. was *not eating properly, was losing weight, and seemed to be isolating herself* more and more. She had not left her apartment in weeks. Her physician referred her to psychiatric home health care.

On her initial visit, Carol, the psychiatric home health nurse, conducted a preliminary assessment revealing the following information about Mrs. C.:

1. Blood pressure *90/60* mm Hg
2. Height 5 feet, 5 inches; weight *102 pounds*
3. Poor skin turgor; *dehydration*
4. Subjective report of occasional *dizziness*
5. Subjective report of *loss of 20 pounds since the death of her husband*
6. Oriented to time, place, person, and situation
7. Memory (remote and recent) intact
8. *Flat affect*
9. Mood is *dysphoric and tearful* at times, but client is cooperative
10. *Denies thoughts to harm self*, but states, "I feel so alone; so useless"
11. Subjective report of *difficulty sleeping*
12. Subjective report of *constipation*

Analyzing cues: The nurse must be able to interpret the information (NCSBN, 2021).

The nurse recognizes that several symptoms of depression, including anorexia, are significant enough to be threatening Mrs. C.'s physical health. Having ruled out an immediate concern for risk of suicide, the nurse recognizes that Mrs. C.'s recent loss of her husband is associated with the symptoms of clinical depression. The nurse notes that Mrs. C.'s support system is limited, and she has been isolating, which may also be associated with depression.

Prioritize hypotheses: The nurse must be able to identify the client's most important needs (NCSBN, 2021).

The nurse concludes that Mrs. C.'s poor nutritional status, depression associated with the loss of her husband, and social isolation are the three priority needs.

NURSING DIAGNOSES AND OUTCOME IDENTIFICATION

Generate solutions: The nurse must be able to connect their prioritized understanding of client needs to a course of action or plan of care (NCSBN, 2021).

The following nursing diagnoses were formulated for Mrs. C.:

1. Maladaptive grieving related to the death of her husband evidenced by symptoms of depression such as withdrawal, anorexia, weight loss, difficulty sleeping, and dysphoric/tearful mood
2. Risk for injury related to dizziness and weakness from lack of activity, low blood pressure, and poor nutritional status
3. Social isolation related to depressed mood and feelings of worthlessness, evidenced by staying home alone and refusing to leave her apartment

Outcome Criteria

The following criteria were selected as measurement outcomes in the care of Mrs. C.:

1. Experiences no physical harm/injury
2. Is able to discuss feelings about husband's death with nurse

CLINICAL JUDGMENT IN ACTION: CASE STUDY AND SAMPLE CARE PLAN—cont'd

3. Sets realistic goals for self
4. Is able to participate in problem-solving regarding her future
5. Eats a well-balanced diet with snacks to restore nutritional status and gain weight
6. Drinks adequate fluids daily
7. Sleeps at least 6 hours per night and verbalizes feeling well rested
8. Shows interest in personal appearance and hygiene and is able to accomplish self-care independently
9. Seeks to renew contact with previous friends and acquaintances
10. Verbalizes interest in participating in social activities

PLANNING AND IMPLEMENTATION

Take action: The nurse must be able to identify what actions need to be taken and how they will be implemented (NCSBN, 2021).

A plan of care for Mrs. C. is presented in Table 35–1.

EVALUATION

Evaluate outcomes: The nurse must be able to evaluate actions taken and determine whether they have had a positive, neutral, or negative impact (NCSBN, 2021).

Mrs. C. started the second week taking trazodone (Desyrel) 150 mg at bedtime. Her sleep was enhanced, and within 2 weeks she showed a noticeable improvement in mood. She began to discuss how angry she felt about being all alone in the world. She admitted that she had felt anger toward her husband but experienced guilt and tried to suppress that anger. As she was assured that these feelings were normal, they became easier for her to express.

The nurse arranged for a local teenager to do some weekly grocery shopping for Mrs. C. and contacted the local Meals on Wheels program, which delivered her noon meal to her every day. Mrs. C. began to eat more and slowly gained a few pounds. She still has an occasional problem with constipation but verbalizes improvement with the addition of vegetables, fruit, and a daily stool softener prescribed by her physician.

Mrs. C. used her walker until she felt she was able to ambulate without assistance. She reports that she no longer experiences dizziness, and her blood pressure has stabilized at around 100/70 mm Hg.

Mrs. C. has joined a senior citizens' group and attends activities weekly. She has renewed previous friendships and formed new acquaintances. She sees her physician monthly for medication management and visits a local adult day health center for regular blood pressure and weight checks. Her niece still visits regularly, but her favorite relationship is the one she has formed with her constant canine companion, Molly, whom Mrs. C. rescued from the local animal shelter and who continually demonstrates her unconditional love and gratitude.

Table 35–1 │ CARE PLAN FOR PSYCHIATRIC HOME HEALTH CARE OF DEPRESSED OLDER ADULT (MRS. C.)		

NURSING DIAGNOSIS: MALADAPTIVE GRIEVING

RELATED TO: Death of husband

EVIDENCED BY: Symptoms of depression such as withdrawal, anorexia, weight loss, difficulty sleeping, and dysphoric/tearful mood

OUTCOME CRITERIA	NURSING INTERVENTIONS	RATIONALE
Short-Term Goal: ■ Mrs. C. discusses any angry feelings she has about the loss of her husband. **Long-Term Goal:** ■ Mrs. C. demonstrates adaptive grieving behaviors and evidence of progress toward resolution.	1. Assess Mrs. C.'s position in the grief process. 2. Develop a trusting relationship by showing empathy and caring. Be honest and keep all promises. Show genuine positive regard. 3. Explore feelings of anger and help Mrs. C. direct them toward the source. Help her understand it is appropriate and acceptable to have feelings of anger and guilt about her husband's death.	1. Accurate baseline data are required to plan accurate care for Mrs. C. 2. These interventions provide the basis for a therapeutic relationship. 3. Knowledge of acceptability of the feelings associated with normal grieving may help to relieve some of the guilt that these responses generate.

Continued

Table 35–1 | CARE PLAN FOR PSYCHIATRIC HOME HEALTH CARE OF DEPRESSED OLDER ADULT (MRS. C.)—cont'd

OUTCOME CRITERIA	NURSING INTERVENTIONS	RATIONALE
	4. Encourage Mrs. C. to review honestly the relationship she had with her husband. With support and sensitivity, point out the reality of the situation in areas where misrepresentations may be expressed.	4. Mrs. C. must give up an idealized perception of her husband. Only when she is able to see both positive and negative aspects about the relationship will the grieving process be complete.
	5. Determine whether Mrs. C. has spiritual needs that are going unfulfilled. If so, contact spiritual leader for intervention with Mrs. C.	5. Recovery may be blocked if spiritual distress is present and care is not provided.
	6. Refer Mrs. C. to physician for medication evaluation.	6. Antidepressant therapy may help Mrs. C. to function while confronting the dynamics of her depression.

NURSING DIAGNOSIS: RISK FOR INJURY

RELATED TO: Dizziness and weakness from lack of activity, low blood pressure, and poor nutritional status

OUTCOME CRITERIA	NURSING INTERVENTIONS	RATIONALE
Short-Term Goals: ■ Mrs. C. uses walker when ambulating. ■ Mrs. C. does not experience physical harm or injury. Long-Term Goal: ■ Mrs. C. does not experience physical harm or injury.	1. Assess vital signs at every visit. Report to physician should they fall below baseline.	1. Patient safety is a nursing priority.
	2. Encourage Mrs. C. to use walker until strength has returned.	2. The walker will help prevent Mrs. C. from falling.
	3. Visit Mrs. C. during mealtimes and sit with her while she eats. Encourage her niece to do the same. Ensure that easy-to-prepare, nutritious foods for meals and snacks are available in the house and that they are items that Mrs. C. likes.	3. She is more likely to eat what is convenient and what she enjoys.
	4. Contact local meal delivery service (e.g., Meals on Wheels) to deliver some of Mrs. C.'s meals.	4. Engaging this service ensures that she receives at least one complete and nutritious meal each day.
	5. Weigh Mrs. C. each week.	5. Weight gain is a measurable, objective means of assessing whether Mrs. C. is eating.
	6. Ensure that diet contains sufficient fluid and fiber.	6. Adequate dietary fluid and fiber will help to alleviate constipation. She may also benefit from a daily stool softener.

| **Table 35–1 ❘ CARE PLAN FOR PSYCHIATRIC HOME HEALTH CARE OF DEPRESSED OLDER ADULT (MRS. C.)–cont'd** | | |

NURSING DIAGNOSIS: SOCIAL ISOLATION

RELATED TO: Depressed mood and feelings of worthlessness

EVIDENCED BY: Staying home alone, refusing to leave apartment

OUTCOME CRITERIA	NURSING INTERVENTIONS	RATIONALE
Short-Term Goal: ■ Mrs. C. discusses with nurse feelings about past social relationships and those she may like to renew. **Long-Term Goal:** ■ Mrs. C. renews contact with friends and participates in social activities.	1. As nutritional status is improving and strength is gained, encourage Mrs. C. to become more active. Take walks with her; help her perform simple tasks around her house.	1. Increased activity enhances both physical and mental status.
	2. Assess lifelong patterns of relationships.	2. Basic personality characteristics will not change. Mrs. C. will likely keep the same style of relationship development that she had in the past.
	3. Help her identify present relationships that are satisfying and activities that she considers interesting.	3. She is the person who truly knows what she likes, and these personal preferences will facilitate success in reversing social isolation.
	4. Consider the feasibility of a pet.	4. There are many documented studies of the benefits of companion pets for older adults.
	5. Suggest possible alternatives that Mrs. C. may consider as she seeks to participate in social activities. These may include foster grandparent programs, senior citizens centers, church activities, craft groups, and volunteer activities. Help her to locate individuals with whom she may attend some of these activities.	5. She is more likely to attend and participate if she does not have to do so alone.

Care for the Caregivers

Psychiatric home health care also provides support and assistance to primary caregivers. When family members provide care on a 24/7 schedule for a loved one with a serious and persistent mental disorder, it can be exhausting and frustrating. A care plan for primary caregivers is presented in Table 35–2.

The Homeless Population

History and Epidemiology

In 1993 Dr. Richard Lamb, a recognized expert in the field of serious and persistent mental illness, wrote:

> Alec Guinness, in his memorable role as a British Army colonel in *Bridge on the River Kwai*, exclaims at the end of the film when he finally realizes he

Table 35–2 | CARE PLAN FOR PRIMARY CAREGIVER OF PATIENT WITH SERIOUS AND PERSISTENT MENTAL ILLNESS

NURSING DIAGNOSIS: CAREGIVER ROLE STRAIN

RELATED TO: Severity and duration of the care receiver's illness and lack of respite and recreation for the caregiver

EVIDENCED BY: Feelings of stress in relationship with care receiver, feelings of depression and anger, family conflict around issues of providing care

OUTCOME CRITERIA	NURSING INTERVENTIONS	RATIONALE
Short-Term Goal: ■ Caregivers verbalize understanding of ways to facilitate the caregiver role. Long-Term Goal: ■ Caregivers demonstrate effective problem-solving skills and develop adaptive coping mechanisms to regain equilibrium.	1. Assess caregivers' abilities to anticipate and fulfill client's unmet needs. Provide information to assist caregivers with this responsibility. Ensure that caregivers encourage client to be as independent as possible. 2. Ensure that caregivers are aware of available community support systems from which they may seek assistance when required. Examples include respite care services, day treatment centers, and adult day-care centers. 3. Encourage caregivers to express feelings, particularly anger. 4. Encourage participation in support groups composed of members with similar life situations. Provide information about individual and group support that may be helpful: a. National Alliance on Mental Illness (NAMI) b. American Association on Intellectual and Developmental Disabilities (AAIDD) c. Alzheimer's Association	1. Caregivers may be unaware of what the client can realistically accomplish. They may be unaware of the nature of the illness. 2. Caregivers require relief from the pressures and strain of providing 24-hour care for their loved one. Studies have shown that abuse risk increases in situations where the caregiver is highly stressed and overwhelmed (Patel et al., 2021). 3. Release of these emotions can serve to prevent psychopathology, such as depression or psychophysiological disorders, from occurring. 4. Hearing others who are experiencing the same problems discuss ways in which they have coped may help the caregiver adopt more adaptive strategies. Individuals who are experiencing similar life situations provide empathy and support for each other.

has been working to help the enemy, "What have I done?" As a vocal advocate and spokesman for deinstitutionalization and community treatment of severely mentally ill patients for well over two decades, I often find myself asking that same question. (p. 1209)

Individuals with SMI are a high-risk population for homelessness, and substance misuse is a common comorbidity. It is difficult to determine the true scope of the problem because a consistent definition of homeless persons is lacking. They have sometimes been identified as "those people who sleep in shelters or public spaces." Because not all those who are homeless are able to access shelters, and public spaces are difficult to define, statistics about the number of homeless individuals with SMI are underestimated.

According to the Stewart B. McKinney Act (GovTrack, 1987), a person is considered homeless who

lacks a fixed, regular, and adequate nighttime residence; and ... has a primary nighttime residency that is: (A) a supervised publicly or privately operated shelter designed to provide temporary living accommodations, (B) an institution that provides a temporary residence for individuals intended to be institutionalized, or (C) a public or private place not designed for, or ordinarily used as, a regular sleeping accommodation for human beings.

The National Alliance to End Homelessness (2021) reports that from 2007 to 2020, homelessness overall declined by 10%, with the most dramatic decreases among veterans. Despite the overall decline in homelessness since 2007, the last 4 years have been a period of incremental growth in this population (with a 2% growth between 2019 and 2020). Current reports have not yet been able to measure the impact of the COVID-19 pandemic with its associated unemployment and evictions, but it is expected that it will also influence the numbers of those who are homeless. Reports indicate that mental illness precedes homelessness in approximately 75% of the cases (Balisuriya et al., 2020) and about 16% of the single adult homeless population suffers from some form of serious and persistent mental illness (National Coalition for the Homeless [NCH], 2020b). One of the cited contributing factors is limited access to inpatient psychiatric treatment. Homelessness among the mentally ill continues to be a significant concern for this vulnerable population.

Many homeless individuals are children and young adults. Some are homeless because of their dependence on a parent who is homeless, but many are trauma victims who have left their homes to avoid physical or sexual abuse and neglect. Some are lesbian, gay, bisexual, transgender, or questioning (LGBTQ) youth who have become homeless secondary to family intolerance about their sexual orientation and identity (Safe Horizon, 2022).

On a single night in 2021, 15,763 people under the age of 25 experienced sheltered homelessness on their own as "unaccompanied youth" (U.S. Department of Housing and Urban Development [HUD], 2022). Although the number of homeless youth and young adults represents an overall decline, within this group the percentages of those who are transgender, gender nonconforming, or Native American have increased. Many initiatives have sought to reduce the numbers of homeless youth and to provide resources to minimize disruptions posed by homelessness. In October 2016 amendments to the McKinney-Vento Act went into effect that include provisions for homeless children and young adults to receive adequate and accessible education. However, these provisions do not address the child who is "on the run." These children remain a high-risk, vulnerable population who often have a history of trauma, in addition to the trauma posed by homelessness and sex trafficking.

Mental Illness and Homelessness

The prevalence of SMI among the homeless population is difficult to clarify. SAMHSA (2022a) provides the following demographics through statistics gathered from Projects for Assistance in Transition from Homelessness (PATH), which was specifically established for funding services to people with SMI. Thus these statistics are based on the makeup of PATH clients.

Age

Almost 19% of clients with SMI are younger than age 30; individuals between the ages of 31 and 61 make up the bulk of this population at 72.5%; about 8.1% are age 62 years or older.

Gender

Male individuals with SMI comprise 58.2% of the homeless population, and 40.4% are female. Another 0.7% are transgender or gender nonconforming.

Ethnicity and Race

The homeless SMI population is estimated to be 54.5% Caucasian, 34.7% African American, 14.6% Hispanic, 4.2% American Indian or Alaska Native, and 2% other racial/ethnic groups (SAMHSA, 2022a). The ethnic makeup of homeless populations varies according to geographical location.

Types of Mental Illness Among the Homeless

Several studies have been conducted, primarily in large urban areas, that have addressed the most common types of mental illness among homeless individuals. Schizophrenia is frequently described as the most common diagnosis. Other prevalent disorders include bipolar disorder, substance addiction, depression, personality disorders, and neurocognitive disorders. Many exhibit psychotic symptoms, many are former residents of long-term care institutions for the mentally ill, and many have such a strong desire for independence that they isolate themselves to avoid identification by the mental health system. Many are a danger to themselves or others, yet they often do not even see themselves as ill. SAMHSA (2022a) identifies that in 2020, 38.8% of clients receiving PATH services had a co-occurring substance use disorder.

Contributing Factors to Homelessness Among Individuals With Mental Illness

Deinstitutionalization

As previously stated, deinstitutionalization is frequently implicated as a contributing factor to homelessness among individuals with mental illness. Deinstitutionalization began out of expressed concern by mental health professionals and others who described the "deplorable conditions" under which mentally ill individuals were housed.

The advent of psychotropic medications and the community mental health movement began to foster the philosophical view that individuals with mental illness receive better and more humanitarian treatment in the community than in state hospitals far removed from their homes. It was believed that commitment and institutionalization in many ways deprived these individuals of their civil rights. Not the least of the motivating factors for deinstitutionalization was the financial burden these clients placed on state governments.

Although the deinstitutionalization movement has prompted an expansion of community mental health resources, the number of people with mental illness incarcerated in correctional facilities has skyrocketed and is now estimated to be two to four times that of the general population (National Institute of Corrections, n.d.). Supporters of the community mental health movement have argued that ongoing problems for those with serious mental illness are related to lack of compliance with medications, but critics have argued that the community mental health model is too narrowly focused on a biomedical approach and needs to revise and expand its services to meet the complex needs of this population going forward.

The Treatment Advocacy Center (2018) reports that roughly 33% of the homeless population are those with untreated SMI. Who are these individuals, and why are they homeless? Some blame the deinstitutionalization movement. People with mental illness who were released from state and county mental hospitals and did not have families with whom they could reside sought residence in board-and-care homes of varying quality. Halfway houses and supportive group living arrangements were helpful but scarce. Many of those with families returned to their homes, but because families received little, if any, instruction or support, the environment was frequently turbulent, and individuals with mental illness often went on to leave these homes.

Deinstitutionalization has been criticized for contributing to both homelessness rates and criminalization of people with mental illnesses, but several other factors have been implicated as well.

Poverty

Cuts in various government entitlement programs have depleted the allotments available for individuals with serious and persistent mental illness living in the community. The job market is prohibitive for individuals whose behavior is incomprehensible or even frightening to many. The stigma and discrimination associated with mental illness may be diminishing slowly, but they remain highly visible.

Scarcity of Affordable Housing

Not only is there a scarcity of affordable housing but the number of single-room-occupancy (SRO) hotels has diminished drastically. SRO hotels provided a means of relatively inexpensive housing, and although some people believe that these facilities nurtured isolation, they provided adequate shelter from the elements for their occupants. So many individuals currently frequent the shelters of our cities that there is concern they are becoming mini-institutions for individuals with SMI.

Other Factors

Several other factors that may contribute to homelessness have been identified:

- **Lack of affordable health care:** For families barely able to afford day-to-day living expenses, a catastrophic illness can create a level of poverty that starts the downward spiral to homelessness.
- **Domestic violence:** According to a Family and Youth Services Bureau report (2016), up to 57% of homeless women identify domestic violence as the primary reason for homelessness. Other research found that 93% of homeless mothers had a history of trauma, 79% experienced trauma as children, and 81% experienced multiple traumatic events (NCH, 2015). The need for trauma-informed care in this population cannot be overstated.
- **Substance use disorders:** Individuals with untreated alcohol or drug addictions are at increased risk for homelessness. The following have been cited as obstacles to addiction treatment for homeless persons: lack of health insurance, lack of documentation, waiting lists, scheduling difficulties, daily contact requirements, lack of transportation, ineffective treatment methods, lack of supportive services, and cultural insensitivity.

Community Resources for the Homeless
Interfering Factors

Among the many issues that complicate service planning for homeless individuals with mental illness is this population's mobility. Frequent relocation confounds service delivery and interferes with providers' efforts to ensure appropriate care. Some individuals with SMI may be affected by homelessness only temporarily or intermittently. These individuals are sometimes called the "episodically homeless." Others move around within neighborhoods or cities as needs and availability of services change. A large number of the homeless mentally ill population exhibits continuous unbounded movement over wide geographical areas.

Not all homeless individuals with mental illness are mobile. Some studies have indicated that a large percentage remain in the same location over several years. Health-care workers must identify movement patterns of homeless people in their area to at least try to bring the best care possible to this unique population. This effort may mean delivering services to those individuals who do not seek out services on their own.

Health Issues

Life as a homeless person can have severe consequences in terms of health. Exposure to the elements, poor diet, sleep deprivation, risk of violence, injuries, and lack of health care lead to a precarious state of health and exacerbate preexisting illnesses. Compared with other homeless individuals, those who abuse alcohol are at greater risk for neurological impairment, heart disease and hypertension, chronic lung disease, gastrointestinal disorders, hepatic dysfunction, and trauma.

Thermoregulation is a health problem for all homeless individuals because of their exposure to all kinds of weather. It is a compounded problem for the homeless alcoholic, who spends much time in an altered level of consciousness.

It is difficult to determine whether mental illness is a cause or effect of homelessness. Some behaviors that seem deviant may actually be adaptations to life on the street. Homeless individuals may even seek hospitalization in psychiatric institutions in an attempt to get off the streets for a while.

Whereas tuberculosis (TB) rates in the United States have been on the decline for several years, the homeless remain an at-risk population; 4% of those with TB reported homelessness within the prior year (Centers for Disease Control and Prevention [CDC], 2021). Crowded shelters provide ideal conditions for the spread of respiratory infections among inhabitants. The risk of acquiring TB is also increased by the prevalence of alcoholism, drug addiction, HIV infection, and poor nutrition among homeless individuals. These concerns have been amplified during the global COVID-19 pandemic, prompting the CDC to reinforce the critical need to maintain shelter services for the homeless population and to identify guidelines for minimizing spread of infections, including the recommendation that communities identify the need for overflow sites to maintain safe distancing in shelters (CDC, 2022). (See the feature "Implications of Research for Evidence-Based Practice" for research related to the COVID-19 pandemic.)

Dietary deficiencies are a continuing problem for homeless individuals. Not only is the homeless person commonly in a poor nutritional state but the condition itself exacerbates a number of other health problems. Homeless people have higher mortality rates and a greater number of serious disorders than their counterparts in the general population.

Sexually transmitted infections (STIs), such as gonorrhea and syphilis, are a serious problem for the homeless. One of the most serious STIs prevalent among homeless individuals is HIV infection. Street life is precarious for individuals immunosuppressed by HIV. Rummaged food scraps are often spoiled, and exposure to the elements is a continuous threat. Individuals with HIV who stay in shelters often are exposed to the infectious diseases of others, which can be life-threatening in this vulnerable condition.

Homeless children have special health needs. Children without a home are prone to higher rates of asthma, ear infections, stomach problems, and speech problems than their counterparts who are not homeless. They are also more likely to experience mental health problems, such as anxiety, depression, and withdrawal.

A growing problem that has captured national attention is the increasing number of hate crimes perpetrated against the homeless. These attacks do not appear to be specifically directed toward the mentally ill, but rather reflect a primary bias against homeless people. Based on the most recent report by NCH (2020a), almost 47% of these attacks were fatal. Most of the victims (85%) who lost their lives were male and 65% were 40 years of age or older. Seventy-seven percent of the perpetrators were younger than age 40. The NCH adds that there is a documented correlation between criminalization laws and increases in attacks on the homeless, possibly because it sends a message to the public that homeless people "do not matter and are not worthy of living in our city. This message is blatant in the attitudes many cities have toward homeless people and can be used as an internal justification for attacking someone" (2020, p. 16). Less than half of these attacks (NCH, 2020a) are reported to police, and those who survive the attacks are vulnerable to PTSD. Community mental health nurses have an opportunity and a responsibility to assess and intervene for homeless people who are a vulnerable population on so many levels.

Types of Resources Available

Homeless Shelters

Shelters for the homeless in the United States vary from converted warehouses that provide cots or floor space for overnight stays to significant operations that provide a multitude of social and health-care services. They are run by volunteers and paid professionals and sponsored by churches, community governments, and various social agencies.

It is impossible, then, to describe a "typical" shelter. One description is the provision of lodging, food, and clothing to individuals who are in need of these services. Some shelters also provide medical and psychiatric evaluations, first aid and other health-care services, and referral for case management services by nurses or social workers.

Individuals who seek services from the shelter are generally assigned a bed or cot, issued a set of clean linen, provided a place to shower, shown laundry facilities, and offered a meal in the shelter kitchen or dining hall. Most shelters attempt to separate dormitory areas for men and women, with various consequences for those who violate the rules.

Shelters cover expenses through private and corporate donations, church sponsorships, and government grants. From the outset, shelters were conceptualized as "temporary" accommodations. In reality, they have become permanent lodging for homeless individuals with little hope for improving their situations. Some individuals even use their shelters' mailing address.

Shelters provide a safe and supportive environment for homeless individuals who have no other place to go. Some homeless people who inhabit shelters use the resources offered to improve their lot in life, whereas others may become dependent on the shelter's provisions.

Health-Care Centers and Storefront Clinics

Some communities have established "street clinics" to serve the homeless population. Many are operated by nurse practitioners who work in consultation with physicians in the area. In recent years, some of these clinics have provided clinical sites for nursing students in community health rotations. Some have been staffed by nursing school faculties that have established group practices in the community setting.

A wide variety of services are offered at these clinics, including administering medications, assessing vital signs, screening for TB and other communicable diseases, giving immunizations and flu shots, changing dressings, and administering first aid.

Physical and psychosocial assessments, health education, and supportive counseling are also frequent interventions.

Nursing in **storefront clinics** for the homeless provides many special challenges, not the least of which is poor working conditions. These clinics often operate under severe budgetary constraints with inadequate staffing, supplies, and equipment, in rundown facilities located in high-crime neighborhoods. Frustration is often high among nurses who work in these clinics, as they are seldom able to see measurable progress in their homeless clients. Maintenance of health management is virtually impossible for individuals who have no resources outside the health-care setting. If return appointments for preventive care are made, they are often missed.

Mobile Outreach Units

Outreach programs literally reach out to the homeless in their own environments to provide health care. Volunteers and paid professionals form teams to seek out homeless individuals who are in need of assistance. They offer coffee, sandwiches, and blankets to show concern and establish trust. Assistance can be provided at the site if possible. If not, every effort is made to ensure that the individual is linked with a source that can provide the necessary services.

Mobile outreach units provide assistance to homeless individuals who are in need of physical or psychological care. The emphasis of outreach programs is to accommodate the homeless who refuse to seek treatment elsewhere. Most target the mentally ill segment of the population. When trust has been established and the individual agrees to come to the team's office, medical and psychiatric treatment is initiated. Involuntary hospitalization is initiated when an individual is deemed harmful to self or others or otherwise meets the criteria to be considered "gravely disabled."

The Homeless Client and the Nursing Process

A case study demonstrating the nursing process with a homeless client is presented in Box 35–3.

BOX 35–3 Case Study: Nursing Process With a Homeless Client

ASSESSMENT

Joe, age 68, is brought to the community health clinic by two of his peers, who report, "He just had a fit. He needs a drink bad!" Joe is dirty and unkempt, has visible tremors of the upper extremities, and is weak enough to require assistance when ambulating. He is cooperative as the nurse completes the intake assessment. He is coherent, although thought processes are slow. He is disoriented to

time and place. He appears somewhat frightened as he scans the unfamiliar surroundings. He is unable to tell the nurse when he had his last drink. He reports no physical injury, and none is observable.

Joe carries a small bag with a few personal items inside, including a Department of Veterans Affairs (VA) benefit card, identifying him as a veteran of the Vietnam War. The nurse finds a cot for Joe, ensures that his vital signs are

BOX 35–3 Case Study: Nursing Process With a Homeless Client—cont'd

stable, and telephones the number on the VA card. The clinic nurse discovers that Joe is well known to the admissions personnel at the VA. He has a 35-year history of schizophrenia with numerous hospitalizations. At the time of his last discharge, he was taking fluphenazine (Prolixin) 10 mg twice a day. He told the clinic nurse that he took the medication for a few months after he got out of the hospital but then did not have the prescription refilled. He could not remember when he had last taken fluphenazine.

Joe also has a long history of alcohol-related disorders and has participated in the VA substance rehabilitation program three times. He has no home address and receives his VA disability benefit checks at a shelter address. He reports that he has no family. The nurse makes arrangements for VA personnel to drive Joe from the clinic to the VA hospital, where he is admitted for detoxification. She sets up a case management file for Joe and arranges with the hospital to have Joe return to the clinic after discharge.

DIAGNOSIS AND OUTCOME IDENTIFICATION

The following nursing diagnosis was formulated for Joe:

- Ineffective health maintenance related to ineffective coping skills evidenced by abuse of alcohol, lack of follow-through with antipsychotic medication, and lack of personal hygiene

Ongoing criteria were selected as outcomes for Joe:

- Follows the rules of the group home and maintains his residency status
- Attends weekly sessions of group therapy at the VA day treatment program
- Attends weekly sessions of Alcoholics Anonymous and maintains sobriety
- Reports regularly to the health clinic for injections of fluphenazine
- Volunteers at the VA hospital 3 days a week
- Secures and retains permanent employment

PLANNING AND IMPLEMENTATION

During Joe's hospitalization, the clinic nurse remained in contact with his case. Joe received complete physical and dental examinations and treatment during his hospital stay. The clinic nurse attended the treatment team meeting for Joe as his outpatient case manager. It was decided at the meeting to try giving Joe injections of fluphenazine because of his history of lack of adherence to his daily oral

medication regimen. The clinic nurse would administer the injection every 4 weeks.

At Joe's follow-up clinic visit, the nurse explains to Joe that she has found a group home where he may live with others who have personal circumstances similar to his. At the group home, meals will be provided, and the group home manager will ensure that Joe's basic needs are fulfilled. A criterion for remaining at the residence is for Joe to remain free from alcohol. Joe is agreeable to these living arrangements.

With Joe's concurrence, the clinic nurse also performs the following interventions:

- Goes shopping with Joe to purchase some new clothing, allowing Joe to make decisions as independently as possible
- Helps Joe move into the group home and introduces him to the manager and residents
- Helps Joe change his address from the shelter to the group home so that he may continue to receive his VA benefits
- Enrolls Joe in the weekly group therapy sessions of the day treatment facility connected with the VA hospital
- Helps Joe locate the nearest Alcoholics Anonymous group and identifies a sponsor who will ensure that Joe gets to the meetings
- Sets up a clinic appointment for Joe to return in 4 weeks for his fluphenazine injection; telephones Joe 1 day in advance to remind him of his appointment
- Instructs Joe to return to or call the clinic if any of the following symptoms occur: sore throat, fever, nausea and vomiting, severe headache, difficulty urinating, tremors, skin rash, or yellow skin or eyes
- Assists Joe in securing transportation to and from appointments
- Encourages Joe to set realistic goals for his life and offers recognition for follow-through
- When Joe is ready, discusses employment alternatives with him; suggests the possibility of starting with a volunteer job (perhaps as a VA hospital volunteer)

EVALUATION

Evaluation of the nursing process with homeless individuals who have mental illness must be highly individualized. Statistics show that chances for relapse with this population are high. Therefore it is important that outcome criteria are realistic so as not to set the client up for failure.

Summary and Key Points

- ◢ Psychiatric care has shifted from primarily inpatient hospitalization to a continuum of services within the community. This trend is largely a result of the need for greater cost-effectiveness in the provision of care to individuals with mental illness.

- ◢ The community mental health movement began in the 1960s with the closing of state hospitals and the deinstitutionalization of many individuals with serious and persistent mental illness.
- ◢ Mental health care within the community targets primary prevention (reducing the incidence of mental disorders within the population), secondary

prevention (reducing the prevalence of psychiatric illness by shortening the course of the illness), and tertiary prevention (reducing the residual defects that are associated with serious and persistent mental illness).

■ Primary prevention focuses on the identification of populations at risk for mental illness, increasing their ability to cope with stress, and targeting and diminishing harmful forces within the environment.

■ The focus of secondary prevention is accomplished through early identification of problems and prompt initiation of effective treatment.

■ Tertiary prevention focuses on preventing complications of the illness and promoting rehabilitation

directed toward the achievement of the individual's maximum level of functioning.

■ Registered nurses serve as providers of psychiatric-mental health care in the community setting.

■ Nurses provide outpatient care for individuals with serious and persistent mental illness in community mental health centers, in day and evening treatment programs, in partial hospitalization programs, in community residential facilities, and with psychiatric home health care.

■ Homeless individuals with mental illness provide a special challenge for the community mental health nurse. Care is provided within homeless shelters, at health-care centers or storefront clinics, and through mobile outreach programs.

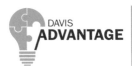

Go to **Davis Advantage** to complete your learning: strengthen understanding, apply your knowledge, and prepare for the Next Gen NCLEX®.

Review Questions

1. Which of the following represents a nursing intervention at the primary level of prevention?
   a. Teaching a class in parent effectiveness training
   b. Leading a group of adolescents in drug rehabilitation
   c. Referring a married couple for sex therapy
   d. Leading a support group for battered women

2. Which of the following represents a nursing intervention at the secondary level of prevention?
   a. Teaching a class about menopause to middle-aged women
   b. Providing support in the emergency department to a rape victim
   c. Leading a support group for women in transition
   d. Making monthly visits to the home of a client with schizophrenia to ensure medication compliance

3. Which of the following represents a nursing intervention at the tertiary level of prevention?
   a. Serving as case manager for a mentally ill homeless client
   b. Leading a support group for newly retired men
   c. Teaching prepared childbirth classes
   d. Caring for a depressed widow in the hospital

4. A 78-year-old widow who lives alone has been diagnosed with depression. Which of the following criteria would qualify this client for home health visits?
   a. The client doesn't like to drive on busy roads.
   b. The client is physically too weak to travel without risk of injury.
   c. The client refuses to seek assistance as suggested by her physician, "because I don't have a psychiatric problem."
   d. The client says she would rather have home visits than go to the physician's office.

5. Which of the following issues have been identified as contributing to the increase in the population of those who are homeless? (Select all that apply.)
   a. Poverty
   b. Lack of affordable health care
   c. Substance misuse
   d. Serious and persistent mental illness
   e. Growth in the number of family members living together

Clinical Judgment Questions

6. A homeless person has just come to live in a shelter. The shelter nurse is assigned to their care. Which of the following is a *priority* intervention on the part of the nurse?
   a. Referring them to a social worker
   b. Developing a plan of care
   c. Conducting a behavioral and needs assessment
   d. Helping them apply for Social Security benefits

7. A psychiatric home health nurse has received an order to begin regular visits to a client diagnosed with depression. Which of these potential problems is a priority to evaluate during the first home visit?
   a. Maladaptive grieving
   b. Social isolation
   c. Risk for injury
   d. Sleep pattern disturbance

8. The home health nurse is assessing an 87-year-old man who states, "I've lived long enough and there's just nothing left for me." Which is the best response on the part of the nurse?
   a. "Of course there is; why would you say such a thing?"
   b. "You seem so sad. I'm going to do my best to cheer you up."
   c. "Let's talk about why you are feeling this way."
   d. "Are you having any thoughts of suicide?"

9. The physician has ordered trazodone (Desyrel) 150 mg to be taken at bedtime for a 75-year-old widow with co-occurring insomnia and a history of depression. Which of the following statements about this medication is a *priority* for the home health nurse to make in teaching the client about trazodone?
   a. "You may feel dizzy when you stand up, so go slowly when you get up from sitting or lying down."
   b. "Make sure you let me know if you're getting adequate sleep. Trazodone sometimes interferes with sleep."
   c. "Don't get out of bed unless someone is available to assist you."
   d. "This medication takes around 4 to 6 weeks before you will notice any therapeutic effect."

10. The community mental health nurse is assessing a homeless woman who left her husband and "had nowhere else to go." She was referred to the clinic from the homeless shelter for an evaluation to rule out depression. Which of the following are priority actions for the nurse to include in the initial assessment? (Select all that apply.)
    a. Ask about trauma history.
    b. Assess risk for suicide.
    c. Assess her comfort level with the accommodations at the homeless shelter.
    d. Explore her financial resources.

IMPLICATIONS OF RESEARCH FOR EVIDENCE-BASED PRACTICE

Moreno, C., Wykes, T., Galderisi, S., Nordentoft, M., Crossley, N., Jones, N., Cannon, M., Correll, U. C., Byrne, L., Carr, S., Chen, E. Y. H., Gorwood, P., Johnson, S., Kärkkäinen, H., Krystal, J. H., Lee, J., Lieberman, J., López-Jaramillo, C., Männikkö, M., … & Arango, C. (2020). How mental health care should change as a consequence of the COVID-19 pandemic. *Lancet Psychiatry, 7*(9), 813–824. https://doi.org/10.1016/S2215-0366(20)30307-2

DESCRIPTION OF THE STUDY: This study was conducted by a panel of experts worldwide and involved a review of available literature on mental health consequences associated with the COVID-19 pandemic with the intent to develop a position paper on emerging mental health priorities going forward. The authors note that most research is preliminary and that longitudinal studies will be needed to confirm the ongoing relevance of current priorities.

RESULTS OF THE STUDY: Several findings relevant to mental health priorities in the COVID-19 pandemic were identified. Selected findings include:

■ Most surveys identified increases in depression, anxiety, and stress related to fear of illness, fear of life disruptions, and fear of economic distress.

Continued

IMPLICATIONS OF RESEARCH FOR EVIDENCE-BASED PRACTICE–cont'd

■ Social media exposure has been associated with increased anxiety and comorbid anxiety and depression.

■ Emerging reports have identified a 33% incidence of dysexecutive syndrome (a syndrome of emotional, behavioral, and cognitive deficits) after discharge among patients hospitalized in the intensive care unit (ICU) with COVID-19.

■ Risk factors for infection and a severe course of illness include those with SMI, substance use disorders, and homelessness.

■ People with preexisting mental health disorders have reported increased symptoms and poorer access to services and supports since the onset of the COVID-19 pandemic.

The authors' conclusions include:

■ Retaining existing services and promoting new practices that expand access and provide cost-effective delivery of effective mental health services to individuals who already have mental disorders or who have developed them during the pandemic should be a priority.

■ Ongoing community assessment to identify post-COVID mental health and neurological issues needs to be systematically conducted.

■ Service provision that targets health needs and reduces disparities, both globally and within individual countries, needs to be put in place.

IMPLICATIONS FOR NURSING PRACTICE: Nurses who work in community mental health can be instrumental in identifying and responding to immediate and long-term mental health needs associated with this pandemic. The findings and position paper that resulted from this study clarified some associated mental health needs and disparities for those with preexisting SMI and for those in the general population.

References

American Nurses Association (ANA), American Psychiatric Nurses Association, & International Society of Psychiatric-Mental Health Nurses. (2022). Psychiatric-mental health nursing: *Scope and standards of practice* (3rd ed.). ANA.

American Psychiatric Association (APA). (2022). *Diagnostic and statistical manual of mental disorders, fifth edition, text revision (DSM-5-TR)*. American Psychiatric Association.

Balisuriya, L., Buelt, E., & Tsai, J. (2020). The never-ending loop: Homelessness, psychiatric disorder, and mortality. *Psychiatric Times, 37*(5). https://www.psychiatrictimes.com/view/never-ending-loop-homelessness-psychiatric-disorder-and-mortality

Case Management Society of America. (2020). *Case management standards of practice & scope of services*. CMSA.

Casper, L. M., & Coritz, A. (2018). Family demography: Continuity and change in North American families. In J. R. Kaakinen, D. P. Coehlo, R. Steele, & M. Robinson (Eds.), *Family health care nursing* (6th ed., pp. 53–81). F.A. Davis.

Centers for Disease Control and Prevention (CDC). (2021). *TB and people experiencing homelessness*. https://www.cdc.gov/tb/topic/populations/Homelessness/default.htm

Centers for Disease Control and Prevention (CDC). (2022). *Interim guidance for homeless service providers to plan and respond to coronavirus disease 2019 (COVID-19)*. https://www.cdc.gov/coronavirus/2019-ncov/community/homeless-shelters/plan-prepare-respond.html

Centers for Medicare & Medicaid Services. (n.d.). *The Mental Health Parity and Addiction Equity Act*. https://www.cms.gov/CCIIO/Programs-and-Initiatives/Other-Insurance-Protections/mhpaea_factsheet.html

Family and Youth Services Bureau. (2016). *Domestic violence and homelessness: Statistics (2016)*. https://www.acf.hhs.gov/fysb/resource/dv-homelessness-stats-2016

Giardino, A. P., & De Jesus, O. (2021). *Case management*. https://www.ncbi.nlm.nih.gov/books/NBK562214/

Mayo Clinic. (2022). *Male menopause: Myth or reality?* https://www.mayoclinic.org/healthy-lifestyle/mens-health/in-depth/male-menopause/art-20048056

McLeod, S. A. (2010). *SRRS—Stress of life events*. www.simplypsychology.org/SRRS.html

Moreno, C., Wykes, T., Galderisi, S., Nordentoft, M., Crossley, N., Jones, N., Cannon, M., Correll, U. C., Byrne, L., Carr, S., Chen, E. Y. H., Gorwood, P., Johnson, S., Kärkkäinen, H., Krystal, J. H., Lee, J., Lieberman, J., López-Jaramillo, C., Männikkö, M., ... Arango, C. (2020). How mental health care should change as a consequence of the COVID-19 pandemic. *Lancet Psychiatry, 7*(9), 813–824. https://doi.org/10.1016/S2215-0366(20)30307-2

National Alliance on Mental Illness. (2022). *Psychosocial treatments: Assertive community treatment*. https://www.nami.org/Learn-More/Treatment/Psychosocial-Treatments

National Alliance to End Homelessness. (2021). *The state of homelessness: 2021 edition*. https://endhomelessness.org/homelessness-in-america/homelessness-statistics/state-of-homelessness-2021/

National Coalition for the Homeless (NCH). (2015). *How trauma informed care is helping homeless families*. http://nationalhomeless.org/category/domestic-violence/

National Coalition for the Homeless (NCH). (2020a). *20 years of hate: National coalition for the homeless hate crimes report 2018–2019*. https://nationalhomeless.org/wp-content/uploads/2020/12/hate-crimes-2018-2019_web.pdf

National Coalition for the Homeless (NCH). (2020b). *Homelessness in America*. https://nationalhomeless.org/about-homelessness/

National Council of State Boards of Nursing (NCSBN). (2021). *Next generation NCLEX®: Comparison between case studies and stand-alone items*. https://www.ncsbn.org/public-files/NGN_Fall21_English_Final.pdf

National Institute of Corrections. (n.d.). *Mentally ill persons in corrections*. http://nicic.gov/mentalillness

National Institutes of Health. (2018). *The Helping to End Addiction Long-term® initiative*. https://heal.nih.gov/

National Institute of Mental Health (NIMH). (2022). *Mental illness*. https://www.nimh.nih.gov/health/statistics/mental-illness.shtml

Patel, K., Bunachita, S., Chiu, H., Suresh, P., & Patel, U. K. (2021). Elder abuse: A comprehensive overview and physician-associated challenges. *Cureus, 13*(4), e14375. https://doi.org/10.7759/cureus.14375

President's New Freedom Commission on Mental Health. (2003). *Achieving the promise: Transforming mental health care in America.* http://govinfo.library.unt.edu/mentalhealthcommission/reports/reports.htm

Safe Horizon. (2022). *Youth homelessness statistics and facts.* https://www.safehorizon.org/get-informed/homelessyouth-statistics-facts/#definition/

Shajani, Z., & Snell, D. (2019). *Nurses and families: A guide to family assessment and intervention* (7th ed.). F.A. Davis.

Spock, B., & Needlman, R. (2018). *Dr. Spock's baby and child care* (10th ed.). Gallery Books.

Substance Abuse and Mental Health Services Administration (SAMHSA). (2016). Behind the term serious mental illness. https://www.hsdl.org/?view&did=801613

Substance Abuse and Mental Health Services Administration (SAMHSA). (2022a). *PATH annual report for FY 2020.* https://pathpdx.samhsa.gov/Content/preGen/national/25/PATH_Annual_Report_For_FY_2020.pdf

Substance Abuse and Mental Health Services Administration (SAMHSA). (2022b). *SAMHSA strategic plan FY2019–FY 2023.* https://www.samhsa.gov/about-us/strategic-plan-fy2019-fy2023

Treatment Advocacy Center. (2018). *Eliminating barriers to the treatment of mental illness.* https://www.treatmentadvocacycenter.org/fixing-the-system/features-and-news/2596-how-many-people-with-serious-mental-illness-are-homeless

U.S. Department of Housing and Urban Development (HUD). (2022). *The 2021 annual homeless assessment report (AHAR) to congress.* https://www.huduser.gov/portal/sites/default/files/pdf/2021-AHAR-Part-1.pdf

Vanderplasschen, W., Rapp, R. C., Pearce, S., Vandevelde, S., & Broekaert, E. (2013). Mental health, recovery, and the community. *The Scientific World Journal, 2013*(4), 1–3. doi: http://dx.doi.org/10.1155/2013/926174

Veltri, L., Wilson-Mitchell, K., & O'Mahony, J. M. (2018). Family nursing with childbearing families. In J. R. Kaakinen, D. P. Coehlo, R. Steele, & M. Robinson (Eds.), *Family health care nursing* (6th ed., pp. 357–387). F.A. Davis.

White, D. L., & Cartwright, J. C. (2018). Family health in mid- and later life. In J. R. Kaakinen, D. P. Coehlo, R. Steele, & M. Robinson (Eds.), *Family health care nursing* (6th ed., pp. 457–496). F.A. Davis.

Classical References

Caplan, G. (1964). *Principles of preventive psychiatry.* Basic Books.

Erikson, E. (1963). *Childhood and society* (2nd ed.). WW Norton.

GovTrack. (1987). *H.R. 558 (100th): Stewart B. McKinney Homeless Assistance Act.* https://www.govtrack.us/congress/bills/100/hr558/text

Lamb, H. R. (1993). Perspectives on effective advocacy for homeless mentally ill persons. *Hospital and Community Psychiatry, 43*(12), 1209–1212. doi: http://dx.doi.org/10.1176/ps.43.12.1209

36

The Bereaved Individual

CORE CONCEPTS

Grief and Loss
Self
Stress and Coping
Clinical Judgment

KEY TERMS

advance directive
anticipatory grieving
bereavement
bereavement overload

grief
hospice
maladaptive grieving
mourning

OBJECTIVES
After reading this chapter, the student will be able to:

1. Describe various types of loss that trigger the grief response in individuals.
2. Discuss theoretical perspectives of grieving as proposed by Elisabeth Kübler-Ross, John Bowlby, George Engel, and J. William Worden.
3. Differentiate between normal and maladaptive responses to loss.
4. Discuss grieving behaviors common to individuals at various stages across the life span.
5. Describe customs associated with grief in individuals of various cultures.
6. Formulate nursing diagnoses and goals of care for individuals experiencing the grief response.
7. Describe appropriate nursing interventions for individuals experiencing the grief response.
8. Identify relevant criteria for evaluating the nursing care of individuals experiencing the grief response.
9. Describe the concept of hospice care for people who are dying and their families.
10. Discuss the use of advance directives for individuals to provide directions about their future medical care.

CORE CONCEPT

Loss
The experience of separation from something of personal importance.

Loss is anything that is perceived as such by the individual. The separation from loved ones or the giving up of treasured possessions, for whatever reason; the experience of failure, either real or perceived; or life events that create change in a familiar pattern of existence—all can be experienced as loss, and all can trigger behaviors associated with the grieving process. Loss and bereavement are universal events encountered by all beings that experience emotions. The following are examples of some notable forms of loss:

■ A significant other (person or pet), through death, divorce, or separation for any reason.

■ Illness or debilitating conditions. Examples include (but are not limited to) diabetes, stroke, cancer, rheumatoid arthritis, multiple sclerosis, Alzheimer's disease, hearing or vision loss, and spinal cord or head injuries. Some of these conditions not only incur a loss of physical or emotional wellness but may also result in the loss of personal independence.

■ Developmental and maturational changes or situations, such as menopause, andropause, infertility, "empty nest," aging, impotence, or hysterectomy.

■ Real or perceived loss of hopes, dreams, and potential for specific accomplishments.

■ Personal possessions that symbolize familiarity and security in a person's life. Separation from these familiar and personally valued external objects represents a loss of material extensions of the self.

CORE CONCEPT
Grief
Deep mental and emotional anguish that is a response to the subjective experience of loss of something significant.

Mourning may be described as the outward signs of one's sorrow at the loss of a loved one. **Grief** may be viewed as the subjective states that accompany mourning or the emotional work involved in the mourning process. Similarly, **bereavement** is described as the period during which grief and mourning occur. Bereavement, grief, and mourning encompass all the mental, physical, emotional, and social reactions to loss. For purposes of this text, grief, bereavement, and the process of mourning are collectively referred to as the *grief response*.

This chapter examines human responses to the experience of loss. Care of bereaved individuals is presented in the context of the nursing process.

Theoretical Perspectives on Loss and Bereavement

Stages of Grief

Behavior patterns associated with the grief response include many individual variations. However, sufficient

similarities have been observed to warrant characterization of the grief response as a syndrome that has a predictable course with an expected resolution. Early theorists, including Kübler-Ross (1969), Bowlby (1961), and Engel (1964), described behavioral stages through which individuals advance in their progression toward resolution. Many variables influence one's progression through the grief process, and it should be viewed as a dynamic rather than a linear process. Some individuals may reach acceptance only to revert to an earlier stage, some may never complete the sequence, and some may never progress beyond the initial stage.

A more contemporary grief specialist, J. William Worden (2009), offers a set of tasks that must be processed in order to complete the grief response. He suggests that it is possible for a person to accomplish some of these tasks and not others, resulting in an incomplete bereavement that impairs further growth and development. A comparison of the similarities among these four models of the normal grief response is presented in Table 36–1.

Elisabeth Kübler-Ross

These well-known stages of the grief process were identified by Kübler-Ross in her extensive work with dying patients. Behaviors associated with each of these stages can be observed in individuals experiencing the loss of any concept of personal value.

■ **Stage I: Denial.** In this stage, the individual has difficulty believing that the loss has occurred. They may say, "No, it can't be true!" or "It's just not possible." This stage may protect the individual against the psychological pain of reality.

■ **Stage II: Anger.** This is the stage when reality sets in. Feelings associated with this stage include sadness, guilt, shame, helplessness, and hopelessness. Self-blame or blaming of others may lead to feelings of anger toward the self and others. The anxiety level may be elevated, and the individual may experience confusion and a decreased ability to function independently. They may be preoccupied with an idealized image of what has been lost. Numerous somatic complaints are common.

■ **Stage III: Bargaining.** At this stage in the grief response, the individual attempts to strike a bargain with God for a second chance or for more time. The person acknowledges the loss or impending loss but holds out hope for additional alternatives, as evidenced by statements such as, "If only I could . . ." or "If only I had . . ."

■ **Stage IV: Depression.** In this stage, the individual mourns for that which has been or will be lost. In this stage, the individual must confront feelings associated with having lost someone or

TABLE 36–1   Stages and Tasks of the Normal Grief Response: A Comparison of Models by Elisabeth Kübler-Ross, John Bowlby, George Engel, and William Worden

STAGES/TASKS				POSSIBLE TIME DIMENSION	BEHAVIORS
KÜBLER-ROSS	BOWLBY	ENGEL	WORDEN		
I. Denial	I. Numbness/protest	I. Shock/disbelief	I. Accepting the reality of the loss	Occurs immediately on experiencing the loss. Usually lasts no more than a few weeks.	Individual has difficulty believing that the loss has occurred.
II. Anger	II. Disequilibrium	II. Developing awareness		In most cases begins within hours of the loss. Peaks within a few weeks.	Anger is directed toward self or others. Ambivalence and guilt may be felt toward the lost entity.
III. Bargaining					The individual fervently seeks alternatives to improve the current situation.
		III. Restitution			Attends to various rituals associated with the culture in which the loss has occurred.
IV. Depression	III. Disorganization and despair	IV. Resolution of the loss	II. Processing the pain of grief	Very individual. Commonly 6–12 months. Longer for some.	The actual work of grieving. Preoccupation with the lost entity. Feelings of helplessness and loneliness occur in response to realization of the loss. Feelings associated with the loss are confronted.
			III. Adjusting to a world without the lost entity	Ongoing.	How the environment changes depends on the roles the lost entity played in the life of the bereaved person. Adaptations will have to be made as the changes are presented in daily life. New coping skills will have to be developed.
V. Acceptance	IV. Reorganization	V. Recovery	IV. Finding an enduring connection with the lost entity in the midst of embarking on a new life		Resolution is complete. The bereaved person experiences a reinvestment in new relationships and new goals. The lost entity is not purged or replaced, but relocated in the life of the bereaved. At this stage, terminally ill persons express a readiness to die.

something of value (called *reactive* depression). An example is an individual who is mourning a change in body image. Feelings associated with an impending loss (called *preparatory* depression) are also confronted. Examples include permanent lifestyle changes related to the altered body image or even an impending loss of life itself. Regression, withdrawal, and social isolation may be observed behaviors with this stage. Therapeutic intervention should be available but not imposed, with guidelines for implementation based on individual readiness.

■ **Stage V: Acceptance.** At this time, the individual has worked through the behaviors associated with the other stages and accepts or is resigned to the loss. Anxiety decreases, and methods for coping with the loss have been established. The individual is less preoccupied with what has been lost and increasingly interested in other aspects of the environment. If the individual is confronting death, they are ready to die. The person may become very quiet and withdrawn, seemingly devoid of feelings. These behaviors are an attempt to facilitate the passage by slowly disengaging from the environment.

David Kessler, who collaborated with Kübler-Ross, recently advanced the concept of a sixth stage of grief, which he labels *finding meaning* (Kessler, 2019). He advances the idea that grief is transformed into peace and a renewed sense of hopefulness when meaning rather than closure is sought.

John Bowlby

John Bowlby hypothesized four stages in the grief process. He suggests that these behaviors can be observed in all individuals who have experienced the loss of something or someone of value, even in babies as young as 6 months of age.

■ **Stage I: Numbness or protest.** This stage is characterized by a feeling of shock and disbelief that the loss has occurred. The reality of the loss is not acknowledged.

■ **Stage II: Disequilibrium.** During this stage, the individual has a profound urge to recover what has been lost. Behaviors associated with this stage include a preoccupation with the loss, intense weeping, expressions of anger toward the self and others, and feelings of ambivalence and guilt associated with the loss.

■ **Stage III: Disorganization and despair.** Feelings of despair occur in response to the realization that the loss has occurred. Activities of daily living become increasingly disorganized, and behavior is characterized by restlessness and aimlessness.

Efforts to regain productive patterns of behavior are ineffective, and the individual experiences fear, helplessness, and hopelessness. Somatic complaints are common. Perceptions of visualizing or being in the presence of that which has been lost may occur. Social isolation is common, and the individual may feel a great deal of loneliness.

■ **Stage IV: Reorganization.** The individual accepts or becomes resigned to the loss. New goals and patterns of organization are established. The individual begins a reinvestment in new relationships and indicates a readiness to move forward within the environment. Grief subsides and recedes into valued remembrances.

George Engel

George Engel hypothesized five stages of the grief process with a greater emphasis on the movement toward grief recovery.

■ **Stage I: Shock and disbelief.** The initial reaction to a loss is a stunned, numb feeling and refusal by the individual to acknowledge the reality of the loss. Engel states that this stage is an attempt by the individual to protect the self from the extreme stress associated with significant loss by defending oneself against it.

■ **Stage II: Developing awareness.** This stage begins within minutes to hours of the loss. Behaviors associated with this stage include excessive crying and regression to a state of helplessness and a childlike manner. Awareness of the loss creates feelings of emptiness, frustration, anguish, and despair. Anger may be directed toward the self or toward others in the environment who are held accountable for the loss.

■ **Stage III: Restitution.** In this stage, the various rituals associated with loss within a culture are performed. Examples include funerals, wakes, special attire, a gathering of friends and family, and religious practices customary to the spiritual beliefs of the bereaved. Participation in these rituals is thought to assist the individual to accept the reality of the loss and facilitate the recovery process.

■ **Stage IV: Resolution of the loss.** This stage is characterized by a preoccupation with the loss. The concept of the loss is idealized, and the individual may even imitate admired qualities of the lost entity. Preoccupation with the loss gradually decreases over a year or more, and the individual eventually begins to reinvest feelings in others.

■ **Stage V: Recovery.** Obsession with the loss has ended, and the individual is able to go on with their life.

J. William Worden

Worden views the bereaved person as active and self-determining rather than a passive participant in the grief process. He proposes that bereavement includes a set of tasks that must be reconciled in order to complete the grief process. Worden's four tasks of mourning include the following:

■ **Task I. Accepting the reality of the loss.** When something of value is lost, it is common for individuals to refuse to believe that the loss has occurred. Behaviors include misidentifying individuals in the environment for their lost loved one, retaining possessions of the lost loved one as though they had not died, and removing all reminders of the lost loved one so as not to have to face the reality of the loss. Worden (2009) stated:

Coming to an acceptance of the reality of the loss takes time since it involves not only an intellectual acceptance but also an emotional one. The bereaved person may be intellectually aware of the finality of the loss long before the emotions allow full acceptance of the information as true. (p. 42)

Belief and denial are intermittent while grappling with this task. It is thought that traditional rituals such as the funeral help some individuals move toward acceptance of the loss.

■ **Task II. Processing the pain of grief.** Pain associated with a loss includes both physical pain and emotional pain. This pain must be acknowledged and worked through. To avoid or suppress it serves only to delay or prolong the grieving process. People do this by refusing to allow themselves to think painful thoughts, by idealizing or avoiding reminders of the lost entity, and by using alcohol or drugs. The intensity of the pain and the manner in which it is experienced are different for all individuals. However, the commonality is that it *must* be experienced. Failure to do so generally results in some form of depression. Individuals who repress the feelings of loss may require therapy to work through the pain of grief that they failed to face at the time of the loss. In this difficult task II, individuals must "allow themselves to process the pain—to feel it and to know that 1 day it will pass" (Worden 2009, p. 45).

■ **Task III. Adjusting to a world without the lost entity.** It usually takes several months for a bereaved person to realize what their world will be like without the lost entity. In the case of a lost loved one, how the environment changes will depend on the types of roles that person fulfilled in life. In the case of a changed lifestyle, the individual will be required to make adaptations to their environment in terms of the changes as they are presented in daily life.

In addition, those individuals who had defined their identity through the lost entity will require an adjustment to their own sense of self. Worden identifies that successful completion of task III entails redefining the loss in a way that is beneficial to the survivor.

If the bereaved person experiences failures in their attempt to adjust in an environment without the lost entity, feelings of low self-esteem may result. Regressed behaviors and feelings of helplessness and inadequacy are not uncommon. Worden states:

[Another] area of adjustment is to one's sense of the world. Loss through death can challenge one's fundamental life values and philosophical beliefs—beliefs that are influenced by our families, peers, education, and religion as well as life experiences. The bereaved person searches for meaning in the loss and its attendant life changes in order to make sense of it and to regain some control of his or her life. (pp. 48–49)

To be successful in task III, bereaved individuals must develop new skills to cope and adapt to their new environment without the lost entity. Achievement of this task determines the outcome of the mourning process—that of continued growth or a state of arrested development.

■ **Task IV. Finding an enduring connection with the lost entity in the midst of embarking on a new life.** This task allows the bereaved person to identify a special place for the lost entity. Individuals need not purge from their history or find a replacement for that which has been lost. Instead, there is a continued presence of the lost entity that becomes *relocated* in the life of the bereaved. Successful completion of task IV involves letting go of past attachments and forming new ones. However, there is also the recognition that although the relationship between the bereaved and what has been lost is changed, it is nonetheless still a relationship. Worden suggests that one never loses memories of a significant relationship. He states:

For many people, Task IV is the most difficult one to accomplish. They get stuck at this point in their grieving and later realize that their life in some way stopped at the point the loss occurred. (p. 52)

■ Worden relates the story of a teenage girl who had a difficult time adjusting to the death of her father. After 2 years, when she began to finally fulfill some of the tasks associated with successful grieving, she wrote these words that express rather clearly what bereaved people in task IV are struggling with: "There are other people to be loved, and it doesn't mean that I love Dad any less" (p. 52).

Length of the Grief Process

Stages of grief allow bereaved persons an orderly approach to the resolution of mourning. Each stage presents tasks that must be overcome through a painful experiential process. Engel (1964) stated that successful resolution of the grief response is thought to have occurred when a bereaved individual is able "to remember comfortably and realistically both the pleasures and disappointments of the lost relationship" (p. 96). The length of the grief process depends on the individual and can last for several years without being maladaptive. The most acute phase of normal grieving usually lasts about 6 to 8 weeks—longer in older adults—but complete resolution of the grief response may take much longer. Boland and Verduin (2022) state:

> Ample evidence suggests that the bereavement process does not end within a prescribed interval; certain aspects persist indefinitely for many otherwise high-functioning, normal individuals. Common manifestations of protracted grief occur intermittently … most grief does not fully resolve or permanently disappear; rather grief becomes circumscribed and submerged only to reemerge in response to certain triggers. (p. 850)

The *Diagnostic and Statistical Manual of Mental Disorders, Fifth Edition, Text Revision (DSM-5-TR)* (American Psychiatric Association [APA], 2022), identifies a new diagnostic category called *prolonged grief disorder*, in which a maladaptive grief response is diagnosed after at least 12 months of time have elapsed since the death of the loved one (at least 6 months in children and adolescents). The authors add, though, that although they believe this time frame to generally discriminate between normal grief and maladaptive grief reactions, "the duration of adaptive grief may vary individually and cross-culturally" (p. 323). In addition, the time frame alone does not dictate a maladaptive grief reaction. The *DSM-5-TR* (APA, 2022, p. 323) identifies several other indicators (of which there must be at least three), which may include a persistent feeling as though part of oneself has died; a marked sense of disbelief about the death; avoidance of reminders about the deceased; intense emotional pain; difficulty reintegrating with other relationships or activities, or planning for the future; emotional numbness; feeling that life is meaningless; and intense loneliness.

A number of factors influence the eventual outcome of the grief response. The grief response can be more difficult if:

- The bereaved person was strongly dependent on or perceived the lost entity as an important means of physical or emotional support.

- The relationship with the lost entity was highly ambivalent. A love–hate relationship may instill feelings of guilt that can interfere with the grief work.
- The individual has experienced other recent losses. Grief tends to be cumulative, and if previous losses have not been resolved, each succeeding grief response becomes more difficult.
- The loss is that of a young person. Grief over the loss of a child is often more intense than that over the loss of an older person. Traumatic death in general increases the likelihood of abnormal grief.
- The state of the person's physical or psychological health is unstable at the time of the loss.
- The bereaved person perceives (whether real or imagined) some responsibility for the loss.
- The loss is secondary to suicide.
- The loss is a traumatic death such as murder.

The grief response may be facilitated if:

- The individual has the support of significant others to assist them through the mourning process.
- The individual has the opportunity to prepare for the loss. Grief work is more intense when the loss is sudden and unexpected. The experience of *anticipatory grieving* is thought to facilitate the grief response that occurs at the time of the actual loss.

Worden (2009) states:

> There is a sense in which mourning can be finished, when people regain an interest in life, feel more hopeful, experience gratification again, and adapt to new roles. There is also a sense in which mourning is never finished. [People must understand] that mourning is a long-term process and that the culmination will not be a pregrief state. (p. 77)

Anticipatory Grief

Anticipatory grieving is the experiencing of the feelings and emotions associated with the normal grief response before the loss actually occurs. It is different in several ways from conventional grief. For example, conventional grief tends to diminish in intensity with time, whereas anticipatory grief can become more intense as the expected loss becomes imminent.

Although anticipatory grief is thought to facilitate the actual mourning process after the loss, it may be problematic. In the case of a dying person, difficulties can arise when the family members complete the process of anticipatory grief and detachment from the dying person occurs prematurely. The person who is dying experiences feelings of loneliness and isolation as the psychological pain of imminent death is faced without family support. Another example of difficulty associated with premature completion of the grief response is the reaction that can occur on the return of persons long absent and presumed dead (e.g., soldiers missing in action or prisoners of war). In this instance, resumption of the previous relationship may be difficult for the bereaved person.

Anticipatory grieving may serve as a defense for some individuals to ease the burden of loss when it actually occurs. It may prove to be less functional for others who, because of interpersonal, psychological, or sociocultural variables, are unable in advance of the actual loss to express the intense feelings that accompany the grief response.

One qualitative study examined the unique process of grief for family caregivers of a relative who has dementia. One common theme was that in addition to anticipatory grief related to the final loss, these family members were, at the same time, grieving actual losses throughout the journey of their family member's illness (Peacock et al., 2014). These included grieving the loss of the ill person's personality, companionship, social self, and cognition as the disease progressed. Another study added that caregiver grief increased as the disease progressed in severity (Li et al., 2021). The grief reactions of these active caregivers were similar to those of bereaved caregivers, although their family member was still alive. These studies highlight the multiplicity of factors that can influence the grieving process.

Maladaptive Responses to Loss

When, then, is the grieving response considered to be maladaptive? Three types of pathological grief reactions are described in the following sections. **Maladaptive grieving** includes delayed or inhibited grief, an exaggerated or distorted grief response, and chronic or prolonged grief.

Delayed or Inhibited Grief

Delayed or inhibited grief refers to the absence of evidence of grief when it ordinarily would be expected. Many times, cultural influences, such as the expectation to keep a "stiff upper lip," contribute to the delayed response.

Delayed or inhibited grief is potentially complicated because the person is not acknowledging the reality of the loss. The individual remains fixed in the denial stage of the grief process, sometimes for many years. When this occurs, the grief response may be triggered, sometimes many years later, when the individual experiences a subsequent loss. Sometimes the grief process is triggered spontaneously or in response to a seemingly insignificant event. Overreaction to another person's loss may be one manifestation of delayed grief.

The recognition of delayed grief is critical because, depending on the profoundness of the loss, the failure of the mourning process may prevent assimilation of the loss and thereby delay a return to satisfying living. Without the lessons that the grief process can provide, subsequent losses may be compounded by previously unresolved grief work. Delayed grieving most commonly occurs because of ambivalent feelings toward the lost entity, outside pressure to resume normal function, or perceived lack of internal and external resources to cope with a profound loss.

Distorted (Exaggerated) Grief Response

In the distorted grief reaction, all of the symptoms associated with normal grieving are exaggerated. Feelings of sadness, helplessness, hopelessness, powerlessness, anger, and guilt, in addition to numerous somatic complaints, render the individual dysfunctional in terms of management of daily living. Morrow (2022) describes this as a state of feeling "trapped" in one's grief and "the usual responses to the death of a loved one do not fade over time and can impair or prevent them from leading their normal lives."

When the exaggerated grief reaction occurs, the individual remains fixed in the anger stage of the grief response. This anger may be directed toward others in the environment to whom the individual may be attributing the loss. However, often the anger is turned inward on the self, resulting in depression. Clinical depressions may be related to exaggerated grief reactions. This should be distinguished, however, from the depression that is considered part of the normal grieving process. A summary of differences between normal grieving and clinical depression is presented in Table 36–2.

Chronic or Prolonged Grieving

Some authors have discussed a chronic or prolonged grief response as a type of maladaptive grief response. Care must be taken in making this determination because, as stated previously, the length of the grief response depends on the individual. An adaptive response may take years for some people. A prolonged process may be considered maladaptive when certain behaviors are exhibited. Prolonged grief may be a problem when behaviors such as those that prevent the bereaved from adaptively performing activities of daily living are in evidence. An example is the widow who refuses to participate in family gatherings after the death of her husband. For many years until her death, she takes a sandwich to the cemetery on holidays, sits on the tombstone, and eats her "holiday meal" with her husband. Whether one's behaviors constitute prolonged or chronic grieving

TABLE 36–2 Normal Grief Reactions Versus Symptoms of Clinical Depression	
NORMAL GRIEF	**CLINICAL DEPRESSION**
Self-esteem intact	Self-esteem is disturbed
May openly express anger	Usually does not directly express anger
Experiences a mixture of "good and bad days"	Persistent state of dysphoria
Able to experience moments of pleasure	Anhedonia is prevalent
Accepts comfort and support from others	Does not respond to social interaction and support from others
Maintains feeling of hope	Feelings of hopelessness prevail
May express guilt feelings over some aspect of the loss	Has generalized feelings of guilt
Relates feelings of depression to specific loss experienced	Does not relate feelings to a particular experience
May experience transient physical symptoms	Expresses chronic physical complaints
	Thoughts of suicide

Sources: Boland, R., & Verduin, M. L. (2022). *Synopsis of psychiatry: Behavioral sciences/clinical psychiatry* (12th ed.). Wolter Kluwer; Corr, C. A., Corr, D. M., & Doka, K. J. (2019). *Death & dying, life & living* (8th ed.). Cengage.

must consider cultural context. In some cultures, establishing a memorial ritual to the deceased is the norm, whereas in other cultures, it might be perceived as prolonged grieving.

Normal Versus Maladaptive Grieving

Although Morrow (2022) identifies that it is difficult to establish a time frame signaling the difference between normal and maladaptive grieving, several symptoms are red flags of maladaptive grieving. These include the following:

■ Episodes of rage or prolonged, unresolved anger
■ Inability to focus on anything but the loss
■ Intense focus or avoidance of any reminders of the lost entity
■ Prolonged difficulty accepting the reality of the loss
■ Self-destructive behavior, including alcohol and drug misuse
■ Suicidal thoughts and actions

A crucial difference between normal and maladaptive grieving is the loss of self-esteem. Marked feelings of worthlessness are indicative of depression rather than uncomplicated, normal bereavement. Hensley and Clayton (2013) found that when clinically depressed inpatients were compared with individuals experiencing depression associated with bereavement, four symptoms were absent in the bereavement population: suicidal thoughts, feeling like they were a burden to others, feeling like they would rather be dead, and psychomotor

retardation. These may be considered associated symptoms of low self-esteem and feelings of worthlessness. The presence of suicidal ideation automatically indicates an abnormal grief reaction and requires careful assessment and immediate intervention to prevent suicide.

It is thought that this major difference between normal grieving and a maladaptive grieving response (the feeling of worthlessness or low self-esteem) ultimately precipitates depression, which can be a progressive situation for some individuals. Clark and associates (2021) identify that prolonged grief disorders occur in about 7% to 10% of bereaved individuals. Hensley and Clayton (2013) note that the incidence of major depressive disorder among the bereaved is around 35% at 1 month after a loss; although incidence tends to decrease over time, 8% to 11% develop chronic depression. The authors add that factors such as poor physical health, poor mental health, and substance use disorders before a loss increase the risk for chronic depression after the loss.

Application of the Nursing Process

Background Assessment Data: Concepts of Death—Developmental Issues

All individuals have their own unique concept of death, which is influenced by past experiences with death in addition to age and level of emotional development. This section addresses the various perceptions of death according to developmental age.

Children

Birth to Age 2

Infants are unable to recognize and understand death, but they can experience feelings of loss and separation. Infants who are separated from their mothers may become quiet, lose weight, and sleep less. Children at this age will likely sense changes in the atmosphere of the home where a death has occurred. They often react to the emotions of adults by becoming more irritable and crying more.

Ages 3 to 5

Preschoolers and kindergartners have some understanding of death but often have difficulty distinguishing between fantasy and reality. They believe death is reversible, and their thoughts about death may include magical thinking. For example, they may believe that their thoughts or behaviors caused a person to become sick or to die.

Children of this age are capable of understanding at least some of what they see and hear from adult conversations or media reports. They become frightened if they feel a threat to themselves or their loved ones. They are concerned with safety issues and require a great deal of personal reassurance that they will be protected. Regressive behaviors, such as loss of bladder or bowel control, thumb sucking, and temper tantrums, are common. Changes in eating and sleeping patterns may also occur.

Ages 6 to 9

Children at this age are beginning to understand the finality of death. They are able to understand a more detailed explanation of why or how a person died, although the concept of death is often associated with old age or with accidents. They may believe that death is contagious and avoid association with individuals who have experienced a loss by death. Death is often personified, in the form of a "bogey man" or a monster—someone who takes people away or someone whom they can avoid if they try hard enough. It is difficult for them to perceive their own death. Normal grief reactions at this age include regressive and aggressive behaviors, withdrawal, school phobias, somatic symptoms, and clinging behaviors.

Ages 10 to 12

Preadolescent children are able to understand that death is final and eventually affects everyone, including themselves. They are interested in the physical aspects of dying and the final disposition of the body. They may ask questions about how the death will affect them personally. Feelings of anger, guilt, and depression are common. Peer relationships and school performance may be disrupted. There may be a preoccupation with the loss and a withdrawal into the self.

Adolescents

Adolescents are usually able to view death on an adult level. They understand death to be universal and inevitable; however, they have difficulty tolerating the intense feelings associated with the death of a loved one. They may or may not cry. They may withdraw into themselves or attempt to go about usual activities to avoid dealing with the pain of the loss. Some teens exhibit acting-out behaviors, such as aggression and defiance. It is often easier for adolescents to discuss their feelings with peers than with their parents or other adults. Some adolescents may show regressive behaviors, whereas others react by trying to take care of their loved ones who are also grieving. In general, individuals of this age-group have an attitude of immortality. Although they can understand that their own death is inevitable, the concept is so far-reaching as to be imperceptible.

Evidence supports (Oosterhoff et al., 2018) that young people who are bereaved, and particularly those having experienced sudden loss, are more likely to have lower academic achievement, lower ability to concentrate and learn, less enjoyment of school, lower school belongingness, and lower beliefs that teachers treat youth fairly. These complications may put them at higher risk for health problems, feelings of hopelessness, and depression. They will require support, flexibility in the management of anger responses, and reassurance of their own safety and self-worth.

Adults

The adult's concept of death is influenced by experiential, cultural, and religious backgrounds. Behaviors associated with grieving in the adult were discussed in the section "Theoretical Perspectives on Loss and Bereavement."

Older Adults

Philosophers and poets have described late adulthood as the "season of loss." By the time individuals reach their 60s and 70s, they have experienced numerous losses, and mourning has become a lifelong process. Those who are most successful at adapting earlier in life will similarly cope better with the losses and grief inherent in aging. Unfortunately, with the aging process comes a convergence of losses, the timing of which makes it impossible for the aging individual to complete the grief process in response to one loss before another occurs. Because grief is cumulative, this can result in **bereavement overload**, in which the person is less able to adapt and reintegrate; complicated grief responses ensue, and mental and physical health may be jeopardized (Tousley, 2022). The COVID-19 pandemic is a relevant example of a circumstance that increases the risk for bereavement overload for all age-groups but particularly among older adults. De Leon Corona and associates (2021) described this as "virulent grief," noting that it has not been uncommon for individuals to have lost multiple loved ones, and for every COVID-associated death, an average of nine people were left bereaved. Bereavement overload has been implicated as a predisposing factor in the development of depressive disorder in older adults.

Some believe that bereavement among older adult couples is also associated with increased risk for mortality. Although many variables influence mortality in this population, evidence suggests that, in cases where the loss is anticipated, there is not an increased risk for mortality, but when the loss was unexpected, there was indeed an increased risk (Chen et al., 2022; Pool et al., 2018; Shah et al., 2013). This research highlights the need for additional assessment and support during the bereavement period when loss, particularly of a spouse, is unexpected.

Background Assessment Data: Bereavement Risk Assessment

Several tools have been developed to assess the risk for maladaptive grief responses. They incorporate many of the issues previously discussed and are framed to identify multiple risk factors commonly associated with complicated grief reactions that may require additional resources and intervention. Some additional aspects to include in an assessment that may signal increased risk for maladaptive grief follow:

■ Financial problems posed by the loss
■ Lack of coping skills or lack of experience in responding to the loss
■ Emotional or physical dependence on the lost person or item
■ History of mental illness or substance use disorders
■ History of trauma, including abuse
■ Multiple losses within a short time

Although formalized tools are more often used in palliative care settings, they constitute an important aspect of assessment for all nurses responding to the needs of the bereaved patient.

Background Assessment Data: Concepts of Death—Cultural Issues

As previously stated, bereavement practices are greatly influenced by cultural and religious backgrounds. It is important for health-care professionals to have an understanding of these individual differences to provide culturally sensitive care to their patients. Clinicians must be able to identify and appreciate what is culturally expected or required, because failure to carry out expected rituals may hinder the grief process and result in unresolved grief for some bereaved individuals. Box 36–1 provides a set of guidelines for assessing individual preferences related to death rituals.

Nursing Diagnosis and Outcome Identification

From the analysis of the assessment data, appropriate nursing diagnoses are formulated for the patient and family experiencing grief and loss. From these identified diagnoses, accurate planning of nursing care is executed. Possible nursing diagnoses for grieving persons include the following:

■ Risk for maladaptive grieving related to loss of a valued entity/concept; loss of a loved one
■ Risk for spiritual distress related to maladaptive grief reactions

The following criteria may be used for the measurement of outcomes in the care of the grieving patient:

The patient:

■ Acknowledges awareness of the loss
■ Is able to express feelings about the loss
■ Verbalizes stages of the grief process and behaviors associated with each
■ Expresses personal satisfaction and support from spiritual practices

Planning and Implementation

Table 36–3 provides a plan of care for the grieving person. Selected nursing diagnoses are presented, along with outcome criteria, appropriate nursing interventions, and rationales for each.

BOX 36–1 Guidelines for Assessing Individual Preferences Related to Death Rituals

DEATH RITUALS AND EXPECTATIONS
1. Identify specific death rituals and expectations.
2. Encourage the individual to describe their preferred death rituals and mourning practices.
3. What are preferences regarding burial practices, such as cremation?

RESPONSES TO DEATH AND GRIEF
4. Identify values and beliefs about death and grief.
5. Explore the individual's perceptions about death, dying, and the afterlife.

Table 36–3 | CARE PLAN FOR THE GRIEVING PERSON

NURSING DIAGNOSIS: RISK FOR MALADAPTIVE GRIEVING

RELATED TO: Loss of a valued entity/concept; loss of a loved one

OUTCOME CRITERIA	NURSING INTERVENTIONS	RATIONALE
Short-Term Goals: ■ Patient acknowledges awareness of the loss. ■ Patient expresses feelings about the loss. ■ Patient verbalizes own position in the grief process. Long-Term Goal: ■ Patient progresses through the grief process in a healthful manner toward resolution.	1. Assess the patient's current grief process. Assess for bereavement risk factors. 2. Develop trust. Show empathy, concern, and unconditional positive regard. 3. Help the patient actualize the loss by talking about it. "When did it happen? How did it happen?" and so forth. 4. Help the patient identify and express feelings. Some of the more problematic feelings include the following: a. *Anger.* The anger may be directed at the deceased, directed at God, displaced onto others, or retroflected inward on the self. Encourage the patient to examine this anger and validate the appropriateness of this feeling. b. *Guilt.* The patient may feel that they did not do enough to prevent the loss. Help the patient by reviewing the circumstances of the loss and the reality that it could not be prevented. c. *Anxiety and helplessness.* Help the patient to recognize the way that life was managed before the loss. Help the patient to put the feelings of helplessness into perspective by pointing out ways that they managed situations effectively without help from others. Role-play life events and assist with decision-making situations.	1. Accurate baseline data are required to provide appropriate assistance. 2. Developing trust provides the basis for a therapeutic relationship. 3. Reviewing the events of the loss can help the patient come to full awareness of the loss. 4. Until the patient can recognize and accept personal feelings regarding the loss, grief work cannot progress. a. Many people will not admit to angry feelings, believing it is inappropriate and unjustified. Expression of this emotion is necessary to prevent fixation in this stage of grief. b. Feelings of guilt prolong resolution of the grief process. c. The patient may have fears that they may not be able to carry on alone.

Table 36-3 | CARE PLAN FOR THE GRIEVING PERSON—cont'd

OUTCOME CRITERIA	NURSING INTERVENTIONS	RATIONALE
	5. Interpret normal behaviors associated with grieving and provide the patient with adequate time to grieve.	5. Understanding of the grief process will help prevent feelings of guilt generated by these responses. Individuals need adequate time to adjust to the loss and all its ramifications. This involves getting past birthdays and anniversaries of which the deceased was a part.
	6. Provide continuing support. If this is not possible by the nurse, offer referrals to support groups. Support groups of individuals going through the same experiences can be very helpful for the grieving individual.	6. The availability of emotional support systems facilitates the grief process.
	7. Identify pathological defenses that the patient may be using (e.g., drug/alcohol use, somatic complaints, social isolation). Assist the patient in understanding why these are not healthy defenses and how they delay the process of grieving.	7. The bereavement process is impaired by behaviors that mask the pain of the loss.
	8. Encourage the patient to make an honest review of the relationship with the lost entity. Journal keeping is a facilitative tool with this intervention.	8. Helping the patient to evaluate positive and negative aspects of the lost relationship facilitates moving through the grief process.

NURSING DIAGNOSIS: RISK FOR SPIRITUAL DISTRESS

RELATED TO: Maladaptive grief process

OUTCOME CRITERIA	NURSING INTERVENTIONS	RATIONALE
Short-Term Goal: ■ Patient identifies meaning and purpose in life, moving forward with hope for the future. Long-Term Goal: ■ Patient expresses achievement of support and personal satisfaction from spiritual practices.	1. Be accepting and nonjudgmental when the patient expresses anger and bitterness (e.g., toward God, the universe). Stay with the patient.	1. The nurse's presence and nonjudgmental attitude promote patient's feelings of self-worth and promote trust in the relationship.
	2. Encourage the patient to ventilate feelings related to the meaning of their own existence in the face of current loss.	2. The patient may believe they cannot go on living without the lost object. Catharsis can provide relief and put life back into a realistic perspective.

Continued

Table 36–3 | CARE PLAN FOR THE GRIEVING PERSON–cont'd

OUTCOME CRITERIA	NURSING INTERVENTIONS	RATIONALE
	3. Encourage the patient as part of grief work to reach out to previously used religious practices for support. Encourage the patient to discuss these practices and how they provided support in the past.	3. The patient may find comfort in religious rituals with which they are familiar.
	4. Assure the patient that they are not alone when feeling inadequate in the search for life's answers.	4. Validation of the patient's feelings and assurance that they are shared by others offer encouragement and an affirmation of acceptability.
	5. Contact spiritual leader of the patient's choice if they request.	5. These individuals serve to provide relief from spiritual distress and often can do so when other support persons cannot.

Evaluation

In the final step of the nursing process, a reassessment is conducted to determine whether the nursing actions have been successful in achieving the objectives of care. Evaluation of the nursing actions for the grieving patient may be facilitated by gathering information using the following types of questions:

■ Has the patient discussed the recent loss with staff and family members?

■ Is the patient able to verbalize feelings and behaviors associated with each stage of the grieving process and recognize their own position in the process?

■ Has obsession with and idealization of the lost entity subsided?

■ Is anger toward the loss expressed appropriately?

■ Is the patient able to participate in usual spiritual practices and feel satisfaction and support from them?

■ Is the patient seeking out interaction with others in an appropriate manner?

■ Is the patient able to verbalize positive aspects about their life, past relationships, and prospects for the future?

Additional Assistance

Hospice

Hospice is a program that provides comfort and supportive care to meet the special needs of people who are dying and their families. Typical services include physical, psychological, spiritual, and social care for the person when aggressive treatment is no longer appropriate. Palliative care is differentiated as a model that provides many comfort care services like hospice care but may be implemented to assist with management of a condition not currently life-threatening and may or may not include aggressive or curative treatment.

Various models of hospice exist, including freestanding institutions that provide both inpatient and home care, those affiliated with hospitals and nursing homes in which hospice services are provided within the institutional setting, and hospice organizations that provide home care only. The hospice movement in the United States has evolved mainly as a system of home-based care.

Hospice helps patients achieve physical and emotional comfort so that they can concentrate on living life as fully as possible. Patients are urged to stay active for as long as they are able, take part in activities they enjoy, and focus on the quality of life.

Hospice follows an interdisciplinary team approach to provide care for the terminally ill individual in the familiar surroundings of the home environment. The interdisciplinary team consists of nurses, attendants (homemakers, home health aides), physicians, social workers, volunteers, and health-care workers from other disciplines as required for individual patients.

The hospice approach is based on seven components:

1. The interdisciplinary team
2. Pain and symptom management
3. Emotional support to the patient and family
4. Pastoral and spiritual care
5. Bereavement counseling
6. 24-hour on-call nurse/counselor
7. Staff support

Not all hospice programs may include all of these services. The National Hospice and Palliative Care Organization (NHPCO) is an organization that publishes standards of care based on principles that are directed at the hospice program concept.

Interdisciplinary Team

Nurses

A registered nurse usually acts as the case manager for care of hospice patients. The nurse assesses the patient's and family's needs; establishes the goals of care; supervises and assists caregivers; evaluates care; serves as the patient's advocate; and provides educational information as needed to patient, family, and caregivers. They also provide physical care when needed, including IV therapy.

Attendants

These individuals are usually the members of the team who spend the most time with the patient. They assist with personal care and all activities of daily living. Without these daily attendants, many individuals would be unable to spend their remaining days in their home. Attendants may be noncertified and provide basic housekeeping services; they may be certified nursing assistants who assist with personal care; or they may be licensed vocational or practical nurses who provide more specialized care, such as dressing changes or tube feedings.

Physicians

The patient's primary physician and the hospice medical consultant give input into the care of the hospice patient. Orders may continue to come from the primary physician, whereas pain and symptom management may come from the hospice consultant. Ideally, these physicians attend weekly patient care conferences and provide in-service education for hospice staff and for others in the medical community.

Social Workers

The social worker assists the patient and family members with psychosocial issues, including those associated with the patient's condition, financial issues, legal needs, and bereavement concerns. The social worker provides information on community resources from which the patient and family may receive support and assistance. Some of the functions of the nurse and social worker may overlap at times.

Trained Volunteers

Volunteers are vital to the hospice concept. They provide services that may otherwise be financially impossible. They are specially selected and extensively trained, and they provide services such as transportation, companionship, respite care, recreational activities, light housekeeping, and sensitivity to the needs of families in stressful situations.

Rehabilitation Therapists

Physical therapists may assist hospice patients to minimize physical disability. They may assist with strengthening exercises and assist with special equipment needs. Occupational therapists may help the debilitated patient learn to accomplish activities of daily living as independently as possible. Other consultants, such as speech therapists, may be called on for the patient with special needs.

Dietitian

A nutritional consultant may be helpful to the hospice patient who is experiencing nausea and vomiting, diarrhea, anorexia, and weight loss. A nutritionist can ensure that the patient is receiving the proper balance of calories and nutrients.

Counseling Services

The hospice patient may require the services of a psychiatrist or psychologist if there is a history of mental illness or if a neurocognitive disorder or depression has become a problem. Other types of counseling services are available to provide assistance in managing the special needs of each patient.

Pain and Symptom Management

Improved quality of life at all times is a primary goal of hospice care. Thus, a major intervention for all caregivers is to ensure that the patient is as comfortable as possible, whether experiencing pain or other types of symptoms common in the terminal stages of an illness.

Emotional Support

Members of the hospice team encourage patients and families to discuss the eventual outcome of the disease process. Some individuals find discussing issues associated with death and dying uncomfortable, and if so, their decision is respected. However, honest discussion of these issues provides a sense of relief for some people, and they are more realistically prepared for the future. It may even draw some patients and families closer together during this stressful time.

Pastoral and Spiritual Care

The hospice philosophy supports the individual's right to seek guidance or comfort in the spiritual practices most suited to that person. The hospice team members help the patient obtain the spiritual support and guidance for which they express a preference.

Bereavement Counseling

Hospice provides a service to surviving family members or significant others after the death of their loved one. These services are usually provided by a bereavement counselor, but when one is not available, volunteers with special training in bereavement care may be of assistance. A grief support group may be helpful for the bereaved and provide a safe place for them to discuss their own fears and concerns about the death of a loved one.

24-Hour On-Call

The standards of care set forth by NHPCO state that care shall be available 24 hours a day, 7 days a week. A nurse or counselor is usually available by phone or for home visits around the clock. The knowledge that emotional or physical support is available at any time should it be required provides considerable support and comfort to significant others or family caregivers.

Staff Support

Team members who work closely and frequently with the patient often experience emotions similar to those of the patient or their family and significant others. They may experience anger, frustration, or fears of death and dying—all of which must be addressed through staff support groups, team conferences, time off, and adequate and effective supervision. Burnout is a common concern among hospice staff. Stress can be reduced, trust enhanced, and team functioning more effective if lines of communication are kept open among all members, if information is readily accessible through staff conferences and in-service education, and if staff know they are appreciated and feel good about what they are doing. Each of these roles and services is designed to promote adaptive coping in loss and bereavement.

Advance Directives

The term **advance directive** refers to a living will (which specifies what types of medical treatment are desired should the individual become incapacitated), a durable power of attorney (which designates who can make and handle financial affairs if the individual is incapacitated), and a health-care proxy (which designates who can make health-care decisions for the person if they are unable to make their wishes known). These legal documents allow individuals to provide directions about their future medical care. Advance directives are legally binding in all 50 states (Boland & Verduin, 2022).

Doctors usually follow clearly stated directives. It is important that the physician be informed that an advance directive exists and the specific wishes of the patient. In 1991 the U.S. Congress passed the *Patient Self-Determination Act*. This legislation requires that all health-care facilities must advise patients of their rights to refuse treatment, to make advance directive forms available to patients on admission, and to keep records of whether a patient has an advance directive or a designated health-care proxy. State laws also define how and under what circumstances individuals can refuse life-sustaining medical interventions. These laws are generally referred to as *natural death acts*. Nurses need to be aware of both federal law and the applicable state laws in the state where they practice nursing.

Despite the laws allowing for an advance directive document, many people have not established this document for themselves—and even when advance directives exist, they may not be honored when circumstances are confusing or unclear. In emergencies, treatment decisions sometimes must be made before information about an advance directive is available. Catalano and Catalano (2020) identify additional reasons why advance directives are sometimes not honored:

■ Advance directives that were formulated long before their implementation may call into question whether the patient understood the ramifications of their decisions for future medical problems and interventions at that time.

■ In general, the language used in standard living-will documents is not specific enough to cover all health-care circumstances. Consequently, health-care providers may lack clarity about how to proceed because the advance directive lacks clarity.

■ Because state laws vary, when a patient is in a state other than the one where the advance directive was established, it may raise questions about the document's legality.

Advance directives are designed to allow the patient to be in control of decisions about their right to live or die. It is also a way to spare family and loved ones the burden of making choices without knowing the wishes of the person who is dying. Nurses can play an active role in discussing advance directives within a culturally sensitive framework and encouraging patients who have advance directives to review and update them periodically to ensure that their wishes remain clear.

Summary and Key Points

- Loss is the experience of separation from something of personal importance.
- Loss is anything that is perceived as such by the individual.
- Loss of any concept of value to an individual can trigger the grief response.
- Elisabeth Kübler-Ross identified five stages that individuals pass through on their way to resolution of a loss: denial, anger, bargaining, depression, and acceptance. David Kessler adds a sixth stage: finding meaning.
- John Bowlby described four stages: stage I, numbness or protest; stage II, disequilibrium; stage III, disorganization and despair; and stage IV, reorganization.
- George Engel's stages include shock and disbelief, developing awareness, restitution, resolution of the loss, and recovery.
- J. William Worden, a more contemporary clinician, has proposed that bereaved individuals must accomplish a set of four tasks in order to complete the grief process: accepting the reality of the loss, processing the pain of grief, adjusting to a world without the lost entity, and finding an enduring connection with the lost entity in the midst of embarking on a new life.
- The length of the grief process is highly individual and can last several years without being maladaptive.
- The acute stage of the grief process typically lasts a couple of months, but resolution usually takes much longer.
- Anticipatory grieving is the experiencing of the feelings and emotions associated with the normal grief process in response to anticipation of the loss.
- Anticipatory grieving is thought to facilitate the grief process when the actual loss occurs.
- Three types of maladaptive grieving have been described:
  1. Delayed or inhibited grief in which there is an absence of grief when it ordinarily would be expected

  2. Distorted or exaggerated grief response in which the individual remains fixed in the anger stage of the grief process and the symptoms associated with normal grieving are exaggerated
  3. Chronic or prolonged grieving in which the individual is unable to let go of grieving behaviors after an extended time and in which behaviors indicate that they are not accepting that the loss has occurred
- Several authors have identified one crucial difference between normal and maladaptive grieving: the loss of self-esteem. Loss of self-esteem is more indicative of clinical depression.
- Feelings of worthlessness, feeling that one is a burden to others, suicidal ideation, and psychomotor retardation are indicative of clinical depression rather than uncomplicated bereavement.
- Very young children do not understand death but often react to the emotions of adults by becoming more irritable and crying more frequently. They often believe death is reversible.
- School-aged children understand the finality of death. Grief behaviors may reflect regression or aggression, school phobias, or sometimes a withdrawal into the self.
- Adolescents are usually able to view death on an adult level. Grieving behaviors may include withdrawal or acting out. Although they understand that their own death is inevitable, the concept is so far-reaching as to be imperceptible.
- By the time a person reaches their 60s or 70s, they have experienced numerous losses. Because grief is cumulative, these losses can result in bereavement overload. Depression is a common response.
- Nurses should assess a patient's bereavement needs within a culturally sensitive context.
- Hospice is a program that provides comfort and supportive care to meet the special needs of people who are dying and their families.
- The term advance directive refers to either a living will or durable power of attorney for health care. Advance directives allow individuals to be in control of decisions at the end of life and spare family and loved ones the burden of making choices without knowing what is most important to the person who is dying.

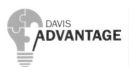

DAVIS ADVANTAGE | Go to **Davis Advantage** to complete your learning: strengthen understanding, apply your knowledge, and prepare for the Next Gen NCLEX®.

Review Questions

1. Which of the following is likely to initiate a grief response in an individual? (Select all that apply.)
   a. Death of a pet dog
   b. Onset of menopause
   c. Failing an examination
   d. Losing a spouse through divorce

2. A client, who is dying of cancer, says to the nurse, "I just want to see my new grandbaby. If only God will let me live until she is born, then I'll be ready to go." This is an example of which of Kübler-Ross's stages of grief?
   a. Denial
   b. Anger
   c. Bargaining
   d. Acceptance

3. A recent widow states, "I'm going to have to learn to pay all the bills. Hank always did that. I don't know if I can handle all of that." This is an example of which of the tasks described by Worden?
   a. Task I: Accepting the reality of the loss
   b. Task II: Processing the pain of grief
   c. Task III: Adjusting to a world without the lost entity
   d. Task IV: Finding an enduring connection with the lost entity in the midst of embarking on a new life

4. Engel identifies which of the following as successful resolution of the grief process?
   a. When the bereaved person can talk about the loss without crying
   b. When the bereaved person no longer talks about the lost entity
   c. When the bereaved person puts all remembrances of the loss out of sight
   d. When the bereaved person can discuss both positive and negative aspects about the lost entity

5. Which of the following is thought to facilitate the grief process?
   a. The ability to grieve in anticipation of the loss
   b. The ability to grieve alone without interference from others
   c. Having recently grieved for another loss
   d. Taking personal responsibility for the loss

Clinical Judgment Questions

6. A client who lost his wife after 35 years of marriage presents at his primary care physician's office 10 months later. He has lost 20 pounds and tells the nurse, "I just don't want to eat or do anything else for that matter." Which of these actions by the nurse is a priority?
   a. Assess the client for depression and suicide risk.
   b. Ask the physician to order gastrointestinal studies.
   c. Encourage the client to talk about his relationship with his deceased wife.
   d. Instruct the client that the doctor will be in shortly, but right now the physical assessment must be completed.

7. An 80-year-old client arrives at the emergency department accompanied by her daughter. The daughter tells the nurse that her mom lost her husband 2 months ago and since then her mom has complained of feeling depressed and anxious. Earlier today, she began complaining of chest pain. Which of these actions by the nurse is a priority?
   a. Instruct the daughter not to worry; these are common grief responses in the elderly.
   b. Assess vital signs and obtain an ECG.
   c. Refer the client to grief support groups in the area.
   d. Educate the client in relaxation and deep breathing exercises and evaluate whether this helps resolve the chest pain.

8. A 10-year-old child returns to school after the death of his mother. The school nurse becomes aware that this child is frequently talking in the classroom about fears that he will die, too. The classroom teacher is asking for recommendations about how to handle this situation. Which of these actions by the nurse is most appropriate?
   a. Instruct the teacher to refer the child for psychological evaluation because this is a warning sign of depression and possible suicide.
   b. Encourage the teacher to redirect the child to activities that are focused on school performance.
   c. Educate the teacher that this a common reaction in children of this age and it is best for the teacher to offer reassurance that he is safe.
   d. Instruct the teacher to prohibit discussion of this topic in class because children in this age-group cannot understand the finality of death.

9. A client whose husband died from cancer 1 month ago attends a grief support group being conducted by the hospice nurse. During the group this client states, "Sometimes I wish I could go be with my husband. I just want to die." Which action by the nurse is a priority?
   a. Ask the client if she is having thoughts of harming or killing herself.
   b. Instruct the client and the other group members that this is a normal part of the grieving process.
   c. Make arrangements for the client to be evaluated by a psychiatrist.
   d. Elicit support from other group members by asking if any of them have had similar feelings.

10. An adolescent who recently lost his brother in a fatal accident is referred to the school nurse after a physical fight with a peer. After attending to the client's bleeding lip, the parents ask the nurse for recommendations because their son has had several physical confrontations after the death of his brother. Which of these actions by the nurse is most beneficial?
    a. Encourage the parents to set more limits because adolescents need more structure as they work through their grief.
    b. Encourage the parents to schedule an appointment with a psychiatrist because his behavior is a sign of a developing conduct disorder.
    c. Provide information about available support groups for adolescents who have also experienced the loss of a loved one.
    d. Instruct the parents that making their son accept legal consequences for his behavior will likely resolve the problem behavior.

IMPLICATIONS OF RESEARCH FOR EVIDENCE-BASED PRACTICE

Cacciatore, J., Thieleman, K., Fretts, R., & Jackson, L. B. (2021). What is good grief support? Exploring the actors and actions in social support after traumatic grief. *PLoS ONE 16*(5), e0252324. https://doi.org/10.1371/journal.pone.0252324

DESCRIPTION OF THE STUDY: The researchers conducted a qualitative study and content analysis (n = 372) to assess bereaved individuals' satisfaction with social support in traumatic grief. Traumatic grief was defined as loss resulting from a violent or sudden death of a close loved one or the death of a child. The evaluation was structured around four constructs of support: informational, instrumental, appraisal, and emotional support. The largest percentage of respondents (75.1%) had experienced the death of a child.

RESULTS OF THE STUDY: Need for emotional support was one of the most common themes identified. Predominant associated actions included a desire for supporters to simply be present, with nonjudgmental, deep listening and quiet understanding. This includes foregoing advice-giving or "needing to fix" something, but rather being actively open to grief. Unsupportive actions that were identified included "use of platitudes; judging or rushing grief; failure to approach or acknowledge loss; feeling abandoned by family, friends, and community members; avoidance of grief and griever; not listening; the perception that others were pretending the person who died had never existed; others' propensity to center their own needs and feelings above the primary griever; and offering unsolicited advice, especially about how to heal grief."

A second, more surprising, theme that emerged from a majority of respondents was the importance of pets as a means of social support. The authors conclude that pet adoption may be an avenue to explore to promote well-being and reduce loneliness, particularly among bereaved individuals who lack strong social support networks.

Continued

IMPLICATIONS OF RESEARCH FOR EVIDENCE-BASED PRACTICE—cont'd

IMPLICATIONS FOR NURSING PRACTICE: The essence of patient-centered care involves listening to patients about their perceived needs. This study informs nurses about what bereaved individuals who experienced traumatic grief perceive as good emotional support. These findings are consistent with other studies that have identified the benefits of pets and pet therapy in promoting well-being and reducing loneliness.

💬 Communication Exercises

1. Jane's husband has been hospitalized for several days in end-stage congestive heart failure, and Jane has just been told that he has died. She begins sobbing and screams at the nurse, "You killed my husband! I should have never brought him to the hospital!"

   What would be an appropriate, empathic response by the nurse?

2. The doctor has shared with John test results revealing that his terminal cancer has not responded to treatment. John looks at the nurse and asks, "Am I dying?"

   What would be an appropriate response by the nurse?

3. Nancy has been told that she has a terminal illness. She says to the nurse, "Why would God do this to me?"

   What response by the nurse would demonstrate sensitivity to Nancy's spiritual distress?

MOVIE CONNECTIONS

Steel Magnolias • *My Girl* • *Up* • *Rabbit Hole* • *Stepmom* • *The Bucket List* • *Tig*

References

American Psychiatric Association. (2022). *Diagnostic and statistical manual of mental disorders, fifth edition, text revision (DSM-5-TR)*. American Psychiatric Association.

Boland, R., & Verduin, M. L. (Eds.). (2022). *Kaplan & Sadock's synopsis of psychiatry* (12th ed.). Wolters Kluwer.

Catalano, J. T., & Catalano, S. (2020). Bioethical issues. In J. T. Catalano (Ed.), *Nursing now! Today's issues, tomorrow's trends*. F.A. Davis.

Cacciatore, J., Thieleman, K., Fretts, R., & Jackson, L. B. (2021). What is good grief support? Exploring the actors and actions in social support after traumatic grief. *PLoS ONE 16*(5), e0252324. https://doi.org/10.1371/journal.pone.0252324

Chen, H., Wei, D., Janszky, I., Dahlström, U., Rostila, M., & László, K. D. (2022). Bereavement and prognosis in heart failure: A Swedish cohort study. *JACC: Heart Failure, 10*(10), 753–764. https://doi.org/10.1016/j.jchf.2022.05.005.

Clark, A., Inglewicz, A., & Zisook, S. (2021). *Bereavement and depression*. https://www.psychiatrictimes.com/view/bereavement-and-depression

Corr, C. A., Corr, D. M., & Doka, K. J. (2019). *Death & dying, life & living* (8th ed.). Cengage.

De Leon Corona, A. G., Chin, J., No, P., & Tom, J. (2021). The virulence of grief in the pandemic: Bereavement overload during COVID. *American Journal of Hospice and Palliative Medicine, 39*(10), 1244–1249. doi:10.1177/10499091211057094

Hensley, P. L., & Clayton, P. J. (2013). Why the bereavement exclusion was introduced in DSM-III. *Psychiatric Annals, 43*(6), 256–260.

Kessler, D. (2019). *Finding meaning: The sixth stage of grief*. Scribner.

Li, J., Li, Y., & Li, P. (2021). Perceived grief among caregivers of patients with dementia in China. *Clinical Nursing Research, 30*(1), 70–81. doi:10.1177/1054773819839265

Morrow, A. (2022). *Differences between normal and complicated grief*. https://www.verywell.com/grief-and-mourning-process-1132545

Oosterhoff, B., Kaplow, J. B., & Layne, C. M. (2018). Links between bereavement due to sudden death and academic functioning: Results from a nationally representative sample of adolescents. *School Psychology Quarterly, 33*(3), 372–380. https://doi.org/10.1037/spq0000254

Peacock, S. C., Hammond-Collins, K., & Ford, D. A. (2014). The journey with dementia from the perspective of bereaved caregivers: A qualitative descriptive study. *BioMed Central Nursing, 13*(42), 1–10. doi:10.1186/s12912-014-0042-x

Pool, L. R., Burgard, S. A., Needham, B. L., Elliott, M. R., Langa, K. M., & Mendes de Leon, C. F. (2018). Association of a negative wealth shock with all-cause mortality in middle-aged and older adults in the United States. *JAMA, 319*(13), 1341–1350. https://doi.org/10.1001/jama.2018.2055

Shah, S. M., Carey, I. M., Harris, T., DeWilde, S., Victor, C. R., & Cook, D. G. (2013). The effect of unexpected bereavement on mortality in older couples. *American Journal of Public Health, 103*(6), 1140–1145. doi:10.2105/AJPH.2012.301050

Tousley, M. (2022). *Coping with cumulative losses*. Grief Healing. www.griefhealingblog.com/2013/02/coping-with-cumulative-losses.html

Worden, J. W. (2009). *Grief counseling and grief therapy: A handbook for the mental health practitioner* (4th ed.). Springer.

Classical References

Bowlby, J. (1961). Processes of mourning. *International Journal of Psychoanalysis, 42*, 22.

Engel, G. (1964). Grief and grieving. *American Journal of Nursing, 64*(9), 93.

Kübler-Ross, E. (1969). *On death and dying*. Macmillan.

Military Families
37

CORE CONCEPTS

Stress and Coping

Mood and Affect

Grief and Loss

Addiction

Professionalism:
Nursing process in the care of military families

KEY TERMS

military deployment

post-traumatic stress disorder (PTSD)

traumatic brain injury (TBI)

veterans

OBJECTIVES
After reading this chapter, the student will be able to:

1. Discuss the history and epidemiology associated with members and veterans of the U.S. military.
2. Describe the lifestyle of career military families.
3. Discuss the impact of deployment on families of service members.
4. Discuss the concerns of women in the military.
5. Describe combat-related illnesses common in members and veterans of the U.S. military.
6. Apply steps of the nursing process in the care of veterans with traumatic brain injury and post-traumatic stress disorder.
7. Discuss various modalities relevant to treatment of traumatic brain injury and post-traumatic stress disorder.

Because of U.S. involvement in Iraq and Afghanistan, perhaps at no time in modern history has so much attention been given to what individuals and families experience as a result of their lives in the military. Services to meet the needs of active duty military personnel and **veterans** (individuals who have served in the military but are no longer serving) are in great demand, and resources for these services will be required for many years to come. More mental health-care practitioners will also be needed as the increasing number of veterans and their family members struggle to cope with the effects of **military deployment** (movement into active tours of duty).

This chapter addresses issues associated with the lives of military families and veterans of military combat. A discussion of nursing care for these individuals is presented, and selected medical treatment modalities are described.

Historical Aspects

"To care for him who shall have borne the battle and for his widow and his orphan."

—Abraham Lincoln, 1865

There is little doubt that individuals who survive military combat return from battle with scars—physical, psychological, or both. Reports of war-related psychological symptoms have existed in writing throughout the centuries, identified by terms such as "shell shock" and "battle fatigue." Many veterans of World War I and World War II were expected to be stoic, to lock up their feelings, and to never speak of the scenes of carnage and combat that they witnessed. The misuse of alcohol became a common way to deal with the emotions that were painful to discuss. **Post-traumatic stress disorder (PTSD)** (a psychiatric disorder associated with exposure to one or more traumatic events) has been associated with high rates of alcoholism among veterans, particularly those who have experienced active-duty combat. Only in recent history have the invisible wounds of combat veterans received the attention they desperately require.

Very little was written about PTSD during the years between 1950 and 1970. This absence was followed in the 1970s and 1980s by a significant increase in the amount of research and writing on the subject. Many of the papers written during this time were about Vietnam veterans. Clearly, the renewed interest in PTSD was linked to the psychological casualties of the Vietnam War. The diagnostic category of PTSD did not appear until the third edition of the *Diagnostic and Statistical Manual of Mental Disorders (DSM-III)* in 1980, after a need was indicated by increasing numbers of problems with Vietnam veterans and victims of multiple disasters.

Epidemiology

Currently, the military comprises more than 1.3 million individuals on active duty in the U.S. armed forces in more than 150 countries around the world. Reserve forces number over 1 million, and the overall total number of military personnel (including civilian personnel) is nearly 3.5 million (Department of Defense [DoD], 2021a). Women represent 17.2% of active-duty members and almost 24% of those are active-duty officers. In 2021, there were 18 million veterans in the United States (U.S. Bureau of Labor Statistics & U.S. Department of Labor, 2021).

In a landmark Institute of Medicine report (2013), *Returning Home from Iraq and Afghanistan: Readjustment Needs of Veterans, Service Members, and Their Families,* 44% of military personnel identified difficulty readjusting to daily living upon return from deployment, and 30% reported unemployment after returning. Current statistics about the incidence of mental illnesses (such as PTSD, substance use disorders [SUDs], and others) vary and may be underreported related to stigma in addition to the impact of acknowledging psychological problems on one's military benefits. The cumulative cost in deaths and physical and psychological injuries cannot be measured.

Application of the Nursing Process

Assessment

The Military Family

The military lifestyle offers both positive and negative aspects for those who choose this way of life. Hall (2011) summarizes the advantages and disadvantages of what is sometimes called the *Warrior Society.* Advantages include the following:

- Early retirement compared with civilian counterparts
- A vast resource system to meet family needs
- Job security with a guaranteed paycheck
- Health-care benefits
- Opportunities to see different areas of the world
- Educational opportunities

Disadvantages include the following:

- Frequent familial separations and reunions
- Regular household relocations
- Living life under the maxim of "the mission must always come first"
- A pattern of rigidity, regimentation, and conformity in family life
- Feelings of detachment from nonmilitary community
- The social effects of "rank"
- The lack of control over pay, promotion, and other benefits

Mary Wertsch (1996), who conducted a vast amount of research on the culture of the military family, stated, "The great paradox of the military is that its members, the self-appointed frontline guardians of our cherished American democratic values, do not live in democracy themselves" (p. 15). The military is maintained by a rigid authoritarian structure, and these characteristics often extend into the structure of the home.

A class system is strikingly evident in the military, with two distinct subcultures: that of the officer and that of the enlisted ranks. Hall (2011) states:

> The United States has made great strides in the past five decades to affirm and equalize the differences in society, but the assumption of all military systems in the world is that it is essential for the functioning of the organization to maintain a rigid hierarchical system based on dominance and subordination. (p. 38)

Isolation and alienation are common facets of military life. To compensate for the extreme mobility, the focus of this lifestyle turns inward to the military world rather than outward to the local community. Children of military families almost always report that no matter what school they attend, they feel "different" from the other students (Wertsch, 1996).

These descriptions apply principally to "career" military families. Another type of military family, those in the all-volunteer military, has become a familiar part of the American culture in recent years. The Operation Enduring Freedom (OEF) and Operation Iraqi Freedom (OIF) military campaigns together make up the longest sustained U.S. military operation since the Vietnam War, and they are the first extended conflicts to depend on an all-volunteer military (IOM, 2013). There has been heavy dependence on the National Guard and Reserves and an escalation in the pace, duration, and number of deployments and redeployments experienced by these individuals. Many joined the National Guard or Reserves as a second job for financial reasons or the educational opportunities available to them. Little thought had been given to the possibility of actually fighting in a war. As one anonymous reservist posted on his blog:

> The active forces have the harder role. They're required to be fully ready 24/7/365, and to deploy and fight on much shorter notice than the Reserve [forces] … it's their livelihood and (for many) their career. They're serving full-time; reservists aren't. But is that really quite true anymore? … Many reservists have already served multiple years on active duty since 9/11, away from home/job/family. And this situation doesn't look to change anytime soon. (Kelly Temps in Uniform, 2012)

In recent years, enlistees in the National Guard and Reserves have been told that they should expect to serve an interval of active duty. The Iraq and Afghanistan conflicts have engaged more National Guard and Reserve forces members than previous conflicts, and more women and parents of young children are being deployed as well (IOM, 2013). Most individuals in the National Guard and Reserves are willing to serve when and where they are needed but consider themselves "part-timers." The extended OEF and OIF campaigns have changed this part-time concept for many who have served multiple tours of duty, creating a hardship on their families and their civilian careers. The IOM reports that, in general, recent military tours of duty are marked by longer deployments and shorter intervals at home. Many of these "temporary citizen soldiers," and their full-time military counterparts, now carry the physical and psychological scars of battle.

Military Spouses and Children

A military spouse inherently knows and lives with the concept of "mission first." Devries and colleagues (2012) state, "While the military works hard to value the family lives of service members and their welfare, the nature of the job is that the mission trumps all other concerns" (p. 11). However, times have changed from the days when life in the military was viewed as a two-person career, in which a woman was expected to "create the right family setting so that her husband's work reflected his life at home, by staying positive, being interested in his duty, and being flexible and adaptable" (Hall, 2012, p. 148). Many of today's military spouses have their own careers or are pursuing higher levels of education. They do not view the military as a joint career with their service member spouse.

The lives of military spouses and children are clearly affected when the service member's active-duty assignments require frequent family moves. In most instances, when the service member receives orders for a new geographical assignment, the spouse's education, career, or both are put on hold, and the entire family is relocated. Other occasions may arise when the family is unable to immediately follow the service member to the new location. In certain instances, such as when a student may be about to complete a semester or is about to graduate, the service member may proceed to the new assignment without the family. This situation is difficult for the military spouse who is left alone to care for the children and to deal with all aspects of the move. Among active-duty members, almost 38% have children (DoD, 2021a).

Military children face unique challenges. In 2020 there were 1,621,473 children and youth in military families, and approximately 41.4% of the children of active-duty members were 5 years of age or younger (DoD, 2021a). School-aged children primarily attend civilian public schools where they form a unique subculture among staff and peers who often do not understand their life experiences. Children who grow up in a career military family learn to adapt to changing situations very quickly and to hide a certain level of fear associated with the nomadic lifestyle. Hall (2008) states:

> It is not just a fear of what might happen to their family or their military parents but a fear of the unknown, of not being accepted, of being behind, of not finding friends, or of not being cool. One of the most common concerns expressed by students when they arrive in a new school is who they will eat lunch with. Another reality for student athletes is that a student could be the star of the basketball team in one school and be sitting on the bench at the next. (p. 103)

The Impact of Deployment

Not since the Vietnam War have so many U.S. military families been affected by deployment-related family separation, combat injury, and death. Many service members have been deployed multiple times. Those who are deployed most frequently describe their greatest fear as having to leave their spouse and children. Lengthy separations pose many challenges to all members of the family. Spouses undertake all the challenges of managing the household in addition to assuming the role of the single parent. The pressure and stress are intense as the spouse attempts to maintain an atmosphere of strength for the children while experiencing the fears and anxiety associated with the life-threatening conditions facing the service member partner.

Millions of American children have experienced the deployment of a parent to Iraq or Afghanistan, and thousands have either lost a parent or have a parent who was wounded in these conflicts. Smith (2012) states:

> The stress that comes when a family member is deployed is significant, and that stress is multiplied when a loved one is wounded or killed. When parents return from deployment, they are not always the same as they were before. Major injuries, such as loss of a limb, traumatic brain injury, or posttraumatic stress disorder are life-altering, and children often have a hard time understanding the reason for a significant change in the appearance, personality, or behavior of a parent.

The following behaviors have been reported in children in response to the deployment of a parent (American Academy of Child & Adolescent Psychiatry, n.d.):

- Infants (birth to 12 months): May respond to disruptions in their schedule with decreased appetite, weight loss, irritability, or apathy.
- Toddlers (1 to 3 years): May become sullen, tearful, throw temper tantrums, or develop sleep problems.
- Preschoolers (3 to 6 years): May regress in areas such as toilet training, sleep, separation fears, physical complaints, or thumb sucking. May assume blame for the parent's departure.
- School-aged children (6 to 12 years): Are more aware of potential dangers to the parent. May exhibit irritable behavior, aggression, or whininess. May become more regressed and fearful about parent's safety.
- Adolescents (13 to 18 years): May be rebellious, irritable, or more challenging of authority.

Parents need to be alert to high-risk behaviors, such as problems with the law, sexual acting out, and drug or alcohol misuse.

A recent meta-analysis (Cunitz et al., 2019) of studies on the impact of deployment as a risk factor for children's mental health issues found that the reduced contact with the deployed parent, concerns about that parent's safety, and the role confusion brought on by taking on too early and possibly age-inappropriate family responsibilities can lead to physical and mental overload and result in less family involvement, reduced emotional warmth and responsiveness, controlling or rejecting behaviors, and even hostility.

Pincus and associates (2022) describe the cycle of deployment in five distinct stages: predeployment, deployment, sustainment, redeployment, and postdeployment.

Predeployment

The time frame for this stage is variable, beginning with the receipt of the orders and ending when the service member departs. Family members alternate between feelings of denial and anticipation of loss. The soldier and family get their affairs in order, extended training periods result in long hours apart, and the anxiety of the anticipated departure promotes stress and irritability among family members.

Deployment

This stage includes the time from actual deployment through the first month of separation. Military spouses report feeling disoriented and overwhelmed and experience a range of emotions, including numbness, sadness, loneliness, and abandonment. It is a time of disorganization as the spouse struggles to take charge of the details of living without their partner. Pincus and associates (2022) note that in the last decade, military downsizing has increased the likelihood of a soldier participating in an extended mission.

Sustainment

Sustainment begins about 1 month into the deployment until about a month before the service member's expected return. During this stage, the spouse and children establish new support systems and institute new family routines. Technology makes it possible for the family and service member to keep in touch with each other by phone, video, and e-mail. Despite the difficulties and obstacles encountered, most military families successfully negotiate this stage and anxiously anticipate their loved one's return.

Redeployment

This stage is defined as the month before the service member is scheduled to return home. There is excitement and apprehension associated with the homecoming. During this stage, concerns arise about how to reestablish relationships and communication and how to navigate family life changes that have occurred during the deployment.

Postdeployment

This stage typically lasts 3 to 6 months and begins with the return of the service member to the home station. There is a period of adjustment beginning with the "honeymoon" period, when the spouses reconnect physically, but not necessarily emotionally. The returning service member may desire to "pick up where they left off," only to encounter resistance from the spouse who expresses a reluctance to relinquish the degree of independence and autonomy to which they have become accustomed during the separation. Pincus and associates (2022) state:

> Postdeployment is probably the most important stage for both soldier and spouse. Patient communication, going slow, lowering expectations, and taking time to get to know each other again is critical to the task of successful reintegration of the soldier back into the family.

Counseling may be required if the service member has been injured or experiences a traumatic stress reaction. In addition, the fact that many service members are redeployed back into active duty creates unique challenges in a family's attempts to reestablish roles and relationships postdeployment. Children may express a variety of emotions and behaviors including numbness, rejection, or hostility.

Women in the Military

Women make up approximately 17.2% of the U.S. military and 21.1% of National Guard and Reserve members (DoD, 2021a). Women have been serving in the military since the time of the Civil War, mostly as nurses, spies, and support persons. Early in 2013 (and put into action in 2015) the Secretary of Defense lifted the ban on combat jobs to women, gradually opening direct combat units to female troops. Since then, over 9,000 women have earned combat action badges, and many have successfully completed the most challenging Navy SEAL officer assessment and selection (DeSimone, 2022). As women's roles in the military are changing and increasing, so may their mental and emotional health concerns in this evolution.

Special Concerns of Women in the Military

A number of issues are of special concern to women in the military, including sexual harassment, sexual assault, differential treatment and conditions, and being a parent.

Sexual Harassment

Sexual harassment includes "unwelcome sexual advances, requests for sexual favors, and other verbal or physical harassment of a sexual nature" (U.S. Equal Employment Opportunity Commission [EEOC], n.d.). In addition to overt sexual behavior, sexual harassment includes making offensive comments about a person's gender. From statements such as "You look nice this morning" or "Hey, you smell good" to blatant suggestions or requests for sexual interactions, Wolfe and associates (1998), in a study of women on active duty during the Persian Gulf War, found that both physical and sexual harassment were higher than typically found in peacetime military samples. Reports by military therapists conveyed that women who were sexually harassed while in the military had higher-than-average rates of a range of problems after discharge, including poor self-image, relationship issues, drug use, depression, and PTSD.

Sexual Assault

The DoD (2021c) reported receiving 7,816 reports of sexual assault in 2020 and 6,290 involved allegations from service members for incidents that occurred during military service (up by 1% from the 6,236 service member reports received in 2019). Both men and women report sexual assault, but 81% of these incidents were reported by women. The DoD defines "sexual assault" as referring to a range of crimes, including rape, sexual assault, forcible sodomy, aggravated sexual contact, abusive sexual contact, and attempts to commit these offenses. Congress requires annual tracking of reported events, and the DoD is also collecting data on reports of sexual assault in military academies as part of an early identification and intervention strategy.

In addition to collecting data on reports of sexual assaults, the DoD began collecting data on reports of retaliation associated with reporting. In its latest report, the DoD (2021c) notes that, in most cases, the reports of retaliation were from women and the retaliation was most often from a superior in the chain of command rather than the perpetrator of the sexual assault. Clearly, the culture within the military continues to reinforce that there are consequences when events such as these are reported. Thus there is concern that incidents are underreported.

Reasons for not reporting include fear of causing trouble in their units, that their commanders and fellow soldiers would turn against them, that they would be passed over for well-deserved promotions, or that they would be transferred and removed from duty altogether (Vlahos, 2012). Some women who have reported incidents to their commanding officers have been told to "forget about it," "suck it up," or "pretend it didn't happen," and are made to feel as though they are perpetrators instead of victims.

In 2000, after incidents of military sexual assaults that were made public, the Veterans Health Administration mandated universal health screening for sexual trauma among military personnel. But despite the efforts within the DoD to identify and correct the problem, incidents continue, suggesting that sexual assault remains a part of military culture. The COVID-19 pandemic raised additional concerns about accessibility to support services when incidents are reported. Many of these services were converted to online services, and the DoD reported that calls to their Safe Help Line (SHL) increased by 35% during this time (DoD, 2021c).

Some women who report their sexual assaults are discharged from the service with psychiatric diagnoses of personality disorder or adjustment disorder. Vlahos (2012) reports:

> For the veteran, getting a personality disorder or adjustment disorder discharge can be catastrophic. Not only does it carry a stigma for future employers, it cuts the veteran off from a series of benefits, including health care and service-related disability compensation.

Survivors of sexual assault in the military report long-lasting effects, including PTSD, depression, suicidal ideation and attempts, eating disorders, anxiety disorders, relationship difficulties, and substance misuse. Women in the military are more than twice as likely as men to experience PTSD (Absher, 2021), and this is, at least in part, related to the greater incidence of sexual assault perpetrated against women. Wolf (2012) notes that among military veterans, the leading cause of PTSD for men is combat trauma, whereas for women it is sexual trauma. She states, "Our women veterans are more likely to be traumatized by a sexual assault by a fellow soldier or a commander than by their own battlefield or war experiences."

Differential Treatment and Conditions

Although their numbers have increased, women still constitute a minority in the military. One female officer recounted that because of the small number of women in any given unit, female officers and enlisted personnel are often housed together. She indicated that she missed being with other officers to discuss work and spend time with her peers. She also reported that the enlisted women were uncomfortable with an officer in their presence. Burgess and associates (2013) add that when sexual trauma occurs among military personnel, it is occurring in the workplace, and as such, the victim often has ongoing contact with the perpetrator and may also be in a dependent position if the perpetrator was in a supervisory role. Fear of additional occupational discrimination may prevent women from reporting sexual harassment and assault.

Parenting Issues

Women's feelings associated with leaving their children often differ from those of men. Women may struggle more with guilt feelings for "abandoning" their children, whereas men have stronger emotions tied to a sense of doing their duty. Although men also experience regret at leaving their children, they often rely on the assurance that the children have their mothers to care for them.

Veterans

Most veterans returning from a combat zone undergo a period of adjustment. A study of young veterans (Pedersen et al., 2016) identified that 70% screened positive for behavioral health problems, less than one-third of whom received adequate psychotherapy or psychotropic treatment. Many veterans experience migraine headaches and cognitive difficulties such as memory loss. Hypervigilance, insomnia, and jitteriness are common. The Substance Abuse and Mental Health Services Administration (SAMHSA) (Pemberton et al., 2016) reported that, particularly in the 18- to 25-year-old age-group of veterans, there is a higher incidence of nonmedical use of pain relievers, amphetamine use, and alcohol misuse or dependence than nonveterans and a higher incidence of mental illness, including major depressive episodes and severe mental illnesses. Plach and Sells (2013) identified in a study of veterans that over 50% screened positive for problem drinking and over 90% had engaged in hazardous drinking.

Traumatic Brain Injury

The incidence of **traumatic brain injury (TBI)** is a significant consequence of the Iraq and Afghanistan conflicts. Mild TBI is so frequent that it has been referred to as the "signature injury" of the wars in these countries (Cogan, 2014). The DoD (2021d) reports a total of 434,618 TBIs since 2000, and over 16,000 in 2020 alone.

The Department of Veterans Affairs (VA) and the DoD (VA & DoD, 2016, p. 6) offer the following definition of TBI:

> A traumatically induced structural injury or physiological disruption of brain function as a result of an external force that is indicated by new onset or worsening of at least one of the following clinical signs, immediately following the event:
>
> - Any period of loss of or a decreased level of consciousness
> - Any loss of memory for events immediately before or after the injury (post-traumatic amnesia)
> - Any alteration in mental state at the time of the injury (e.g., confusion, disorientation, slowed thinking) (alteration of consciousness/mental state)
> - Neurological deficits (e.g., weakness, loss of balance, change in vision, praxis, paresis/plegia, sensory loss, aphasia) that may or may not be transient
> - Intracranial lesion

Symptoms may be classified as mild, moderate, or severe. Head injuries caused by bullet penetration, violent impact, or shock waves from explosive weapons are the main causes of TBI among military members (Kong et al., 2022). Although the mechanism of damage from explosive blasts is not completely understood, researchers believe that it is "the pressure wave passing through the brain that significantly disrupts brain function" (Mayo Clinic, 2022). TBI also results from penetrating wounds, severe blows to the head with shrapnel or debris, and falls or bodily collisions with objects after a blast. Symptoms of TBI according to the level of severity are presented in Table 37–1.

Most soldiers who have sustained a mild TBI improve with no lasting clinical complications (VA/DoD, 2016). Many recover within hours, days, or, at most, weeks. In a small minority, symptoms persist from 6 months to a year. The location and severity of the injury are factors that determine the long-term outcome for individuals with TBI. Severity is determined by the nature, speed, and location of the impact and the presence of complications such as hypoxemia, hypotension, intracranial hemorrhage, or increased intracranial pressure.

The most common long-term consequences of TBI include problems with cognition (e.g., thinking, memory, and reasoning) and behavior or mental health (e.g., depression, anxiety, personality changes, aggression, acting out, and social inappropriateness) (Mayo Clinic, 2022). Seizures occur in about 15% to 20% of individuals with TBI and commonly develop within the first 24 hours after the injury. With mild TBI, seizures usually subside within a week after the initial trauma. The potential for chronic epilepsy increases with severity of the injury.

Language and communication problems, such as aphasia, dysarthria, and dysphasia, can result from TBI (Byers & Jorge, 2017). Difficulties may also exist in the subtle aspects of communication, such as body language and nonverbal expression.

Studies show that TBI has long-term adverse effects on social functioning and productivity. Temkin and associates (2009) stated:

> A penetrating head injury sustained in wartime is clearly associated with increased unemployment. TBI also adversely affects leisure and recreation, social relationships, functional status, quality of life, and independent living. Although there is a dose-response relationship between severity of injury and

TABLE 37–1	Criteria and Symptomatology of Traumatic Brain Injury According to Level of Severity	
MILD/CONCUSSION	**MODERATE**	**SEVERE**
CRITERIA	**CRITERIA**	**CRITERIA**
Structural imaging = normal	Structural imaging = normal or abnormal	Structural imaging = normal or abnormal
Loss of consciousness 0–30 minutes	Loss of consciousness >30 minutes and <24 hours	Loss of consciousness >24 hours
Alteration of consciousness/mental state = a moment up to 24 hours	Alteration of consciousness/mental state = >24 hours. Severity based on other criteria.	Alteration of consciousness/mental state = >24 hours. Severity based on other criteria.
Post-traumatic amnesia = 0–1 day	Post-traumatic amnesia = >1 and <7 days	Post-traumatic amnesia = >7 days
Glasgow Coma Scale = 13–15	Glasgow Coma Scale = 9–12	Glasgow Coma Scale = <9
SYMPTOMS	**SYMPTOMS**	**SYMPTOMS**
Headache	Any of the symptoms of mild TBI	Any of the symptoms of mild TBI
Dizziness, ringing in the ears	Headache that gets worse or does not go away	Headache that gets worse or does not go away
Nausea	Repeated nausea and vomiting	Repeated nausea and vomiting
Trouble concentrating, confusion	Seizures	Seizures
Blurred vision	Difficulty awakening from sleep	Inability to awaken from sleep
Changes in sleep patterns	Dilation of one or both pupils of the eyes	Dilation of one or both pupils of the eyes
Mood changes	Slurred speech	Slurred speech
Sensitivity to light or sound	Weakness or numbness in the extremities	Weakness or numbness in the extremities
	Loss of coordination	Loss of coordination
	Increased confusion	Profound confusion
	Restlessness	Restlessness
	Agitation	Agitation

Source: Compiled from Department of Veterans Affairs & Department of Defense (2016); Mayo Clinic (2022); National Institute of Neurological Disorders and Stroke (2020).
*In 2015, the DoD recommended against using the Glasgow Coma Scale to diagnose TBI.

social outcomes, there is insufficient evidence to determine at what level of severity the adverse effects are demonstrated. (p. 460)

Risk for degenerative brain diseases such as Alzheimer's disease (AD), Parkinson's disease, and dementia pugilistica (dementia associated with repetitive blows to the head) may be increased with severe or repeated TBI (Mayo Clinic, 2022). The risk for AD in individuals with moderate TBI is 2.3 times greater than that of the general population. More research is needed to identify why and how TBI increases these risks.

Several factors have been identified that may worsen the condition of military personnel sustaining a TBI. Being in a high-stress environment, extreme temperatures such as the 120-degree heat common in Iraq, and delay of TBI recognition until the post-deployment period may all interfere with healing (Cogan, 2014). The prevalence of TBI, in addition to potential short- and long-term consequences, suggests that screening for TBI should be conducted for any military personnel returning from active duty who present with physical, cognitive, or emotional symptoms. Emotional symptoms of TBI may be mis-diagnosed (particularly in women) as mental health problems and because there are many service-related injuries beyond exposure to explosive blasts that can result in TBIs, assessment should always attempt to rule out TBI before finalizing a diagnosis (Bolster 2019).

Post-Traumatic Stress Disorder

PTSD is the most common mental disorder among veterans returning from military combat. The lifetime prevalence for PTSD in the general population is 6.8%; among military veterans, estimates range from 13.8% to 30% (Gradus, 2021).

The diagnostic criteria for PTSD from the *Diagnostic and Statistical Manual of Mental Disorders, Fifth Edition, Text Revision (DSM-5-TR)* (APA, 2022) are presented in Chapter 28, "Trauma- and Stressor-Related Disorders," of this text. The disorder can occur when an individual is exposed to an accident or violence in which death or serious injury to others or oneself occurs or is threatened. Symptoms of PTSD include the following:

- Reliving the trauma through flashbacks, nightmares, and intrusive thoughts
- Intensive efforts to avoid activities, people, places, situations, or objects that arouse recollections of the trauma
- Chronic negative emotional state and diminished interest or participation in significant activities
- Aggressive, reckless, or self-destructive behavior
- Hypervigilance and exaggerated startle response

- Angry outbursts, problems with concentration, and sleep disturbances

Symptoms of PTSD may be delayed—in some instances for years. When emotions are constricted, they may suddenly appear in the future after a major life event, stressor, or an accumulation of stressors over time that challenge the person's defenses. Symptoms also may be masked by other physical or mental health problems. In some instances, the symptoms do not appear to be problematic until the individual begins a readjustment to routine occupational or social functioning.

Reports indicate that many veterans, decades after returning from combat, have been diagnosed with PTSD (VA, 2022). At the time of their return, veterans often don't talk about their war experiences. But for many, the visions of horror have seeped to the surface in nightmares, flashbacks, anxiety, and emotional numbness. Langer (2011) reported that the PTSD symptoms for these veterans seemed to become more prominent in midlife, and the most significant precipitant was retirement. For many, their work gave meaning to their lives, and without it the symptoms of depression, anxiety, substance misuse, and PTSD began to emerge. Langer (2011) stated:

> Besides retirement, precipitants [to PTSD in midlife] include the deaths of friends, one's own deteriorating health, children becoming autonomous, divorce, and other losses associated with aging. Other precipitants include current events that trigger memories of one's own combat experience, e.g., 9/11, and other wars.

Soldiers with PTSD, TBI, or depression have all been identified as high risk for partner abuse, and research has identified "severe and pervasive negative effects on marital adjustment, general family functioning, and the mental health of partners" (Price & Stevens, 2021) contributing to parenting problems, caregiver burden, and divorce. In its report on the readjustment needs of veterans, the IOM (2013) identified a significant increase in domestic violence among veterans of the Iraq and Afghanistan wars and recommended this issue as a high priority for assessment and intervention. The burden of caregiving for a partner with PTSD has been noted as an etiological factor in relationship difficulties. Some caregivers may experience what has been termed *secondary trauma* or *vicarious traumatization*, a condition in which somatic symptoms and emotional distress occur as a response to caring for an individual who exhibits the symptoms of PTSD. Secondary symptoms are also common in children of a parent with PTSD. Family members sometimes report having nightmares that mimic the feelings and experiences of the veteran, difficulty sleeping, depression, and even visual hallucinations that are similar to the veteran's flashbacks.

Co-occurring disorders are common in individuals with PTSD, including major depressive disorder, SUDs, and anxiety disorders. Individuals with TBI also may develop PTSD, depending on the degree of amnesia experienced immediately after the cerebral trauma. In addition, evidence supports that PTSD increases the risk for dementia (Desmarais et al., 2020).

Depression and Suicide

Depressive disorder has been identified as one of the most common mental health disorders among veterans, and among those who were diagnosed with depression, 33.2% of them also had a PTSD diagnosis (Close, 2020). Both disorders are associated with impairment in interpersonal relationships, occupational and social functioning, increased risk for SUDs, and increased risk for suicide. Reports by the DoD and VA indicate that the number of suicides among veterans and active-duty military rose dramatically since 2001, the year that detailed record-keeping began, and this number reached an all-time high in 2012 with a rate of 22.7 suicides per 100,000 (319 individuals) active-duty military personnel. In 2020, the most recent report (DoD, 2021b) indicated that the rate was 27.8 suicides per 100,000 and had been significantly increasing since 2015. In contrast, there were no significant changes in suicide rates among National Guard members and Reservists. The highest number of suicides across all branches of the military were among male enlisted members under 30 years of age, and firearms were the primary method of suicide death. The IOM report (2013) identified that the VA policy against restricting access to privately owned weapons compounds suicide risk. Several initiatives have been advanced by the DoD to address these concerns through education and outreach services. In 2014 VA policies were expanded to allow commanders to discuss access to firearms with at-risk populations and provide for voluntary surrender of their firearms if they request it (Kime, 2015). More recent efforts have focused on the importance of safe storage as a deterrent to using a firearm in suicide. In one of its most recent initiatives the DoD (2021b) conducted a survey of members to assess attitudes and behaviors regarding firearm storage and suicide risk. They found a significant percentage of respondents (66%) had misconceptions about the associated risks and identified that more safety education is needed.

Suicide among military personnel is closely associated with the diagnoses of SUD, major depressive disorder, PTSD, and TBI. A common theme among investigations of suicide attempts and completed suicides by military service members is marital/relationship distress. Devries and associates (2012) found that relationship problems were a factor in over 50% of suicides in the Army. A study by Ravindran and associates (2020) found that veterans who were never married or who were divorced, separated, or widowed at the time of transition from active duty were at higher risk for suicide. Conversely, a study of National Guard members (Blow et al., 2018) found that, in the postdeployment period, a strong intimate relationship *decreased* suicide rates in members who had PTSD, depression, and anxiety (a group that has been identified at particularly high risk for suicide).

The multiplicity of factors influencing these dramatic suicide rates makes it difficult to pinpoint a specific cause, but it has captured the attention of the government and the general public. President Obama signed into law the Clay Hunt Suicide Prevention for American Veterans (SAV) Act (2015), which, among other things, intends to expand peer support for troubled veterans, streamline transitions for exiting service members, and mandate annual surveying of VA mental health and suicide prevention programs. Clay Hunt was a decorated Marine who struggled with PTSD and depression after returning home from active duty and took his own life in 2011.

Substance Use Disorder

In addition to rising suicide rates, alcohol and drug misuse is a significant problem in the military, with more than 1 in 10 veterans being diagnosed with an SUD (National Institute on Drug Abuse [NIDA], 2019). About 30% of Army suicides and over 45% of suicide attempts since 2003 involved alcohol or drug use, and an estimated 20% of high-risk behavior deaths were attributed to alcohol or drug overdose (NIDA, 2019). SUD is a common co-occurring condition with PTSD. Among OEF/OIF veterans, 63% diagnosed with an SUD also met criteria for PTSD, and veterans dually diagnosed with PTSD and SUDs are more likely to have additional co-occurring psychiatric and medical conditions, such as seizures, liver disease, HIV, schizophrenia, anxiety disorders, and bipolar disorder (Teeters et al., 2017). The combination of substance use, PTSD, depression, and TBI contributes to a significant risk for mental illness, relationship problems, difficult readjustment to home life, and, in many cases, suicide.

Alcohol use is identified as the most frequent substance of misuse among military members (NIDA, 2019), but opioid pain medication use and abuse among military personnel has increased. NIDA (2019) reported that from 2005 to 2009, prescriptions for pain medications prescribed by military physicians quadrupled, and although prescriptions have declined since 2011 in military and civilian populations, one study found that 46.2% of combat-wounded veterans were misusing opioids and 21.7% were misusing sedatives (Kelley et al., 2019). In addition, according to a 2018 analysis, 30% of veterans and 14% of active-duty members report using tobacco, and e-cigarette use is increasing (U.S. Food and Drug Administration, 2020). Substance misuse is clearly a compounding factor in the physical and mental challenges associated with having served in combat situations. A first-hand account of what it was like for Sean, a soldier who served in Iraq and faced several challenges in his return to civilian life, is presented in "Real People, Real Stories: The Military Experience."

Real People, Real Stories: The Military Experience

(The individual requested that his real name not be used.)

Karyn: What was it like for you when you returned from your tour of duty?

Sean: I was in Iraq for 360 days, and when we landed in the U.S., there was a little welcome home ceremony, and then we went to hang out at the NCO club. The next day, there was a lot of paper to process for benefits and release forms. There was an assessment by a doctor that was about 5 minutes. Basically, they ask if you're okay and they take your word for it. If you say you're not okay, then you can't leave with everyone else. The third day, they encouraged us to join the American Legion and VFW clubs and then bussed us home.

Karyn: You've mentioned before that you had postconcussion headaches and some nightmares. Were you still having these symptoms when you got home?

Sean: Yeah, I had been in an area, during my tour of duty, where a roadside bomb detonated. At the time, I was having extreme headaches, and I got pain medications, but no one talked about what had happened or how I was handling that. The role of the military was to make the soldier mission-capable, so that meant just treating the symptoms. When I got home, I was still having some nightmares and headaches, but I couldn't talk about it. My wife was in the military too, so we had both learned not to talk about emotions. Within a year, I was drinking heavily and separated from my wife. I sought out treatment at the VA, but I only went three times. I felt like they were primarily trying to validate my story as if they wanted to defend themselves against a potential claim. They never asked about alcohol use. I felt angry, and I had some aggression. I felt abandoned. Then I found out my mom had stolen my military checks and had spent them. At that point, I lost faith in everything. All of my core beliefs were gone. The only thing I had faith in was my fellow soldiers, and now that we were back home, they weren't there.

Karyn: Do you get together with any fellow vets?

Sean: Mostly people connect over Facebook, so they don't really get together. The military clubs are all about drinking, so there aren't any healthy options. I do know, though, that sometimes when vets have gotten wind through Facebook that one of us is suicidal, they've traveled across the country to track them down and try to get them help.

Karyn: The suicide rates have been tragically high among vets. Have you ever had thoughts yourself about suicide?

Sean: I have. I was in a very dark place. I thought I was such an awful person that the best option was to kill myself. I was drinking, I was making bad moral decisions, and I was nasty to friends. I didn't care about anything or any consequences. I just wanted momentary relief, so I drank more, but, of course, that increased the depression. And it seems like every time we go to military exercises, we hear of another loss of someone to suicide. Last week, it was a fellow soldier who was a decorated hero for saving the lives of many of our guys. [Tearful.] So how do you rectify that someone saved all those lives and then comes home and takes their own life?

Karyn: It does seem like senseless, tragic loss. What has helped you get out of that dark place?

Sean: I have a brother who, even though he couldn't understand what I was going through, he kept checking in on me and repeatedly told me he was praying for me. He just kept showing up and telling me I had to get God back in my life. I knew he cared. I had a DUI and an accident, but I kept thinking, "I just have to suck it up and be stronger than this." Instead, the drinking just increases exponentially faster than you can respond or try to control it. One night, I went home and trashed my house. I was ripping sinks out of walls. I remember a neighbor came over and told me I just needed to sober up, but I called the police and told them to take me in. I knew I was out of control. When I got to the psych unit, I knew I wanted to be "fixed," but that mainly meant I wanted to be under control. I don't remember being asked if I wanted pills, but they gave me pills, and I didn't want to take them because it just made me feel less in control. There was an LPN there who told me that her husband was a vet and that she knew he was a good person. She said she never let his behavior define who he was. That gave me a lot of hope, like maybe I wasn't such an awful person. I reached out to God, and things started to change. I acknowledged that drinking was a primary issue, I cut ties with several unhealthy relationships, and there were supportive friends who came to visit me in the hospital, so I started to see that there were people who genuinely cared about me.

Karyn: What do you want health-care providers and fellow soldiers to learn from your experience?

Sean: First, a soldier is not who you are; it's a job you do. I wish I had spent more time before my deployment literally writing down all those things that define who I am, like, I'm a loving father and a good friend and what is most important to me; what am I willing to die for. I think it would have helped me, when I came back home, to concretely remind myself of who I am. It's

Real People, Real Stories: The Military Experience—cont'd

easy to lose all sense of that in the military. Second, no mood-altering chemicals. There are a lot of things within the military that promote the use of chemicals such as alcohol and pain medication, and while it may keep people mission-ready or temporarily numb you, it becomes disastrous. Third, reach out for support or, if you are a health-care provider, help someone identify those people who will provide ongoing support. Supportive people and reaching out to God have been my lifelines.

Diagnosis and Outcome Identification

Nursing diagnoses are formulated from the data gathered during the assessment phase and with background knowledge regarding predisposing factors to the disorder. Table 37–2 presents a list of selected patient behaviors and the NANDA-I nursing diagnoses that correspond to those behaviors, which may be used in planning assistance for families as they confront the unique challenges associated with military life. Outcome criteria are presented for each.

Table 37–2 | NURSING DIAGNOSES: PLANNING CARE FOR MILITARY FAMILIES

RISK FACTORS/DEFINING CHARACTERISTICS	NURSING DIAGNOSES	OUTCOME CRITERIA
PTSD		
Rage reactions, aggression, irritability, substance use, flashbacks, startle reaction	Risk for other-directed violence	Patient will demonstrate appropriate coping behaviors. Patient will not harm others.
Depression, perception of lack of social support, physical disabilities from combat injuries, feelings of hopelessness	Risk for suicide	Patient will not harm self.
Anger, aggression, depression, difficulty concentrating, flashbacks, guilt, headaches, hypervigilance, intrusive thoughts and dreams, nightmares, emotional numbness, panic attacks, substance misuse	Post-trauma syndrome related to having experienced the trauma of military combat	Patient will begin a healthy grief resolution, initiating the process of psychological healing. Patient will demonstrate ability to deal with emotional reactions in an individually appropriate manner.
Substance misuse	Ineffective coping; denial	Patient will verbalize understanding of the destructiveness of substance misuse and demonstrate a more adaptive method of coping.
Confusion, fear, and anxiety among family members and their inability to deal with the affected member's unpredictable behavior; ineffective family decision-making process	Interrupted family processes related to crisis associated with veteran member's illness	Family will verbalize understanding of trauma-related illness, demonstrate ability to maintain anxiety at manageable level, and make appropriate decisions to stabilize family functioning.
Traumatic Brain Injury		
Impaired physical mobility, limited range of motion, decreased muscle strength and control, perceptual or cognitive impairment, seizures	Risk for injury	Patient will remain free of physical injury.
Memory deficits; distractibility; altered attention span or concentration; impaired ability to make decisions, problem-solve, reason, or conceptualize; personality changes	Disturbed thought processes	Patient will regain cognitive ability to execute mental functions realistic with the extent of the injury.

Continued

Table 37-2 | NURSING DIAGNOSES: PLANNING CARE FOR MILITARY FAMILIES–cont'd

RISK FACTORS/DEFINING CHARACTERISTICS	NURSING DIAGNOSES	OUTCOME CRITERIA
Inability to perform desired or appropriate activities of daily living	Self-care deficit (specify)	Patient will perform self-care activities within level of own ability.
Confusion, fear, and anxiety among family members and the inability to adapt to changes associated with veteran member's injury; difficulty accepting/receiving help; inability to express or to accept each other's feelings	Interrupted family processes related to situational transition and crisis; uncertainty about expectations and ultimate outcome	Family will verbalize understanding of trauma-related illness, demonstrate ability to maintain anxiety at manageable level, and make appropriate decisions to stabilize family functioning.
Family Members' Issues Regressive behaviors, loss of appetite, temper tantrums, clinging behaviors, guilt and self-blame, sleep problems, irritability, aggression (children)	Risk for delayed development related to feelings of abandonment associated with parent's deployment	Parent/caregiver will identify behaviors at risk and initiate interventions to promote appropriate development. Child will develop healthy coping strategies and resume normal developmental progression.
Rebelliousness, irritability, acting-out behaviors, promiscuity, substance use (adolescents)	Ineffective coping related to feelings of abandonment associated with parent's deployment	Patient will work through stages of grief associated with the perceived loss and demonstrate healthy, age-appropriate coping strategies.
Depression, anxiety, loneliness, fear, feeling overwhelmed and powerless, anger (spouse/partner)	Risk for maladaptive grieving related to military deployment of spouse/partner	Patient will work through stages of grief, achieve a healthy acceptance, and express a sense of control over the present situation and future outcome.
Anger, anxiety, frustration, ineffective coping, sleep deprivation, somatic symptoms, fatigue (spouse/partner/caregiver)	Caregiver role strain related to complexity of care-giving responsibilities; lack of respite	Caregiver will demonstrate effective problem-solving skills and develop adaptive coping mechanisms to regain equilibrium.

Planning, Implementation, and Evaluation

Nurses provide care for service members, veterans, and their families in a variety of settings, including general hospitals, VA hospitals, community health centers, doctors' offices, long-term care centers, and community-based clinics. The care required by veterans returning from combat in the war on terrorism is complex and multifaceted. War-related physical injuries are often striking and conspicuous in their visibility. However, it is the veterans' *invisible* injuries that psychiatric–mental health nurses are most often called on to treat. The need for nurses to provide care for the increasing number of veterans with these invisible injuries is intensifying, and the VA continues to search for more effective ways to ensure that military veterans and families receive the care that they desperately need and deserve. Clever and Segal (2013) caution that although military families have unique challenges, including compounding issues when both spouses are in the military, they are a diverse group, and their needs are dynamic as they move through transitions in their military career and family life.

Interventions for a selected number of nursing diagnoses relevant to veterans and military families are presented in Table 37–3. Evaluation is conducted by reassessing to determine whether the nursing actions have been successful in meeting the outcome criteria.

Treatment Modalities

Treatment for PTSD and TBI includes psychosocial, rehabilitative, and medical approaches, which often can be combined for optimal response. Selection of appropriate therapy depends on accurate diagnosis and symptom assessment.

TABLE 37–3 Nursing Interventions for Veteran Patients and Military Families

Post-trauma syndrome (PTSD)	Stay with the patient during periods of flashbacks and nightmares and offer reassurance of personal safety.
	Encourage the patient to talk about the traumatic experience at their own pace.
	Discuss maladaptive coping mechanisms being employed. Assist the patient in their effort to use more adaptive strategies.
	Include available support systems, and make referrals for additional assistance where required.
	Help patient understand that use of substances numbs feelings and delays healing. Refer for treatment of substance use disorder.
	Discuss use of stress-management techniques, such as deep breathing, meditation, relaxation, and exercise.
	Administer medications as prescribed, and provide medication education.
	Provide trauma-informed care and refer the patient as needed to specialized trauma recovery treatment programs.
Risk for suicide (PTSD, TBI)	Assess degree of risk according to seriousness of threat, existence of a plan, and availability and lethality of the means.
	Ask directly if person is thinking of acting on thoughts or feelings.
	Ascertain presence of significant others for support.
	Determine whether substance use is a factor.
	Encourage expression of feelings, including appropriate expression of anger.
	Ensure that environment is safe.
	Help patient identify more appropriate solutions and offer hope for the future.
	Collaborate with the patient to develop a plan for ongoing safety.
	Involve family/significant others in the planning.
Disturbed thought processes (TBI)	Evaluate mental status, including extent of impairment in thinking ability; remote and recent memory; orientation to person, place, and time; insight and judgment; changes in personality; attention span, distractibility, and ability to make decisions or problem-solve; ability to communicate appropriately; anxiety level; evidence of psychotic behavior.
	Report to physician any cognitive changes that become obvious.
	Note behavior indicative of potential for violence and take appropriate action to prevent harm to patient and others.
	Provide safety measures as required. Institute seizure precautions if indicated. Assist with limited mobility issues.
	Monitor medication regimen.
	Refer to appropriate rehabilitation providers.
Interrupted family processes (PTSD, TBI)	Encourage the importance of continuous, open communication between family members to facilitate ongoing problem-solving.
	Assist the family in identifying and using previously successful coping strategies.
	Encourage family participation in multidisciplinary team conference or group therapy.
	Involve family members in social support and community activities of their interest and choice.
	Encourage use of stress-management techniques.
	Make necessary referrals (e.g., parent effectiveness training, specific disease or disability support groups, self-help groups, clergy, psychological counseling, or family therapy).
	Assist family in identifying situations that may lead to fear or anxiety.
	Involve family in mutual goal-setting to plan for the future.
	Identify community agencies from which family may seek assistance (e.g., Meals on Wheels, visiting nurse, trauma support group, American Cancer Society, Veterans Administration).
Risk for maladaptive grieving (family of deployed service member)	Help family members to realize that all of the feelings they are having are a normal part of the grieving process.
	Validate their feelings of anger, loneliness, fear, powerlessness, dysphoria, and distress at separation from their loved one.
	Help parent to understand that children's and adolescents' problematic behaviors are symptoms of grieving and that these behaviors should not be deemed unacceptable and result in punishment, but rather recognized as having their basis in grief.

Continued

TABLE 37–3	Nursing Interventions for Veteran Patients and Military Families–cont'd
	Children should be allowed an appropriate amount of time to grieve. Research shows that children need at least 6 weeks to adjust to a parent's deployment (Morin, 2020). Refer for professional help if improvement is not observed in a reasonable period of time.
	Assess if maladaptive coping strategies, such as substance misuse, are being used.
	Identify and encourage family members to employ previously used successful coping strategies.
	Encourage resumption of involvement in usual activities.
	Caution against spending too much time alone.
	Suggest keeping a journal of experiences and feelings.
	Refer to other resources, as needed, such as psychotherapy, family counseling, religious references or pastor, or grief support group.
Caregiver role strain (spouse/caregiver of injured service member)	Assess the spouse/caregiver's ability to anticipate and fulfill the injured service member's unmet needs. Provide information to assist the caregiver with this responsibility.
	Ensure that the caregiver encourages the injured service member to be as independent as possible.
	Encourage the caregiver to express feelings and to participate in a support group.
	Provide information or demonstrate techniques for dealing with acting-out or violent or disoriented behavior by the injured service member.
	Identify additional needs and ensure that resources are provided (e.g., physical therapy, occupational therapy, nutritionist, financial and legal help, and respite care).
	Assess for misuse of substances as a coping strategy.
	Refer to counseling or psychotherapy as needed.

PTSD, Post-traumatic stress disorder; *TBI,* traumatic brain injury.

Post-Traumatic Stress Disorder

Psychosocial Therapies

Cognitive behavior therapy (CBT), prolonged exposure therapy, group and family therapy, and eye movement desensitization and reprocessing have all been used successfully in the treatment of PTSD.

Psychopharmacology

Selective serotonin reuptake inhibitors (SSRIs) are now considered the first-line treatment for PTSD because of their efficacy, tolerability, and safety ratings. Other antidepressants that have been effective include trazodone, the tricyclics amitriptyline and imipramine, and the monoamine oxidase inhibitor phenelzine. Benzodiazepines are sometimes prescribed for their antipanic effects, although their addictive properties make them less desirable. Antihypertensives, such as propranolol and clonidine, have been successful in alleviating symptoms such as nightmares, intrusive recollections, hypervigilance, insomnia, startle responses, and angry outbursts. More recently, intravenous ketamine, an N-methyl-D-aspartate receptor antagonist, has demonstrated efficacy (along with psychotherapy) in treating PTSD (Greenway et al., 2020). Das and associates (2019), in their research on ketamine as a pharmacological treatment for problem drinking, found that ketamine was able to disrupt maladaptive memories when administered immediately after those memories were retrieved. Such findings offer hope for the same benefits in the treatment of PTSD. Although the mechanisms of action are not yet clearly understood, research supports that it may be a highly beneficial treatment option for PTSD (Feder et al., 2021).

Complementary Therapies

Several complementary and alternative medicine therapies have demonstrated some efficacy in treating symptoms of PTSD including acupuncture, moxibustion (a type of traditional Chinese medicine that involves burning moxa, a cone or stick made of ground mugwort leaves, on or near acupuncture points), Chinese herbal medicines, meditation, yoga, deep-breathing exercises, progressive relaxation, and tai chi (Song et al., 2020). The authors note, though, that more research is needed.

Pet therapy (also called *animal-assisted therapy*) has been used with some reported success. In a systematic review of studies on the effectiveness of this treatment (O'Haire et al., 2015), the authors found evidence that pet therapy contributed to a reduction in symptoms of anxiety, depression, and PTSD. They note, though, that methodological rigor was absent in most studies, indicating the need for more research.

Traumatic Brain Injury

The type of care for the individual with TBI depends on severity of the injury and area of the brain involved. Those with mild TBI most often achieve full recovery without ongoing treatment. Symptom treatment and rest may be adequate for a full recovery. For those with moderate or severe TBI, several treatment options are listed next.

Psychosocial Therapies

In a systematic review (Gomez de Regil et al., 2019), researchers found that CBT stands out as the primary psychological treatment for patients with TBIs; several studies support improvement in a variety of symptoms including depression, anxiety, coping, cognitive, and social functioning.

Rehabilitation Therapies

Rehabilitation therapy is multifaceted and determined by the severity and location of the brain damage. Cognitive rehabilitation therapy (CRT) is one strategy designed to help individuals regain their normal brain function through an individualized training program that incorporates learning compensatory strategies for coping with persistent deficiencies involving memory, problem-solving, and the thinking skills to get things done (National Institute of Neurological Disorders and Stroke [NINDS], 2020). Specialists in the care of the individual with TBI may include any or all of the following (Mayo Clinic, 2022):

- **Physiatrist:** A physician trained in the medical specialty of physical medicine and rehabilitation. This physician oversees other professionals involved in the rehabilitation process.
- **Occupational therapist:** Helps the individual learn, relearn, or improve skills for everyday living.
- **Physical therapist:** Assists the veteran with mobility and relearning movement patterns, balance, and walking.
- **Recreational therapist:** Assists with leisure activities.
- **Speech and language pathologist:** Helps the person improve communication skills and use assistive communication devices, if necessary.
- **Neuropsychologist or psychiatrist:** Helps the veteran manage behaviors or learn coping strategies, provides talk therapy as needed for emotional and psychological well-being, and prescribes medication as needed.
- **Social worker or case manager:** Coordinates access to services; assists with care decisions and planning; and facilitates communication among various professionals, care providers, and family members.
- **Rehabilitation nurse:** Provides ongoing rehabilitation care and helps with discharge planning.

- **Traumatic brain injury nurse specialist:** Coordinates care and provides family education.
- **Vocational counselor:** Assesses occupation issues or barriers and provides resources to facilitate returning to work.

Psychopharmacology

Medications for the individual with TBI are given to ameliorate specific symptoms. Antidepressants are prescribed for depression, which is common in individuals with TBI. SSRIs are the antidepressants of choice, although tricyclics and others, such as venlafaxine, trazodone, bupropion, and duloxetine, are also used. Benzodiazepines or SSRIs may be administered for treatment of anxiety symptoms, and antipsychotics are prescribed if aggression, agitation, or psychotic behaviors occur. Anticonvulsants are given if seizures are a problem, and the physician may prescribe skeletal muscle relaxants for muscle spasms or spasticity. Methylphenidate or modafinil has demonstrated effectiveness in treating attention deficits (Huang et al., 2016), and donepezil has been shown to be effective in enhancing cognitive performance of individuals with TBI (Yu et al., 2015).

Summary and Key Points

- Over 3 million individuals are serving in the U.S. armed forces in more than 150 countries around the world.
- Veterans currently number 18 million.
- The military lifestyle offers both positive and negative aspects for those who choose this way of life.
- To compensate for the extreme mobility, the focus of the military lifestyle turns inward to the military world rather than outward to the local community.
- In the OEF and OIF campaigns, there has been heavy dependence on the National Guard and Reserves and an escalation in the pace, duration, and number of deployments and redeployments experienced by these individuals.
- Military families face unique challenges, including frequent moves and many separations.
- Children and adolescents may exhibit several problematic behaviors in response to the separation from a deployed parent.
- The cycle of deployment is described in five distinct stages: predeployment, deployment, sustainment, redeployment, and postdeployment.
- Special concerns of women in the military include sexual harassment, sexual assault (although a smaller percentage of men are also victims of sexual assault in the military), differential treatment and conditions, and issues related to being a parent.
- Evidence supports that a majority of young veterans screen positive for behavioral health problems, and

one-third or less of these veterans have had adequate health-care treatment. Returning from a combat zone causes feelings and reactions that may contribute to difficulties with reintegration into civilian life.

■ TBI is a trauma-induced structural injury or physiological disruption of brain function as a result of an external force to the head.

■ Symptoms of TBI are related to the severity of the injury and the area of the brain that has been injured.

■ The most common long-term consequences of TBI include problems with cognition and behavior or mental health.

■ PTSD is the most common mental health disorder among veterans returning from military combat.

■ Symptoms of PTSD may occur shortly after the trauma or may be delayed, in some instances for years.

■ Depression among military veterans is common, and suicide rates among veterans and active-duty service members have continued to rise.

■ SUD is a common co-occurring condition with PTSD.

■ Nursing care of military families and veterans is multifaceted and requires reassessment over time using the six steps of the nursing process. Treatment modalities for PTSD and TBI include psychosocial therapies, psychopharmacology, complementary therapies, and rehabilitation therapies.

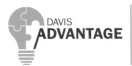 Go to **Davis Advantage** to complete your learning: strengthen understanding, apply your knowledge, and prepare for the Next Gen NCLEX®.

Review Questions

1. Which of the following postdeployment situations have been identified as likely to occur during the first few months of a soldier's return home? (Select all that apply.)
   a. A honeymoon period of physical reconnection
   b. Resistance from the spouse regarding possible loss of autonomy
   c. Rejection by the children for perceived abandonment
   d. A period of adjustment to reconnect emotionally

2. Which of the following is the leading cause of TBI in active-duty military personnel in combat?
   a. Military vehicle accidents
   b. Blasts from explosive devices
   c. Falls
   d. Blows to the head from falling debris

3. Which of the following medications may be prescribed to treat panic anxiety attacks associated with PTSD?
   a. Alprazolam
   b. Lithium
   c. Carbamazepine
   d. Haldol

4. Which of the following psychosocial therapies has been shown to be helpful for clients with TBI?
   a. Eye movement desensitization
   b. Psychoanalysis
   c. Reality therapy
   d. Cognitive behavior therapy

5. A client who was injured during combat in Afghanistan has a diagnosis of TBI. Which of the following medications might the physician prescribe to improve his memory and thinking capability?
   a. Carbamazepine
   b. Duloxetine
   c. Donepezil
   d. Bupropion

Clinical Judgment Questions

6. A veteran of the war in Iraq has been diagnosed with PTSD. He has been hospitalized after swallowing a handful of his antipanic medication. His physical condition was stabilized in the emergency department, and he has been admitted to the psychiatric unit. In developing his initial plan of care, which of the following should the nurse identify as the priority nursing diagnosis?
   a. Post-trauma syndrome
   b. Risk for suicide
   c. Maladaptive grieving
   d. Disturbed thought processes

7. A veteran of the war in Iraq has been diagnosed with PTSD. He has been hospitalized on the psychiatric unit after an attempted suicide. In the middle of the night, he wakes up yelling and tells the nurse he was having a flashback to when his unit transport drove over an improvised explosive device (IED) and most of his fellow soldiers were killed. He is breathing heavily, is perspiring, and his heart is pounding. The nurse's most appropriate *initial* intervention is which of the following?
   a. Contact the doctor on call to report the incident.
   b. Administer the prn order for chlorpromazine.
   c. Stay with the client and reassure him of his safety.
   d. Instruct him to sit outside the nurses' station until he is calm.

8. Mike, a veteran of combat in Afghanistan, has a diagnosis of mild TBI. The psychiatric home health nurse from the VA medical center is assigned to make home visits to Mike and his wife, Marissa, who is his caregiver. Which of the following would be an appropriate nursing intervention by the home health nurse? (Select all that apply.)
   a. Assess for the use of substances by Mike or Marissa.
   b. Encourage Marissa to do everything for Mike to prevent further deterioration in his condition.
   c. Assess Marissa's level of stress and potential for burnout.
   d. Encourage Marissa to allow Mike to be as independent as possible.
   e. Suggest that Marissa ask the physician for a nursing home placement for Mike.

9. A veteran who has returned 6 months ago reports to the mental health clinic, stating, "I'm falling apart. I think I'm losing it." Based on an understanding of common problems among military personnel and veterans, which of the following items should the nurse prioritize in conducting an assessment? (Select all that apply.)
   a. Screen for alcohol and other drug misuse.
   b. Assess for suicide risk.
   c. Evaluate for evidence of TBI.
   d. Assess for signs and symptoms of PTSD.
   e. Assess whether the client had evidence of any mental illness symptoms before entry in the military.

 MOVIE CONNECTIONS

The Best Years of Our Lives (1946) • *The Deer Hunter* (1978) • *Jarhead* (2005) • *In the Valley of Elah* (2007) • *The Lucky Ones* (2008) • *A Walk in My Shoes* (2010) • *Thank-You for Your Service* (2017) • *The Outpost* (2020)

REFERENCES

Absher, J. (2021). *VA finds PTSD affects women differently than men.* https://www.military.com/benefits/veterans-health-care/va-finds-ptsd-affects-women-differently-then-men.html

American Academy of Child & Adolescent Psychiatry. (n.d.). *Military families resource center.* www.aacap.org/aacap/families_and_youth/resource_centers/Military_Families_Resource_Center/FAQ.aspx#question4

American Psychiatric Association (APA). (2022). *Diagnostic and statistical manual of mental disorders, fifth edition, text revision (DSM-5-TR).* American Psychiatric Association.

Blow, A. J., Farero, A., Ganoczy, D., Walters, H., & Valenstein, M. (2018). Intimate relationships buffer suicidality in National Guard service members: A longitudinal study. *Suicide and Life-Threatening Behavior, 49*(6), 1523–1540. https://doi.org/10.1111/sltb.12537

Bolster, M. (2019). Moving ahead. *Brain & Life* (October/November), 38.

Burgess, A. W., Slattery, D. M., & Herlihy, P. A. (2013). Military sexual trauma: A silent syndrome. *Journal of Psychosocial Nursing, 51*(2), 20–26. doi:10.3928/02793695-20130109-03

Byers, J. A., & Jorge, R. E. (2017). Neuropsychiatric consequences of traumatic brain injury. In B. J. Sadock, V. A. Sadock, &

P. Ruiz (Eds.), *Comprehensive textbook of psychiatry* (pp. 522–540). Wolters Kluwer.

Clay Hunt Suicide Prevention for American Veterans Act of 2015, 38 U.S.C. § 1709B et seq. (2015). https://www.congress.gov/bill/114th-congress/house-bill/203

Clever, M., & Segal, D. R. (2013). The demographics of military children and families. *The Future of Children, 23*(2), 13–39. doi:10.1353/foc.2013.0018

Close, L. (2020). *Veterans' mental health issues.* https://veteran addiction.org/veterans-mental- health-issues/#:~:text = PTSD

Cogan, A. M. (2014). Occupational needs and intervention strategies for military personnel with mild traumatic brain injury and persistent postconcussion symptoms: A review. *OTJR: Occupation, Participation, and Health, 34*(3), 150–159. doi:10.3928/15394492-20140617-01

Cunitz, K., Dölitzsch, C., Kösters, M., Willmund, G. D., Zimmermann, P., Bühler, A. H., Fegert, J. M., Ziegenhain, U., & Kölch, M. (2019). Parental military deployment as risk factor for children's mental health: A meta-analytical review. *Child and Adolescent Psychiatry and Mental Health, 13*(26). https://doi.org/10.1186/s13034-019-0287-y

Das, R. K., Gale, G., Walsh, K., Hennessy, V. E., Iskandar, G., Mordecai, L. A., Brandner, B., Kindt, M., Curran, H. V., & Kamboj, S. K. (2019). Ketamine can reduce harmful drinking by pharmacologically rewriting drinking memories. *Nature Communications, 10*(1), 5187. https://doi.org/10.1038/s41467-019-13162

Department of Defense (DoD). (2021a). *2020 demographics: Profile of the military community.* https://download.militaryonesource.mil/12038/MOS/Reports/2020-demographics-report.pdf

Department of Defense (DoD). (2021b). *Annual suicide report: 2020.* https://www.dspo.mil/Portals/113/Documents/CY%20%20Suicide%20Report/CY%202020%20Annual%20Suicide%20Report.pdf?ver = 0OwlvDd-PJuA-igow5fBFA%3d%3d

Department of Defense (DoD). (2021c). *Department of Defense annual report on sexual assault in the military for fiscal year 2020.* Department of Defense.

Department of Defense (DoD). (2021d). *DoD worldwide numbers for TBI.* https://health.mil/About-MHS/OASDHA/Defense-Health-Agency/Research-and-Development/Traumatic-Brain-Injury-Center-of-Excellence/DOD-TBI-Worldwide-Numbers

Department of Veteran Affairs (VA). (2022). *Depression, trauma, and PTSD.* https://www.ptsd.va.gov/understand/related/depression_trauma.asp

Department of Veterans Affairs & Department of Defense (VA/DoD). (2016). *Clinical practice guideline for management of concussion/mild traumatic brain injury.* www.healthquality.va.gov/guidelines/Rehab/mtbi/mTBICPGClinicianSummary50821816.pdf

Desimone, D. (2022). *Over 200 years of service: The history of women in the U.S. military.* https://www.uso.org/stories/3005-over-200-years-of-service-the-history-of-women-in-the-us-military

Desmarais, P., Weidman, D., Wassef, A., Bruneau, M. A., Friedland, J., Bajsarowicz, P., Thibodeau, M. P., Herrmann, N., & Nguyen, Q. D. (2020). The interplay between post-traumatic stress disorder and dementia: A systematic review. *The American Journal of Geriatric Psychiatry, 28*(1), 48–60. https://doi.org/10.1016/j.jagp.2019.08.006

Devries, M. R., Hughes, H. K., Watson, H., & Moore, B. A. (2012). Understanding the military culture. In B. A. Moore (Ed.), *Handbook of counseling military couples* (pp. 7–18). Routledge.

Feder, A., Costi, S., Rutter, S. B., Collins, A. B., Govindarajulu, U., Jha, M. K., Horn, S. R., Kautz, M., Corniquel, M., Collins, K. A., Bevilacqua, L., Glasgow, A. M., Brallier, J., Pietrzak, R. H.,

Murrough, J. W., & Charney, D. S. (2021). A randomized controlled trial of repeated ketamine administration for chronic posttraumatic stress disorder. *American Journal of Psychiatry, 178*(2), 193–202. https://doi.org/10.1176/appi.ajp.2020.20050596

Gómez-de-Regil, L., Estrella-Castillo, D. F., & Vega-Cauich, J. (2019). Psychological intervention in traumatic brain injury patients. *Behavioural Neurology.* https://doi.org/10.1155/2019/6937832

Gradus, J. L. (2021). *Epidemiology of PTSD.* www.ptsd.va.gov/professional/PTSD-overview/epidemiological-facts-ptsd.asp

Greenway, K. T., Garel, N., Jerome, L., & Feduccia, A. A. (2020). Integrating psychotherapy and psychopharmacology: Psychedelic-assisted psychotherapy and other combined treatments. *Expert Review of Clinical Pharmacology, 13*(6), 655–670. https://doi.org/10.1080/17512433.2020.1772054.

Hall, L. K. (2008). *Counseling military families.* Taylor & Francis.

Hall, L. K. (2011). The military culture, language, and lifestyle. In R. B. Everson & C. R. Figley (Eds.), *Families under fire* (pp. 31–52). Routledge.

Hall, L. K. (2012). The military lifestyle and the relationship. In B. A. Moore (Ed.), *Handbook of counseling military couples* (pp. 137–156). Routledge.

Huang, C. H., Huang, C. C., Sun, C. K., Lin, G. H., & Hou, W. H. (2016). Methylphenidate on cognitive improvement in patients with traumatic brain injury: A meta-analysis. *Current Neuropharmacology, 14*(3), 272–281. doi:10.2174/1570159X13666150514233033

Institute of Medicine (IOM). (2013). *Returning home from Iraq and Afghanistan: Readjustment needs of veterans, service members, and their families.* http://iom.nationalacademies.org/~/media/Files/Report%20Files/2013/Returning-Home-Iraq-Afghanistan/Returning-Home-Iraq-Afghanistan-RB.pdf

Kelley, M. L., Bravo, A. J., Votaw, V. R., Stein, E., Redman, J. C., & Witkiewitz, K. (2019). Opioid and sedative misuse among veterans wounded in combat. *Addictive Behaviors, 92*, 168–172. https://doi.org/10.1016/j.addbeh.2018.12.007

Kelly Temps in Uniform. (2012). *This ain't Hell, but you can see it from here.* http://thisainthell.us/blog/?p=30410

Kime, P. (2015). *DoD military suicide rate declining.* Military Times. www.militarytimes.com/story/military/pentagon/2015/01/16/defense-department-suicides-2013-report/21865977/

Kong, L. Z., Zhang, R. L., Hu, S. H., & Lai, J. B. (2022). Military traumatic brain injury: A challenge straddling neurology and psychiatry. *Military Medical Research 9*(2). https://doi.org/10.1186/s40779-021-00363-y

Langer, R. (2011). Combat trauma, memory, and the World War II veteran. *War, Literature & the Arts, 23*(1). http://wlajournal.com/23_1/images/langer.pdf

Mayo Clinic. (2022). *Traumatic brain injury.* www.mayoclinic.com/health/traumatic-brain-injury/DS00552

Morin, A. (2020). *Effects of military deployment on children.* https://www.verywellfamily.com/the-effects-of-military-deployment-on-children-4150518#

National Institute of Neurological Disorders and Stroke (NINDS). (2020). *Traumatic brain injury: Hope through research.* https://www.ninds.nih.gov/Disorders/Patient-Caregiver-Education/Hope-Through-Research/Traumatic-Brain-Injury-Hope-Through

National Institute on Drug Abuse (NIDA). (2019). *Substance use and military life.* https://www.drugabuse.gov/related-topics/military

O'Haire, M. E., Guérin, N. A., & Kirkham, A. C. (2015). Animal-assisted intervention for trauma: A systematic literature review. *Frontiers in Psychology 6*, 1121. doi: 10.3389/fpsyg.2015.01121

Pedersen, E. R., Marshall, G. N., & Kurz, J. (2016). Behavioral health treatment receipt among a community sample of young adult veterans. *Journal of Behavioral Health Services & Research*. doi:10.1007/s11414-016-9534-7

Pemberton, M. R., Forman-Hoffman, V. L., Lipari, R. N., Ashley, O. S., Heller, D. C., & Williams, M. R. (2016). *Prevalence of past year substance use and mental illness by veteran status in a nationally representative sample.* https://www.samhsa.gov/data/sites/default/files/NSDUH-DR-VeteranTrends-2016/NSDUH-DR-VeteranTrends-2016.htm

Pincus, S. H., House, R., Christenson, J., & Alder, L. E. (2022). *The emotional cycle of deployment: A military family perspective.* https://www.military.com/spouse/military-deployment/emotional-cycle-of-deployment-military-family.html

Plach, H. L., & Sells, C. H. (2013). Occupational performance needs of young veterans. *American Journal of Occupational Therapy, 67*, 73–81. doi:10.5014/ajot.2013.003871

Price, J. L., & Stevens, S. P. (2021). *Partners of veterans with PTSD: Research findings.* https://www.ptsd.va.gov/professional/treat/specific/vet_partners_research.asp

Ravindran, C., Morley, S. W., Stephens, B. M., Stanley, I. H., & Reger, M. A. (2020). Association of suicide risk with transition to civilian life among us military service members. *JAMA Network Open, 3*(9), e2016261. https://doi.org/10.1001/jamanetworkopen.2020.16261

Smith, R. (2012). *Military children and families.* Helping Hands for Freedom. http://helpinghandsforfreedom.org/remaining-programs-2012-arizona-military-children-families/#more-567

Song, K., Xiong, F. M., Ding, N., Huang, A., & Zhang, H. (2020). Complementary and alternative therapies for post-traumatic stress disorder: A protocol for systematic review and network meta-analysis. *Medicine, 99*(28), e21142. https://doi.org/10.1097/MD.0000000000021142

Teeters, J. B., Lancaster, C. L., Brown, D. G., & Back, S. E. (2017). Substance use disorders in military veterans: Prevalence and treatment challenges. *Substance Abuse and Rehabilitation, 8*, 69–77. https://doi.org/10.2147/SAR.S116720

Temkin, N. R., Corrigan, J. D., Dikmen, S. S., & Machamer, J. (2009). Social functioning after traumatic brain injury. *Journal of Head Trauma Rehabilitation, 24*(6), 460–467. doi:10.1097/HTR.0b013e3181c13413

U.S. Bureau of Labor Statistics, & U.S. Department of Labor. (2021). *The Economics Daily, Labor force participation rate for veterans was 46.8% in October 2021.* https://www.bls.gov/opub/ted/2021/labor-force-participation-rate-for-veterans-was-46-8-percent-in-october-2021.htm

U.S. Equal Employment Opportunity Commission (EEOC). (n.d.). *Sexual harassment.* https://www.eeoc.gov/laws/types/sexual_harassment.cfm

U.S. Food and Drug Administration. (2020). *Tobacco use in the military: A danger for those who keep us safe.* https://www.fda.gov/tobacco-products/health-information/tobacco-use-military-danger-those-who-keep-us-safe

Vlahos, K. B. (2012). *The rape of our military women.* Anti-war.com. http://original.antiwar.com/vlahos/2012/05/14/the-rape-of-our-military-women

Wolf, N. (2012). *A culture of cover-up: Rape in the ranks of the U.S. military.* The Guardian. www.guardian.co.uk/commentisfree/2012/jun/14/culture-coverup-rape-ranks-us-military

Yu, T. S., Kim, A., & Kernie, S. G. (2015). Donepezil rescues spatial learning and memory deficits following traumatic brain injury independent of its effects on neurogenesis. *PLOS ONE.* https://doi.org/10.1371/journal.pone.0118793

Classical References

Wertsch, M. E. (1996). *Military brats: Legacies of childhood inside the fortress.* Brightwell.

Wolfe, J., Sharkansky, E. J., Read, J. P., Dawson, R., Martin, J. A., & Oimette, P. C. (1998). Sexual harassment and assault as predictors of PTSD symptomatology among U.S. female Persian Gulf military personnel. *Journal of Interpersonal Violence, 13*(1), 40–57. doi:10.1177/088626098013001003

Appendix A

Answers to Chapter Review and Clinical Judgment Questions

CHAPTER 1. The Concept of Stress Adaptation
1. a **2.** b **3.** c **4.** b **5.** b **6.** b, c, d **7.** a, b, c
8. d **9.** d **10.** b

CHAPTER 2. Mental Health and Mental Illness: Historical and Theoretical Concepts
1. a **2.** c **3.** d **4.** b **5.** d **6.** c **7.** b **8.** c
9. a **10.** b

CHAPTER 3. Concepts of Psychobiology
1. d **2.** d **3.** a **4.** b **5.** c **6.** a **7.** d **8.** c
9. b **10.** a **11.** a, b, c **12.** b, c, d

CHAPTER 4. Psychopharmacology
1. a **2.** b **3.** c **4.** b **5.** a **6.** b **7.** a **8.** b
9. d **10.** b

CHAPTER 5. Ethical and Legal Issues
1. b **2.** a **3.** c **4.** b **5.** c **6.** d **7.** d **8.** b
9. a **10.** a

CHAPTER 6. Relationship Development
1. a, b, c **2.** b **3.** b, e **4.** d **5.** c **6.** b **7.** c
8. a **9.** b **10.** a **11.** a

CHAPTER 7. Therapeutic Communication
1. d **2.** a **3.** a, b, d **4.** b **5.** d **6.** d **7.** b
8. a **9.** d **10.** c **11.** a **12.** b

CHAPTER 8. The Nursing Process in Psychiatric-Mental Health Nursing
1. b **2.** a **3.** d **4.** a **5.** c **6.** b **7.** a, b, c, d **8.** d
9. c **10.** a

CHAPTER 9. Therapeutic Groups
1. b **2.** d **3.** a **4.** c **5.** c **6.** b **7.** a **8.** c
9. b **10.** d

CHAPTER 10. Intervention With Families
1. b **2.** c **3.** a **4.** b **5.** a **6.** b **7.** c **8.** b
9. d

CHAPTER 11. Psychosocial Interventions and Spiritual Care
1. c **2.** a, b, c **3.** a, b, d, e **4.** b **5.** b **6.** a
7. b **8.** d **9.** c **10.** d **11.** a **12.** d

CHAPTER 12. Crisis Intervention
1. c **2.** d **3.** a, c, d **4.** c **5.** c **6.** b **7.** a
8. b **9.** c **10.** b

CHAPTER 13. Assertiveness Training
1. a **2.** a **3.** b **4.** a **5.** a **6.** c **7.** d **8.** a
9. d **10.** b

CHAPTER 14. Promoting Self-Esteem
1. a **2.** c **3.** b **4.** d **5.** b **6.** a **7.** a, b, d, e
8. d **9.** b **10.** a

CHAPTER 15. Anger and Aggression Management
1. b, c **2.** a, b, d **3.** a, b, c **4.** b **5.** b, c, d, e
6. c **7.** a **8.** c **9.** c **10.** b

CHAPTER 16. Suicide Prevention
1. a **2.** a, c, d, e **3.** d **4.** a, b, c **5.** b **6.** c
7. a **8.** c **9.** b **10.** b, e

CHAPTER 17. Behavior Therapy
1. a **2.** a **3.** b **4.** c **5.** a **6.** b **7.** d **8.** f, b, d, a, e, c **9.** b

CHAPTER 18. Cognitive Behavior Therapy
1. c **2.** a **3.** d **4.** b **5.** c **6.** a **7.** b **8.** a
9. b

CHAPTER 19. Electroconvulsive Therapy
1. c **2.** b **3.** a, b, c, d **4.** d **5.** b **6.** c
7. b **8.** a **9.** c **10.** d

CHAPTER 20. The Recovery Model
1. b, d **2.** c **3.** d **4.** a **5.** c **6.** d **7.** b

CHAPTER 21. Caring for Patients With Mental Illness and Substance Use Disorders in General Practice Settings
1. c **2.** d **3.** a **4.** d **5.** a, b, c **6.** a, d **7.** b
8. d

CHAPTER 22. Neurocognitive Disorders
1. c, e **2.** d **3.** a, b, e **4.** a **5.** a, c, e **6.** b
7. d **8.** c **9.** b **10.** c

CHAPTER 23. Substance-Related and Addictive Disorders
1. a **2.** c **3.** b **4.** a **5.** b **6.** c **7.** d **8.** c
9. a **10.** a, b, c, d, e

CHAPTER 24. Schizophrenia Spectrum and Other Psychotic Disorders
1. a, b, e **2.** b **3.** a **4.** a **5.** d **6.** c **7.** d **8.** d **9.** c **10.** b **11.** c **12.** b

CHAPTER 25. Depressive Disorders
1. c **2.** a **3.** a, b, d **4.** a, c, e **5.** a **6.** b **7.** b **8.** d **9.** c **10.** a, b, d

CHAPTER 26. Bipolar and Related Disorders
1. c **2.** a **3.** a, c, d **4.** a **5.** d **6.** b **7.** b **8.** c **9.** a, c, d **10.** b

CHAPTER 27. Anxiety, Obsessive-Compulsive, and Related Disorders
1. d **2.** c **3.** d **4.** a **5.** a, b, c **6.** b **7.** c **8.** c **9.** a **10.** b

CHAPTER 28. Trauma- and Stressor-Related Disorders
1. b **2.** a **3.** d **4.** c **5.** a **6.** a, c **7.** c **8.** d **9.** b **10.** d

CHAPTER 29. Somatic Symptom and Dissociative Disorders
1. a **2.** b **3.** d **4.** b **5.** a **6.** b **7.** d **8.** c **9.** d **10.** b

CHAPTER 30. Eating Disorders
1. c **2.** a **3.** b **4.** c **5.** c **6.** b **7.** b **8.** b **9.** c **10.** a, b, c, d

CHAPTER 31. Personality Disorders
1. a **2.** a **3.** b **4.** d **5.** a **6.** b **7.** d **8.** d **9.** c **10.** b

CHAPTER 32. Children and Adolescents
1. b **2.** c **3.** d **4.** a **5.** b **6.** b, c, d **7.** b **8.** c **9.** a **10.** b

CHAPTER 33. The Aging Individual
1. c **2.** d **3.** b **4.** a **5.** d **6.** a **7.** d **8.** b **9.** a **10.** c

CHAPTER 34. Survivors of Abuse or Neglect
1. c **2.** a **3.** b **4.** d **5.** d **6.** b **7.** d **8.** a **9.** b **10.** b

CHAPTER 35. Community Mental Health Nursing
1. a **2.** b **3.** a **4.** b **5.** a, b, c, d **6.** c **7.** c **8.** d **9.** a **10.** a, b

CHAPTER 36. The Bereaved Individual
1. a, b, c, d **2.** c **3.** c **4.** d **5.** a **6.** a **7.** b **8.** c **9.** a **10.** c

CHAPTER 37. Military Families
1. a, b, c, d **2.** b **3.** a **4.** d **5.** c **6.** b **7.** c **8.** a, c, d **9.** a, b, c, d

eBook Bonus Chapters

CHAPTER 38. Theoretical Models of Personality Development
1. b **2.** c **3.** d **4.** b **5.** b **6.** b **7.** a **8.** c **9.** a **10.** b

CHAPTER 39. Cultural Concepts Relevant to Psychiatric-Mental Health Nursing
1. c **2.** d **3.** a **4.** d **5.** b **6.** c **7.** b **8.** b **9.** d **10.** c

CHAPTER 40. Complementary Therapies and Integrative Health
1. a, c, e, f **2.** a, b, d **3.** c, d **4.** a, d, e **5.** c **6.** d **7.** c **8.** b **9.** b **10.** c

CHAPTER 41. Issues Related to Human Sexuality and Gender Dysphoria
1. d **2.** b **3.** a, b, d, e **4.** a **5.** c **6.** a, b, c, d **7.** b **8.** b **9.** c

Examples of Answers to Communication Exercises

Chapter 12. Crisis Intervention

1. "I'll try to help you to the best of my ability. Please tell me what is upsetting you." Establish rapport, convey respect, and assess precipitating events.
2. "Hi Shelley, my name is Mrs. Smith, and I am a registered nurse here to help you. I'm so glad you came in to seek help. I'd like to ask you some questions about the events you've experienced. All right?" (Convey respect, provide reassurance of help, and empower the patient to be involved in decision making.)
3. "Thomas, last evening you became very upset, stating you thought the FBI was trying to kill you, and you struck another patient." (Giving information.) "Do you remember any of those events?" (Assessing the patient's perception and memory.) "Restraint is an intervention that we only use when other efforts have failed to protect your safety and the safety of others." (Giving information.) "Let's talk about what you think would be helpful in preventing that from happening again." (Formulating a plan, empowering the patient to be involved in problem-solving.)

Chapter 16. Suicide Prevention

1. "Mr. J., it sounds like you have been feeling hopeless; this is a common symptom of depression." (Giving information.) "Have you been having any thoughts of taking your own life?" (Closed-ended, directive questioning to assess for the presence of suicide ideation.)
2. Communication at this point should be focused on thorough assessment of Mr. J.'s expressed suicide ideas. Assessment questions include the following (but are not comprehensive): "When you have these ideas, do you have a plan in mind?" "How strong is your intention to die?" "Do you have access to the means for implementing this plan?"
3. "It sounds like you are grieving. That must be very painful. Tell me more about your experience and feelings related to losing your wife." (Empathy, exploring and encouraging description.)

Chapter 20. The Recovery Model

1. Because inability to sit still may be a side effect of many antipsychotic medications, one response is to assess the patient's medications and symptoms and educate him about akathisia as appropriate. This response supports the principle that recovery should empower the patient to make informed decisions through providing information and resources. Asking the patient how he wishes to proceed supports the principle that recovery is person-driven.
   For example:
   "Joshua, I see that you are taking Thorazine, and the inability to sit still may be a side effect of this medication. There are other medications that will treat your symptoms and that don't have the same risk for this side effect. Would you like to explore these options further?"
2. Using the recovery model principles of respect and the importance of support through peers and allies, one possible response may be, "Kelly, I haven't been in an active combat situation, but I hope to earn your trust as a mental health professional and try to understand, to the best of my ability, the issues you've been struggling with. Many veterans identify, as you have, that fellow veterans are better able to provide ongoing support with an appreciation for the shared experiences you've endured. Are you interested in exploring some of those options, too?"

Chapter 22. Neurocognitive Disorders

1. "Mrs. B., you are not in a restaurant. This is the General Hospital. I am your nurse, Mary. How may I help you?" (Reality orientation.)
2. "Mrs. B., you have already eaten your breakfast. Would you like a snack?"
   "Please tell me what it was like when you lived on the farm." (Reminiscing.)

Chapter 23. Substance-Related and Addictive Disorders

1. "Tom, you are here because it has been determined that drinking alcohol is causing problems for you at home and at your work." (Confronting reality.)
2. "Tom, you are experiencing symptoms related to your body's withdrawal from alcohol. When did you have your last drink?" (Confrontation with caring.)

3. "You are feeling angry toward your boss and your wife, but your drinking is apparently interfering with your job and your marriage. Unless you abstain from alcohol, you are at risk of losing both." (Confronting reality.)

Chapter 24. Schizophrenia Spectrum and Other Psychotic Disorders

1. "I know that you believe what you are saying is true, but I find it very hard to accept." (Voicing doubt.)

"Please understand that you are safe here." (Reassurance of safety.)

2. The nurse should slowly and carefully approach Hal so that he is not startled by the nurse's presence. "Hal, are you hearing the voices again? What do you hear the voices saying to you?" (Encouraging description of perceptions. This type of information may help to protect the patient and others from potential violence associated with command hallucinations.)

"I know the voices seem real to you, but I do not hear any voices speaking." (Presenting reality.)

3. "I don't understand what you are saying, Hal. What message do you want to give me? Might you be telling me that you are lonely?" (Seeking clarification; attempting to translate words into feelings.)

Chapter 25. Depressive Disorders

1. "You have had a lot of losses. You are feeling very much alone right now." (Verbalizing the implied.)

2. "You feel sad because you can no longer do the things that you used to do ... the things that made you feel good about yourself." (Statement that focuses on feelings.)

3. Direct questions assessing suicide potential: "Are you or have you been thinking about harming yourself? Do you have a plan for doing so? Have you ever acted on that plan?"

Demonstrations of genuine concern and caring: "I care about you, Carrie. I will stay here with you." Expressions of empathy: "It must be frightening to feel so all alone. But you are not alone. There are many people who care about you, and I am one of those people."

Chapter 26. Bipolar and Related Disorders

1. "Bob, I'm not sure I understand what you are saying. Are your thoughts racing?" (Clarifying, assessing.)

2. "John, I have an activity in the next room that I could use your help with. Would you please come with me?" (Offering an alternative activity, redirecting, reducing stimulation.)

Chapter 27. Anxiety, Obsessive-Compulsive, and Related Disorders

1. "John, I'd like to check your vital signs and then discuss how I can best help you feel more comfortable." (Giving information, physical assessment is a priority. Informing the patient about nursing intervention with a matter-of-fact approach may facilitate anxiety reduction; offering self.)

2. "Often, when people become very anxious, they develop irrational thinking patterns that contribute to worsening their mood and affecting their behavior in negative ways. By becoming aware of thought patterns that increase your anxiety, you can learn how to replace those automatic thoughts with more rational patterns in a way that improves your mood, symptoms, and behavior." (Giving information. The nurse in this example provides information and identifies how that is relevant to the patient's recovery.)

Chapter 30. Eating Disorders

1. "Helena, we've established a treatment plan that limits going to the restroom immediately after a meal because we are trying to help you avoid the urge to purge the food you just ate. Let's talk about how you are feeling right now and see if we can identify some other options for your behaviors before and after meals." (Setting limits, formulating a plan.)

2. "John, many people with this kind of eating disorder report feeling a loss of control, and I understand how that can alter your self-esteem. These are symptoms of an illness with many contributing factors. I want to support you in your efforts to manage this illness, and there is good evidence that recovery is achievable." (Validation of patient's feelings, empathy, giving information, offering self.)

Chapter 31. Personality Disorders

1. "My name is Nancy. I am your nurse on this shift, and you will be in my care until 11 p.m. You may ask for me by my name if you have any requests." (Giving information.)

2. "You were arrested because you broke the law." (Confronting reality.)

3. "I do not give out personal information to patients, and I do not go out with patients. I hope that you will be able to remain focused on making decisions that support your recovery." (Confrontation with caring.)

Chapter 34. Survivors of Abuse or Neglect

1. "You are not to blame, Sarah. You do not deserve to be abused in this way. He is responsible for his behavior." (Presenting reality, empathy.)

2. "There are places you can go where you and your children will be safe. I will give you that information." (Giving information.)

"You will need to consider whether you want to press charges against him." (Encouraging formulation of a plan.)

3. "You must consider the safety of yourself and your children. You have the phone number of the Safe House. It is your decision what to do now." (Patient-centered care involves communicating important information and empowering patients to make their own decisions.)

Chapter 36. The Bereaved Individual

1. "I believe we did everything we could to provide care for your husband, and it's so hard to lose someone you love to a terminal illness. I'll stay with you and try to answer any questions you have." (The nurse uses "I" communication to respond assertively with empathy; offering self.)

2. "Yes, John, it's probable that you are in the end stage of life. Let's talk about how to prepare for this." (Giving information; offering self; encouraging formulation of a plan.)

3. "Nancy, those are difficult spiritual questions. Would you like to talk more with the chaplain?" (Verbalizing the implied; formulating a plan.)

Online Chapter 41. Issues Related to Human Sexuality and Gender Dysphoria

1. "Are you having thoughts of taking your own life?" (Assessment for suicide ideation and intentions are the priority because Jamie has expressed feeling that he wants to die.)

2. "I'd be glad to discuss with you the benefits and disadvantages of this option. What do you already know about hormone treatments?" (Conveys respect, collaboration, assessment.)

Appendix C

Mental Status Assessment

Gathering the correct information about the patient's mental status is essential to the development of an appropriate plan of care. The mental status examination is a description of all the areas of the patient's mental functioning. The following components are considered critical in the assessment of a patient's mental status. Examples of interview questions and criteria for assessment are included.

Identifying Data

1. Name
2. Gender
3. Age
   a. How old are you?
   b. When were you born?
4. Race/culture
   a. What country did you (your ancestors) come from?
   b. Are there cultural practices that are important to you?
5. Occupational/financial status
   a. How do you make your living?
   b. How do you obtain money for your needs?
6. Educational level
   a. What was the highest grade level you completed in school?
7. Significant other
   a. Are you married?
   b. Do you have a significant relationship with another person?
8. Living arrangements
   a. Do you live alone?
   b. With whom do you share your home?
9. Religious preference
   a. Do you have a religious preference?
   b. Is religion something that is important to you?
10. Allergies
    a. Are you allergic to anything?
    b. Foods? Medications?
11. Special diet considerations
    a. Do you have any special diet requirements?
    b. Diabetic? Low sodium?
12. Chief complaint
    a. For what reason did you come for help today?
    b. What seems to be the problem?
13. Medical diagnosis

General Description

Appearance

1. Grooming and dress
   a. Note unusual modes of dress.
   b. Evidence of soiled clothing?
   c. Use of makeup?
   d. Neat; unkempt?
2. Hygiene
   a. Note evidence of body or breath odor.
   b. Note condition of skin, fingernails.
3. Posture
   a. Note if standing upright, rigid, slumped over.
4. Height and weight
   a. Perform accurate measurements.
5. Level of eye contact
   a. Intermittent?
   b. Occasional and fleeting?
   c. Sustained and intense?
   d. No eye contact?
6. Hair color and texture
   a. Is hair clean and healthy looking?
   b. Greasy, matted, tangled?
7. Evidence of scars, tattoos, or other distinguishing skin marks
   a. Note any evidence of swelling or bruises.
   b. Birth marks?
   c. Rashes?
8. Evaluation of patient's appearance compared with chronological age

Motor Activity

1. Tremors
   a. Do hands or legs tremble?
      • Continuously?
      • At specific times?
2. Tics or other stereotypical movements
   a. Any evidence of facial tics?
   b. Jerking or spastic movements?
3. Mannerisms and gestures
   a. Specific facial or body movements during conversation?
   b. Nail biting?
   c. Covering face with hands?
   d. Grimacing?
4. Hyperactivity
   a. Gets up and down out of chair.
   b. Paces.
   c. Unable to sit still.

5. Restlessness or agitation
   a. Lots of fidgeting.
   b. Clenching hands.
6. Aggressiveness
   a. Overtly angry and hostile.
   b. Threatening.
   c. Uses sarcasm.
7. Rigidity
   a. Sits or stands in a rigid position.
   b. Arms and legs appear stiff and unyielding.
8. Gait patterns
   a. Any evidence of limping?
   b. Limitation of range of motion?
   c. Ataxia?
   d. Shuffling?
9. Echopraxia
   a. Evidence of mimicking the actions of others?
10. Psychomotor retardation
    a. Movements are very slow.
    b. Thinking and speech are very slow.
    c. Posture is slumped.
11. Freedom of movement (range of motion)
    a. Note any limitation in ability to move.
12. Apraxia
    a. Evidence of difficulty performing tasks or movements when asked, even though the request is understood.

Speech Patterns

1. Slowness or rapidity of speech
   a. Note whether speech seems very rapid or slower than normal.
2. Pressured speech
   a. Note whether speech seems frenzied.
   b. Unable to be interrupted?
3. Intonation
   a. Are words spoken with appropriate emphasis?
   b. Are words spoken in monotone, without emphasis?
4. Volume
   a. Is speech very loud? Soft?
   b. Is speech low-pitched? High-pitched?
5. Stuttering or other speech impairments
   a. Hoarseness?
   b. Slurred speech?
6. Aphasia
   a. Difficulty forming words.
   b. Use of incorrect words.
   c. Difficulty thinking of specific words.
   d. Making up words (neologisms).

General Attitude

1. Cooperative/uncooperative
   a. Answers questions willingly.
   b. Refuses to answer questions.
2. Friendly/hostile/defensive
   a. Is sociable and responsive.
   b. Is sarcastic and irritable.
3. Uninterested/apathetic
   a. Refuses to participate in interview process.
4. Attentive/interested
   a. Actively participates in interview process.
5. Guarded/suspicious
   a. Continuously scans the environment.
   b. Questions motives of interviewer.
   c. Refuses to answer questions.

Emotions

Mood

1. Depressed; despairing
   a. Do you have overwhelming feelings of sadness?
   b. Have you experienced a loss of interest in regular activities?
2. Irritable
   a. Are you easily annoyed or provoked to anger?
3. Anxious
   a. Are you feeling anxious, apprehensive, or worried?
   b. Does the patient appear anxious?
4. Elated
   a. Expresses feelings of joy and intense pleasure.
   b. Is intensely optimistic.
5. Euphoric
   a. Demonstrates a heightened sense of elation.
   b. Expresses feelings of heightened elation ("Everything is wonderful!").
6. Fearful
   a. Demonstrates or verbalizes feeling of apprehension associated with real or perceived danger.
7. Guilty
   a. Expresses a feeling of discomfort associated with real or perceived wrongdoing.
   b. May be associated with feelings of sadness and despair.
8. Labile
   a. Exhibits mood swings that range from euphoria to depression or anxiety.

Affect

1. Congruence with mood
   a. Outward emotional expression is consistent with mood (e.g., if depressed, emotional expression is sadness, eyes downcast, may be crying).
2. Constricted or blunted
   a. Minimal outward emotional expression is observed.
3. Flat
   a. There is an absence of outward emotional expression.

4. Appropriate
   a. The outward emotional expression is what would be expected in a certain situation (e.g., crying upon hearing of a death).
5. Inappropriate
   a. The outward emotional expression is incompatible with the situation (e.g., laughing upon hearing of a death).

Thought Processes

Form of Thought

1. Flight of ideas
   a. Verbalizations are continuous and rapid, and flow from one to another.
2. Loose association
   a. Verbalizations shift from one unrelated topic to another.
3. Circumstantiality
   a. Verbalizations are lengthy and tedious, and because of numerous details, are delayed reaching the intended point.
4. Tangentiality
   a. Verbalizations that are lengthy and tedious, and never reach an intended point.
5. Neologisms
   a. The individual is making up nonsensical-sounding words, which only have meaning to him or her.
6. Concrete thinking
   a. Thinking is literal; elemental.
   b. Absence of ability to think abstractly.
   c. Unable to translate simple proverbs.
7. Clang associations
   a. Speaking in puns or rhymes; using words that sound alike but have different meanings.
8. Word salad
   a. Using a mixture of words that have no meaning together; sounding incoherent.
9. Perseveration
   a. Repetition of words or phrases in the absence or cessation of socially appropriate context.
10. Echolalia
    a. Persistently repeating what another person says.
11. Mutism
    a. Does not speak (either cannot or will not).
12. Poverty of speech
    a. Speaks very little; may respond in monosyllables.
13. Ability to concentrate and disturbance of attention
    a. Does the person hold attention to the topic at hand?
    b. Is the person easily distractible?
    c. Is there selective attention (e.g., blocks out topics that create anxiety)?

Content of Thought

1. Delusions: Does the person have unrealistic ideas or beliefs?
   a. Persecutory: A belief that someone is out to get him or her in some way (e.g., "The FBI will be here at any time to take me away").
   b. Grandiose: An idea that he or she is all-powerful or of great importance (e.g., "I am the king—and this is my kingdom! I can do anything!").
   c. Reference: An idea that whatever is happening in the environment is about him or her (e.g., "Just watch the movie on TV tonight. It is about my life").
   d. Control or influence: A belief that their behavior and thoughts are being controlled by external forces (e.g., "I get my orders from Channel 27. I do only what the forces dictate").
   e. Somatic: A belief that he or she has a dysfunctional body part (e.g., "My heart is at a standstill. It is no longer beating").
   f. Nihilistic: A belief that he or she, or a part of the body, or even the world does not exist or has been destroyed (e.g., "I am no longer alive").
2. Suicidal or homicidal ideas
   a. Is the individual expressing ideas of harming self or others?
   b. Does the individual express plans and intentions to die? Or plans and intentions to harm another? How strong are these intentions?
   c. Does the individual have access to their chosen means of suicide?
3. Obsessions
   a. Is the person verbalizing about a persistent thought or feeling that he or she is unable to eliminate from their consciousness?
4. Paranoia/suspiciousness
   a. Continuously scans the environment.
   b. Questions motives of interviewer.
   c. Refuses to answer questions.
5. Magical thinking
   a. Is the person speaking in a way that indicates they think their words or actions have power (e.g., "If you step on a crack, you break your mother's back!")?
6. Impaired religiosity
   a. Is the individual demonstrating obsession with religious ideas and behavior that is causing marked distress and impairing ability to function?
7. Phobias
   a. Is there evidence of irrational fears (of a specific object, or a social situation)?
8. Poverty of content
   a. Is the individual vague, stereotypical, or limited in ability to share information? Does the patient express feelings of emptiness or being devoid of thought?

Perceptual Disturbances

1. Hallucinations (Is the person experiencing unrealistic sensory perceptions?)
   a. Auditory (Is the individual hearing voices or other sounds that do not exist?)
   b. Visual (Is the individual seeing images that do not exist?)
   c. Tactile (Does the individual feel unrealistic sensations on the skin?)
   d. Olfactory (Does the individual smell odors that do not exist?)
   e. Gustatory (Does the individual have a false perception of an unpleasant taste?)
2. Illusions
   a. Does the individual misperceive or misinterpret real stimuli within the environment? (Sees something and thinks it is something else?)
3. Depersonalization (altered perception of the self)
   a. Does the individual verbalize feeling "outside the body," visualizing himself or herself from afar?
4. Derealization (altered perception of the environment)
   a. Does the individual verbalize that the environment feels "strange or unreal"? A feeling that the surroundings have changed?

Sensorium and Cognitive Ability

1. Level of alertness/consciousness
   a. Is the individual clear-minded and attentive to the environment?
   b. Or is there disturbance in perception and awareness of the surroundings?
2. Orientation. Is the person oriented to:
   a. Time?
   b. Place?
   c. Person?
   d. Circumstances?
3. Memory
   a. Recent (Is the individual able to remember occurrences of the past few days?)
   b. Remote (Is the individual able to remember occurrences of the distant past?)
   c. Confabulation (Does the individual fill in memory gaps with experiences that have no basis in fact?)
4. Capacity for abstract thought
   a. Can the individual interpret proverbs correctly?
      • "What does 'no use crying over spilled milk' mean?"

Impulse Control

1. Ability to control impulses (Does psychosocial history reveal problems with any of the following?)
   a. Aggression
   b. Hostility
   c. Fear
   d. Guilt
   e. Affection
   f. Sexual feelings

Judgment

1. Ability to solve problems and make decisions
   a. What are your plans for the future?
   b. What do you plan to do to reach your goals?
2. Adaptive versus maladaptive coping strategies

Insight

1. Knowledge about self
   a. Awareness of limitations.
   b. Awareness of consequences of actions.
   c. Awareness of illness.
      • "Do you think you have a problem?"
      • "Do you think you need treatment?"
2. Awareness or lack of awareness of adaptive/maladaptive use of coping strategies and ego defense mechanisms (e.g., rationalizing maladaptive behaviors, projection of blame, displacement of anger)

Glossary

A

abandonment. A unilateral severance of the professional relationship between a health-care provider and a client without reasonable notice at a time when there is still a need for continuing health care.

abreaction. "Remembering with feeling"; bringing into conscious awareness painful events that have been repressed and reexperiencing the emotions that were associated with the events.

abuse. To use wrongfully or in a harmful way. Improper treatment or conduct that may result in injury.

acculturation. To change one's cultural beliefs, behaviors, and/or values as a result of engagement with people of a different culture.

acquaintance rape. Rape perpetrated by someone with whom the victim has met or priorly been acquainted.

acupoints. In Chinese medicine, areas along the body that link pathways of healing energy.

acupressure. A technique in which the fingers, thumbs, palms, or elbows are used to apply pressure to certain points along the body. This pressure is thought to dissolve any obstructions in the flow of healing energy and to restore the body to a healthier functioning.

acupuncture. A technique in which hair-thin, sterile, disposable, stainless steel needles are inserted into points along the body to dissolve obstructions in the flow of healing energy and restore the body to a healthier functioning.

acute mania. A primary symptom of bipolar disorder characterized by euphoria and elation. The person may appear to be on a continuous "high." However, the mood is always subject to frequent variation, easily changing to irritability and anger or even to sadness and crying.

acute stress disorder. The *DSM-5-TR* diagnostic category describing a trauma and stressor-related disorder that is short term (from 3 days to 1-month duration) and results in significant distress or impairment in function. (For a complete list of diagnostic criteria, refer to Chapter 28, Trauma- and Stressor-Related Disorders.)

adaptation. Restoration of the body to homeostasis after a physiological and/or psychological response to stress.

addiction. A compulsive or chronic requirement. The need is so strong it generates distress (either physical or psychological) if left unfulfilled.

adjustment. The process of modifying one's behavior in changed circumstances or an altered environment to fulfill psychological, physiological, and social needs.

adjustment disorder. A maladaptive reaction to an identifiable psychosocial stressor that occurs within 3 months after onset of the stressor. The individual shows impairment in social and occupational functioning or exhibits symptoms that are in excess of a normal and expectable reaction to the stressor.

advance directive. A legal document that a competent individual may sign to convey wishes regarding future health-care decisions intended for a time when the individual is no longer capable of informed consent. It may include one or both of the following: (1) a living will, in which the individual identifies the type of care that they do or do not wish to have performed and (2) a durable power of attorney for health care, in which the individual names another person who is given the right to make health-care decisions for the individual who is incapable of doing so.

adverse childhood experiences (ACEs). Traumatic events including abuse, neglect, and other exposures to violence that are linked to future chronic health problems, mental illness, and substance use disorders.

advocacy. The act of pleading for, supporting, or representing a cause or individual. Advocacy in nursing applies to any act in which the nurse is serving in the best interests of the patient, from simple procedures such as hand washing to protect the patient from infection to complex ethically and morally charged issues in which certain clients are unable to advocate for themselves. Nurses also advocate for their patients indirectly by serving in organizations that support and serve to improve health care for all individuals and by participating in policy-making legislation that affects health care of the public.

affect. The behavioral expression of emotion; may be appropriate (congruent with the situation), inappropriate (incongruent with the situation), constricted or blunted (diminished range and intensity), or flat (absence of emotional expression).

affective domain. A category of learning that includes attitudes, feelings, and values.

aggression. Harsh physical or verbal actions intended (either consciously or unconsciously) to harm or injure another.

aggressive. Behavior that defends an individual's own basic rights by violating the basic rights of others (as contrasted with **assertiveness**).

agonist. A drug that activates specific receptors in the brain thereby increasing a biological reaction.

agoraphobia. The fear of being in places or situations from which escape might be difficult (or embarrassing) or in which help might not be available in the event of a panic attack.

agranulocytosis. Extremely low levels of white blood cells. Symptoms include sore throat, fever, and malaise. This may be a side effect of long-term therapy with some antipsychotic medications.

akathisia. Restlessness; an urgent need for movement; a type of extrapyramidal side effect associated with some antipsychotic medications.

akinesia. Muscular weakness or a loss or partial loss of muscle movement; a type of extrapyramidal side effect associated with some antipsychotic medications.

Alcoholics Anonymous (AA). A major self-help organization for the treatment of alcoholism. It is based on a 12-step program to help members attain and maintain sobriety. Once individuals have achieved sobriety, they in turn are expected to help other alcoholics.

allopathic medicine. Traditional medicine; the type of medicine traditionally and currently practiced in the United States and taught in U.S. medical schools.

alternative medicine. Practices that differ from usual traditional (allopathic) medicine.

altruism. One therapeutic factor of group therapy (identified by Irvin Yalom) in which individuals gain self-esteem through mutual sharing and concern. Providing assistance and support to others creates a positive self-image and promotes self-growth.

altruistic suicide. Suicide based on behavior of a group in which an individual is excessively integrated.

amenorrhea. Cessation of the menses; may be a side effect of some antipsychotic medications and may be a symptom in anorexia nervosa.

amnesia. An inability to recall important personal information that is too extensive to be explained by ordinary forgetfulness.

amnesia, generalized. The inability to recall anything that has happened during the individual's entire lifetime.

amnesia, localized. The inability to recall all incidents associated with a traumatic event for a specific time period after the event.

amnesia, selective. The inability to recall only certain incidents associated with a traumatic event for a specific time period after the event.

amphetamine. A racemic sympathomimetic amine that acts as a central nervous system stimulant. It (and its derivatives such as methamphetamine and dextroamphetamine) is a commonly misused substance but has therapeutic use in the treatment of narcolepsy and attention deficit-hyperactivity disorder.

andropause. Also called *male menopause*. A syndrome of symptoms related to the decline of testosterone levels in men. Some symptoms include depression, weight gain, insomnia, hot flashes, decreased libido, mood swings, decreased strength, and erectile dysfunction.

anger. An emotional response to one's perception of a situation. Anger has both positive and negative functions.

anger management. The use of various techniques and strategies to control responses to anger-provoking situations. The goal of anger management is to reduce both the emotional feelings and the physiological arousal that anger engenders.

anhedonia. The inability to experience or even imagine any pleasant emotion.

anomic suicide. Suicide that occurs in response to changes that occur in an individual's life that disrupt cohesiveness from a group and cause that person to feel without support from the formerly cohesive group.

anorexia nervosa. An illness characterized by morbid fear of obesity, distorted body image, preoccupation with food, and refusal to eat.

anorexiants. Drugs that suppress appetite.

anorgasmia. Inability to achieve orgasm.

anosmia. Inability to smell.

anosognosia. A symptom of some mental illnesses, such as schizophrenia, in which the individual is manifesting overt symptoms of illness but is unaware of the presence of symptoms/unaware that there is anything wrong.

antagonist. A drug that blocks a receptor thereby dampening a biological reaction.

anticipatory grief. A subjective state of emotional, physical, and social responses to an anticipated loss of a valued entity. The grief response is repeated once the loss actually occurs, but it may not be as intense as it might have been if anticipatory grieving has not occurred.

antisocial personality disorder. A pattern of socially irresponsible, exploitative, and guiltless behavior, evident in the tendency to fail to conform to the law, develop stable relationships, or sustain consistent employment; exploitation and manipulation of others for personal gain is common.

anxiety. Vague, diffuse apprehension that is associated with feelings of uncertainty and helplessness.

aphasia. Inability to communicate through speech, writing, or signs, caused by dysfunction of brain centers.

aphonia. Inability to speak.

apraxia. Inability to carry out motor activities despite intact motor function or inability to use objects properly.

arbitrary inference. In cognitive therapy this is a type of thinking error in which the individual automatically comes to a conclusion about an incident without the facts to support it or even sometimes despite contradictory evidence to support it.

ascites. Excessive accumulation of serous fluid in the abdominal cavity, occurring in response to portal hypertension caused by cirrhosis of the liver.

assault. An act that results in a person's genuine fear and apprehension that he or she will be touched without consent. Nurses may be guilty of assault for threatening to place an individual in restraints against their will.

assertive. Behavior that enables individuals to act in their own best interests, to stand up for themselves without undue anxiety, to express their honest feelings comfortably, or to exercise their own rights without denying those of others.

assimilation. Adopting the behaviors, beliefs, and values of the majority culture.

associative looseness. Sometimes called *loose associations*, a thinking process characterized by speech in which ideas shift from one unrelated subject to another. The individual is unaware that the topics are unconnected.

ataxia. Muscular incoordination.

attachment. Connectedness with others in interpersonal relationship.

attachment theory. The hypothesis that individuals who maintain close relationships with others into old age are more likely to remain independent and less likely to be institutionalized than those who do not.

attention deficit-hyperactivity disorder (ADHD). A disorder characterized by inattention and/or hyperactivity and impulsivity. Frequently the disorder is not recognized until a child begins attending school.

attitude. A frame of reference around which an individual organizes knowledge about their world. It includes an emotional element and can have a positive or negative connotation.

autism spectrum disorder. A disorder that is characterized by impairment in social interaction skills and interpersonal communication and a restricted repertoire of activities and interests.

autocratic. A leadership style in which the leader makes all decisions for the group. Productivity is very high with this type of leadership, but morale is often low because of the lack of member input and creativity.

autoimmunity. A condition in which the body produces a disordered immunological response against itself. In this situation, the body fails to differentiate between what is normal and what is a foreign substance. When this occurs, the body produces antibodies against normal parts of the body to such an extent as to cause tissue injury.

automatic thoughts. Thoughts that occur rapidly in response to a situation and without rational analysis. They are often negative and based on erroneous logic.

autonomy. Independence; self-governance. An ethical principle that emphasizes the status of persons as autonomous moral agents whose right to determine their destinies should always be respected.

aversive stimulus. A stimulus that follows a behavioral response and decreases the probability that the behavior will recur; also called punishment.

avoidant personality disorder. A personality disorder characterized by social withdrawal rooted in extreme fear of rejection and feelings of inadequacy.

axon. The cellular process of a neuron that carries impulses away from the cell body.

B

battering. A pattern of repeated physical assault, usually of a woman by her spouse or intimate partner. Men are also battered, although this occurs much less frequently.

battery. The unconsented touching of another person. Nurses may be charged with battery should they participate in the treatment of a client without their consent and outside of an emergency situation.

behavior modification. A treatment modality aimed at changing undesirable behaviors using a system of reinforcement to bring about the modifications desired.

behavior therapy. A form of psychotherapy, the goal of which is to modify maladaptive behavior patterns by reinforcing more adaptive behaviors.

behavioral objectives. Statements that indicate to an individual what is expected of them. Behavioral objectives are a way of measuring learning outcomes and are based on the affective, cognitive, and psychomotor domains of learning.

belief. A belief is an idea that one holds to be true. It can be rational, irrational, taken on faith, or a stereotypical idea.

beneficence. An ethical principle that refers to one's duty to benefit or promote the good of others.

bereavement. The period of grief and sadness that is the normal process of reacting to a loss and may include mental, physical, social, and emotional reactions.

bereavement overload. An accumulation of grief that occurs when an individual experiences many losses over a short period and is unable to resolve one before another is experienced. This phenomenon is common among the elderly.

binge eating disorder. An illness characterized by recurrent episodes of binging on food.

binging. A symptom of some eating disorders, notably binge eating disorder and bulimia nervosa, in which an individual consumes thousands of calories at one sitting.

bioethics. The term used with ethical principles that refer to concepts within the scope of medicine, nursing, and allied health.

biofeedback. The use of instrumentation to become aware of processes in the body that usually go unnoticed and to bring them under voluntary control (e.g., the blood pressure or pulse); used as a method of stress reduction.

bipolar disorder. Characterized by mood swings from profound depression to extreme euphoria (mania) with intervening periods of normalcy. Psychotic symptoms may or may not be present.

black box warning. Formally called a boxed warning by the U.S. Food and Drug Administration (FDA), this is a designation which appears on a prescription drug label to call attention to serious or life-threatening risks.

body dysmorphic disorder. An exaggerated belief that the body is deformed or defective in some specific way.

body image. One's perception of their own body. It may also be how one believes others perceive their body. See **physical self**.

borderline personality disorder. A disorder characterized by a pattern of intense and chaotic relationships with affective instability; fluctuating and extreme attitudes regarding other people; impulsivity; direct and indirect self-destructive behavior; and lack of a clear or certain sense of identity, life plan, or values.

boundaries. The level of participation and interaction between individuals and between subsystems. Boundaries denote physical and psychological space that individuals identify as their own. They are sometimes referred to as *limits*. Boundaries are appropriate when they permit appropriate contact with others while preventing excessive interference. Boundaries may be clearly defined (healthy) or rigid or diffuse (unhealthy).

bulimia nervosa. An illness characterized by recurrent binge eating followed by compensatory purging behaviors, such as vomiting, laxative use, excessive exercise, medication use, and others, to prevent weight gain.

C

cachexia. A state of ill health, malnutrition, and wasting; extreme emaciation.

cannabis. The dried flowering tops of the hemp plant. It produces euphoric effects when ingested or smoked and is commonly used in the form of marijuana or hashish.

case management. A health-care delivery process, the goals of which are to provide quality health care, decrease fragmentation, enhance the client's quality of life, and contain costs. A case manager coordinates the client's care from admission to discharge and sometimes after discharge. Critical pathways of care are the tools used for the provision of care in a case management system.

case manager. The individual responsible for negotiating with multiple health-care providers to obtain a variety of services for a client.

catastrophic thinking. Always thinking that the worst will occur without considering the possibility of more likely, positive outcomes.

catatonia. A type of psychological disturbance that is typified by stupor or excitement. Stupor is characterized by extreme psychomotor retardation, mutism, negativism, and posturing; excitement, by psychomotor agitation, in which the movements are frenzied and purposeless. Catatonic symptoms may be associated with other mental or physical disorders.

catharsis. One curative factor of group therapy (identified by Irvin Yalom), in which members in a group can express both positive and negative feelings in a nonthreatening atmosphere.

cell body. The part of the neuron that contains the nucleus and is essential for the continued life of the neuron.

child abuse. Physical or sexual abuse, psychological maltreatment, or neglect of a child.

child sexual abuse. Any sexual act, from indecent exposure or improper touching to penetration (sexual intercourse), that is carried out with a child.

chiropractic medicine. A system of alternative medicine based on the premise that the relationship between structure and function in the human body is a significant health factor and that such relationships between the spinal column and the nervous system are important because the normal transmission and expression of nerve energy are essential to the restoration and maintenance of health.

Christian ethics. The ethical philosophy, based on Christian doctrine stating that we should treat others as moral equals and treat others as we would want to be treated were we in similar situations; sometimes referred to as *the ethic of the golden rule.*

circadian rhythm. A 24-hour biological rhythm controlled by a "pacemaker" in the brain that sends messages to other systems in the body. Circadian rhythm influences various regulatory functions, including the sleep–wake cycle, body temperature regulation, patterns of activity such as eating and drinking, and hormonal and neurotransmitter secretion.

circumstantiality. In speaking, the delay of an individual to reach the point of a communication, due to unnecessary and tedious details.

cisgender. Describes individuals whose gender identity matches their assigned sex at birth.

civil law. Law that protects the private and property rights of individuals and businesses.

clang association. A pattern of speech in which the choice of words is governed by sounds. Clang associations often take the form of rhyming.

classical conditioning. A type of learning that occurs when an unconditioned stimulus (UCS) that produces an unconditioned response (UCR) is paired with a conditioned stimulus (CS), until the CS alone produces the same response, which is then called a conditioned response (CR). Pavlov's example: food (i.e., UCS) causes salivation (i.e., UCR); ringing bell (i.e., CS) with food (i.e., UCS) causes salivation (i.e., UCR), ringing bell alone (i.e., CS) causes salivation (i.e., CR).

clinging. A common symptom of separation anxiety disorders in which the child excessively clings to the mother or other individual from whom the child fears being separated.

codependency. An exaggerated dependent pattern of learned behaviors, beliefs, and feelings that make life painful. It is a dependence on people and things outside the self, along with neglect of the self to the point of having little self-identity.

cognition. Mental operations that relate to logic, awareness, intellect, memory, language, and reasoning powers.

cognitive. Relating to the mental processes of thinking and reasoning.

cognitive development. A series of stages described by Piaget through which individuals progress, demonstrating at each successive stage a higher level of logical organization than at each previous stage.

cognitive domain. A category of learning that involves knowledge and thought processes within the individual's intellectual ability. The individual must be able to synthesize information at an intellectual level before the actual behaviors are performed.

cognitive maturity. The capability to perform all mental operations needed for adulthood.

cognitive therapy. A type of therapy in which the individual is taught to control thought distortions that are considered to be a factor in the development and maintenance of emotional disorders. Commonly referred to as cognitive behavior therapy (CBT).

collaborative safety plan. A plan that is developed in collaboration with a suicidal patient to identify strategies for maintaining ongoing safety and prevention of suicide.

collectivist culture. A type of culture that highly values interdependence among its members.

colposcope. An instrument that contains a magnifying lens and to which a 35-mm camera can be attached. A colposcope is used to examine for tears and abrasions inside the vaginal area of a sexual assault victim.

common law. Laws that are derived from decisions made in previous cases.

communication. An interactive process of transmitting information between two or more entities.

community. One of the four major dimensions of The Recovery Model identified by Substance Abuse and Mental Health Services Administration (SAMHSA) as essential to promoting wellness in individuals with mental illness. Community entails relationships and social networks that provide support, friendship, love, and hope.

compensation. An ego defense mechanism in which an individual covers up a real or perceived weakness by emphasizing a trait that one considers more desirable.

complementary medicine. Practices that differ from usual traditional (allopathic) medicine but may in fact supplement it in a positive way.

compounded rape reaction. Symptoms that are in addition to the typical rape response of physical complaints, rage, humiliation, fear, and sleep disturbances. They include depression and suicide, substance misuse and even psychotic behaviors.

compulsions. Unwanted repetitive behavior patterns or mental acts that are intended to reduce anxiety. They may be performed in response to an obsession or in a stereotyped fashion.

concept mapping. A diagrammatic teaching and learning strategy that allows students and faculty to visualize interrelationships between medical diagnoses, nursing diagnoses, assessment data, and treatments. A diagram of client problems and interventions.

concrete thinking. Thought processes that are focused on specifics rather than on generalities and immediate issues rather than eventual outcomes. Individuals who are experiencing concrete thinking are unable to comprehend abstract terminology.

conditioned response. In classical conditioning, a response that is a *learned* response (not reflexive) after repeated exposure to a target stimulus.

conditioned stimulus. In classical conditioning, an unrelated stimulus that is presented to a subject with a target stimulus and that, with repeated exposure, comes to elicit the same response as the original target stimulus.

confabulation. Creating imaginary events to fill in memory gaps.

confidentiality. The right of an individual to the assurance that their case will not be discussed outside the boundaries of the health-care team.

conscientiousness. A personality trait that includes features such as a sense of personal responsibility, one's belief in their ability to control their own behavior, and sense of themselves as hardworking. Conscientiousness has been found to be associated with decreased risk for cognitive impairment and dementia in older adulthood.

contextual stimuli. Conditions present in the environment that support a focal stimulus and influence a threat to self-esteem.

contingency contracting. A written contract between individuals used to modify behavior. Benefits and consequences for fulfilling the terms of the contract are delineated.

controlled response pattern. The response to rape in which feelings are masked or hidden, and a calm, composed, or subdued affect is seen.

counselor. One who listens as the client reviews feelings related to difficulties he or she is experiencing in any aspect of life; one of the nursing roles identified by H. Peplau.

countertransference. In psychoanalytic theory, countertransference refers to the counselor's behavioral and emotional response to the client. These responses may be related to unresolved feelings toward significant others from the counselor's past or they may be generated in response to the client's behavior toward the counselor.

covert sensitization. An aversion technique used to modify behavior that relies on the individual's imagination to produce unpleasant symptoms. When the individual is about to succumb to undesirable

behavior, he or she visualizes something that is offensive or even nauseating in an effort to block the behavior.

criminal law. Law that provides protection from conduct deemed injurious to the public welfare. It provides for punishment of those found to have engaged in such conduct.

crisis. Psychological disequilibrium in a person who confronts a hazardous circumstance that constitutes an important problem that he or she can neither escape nor solve with usual problem-solving resources.

crisis intervention. An emergency type of assistance in which the intervener becomes a part of the individual's life situation. The focus is to provide guidance and support to help mobilize the resources needed to resolve the crisis and restore or generate an improvement in previous level of functioning. Usually lasts no longer than 6 to 8 weeks.

critical pathways of care (CPCs). An abbreviated plan of care that provides outcome-based guidelines for goal achievement within a designated length of time.

cultural syndromes. Syndromes that are specific to a cultural group.

culture. A particular society's entire way of living, encompassing shared patterns of belief, feeling, and knowledge that guide people's conduct and are passed down from generation to generation.

cycle of battering. Three phases of predictable behaviors that are repeated over time in a relationship between a batterer and a victim: tension-building phase; the acute battering incident; and the calm, loving, respite (honeymoon) phase.

cyclothymic disorder. A chronic mood disturbance involving numerous episodes of hypomania and depressed mood of insufficient severity or duration to meet the criteria for bipolar disorder.

D

date rape. A situation in which the rapist is known to the victim. This may occur during dating or with acquaintances or schoolmates. (Also called *acquaintance rape.*)

decatastrophizing. In cognitive therapy, with this technique the therapist assists the client to examine the validity of a negative automatic thought. Even if some validity exists, the client is then encouraged to review ways to cope adaptively, moving beyond the current crisis situation.

defamation of character. An individual may be liable for defamation of character by sharing with others information about a person that is detrimental to that person's reputation.

deinstitutionalization. The removal of mentally ill individuals from institutions and the subsequent plan to provide care for these individuals in the community setting.

delayed ejaculation. Delayed or absent ejaculation, even though the man has a firm erection and has had more than adequate stimulation.

delayed grief. The absence of evidence of grief when it ordinarily would be expected.

delirious mania. A grave form of mania characterized by severe clouding of consciousness and representing an intensification of the symptoms associated with mania. The symptoms of delirious mania have become relatively rare since the availability of antipsychotic medications.

delirium. A state of mental confusion and excitement characterized by disorientation for time and place, often with hallucinations, incoherent speech, and a continual state of aimless physical activity.

delusions. False personal beliefs not consistent with a person's intelligence or cultural background. The individual continues to have the belief in spite of obvious proof that it is false and/or irrational.

dementia. A general term to describe the impaired ability to remember, think, or make decisions that that is severe enough to interfere with social, behavioral, occupational, and emotional functioning. Several different disease processes can culminate in dementia. Unlike delirium, the progression of cognitive decline occurs slowly, over time and is, in most cases, irreversible.

democratic leadership. A leadership style employed in group interventions that focuses on full participation of the members in decision making and problem-solving.

dendrites. The cellular processes of a neuron that carry impulses toward the cell body.

denial. Refusal to acknowledge the existence of a real situation and/or the feelings associated with it.

density. The number of people in a given environmental space, influencing interpersonal interaction.

dependent personality disorder. A personality disorder characterized by pervasive, excessive dependency needs, submissiveness, and exaggerated fears of inability to care for oneself.

depersonalization. An alteration in the perception or experience of the self so that the feeling of one's own reality is temporarily lost.

deployment. A term used in the military to describe movement of troops into an active-duty environment.

depression. An alteration in mood that is expressed by feelings of sadness, despair, and pessimism. There is a loss of interest in usual activities, and somatic symptoms may be evident. Changes in appetite and sleep patterns are common.

derealization. An alteration in the perception or experience of the external world so that it seems strange or unreal.

detoxification. The process of managed withdrawal from a substance to which one has become addicted.

diagnosis related groups (DRGs). A system used to determine prospective payment rates for reimbursement of hospital care based on the client's diagnosis.

Diagnostic and Statistical Manual of Mental Disorders, Fifth Edition, Text Revision (DSM-5-TR). The most current version of the standard nomenclature of emotional illness published by the American Psychiatric Association (APA) and used by all health-care practitioners. It classifies mental illness and presents guidelines and diagnostic criteria for various mental disorders.

diagnostic overshadowing. A phenomenon in which a person's physical symptoms are assumed to be attributed to their mental illness.

dichotomous thinking. In this type of thinking, situations are viewed in all-or-nothing, black-or-white, good-or-bad terms.

directed association. A technique used to help clients bring into consciousness events that have been repressed. Specific thoughts are guided and directed by the psychoanalyst.

disaster. A natural or man-made occurrence that overwhelms the resources of an individual or community and increases the need for emergency evacuation and medical services.

discriminative stimulus. A stimulus that precedes a behavioral response and predicts that a particular reinforcement will occur. Individuals learn to discriminate between various stimuli that will produce the responses they desire.

disengagement. In family theory, disengagement refers to extreme separateness among family members. It is promoted by rigid boundaries or lack of communication among family members.

disengagement theory. This theory suggests there is a process of mutual withdrawal of aging persons and society from each other that is correlated with successful aging. This theory has been challenged by many investigators.

displacement. Feelings that are transferred from one target to another that is considered less threatening or neutral.

dissociation. The splitting off of clusters of mental contents from conscious awareness, a mechanism central to hysterical conversion and dissociative disorder.

distance. A cultural characteristic that defines the means by which various cultures use interpersonal space to communicate.

distraction. In cognitive therapy, when dysfunctional cognitions have been recognized, activities are identified that can be used to distract the client and divert him or her from the intrusive thoughts or depressive ruminations that are contributing to the client's maladaptive responses.

disulfiram. A drug that is administered to individuals who misuse alcohol as a deterrent to drinking. Ingestion of alcohol while disulfiram is in the body results in a syndrome of symptoms that can produce a great deal of discomfort and can even result in death if the blood alcohol level is high.

domains of learning. Categories in which individuals learn or gain knowledge and demonstrate behavior. There are three domains of learning: affective, cognitive, and psychomotor.

double-bind communication. An emotionally distressing situation in which an individual receives conflicting messages in the communication process, whereby one message is negated by another. This creates a condition in which a successful response to one message results in a failed response to the other.

dual diagnosis. A client has a dual diagnosis when it is determined that he or she has a coexisting substance disorder and mental illness. Treatment is designed to target both problems.

dysthymia. A depressive neurosis. The symptoms are similar to, if somewhat milder than, those ascribed to major depressive disorder. There is no loss of contact with reality.

dystonia. Involuntary muscular movements (spasms) of the face, arms, legs, and neck; may occur as an extrapyramidal side effect of some antipsychotic medications.

E

echolalia. The parrot-like repetition, by an individual with loose ego boundaries, of the words spoken by another.

echopraxia. An individual with loose ego boundaries attempting to identify with another person by imitating movements that the other person makes.

ego. One of the three elements of the personality identified by Freud as the rational self or "reality principle." The ego seeks to maintain harmony between the external world, the id, and the superego.

ego defense mechanisms. Strategies employed by the ego for protection in the face of threat to biological or psychological integrity. See **compensation, denial, displacement, identification, intellectualization, introjection, isolation, projection, rationalization, reaction formation, regression, repression, sublimation, suppression, and undoing**.

elder abuse. Abuse perpetrated against older adults (typically defined as 65 years of age and older) that may include physical, psychological, sexual, or financial abuse and intentional or unintentional neglect.

electroconvulsive therapy (ECT). A type of somatic treatment in which electric current is applied to the brain through electrodes placed on the temples. A grand mal seizure produces the desired effect. This is used with severely depressed patients refractory to antidepressant medications.

emaciated. The state of being excessively thin or physically wasted.

emotional abuse. A pattern of behavior on the part of the parent or caretaker that results in serious impairment of the victim's social, emotional, or intellectual functioning.

emotional neglect. A chronic failure by the parent or caretaker to provide the child with the hope, love, and support necessary for the development of a sound, healthy personality.

empathy. The ability to see beyond outward behavior and sense accurately another's inner experiencing. With empathy, one can accurately perceive and understand the meaning and relevance in the thoughts and feelings of another.

enculturation. The process of learning the norms within a culture.

enmeshment. Exaggerated connectedness among family members. It occurs in response to diffuse boundaries in which there is overinvestment, overinvolvement, and lack of differentiation between individuals or subsystems.

esophageal varices. Veins in the esophagus that become distended because of excessive pressure from defective blood flow through a cirrhotic liver.

essential hypertension. Persistent elevation of blood pressure for which there is no apparent cause or associated underlying disease.

ethical dilemma. A situation that arises when, based on moral considerations, an appeal can be made for taking each of two opposing courses of action.

ethical egoism. An ethical theory espousing that what is "right" and "good" is what is best for the individual making the decision.

ethics. A branch of philosophy dealing with values related to human conduct, to the rightness and wrongness of certain actions, and to the goodness and badness of the motives and ends of such actions.

ethnicity. The concept of people identifying with each other because of a shared heritage.

exhibitionistic disorder. A paraphilic disorder characterized by a recurrent urge to expose one's genitals to a stranger.

expressed response pattern. Pattern of behavior in which the victim of rape expresses feelings of fear, anger, and anxiety through such behavior as crying, sobbing, restlessness, and tenseness; in contrast to the rape victim who withholds feelings in the controlled response pattern.

extinction. In behavior therapy, the gradual decrease in frequency or disappearance of a response when the positive reinforcement is withheld.

extrapyramidal symptoms (EPS). A variety of responses that originate outside the pyramidal tracts and in the basal ganglion of the brain. Symptoms may include tremors, chorea, dystonia, akinesia, akathisia, and others. May occur as a side effect of some antipsychotic medications.

F

factitious disorder. Disorders that involve conscious, intentional feigning of physical or psychological symptoms. Individuals with factitious disorder pretend to be ill to receive emotional care and support commonly associated with the role of "patient."

false imprisonment. The deliberate and unauthorized confinement of a person within fixed limits by the use of threat or force. A nurse may be charged with false imprisonment by placing a patient in restraints against their will in a nonemergency situation.

family. Two or more individuals who depend on one another for emotional, physical, and economical support. The members of the family are self-defined.

family structure. A set of invisible principles that influence the interaction among family members. These principles are established over time and become the "laws" that govern the conduct of various family members.

family system. A system in which the parts of the whole may be the marital dyad, parent-child dyad, or sibling groups. Each of these subsystems is further divided into subsystems of individuals.

family therapy. A type of therapy in which the focus is on relationships within the family. The family is viewed as a system in which the members are interdependent, and a change in one creates change in all.

fetishistic disorder. A paraphilic disorder characterized by recurrent sexual urges and sexually arousing fantasies involving the use of nonliving objects.

"fight-or-flight" syndrome. A syndrome of physical symptoms that results from an individual's real or perceived notion that harm or danger is imminent.

flexible boundary. A personal boundary is flexible when, because of unusual circumstances, individuals can alter limits that they have set for themselves. Flexible boundaries are healthy boundaries.

flight of ideas. A symptom common in bipolar manic episodes in which the individual's thoughts are racing and they rapidly switch topics when communicating.

flooding. Sometimes called *implosion therapy,* this technique is used to desensitize individuals to phobic stimuli. The individual is "flooded" with a continuous presentation (usually through mental imagery) of the phobic stimulus until it no longer elicits anxiety.

focal stimulus. A situation of immediate concern that results in a threat to self-esteem.

Focus Charting. A type of documentation that follows a data, action, and response (DAR) format. The main perspective is a client "focus," which can be a nursing diagnosis, a client's concern, a change in status, or a significant event in the client's therapy. The focus cannot be a medical diagnosis.

forensic. Pertaining to the law; legal.

forensic nursing. The application of forensic science combined with the biopsychological education of the registered nurse in the scientific investigation, evidence collection and preservation, analysis, prevention, and treatment of trauma and/or death-related medical-legal issues.

free association. A technique used to help individuals bring to consciousness material that has been repressed. The individual is encouraged to verbalize whatever comes into their mind, drifting naturally from one thought to another.

frotteuristic disorder. A paraphilic disorder characterized by the recurrent preoccupation with intense sexual urges or fantasies involving touching or rubbing against a nonconsenting person.

fugue. A sudden, unexpected travel away from home or customary work locale with the assumption of a new identity and an inability to recall one's previous identity; usually occurring in response to severe psychosocial stress.

G

gains. The reinforcements an individual receives for somaticizing.

Gamblers Anonymous (GA). An organization of inspirational group therapy, modeled after Alcoholics Anonymous (AA), for individuals who desire to, but cannot, stop gambling.

gender. The condition of being either male or female, particularly as differentiated by social and cultural roles and behavior.

gender dysphoria. A sense of marked distress and mood disturbances associated with an incongruence between biologically assigned gender and subjectively experienced gender.

general adaptation syndrome. The general biological reaction of the body to a stressful situation, as described by Hans Selye. It occurs in three stages: the alarm reaction stage, the stage of resistance, and the stage of exhaustion.

generalized anxiety disorder. A disorder characterized by chronic (at least 6 months), unrealistic, and excessive anxiety and worry.

genetics. Study of the biological transmission of certain characteristics (physical and/or behavioral) from parent to offspring.

genogram. A graphic representation of a family system. It may cover several generations. Emphasis is on family roles and emotional relatedness among members. Genograms facilitate recognition of areas requiring change.

genotype. The total set of genes present in an individual at the time of conception and coded in the DNA.

genuineness. The ability to be open, honest, and "real" in interactions with others; the awareness of what one is experiencing internally and the ability to project the quality of this inner experiencing in a relationship.

geriatrics. The branch of clinical medicine specializing in the care of the elderly and concerned with the problems of aging.

gerontology. The study of normal aging.

geropsychiatry. The branch of clinical medicine specializing in psychopathology of the elderly.

grief. A subjective state of emotional, physical, and social responses to the real or perceived loss of a valued entity. Change and failure can also be perceived as losses. The grief response consists of a set of relatively predictable behaviors that describe the subjective state that accompanies mourning.

grief, maladaptive. A grief process that is delayed, exaggerated, or chronic and interferes with an individual's ability to function socially, emotionally, and in activities of daily living.

group. A collection of individuals whose association is founded on shared commonalities of interest, values, norms, or purpose. Membership in a group is generally by chance (born into the group), by choice (voluntary affiliation), or by circumstance (the result of life cycle events over which an individual may or may not have control).

group therapy. A therapy group, founded in a specific theoretical framework, led by a person with an advanced degree in psychology, social work, nursing, or medicine. The goal is to encourage improvement in interpersonal functioning.

gynecomastia. Enlargement of the breasts in men; may be a side effect of some antipsychotic medications.

H

habit-reversal therapy. A type of behavior therapy in which the individual develops awareness of unhealthy habits and learns to substitute more adaptive coping strategies in an effort to extinguish unwanted behaviors.

hallucinations. False sensory perceptions not associated with real external stimuli. Hallucinations may involve any of the five senses.

health. One of the four major dimensions of The Recovery Model identified by Substance Abuse and Mental Health Services Administration (SAMHSA) as essential to promoting wellness in individuals with mental illness. Health entails overcoming or managing one's disease as well as living in a physically and emotionally healthy way.

hepatic encephalopathy. A brain disorder resulting from the inability of the cirrhotic liver to convert ammonia to urea for excretion. The continued rise in serum ammonia results in progressively impaired mental functioning, apathy, euphoria or depression, sleep disturbances, increasing confusion, and progression to coma and eventual death.

histrionic personality disorder. A type of personality disorder characterized by excessively emotional and attention-seeking behavior, often presented in a very colorful and dramatic fashion.

HIV-associated neurocognitive disorder. A neuropathological syndrome, possibly caused by chronic HIV encephalitis and myelitis and manifested by cognitive, behavioral, and motor symptoms that become more severe with progression of the disease.

hoarding disorder. A disorder in which the individual has extreme difficulty parting with possessions, regardless of their value, and may also be accompanied by excessive acquisition of material possessions.

home. One of the four major dimensions of The Recovery Model identified by Substance Abuse and Mental Health Services Administration (SAMHSA) as essential to promoting wellness in individuals with mental illness. This entails having a stable and safe place to live.

home care. A wide range of health and social services that are delivered at home to recovering, disabled, and chronically or terminally ill persons in need of medical, nursing, social, or therapeutic treatment and/or assistance with essential activities of daily living.

homocysteine. An amino acid produced by the catabolism of methionine. Elevated levels may be linked to increased risk of cardiovascular disease.

hope. A guiding principle of The Recovery Model that stresses potential for improved quality of life and recovery from illness.

hospice. A program that provides palliative and supportive care to meet the special needs arising out of the physical, psychosocial, spiritual, social, and economic stresses that are experienced during the final stages of illness and during bereavement.

hyperactivity. Excessive psychomotor activity that may be purposeful or aimless, accompanied by physical movements and verbal utterances that are usually more rapid than normal. Inattention and distractibility are common with hyperactive behavior.

hypersomnia. Excessive sleepiness or seeking excessive amounts of sleep.

hypertensive crisis. A potentially life-threatening syndrome that results when an individual taking monoamine oxidase inhibitors (MAOIs) eats a product high in tyramine. Symptoms include severe occipital headache, palpitations, nausea and vomiting, nuchal rigidity, fever, sweating, marked increase in blood pressure, chest pain, and coma. Foods with tyramine include aged cheeses or other aged, overripe, and fermented foods; broad beans; pickled herring; beef or chicken liver; preserved meats; beer and wine; yeast products; chocolate; caffeinated drinks; canned figs; sour cream; yogurt; soy sauce; and some over-the-counter cold medications and diet pills.

hypnosis. A treatment for disorders brought on by repressed anxiety. The individual is directed into a state of subconsciousness and assisted, through suggestions, to recall certain events that he or she cannot recall while conscious.

hypomanic episode. A mild form of mania. Symptoms are excessive hyperactivity but not severe enough to cause marked impairment in social or occupational functioning or to require hospitalization.

I

id. One of the three components of the personality identified by Freud as the "pleasure principle." The id is the locus of instinctual drives, is present at birth, and compels the infant to satisfy needs and seek immediate gratification.

identification. An attempt to increase self-worth by acquiring certain attributes and characteristics of an individual one admires.

illusion. A misperception of a real external stimulus.

implosion therapy. See **flooding.**

impulsivity. The urge or inclination to act without consideration of the possible consequences of one's behavior.

incest. Sexual exploitation of a child under 18 years of age by a relative or nonrelative who holds a position of trust in the family.

informed consent. Permission granted to a physician by a client to perform a therapeutic procedure, before which information about the procedure has been presented to the client with adequate time given for consideration about the pros and cons.

insomnia. Difficulty initiating or maintaining sleep.

integration. The process used with individuals with dissociative identity disorder in an effort to bring all the subpersonalities together into one; usually achieved through hypnosis.

integrative health. A holistic approach that incorporates complementary and conventional practices in a coordinated, comprehensive treatment plan.

intellectualization. An attempt to avoid expressing actual emotions associated with a stressful situation by using the intellectual processes of logic, reasoning, and analysis.

interdisciplinary care. A concept of providing care for a client in which members of various disciplines work together with common goals and shared responsibilities for meeting those goals.

intimate distance. The closest distance that individuals will allow between themselves and others. In the United States, this distance is 0 to 18 inches.

intimate partner violence. A pattern of abusive behavior that is used by an intimate partner to gain or maintain power and control over the other intimate partner.

intoxication. A physical and mental state of exhilaration and emotional frenzy or lethargy and stupor.

introjection. The beliefs and values of another individual are internalized and symbolically become a part of the self to the extent that the feeling of separateness or distinctness is lost.

isolation. The separation of a thought or a memory from the feeling, tone, or emotions associated with it (sometimes called *emotional isolation*).

J

justice. An ethical principle reflecting that all individuals should be treated equally and fairly.

K

Kantianism. The ethical principle espousing that decisions should be made and actions taken out of a sense of duty.

kleptomania. A recurrent failure to resist impulses to steal objects not needed for personal use or monetary value.

Korsakoff's psychosis. A syndrome of confusion, loss of recent memory, and confabulation in alcoholics caused by a deficiency of thiamine. It often occurs together with Wernicke's encephalopathy and may be termed *Wernicke-Korsakoff syndrome.*

L

laissez-faire leadership. A leadership type in which the leader lets group members do as they please. There is no direction from the leader. Member productivity and morale may be low due to frustration from lack of direction.

lanugo. Fine, neonatal-like hair growth on the body and a symptom sometimes seen in individuals with anorexia nervosa.

lesbian. A female homosexual.

libel. An action with which an individual may be charged for sharing with another individual, in writing, information that is detrimental to someone's reputation.

libido. Freud's term for the psychic energy used to fulfill basic physiological needs or instinctual drives, such as hunger, thirst, and sexuality.

limbic system. Parts of the brain that collectively make up what is often called the *emotional brain*. The limbic system is associated with feelings such as fear, anger, love, joy, hope, and with sexuality, and social behavior. As research has progressed it has become more difficult to define the boundaries of the limbic system.

long-term memory. Memory for remote events or those that occurred many years ago. The type of memory that is preserved in the elderly individual.

loose association. A thinking process characterized by speech in which ideas shift from one unrelated topic to another. The individual is unaware that topics are unconnected. See also **associative looseness**.

loss. The experience of separation from something of personal importance.

M

magical thinking. A primitive form of thinking in which an individual believes that thinking about a possible occurrence can make it happen.

magnification. A type of thinking in which the negative significance of an event is exaggerated.

maladaptation. A failure of the body to return to homeostasis after a physiological and/or psychological response to stress, disrupting the individual's integrity.

maladaptive grief. A grief process that it delayed, exaggerated, or chronic and interferes with an individual's ability to function socially, emotionally, and in activities of daily living.

malpractice. The failure of one rendering professional services to exercise that degree of skill and learning commonly applied under all the circumstances in the community by the average prudent reputable member of the profession, with the result of injury, loss, or damage to the recipient of those services or to those entitled to rely upon them.

managed care. A concept purposefully designed to control the balance between cost and quality of care. Examples of managed care are health maintenance organizations (HMOs) and preferred provider organizations (PPOs). The amount and type of health care that the individual receives is determined by the organization providing the managed care.

mania. A manifestation of bipolar disorder in which the predominant mood is elevated, expansive, or irritable. Motor activity is frenzied and excessive. Psychotic features may or may not be present.

marital rape. Sexual violence directed at a marital partner against that person's will.

marital schism. A state of severe chronic disequilibrium and discord within the marital dyad with recurrent threats of separation.

marital skew. A marital relationship in which there is lack of equal partnership. One partner dominates the relationship and the other partner.

Medicaid. A system established by the federal government to provide medical care benefits for indigent Americans. The Medicaid program is jointly funded by state and federal governments, and coverage varies significantly from state to state.

Medicare. A system established by the federal government to provide medical care benefits for older adult Americans.

medication-assisted treatment. The use of various medications to decrease the intensity of symptoms in an individual who is withdrawing from, or who is experiencing the effects of excessive use of, alcohol and other drugs and to decrease cravings by administering a controlled dose of another medication.

meditation. A method of relaxation in which an individual sits in a quiet place and focuses total concentration on an object, a word, or a thought.

melancholia. A severe form of major depressive episode. Symptoms are exaggerated, and interest or pleasure in virtually all activities is lost.

mental health. The successful adaptation to stressors from the internal or external environment, evidenced by thoughts, feelings, and behaviors that are age-appropriate and congruent with local and cultural norms.

mental illness. Maladaptive responses to stressors from the internal or external environment, evidenced by thoughts, feelings, and behaviors that are incongruent with the local and cultural norms and interfere with the individual's social, occupational, and/or physical functioning.

mental imagery. A method of stress reduction that employs the imagination. The individual focuses imagination on a scenario that is particularly relaxing to them (e.g., a scene on a quiet seashore, a mountain atmosphere, or floating through the air on a fluffy white cloud).

meridians. In Chinese medicine, pathways along the body in which the healing energy (qi) flows and which are links between acupoints.

milieu. French for "middle"; the English translation connotes "surroundings or environment."

milieu therapy. Also called therapeutic community or therapeutic environment, this type of therapy consists of a scientific structuring of the environment to effect behavioral changes and to improve the individual's psychological health and functioning.

minimization. A type of thinking in which the positive significance of an event is minimized or undervalued.

misuse (of substances). Overuse of substances with potential for harmful consequences. Equivalent to the term abuse but preferred in some contexts to reduce the shaming and stigma associated with referring to individuals as "abusers."

mobile outreach units. Programs in which volunteers and paid professionals drive or walk around and seek out homeless individuals who need assistance with physical or psychological care.

modeling. Learning new behaviors by imitating the behaviors of others.

mood. An individual's sustained emotional tone, which significantly influences behavior, personality, and perception.

moral behavior. Conduct that results from serious critical thinking about how individuals ought to treat others; reflects respect for human life, freedom, justice, or confidentiality.

moral-ethical self. That aspect of the personal identity that functions as observer, standard setter, dreamer, comparer, and most of all evaluator of who the individual says he or she is. This component of the personal identity makes judgments that influence an individual's self-evaluation.

mourning. The psychological process (or stages) through which the individual passes on the way to successful adaptation to the loss of a valued entity.

multidisciplinary care. A concept of providing care for a client in which individual disciplines provide specific services for the client without formal arrangement for interaction between the disciplines.

Munchausen syndrome. See **factitious disorder.**

N

narcissism. Self-love or self-admiration.

narcissistic personality disorder. A disorder characterized by an exaggerated sense of self-worth. These individuals lack empathy and are hypersensitive to the evaluation of others.

narcolepsy. A disorder in which the characteristic manifestation is sleep attacks. The individual cannot prevent falling asleep even in the middle of a sentence or performing a task.

National Standards for Culturally and Linguistically Appropriate Services (NCLAS). A set of standards established by the U.S. Department of Health and Human Services Office of Minority Health for health-care organizations and providers focusing on culturally competent care.

natural law theory. The ethical theory that has as its moral precept to "do good and avoid evil" at all costs. Natural law ethics are grounded in a concern for the human good that is based on people's ability to live according to the dictates of reason.

negative reinforcement. Increasing the probability that a behavior will recur by removal of an undesirable reinforcing stimulus.

negativism. Strong resistance to suggestions or directions; exhibiting behaviors contrary to what is expected.

neglect of a child. *Physical neglect* of a child includes refusal of or delay in seeking health care, abandonment, expulsion from the home or refusal to allow a runaway to return home, and inadequate supervision. *Emotional neglect* refers to a chronic failure by the parent or caretaker to provide the child with the hope, love, and support necessary for the development of a sound, healthy personality.

negligence. The failure to do something that a reasonable person, guided by those considerations that ordinarily regulate human affairs, would do or doing something that a prudent and reasonable person would not do.

neologism. New words that an individual invents that are meaningless to others but have symbolic meaning to the psychotic person.

neurocognitive disorder (NCD). The *DSM-5-TR* diagnostic label for disorders of global impairment of cognitive functioning that is progressive and interferes with social and occupational abilities. These disorders include Alzheimer's disease and Lewy body dementia, among others.

neuroendocrinology. The study of hormones functioning within the neurological system.

neuroleptic. Antipsychotic medication used to prevent or control psychotic symptoms.

neuroleptic malignant syndrome (NMS). A rare but potentially fatal complication of treatment with neuroleptic drugs. Symptoms include severe muscle rigidity, high fever, tachycardia, fluctuations in blood pressure, diaphoresis, and rapid deterioration of mental status to stupor and coma.

neuron. A nerve cell; consists of a cell body, an axon, and dendrites.

neurosis. An unconscious conflict that produces anxiety and other symptoms and leads to maladaptive use of defense mechanisms.

neurotransmitter. A chemical that is stored in the axon terminals of the presynaptic neuron. An electrical impulse through the neuron stimulates the release of the neurotransmitter into the synaptic cleft, which in turn determines whether or not another electrical impulse is generated.

nonassertive. Individuals who are nonassertive (sometimes called *passive*) seek to please others at the expense of denying their own basic human rights.

nonmaleficence. The ethical principle that espouses abstaining from negative acts toward another, including acting carefully to avoid harm.

nonsuicidal self-injuring behavior (NSSIB). Repetitive, nonlethal forms of self-injury that are not intended to end one's life but instead are intended to reduce emotional distress. Examples of NSSIB include "cutting" (cutting oneself with a sharp object), burning, self-hitting, or head banging.

nursing diagnosis. A clinical judgment about individual, family, or community responses to actual and potential health problems/life processes. Nursing diagnoses provide the basis for selection of nursing interventions to achieve outcomes for which the nurse is accountable.

Nursing Interventions Classification (NIC). A comprehensive, research-based, standardized classification of interventions that nurses perform.

Nursing Outcomes Classification (NOC). A comprehensive, standardized classification of patient/client outcomes developed to evaluate the effects of nursing interventions.

nursing process. A dynamic, systematic process by which nurses assess, diagnose, identify outcomes, plan, implement, and evaluate nursing care. It has been called "nursing's scientific methodology." Nursing process gives order and consistency to nursing intervention.

O

obesity. The state of having a body mass index of 30 or greater.

object constancy. The phase in the separation/individuation process when the child learns to relate to objects in an effective, constant manner. A sense of separateness is established, and the child is able to internalize a sustained image of the loved object or person when out of sight.

obsessions. Unwanted, intrusive, persistent ideas, thoughts, impulses, or images that cause marked anxiety or distress

obsessive-compulsive disorder. Recurrent thoughts or ideas (obsessions) that an individual is unable to put out of their mind and actions that an individual is unable to refrain from performing (compulsions). The obsessions and compulsions are severe enough to interfere with social and occupational functioning.

obsessive-compulsive personality disorder. A type of personality disorder in which the individual has an intense fear of making mistakes, which manifests in inflexible and perfectionistic behavior. It is differentiated from obsessive-compulsive disorder in that there is no evidence of the obsessive-compulsive rituals in the individual with this personality disorder.

oculogyric crisis. An attack of involuntary deviation and fixation of the eyeballs, usually in the upward position. It may last for several minutes or hours and may occur as an extrapyramidal side effect of some antipsychotic medications.

operant conditioning. The learning of a particular action or type of behavior that is followed by a reinforcement.

opioids. A synthetic or naturally occurring substance that acts on opiate receptors to produce opiate-like effects.

oppositional defiant disorder (ODD). A disorder characterized by a persistent pattern of angry mood and defiant behavior that interferes with social, educational, occupational, or other important areas of functioning. The age of onset is typically around 8 years of age.

orgasm. A peaking of sexual pleasure with release of sexual tension and rhythmic contraction of the perineal muscles and pelvic reproductive organs.

outcomes. End results that are measurable, desirable, and observable and translate into observable behaviors.

overgeneralization. Also called *absolutistic thinking*. In cognitive therapy, this refers to a distorted thinking pattern in which sweeping conclusions are made based on one incident—an "all-or-nothing" type of thinking.

overt sensitization. A type of aversion therapy that produces unpleasant consequences for undesirable behavior. An example is the use of disulfiram therapy with alcoholics, which induces an undesirable physical response if the individual has consumed any alcohol.

P

palilalia. Repeating one's own sounds or words (a type of vocal tic associated with Tourette's disorder).

panic. A sudden overwhelming feeling of terror or impending doom. This most severe form of emotional anxiety is usually accompanied by behavioral, cognitive, and physiological signs and symptoms considered to be outside the expected range of normalcy.

panic disorder. A disorder characterized by recurrent panic attacks, the onset of which are unpredictable and manifested by intense apprehension, fear, or terror, often associated with feelings of impending doom and accompanied by intense physical discomfort.

paradoxical intervention. In family therapy, "prescribing the symptom." The therapist requests that the family continue to engage in the behavior that they are trying to change. Tension is relieved, and the family is able to view more clearly the possible solutions to their problem.

paralanguage. The gestural component of the spoken word. It consists of pitch, tone, loudness of spoken messages, the rate of speaking, expressively placed pauses, and emphasis assigned to certain words.

paranoia. A term that implies extreme suspiciousness. In schizophrenia, paranoia is characterized by persecutory delusions and hallucinations of a threatening nature.

paranoid personality disorder. A type of personality disorder in which the individual intensely mistrusts others and assumes that they have malevolent intentions toward them.

paraphilic disorder. Repetitive behaviors or fantasies that involve nonhuman objects, real or simulated suffering or humiliation, or nonconsenting partners.

parasomnia. Unusual or undesirable behaviors that occur during sleep (e.g., nightmares, sleep terrors, and sleepwalking).

passive-aggressive. Behavior that defends an individual's own basic rights by expressing resistance to social and occupational demands. Sometimes called *indirect aggression*, this behavior takes the form of sly, devious, and undermining actions that express the opposite of what the person is really feeling.

pathological gambling. A failure to resist impulses to gamble and gambling behavior that compromises; disrupts; or damages personal, family, or vocational pursuits.

patient-centered care. An approach to patient care that focuses on listening to the patient, empowering them as central to decision making about their care, developing a collaborative partnership, and only making decisions for the patient (such as involuntary hospitalization) when he or she is clearly unable to and when it is necessary to protect the patient's safety.

pedophilic disorder. Recurrent urges and sexually arousing fantasies involving sexual activity with a prepubescent child.

peer assistance programs. Programs established by the American Nurses Association to assist impaired nurses. The individuals who administer these efforts are nurse members of the state associations as well as nurses who are in recovery themselves.

perseveration. Persistent repetition of the same word or idea in response to different questions.

personal distance. The distance between individuals who are having interactions of a personal nature, such as a close conversation. In the U.S. culture, personal distance is approximately 18 to 40 inches.

personal identity. An individual's self-perception that defines their functions as observer, standard setter, and self-evaluator. It strives to maintain a stable self-image and relates to what the individual strives to become.

personal self. See **personal identity.**

personality. Deeply ingrained patterns of behavior, which include the way one relates to, perceives, and thinks about the environment and oneself.

personalization. Taking complete responsibility for situations without considering that other circumstances may have contributed to the outcome.

phencyclidine. An anesthetic used in veterinary medicine; used illegally as a hallucinogen, referred to as *PCP* or *angel dust.*

phenotype. Characteristics of physical manifestations that identify a particular genotype. Examples of phenotypes include eye color, height, blood type, language, and hairstyle. Phenotypes may be genetic or acquired.

phobia. An irrational fear.

physical neglect of a child. The failure on the part of the parent or caregiver to provide for a child's basic needs, such as food, clothing, shelter, medical and dental care, and supervision.

physical self. A personal appraisal by an individual of their physical being; includes physical attributes, functioning, sexuality, wellness-illness state, and appearance.

physical violence. In the context of intimate partner violence (IPV), physical violence is when a person hurts or tries to hurt a partner by hitting, kicking, or using another type of physical force.

PIE charting. More specifically called *APIE,* this method of documentation has an assessment, problem, intervention, and evaluation (APIE) format and is a problem-oriented system used to document nursing process.

positive reinforcement. A reinforcement stimulus that increases the probability that the behavior will recur.

positive symptoms. A group of symptoms in schizophrenia that are present because of the disorder. Examples include delusions, hallucinations, and disorganized thinking, speech, and behavior.

postpartum depression. Depression that occurs during the postpartum period. It may be related to hormonal changes, tryptophan metabolism, or alterations in membrane transport during the early postpartum period. Other predisposing factors may also be influential.

post-traumatic stress disorder (PTSD). A syndrome of symptoms that develops after a psychologically distressing event that is outside the range of usual human experience (e.g., rape, war). The individual is unable to cope with the associated anxiety and has nightmares, flashbacks, and panic attacks.

posturing. The voluntary assumption of inappropriate or bizarre postures.

preassaultive tension state. Behaviors predictive of potential violence. They include excessive motor activity; tense posture; defiant affect; clenched teeth and fists; and other arguing, demanding, and threatening behaviors.

precipitating event. A stimulus arising from the internal or external environment that is perceived by an individual as taxing or exceeding their resources and endangering their well-being.

predisposing factors. A variety of elements that influence how an individual perceives and responds to a stressful event. Types of predisposing factors include genetic influences, past experiences, and existing conditions.

Premack principle. This principle states that a frequently occurring response (R1) can serve as a positive reinforcement for a response (R2) that occurs less frequently. For example, a girl may talk to friends on the phone (R2) only if she does her homework (R1).

premature ejaculation. Ejaculation that occurs with minimal sexual stimulation or before, upon, or shortly after penetration and before the person wishes it.

premenstrual dysphoric disorder. A disorder that is characterized by depressed mood, anxiety, mood swings, and decreased interest in activities during the week before menses and subsiding shortly after the onset of menstruation.

pressured speech. Rapid, frenetic speech that often occurs as a symptom of bipolar disorder.

priapism. Prolonged painful penile erection, may occur as an adverse effect of some antidepressant medications, particularly trazodone.

primary gain. The receipt of positive reinforcement for somaticizing by being able to avoid difficult situations because of physical complaint.

primary neurocognitive disorder (NCD). NCD, such as Alzheimer's disease, in which the NCD itself is the major sign of some organic brain disease not directly related to any other organic illness.

primary prevention. Reduction of the incidence of mental disorders within the population by helping individuals to cope more effectively with stress and by trying to diminish stressors within the environment.

privileged communication. A doctrine common to most states that grants certain privileges under which health-care professionals may refuse to reveal information about and communications with clients.

problem-oriented recording (POR). A system of documentation that follows a subjective data, objective data, assessment, plan, implementation, and evaluation (SOAPIE) format. It is based on a list of identified patient problems to which each entry is directed.

prodromal syndrome. A syndrome of symptoms that often precede the onset of aggressive or violent behavior. These symptoms include anxiety and tension, verbal abuse and profanity, and increasing hyperactivity.

progressive relaxation. A method of deep muscle relaxation in which each muscle group is alternately tensed and relaxed in a systematic order with the person concentrating on the contrast of sensations experienced from tensing and relaxing.

projection. Attributing to another person's feelings or impulses unacceptable to oneself.

prospective payment. The program of cost containment within the health-care profession directed at setting forth preestablished amounts that would be reimbursed for specific diagnoses.

pseudocyesis. A condition in which an individual has nearly all the signs and symptoms of pregnancy but is not pregnant; a conversion reaction.

pseudodementia. Symptoms of depression that mimic those of neurocognitive disorder.

pseudohostility. A family interaction pattern characterized by a state of chronic conflict and alienation among family members. This relationship pattern allows family members to deny underlying fears of tenderness and intimacy.

pseudomutuality. A family interaction pattern characterized by a facade of mutual regard with the purpose of denying underlying fears of separation and hostility.

pseudoparkinsonism. A side effect of some antipsychotic medications. Symptoms mimic those of Parkinson's disease, such as tremor, shuffling gait, drooling, and rigidity.

psychiatric home care. Care provided by psychiatric nurses in the client's home. Psychiatric home-care nurses must have physical and psychosocial nursing skills to meet the demands of the client population they serve.

psychoanalysis. An approach to treatment of mental and emotional distress, originated by Sigmund Freud, that focuses on bringing unconscious thoughts and drives into conscious awareness.

psychobiology. The study of the biological foundations of cognitive, emotional, and behavioral processes.

psychodrama. A specialized type of group therapy that employs a dramatic approach in which patients become "actors" in life situation scenarios. The goal is to resolve interpersonal conflicts in a less-threatening atmosphere than the real-life situation would present.

psychodynamic nursing. Being able to understand one's own behavior, to help others identify felt difficulties, and to apply principles of human relations to the problems that arise at all levels of experience.

psychoimmunology. The study of the implications of the immune system in psychiatry.

psychological aggression. In the context of intimate partner violence (IPV), psychological aggression is the use of verbal and nonverbal communication with the intent to harm another person mentally or emotionally and/or to exert control over another person.

Psychological Recovery Model. A model of treatment that focuses on the importance of hopefulness, self-determination, and positive self-concept in recovery from mental illnesses or emotional stress.

psychomotor domain. A category of learning in which the behaviors are processed and demonstrated. The information has been intellectually processed, and the individual is displaying motor behaviors.

psychomotor retardation. Extreme slowdown of physical movements. Posture slumps, speech is slowed, and digestion becomes sluggish. Common in severe depression.

psychophysiological. Referring to psychological factors contributing to the initiation or exacerbation of a physical condition. Either a demonstrable organic pathology or a known pathophysiological process is involved.

psychosis. A mental state in which there is a severe loss of contact with reality. Symptoms may include delusions, hallucinations, disorganized speech patterns, and bizarre or catatonic behaviors.

psychosomatic. See **psychophysiological.**

psychotic disorder. A serious psychiatric disorder in which there is a gross disorganization of the personality, a marked disturbance in reality testing, and the impairment of interpersonal functioning and relationship to the external world.

psychotropic medication. Medication that affects psychic function, behavior, or experience.

public distance. Appropriate interactional distance for speaking in public or yelling to someone some distance away. U.S. culture defines this distance as 12 feet or more.

purging. The act of attempting to rid the body of calories by self-induced vomiting or excessive use of laxatives or diuretics.

purpose. A guiding principle in The Recovery Model that stresses the importance of finding purpose in life for the process of recovery from mental illness.

pyromania. An inability to resist the impulse to set fires.

Q

qi. In Chinese medicine, the healing energy that flows through pathways in the body called *meridians.* (Also called *chi.*)

R

rape. The expression of power and dominance by means of sexual violence, most commonly by men over women, although men may also be rape victims. Rape is considered an act of aggression, not of passion.

rape trauma syndrome. A variable group of symptoms that are indicative of the trauma associated with rape. Symptoms may include expressed response patterns, controlled responses, or silent reactions.

rapport. The development between two people in a relationship of special feelings based on mutual acceptance, warmth, friendliness, common interest, a sense of trust, and a nonjudgmental attitude.

rationalization. Attempting to make excuses or formulate logical reasons to justify unacceptable feelings or behaviors.

reaction formation. Preventing unacceptable or undesirable thoughts or behaviors from being expressed by exaggerating opposite thoughts or types of behaviors.

reality therapy. A type of therapy developed by William Glasser, rooted in control theory, which stresses individual responsibility for choosing how to respond to present situations.

receptor sites. Molecules that are situated on the cell membrane of the postsynaptic neuron that will accept only molecules with a complementary shape. These complementary molecules are specific to certain neurotransmitters that determine whether an electrical impulse will be excited or inhibited.

reciprocal inhibition. Also called *counterconditioning,* this technique serves to decrease or eliminate a behavior by introducing a more adaptive behavior but one that is incompatible with the unacceptable behavior (e.g., introducing relaxation techniques to an anxious person; relaxation and anxiety are incompatible behaviors).

recovery. An ongoing process of movement toward improvement in health and quality of life. Originally used to describe the lifelong process of recovering from an addiction, recovery has evolved into a similar ongoing process for those with serious mental illness.

Recovery Model. Refers to several approaches to treatment that share in common a focus on connectedness, hope, optimism about the future, identity, meaning in life, and empowerment in recovery from mental illnesses or emotional stress.

reframing. Changing the conceptual or emotional setting or viewpoint in relation to which a situation is experienced and placing it in another frame that fits the "facts" of the same concrete situation equally well or even better and thereby changing its entire meaning. Reframing is often used as an intervention to challenge irrational thoughts and cognitive distortions.

regression. A retreat to an earlier level of development and the comfort measures associated with that level of functioning.

relaxation. A decrease in tension or intensity, resulting in refreshment of body and mind. A state of refreshing tranquility.

religion. A set of beliefs, values, rites, and rituals adopted by a group of people. The practices are usually grounded in the teachings of a spiritual leader.

religiosity, *impaired.* When identified as a symptom of illness, refers to excessive demonstration of or obsession with religious ideas and behavior that causes marked distress and impairs ability to function; common in schizophrenia.

reminiscence therapy. A process of life review by elderly individuals that promotes self-esteem and provides assistance in working through unresolved conflicts from the past.

repression. The involuntary blocking of unpleasant feelings and experiences from one's awareness.

residual stimuli. Certain beliefs, attitudes, experiences, or traits that may contribute to an individual's low self-esteem.

retraumatization. Any situation that consciously or unconsciously triggers a reminder of previous trauma and associated symptoms such as anxiety, fear, and feeling unsafe. Retraumatization can exacerbate physical, mental, and emotional consequences of previous trauma.

retrograde ejaculation. Ejaculation of the seminal fluid backward into the bladder; may occur as a side effect of antipsychotic medications.

reuptake. The process of neurotransmitter inactivation by which the neurotransmitter is reabsorbed into the presynaptic neuron from which it had been released.

right. That which an individual is entitled (by ethical, legal, or moral standards) to have, or to do, or to receive from others within the limits of the law.

rigid boundaries. A person with rigid boundaries is "closed" and difficult to bond with. Such a person has a narrow perspective on life, sees things one way, and cannot discuss matters that lie outside their perspective.

ritualistic behavior. Purposeless activities that an individual performs repeatedly in an effort to decrease anxiety (e.g., hand washing); common in obsessive-compulsive disorder.

S

safe house or shelter. An establishment set up by many cities to provide protection for battered women and their children.

SBIRT. An acronym for Screening, Brief Intervention, and Referral for Treatment, SBIRT is an evidence-based approach that can be used in emergency departments, trauma centers, primary care, and other community settings to quickly identify the severity of substance use disorders and refer for treatment as necessary.

scapegoating. Occurs when hostility exists in a marriage dyad and an innocent third person (usually a child) becomes the target of blame for the problem.

schemas. Also called *core beliefs,* cognitive structures that consist of the individual's fundamental beliefs and assumptions, which develop early in life from personal experiences and identification with significant others. These concepts are reinforced by further learning experiences and, in turn, influence the formation of other beliefs, values, and attitudes.

schizoid personality disorder. A type of personality disorder characterized by extreme detachment from personal relationships and restricted expression of emotions.

schizophrenia. One of the schizophrenia spectrum disorders characterized by disturbance in thinking, cognition, emotions, and behavior. Considered a serious mental illness, the course is chronic with episodes of exacerbation and remission. Its causes are likely a combination of genetic, neurodevelopmental, and environmental factors.

schizotypal personality disorder. A disorder characterized by odd and eccentric behavior, not decompensating to the level of schizophrenia.

screening. An aspect of the assessment process in which broad questions are used to identify issues requiring further evaluation.

secondary gain. The receipt of positive reinforcement for somaticizing through added attention, sympathy, and nurturing.

secondary neurocognitive disorder (NCD). Neurocognitive disorder that is caused by or related to another disease or condition, such as HIV disease or a cerebral trauma.

secondary prevention. Health care that is directed at reduction of the prevalence of psychiatric illness by shortening the course (duration) of the illness. This is accomplished through early identification of problems and prompt initiation of treatment.

selective abstraction. Sometimes called *mental filter*, a type of thinking in which a conclusion is drawn based on only a selected portion of the evidence.

self-concept. The composite of beliefs and feelings that one holds about oneself at a given time, formed from perceptions of others' reactions. The self-concept consists of the physical self or body image, the personal self or identity, and the self-esteem.

self-consistency. The component of the personal identity that strives to maintain a stable self-image.

self-esteem. The degree of regard or respect that individuals have for themselves. It is a measure of worth that they place on their abilities and judgments.

self-expectancy. The component of the personal identity that is the individual's perception of what he or she wants to be, to do, or to become.

self-ideal. See **self-expectancy.**

sensate focus. A therapeutic technique used to treat individuals and couples with sexual dysfunction. The technique involves touching and being touched by another and focusing attention on the physical sensations encountered thereby. Clients gradually move through various levels of sensate focus that progress from nongenital touching to touching that includes the breasts and genitals; touching done in a simultaneous, mutual format rather than by one person at a time; and touching that extends to and allows eventually for the possibility of intercourse.

separation anxiety disorder. A disorder characterized by excessive fear or anxiety concerning separation from those to whom the individual is attached. Its onset may occur at any age but is most commonly diagnosed around the age of 5 or 6 when a child begins attending school.

serious mental illness (SMI). A mental, behavioral, or emotional disorder resulting in serious functional impairment that substantially interferes with or limits one or more major life activities.

serotonin syndrome. A syndrome that is an adverse reaction to serotonergic medications. It may range from mild to severe and is potentially fatal. Symptoms may include significantly elevated temperature, agitation, muscle rigidity or twitching, sweating, irregular heartbeat, and seizures.

sexual assault nurse examiner (SANE). A clinical forensic registered nurse who has received specialized training to provide care to the sexual assault victim.

sexual exploitation of a child. The inducement or coercion of a child into engaging in sexually explicit conduct for the purpose of promoting any performance (e.g., child pornography).

sexual masochism disorder. Sexual stimulation derived from being humiliated, beaten, bound, or otherwise made to suffer.

sexual sadism disorder. Recurrent urges and sexually arousing fantasies involving acts (real, not simulated) in which the psychological or physical suffering (including humiliation) of the victim is sexually exciting.

sexual violence. In the context of intimate partner violence, sexual violence is forcing or attempting to force a partner to take part in a sex act, sexual touching, or a nonphysical sexual event (e.g., sexting) when the partner does not or cannot consent.

sexuality. Sexuality is the constitution and life of an individual relative to characteristics regarding intimacy. It reflects the totality of the person and does not relate exclusively to the sex organs or sexual behavior.

shaping. In learning, one shapes the behavior of another by giving reinforcements for increasingly closer approximations to the desired behavior.

shelters. A variety of places designed to help the homeless, ranging from converted warehouses that provide cots or floor space on which to sleep overnight to significant operations that provide a multitude of social and health-care services.

short-term memory. The ability to remember events that occurred very recently. This ability deteriorates with age.

silent rape reaction. The response of a rape victim in which he or she tells no one about the assault.

slander. An action with which an individual may be charged for orally sharing information that is detrimental to a person's reputation.

social anxiety disorder. A disorder in which the individual experiences extreme fear of doing something embarrassing or being negatively evaluated by others in a social situation.

social distance. The distance considered acceptable in interactions with strangers or acquaintances, such as at a cocktail party or in a public building. U.S. culture defines this distance as 4 to 12 feet.

social distancing. An aspect of stigma that refers to the tendency of health-care workers and others to avoid people with mental illness or addiction.

social phobia. The fear of being humiliated in social situations.

social skills training. Educational opportunities through role play for the person with schizophrenia to learn appropriate social interaction skills and functional skills that are relevant to daily living.

Socratic questioning. When the therapist questions the client with Socratic questioning (also called *guided discovery*), the client is asked to describe feelings associated with specific situations. Questions are stated in a way that may stimulate in the client a recognition of possible dysfunctional thinking and may produce a dissonance about the validity of the thoughts.

somatization. A method of coping with psychosocial stress by developing physical symptoms.

specific phobia. A persistent fear of a specific object or situation, other than the fear of being unable to escape from a situation (agoraphobia) or the fear of being humiliated in social situations (social phobia).

spirituality. The human quality that gives meaning and sense of purpose to an individual's existence. Spirituality exists within each individual regardless of belief system and serves as a force for interconnectedness between the self and others, the environment, and a higher power.

splitting. A primitive ego defense mechanism in which the person is unable to integrate and accept both positive and negative feelings. In the view of these individuals, people—including themselves—and life situations are either all good or all bad. This trait is common in borderline personality disorder.

stalking. In the context of intimate partner violence (IPV), stalking is a pattern of repeated, unwanted attention and contact by a partner that causes fear or concern for one's own safety or the safety of someone close to the victim.

statutory law. A law that has been enacted by legislative bodies, such as a county or city council, state legislature, or the U.S. Congress.

statutory rape. Unlawful intercourse between a person who is over the age of consent and a person who is under the age of consent. Legal age of consent varies from state to state. An individual can be arrested for statutory rape even when the interaction has occurred between consenting individuals.

stereotyping. The process of classifying all individuals from the same culture or ethnic group as identical.

stigmatization. The devaluing, marginalizing, and disenfranchising of certain patients because of symptoms or conditions.

stimulus. In classical conditioning, that which elicits a response.

stimulus generalization. The process by which a conditioned response is elicited from all stimuli *similar* to the one from which the response was learned.

store-front clinics. Establishments that have been converted into clinics that serve the homeless population.

stress. A state of disequilibrium that occurs when there is a disharmony between demands occurring within an individual's internal or external environment and their ability to cope with those demands.

stress management. Various methods used by individuals to reduce tension and other maladaptive responses to stress in their lives; includes relaxation exercises, physical exercise, music, mental imagery, or any other technique that is successful for a person.

stressor. A demand from within an individual's internal or external environment that elicits a physiological and/or psychological response.

sublimation. The rechanneling of personally and/or socially unacceptable drives or impulses into activities that are more tolerable and constructive.

subluxation. The term used in chiropractic medicine to describe vertebrae in the spinal column that have become displaced, possibly pressing on nerves and interfering with normal nerve transmission.

substance addiction. Physical addiction is identified by the inability to stop using a substance despite attempts to do so, a continual use of the substance despite adverse consequences, a developing tolerance, and the development of withdrawal symptoms upon cessation or decreased intake. Psychological addiction is said to exist when a substance is perceived by the user to be necessary to maintain an optimal state of personal well-being, interpersonal relations, or skill performance.

substance misuse. Use of psychoactive drugs that poses significant hazards to health and interferes with social, occupational, psychological, or physical functioning.

substitution therapy. The use of various medications to decrease the intensity of symptoms in an individual who is withdrawing from, or experiencing the effects of excessive use of, substances.

subsystems. The smaller units of which a system is composed. In family systems theory, the subsystems are composed of husband-wife, parent-child(ren), or sibling-sibling.

suicide. The act of taking one's own life. Suicide is most often associated with severe depression, but there is increased risk of suicide in many mental illnesses including substance use disorders, bipolar disorders, schizophrenia, anxiety disorders, and eating disorders.

suicide prevention. The collective efforts including screening, assessment, referral for treatment, and collaborative partnership with the patient to prevent suicide as an outcome.

suicide risk factors. Situations, stressors, or demographics that have been statistically related to increased vulnerability toward suicide.

suicide warning signs. Behaviors and communication that are associated with more imminent risk for suicide and requiring immediate intervention. These include threats of suicide, a plan with access to means, hopelessness, and others.

sundowning. A phenomenon in neurocognitive disorder in which the symptoms seem to worsen in the late afternoon and evening.

superego. One of the three elements of the personality identified by Freud that represents the conscience and the culturally determined restrictions that are placed on an individual.

suppression. The voluntary blocking from one's awareness of unpleasant feelings and experiences.

surrogate. One who serves as a substitute figure for another.

symbiosis. One of the stages of development in Object Relations Theory in which the child views himself or herself as an extension of their mother rather than a separate entity.

symbiotic relationship. A type of "psychic fusion" that occurs between two people; it is unhealthy in that severe anxiety is generated in either or both if separation is indicated. A symbiotic relationship is normal between infant and mother.

sympathy. The actual sharing of another's thoughts and behaviors. Differs from **empathy** in that with empathy one experiences an objective understanding of what another is feeling rather than actually sharing those feelings.

synapse. The junction between two neurons. The small space between the axon terminals of one neuron and the cell body or dendrites of another is called the synaptic cleft.

systematic desensitization. A treatment for phobias in which the individual is taught to relax and then asked to imagine various components of the phobic stimulus on a graded hierarchy, moving from that which produces the least fear to that which produces the most.

T

tangentiality. The inability to get to the point of a story. The speaker introduces many unrelated topics until the original topic of discussion is lost. Tangentiality can be symptomatic of cognitive disruptions common in schizophrenia.

tardive dyskinesia. Syndrome of symptoms characterized by bizarre facial and tongue movements, a stiff neck, and difficulty swallowing. It may occur as an adverse effect of long-term therapy with some antipsychotic medications.

technical expert. Peplau's term for one who understands various professional devices and possesses the clinical skills necessary to perform the interventions that are in the best interest of the client.

temperament. A set of inborn personality characteristics that influence an individual's manner of reacting to the environment and ultimately influences their developmental progression.

territoriality. The innate tendency of individuals to own space. Individuals lay claim to areas around them as their own. This phenomenon can have an influence on interpersonal communication.

tertiary gain. The receipt of positive reinforcement for somaticizing by causing the focus of the family to switch to the individual and away from conflict that may be occurring within the family.

tertiary prevention. Health care that is directed toward reduction of the residual effects associated with severe or chronic physical or mental illness.

therapeutic communication. Caregiver verbal and nonverbal techniques that focus on the care receiver's needs and advance the promotion of healing and change. Therapeutic communication encourages exploration of feelings and fosters understanding of behavioral motivation. It is nonjudgmental, discourages defensiveness, and promotes trust.

therapeutic community. Also called *milieu therapy*, this approach strives to manipulate the environment so that all aspects of the client's hospital experience are considered therapeutic.

therapeutic group. Differs from group therapy in that there is a lesser degree of theoretical foundation. Focus is on group relations, interactions between group members, and the consideration of a selected issue. Leaders of therapeutic groups do not require the degree of educational preparation required of group therapy leaders.

therapeutic relationship. An interaction between two people (usually a caregiver and a care receiver) in which input from both participants contributes to a climate of healing, growth promotion, and/or illness prevention.

thought-stopping technique. A self-taught technique that an individual uses each time they wish to eliminate intrusive or negative, unwanted thoughts from awareness.

Tidal Model. A nursing-developed, person-centered approach to the recovery model, which stresses the individual's personal story as significant to working on recovery.

time out. An aversive stimulus or punishment during which the individual is removed from the environment where the unacceptable behavior is being exhibited.

token economy. In behavior modification, a type of contracting in which the reinforcers for desired behaviors are presented in the form of tokens, which may then be exchanged for designated privileges.

tolerance. The need for increasingly larger or more frequent doses of a substance to obtain the desired effects originally produced by a lower dose.

tort. The violation of a civil law in which an individual has been wronged. In a tort action, one party asserts that wrongful conduct on the part of the other has caused harm, and compensation for harm suffered is sought.

transcendence. A developmental task more recently identified by Eric Erikson and associates in which the older adult must learn to move from materialistic, rational thinking to a broader worldview that includes increased sense of meaning in life, well-being, and a sense of satisfaction.

transference. Transference occurs when a client unconsciously displaces (or "transfers") to the nurse or therapist feelings formed toward a person from their past.

transgender. An individual, despite having the anatomical characteristics of a given gender, has the self-perception of being of the opposite gender and may seek to have gender changed through surgical intervention.

transvestic disorder. A *DSM-5-TR* diagnostic category identified as one of a group of paraphilic disorders in which recurrent sexual urges, sexually arousing fantasies, or behaviors arise from dressing in the clothes of the opposite gender *and* the outcome is clinically significant distress or impairment in social, occupational, or other important areas of functioning.

trauma-informed care. An approach to care that assesses for history of physical, sexual, or psychosocial trauma and provides care with consideration for how trauma history may influence an individual's response to interventions and treatments.

traumatic brain injury. Injury to the brain that is the result of head trauma.

triangles. A three-person emotional configuration that is considered the basic building block of the family system. When anxiety becomes too great between two family members, a third person is brought in to form a triangle. Triangles are dysfunctional in that they offer relief from anxiety through diversion rather than through resolution of the issue.

trichotillomania (hair-pulling disorder). The recurrent failure to resist impulses to pull out one's own hair.

type A personality. The personality characteristics attributed to individuals prone to coronary heart disease, including excessive competitive drive, chronic sense of time urgency, easy anger, aggressiveness, excessive ambition, and inability to enjoy leisure time.

type B personality. The personality characteristics attributed to individuals who are not prone to coronary heart disease; includes characteristics such as ability to perform even under pressure but without the competitive drive and constant sense of time urgency experienced by the type A personality. Type Bs can enjoy their leisure time without feeling guilty, and they are much less impulsive than type A individuals; that is, they think things through before making decisions.

type C personality. The personality characteristics attributed to the cancer-prone individual. Includes characteristics such as suppression of anger, calm, passive, puts the needs of others before their own but holds resentment toward others for perceived "wrongs."

type D personality. Personality characteristics attributed to individuals who are at increased risk of cardiovascular morbidity and mortality. The characteristics include a combination of negative emotions and social inhibition.

tyramine. An amino acid found in aged cheeses or other aged, overripe, and fermented foods; broad beans; pickled herring; beef or chicken liver; preserved meats; beer and wine; yeast products; chocolate; caffeinated drinks; canned figs; sour cream; yogurt; soy sauce; and some over-the-counter cold medications and diet pills. If foods high in tyramine content are consumed while an individual is taking monoamine oxidase inhibitors, a potentially life-threatening syndrome called *hypertensive crisis* can result.

U

unconditional positive regard. Carl Rogers's term for the respect and dignity of an individual regardless of their unacceptable behavior.

unconditioned response. In classical conditioning, an unconditioned response refers to a reflexive response to a specific target stimulus.

unconditioned stimulus. In classical conditioning, a specific stimulus that elicits an unconditioned, reflexive response.

undoing. A mechanism used to symbolically negate or cancel out a previous action or experience that one finds intolerable.

universality. One therapeutic factor of groups (identified by Irvin Yalom) in which individuals realize that they are not alone in a problem and in the thoughts and feelings they are experiencing. Anxiety is relieved by the support and understanding of others in the group who share similar experiences.

utilitarianism. The ethical theory that espouses the greatest happiness for the greatest number. Under this theory, action would be taken based on the end results that will produce the most good (happiness) for the most people.

V

values. Personal beliefs about the truth; beauty; or worth of a thought, object, or behavior that influences an individual's actions.

values clarification. A process of self-discovery by which people identify their personal values and their value rankings. This process increases awareness about why individuals behave in certain ways.

veracity. An ethical principle that refers to one's duty to always be truthful.

veterans. Individuals who have served in the military.

voyeuristic disorder. Recurrent urges and sexually arousing fantasies involving the act of observing unsuspecting people, usually strangers, who are either naked, in the process of disrobing, or engaging in sexual activity.

W

waxy flexibility. A condition by which the individual with schizophrenia passively yields all movable parts of the body to any efforts made at placing them in certain positions.

Wernicke's encephalopathy. A brain disorder caused by thiamine deficiency and characterized by visual disturbances, ataxia, somnolence, stupor, and, without thiamine replacement, death.

withdrawal. The physiological and mental readjustment that accompanies the discontinuation of an addictive substance.

word salad. A group of words that are put together in a random fashion without any logical connection.

WRAP Model. An approach to the recovery model (Wellness Recovery Action Plan) that stresses learning a distinct set of skills necessary for managing symptoms of mental illness or emotional distress in everyday life.

Y

yin and yang. The fundamental concept of Asian health practices. Yin and yang are opposite forces of energy, such as negative/positive, dark/light, cold/hot, hard/soft, and feminine/masculine. Food, medicines, and herbs are classified according to their yin and yang properties and are used to restore a balance, thereby restoring health.

yoga. A system of beliefs and practices, the ultimate goal of which is to unite the human soul with the universal spirit. In Western countries, yoga uses body postures, along with meditation and breathing exercises, to achieve a balanced, disciplined workout that releases muscle tension; tones the internal organs; and energizes the mind, body, and spirit so that natural healing can occur.

Index